BNF for children 2006

The essential resource for clinical use of medicines in children

bnfc.org

Published by
BMJ Publishing Group Ltd
Tavistock Square, London WC1H 9JP, UK

RPS Publishing
RPS Publishing is the wholly-owned publishing organisation of the Royal Pharmaceutical Society of Great Britain
1 Lambeth High Street, London, SE1 7JN, UK

RCPCH Publications Ltd
50 Hallam Street, London W1W 6DE, UK

ISBN: 0 85369 676 4 (Royal Pharmaceutical Society of Great Britain)

ISSN: 1747–5503

Printed in Germany by Clausen & Bosse, CPI Books, Leck

A catalogue record for this book is available from the British Library.

Copies may be obtained through any bookseller or direct from:

RPS Publishing
c/o Turpin Distribution
Stratton Business Park
Pegasus Drive
Biggleswade
Bedfordshire
SG18 8TQ
UK
Tel: +44 (0) 1767 604 971
Fax: +44 (0) 1767 601 640
E-mail: custserv@turpin-distribution.com
www.pharmpress.com

RPS Publishing also supplies *BNF for Children* in digital formats suitable for standalone use or for small networks and for use over an intranet.

Copies for NHS primary healthcare
General practitioners and community pharmacies in **England** can telephone the DH Publication Orderline for enquiries concerning the direct mailing of the *BNF for Children*
Tel: 08701 555 455
In **Wales** telephone the Business Services Centre
Tel: 01495 332 000

The *BNF for Children* is for use by health professionals engaged in prescribing, dispensing, and administering medicines to children. It has been prepared under the guidance of the Paediatric Formulary Committee.

BNF for Children has been constructed using robust procedures for gathering, assessing and assimilating information on paediatric drug treatment. It is, however, expected that the reader will be relying on appropriate professional knowledge and expertise to interpret the contents in the context of the circumstances of the individual child. *BNF for Children* should be used in conjunction with other appropriate and up-to-date literature and, where necessary, supplemented by expert advice. *Special care is required in managing childhood conditions with unlicensed medicines or with licensed medicines for unlicensed uses.*

Responsibility for the appropriate use of medicines lies solely with the individual health professional.

Contents

Preface

BNF for Children aims to provide prescribers, pharmacists and other healthcare professionals with sound up-to-date information on the use of medicines for treating children.

A joint publication of the British Medical Association, the Royal Pharmaceutical Society of Great Britain, the Royal College of Paediatrics and Child Health, and the Neonatal and Paediatric Pharmacists Group, *BNF for Children* ('BNFC') is published under the authority of a Paediatric Formulary Committee.

Many areas of paediatric practice have suffered from inadequate information on effective medicines. BNFC addresses this significant knowledge gap by providing practical information on the use of medicines in children of all ages from birth to adolescence. *Medicines for Children* (RCPCH Publications Ltd) and the *British National Formulary* itself form the basis for BNFC. Information in BNFC has been validated against emerging evidence, best-practice guidelines, and crucially, advice from a network of clinical experts.

Drawing information from manufacturers' literature where appropriate, BNFC also includes a great deal of advice that goes beyond marketing authorisations (product licences). This is necessary because licensed indications frequently do not cover the clinical needs of children; in some cases, products for use in children need to be specially manufactured or imported. Careful consideration has been given to establishing the clinical need for unlicensed interventions with respect to the evidence and experience of their safety and efficacy; local paediatric formularies, clinical literature and national information resources have been invaluable in this process.

BNFC has been designed for rapid reference and the information presented has been carefully selected to aid decisions on prescribing, dispensing and administration of medicines. Less detail is given on areas such as malignant disease and the very specialist use of medicines generally undertaken in tertiary centres. BNFC should be interpreted in the light of professional knowledge and it should be supplemented as necessary by specialised publications. Information is also available from medicines information services (see inside front cover).

The website (bnfc.org) includes additional information of relevance to healthcare professionals. BNFC is also available on other digital platforms.

Acknowledgements

The Paediatric Formulary Committee is grateful to individuals and organisations that have provided advice and information to the *BNF for Children*.

The principal contributors for this edition were:

K. W. Ah-See, A. J. Baker, T. G. Barrett, D. N. Bateman, G. D. L. Bates, R. M. Bingham, I. W. Booth, L. Brook, K. G. Brownlee, R. J. Buckley, R. H. Bull, I. F. Burgess, J. B. S. Coulter, B. G. Craig, J. H. Cross, A. Dhawan, M. J. Dillon, A. Durward, O. B. Eden, J. Edge, D. A. C. Elliman, J. Gray, J. W. Gregory, J. Harcourt, R. J. Hay, S. Haworth, P. J. Helms, B. G. Higgins, R. Hull, H. R. Jenkins, C. J. H. Kelnar, D. Kwiatkowski, P. Lee, H. Lyall, A. Macdonald, D. Macrae, A. G. Marson, N. Mayne, N. McIntosh, N. S. Morton, C. Moss, C. Ng, A. J. Nunn, D. J. Nutt, J. Y. Paton, G. A. Pearson, J. F. Price, J. M. Rennie, I. Roberts, J. Rogers, J. W. Sander, M. R. Sharland, N. Shaw, O. Stumper, A. Sutcliffe, E. A. Taylor, M. A. Thomson, P. K. Thompson, J. O. Warner, N. J. A. Webb, R. Welbury, P. H. Weller, C. Wren, A. Wright.

Members of the Advisory Committee on Malaria Prevention, B. A. Bannister, R. H. Behrens, P. L. Chiodini, A. D. Green, D. Hill, G. Kassianos, D. G. Lalloo, G. Lea, G. Pasvol, M. Povell, E. Walker, D. A. Warrell, C. J. M. Whitty, P. A. Winstanley, and C. A. Swales (Secretariat) have also provided valuable advice.

The *BNF for Children* has valuable access to the *Martindale* data banks by courtesy of S. Sweetman and staff.

E. M. Carranza-Pitcher provided considerable assistance during the production of this edition of *BNF for Children*.

Xpage and CSW Informatics Ltd have provided technical assistance with the editorial database and typesetting software.

BNFC aims to provide information suited to the needs of the clinician and recognises that, although this edition represents a considerable advance in the content and presentation of information on the paediatric use of medicines, further changes will be necessary. Comments from healthcare professionals are therefore very welcome and should be sent to:

Executive Editor, British National Formulary Publications, Royal Pharmaceutical Society of Great Britain, 1 Lambeth High Street, London SE1 7JN.

Email: bnfc@bnf.org

Paediatric Formulary Committee 2004–2005

Chairman
George Rylance
MB, FRCPCH

Committee Members
Jeffrey K Aronson
MA, MBChB, DPhil, FRCP, FBPharmacolS
Catherine M. Baldridge
BSc, DipClinPharm, MSc, MRPharmS
Anne M. Burns
BSc, MPS, SP
Judith H Cope
MSc, BPharm, MRPharmS
Julia Dunne
MA, MBBS, MRCP
Martin J. Kendall
MB, ChB, MD, FRCP
(Chairman, Formulary Development Committee)
Neena Modi
MB, ChB, MD, FRCP, FRCPCH
Stuart Tanner
MB, BS, MSc, FRCP(Lond & Glas), FRCPCH
David W. Wall
MB, ChB, PCME, MMEd, FRCP, FRCGP
Edward R. Wozniak
BSc, MB, BS, FRCP, FRCPCH, DCH

Executive Secretary
Tracy L. South
BTEC

Editorial Staff

Executive Editor
Dinesh K. Mehta *BPharm, MSc, FRPharmS*

Senior Assistant Editor
John Martin *BPharm, PhD, MRPharmS*

Lead Editor: BNF for Children
Ian Costello *BPharm, MSc, MRPharmS*

Assistant Editors
Bryony Jordan *BSc, DipPharmPract, MRPharmS*
Colin R. Macfarlane *BPharm, MSc, MRPharmS*
Rachel S. M. Ryan *BPharm, MRPharmS*
Shama M. S. Wagle *BPharm, DipPharmPract, MRPharmS*

Staff Editors
Leigh Anne Claase *BSc, PhD, MRPharmS*
Allison F. Corbett *BPharm, MRPharmS*
Laura K. Glancy *MPharm, MRPharmS*
Trinh Huynh *BPharm, MRPharmS*
Maria Kouimtzi *BPharm, PhD, MRPharmS*
Helen M. N. Neill *MPharm, MRPharmS*
Elizabeth Nix *DipPharm(NZ), MRPharmS*
Shaistah J. Qureshi *MPharm, MRPharmS*
Benjamin Rehman *BPharm, MRPharmS*
Vinaya K. Sharma *BPharm, MSc, PGDipPIM, MRPharmS*

Editorial Assistant
Gerard P. Gallagher *MSc, MRSH, MRIPH*

Knowledge Systems
Eric I. Connor *BSc(Econ), MSc, DIC, MBCS*
Knowledge Systems Manager
Simon N. Dunton *BA, PhDr*
Editorial Production Assistant
Philip D. Lee *BSc, PhD*
Digital Development Editor
Karl A. Parsons *BSc*
Knowledge Systems Administrator
Candace C. Partridge *BA*
Digital Quality Specialist

Head of Publishing Services
John Wilson

Director of Publications
Charles Fry

How to use *BNF for Children*

The *BNF for Children* provides information on the use of medicines in children ranging from neonates (including preterm neonates) to adolescents. The terms infant, child, and adolescent are not used consistently in the literature; to avoid ambiguity actual ages are used in the dose statements in *BNF for Children*. The term neonate is used to describe a newborn infant aged 0–28 days. The terms child or children are used generically to describe the entire range from infant to adolescent in *BNF for Children*.

BNF for Children is divided into the following broad areas.

General Guidance

The section on general guidance includes general advice on the use of medicines for managing childhood conditions. It also includes information on prescribing controlled drugs and the management of palliative care. Advice is given on the reporting of adverse reactions. General principles on the use of medicines in hepatic impairment, renal impairment, pregnancy, and breast-feeding are also included in this section.

Notes on conditions, drugs and preparations

The main text consists of classified notes on clinical conditions, drugs and preparations. These notes are divided into 15 chapters, each of which is related

DRUG NAME ◢

Cautions details of precautions required and also any monitoring required
Hepatic impairment advice for use of drug in these circumstances
Renal impairment
Pregnancy
Breast-feeding
Counselling Verbal explanation to the patient of specific details of the drug treatment (e.g. posture when taking a medicine)
Contra-indications details of any contra-indications to use of drug
Side-effects details of common and more serious side-effects
Licensed use licensing status where this is of clinical relevance
Indications and dose
Details of uses and indications
- By route
  Child dose and frequency of administration (max. dose) for specific age group
- By alternative route
  Child dose and frequency

*** Approved Name (Non-proprietary)** PoM
Pharmaceutical form colour, coating, active ingredient and amount in dosage form, net price, pack size = basic NHS price. Label: (as in Appendix 3)

Proprietary Name® (Manufacturer) PoM NHS
Pharmaceutical form sugar-free, active ingredient mg/mL, net price, pack size = basic NHS price. Label: (as in Appendix 3)
Excipients: includes clinically important excipients or electrolytes
* exceptions to the prescribing status indicated by a footnote.
Note Specific notes about the product e.g. handling

Preparations

Preparations usually follow immediately after the drug which is their main ingredient.

Preparations are included under a non-proprietary title, if they are marketed under such a title, if they are not otherwise prescribable under the NHS, or if they may be prepared extemporaneously.

If proprietary preparations are of a distinctive colour this is stated.

In the case of compound preparations the indications, cautions, contra-indications, side-effects, and interactions of all constituents should be taken into account for prescribing.

When no suitable licensed preparation is available details of preparations that may be imported or formulations available as manufactured specials or extemporaneous preparations are included.

Drugs

The symbol ◢ is used to denote those preparations considered to be less suitable for prescribing. Although such preparations may not be considered as drugs of first choice, their use may be justifiable in certain circumstances.

Prescription-only medicines PoM

This symbol has been placed against preparations that are available only on a prescription from an appropriate practitioner.

The symbol CD indicates that the preparation is subject to the prescription requirements of the Misuse of Drugs Act. For advice on prescribing such preparations see Controlled drugs.

Preparations not available for NHS prescription NHS

This symbol has been placed against preparations that are not prescribable under the NHS. Those prescribable only for specific disorders have a footnote specifying the condition(s) for which the preparation remains available. Some preparations which are not *prescribable* by brand name under the NHS may nevertheless be *dispensed* using the brand name provided that the prescription shows an appropriate non-proprietary name.

Prices

Prices have been calculated from the basic cost used in pricing NHS prescriptions. The price for an extemporaneously prepared preparation has been omitted where the net cost of the ingredients used to make it would give a misleadingly low impression of the final price. Since the prices shown in the *BNF for Children* do not include professional fees and overhead allowances, they are not suitable for quoting to patients seeking private prescriptions or contemplating over-the-counter purchase.

to a particular system of the body or to an aspect of neonatal and paediatric medical care. Each chapter is then divided into sections which begin with *notes* on the selection and use of medicines. Guidance on dental and oral conditions is identified by means of a relevant heading (e.g. Dental and Orofacial pain) in the appropriate sections. The notes are followed by details of relevant drugs and preparations.

Drug entries

Drugs appear under pharmacopoeial or other non-proprietary titles. When there is an *appropriate current monograph* (Medicines Act 1968, Section 65) preference is given to a name at the head of that monograph; otherwise a British Approved Name (BAN), if available, is used. Information on the properties of each drug is organised as shown in the illustration below; the information on cautions, contra-indications, side-effects, dose and indications reflects, as far as possible, the manufacturer's summary of product characteristics.

Side-effects are generally listed in order of frequency and arranged broadly by body systems. Occasionally a rare side-effect might be listed first if it is considered to be particularly important because of its seriousness.

For the majority of drugs, *doses* are expressed in terms of body-weight (i.e. standardised by weight). To calculate the dose for a given child the weight-standardised dose is multiplied by the child's weight (or occasionally by the child's ideal body-weight). The calculated dose should not normally exceed the maximum recommended dose for an adult. For example if the dose is 8 mg/kg (max. 300 mg) a child of 10 kg body-weight should receive 80 mg but a child of 40 kg body-weight should receive 300 mg (rather than 320 mg).

Doses are expressed for specific age ranges; neonatal doses are preceded by the word Neonate, all other doses are preceded by the word Child. Age ranges in the BNF for Children are described as follows:

Child 1 month–4 years refers to a child from 1 month old up to their 4th birthday;

Child 4–10 years refers to a child from the day of their 4th birthday up to their 10th birthday.

However, a pragmatic approach should be applied to these cut-off points depending on the child's physiological development, condition, and if weight is appropriate for the child's age.

Emergency treatment of poisoning

This chapter provides information on the management of acute poisoning when first seen, although aspects of hospital-based treatment are mentioned.

Appendixes and indexes

The appendixes include information on interactions, borderline substances, and cautionary and advisory labels for dispensed medicines. They are designed for use in association with the main body of the text.

The Dental Practitioners' List and the Nurse Prescribers' List are also included in this section. The indexes consist of the Index of Manufacturers and the Main Index.

Patient Packs

Directive 92/27/EEC specifies the requirements for the labelling of medicines and outlines the format and content of patient information leaflets to be supplied with every medicine; the directive also requires the use of Recommended International Non-proprietary Names for drugs (see p. xii).

All medicines have approved labelling and patient information leaflets; anyone who supplies a medicine is responsible for providing the relevant information to the patient (see also Appendix 3).

Many medicines are available in manufacturers' original packs complete with patient information leaflets. Where patient packs are available, the *BNF for Children* shows the number of dose units in the packs. In particular clinical circumstances, where patient packs need to be split or medicines are provided in bulk dispensing packs, manufacturers will provide additional supplies of patient information leaflets on request.

During the revision of each edition of this publication careful note is taken of the information that appears on the patient information leaflets. Where it is considered appropriate to alert a prescriber to some specific limitation appearing on the patient information leaflet (for example, in relation to pregnancy) this advice now appears in the *BNF for Children*, see also General guidance, patient information leaflets.

The patient information leaflet also includes details of all inactive ingredients in the medicine. A list of common E numbers and the inactive ingredients to which they correspond is now therefore included in the *BNF for Children* (see inside back cover).

PACT and SPA

PACT (Prescribing Analyses and Cost) and SPA (Scottish Prescribing Analysis) provide prescribers with information about their prescribing.

The *PACT Standard Report*, or in Scotland SPA *Level 1 Report*, is sent to all general practitioners on a quarterly basis. The PACT Standard Report contains an analysis of the practitioner's prescribing and the practice prescribing over the last 3 months, and gives comparisons with the local Primary Care Trust equivalent practice and with a national equivalent. The report also contains details of the practice prescribing for a specific topic; a different topic is chosen each quarter.

The *PACT Catalogue*, or in Scotland SPA *Level 2 Report*, provides a full inventory of the prescriptions issued by a prescriber. The PACT catalogue is available on request for periods between 1 and 24 months. To allow the prescriber to target specific areas of prescribing, a Catalogue may be requested to cover individual preparations, BNF sections, or combinations of BNF chapters.

PACT is also available electronically (ePACT.net). This system gives users on-line access through NHSnet to the 3 years' prescribing data held on the Prescription Pricing Authority's database; tools for analysing the data are also provided.

Prices in the *BNF for Children*

Basic **net prices** are given in the *BNF for Children* to provide an indication of relative cost. Where there is a choice of suitable preparations for a particular disease or condition the relative cost may be used in making a selection. Cost-effective prescribing must, however, take into account other factors (such as dose frequency and duration of treatment) that affect the total cost. The use of more expensive drugs is justified if it will result in better treatment of the patient or a reduction of the length of an illness or the time spent in hospital.

Prices have generally been calculated from the net cost used in pricing NHS prescriptions dispensed in September 2005, but where available later prices have been included; unless an original pack is available these prices are based on the largest pack size of the preparation in use in community pharmacies. The price for an extemporaneously prepared preparation has been omitted where the net cost of the ingredients used to make it would give a misleadingly low impression of the final price.

The unit of 20 is still sometimes used as a basis for comparison, but where suitable original packs or patient packs are available these are priced instead.

Gross prices vary as follows:

1. Costs to the NHS are greater than the net prices quoted and include professional fees and overhead allowances;
2. Private prescription charges are calculated on a separate basis;
3. Over-the-counter sales are at retail price, as opposed to basic net price, and include VAT.

***BNF for Children** prices are NOT, therefore, suitable for quoting to patients seeking private prescriptions or contemplating over-the-counter purchases.*

A fuller explanation of costs to the NHS may be obtained from the Drug Tariff.

It should be noted that separate Drug Tariffs are applicable to England and Wales, Scotland, and Northern Ireland. Prices in the different tariffs may vary.

Changes for this edition

Significant changes

The *BNF for Children* is revised yearly and numerous changes are made between issues. All copies of *BNF for Children 2005* should therefore be withdrawn and replaced by *BNF for Children 2006*. Significant changes have been made in the following sections for *BNF for Children 2006*:

Newborn and paediatric basic and advanced life support algorithms, inside back cover

BNF for Children and marketing authorisation, General guidance

Emergency supply of medicines, Guidance on prescribing

Prescribing of controlled drugs, Guidance on prescribing

Prescribing in palliative care, Guidance on prescribing

Gastro-oesophageal reflux, section 1.1.1

Laxatives, section 1.6

Stimulant laxatives, section 1.6.2

Cardiac glycosides, section 2.1.1

ACE inhibitors in heart failure, section 2.2

Centrally acting antihypertensive drugs, section 2.5.2

Tolerance to nitrates, section 2.6.1

Heparinoids, section 2.8.1

Kawasaki syndrome, section 2.9

Lipid-regulating drugs, section 2.12

Management of acute asthma, section 3.1

Treatment of croup, section 3.1

Selective beta$_2$ agonists [reorganised], section 3.1.1.1

Oxygen, section 3.6

Melatonin [updated text], section 4.1.1

Attention deficit hyperactivity disorder, section 4.4

Atomoxetine [CSM warning about risk of suicidal ideation], section 4.4

Epilepsy [updated advice on partial seizures and generalised seizures], section 4.8.1

Drugs used in status epilepticus, section 4.8.2

Nicotine replacement therapy, section 4.10

Treatment of bacterial infections [Updated advice on the initial treatment of salmonella, typhoid fever, shigellosis, respiratory-tract infections in cystic fibrosis, hospital-acquired septicaemia, conjunctivitis, otitis media, impetigo, and erysipelas], Table 1, section 5.1

Prevention of secondary case of group A streptococcal infection [new], Table 2, section 5.1

Prevention of Staphylococcus aureus lung infection in cystic fibrosis, Table 2, section 5.1

Prevention of endocarditis, Table 2, section 5.1

Antibacterial treatment of tuberculosis, section 5.1.9

Antifungal treatment of cryptococcosis, section 5.2

Management of chronic hepatitis B and chronic hepatitis C, section 5.3.3

Palivizumab, section 5.3.5

Treatment of falciparum malaria, section 5.4.1

Malaria prophylaxis [updated advice for Mauritania and South Asia], section 5.4.1

Insulins [updated advice on diabetes and surgery, use of intravenous fluids, and continuous insulin infusion], section 6.1.1

Sulphonylureas [updated advice on the treatment of maturity-onset diabetes of the young], section 6.1.2.1

Diabetic ketoacidosis [reorganised], section 6.1.3

Potassium removal, section 9.2.1.1

Electrolytes and water, section 9.2.2.1

Dental prescribing of fluoride preparations on the NHS, section 9.5.3 and Dental Practitioners' Formulary

Treatment of neonatal gonococcal and chlamydial eye infections, section 11.3.1

Recurrent acute otitis media, section 12.1.2

Desloughing agents, section 13.11.7

BCG vaccines, section 14.4

Hepatitis A vaccine, section 14.4

Hepatitis B vaccine, section 14.4

Anaesthesia, sedation and resuscitation in dental practice, section 15.1

Intravenous anaesthetics, section 15.1.1

Benzodiazepines for dental procedures, section 15.1.4.1

Local anaesthesia [use of vasoconstrictors], section 15.2

Dose changes

Changes in dose statements introduced into *BNF for Children 2006*:

Adenosine, p. 107
ACWY Vax®, p. 692
Alfentanil, p. 719
Allopurinol, p. 459
Ametop®, p. 733
Amiodarone, p. 108
Aspirin [Kawasaki syndrome], p. 149
Atracurium, p. 722
Atropine, p. 713
Benzylpenicillin [endocarditis], p. 294
Bezafibrate, p. 156
Bumetanide, p. 102
Caspofungin, p. 349
Chloral hydrate, p. 203
Ciclosporin, p. 73
Ciprofloxacin, p. 343
Cisatracurium, p. 723
Desflurane [induction of anaesthesia], p. 711
Dexamfetamine, p. 225
Diazepam [for clinical procedures], p. 716
Epoprostenol, p. 121
Fentanyl, p. 720
Flixotide® Nebules®, p. 181
Fluconazole [cryptococcal meningitis], p. 350
Flucytosine, p. 351
FSME-IMMUN®, p. 697
Furosemide, p. 101
Griseofulvin, p. 351
Haloperidol [palliative care], p. 210
Hydrocortisone [severe acute asthma, acute hypersensitivity reactions], p. 429
Ibuprofen, p. 551
Labetalol, p. 114
Levetiracetam, p. 260
Levothyroxine, p. 417
Lidocaine, p. 730
Malarone® Paediatric, p. 385
Methylphenidate, p. 226
Methylprednisolone, p. 430
Midazolam, p. 717
Milrinone, p. 98
Nalidixic acid, p. 343
Netilmicin, p. 319
Nitrous oxide [analgesia], p. 713
Oxis®, p. 170
Oseltamivir, p. 372
Pentasa®, p. 70
Primodine, p. 261
Propofol, p. 709
Propranolol, p. 112
Rabies Immunoglobulin, p. 701
Ranitidine, p. 61
Remifentanil, p. 720
Ribavirin [life-threatening infections in immunocompromised], p. 374
Salbutamol, p. 167
Sumatriptan, p. 251
Terbutaline, p. 169
Tinadazole, p. 388
Tobramycin, p. 319
Voriconazole, p. 355

Classification changes

Classification changes have been made in the following sections of *BNF for Children 2006*:

Section 1.7.4 Management of anal fissures [new subsection]

Section 2.5 Hypertension [title change]

Section 2.6 Nitrates, calcium-channel blockers, and other antianginal drugs [title change]

Section 2.8.1 Heparinoids [new subsection]

Section 3.3 Cromoglicate and related therapy, leukotriene receptor antagonists, and omalizumab [title change]

Section 3.3.1 Cromoglicate and related therapy [title change]

Section 3.3.2 Leukotriene receptor antagonists and omalizumab [title change]

Section 4.3.1 Tricyclic antidepressants [title change]

Section 4.7.3 Neuropathic pain [title change]

Section 6.5.2 Desmopressin [moved from section 7.4.2]

Section 9.1.4 Drugs used in platelet disorders [title change]

Section 12.2.3 Nasal preparations for infection [title change]

Section 13.3 Topical antipruritics [title change]

Discontinued preparations

Preparations discontinued during the compilation of *BNF for Children 2006*:

Aluminium hydroxide oral suspension
Arythmol®
Bioplex®
Bricanyl® aerosol inhalation
Bricanyl® respirator solution
Bricanyl SA®
Cefrom®
Colofac® liquid
Colomycin® powder
Dermovate-NN® ointment
Fluvirin®
Fortovase®
Fungilin® tablets
Gaviscon® liquid and tablets
Hypotears®
Inflexal® V
Intal® nebuliser solution
Konakion® Neonatal
Kytril® Paediatric liquid
LactiCare®
Levocabastine
Lignostab® A
Lipofundin N®
Locabiotal®
Marcain® with Adrenaline
Monovent®
Monotard®
Narcan®
Narcan Neonatal®
Neo-Cortef® eye/ear drops
Nivaquine® tablets
Ossopan®
Phyllocontin Continus® Paediatric
Plesmet®
Pragmatar®
Serevent® aerosol inhalation
Soframycin® eye ointment
Sultrin®
Tetabulin®
Tilade®
Tofranil®
Ultratard®
Zarontin® capsules

New preparations included in this edition

Preparations included in the relevant sections of *BNF for Children 2006*:

Name changes

European Law requires use of the Recommended International Non-proprietary Name (rINN) for medicinal substances. In most cases the British Approved Name (BAN) and rINN were identical. Where the two differed, the BAN was modified to accord with the rINN.

The following list shows those substances for which the former BAN has been modified to accord with the rINN. Former BANs have been retained as synonyms in *BNF for Children.*

Adrenaline and noradrenaline Adrenaline and noradrenaline are the terms used in the titles of monographs in the European Pharmacopoeia and are thus the official names in the member states. For these substances, BP 2005 shows the European Pharmacopoeia names and the rINNs at the head of the monographs; *BNF for Children* has adopted a similar style.

Former BAN	New BAN
adrenaline	see above
amethocaine	tetracaine
aminacrine	aminoacridine
amoxycillin	amoxicillin
amphetamine	amfetamine
amylobarbitone	amobarbital
amylobarbitone sodium	amobarbital sodium
beclomethasone	beclometasone
bendrofluazide	bendroflumethiazide
benzhexol	trihexyphenidyl
benzphetamine	benzfetamine
benztropine	benzatropine
busulphan	busulfan
butobarbitone	butobarbital
carticaine	articaine
cephalexin	cefalexin
cephradine	cefradine
chloral betaine	cloral betaine
chlorbutol	chlorobutanol
chlormethiazole	clomethiazole
chlorpheniramine	chlorphenamine
chlorthalidone	chlortalidone
cholecalciferol	colecalciferol
cholestyramine	colestyramine
clomiphene	clomifene
colistin sulphomethate sodium	colistimethate sodium
corticotrophin	corticotropin
cyclosporin	ciclosporin
cysteamine	mercaptamine
danthron	dantron
dexamphetamine	dexamfetamine
dibromopropamidine	dibrompropamidine
dicyclomine	dicycloverine
dienoestrol	dienestrol
dimethicone(s)	dimeticone
dimethyl sulphoxide	dimethyl sulfoxide
dothiepin	dosulepin
doxycycline hydrochloride (hemihydrate hemiethanolate)	doxycycline hyclate
eformoterol	formoterol
ethamsylate	etamsylate
ethinyloestradiol	ethinylestradiol
ethynodiol	etynodiol
flumethasone	flumetasone
flupenthixol	flupentixol
flurandrenolone	fludroxycortide
frusemide	furosemide
guaiphenesin	guaifenesin
hexachlorophane	hexachlorophene
hexamine hippurate	methenamine hippurate
hydroxyurea	hydroxycarbamide
indomethacin	indometacin
lignocaine	lidocaine
lysuride	lisuride
methotrimeprazine	levomepromazine
methyl cysteine	mecysteine
methylene blue	methylthioninium chloride
methicillin	meticillin
mitozantrone	mitoxantrone
nicoumalone	acenocoumarol
noradrenaline	*see above*
oestradiol	estradiol
oestriol	estriol
oestrone	estrone
oxpentifylline	pentoxifylline
phenobarbitone	phenobarbital
pipothiazine	pipotiazine
polyhexanide	polihexanide
pramoxine	pramocaine
procaine penicillin	procaine benzylpenicillin
prothionamide	protionamide
quinalbarbitone	secobarbital
riboflavine	riboflavin
salcatonin	calcitonin (salmon)
sodium calciumedetate	sodium calcium edetate
sodium cromoglycate	sodium cromoglicate
sodium ironedetate	sodium feredetate
sodium picosulphate	sodium picosulfate
sorbitan monostearate	sorbitan stearate
stibocaptate	sodium stibocaptate
stilboestrol	diethylstilbestrol
sulphacetamide	sulfacetamide
sulphadiazine	sulfadiazine
sulphamethoxazole	sulfamethoxazole
sulphapyridine	sulfapyridine
sulphasalazine	sulfasalazine
sulphathiazole	sulfathiazole
sulphinpyrazone	sulfinpyrazone
tetracosactrin	tetracosactide
thiabendazole	tiabendazole
thioguanine	tioguanine
thiopentone	thiopental
thymoxamine	moxisylyte
thyroxine sodium	levothyroxine sodium
tribavirin	ribavirin
trimeprazine	alimemazine
urofollitrophin	urofollitropin

General guidance

Medicines should be given to children only when they are necessary, and in all cases the benefit of administering the medicine should be considered in relation to the risk involved. This is particularly important during pregnancy where the risk to both mother and fetus must be considered (for further details see Prescribing in Pregnancy).

It is important to discuss treatment options carefully with the child and the child's carer (see also Taking Medicines to Best Effect, below). In particular, the child and the child's carer should be helped to distinguish the side-effects of prescribed drugs from the effects of the medical disorder. Where the beneficial effects of the medicine are likely to be delayed, this should be highlighted.

Taking medicines to best effect Difficulties in adherence to drug treatment occur regardless of age. Factors that contribute to poor compliance with prescribed medicines include:

- Difficulty in taking the medicine (e.g. inability to swallow the medicine)
- Unattractive formulation (e.g. unpleasant taste)
- Prescription not collected or not dispensed
- Purpose of medicine not clear
- Perceived lack of efficacy
- Real or perceived side-effects
- Carers' or child's perception of the risk and severity of side-effects may differ from that of the prescriber
- Ambiguous instructions for administration

The prescriber, the child's carer and the child (if appropriate) should agree on the health outcomes desired and on the strategy for achieving them ('concordance'). The prescriber should be sensitive to religious, cultural, and personal beliefs of the child's family that can affect acceptance of medicines. Further information on concordance is available on the Internet (www.medicines-partnership.org).

Taking the time to explain to the child (and relatives) the rationale and the potential adverse effects of treatment may improve compliance. Reinforcement and elaboration of the physician's instructions by the pharmacist and other members of the healthcare team can be important. Giving advice on the management of side-effects and the possibility of alternative treatments may encourage carers and children to seek advice rather than merely abandon unacceptable treatment.

Simplifying the drug regimen may help; the need for frequent administration may reduce compliance although there appears to be little difference in compliance between once-daily and twice-daily administration.

Administration of medicines to children Children should be involved in decisions about taking medicines and encouraged to take responsibility for using them correctly. The degree of such involvement will depend on the child's age, understanding, and personal circumstances.

Occasionally a medicine or its taste has to be disguised or masked with small quantities of food. However, unless specifically permitted (e.g. some formulations of pancreatin), a medicine should **not** be mixed with large quantities of food because the full dose might not be taken and the child might develop an aversion to food if the medicine imparts an unpleasant taste. Medicines should **not** be mixed or administered in a baby's feeding bottle.

Children under 5 years (and even older children) find a liquid formulation more acceptable than tablets or capsules. However, for long-term treatment it may be possible for a child to be taught to take tablets or capsules.

An oral syringe (see below) should be used for accurate measurement and controlled administration of an oral liquid medicine. Unpleasant taste of an oral liquid may be disguised by flavouring it or by giving a favourite food or drink immediately afterwards but the potential for food-drug interactions should be considered.

Advice should be given on dental hygiene to those receiving medicines containing cariogenic sugars for long term treatment; sugar-free medicines should be provided whenever possible.

Children with nasal feeding tubes in place for prolonged periods should be encouraged to take medicines by mouth where possible; enteric feeding should generally be interrupted before the medicine is given (particularly if enteral feeds reduce the absorption of a particular drug). Oral liquids may be given through the tube provided that precautions are taken to guard against blockage; the dose should be washed down with warm water. If a medicine is given through a nasogastric tube to a neonate then only **sterile water** must be used to accompany the medicine or to wash it down.

The intravenous route is generally chosen when a medicine cannot be given by mouth; reliable access, often a central vein, should be used for children whose treatment involves irritant or inotropic drugs or who need to receive the medicine over a long period or for home therapy. Intramuscular injections should preferably be **avoided** in children, particularly neonates, infants, and young children. However, the intramuscular route may be advantageous for administration of single doses of medicines when intravenous cannulation would be more problematic or painful to the child. Certain drugs, e.g. vaccines, are only administered intramuscularly.

The intrathecal, epidural and intraosseous routes should be used **only** by staff specially trained to administer medicines by these routes. Local protocols for the management of intrathecal injections must be in place (section 8.1.3).

Managing medicines in school Administration of a medicine during schooltime should be avoided if possible; medicines should be prescribed for once or twice-daily administration whenever practicable. If the medicine needs to be taken in school, this should be discussed with parents or carers and the necessary arrangements made in advance; where appropriate, involvement of a school nurse should be sought. *Managing Medicines in Schools and Early Years Settings* produced by the Department of Health provides guidance on access to medicines whilst at school (www.dh.gov.uk).

Patient information leaflets Manufacturers' patient information leaflets that accompany a medicine cover only the licensed use of the medicine (see *BNF for Children* and Marketing Authorisation, below). Therefore, when a medicine is used outside its licence, it may be appropriate to advise the child and the child's parent or carer that some of the information in the leaflet might not apply to the child's treatment. Where necessary, the inappropriate advice in the patient information leaflet should be identified and reassurance provided about the correct use in the context of the child's condition.

Complementary medicine An increasing amount of information on complementary ('alternative') medicine is becoming available. Where appropriate, the child and the child's carers should be asked about the use of complementary medicines, including dietary supplements and topical products. However, the scope of *BNF for Children* is restricted to the discussion of conventional medicines but reference is made to complementary treatments if they affect conventional therapy (e.g. interactions with St John's wort—see Appendix 1). Further information on herbal medicines is available at www.mhra.gov.uk

***BNF for Children* and Marketing Authorisation** Where appropriate the *doses, indications, cautions, contra-indications and side-effects* in *BNF for Children* reflect those in the manufacturers' summaries of product characteristics (SPCs) which, in turn, reflect those in the corresponding marketing authorisations (formerly known as Product Licences). *BNF for Children* does not generally include proprietary medicines that are not supported by a valid summary of product characteristics or where the marketing authorisation holder has not been able to supply essential information.

As far as possible, medicines should be prescribed within the terms of the marketing authorisation. However, many children require medicines not specifically licensed for paediatric use. Although medicines cannot be promoted outside the limits of the licence, the Medicines Act does not prohibit the use of unlicensed medicines.

BNF for Children includes advice involving the use of unlicensed medicines or of licensed medicines for unlicensed uses ('off-label' use). Such advice reflects careful consideration of the options available to manage a given condition and the weight of evidence and experience of the unlicensed intervention (see also Unlicensed Medicines, p. 7). Where the advice falls outside a drug's marketing authorisation, *BNF for Children* shows the licensing status in the drug entry. However, limitations of the marketing authorisation should not preclude unlicensed use where clinically appropriate.

> Prescribing unlicensed medicines or medicines outside the recommendations of their marketing authorisation alters (and probably increases) the prescriber's professional responsibility and potential liability. The prescriber should be able to justify and feel competent in using such medicines.

When a preparation is available from more than one manufacturer, *BNF for Children* reflects advice that is the most clinically relevant regardless of any variation in the marketing authorisation.

Drugs and skilled tasks Prescribers should advise children and their carers if treatment is likely to affect their ability to perform skilled tasks. This applies especially to drugs with sedative effects; patients should be warned that these effects are increased by alcohol.

Oral syringes An **oral syringe** is supplied when oral liquid medicines are prescribed in doses other than multiples of 5 mL. The oral syringe is marked in 0.5-mL divisions from 1 to 5 mL to measure doses of less than 5 mL. It is provided with an adaptor and an instruction leaflet. The *5-mL spoon* is used for doses of 5 mL (or multiples thereof). Different sizes of oral syringe are available for the accurate measurement of smaller volumes, although these can not be prescribed.

Excipients Oral liquid preparations that do not contain *fructose, glucose* or *sucrose* are described as 'sugar-free' in *BNF for Children*. Preparations containing hydrogenated glucose syrup, mannitol, maltitol, sorbitol or xylitol are also marked 'sugar-free' since they do not cause dental caries. Children receiving medicines containing cariogenic sugars, or their carers, should be advised of dental hygiene measures to prevent caries. Sugar-free preparations should be used whenever possible, particularly if treatment is required for a long period.

Where information on the presence of alcohol, *aspartame, gluten, tartrazine, arachis (peanut) oil* or *sesame oil* is available, this is indicated in *BNF for Children* against the relevant preparation.

Information is provided on *selected excipients* in skin preparations (see section 13.1.3), vaccines (see section 14.1) and on *selected preservatives* and *excipients* in eye drops and injections. Pressurised metered aerosols containing *chlorofluorocarbons* (CFCs) have also been identified.

The presence of *benzyl alcohol* and *polyoxyl castor oil* (polyethoxylated castor oil) in injections is indicated in *BNF for Children*. Benzyl alcohol has been associated with a fatal toxic syndrome in preterm neonates, and therefore parenteral preparations containing the preservative should not be used in neonates. Polyoxyl castor oils, used as vehicles in intravenous injections, have been associated with severe anaphylactoid reactions.

The presence of *propylene glycol* in oral or parenteral medicines is indicated in *BNF for Children*; it can cause adverse effects if its elimination is impaired, e.g. in renal failure, in neonates and young children, and in slow metabolisers of the substance. It may interact with metronidazole.

> In the absence of information on excipients in *BNF for Children* and in the product literature, contact the manufacturer (see Index of Manufacturers) if it is essential to check details.

The European Commission guidance, *Excipients in the Label and Package leaflet of Medicinal Products for Human Use* is available at http://europa.eu.int/comm/enterprise/pharmaceuticals/index_en.htm.

Health and safety When handling chemical or biological materials particular attention should be given to the possibility of allergy, fire, explosion, radiation, or poisoning. Care is required to avoid sources of heat (including hair dryers) when flammable substances are used on the skin or hair. Substances, including corticosteroids, some antimicrobials, phenothiazines, and many cytotoxics, are irritant or very potent and should be handled with caution; contact with the skin and inhalation of dust should be avoided. Health care professionals and carers should guard against exposure to sensitising, toxic or irritant substances if it is necessary to crush tablets or open capsules.

Security of prescriptions The Councils of the British Medical Association and the Royal Pharmaceutical Society have issued a joint statement on the security and validity of prescriptions.

In particular, prescription forms should:

- not be left unattended at reception desks;
- not be left in a car where they may be visible; and
- when not in use, be kept in a locked drawer within the surgery and at home.

Patient group direction (PGD) In most cases, the most appropriate clinical care will be provided on an individual basis by a prescriber to a specific child. However, a Patient Group Direction for supply and administration of medicines by other healthcare professionals can be used where it would benefit the child's care without compromising safety.

A Patient Group Direction is a written direction relating to supply and administration (or administration only) of a prescription-only medicine by certain classes of healthcare professionals; the Direction is signed by a doctor (or dentist), and by a pharmacist. Further information on Patient Group Directions is available in Health Service Circular HSC 2000/026 (England), HDL (2001) 7 (Scotland), and WHC (2000) 116 (Wales).

NICE and Scottish Medicines Consortium Advice issued by the National Institute for Health and Clinical Excellence (NICE) and by the Scottish Medicines Consortium (SMC) is included in *BNF for Children* where relevant. Details of the advice together with updates may be obtained from www.nice.org.uk and from www.scottishmedicines.org.uk.

Prescription writing

> **Shared care**
> In its guidelines on responsibility for prescribing (circular EL (91) 127) between hospitals and general practitioners, the Department of Health has advised that legal responsibility for prescribing lies with the doctor who signs the prescription.

Prescriptions[1] should be written legibly in ink or otherwise so as to be indelible[2], should be dated, should state the full name and address of the patient, and should be signed in ink by the prescriber[3]. The age and the date of birth of the child should preferably be stated, and it is a legal requirement in the case of prescription-only medicines to state the age for children under 12 years.

Wherever appropriate the prescriber should state the current weight of the child to enable the dose prescribed to be checked. Consideration should also be given to including the dose per unit mass e.g. mg/kg or the dose per m^2 body-surface area e.g. mg/m^2 where this would reduce error.

The following should be noted:

(a) The unnecessary use of decimal points should be avoided, e.g. 3 mg, not 3.0 mg.
Quantities of 1 gram or more should be written as 1 g, etc.
Quantities less than 1 gram should be written in milligrams, e.g. 500 mg, not 0.5 g.
Quantities less than 1 mg should be written in micrograms, e.g. 100 micrograms, not 0.1 mg.
When decimals are unavoidable a zero should be written in front of the decimal point where there is no other figure, e.g. 0.5 mL, not .5 mL.
Use of the decimal point is acceptable to express a range, e.g. 0.5 to 1 g.

(b) 'Micrograms' and 'nanograms' should **not** be abbreviated. Similarly 'units' should **not** be abbreviated.

(c) The term 'millilitre' (ml or mL)[4] is used in medicine and pharmacy, and cubic centimetre, c.c., or cm^3 should not be used.

(d) Dose and dose frequency should be stated; in the case of preparations to be taken 'as required' a **minimum dose interval** should be specified.
Care should be taken to ensure the child receives the correct dose of the active drug. Therefore, the dose should normally be stated in terms of the mass of the active drug (e.g. '125 mg 3 times daily); terms such as '5 mL' or '1 tablet' should be avoided except for compound preparations.
When doses other than multiples of 5 mL are prescribed for *oral liquid preparations* the dose-volume will be provided by means of an **oral syringe**, see p. 3 (except for preparations intended to be measured with a pipette).

(e) The names of drugs and preparations should be written clearly and **not** abbreviated, using approved titles **only** (see also advice in box on p. 6 to **avoid** creating generic titles for modified-release preparations).

(f) The quantity to be supplied may be stated by indicating the number of days of treatment required in the box provided on NHS forms. In most cases the exact amount will be supplied. This does not apply to items directed to be used as required—if the dose and frequency are not given the quantity to be supplied needs to be stated.
When several items are ordered on one form the box can be marked with the number of days of treatment provided the quantity is added for any item for which the amount cannot be calculated.

(g) Although directions should preferably be in **English without abbreviation**, it is recognised that some Latin abbreviations are used (for details see Inside Back Cover).

---

1. The above recommendations are acceptable for **prescription-only medicines** (PoM). For items marked CD see also Prescribing Controlled Drugs p. 17.
2. It is permissible to issue carbon copies of NHS prescriptions as long as they are signed in ink.
3. Computer-generated facsimile signatures do not meet the legal requirement.
4. The use of capital 'L' in mL is a printing convention throughout *BNF for Children*; both 'mL' and 'ml' are recognised SI abbreviations.

Abbreviation of titles In general, titles of drugs and preparations should be written *in full*. Unofficial abbreviations should **not** be used as they may be misinterpreted.

Non-proprietary titles Where non-proprietary ('generic') titles are given, they should be used for prescribing. This will enable any suitable product to be dispensed, thereby saving delay to the patient and sometimes expense to the health service. The only exception is where bioavailability problems are so important that the child should always receive the same brand; in such cases, the brand name or the manufacturer should be stated.

> Non-proprietary names of **compound preparations** e.g. co-codamol which appear in *BNF for Children* are those that have been compiled by the British Pharmacopoeia Commission or another recognised body; whenever possible they reflect the names of the active ingredients.
>
> Prescribers should avoid creating their own compound names for the purposes of generic prescribing; such names do not have an approved definition and can be misinterpreted.
>
> Special care should be taken to avoid errors when prescribing compound preparations; in particular the hyphen in the prefix 'co-' should be retained.
>
> Special care should also be taken to avoid creating generic names for **modified-release** preparations where the use of these names could lead to confusion between formulations with different duration of action.

Strengths and quantities The strength or quantity to be contained in capsules, lozenges, tablets, etc. should be stated by the prescriber. In particular, strengths of liquid preparations should be clearly stated (e.g. 125 mg/5 mL)

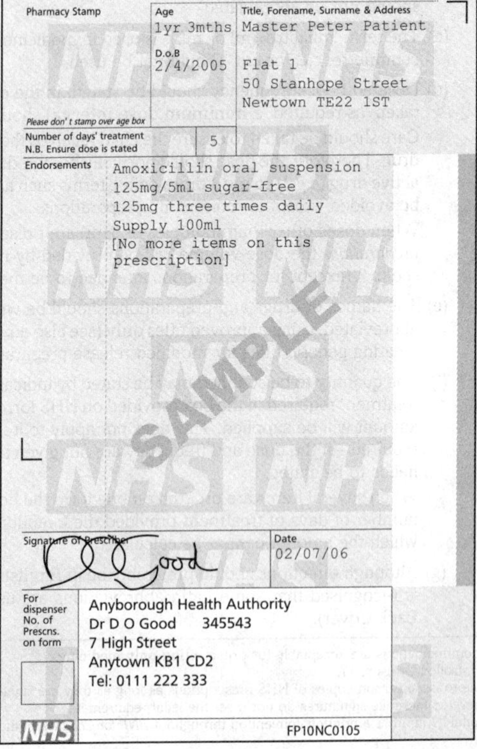
Pharmacy Stamp
Age: 1yr 3mths
D.o.B: 2/4/2005
Title, Forename, Surname & Address: Master Peter Patient, Flat 1, 50 Stanhope Street, Newtown TE22 1ST
Please don't stamp over age box
Number of days' treatment N.B. Ensure dose is stated: 5
Endorsements
Amoxicillin oral suspension
125mg/5ml sugar-free
125mg three times daily
Supply 100ml
[No more items on this prescription]
SAMPLE
Signature of Prescriber: D O Good
Date: 02/07/06
For dispenser No. of Prescns. on form
Anyborough Health Authority
Dr D O Good 345543
7 High Street
Anytown KB1 CD2
Tel: 0111 222 333
NHS
FP10NC0105

Supply of medicines

When supplying a medicine for a child, the pharmacist should ensure that the child and the child's carer understand the nature and identity of the medicine and how it should be used. The child and the carer should be provided with appropriate information (e.g. how long the medicine should be taken for and what to do if a dose is missed or the child vomits soon after the dose is given).

Safety in the home Carers and relatives of children must be warned to keep all medicines out of the reach and sight of children. Tablets, capsules and oral and external liquid preparations must be dispensed in a reclosable *child-resistant container* unless:

- the medicine is in an original pack or patient pack such as to make this inadvisable;
- the child's carer will have difficulty in opening a child-resistant container;
- a specific request is made that the product shall not be dispensed in a child-resistant container;
- no suitable child-resistant container exists for a particular liquid preparation.

All patients should be advised to dispose of *unwanted medicines* by returning them to a pharmacy for destruction.

Validity of prescriptions Where there is any doubt about the authenticity of a prescription, the pharmacist should contact the prescriber. If this is done by telephone, the number should be obtained from the directory rather than relying on the information on the prescription form, which may be false.

Strength and quantities If a pharmacist receives an incomplete prescription for a systemically administered preparation[1] and considers it would not be appropriate for the patient to return to the prescriber, the following procedures will apply:

(a) an attempt must always be made to contact the prescriber to ascertain the intention;

(b) if the attempt is successful the pharmacist must, where practicable, subsequently arrange for details of quantity, strength where applicable, and dosage to be inserted by the prescriber on the incomplete form;

(c) where, although the prescriber has been contacted, it has not proved possible to obtain the written intention regarding an incomplete prescription, the pharmacist may endorse the form 'p.c.' (prescriber contacted) and add details of the quantity and strength where applicable of the preparation supplied, and of the dose indicated. The endorsement should be initialled and dated by the pharmacist;

(d) where the prescriber cannot be contacted and the pharmacist has sufficient information to make a professional judgment the preparation may be dispensed. If the quantity is missing the pharmacist may supply sufficient to complete up to 5 days' treatment; except that where a combination pack (i.e. a proprietary pack containing more than one medicinal product) or oral contraceptive is prescribed by name only, the smallest pack shall be dispensed. In all cases the prescription must be endorsed 'p.n.c.' (prescriber not contacted), the quantity, the dose, and the strength (where applicable) of the preparation supplied must be indicated, and the endorsement must be initialled and dated;

(e) if the pharmacist has any doubt about exercising discretion, an incomplete prescription must be referred back to the prescriber.

Unlicensed medicines A drug or formulation that is not covered by a Marketing Authorisation (see also *BNF for Children* and Marketing Authorisation) may be obtained from a pharmaceutical company, imported by a specialist importer, manufactured by a commercial or hospital licensed manufacturing unit, or prepared extemporaneously (see below) against a prescription.

1. With the exception of temazepam, an incomplete prescription is **not** acceptable for controlled drugs in schedules 2 and 3 of the Misuse of Drugs Regulations 2001

The safeguards that apply to products with Marketing Authorisation should be extended, as far as possible, to the use of unlicensed medicines. The safety, efficacy and quality (including labelling) of unlicensed medicines should be assured by means of clear policies on their prescribing, purchase, supply and administration. Extra care is required with unlicensed medicines because less information may be available on the drug and any formulation of the drug.

The following should be agreed with the supplier when ordering an unlicensed or extemporaneously prepared medicine:

- the specification of the formulation
- documentation confirming the specification and quality of the product supplied (e.g. a certificate of conformity or of analysis)
- for imported preparations product and licensing information should be supplied in English

Extemporaneous preparations A product should be dispensed extemporaneously only when no product with a marketing authorisation is available. Every effort should be made to ensure that an extemporaneously prepared product is stable and that it delivers the requisite dose reliably; the child should be provided with a consistent formulation regardless of where the medicine is supplied to minimise variations in quality. Where there is doubt about the formulation, advice should be sought from a medicines information centre, the pharmacy at a children's hospital, a hospital production unit, a hospital quality control department, or the manufacturer.

In many cases it is preferable to give a licensed product by an unlicensed route (e.g. an injection solution given by mouth) than to prepare a special formulation. Where tablets or capsules are cut, dispersed or used for preparing liquids immediately prior to administration, it is important to confirm uniform dispersal of the active ingredient, especially if only a portion of the solid content (e.g. a tablet segment) is used or if only an aliquot of the liquid is to be administered.

In some cases the child's clinical condition may require a dose to be administered in the absence of full information on the method of administration. It is important to ensure that the appropriate supporting information is available at the earliest opportunity.

Preparation of products that produce harmful dust (e.g. cytotoxic drugs, hormones, or potentially sensitising drugs such as neomycin) should be **avoided** or undertaken with appropriate precautions to protect staff and carers (see also Safety in the Home, above).

The BP direction that a preparation must be *freshly prepared* indicates that it must be made not more than 24 hours before it is issued for use. The direction that a preparation should be *recently prepared* indicates that deterioration is likely if the preparation is stored for longer than about 4 weeks at 15–25° C.

The term **water** used without qualification means either potable water freshly drawn direct from the public supply and suitable for drinking or freshly boiled and cooled purified water. The latter should be used if the public supply is from a local storage tank or if the potable water is unsuitable for a particular preparation (Water for injections, section 9.2.2).

Labelling medicines The *name* of the medicine should appear on the label unless the prescriber indicates otherwise; the name shown on the label should be that written on the prescription. The *strength* should also be stated on the label in the case of preparations that are available in different strengths.

Labels should indicate the *total quantity* of the product dispensed in the container to which the label refers. This requirement applies equally to solid, liquid, internal, and external preparations. If a product is dispensed in more than one container, the reference should be to the amount in each container.

Emergency supply of medicines

Emergency supply requested by member of the public

Pharmacists are sometimes called upon by members of the public to make an emergency supply of medicines. The Prescription Only Medicines (Human Use) Order 1997 allows exemptions from the Prescription Only requirements for emergency supply to be made by a person lawfully conducting a retail pharmacy business provided:

(a) that the pharmacist has interviewed the person requesting the prescription-only medicine and is satisfied:

  (i) that there is immediate need for the prescription-only medicine and that it is impracticable in the circumstances to obtain a prescription without undue delay;

  (ii) that treatment with the prescription-only medicine has on a previous occasion been prescribed by a doctor[1], a supplementary prescriber, a district nurse or health visitor prescriber or an independent nurse prescriber for the person for whom it is being requested;

  (iii) as to the dose which it would be appropriate for the person to take;

(b) that no greater quantity shall be supplied than will provide 5 days' treatment except when the prescription-only medicine is:

  (i) insulin, an ointment or, cream, or a preparation for the relief of asthma in an aerosol dispenser when the smallest pack can be supplied;

  (ii) an oral contraceptive when a full cycle may be supplied;

  (iii) an antibiotic in liquid form for oral administration when the smallest quantity that will provide a full course of treatment can be supplied;

(c) that an entry shall be made by the pharmacist in the prescription book stating:

  (i) the date of supply;

  (ii) the name, quantity and, where appropriate, the pharmaceutical form and strength;

  (iii) the name and address of the patient;

  (iv) the nature of the emergency;

(d) that the container or package must be labelled to show:

  (i) the date of supply;

  (ii) the name, quantity and, where appropriate, the pharmaceutical form and strength;

  (iii) the name of the patient;

  (iv) the name and address of the pharmacy;

  (v) the words 'Emergency supply';

  (vi) the words 'Keep out of the reach of children' (or similar warning).

(e) that the prescription-only medicine is not a substance specifically excluded from the emergency supply provision, and does not contain a Controlled Drug specified in schedules 1, 2, or 3 to the Misuse of Drugs Regulations 2001 except for phenobarbital or phenobarbital sodium for the treatment of epilepsy: for details see *Medicines, Ethics and Practice*, No. 30, London, Pharmaceutical Press, 2006 (and subsequent editions as available).

Emergency supply requested by prescriber

Emergency supply of a prescription-only medicine may also be made at the request of a doctor, a supplementary prescriber, a district nurse or health visitor prescriber, or an independent nurse prescriber provided:

(a) that the pharmacist is satisfied that the prescriber by reason of some emergency is unable to furnish a prescription immediately;

1. The doctor must be a UK-registered doctor.

(b) that the prescriber has undertaken to furnish a prescription within 72 hours;

(c) that the medicine is supplied in accordance with the directions of the prescriber requesting it;

(d) that the medicine is not a substance specifically excluded from the emergency supply provision, and does not contain a Controlled Drug specified in schedules 1, 2, or 3 to the Misuse of Drugs Regulations 2001 except for phenobarbital or phenobarbital sodium for the treatment of epilepsy: for details see *Medicines, Ethics and Practice*, No. 30, London, Pharmaceutical Press, 2006 (and subsequent editions as available);

(e) that an entry shall be made in the prescription book stating:

(i) the date of supply;

(ii) the name, quantity and, where appropriate, the pharmaceutical form and strength;

(iii) the name and address of the practitioner requesting the emergency supply;

(iv) the name and address of the patient;

(v) the date on the prescription;

(vi) when the prescription is received the entry should be amended to include the date on which it is received.

Royal Pharmaceutical Society's Guidelines

1. The pharmacist should consider the medical consequences of *not* supplying a medicine in an emergency.
2. If the pharmacist is unable to make an emergency supply of a medicine the pharmacist should advise the patient how to obtain essential medical care.

For conditions that apply to supplies made at the request of a patient see *Medicines, Ethics and Practice*, No. 30, London Pharmaceutical Press, 2006 (and subsequent editions).

Drug treatment in children

Children, and particularly neonates, differ from adults in their response to drugs. Special care is needed in the neonatal period (first 28 days of life) and doses should always be calculated with care; the risk of toxicity is increased by reduced rate of drug clearance and differing target organ sensitivity.

Many children's doses in *BNF for Children* are standardised by **weight** (and therefore require multiplying by the body-weight in kilograms to determine the child's dose); occasionally, the doses have been standardised by **body surface area** (in m^2) (see also How to Use *BNF for Children*, p. vi). These methods should be used rather than attempting to calculate a child's dose on the basis of doses used in adults. If a dose is not stated, prescribers should seek advice from a medicines information centre.

For most drugs the adult maximum dose should not be exceeded. For example if the dose is 8 mg/kg (max. 300 mg) a child of 10 kg body-weight should receive 80 mg but a child of 40 kg body-weight should receive 300 mg (rather than 320 mg). For certain drugs, young children may require a higher dose per kilogram than adults because of their higher metabolic rates. Calculation by body-weight in the overweight child may result in much higher doses being administered than necessary; in such cases, the dose should be calculated from an ideal weight, related to height and age.

Body-surface area (BSA) estimates are more accurate for calculating paediatric doses than body-weight since many physiological phenomena correlate better to body-surface area.

Body-surface area may be calculated from height and weight by means of a nomogram; see also inside back cover.

Where the dose for children is not stated, prescribers should seek advice from a medicines information centre.

Dose frequency Most drugs can be administered at slightly irregular intervals during the day. Some drugs e.g. antimicrobials are best given at regular intervals. Some flexibility should be allowed in children to avoid waking them during the night. For example, the night-time dose may be given at the parent's bedtime.

Prescribing in hepatic impairment

Children have a large reserve of hepatic metabolic capacity and modification of the choice and dosage of drugs is usually unnecessary even in apparently severe liver disease. However, special consideration is required in the following situations:

- liver failure characterised by severe derangement of liver enzymes and profound jaundice; the use of sedative drugs, opioids and drugs such as diuretics and amphotericin which produce hypokalaemia may precipitate hepatic encephalopathy
- impaired coagulation, which can affect response to oral anticoagulants;
- in cholestatic jaundice elimination may be impaired of drugs such as fusidic acid and rifampicin which are excreted in the bile
- in hypoproteinaemia, the effect of highly protein-bound drugs such as phenytoin, prednisolone, warfarin, and benzodiazepines may be increased;
- use of hepatotoxic drugs is more likely to cause toxicity in children with liver disease; such drugs should be avoided if possible;
- in neonates, particularly pre-term neonates, and also in infants metabolic pathways may differ from older children and adults because liver enzyme pathways may be immature;

Where care is needed in hepatic impairment, this is indicated under the relevant drug in *BNF for Children*.

Prescribing in renal impairment

The use of drugs in children with reduced renal function can give rise to problems for several reasons:

- failure to excrete a drug or its metabolites may produce toxicity;
- sensitivity to some drugs is increased even if elimination is unimpaired;
- many side-effects are tolerated poorly by children in renal failure;
- some drugs cease to be effective when renal function is reduced;
- neonates, particularly pre-term, may have immature renal function.

Many of these problems can be avoided by reducing the dose or by using alternative drugs.

Principles of dose adjustment in renal impairment

The level of renal function below which the dose must be reduced depends on whether the drug is eliminated entirely by renal excretion or is partly metabolised, and on how toxic it is. For many drugs with only minor or no dose-related side-effects very precise modification of the dose regimen in renal impairment is unnecessary and a simple scheme for dose reduction is sufficient.
For more toxic drugs with a small safety margin dose regimens based on glomerular filtration rate should be used. For those where both efficacy and toxicity are closely related to plasma-drug concentrations recommended regimens should be seen only as a guide to initial treatment; subsequent treatment must be adjusted according to clinical response and plasma-drug concentration.

The total daily maintenance dose of a drug can be reduced either by reducing the size of the individual doses or by increasing the interval between doses. For some drugs, if the size of the maintenance dose is reduced it will be important to give a loading dose if an immediate effect is required. This is because when a child is given a regular dose of any drug it takes more than four times the half-life to achieve steady-state plasma concentrations. As the plasma half-life of drugs excreted by the kidney is prolonged in renal failure it may take many days for the reduced dosage to achieve a therapeutic plasma concentration. For most drugs the loading dose should usually be the same size as the initial dose for a child with normal renal function.

Nephrotoxic drugs should, if possible, be avoided in children with renal disease because the consequences of nephrotoxicity are likely to be more serious when the renal reserve is already reduced.

Doses are adjusted according to the severity of renal impairment. This is expressed in terms of glomerular filtration rate (GFR), usually measured by the **creatinine clearance** (mL/minute/1.73m^2). The serum-creatinine concentration is often used as a measure of renal function but is only a **rough guide** even when corrected for age, weight, and sex. Nomograms and equations are available for making the correction and should be used where accuracy is important.

For a child over 1 year, the following equation provides a guide to the creatinine clearance:
Approximate creatinine clearance (mL/minute/1.73 m^2)
= 40 × height (cm)/serum creatinine (micromol/litre)

For a neonate, the following equation provides a guide to creatinine clearance:
Approximate creatinine clearance (mL/minute/1.73 m^2)
= 30 × height (cm)/serum creatinine (micromol/litre)

For *prescribing purposes* renal impairment is arbitrarily divided into 3 grades (definitions vary for grades of renal impairment; therefore, where the product literature does not correspond with this grading, values for creatinine clearance or another measure of renal function are included):

Grades of renal impairment

Grade	GFR	Serum creatinine (approx.) (but see above)
Mild	20–50 mL/minute/1.73 m^2	150–300 micromol/litre
Moderate	10–20 mL/minute/1.73 m^2	300–700 micromol/litre
Severe	$<$ 10 mL/minute/1.73 m^2	$>$ 700 micromol/litre

> **Dialysis**
> For prescribing in children on renal replacement therapy consult specialist literature.

Drug prescribing should be kept to the minimum in all children with severe renal disease.

If even mild renal impairment is considered likely on clinical grounds, renal function should be checked before prescribing **any** drug which requires dose modification.

Where care is needed in renal impairment, this is indicated under the relevant drug in *BNF for Children*.

Prescribing in pregnancy

Drugs can have harmful effects on the fetus at any time during pregnancy. It is important to bear this in mind when prescribing for a female of *childbearing age* or for men *trying to father* a child.

During the *first trimester* drugs may produce congenital malformations (teratogenesis), and the period of greatest risk is from the third to the eleventh week of pregnancy.

During the *second* and *third trimesters* drugs may affect the growth and functional development of the fetus or have toxic effects on fetal tissues; and drugs given shortly before term or during labour may have adverse effects on labour or on the neonate after delivery.

BNF for Children identifies drugs which:

- may have harmful effects in pregnancy and indicates the trimester of risk
- are not known to be harmful in pregnancy

The information is based on human data but information on *animal* studies has been included for some drugs when its omission might be misleading. Maternal drug doses may require adjustment during pregnancy due to changes in maternal physiology but this is beyond the scope of *BNF for Children*.

Drugs should be prescribed in pregnancy only if the expected benefit to the mother is thought to be greater than the risk to the fetus, and all drugs should be avoided if possible during the first trimester. Drugs which have been extensively used in pregnancy and appear to be usually safe should be prescribed in preference to new or untried drugs; and the smallest effective dose should be used.

Few drugs have been shown conclusively to be teratogenic in humans but no drug is safe beyond all doubt in early pregnancy. Screening procedures are available where there is a known risk of certain defects.

Absence of a drug from the list does not imply safety. It should be noted that *BNF for Children* provides independent advice and may not always agree with the product literature.

Information on drugs and pregnancy is also available from the National Teratology Information Service Telephone:

Tel: (0191) 232 1525

Tel: (0191) 223 1307 (out of hours emergency only)

www.nyrdtc.nhs.uk/Services/teratology/teratology.html

Prescribing in breast-feeding

Most medicines given to a mother cause no harm to breast-fed infants and there are few contra-indications to breast-feeding when maternal medicines are necessary. However, administration of some drugs (e.g. ergotamine) to nursing mothers may harm the infant. In the first week of life, some such as preterm or jaundiced infants are at a slightly higher risk of toxicity. Infants with glucose-6-phosphate dehydrogenase (G6PD) deficiency (section 9.1.5) and atopic infants may also be at increased risk of toxicity.

Toxicity to the infant can occur if the drug enters the milk in pharmacologically significant quantities. The concentration in milk of some drugs (e.g. iodides) may exceed the concentration in maternal plasma so that therapeutic doses in the mother may cause toxicity to the infant. Some drugs inhibit the infant's sucking reflex (e.g. phenobarbital). Drugs in breast milk may, at least theoretically, cause hypersensitivity in the infant even when concentration is too low for a pharmacological effect. *BNF for Children* identifies drugs:

- which should be used with caution or which are contra-indicated in breast-feeding for the reasons given above;
- which, on present evidence, may be given to the mother during breast-feeding, because they appear in milk in amounts which are too small to be harmful to the infant;
- which are not known to be harmful to the infant although they are present in milk in significant amounts.

For many drugs insufficient evidence is available to provide guidance and it is advisable to administer only essential drugs to a mother during breast-feeding. Because of the inadequacy of information on drugs in breast milk information in *BNF for Children* should be used only as a guide; absence of information does not imply safety.

Prescribing controlled drugs

Prescriptions Preparations which are subject to the prescription requirements of the Misuse of Drugs Regulations 2001 (and subsequent amendments), i.e. preparations specified in schedules 2 and 3, are distinguished throughout this publication by the symbol CD (Controlled Drug). The principal legal requirements relating to medical prescriptions are listed below. Additional requirements on the prescribing and dispensing of Controlled Drugs are shown under Department of Health guidance, below.

Prescriptions for Controlled Drugs which are subject to prescription requirements must be indelible[1] and must be *signed* by the prescriber, *be dated*, and specify the prescriber's *address*. The prescription must always state[2]:

- The name and address of the patient;
- In the case of a preparation, the form[3] and where appropriate the strength[4] of the preparation;
- The total quantity of the preparation, or the number of dose units, *in both words and figures;*[2]
- The dose;[5]
- The words 'for dental treatment only' if issued by a dentist.

A prescription may order a Controlled Drug to be dispensed by instalments; the amount of the instalments and the intervals to be observed must be specified.[6] Prescriptions ordering 'repeats' on the same form are **not** permitted. A prescription is valid for 13 weeks from the date stated thereon (but see Department of Health guidance, below).

It is an offence for a prescriber to issue an incomplete prescription and a pharmacist is **not** allowed to dispense a Controlled Drug unless all the information required by law is given on the prescription. Failure to comply with the regulations concerning the writing of prescriptions will result in inconvenience to patients and carers and delay in supply of the necessary medicine.

Department of Health guidance Interim guidance issued by the Department of Health in England on prescribing and dispensing of controlled drugs (consult www.dh.gov.uk/controlleddrug for full guidance) requires:

- that prescriptions of Controlled Drugs in Schedules 2, 3 and 4 will be valid for up to 28 days after the date of issue
- in general, prescriptions for Controlled Drugs in Schedules 2, 3 and 4 to be limited to a supply of up to 30 days' treatment; exceptionally, to cover a justifiable clinical need and after consideration of any risk, a prescription can be issued for a longer period, but the reasons for the decision should be recorded on the patient's notes
- use of a specially designated form (FP10PCD) for private prescriptions of Controlled Drugs in Schedules 2 and 3
- a unique identifier, allocated to those who issue private prescriptions, to be shown on private prescriptions for Controlled Drugs in Schedules 2 and 3
- the patient's NHS number to be shown on NHS and private prescriptions for Controlled Drugs in Schedules 2 and 3
- patients, or those collecting medicines on the patient's behalf, to sign for Controlled Drugs in Schedules 2 and 3.

---

1. A machine written prescription is acceptable. The prescriber's signature must be handwritten.
2. Does not apply to prescriptions for temazepam.
3. The dosage form (e.g. tablets) must be included on a Controlled Drugs prescription irrespective of whether it is implicit in the proprietary name (e.g. *MST Continus*) or of whether only one form is available.
4. When more than one strength of a preparation exists the strength required must be specified.
5. The instruction 'one as directed' constitutes a dose but 'as directed' does not.
6. A total of 14 days' treatment by instalment of any drug listed in Schedule 2 of the Misuse of Drugs Regulations and buprenorphine may be prescribed in England. In *England*, form FP10MDA-SS (blue) or occasionally form FP10MDA (blue) should be used; in hospital, form FP10HP(AD) is being replaced by form FP10MDA-SS. In *Scotland* forms HBP(A) (hospital-based prescribers) or GP10 (general practitioners) should be used. In *Wales* a total of 14 days treatment by instalment of any drug listed in Schedules 2–5 of the Misuse of Drugs Regulations may be prescribed. In Wales form WP10(MDA) or form WP10HP(AD) for hospital prescribers should be used.

Dependence and misuse The most serious drugs of addiction are **cocaine**, **diamorphine** (heroin), **morphine**, and the **synthetic opioids**.

Despite marked reduction in the prescribing of **amphetamines** the abuse of illicit amfetamine and related compounds is widespread.

Temazepam is subject to the requirement for safe custody of controlled drugs because of problems with abuse, but it is exempt from the prescription requirements for Controlled Drugs. A prescription for temazepam is valid for 13 weeks from the date stated thereon (but see Department of Health guidance, above).

The principal **barbiturates** are Controlled Drugs and must fulfil all Controlled Drug prescription requirements; for the treatment of epilepsy phenobarbital and phenobarbital sodium are available under the emergency supply regulations (p. 9).

Cannabis (Indian hemp) has no approved medicinal use and cannot be prescribed by doctors. Its use is illegal but has become widespread. Cannabis is a mild hallucinogen seldom accompanied by a desire to increase the dose; withdrawal symptoms are unusual. **Lysergide** (lysergic acid diethylamide, LSD) is a much more potent hallucinogen; its use can lead to severe psychotic states in which life may be at risk.

Prescribing drugs likely to cause dependence or misuse The prescriber has three main responsibilities:

- To avoid creating dependence by introducing drugs to patients without sufficient reason. In this context, the proper use of the morphine-like drugs is well understood. The dangers of other controlled drugs are less clear because

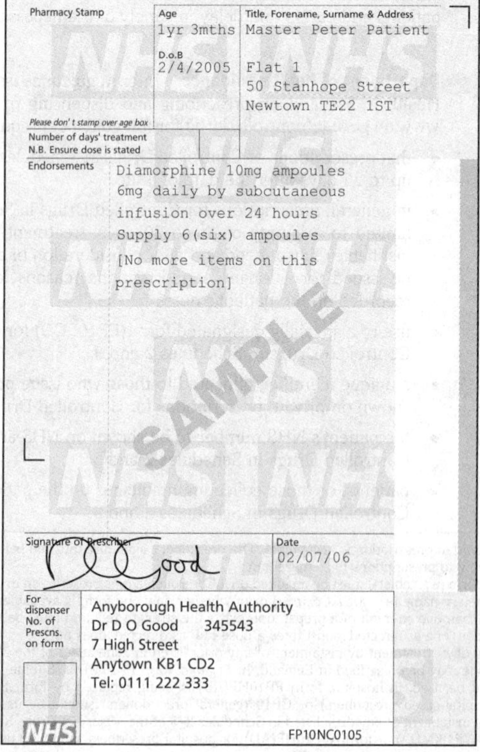

Pharmacy Stamp

Age
1yr 3mths

D.o.B
2/4/2005

Title, Forename, Surname & Address
Master Peter Patient
Flat 1
50 Stanhope Street
Newtown TE22 1ST

Please don't stamp over age box

Number of days' treatment
N.B. Ensure dose is stated

Endorsements

Diamorphine 10mg ampoules
6mg daily by subcutaneous
infusion over 24 hours
Supply 6(six) ampoules
[No more items on this
prescription]

SAMPLE

Signature of Prescriber
D O Good

Date
02/07/06

For dispenser
No. of Prescns. on form

Anyborough Health Authority
Dr D O Good 345543
7 High Street
Anytown KB1 CD2
Tel: 0111 222 333

NHS

FP10NC0105

recognition of dependence is not easy and its effects, and those of withdrawal, are less obvious.

- To see that the patient does not gradually increase the dose of a drug, given for good medical reasons, to the point where dependence becomes more likely. The prescriber should keep a close eye on the amount prescribed to prevent patients or their carers from accumulating stocks. A minimal amount should be prescribed in the first instance, or when seeing a new patient for the first time.
- To avoid being used as an unwitting source of supply for addicts and being vigilant to methods for obtaining medicines which include visiting more than one doctor, fabricating stories, and forging prescriptions.

Patients under temporary care should be given only small supplies of drugs unless they present an unequivocal letter from their own doctors. It is sensible to decrease dosages steadily or to issue weekly or even daily prescriptions for small amounts if dependence is suspected.

The stealing and misuse of prescription forms could be minimised by the following precautions:

(a) do not leave unattended if called away from the consulting room or at reception desks; do not leave in a car where they may be visible; when not in use, keep in a locked drawer within the surgery and at home;

(b) draw a diagonal line across the blank part of the form under the prescription;

(c) the quantity should be shown in words and figures when prescribing drugs prone to abuse; this is obligatory for controlled drugs (see Prescriptions, above);

(d) alterations are best avoided but if any are made they should be clear and unambiguous; add initials against altered items;

(e) if prescriptions are left for collection they should be left in a safe place in a sealed envelope.

Travelling abroad Prescribed drugs listed in schedule 4 Part II (CD Anab) [only when in the form of a medicinal product and for self-administration] and schedule 5 of the Misuse of Drugs Regulations 2001 are not subject to import or export licensing, but doctors are advised that patients intending to carry Schedule 2, 3, and 4 Part I (CD Benz) and part II (CD Anab) drugs abroad may require an export licence (subject to the above exemption for schedule 4 Part II). This is dependent upon the amount of drug to be exported and further details may be obtained from the Home Office by contacting (020) 7035 0472 or licensing_enquiry.aadu@homeoffice.gsi.gov.uk. Applications for licences should be sent to the Home Office, Drugs Licensing Section, 6th Floor, Peel Building, 2 Marsham Street, London, SW1P 4DF.

Applications must be supported by a letter from a doctor giving details of:

- the patient's name and current address;
- the quantities of drugs to be carried;
- the strength and form in which the drugs will be dispensed;
- the dates of travel to and from the United Kingdom.

Ten days should be allowed for processing the application.

Individual doctors who wish to take Controlled Drugs abroad while accompanying patients may similarly be issued with licences. Licences are not normally issued to doctors who wish to take Controlled Drugs abroad solely in case a family emergency should arise.

These import/export licences for named individuals do not have any legal status outside the UK and are only issued to comply with the Misuse of Drugs Act and facilitate passage through UK Customs and Excise control. For clearance in the country to be visited it would be necessary to approach that country's consulate in the UK.

Misuse of Drugs Act

The Misuse of Drugs Act, 1971 prohibits certain activities in relation to 'Controlled Drugs', in particular their manufacture, supply, and possession. The penalties applicable to offences involving the different drugs are graded broadly according to the *harmfulness attributable to a drug when it is misused* and for this purpose the drugs are defined in the following three classes:

Class A includes: alfentanil, cocaine, diamorphine (heroin), dipipanone, lysergide (LSD), methadone, methylenedioxymethamfetamine (MDMA, 'ecstasy'), morphine, opium, pethidine, phencyclidine, remifentanil, and class B substances when prepared for injection

Class B includes: oral amphetamines, barbiturates, codeine, ethylmorphine, glutethimide, pentazocine, phenmetrazine, and pholcodine

Class C includes: certain drugs related to the amphetamines such as benzfetamine and chlorphentermine, buprenorphine, cannabis, cannabis resin, diethylpropion, mazindol, meprobamate, pemoline, pipradrol, most benzodiazepines, zolpidem, androgenic and anabolic steroids, clenbuterol, chorionic gonadotrophin (HCG), non-human chorionic gonadotrophin, somatotropin, somatrem, and somatropin

The Misuse of Drugs Regulations 2001 define the classes of person who are authorised to supply and possess controlled drugs while acting in their professional capacities and lay down the conditions under which these activities may be carried out. In the regulations drugs are divided into five schedules each specifying the requirements governing such activities as import, export, production, supply, possession, prescribing, and record keeping which apply to them.

Schedule 1 includes drugs such as cannabis and lysergide which are not used medicinally. Possession and supply are prohibited except in accordance with Home Office authority.

Schedule 2 includes drugs such as diamorphine (heroin), morphine, remifentanil, pethidine, secobarbital, glutethimide, amfetamine, and cocaine and are subject to the full controlled drug requirements relating to prescriptions, safe custody (except for secobarbital), the need to keep registers, etc. (unless exempted in schedule 5).

Schedule 3 includes the barbiturates (except secobarbital, now schedule 2), buprenorphine, diethylpropion, mazindol, meprobamate, pentazocine, phentermine, and temazepam. They are subject to the special prescription requirements (except for temazepam, see p. 17) but not to the safe custody requirements (except for buprenorphine, diethylpropion, flunitrazepam, and temazepam) nor to the need to keep registers (although there are requirements for the retention of invoices for 2 years).

Schedule 4 includes in Part I benzodiazepines (except temazepam which is in schedule 3) and zolpidem, which are subject to minimal control. Part II includes androgenic and anabolic steroids, clenbuterol, chorionic gonadotrophin (HCG), non-human chorionic gonadotrophin, somatotropin, somatrem, and somatropin. Controlled Drug prescription requirements do not apply (but see Department of Health guidance, p. 17) and Schedule 4 Controlled Drugs are not subject to safe custody requirements.

Schedule 5 includes those preparations which, because of their strength, are exempt from virtually all Controlled Drug requirements other than retention of invoices for two years.

Notification of drug misusers

Doctors are expected to report on a standard form cases of drug misuse to their regional or national drug misuse database or centre—for further advice and contact telephone numbers consult the BNF.

Adverse reactions to drugs

Any drug may produce unwanted or unexpected adverse reactions. Detection and recording of these is vital. Doctors, dentists, coroners, pharmacists and nurses (see also self-reporting, below) are urged to help by reporting suspected adverse reactions on yellow cards to:

Medicines and Healthcare products Regulatory Agency (MHRA)
[1]CSM
Freepost
London, SW8 5BR.
Tel: (0800 731 6789)

The reporting of **all** suspected adverse drug reactions in children, including those relating to unlicensed or off-label use of medicines, is **strongly encouraged** through the Yellow Card scheme (see below) even if the intensive monitoring symbol (▼) has been removed, because experience in children may still be limited.

The identification and reporting of adverse reactions to drugs in children is particularly important because:

- the action of the drug and its pharmacokinetics in children (especially in the very young) may be different from that in adults
- drugs may not be extensively tested in children
- children may be more susceptible to developmental disorders or they may have delayed adverse reactions which do not occur in adults
- many drugs are not specifically licensed for use in children and are used 'off-label'
- suitable formulations may not be available to allow precise dosing in children
- the nature and course of illnesses and adverse drug reactions may differ between adults and children.

Suspected adverse reactions to *any* therapeutic agent should be reported, including drugs *(self-medication* as well as those *prescribed)*, blood products, vaccines, radiographic contrast media and herbal products. Prepaid Yellow Cards for reporting are available from the above address and are also bound in this book (inside back cover). Adverse reactions can also be reported at www.yellowcard.gov.uk.

Spontaneous reporting is particularly valuable for recognising possible new hazards rapidly. An adverse reaction should be reported even if it is not certain that the drug has caused it, or if the reaction is well recognised, or if other drugs have been given at the same time. Reports of overdoses (deliberate or accidental) can complicate the assessment of adverse drug reactions, but provide important information on the potential toxicity of drugs.

A 24-hour Freefone service is available to all parts of the UK for advice and information on suspected adverse drug reactions; contact the National Yellow Card Information Service at the MHRA on 0800 731 6789. Outside office hours a telephone-answering machine will take messages.

The following regional centres also collect data:

Yellow Card Centre, Mersey
Freepost
Liverpool, L3 3AB.
Tel: (0151) 794 8206

Yellow Card Centre, Wales
Freepost
Cardiff, CF4 1ZZ.
Tel: (029) 2074 4181 (direct line)

Yellow Card Centre, Northern & Yorkshire
Freepost 1085
Newcastle upon Tyne, NE1 1BR.
Tel: (0191) 232 1525 (direct line)

1. CSM now subsumed under Commission on Human Medicines (CHM).

Yellow Card Centre, West Midlands
Freepost SW2991
Birmingham, B18 7BR.
Tel: (0121) 507 5672

Yellow Card Centre, Scotland
CARDS
Freepost NAT3271
Edinburgh, EH16 4BR.
Tel: (0131) 242 2919

The MHRA's Adverse Drug Reactions On-line Information Tracking (ADROIT) facilitates the monitoring of adverse drug reactions.

More detailed information on reporting and a list of products currently under intensive monitoring can be found on the MHRA website: (www.mhra.gov.uk).

Self-reporting Patients, parents, and carers can also report suspected adverse reactions as part of a pilot scheme. The reports can cover side-effects of prescribed medicines as well as of over-the-counter and complimentary medicines. For this purpose, yellow cards for patients are available from pharmacies, general practice surgeries and other NHS outlets. Reports can also be submitted on-line to www.yellowcard.gov.uk or by telephone on 0808 100 3352.

Adverse reactions to medical devices Suspected adverse reactions to medical devices including dental or surgical materials, intra-uterine devices and contact lens fluids should be reported. Information on reporting these can be found at: devices.mhra.gov.uk

Prescription-event monitoring In addition to the MHRA's Yellow Card scheme, an independent scheme monitors the safety of new medicines using a different approach. The Drug Safety Research Unit identifies patients who have been prescribed selected new medicines and collects data on clinical events in these patients. The data are submitted on a voluntary basis by general practitioners on green forms. More information about the scheme and the Unit's educational material is available from www.dsru.org.

Side-effects in the *BNF for Children* The *BNF for Children* includes clinically relevant side-effects for most drugs; an exhaustive list is not included for drugs that are used by specialists (e.g. cytotoxics and drugs used in anaesthesia). Side-effects in the manufacturers' literature whose causality has not been established may be omitted from the *BNF for Children*.

In the product literature the frequency of side-effects is generally described as follows:

Very common	greater than 1 in 10
Common	1 in 100 to 1 in 10
Uncommon	1 in 1000 to 1 in 100
Rare	1 in 10 000 to 1 in 1000
Very rare	less than 1 in 10 000

Special problems

Symptoms. Children may be poor at expressing the symptoms of an adverse drug reaction and parental opinion may be required.

Delayed drug effects. Some reactions (e.g. cancers, and effects on development) may become manifest months or years after exposure. Any suspicion of such an association should be reported.

Congenital abnormalities. When an infant is born with a congenital abnormality or there is a malformed aborted fetus doctors are asked to consider whether this might be an adverse reaction to a drug and to report all drugs (including self-medication) taken during pregnancy.

Prevention of adverse reactions

Adverse reactions may be prevented as follows:

- never use any drug unless there is a good indication. If the patient is pregnant do not use a drug unless the need for it is imperative;
- allergy and idiosyncrasy are important causes of adverse drug reactions. Ask if the child has had previous reactions to the drug or formulation;
- prescribe as few drugs as possible and give very clear instructions to the child, parent or carer;
- when possible use a familiar drug. With a new drug be particularly alert for adverse reactions or unexpected events;
- consider if excipients (e.g. colouring agents) may be contributing to the adverse reaction. If the reaction is minor, a trial of an alternative formulation of the same drug may be considered before abandoning the drug;
- obtain a full drug history including asking if the child is already taking other drugs *including over-the-counter medicines*; interactions may occur;
- age and hepatic or renal disease may alter the metabolism or excretion of drugs, particularly in neonates, which can affect the potential for adverse effects. Genetic factors may also be responsible for variations in metabolism, and therefore for the adverse effects of the drug;
- if serious adverse reactions are liable to occur warn the child, parent or carer.

Defective medicines

During the manufacture or distribution of a medicine an error or accident may occur whereby the finished product does not conform to its specification. While such a defect may impair the therapeutic effect of the product and could adversely affect the health of a patient, it should **not** be confused with an Adverse Drug Reaction where the product conforms to its specification.

The Defective Medicines Report Centre assists with the investigation of problems arising from licensed medicinal products thought to be defective and co-ordinates any necessary protective action. Reports on suspect defective medicinal products should include the brand or the non-proprietary name, the name of the manufacturer or supplier, the strength and dosage form of the product, the product licence number, the batch number or numbers of the product, the nature of the defect, and an account of any action already taken in consequence. The Centre can be contacted at:

The Defective Medicines Report Centre

Medicines and Healthcare products Regulatory Agency

Room 1801, Market Towers

1 Nine Elms Lane

London SW8 5NQ

(020) 7273 0574 (weekdays 9.00 am–5.00 pm)

or (020) 7210 3000 or 5371 (any other time)

General guidance

Prescribing in palliative care

Palliative care is the active total care of children and young adults who have incurable, life-limiting conditions and are not expected to survive beyond young adulthood.

The child may be cared for in a hospice or at home according to the needs of the child and the child's family. In all cases, children should receive total care of their physical, emotional, social, and spiritual needs, and their families should be supported throughout. In particular, specialist palliative care is essential for end-of-life care of the child and for supporting the family through death and bereavement.

Drug treatment The number of drugs should be as few as possible. Oral medication is usually appropriate unless there is severe nausea and vomiting, dysphagia, weakness, or coma, in which case parenteral medication may be necessary.

Pain

Analgesics are more effective in preventing pain than in the relief of established pain; it is important that they are given regularly.

The non-opioid analgesics **paracetamol** or an **NSAID** (section 10.1.1) given regularly will often make the use of opioids unnecessary. The NSAID may also control the pain of *bone secondaries.* Radiotherapy and bisphosphonates (section 6.6.2) may also be useful for pain due to bone metastases.

An opioid such as **codeine** or **dihydrocodeine**, alone or in combination with a non-opioid analgesic at adequate dosage, may be helpful in the control of moderate pain if non-opioids alone are not sufficient. If these preparations are not controlling the pain, **morphine** is the most useful opioid analgesic. Alternatives to morphine, including transdermal **fentanyl** (see below and section 4.7.2), are best initiated by those with experience in palliative care. Initiation of an opioid analgesic should not be delayed by concern over a theoretical likelihood of psychological or physical dependence (addiction).

Equivalent single doses of strong analgesics

These equivalences are intended **only** as an approximate guide; patients should be carefully monitored after **any** change in medication and dose titration may be required

Analgesic	Dose
Morphine salts (oral)	10 mg
Diamorphine hydrochloride (subcutaneous)	3 mg
Hydromorphone hydrochloride	1.3 mg
Oxycodone (oral)	5 mg

Oral route Morphine is given *by mouth* as an oral solution or as standard ('immediate release') tablets regularly every 4 hours, the initial dose depending largely on the patient's previous treatment. If the first dose of morphine is no more effective than the previous analgesic, the next dose should be increased by about 50%, the aim being to choose the lowest dose which prevents pain. The dose should be adjusted with careful assessment of the pain and the use of adjuvant analgesics (such as NSAIDs) should also be considered. Although low doses of morphine are usually adequate there should be no hesitation in increasing the dose stepwise according to response if necessary.

If pain occurs between regular doses of morphine ('breakthrough pain'), an additional dose ('rescue dose') should be given. An additional dose should also be given 30 minutes before an activity that causes pain (e.g. wound dressing).

When the pain is controlled and the patient's 24–hour morphine requirement is established, the daily dose can be given as a single dose or in 2 divided doses as a *modified-release preparation.* The first dose of the modified-release preparation is given within 4 hours of the last dose of the oral solution.[1]

1. Studies have indicated that administration of the last dose of the *oral solution* with the first dose of the *modified-release tablets* is not necessary.

Alternatively, a *modified-release preparation* may be commenced immediately and the dose adjusted according to pain control.

Preparations suitable for twice daily administration include *MST Continus®* tablets or suspension, and *Zomorph®* capsules. Preparations that allow administration of the total daily morphine requirement as a single dose include *MXL®* capsules. *Morcap SR®* capsules may be given either twice daily or as a single daily dose.

The starting dose of modified-release preparations designed for twice daily administration is usually 200–800 micrograms/kg every 12 hours if no other analgesic (or only paracetamol) has been taken previously, but to replace a weaker opioid analgesic (such as codeine) the starting dose is usually higher. Increments should be made to the dose, not to the frequency of administration, which should remain at every 12 hours.

Morphine, as oral solution or standard formulation tablets, should be prescribed for breakthrough pain; the dose should be about one-sixth of the total daily dose of oral morphine repeated every 4 hours if necessary (review pain management if analgesic required more frequently). Children often require a higher dose of morphine in proportion to their body-weight compared to adults. Children are more susceptible to certain adverse effects of opioids such as urinary retention (which can be eased by carbachol or bethanechol), and opioid-induced pruritus.

Oxycodone (p. 246) is used in a child who requires an opioid but cannot tolerate morphine. If the child is already receiving an opioid, oxycodone should be started at a dose equivalent to the current analgesic (see p. 24).

Parenteral route **Diamorphine** is preferred for injection because, being more soluble, it can be given in a smaller volume. The equivalent subcutaneous dose is approximately a third of the oral dose of morphine. *Subcutaneous infusion* of diamorphine via syringe driver can be useful (for details, see p. 28).

If the child can resume taking medicines by mouth, then oral morphine may be substituted for subcutaneous infusion of diamorphine; see table of equivalent doses of morphine (p. 28) for equivalences between the two opioids.

Rectal route Morphine is also available for *rectal administration* as suppositories.

Transdermal route Transdermal preparations of fentanyl are available (section 4.7.2). Careful conversion from oral morphine to transdermal fentanyl is necessary. The following 24-hour doses of morphine are considered to be equivalent to the fentanyl patches shown:

Morphine salt 90 mg daily ≡ fentanyl '25' patch
Morphine salt 180 mg daily ≡ fentanyl '50' patch
Morphine salt 270 mg daily ≡ fentanyl '75' patch
Morphine salt 360 mg daily ≡ fentanyl '100' patch

Morphine (as oral solution or standard formulation tablets) is given for breakthrough pain.

Gastro-intestinal pain The pain of *bowel colic* may be reduced by loperamide. Hyoscine hydrobromide may also be helpful in reducing the frequency of spasms; it is given sublingually at a dose of 10 micrograms/kg (max. 300 micrograms) 3 times daily as *Kwells®* (Roche Consumer Health) tablets. For the dose by subcutaneous infusion using a syringe driver, see p. 28).

Gastric distension pain due to pressure on the stomach may be helped by a preparation incorporating an antacid with an antiflatulent (p. 51) and by domperidone before meals.

Muscle spasm The pain of muscle spasm can be helped by a muscle relaxant such as diazepam or baclofen.

Neuropathic pain Patients with neuropathic pain (p. 249) may benefit from a trial of a tricyclic antidepressant, most commonly amitriptyline (p. 220), for several weeks. An anticonvulsant, most commonly carbamazepine (p. 256), may be added or substituted if pain persists; gabapentin is licensed for neuropathic pain in adults.

Pain due to nerve compression may be reduced by a corticosteroid such as dexamethasone, which reduces oedema around the tumour, thus reducing compression.

Nerve blocks may be considered when pain is localised to a specific area. **Transcutaneous electrical nerve stimulation** (TENS) may also help.

Miscellaneous conditions

> Non-licensed indications or routes
> Several recommendations in this section involve non-licensed indications or routes.

Raised intracranial pressure Headache due to raised intracranial pressure often responds to a high dose of a corticosteroid, such as dexamethasone, for 4 to 5 days, subsequently reduced if possible; dexamethasone should be given before 6 p.m. to reduce the risk of insomnia. Treatment of headache and of associated nausea and vomiting should also be considered.

Intractable cough Intractable cough may be relieved by moist inhalations or by regular administration of oral morphine every 4 hours. Methadone linctus should be avoided because it has a long duration of action and tends to accumulate.

Dyspnoea Breathlessness at rest may be relieved by regular oral morphine in carefully titrated doses. Diazepam may be helpful for dyspnoea associated with anxiety. Sublingual lorazepam or subcutaneous or intranasal midazolam are alternatives. A nebulised short-acting beta$_2$ agonist or a corticosteroid, such as dexamethasone or prednisolone, may also be helpful for bronchospasm or partial obstruction.

Excessive respiratory secretion Excessive respiratory secretion (death rattle) may be reduced by hyoscine hydrobromide patches (p. 234) or by subcutaneous or intravenous injection of hyoscine hydrobromide 10 micrograms/kg (max. 600 micrograms) every 4 to 8 hours; care must however be taken to avoid the discomfort of dry mouth. Alternatively glycopyrronium may be given by mouth (see p. 714). Benzodiazepines such as rectal diazepam or subcutaneous midazolam may be helpful in the final stages.

Restlessness and confusion Restlessness and confusion may require treatment with haloperidol 10–20 micrograms/kg by mouth every 8–12 hours. Levomepromazine (methotrimeprazine, p. 210) is also used occasionally for restlessness.

Anxiety Anxiety can be treated with a long-acting benzodiazepine such as diazepam, or by continuous infusion of the short-acting benzodiazepine midazolam. Interventions for more acute episodes of anxiety (such as panic attacks) include short-acting benzodiazepines such as lorazepam given sublingually or midazolam given subcutaneously. Temazepam provides useful night-time sedation in some children.

Hiccup Hiccup due to gastric distension may be helped by a preparation incorporating an antacid with an antiflatulent (p. 51).

Anorexia Anorexia may be helped by prednisolone or dexamethasone.

Constipation Constipation is a very common cause of distress and is almost invariable after administration of an opioid. It should be prevented if possible by the regular administration of laxatives. Suitable laxatives include macrogol (p. 82), co-danthramer (p. 79), or a combination of lactulose (p. 82) with a senna preparation (p. 80). Naloxone given by mouth may help relieve opioid-induced constipation; it is poorly absorbed and there is little risk of it reversing opioid analgesia.

Fungating growth Fungating growth may be treated by regular dressing and oral administration of metronidazole; topical application of metronidazole is also used.

Capillary bleeding Capillary bleeding may be reduced by applying gauze soaked in adrenaline (epinephrine) solution 1 mg/mL (1 in 1000). Vitamin K may be useful in bleeding associated with liver dysfunction.

Mucosal bleeding Mucosal bleeding from the mouth and nose occurs commonly in the terminal phase, particularly in a child suffering from haemopoeitic malignancy. Bleeding from the nose caused by a single bleeding point can be arrested by cauterisation or by dressing it. Tranexamic acid may be effective applied topically or given systemically.

Dry mouth Dry mouth may be caused by certain medication including opioids, antimuscarinic drugs (e.g. hyoscine), antidepressants and some anti-emetics; if possible, an alternative preparation should be considered. Dry mouth may be relieved by good mouth care and measures such as sucking ice or pineapple chunks or the use of artificial saliva (p. 609); dry mouth associated with candidiasis can be treated by oral preparations of nystatin or miconazole (p. 604); alternatively, fluconazole can be given by mouth (p. 350).

Pruritus Pruritus, even when associated with obstructive jaundice, often responds to simple measures such as application of emollients (p. 614). Ondansetron may be effective in some children. Where opioids cause pruritus it may be appropriate to review the dose or to switch to an alternative opioid. In the case of obstructive jaundice, further measures include administration of colestyramine (p. 91).

Convulsions Intractable seizures are relatively common in children dying from non-malignant conditions. Phenobarbital by mouth or as a continuous subcutaneous infusion may be beneficial; continuous infusion of midazolam is an alternative. Both cause drowsiness, but this is rarely a concern in the context of intractable seizures. For breakthrough convulsions diazepam given rectally (as a solution), buccal midazolam, or paraldehyde as an enema may be appropriate (section 4.8.2).

For the use of midazolam by subcutaneous infusion using a syringe driver, see below.

Dysphagia A corticosteroid such as dexamethasone may help, temporarily, if there is an obstruction due to tumour. See also under Dry Mouth above.

Nausea and vomiting Nausea and vomiting are common in patients with advanced cancer. Ideally, the cause should be determined before treatment with an anti-emetic (section 4.6) is started.

Nausea and vomiting with opioid therapy are less common in children but may occur particularly in the initial stages and can be prevented by giving an anti-emetic. An anti-emetic is usually necessary only for the first 4 or 5 days and therefore combined preparations containing an opioid with an anti-emetic are not recommended because they lead to unnecessary anti-emetic therapy (and associated side-effects when used long-term).

Metoclopramide has a prokinetic action and is used by mouth for nausea and vomiting associated with gastritis, gastric stasis, and functional bowel obstruction. Drugs with antimuscarinic effects antagonise prokinetic drugs and, where possible, should not therefore be used concurrently.

Haloperidol (p. 210) is used by mouth for most chemical causes of vomiting (e.g. hypercalcaemia, renal failure).

Cyclizine (p. 229) is used for nausea and vomiting due to mechanical bowel obstruction, raised intracranial pressure, and motion sickness.

Ondansetron (p. 233) is most effective when the vomiting is due to damaged or irritated gut mucosa (e.g. after chemotherapy or radiotherapy).

Anti-emetic therapy should be reviewed every 24 hours; it may be necessary to substitute the anti-emetic or to add another one.

Levomepromazine (methotrimeprazine) may be used if first-line anti-emetics are inadequate. Dexamethasone by mouth may be used as an adjunct.

For the administration of anti-emetics by subcutaneous infusion using a syringe driver, see below.

For the treatment of nausea and vomiting associated with cancer chemotherapy, see section 8.1.

Insomnia Children with advanced cancer may not sleep because of discomfort, cramps, night sweats, joint stiffness, or fear. There should be appropriate treatment of these problems before hypnotics (p. 203) are used. Benzodiazepines, such as temazepam, may be useful.

Hypercalcaemia See section 9.5.1.2.

Syringe drivers

Although drugs can usually be administered *by mouth* to control symptoms in palliative care, the parenteral route may sometimes be necessary. Repeated administration of *intramuscular injections* should be avoided in children, particularly if cachectic. This has led to the use of a portable syringe driver to give a *continuous subcutaneous infusion*, which can provide good control of symptoms with little discomfort or inconvenience to the patient.

> Syringe driver rate settings
> Staff using syringe drivers should be **adequately trained** and different rate settings should be **clearly identified** and **differentiated**; incorrect use of syringe drivers is a common cause of drug errors.

Indications for the **parenteral route** are:

- inability to take medicines by mouth owing to *nausea and vomiting, dysphagia, severe weakness,* or *coma;*
- *malignant bowel obstruction* for which surgery is inappropriate (avoiding the need for an intravenous infusion or for insertion of a nasogastric tube);
- refusal by the child to take regular medication by mouth.

Nausea and vomiting Levomepromazine (methotrimeprazine, p. 210) causes sedation in about 50% of patients. Haloperidol (p. 210) has little sedative effect.

Cyclizine is particularly liable to precipitate if mixed with diamorphine or other drugs (see under Mixing and Compatibility, below); it is given by *subcutaneous infusion.*

Bowel colic and excessive respiratory secretions Hyoscine hydrobromide effectively reduces respiratory secretions and is sedative (but occasionally causes paradoxical agitation); it is given in a *subcutaneous* or *intravenous infusion dose* of 40–60 micrograms/kg/24 hours. Glycopyrronium may also be used.

Hyoscine butylbromide is effective in bowel colic, is less sedative than hyoscine hydrobromide, but is not always adequate for the control of respiratory secretions; it is given by *subcutaneous infusion* (**important:** *hyoscine butylbromide* must not be confused with *hyoscine hydrobromide*, above).

Restlessness and confusion Haloperidol has little sedative effect. Levomepromazine (methotrimeprazine, p. 210) has a sedative effect. Midazolam is a sedative and an antiepileptic, which may be suitable for a very restless patient.

Convulsions If a child has previously been receiving an antiepileptic *or* has a primary or secondary cerebral tumour *or* is at risk of convulsion (e.g. owing to uraemia) antiepileptic medication should not be stopped. Midazolam is the benzodiazepine antiepileptic of choice for *continuous subcutaneous infusion.*

Pain control Diamorphine is the preferred opioid since its high solubility permits a large dose to be given in a small volume (see under Mixing and Compatibility, below). The table below gives the approximate doses of *morphine by mouth* (as oral solution or standard formulation tablets or as modified-release tablets) equivalent to *diamorphine by injection* (by subcutaneous infusion).

Mixing and compatibility The general principle that injections should be given into separate sites (and should not be mixed) does not apply to the use of syringe drivers in palliative care. Provided that there is evidence of compatibility, selected injections can be mixed in syringe drivers. Not all types of medication can be used in a subcutaneous infusion. In particular, chlorpromazine, prochlorperazine and diazepam are **contra-indicated** as they cause skin reactions at the injection site; to a lesser extent cyclizine and levomepromazine (methotrimeprazine) may also sometimes cause local irritation.

In theory injections dissolved in water for injections are more likely to be associated with pain (possibly owing to their hypotonicity). The use of physiological saline (sodium chloride 0.9%) however increases the likelihood of precipitation when more than one drug is used; moreover subcutaneous infusion rates are so slow (0.1–0.3 mL/hour) that pain is not usually a problem when water is used as a diluent.

Diamorphine can be given by subcutaneous infusion in a strength of up to 250 mg/mL; up to a strength of 40 mg/mL either *water for injections* or *physiological saline* (sodium chloride 0.9%) is a suitable diluent—above that strength only *water for injections* is used (to avoid precipitation).

The following can be mixed with *diamorphine*:

Cyclizine[1]
Dexamethasone[2]
Haloperidol[3]
Hyoscine butylbromide
Hyoscine hydrobromide
Levomepromazine
Metoclopramide[4]
Midazolam

Subcutaneous infusion solution should be monitored regularly both to check for precipitation (and discoloration) and to ensure that the infusion is running at the correct rate

Problems encountered with syringe drivers The following are problems that may be encountered with syringe drivers and the action that should be taken:

- if the subcutaneous infusion runs *too quickly* check the rate setting and the calculation;
- if the subcutaneous infusion runs *too slowly* check the start button, the battery, the syringe driver, the cannula, and make sure that the injection site is not inflamed;
- if there is an *injection site reaction* make sure that the site does not need to be changed—firmness or swelling at the site of injection is not in itself an indication for change, but pain or obvious inflammation is.

Equivalent doses of morphine sulphate by mouth or of diamorphine hydrochloride by subcutaneous infusion

These equivalences are approximate only and may need to be adjusted according to response

ORAL MORPHINE		PARENTERAL DIAMORPHINE
Morphine sulphate oral solution or standard tablets	Morphine sulphate modified-release tablets	Diamorphine hydrochloride by subcutaneous infusion
every 4 hours	**every 12 hours**	**every 24 hours**
5 mg	20 mg	15 mg
10 mg	30 mg	20 mg
15 mg	50 mg	30 mg
20 mg	60 mg	45 mg
30 mg	90 mg	60 mg
40 mg	120 mg	90 mg
60 mg	180 mg	120 mg
80 mg	240 mg	180 mg
100 mg	300 mg	240 mg
130 mg	400 mg	300 mg
160 mg	500 mg	360 mg
200 mg	600 mg	400 mg

If breakthrough pain occurs give a subcutaneous injection of diamorphine equivalent to one-sixth of the total 24-hour subcutaneous infusion dose. With an intermittent subcutaneous injection absorption is smoother so that the risk of adverse effects at peak absorption is avoided (an even better method is to use a subcutaneous butterfly needle).
To minimise the risk of infection no subcutaneous infusion solution should be used for longer than 24 hours.

1. Cyclizine may precipitate at concentrations above 10 mg/mL *or* in the presence of physiological saline *or* as the concentration of diamorphine relative to cyclizine increases; mixtures of diamorphine and cyclizine are also liable to precipitate after 24 hours.
2. Special care is needed to avoid precipitation of dexamethasone when preparing.
3. Mixtures of haloperidol and diamorphine are liable to precipitate after 24 hours if haloperidol concentration is above 2 mg/mL.
4. Under some conditions metoclopramide may become discoloured; such solutions should be discarded.

Prescribing in dental practice

Advice on the drug management of dental and oral conditions is covered in the main text. For ease of access, guidance on such conditions is usually identified by means of a relevant heading (e.g. Dental and Orofacial Pain) in the appropriate sections.

The following is a list of topics of particular relevance to dental surgeons.

General guidance

Drugs and sport

UK Sport advises that athletes are personally responsible should a prohibited substance be detected in their body. Information and advice, including the status of specific drugs in sport, can be obtained from UK Sport's Drug Information Database at www.didglobal.com. Alternatively, an advice card listing examples of permitted and prohibited substances is available from:

Drug-Free Sport
UK Sport
40 Bernard Street
London, WC1N 1ST.
drug-free@uksport.gov.uk
Tel: 0800 528 0004
www.uksport.gov.uk

A similar card detailing classes of drugs and doping methods prohibited in football is available from the Football Association.

General Medical Council's advice
Doctors who prescribe or collude in the provision of drugs or treatment with the intention of improperly enhancing an individual's performance in sport would be contravening the GMC's guidance, and such actions would usually raise a question of a doctor's continued registration. This does not preclude the provision of any care or treatment where the doctor's intention is to protect or improve the patient's health.

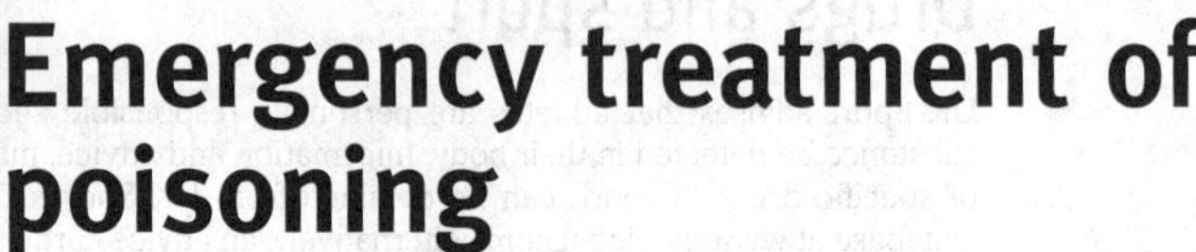

Emergency treatment of poisoning

These notes provide only an overview of the treatment of poisoning and it is strongly recommended that either a **poisons information centre** or **TOXBASE** (see below) be consulted in cases where there is doubt about the degree of risk or about appropriate management.

Most childhood poisoning is accidental. Other causes include intentional overdose, drug abuse, iatrogenic and deliberate poisoning. The drugs most commonly involved in childhood poisoning are paracetamol, ibuprofen, orally ingested creams, aspirin, iron preparations, cough medicines and the contraceptive pill.

Hospital admission All children who show features of poisoning should generally be admitted to hospital. Children who have taken poisons with delayed actions should also be admitted, even if they appear well. Delayed-action poisons include aspirin, iron, paracetamol, tricyclic antidepressants, co-phenotrope (diphenoxylate with atropine, *Lomotil*®), and paraquat; the effects of modified-release preparations are also delayed. A note of all relevant information including what treatment has been given should accompany the patient to hospital.

Further information and advice

TOXBASE, the primary clinical toxicology database of the National Poisons Information Service, is available on the Internet to registered users at www.spib.axl.co.uk. It provides information about routine diagnosis, treatment and management of patients exposed to drugs, household products, and industrial and agricultural chemicals.

Specialist information and advice on the treatment of poisoning is available from the **UK National Poisons Information Service** through the local poisons information centre on the following number:
Tel: 0870 600 6266

Advice on laboratory analytical services can be obtained from TOXBASE or from a poisons information centre.

Help on identifying capsules or tablets may be available from a regional medicines information centre (see inside front cover).

> The **poisons information centres** (Tel: 0870 600 6266) will provide specialist advice on all aspects of poisoning day and night

General care

It is often impossible to establish with certainty the identity of the poison and the size of the dose. Fortunately this is not usually important because only a few poisons (such as opioids, paracetamol, and iron) have specific antidotes; few children require active removal of the poison. In most children, treatment is directed at managing symptoms as they arise. Nevertheless, knowledge of the type and timing of poisoning can help in anticipating the course of events. All relevant information should be sought from the poisoned child and from their carers. However, such information should be interpreted with care because it may not be complete or entirely reliable. Sometimes symptoms arise from other illnesses and children should be assessed carefully. Accidents may involve a number of domestic and industrial products (the contents of which are not generally known). A **poisons information centre** should be consulted where there is doubt about any aspect of suspected poisoning.

Respiration

Respiration is often impaired in unconscious children. An obstructed airway requires immediate attention. In the absence of trauma, the airway should be opened with simple measures such as chin lift or jaw thrust. An oropharyngeal or nasopharyngeal airway may be useful in children with reduced consciousness to prevent obstruction, provided ventilation is adequate. Intubation and ventilation should be considered in children whose airway cannot be protected or who have inadequate ventilation because of respiratory acidosis; such children should be monitored in a critical care area.

Most poisons that impair consciousness also depress respiration. Assisted ventilation by mouth-to-mouth or *Ambu-bag* inflation may be needed. Oxygen is not a substitute for adequate ventilation, though it should be given in the highest concentration possible in poisoning with carbon monoxide and irritant gases.

Respiratory stimulants do not help and should be **avoided**.

The potential for pulmonary aspiration of gastric contents should be considered.

Blood pressure

Hypotension is common in severe poisoning with central nervous system depressants; if severe this may lead to irreversible brain damage or renal tubular necrosis. Hypotension should be corrected initially by tilting down the head of the bed and administration of either sodium chloride intravenous infusion or a colloidal infusion. Vasoconstrictor sympathomimetics (section 2.7.2) are rarely required and their use may be discussed with a poisons information centre.

Fluid depletion without hypotension is common after prolonged coma and after aspirin poisoning due to vomiting, sweating, and hyperpnoea.

Hypertension, often transient, occurs less frequently than hypotension in poisoning; it may be associated with sympathomimetic drugs such as amphetamines, phencyclidine, and cocaine.

Heart

Cardiac conduction defects and arrhythmias may occur in acute poisoning, notably with tricyclic antidepressants, some antipsychotics, some antihistamines, and co-proxamol. Arrhythmias often respond to correction of underlying hypoxia, acidosis, or other biochemical abnormalities. Ventricular arrhythmias that cause serious hypotension may require treatment. If the QT interval is prolonged, specialist advice should be sought because the use of some anti-arrhythmic drugs may be inappropriate. Supraventricular arrhythmias are seldom life-threatening and drug treatment is best withheld until the child reaches hospital.

Body temperature

Hypothermia may develop in patients of any age who have been deeply unconscious for some hours particularly following overdose with barbiturates or phenothiazines. It may be missed unless core temperature is measured using a low-reading rectal thermometer or by some other means. Hypothermia is best treated by wrapping the patient (e.g. in a 'space blanket') to conserve body heat.

Hyperthermia can develop in children taking CNS stimulants; children are also at risk when taking therapeutic doses of drugs with antimuscarinic properties. Hyperthermia is initially managed by removing all unnecessary clothing and using a fan. Sponging with tepid water will promote evaporation; iced water should **not** be used. Advice should be sought from a poisons information centre on the management of severe hyperthermia resulting from conditions such as the serotonin syndrome.

Both hypothermia and hyperthermia require **urgent** hospitalisation for assessment and supportive treatment.

Convulsions

Single short-lived convulsions do not require treatment. If convulsions are protracted or recur frequently, lorazepam 100 micrograms/kg (max. 4 mg) or diazepam (preferably as emulsion) 300–400 micrograms/kg (max. 20 mg) should be given by slow intravenous injection into a large vein. Buccal midazolam 200–300 micrograms/kg (max. 10 mg) may also be used. The benzodiazepines should not be given intramuscularly.

Removal and elimination

Removal from the gastro-intestinal tract

Gastric lavage is rarely required as benefit rarely outweighs risk and should be considered only if a life-threatening amount of a drug has been ingested within the previous hour. It should be carried out only if the airway can be protected adequately to prevent pulmonary aspiration. Gastric lavage is contra-indicated if a corrosive substance or a petroleum distillate has been ingested but it may occasionally be considered in children who have ingested drugs that are not absorbed by charcoal, such as iron or lithium. Induction of *emesis* (e.g. with ipecacuanha) is **not** recommended because there is no evidence that it affects absorption and it may increase the risk of aspiration.

Whole bowel irrigation (by means of a bowel cleansing solution) has been used in poisoning with certain modified-release or enteric-coated formulations, in severe poisoning with iron and lithium salts, and if illicit drugs are carried in the gastro-intestinal tract ('body-packing'). However, it is not clear that the procedure improves outcome and advice should be sought from a poisons information centre.

The administration of **laxatives** alone has no role in the management of the poisoned child and is not a recommended method of gut decontamination. The routine use of a laxative in combination with activated charcoal has mostly been abandoned. Laxatives should not be administered to young children because of the likelihood of fluid and electrolyte imbalance.

Prevention of absorption

Given by mouth, **activated charcoal** can adsorb many poisons in the gastro-intestinal system, thereby *reducing their absorption*. The **sooner** it is given the **more effective** it is, but it may still be effective up to 1 hour after ingestion of the poison—longer in the case of modified-release preparations or of drugs with antimuscarinic (anticholinergic) properties. It is relatively safe and is particularly useful for the prevention of absorption of poisons which are toxic in small amounts, e.g. antidepressants.

A second dose may be required when blood-drug concentration continues to rise suggesting delayed drug release or delayed gastric emptying.

For the use of charcoal in active elimination techniques, see below.

CHARCOAL, ACTIVATED

Cautions drowsy or comatose child (risk of aspiration); reduced gastro-intestinal motility (risk of obstruction); **not** for poisoning with petroleum distillates, corrosive substances, alcohols, clofenotane (dicophane, DDT), malathion, and metal salts including iron and lithium salts

Contra-indications unprotected airway; gastro-intestinal tract not intact

Side-effects black stools

Indication and dose

Adsorption of poisons in the gastro-intestinal system See under individual preparations below

Actidose-Aqua® Advance (Cambridge)
Oral suspension, activated charcoal, net price 50-g pack (240 mL) = £11.63
Note The brand name *Actidose-Aqua®* was formerly used

Dose

Reduction of absorption
- **By mouth**
  - **Child 1 month–1 year** 1 g/kg (approx. 5 mL/kg)
  - **Child 1–12 years** 25–50 g
  - **Child 12–18 years** 50–100 g

Active elimination Repeat above doses every 4–6 hours

Carbomix® (Meadow)
Powder, activated charcoal, net price 25-g pack = £8.50, 50-g pack = £11.90

Dose

Reduction of absorption
- **By mouth**
  - **Child under 12 years** 25 g (50 g in severe poisoning)
  - **Child 12–18 years** 50 g

Active elimination Repeat above doses every 4 hours

Charcodote® (PLIVA)
Oral suspension, activated charcoal, net price 50-g pack = £11.88

Dose

Reduction of absorption
- **By mouth**
  - **Child under 12 years** 25 g (50 g in severe poisoning)
  - **Child 12–18 years** 50 g

Active elimination Repeat above doses every 4 hours

Active elimination techniques

Repeated doses of **activated charcoal** by mouth may *enhance the elimination* of some drugs after they have been absorbed; repeated doses are given after overdosage with:

Carbamazepine
Dapsone
Phenobarbital
Quinine
Theophylline

Vomiting should be treated (e.g. with an anti-emetic drug) since it may reduce the efficacy of charcoal treatment. In cases of intolerance, the dose may be reduced and the frequency increased but this may compromise efficacy.

Other techniques intended to enhance the elimination of poisons after absorption are only practicable in hospital and are only suitable for a small number of severely poisoned patients. Moreover, they only apply to a limited number of poisons. Examples include:

- haemodialysis for salicylates, phenobarbital, methyl alcohol (methanol), ethylene glycol, and lithium
- alkanisation of the urine for salicylates and phenoxyacetate herbicides (e.g. 2,4-dichloro-phenoxyacetic acid).

Forced alkaline diuresis is no longer recommended.

Specific drugs

Alcohol

Acute intoxication with alcohol (ethanol) is common in adults but also occurs in children. The features include ataxia, dysarthria, nystagmus, and drowsiness, which may progress to coma, with hypotension and acidosis. Aspiration of vomit is a special hazard and hypoglycaemia may occur in children and some adults. Patients are managed supportively with particular attention to maintaining a clear airway and measures to reduce the risk of aspiration of gastric contents. The blood glucose is measured and glucose given if indicated.

The **poisons information centres** (Tel: 0870 600 6266) will provide specialist advice on all aspects of poisoning day and night

Analgesics (non-opioid)

Aspirin The chief features of salicylate poisoning are hyperventilation, tinnitus, deafness, vasodilatation, and sweating. Coma is uncommon but indicates very severe poisoning. The associated acid-base disturbances are complex.

Treatment must be in hospital where plasma salicylate, pH, and electrolytes (particularly potassium) can be measured; absorption of aspirin may be slow and the plasma-salicylate concentration may continue to rise for several hours, requiring repeated measurement of plasma-salicylate concentration. Fluid losses are replaced and sodium bicarbonate is administered intravenously to enhance urinary salicylate excretion (optimum urinary pH 7.5–8.5) when the plasma-salicylate concentration is greater than:

350 mg/litre (2.5 mmol/litre) in children.

Plasma-potassium concentration should be corrected before giving sodium bicarbonate as hypokalaemia may complicate alkalinisation of the urine.

Haemodialysis is the treatment of choice for severe salicylate poisoning and should be considered when the plasma-salicylate concentration exceeds 700 mg/litre (5.1 mmol/litre) or in the presence of severe metabolic acidosis, convulsions, renal failure, pulmonary oedema or persistently high plasma-salicylate concentrations unresponsive to urinary alkalinisation.

NSAIDs Mefenamic acid has important consequences in overdosage because it can cause convulsions, which if prolonged or recurrent, require treatment with intravenous lorazepam or diazepam.

Ibuprofen may cause nausea, vomiting, and tinnitus, but more serious toxicity is very uncommon. Activated charcoal followed by symptomatic measures are indicated if more than 400 mg/kg has been ingested within the preceding hour, followed by symptomatic measures.

Paracetamol As little as 150 mg/kg of paracetamol taken within 24 hours may cause severe hepatocellular necrosis and, much less frequently, renal tubular necrosis. Nausea and vomiting, the only early features of poisoning, usually settle within 24 hours. Persistence beyond this time, often associated with the onset of right subcostal pain and tenderness, usually indicates development of hepatic necrosis. Liver damage is maximal 3–4 days after ingestion and may lead to encephalopathy, haemorrhage, hypoglycaemia, cerebral oedema, and death.

Therefore, despite a lack of significant early symptoms, patients who have taken an overdose of paracetamol should be transferred to hospital urgently.

Administration of activated charcoal should be considered if paracetamol in excess of 150 mg/kg or 12 g **whichever is the smaller**, is thought to have been ingested within the previous hour.

Acetylcysteine protects the liver if infused within 24 hours of ingesting paracetamol. It is most effective if given within 8 hours of ingestion after which effectiveness declines sharply and if more than 24 hours have elapsed advice should be sought from a poisons information centre or from a liver unit on the management of serious liver damage. In remote areas **methionine** by mouth is an alternative if acetylcysteine cannot be given promptly. Once the child reaches hospital the need to continue treatment with the antidote will be assessed from the plasma-paracetamol concentration (related to the time from ingestion).

Children at risk of liver damage and therefore requiring treatment can be identified from a single measurement of the plasma-paracetamol concentration, related to the time from ingestion, provided this time interval is not less than 4 hours; earlier samples may be misleading. The concentration is plotted on a paracetamol treatment graph of a reference line ('normal treatment line') joining plots of 200 mg/litre (1.32 mmol/litre) at 4 hours and 6.25 mg/litre (0.04 mmol/litre) at 24 hours (see below). Those whose plasma-paracetamol concentration is above the *normal treatment line* are treated with acetylcysteine by intravenous infusion (or, if acetylcysteine is not available, with methionine by mouth, provided the overdose has been taken **within 10–12 hours** *and* the child is not vomiting). Children on enzyme-inducing drugs (e.g. carbamazepine, phenobarbital, phenytoin, primidone, rifampicin, alcohol, and St John's wort) or who are malnourished (e.g. in anorexia, in underweight children with 'failure to thrive', or those who are HIV-positive) may develop toxicity at **lower** plasma-paracetamol concentrations and should be treated if the concentration is above the *high-risk treatment line* (which joins plots that are at 50% of the plasma-paracetamol concentrations of the normal treatment line).

The prognostic accuracy of plasma-paracetamol concentration taken after 15 hours is uncertain but a concentration above the relevant treatment line should be regarded as carrying a serious risk of liver damage.

Plasma-paracetamol concentration may be difficult to interpret when paracetamol has been ingested over several hours (staggered overdose). If there is doubt about timing or the need for treatment then the child should be treated with acetylcysteine.

In remote areas methionine (child under 6 years 1 g, 6 years and over 2.5 g) should be given by mouth since it is seldom practicable to give acetylcysteine outside hospital. Once the patient reaches hospital the need to continue treatment with the antidote will be assessed from the plasma-paracetamol concentration (related to the time from ingestion).

See also Co-proxamol, under Analgesics (opioid).

> The **poisons information centres** (Tel: 0870 600 6266) will provide specialist advice on all aspects of poisoning day and night

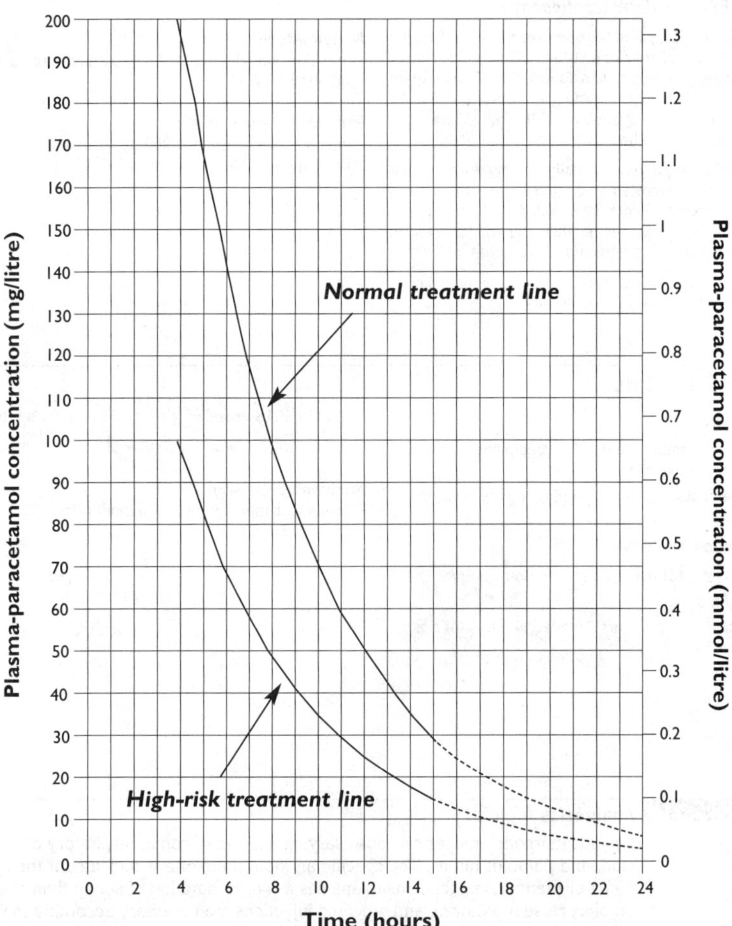

Patients whose plasma-paracetamol concentrations are above the **normal treatment line** should be treated with acetylcysteine by intravenous infusion (or, if acetylcysteine cannot be used, with methionine by mouth, provided the overdose has been taken **within 10–12 hours** and the patient is not vomiting).

Patients on enzyme-inducing drugs (e.g. carbamazepine, phenobarbital, phenytoin, primidone, rifampicin, alcohol, and St John's wort), or who are malnourished (e.g. in anorexia, in alcoholism, or those who are HIV-positive), or underweight due to failure to thrive should be treated if their plasma-paracetamol concentration is above the **high-risk treatment line**.

The prognostic accuracy after 15 hours is uncertain but a plasma-paracetamol concentration above the relevant treatment line should be regarded as carrying a serious risk of liver damage.

Graph reproduced courtesy of University of Wales College of Medicine Therapeutics and Toxicology Centre

ACETYLCYSTEINE

Cautions asthma (see side-effects below, but do not delay acetylcysteine treatment)

Side-effects hypersensitivity-like reactions managed by reducing infusion rate or suspending until reaction settled—contact poisons information centre if reactions severe (rash also managed by giving antihistamine; acute asthma by giving nebulised short-acting $beta_2$ agonist)

Indication and dose

Paracetamol overdosage see notes above

- **By intravenous infusion in glucose intravenous infusion 5%**

  Child 1 month–5 years (or body-weight under 20 kg) initially 150 mg/kg in 3 mL/kg Glucose 5% and given over 15 minutes, followed by 50 mg/kg in 7 mL/kg Glucose 5% and given over 4 hours, then 100 mg/kg in 14 mL/kg Glucose 5% and given over 16 hours

ACETYLCYSTEINE (*continued*)

Child 5–12 years (or body-weight over 20 kg) initially 150 mg/kg in 100 mL Glucose 5% and given over 15 minutes, followed by 50 mg/kg in 250 mL Glucose 5% and given over 4 hours, then 100 mg/kg in 500 mL Glucose 5% and given over 16 hours

Child 12–18 years initially 150 mg/kg in 200 mL Glucose 5% and given over 15 minutes, followed by 50 mg/kg in 500 mL Glucose 5% and given over 4 hours, then 100 mg/kg in 1 litre Glucose 5% and given over 16 hours

Note Manufacturer also recommends other infusion fluids, but Glucose 5% is preferable

Acetylcysteine (Non-proprietary) PoM
Injection, acetylcysteine 200 mg/mL, net price 10-mL amp = £2.50

Parvolex® (Celltech) PoM
Injection, acetylcysteine 200 mg/mL, net price 10-mL amp = £2.50

METHIONINE

Cautions

Hepatic impairment May precipitate coma in hepatic impairment

Side-effects nausea, vomiting, drowsiness, irritability

Indication and dose

Paracetamol overdosage see notes above

- By mouth

Child under 6 years 1 g every 4 hours for a total of 4 doses

Child 6–18 years 2.5 g every 4 hours for a total of 4 doses

Methionine (Celltech)
Tablets, DL-methionine 250 mg, net price 200-tab pack = £66.05

Analgesics (opioid)

Opioids (narcotic analgesics) cause varying degrees of coma, respiratory depression, and pinpoint pupils. The specific antidote **naloxone** is indicated if there is coma or bradypnoea. Since naloxone has a shorter duration of action than many opioids, close monitoring and repeated injections are necessary according to the respiratory rate and depth of coma. Where repeated administration of naloxone is required, it may be given by continuous intravenous infusion instead and the rate of infusion adjusted according to vital signs. All children should be observed for at least 6 hours after the last dose of naloxone. The effects of some opioids, such as buprenorphine, are only partially reversed by naloxone. Dextropropoxyphene and methadone have very long durations of action; patients may need to be monitored for long periods following large overdoses.

Co-proxamol A combination of dextropropoxyphene and paracetamol (co-proxamol) is frequently taken in overdosage and is the most frequent prescription product to cause death in adults. The initial features are those of acute opioid overdosage with coma, respiratory depression, and pinpoint pupils. Patients may die of acute cardiovascular collapse before reaching hospital (particularly if alcohol has also been consumed) unless adequately resuscitated.

Naloxone reverses the opioid effects of dextropropoxyphene; the long duration of action of dextropropoxyphene calls for prolonged monitoring and further doses of naloxone may be required. Norpropoxyphene, a metabolite of dextropropoxyphene, also has cardiotoxic effects which may require treatment with **sodium bicarbonate**, or **magnesium sulphate**, or both; arrhythmias may occur for up to 12 hours. Paracetamol hepatotoxicity may develop later and should be anticipated and treated as indicated above.

> The **poisons information centres** (Tel: 0870 600 6266) will provide specialist advice on all aspects of poisoning day and night

NALOXONE HYDROCHLORIDE

Cautions physical dependence on opioids; cardiac irritability; naloxone is short-acting, see notes above

Indication and dose

Safe Practice Doses used in acute opioid overdosage may not be appropriate for the management of opioid-induced respiratory depression and sedation in those receiving palliative care and in chronic opioid use, see also section 15.1.7 for management of postoperative respiratory depression

Overdosage with opioids

- **By intravenous injection**

  Child 1 month–12 years 10 micrograms/kg, subsequent dose of 100 micrograms/kg if no response

  Child 12–18 years 0.4–2 mg repeated at intervals of 2–3 minutes to a max. of 10 mg if respiratory function does not improve (then question diagnosis)

- **By subcutaneous or intramuscular injection**

  As intravenous injection but only if intravenous route not feasible (onset of action slower)

- **By continuous intravenous infusion using an infusion pump**

  Child 1 month–12 years 5–20 micrograms/kg/hour, adjusted according to response

  Child 12–18 years initially 0.24–1.2 mg infused over 1 hour, then using a solution of 4 micrograms/mL infuse at a rate adjusted according to response

Postoperative respiratory depression section 15.1.7

Administration for *continuous intravenous infusion*, dilute to a concentration of 4 micrograms/mL with Glucose 5% *or* Sodium Chloride 0.9% infusion

Naloxone (Non-proprietary) PoM

Injection, naloxone hydrochloride 400 micrograms/mL, net price 1-mL amp = £4.10; 1 mg/mL, 2-mL prefilled syringe = £6.61

Minijet® Naloxone (Celltech) PoM

Injection, naloxone hydrochloride 400 micrograms/mL, net price 1-mL disposable syringe = £5.57, 2-mL disposable syringe = £10.71, 5-mL disposable syringe = £10.20

Antidepressants

Tricyclic and related antidepressants Tricyclic and related antidepressants cause dry mouth, coma of varying degree, hypotension, hypothermia, hyperreflexia, extensor plantar responses, convulsions, respiratory failure, cardiac conduction defects, and arrhythmias. Dilated pupils and urinary retention also occur. Metabolic acidosis may complicate severe poisoning; delirium with confusion, agitation, and visual and auditory hallucinations, are common during recovery.

Transfer to hospital is strongly advised in case of poisoning by *tricyclic and related antidepressants* but symptomatic treatment and activated charcoal may be given before transfer. Supportive measures to ensure a clear airway and adequate ventilation during transfer are mandatory. Intravenous lorazepam or diazepam (preferably in emulsion form) may be required for control of convulsions. Although arrhythmias are worrying, some will respond to correction of hypoxia and acidosis. The use of anti-arrhythmic drugs is best avoided but intravenous infusion of sodium bicarbonate can arrest arrhythmias or prevent them in those with an extended QRS duration. Diazepam given by mouth is usually adequate to sedate delirious children but large doses may be required.

Selective serotonin re-uptake inhibitors (SSRIs) Symptoms of poisoning by selective serotonin re-uptake inhibitors include nausea, vomiting, agitation, tremor, nystagmus, drowsiness, and sinus tachycardia; convulsions may occur. Rarely, severe poisoning could result in the serotonin syndrome, with marked neuropsychiatric effects, neuromuscular hyperactivity, and autonomic instability; hyperthermia, rhabdomyolysis, renal failure, and coagulopathies may develop.

Management of SSRI poisoning is supportive. Activated charcoal given within 1 hour of the overdose reduces absorption of the drug. Convulsions may be prevented with lorazepam or diazepam (see p. 33). Contact a poisons information centre for the management of hyperthermia or the serotonin syndrome.

Antimalarials

Overdosage with chloroquine and hydroxychloroquine is extremely hazardous and difficult to treat. Urgent advice from a poisons information centre is essential. Life-threatening features include arrhythmias (which can have a very rapid onset)

and convulsions (which can be intractable). Quinine overdosage is also a severe hazard and calls for urgent advice from a poisons information centre.

Beta-blockers

Therapeutic overdosages with beta-blockers may cause lightheadedness, dizziness, and possibly syncope as a result of bradycardia and hypotension; heart failure may be precipitated or exacerbated. These complications are most likely in children with conduction system disorders or impaired myocardial function. Bradycardia is the most common arrhythmia caused by beta-blockers, but sotalol may induce ventricular tachyarrhythmias (sometimes of the torsades de pointes type). The effects of massive overdosage may vary from one beta-blocker to another; propranolol overdosage in particular may cause coma and convulsions.

Acute massive overdosage must be managed in hospital and expert advice should be obtained. Maintenance of a clear airway and adequate ventilation is mandatory. An intravenous injection of atropine is required to treat bradycardia and hypotension (40 micrograms/kg, max. 3 mg). Cardiogenic shock unresponsive to atropine is probably best treated with an intravenous injection of glucagon (50–150 micrograms/kg, max. 10 mg) [unlicensed indication and dose] in glucose 5% (with precautions to protect the airway in case of vomiting) followed by an intravenous infusion of 50 micrograms/kg/hour. If glucagon is not available, intravenous isoprenaline [special order only] is an alternative. A cardiac pacemaker may be used to increase the heart rate.

Calcium-channel blockers

Features of calcium-channel blocker poisoning include nausea, vomiting, dizziness, agitation, confusion, and coma in severe poisoning. Metabolic acidosis and hyperglycaemia may occur. Verapamil and diltiazem have a profound cardiac depressant effect causing hypotension and arrhythmias including complete heart block and asystole. The dihydropyridine calcium-channel blockers cause severe hypotension secondary to profound peripheral vasodilatation.

Activated charcoal is given if the child presents within 1 hour of overdosage with a calcium-channel blocker; repeated doses of activated charcoal are considered if a modified-release preparation is involved (although activated charcoal may be effective beyond 1 hour with modified-release preparations). In children with significant features of poisoning, calcium chloride or calcium gluconate (section 9.5.1.1) is given by injection; atropine is given to correct symptomatic bradycardia. For the management of hypotension, the choice of inotropic sympathomimetic depends on whether hypotension is secondary to vasodilation or to myocardial depression and advice should be sought from a poisons information centre.

Hypnotics and anxiolytics

Benzodiazepines Benzodiazepines taken alone cause drowsiness, ataxia, dysarthria, and occasionally minor and short-lived depression of consciousness. They potentiate the effects of other central nervous system depressants taken concomitantly. Use of the benzodiazepine antagonist flumazenil can be hazardous, particularly in mixed overdoses involving tricyclic antidepressants or in benzodiazepine-dependent patients. Flumazenil should be used on **expert advice** only.

Iron salts

Iron poisoning is commonest in childhood and is usually accidental. The symptoms are nausea, vomiting, abdominal pain, diarrhoea, haematemesis, and rectal bleeding. Hypotension, coma and hepatocellular necrosis occur later. Coma and shock indicate severe poisoning. Mortality is reduced with intensive and specific therapy with **desferrioxamine**, which chelates iron. The stomach should be emptied by gastric lavage (with a wide-bore tube) within 1 hour of ingesting a significant quantity of iron or if radiography reveals tablets in the stomach; whole bowel irrigation may be considered in severe poisoning but advice should be sought from a poisons information centre. The serum-iron concentration is measured as an emergency and intravenous desferrioxamine given to chelate absorbed iron in excess of the expected iron binding capacity. In **severe toxicity** intravenous desferrioxamine should be given *immediately* without waiting for the result of the serum-iron measurement (contact a poisons information centre for advice).

DESFERRIOXAMINE MESILATE

(Deferoxamine Mesilate)

Cautions section 9.1.3

Side-effects section 9.1.3

Licensed use licensed for use in children (age range not specified by manufacturer)

Indication and dose

Iron poisoning

• **By continuous intravenous infusion**

Child 1 month–18 years up to 15 mg/kg/hour, reduced after 4–6 hours; max. 80 mg/kg in 24 hours (in severe cases, higher doses on advice from a poisons information centre)

Chronic iron overload section 9.1.3

Preparations

Section 9.1.3

Lithium

Most cases of lithium intoxication occur as a complication of long-term therapy and are caused by reduced excretion of the drug due to a variety of factors including dehydration, deterioration of renal function, infections, and co-administration of diuretics or NSAIDs (or other drugs that interact). Acute deliberate overdoses may also occur with delayed onset of symptoms (12 hours or more) due to slow entry of lithium into the tissues and continuing absorption from modified-release formulations.

The early clinical features are non-specific and may include apathy and restlessness which could be confused with mental changes due to the child's depressive illness. Vomiting, diarrhoea, ataxia, weakness, dysarthria, muscle twitching, and tremor may follow. Severe poisoning is associated with convulsions, coma, renal failure, electrolyte imbalance, dehydration, and hypotension.

Therapeutic lithium concentrations are within the range of 0.4–1.0 mmol/litre; concentrations in excess of 2.0 mmol/litre are usually associated with serious toxicity and such cases may need treatment with haemodialysis (if there is renal failure). In acute overdosage much higher serum concentrations may be present without features of toxicity and all that is usually necessary is to take measures to increase urine production (e.g. by ensuring adequate fluid intake; but avoid diuretics). Otherwise treatment is supportive with special regard to electrolyte balance, renal function, and control of convulsions. Whole bowel irrigation should be considered for significant ingestion, but advice should be sought from a poisons information centre, p. 32.

The **poisons information centres** (Tel: 0870 600 6266) will provide specialist advice on all aspects of poisoning day and night

Phenothiazines and related drugs

Phenothiazines cause less depression of consciousness and respiration than other sedatives. Hypotension, hypothermia, sinus tachycardia, and arrhythmias may complicate poisoning. Dystonic reactions can occur with therapeutic doses, (particularly with prochlorperazine and trifluoperazine) and convulsions may occur in severe cases. Arrhythmias may respond to correction of hypoxia, acidosis and other biochemical abnormalities but specialist advice should be sought if arrhythmias result from a prolonged QT interval; the use of some anti-arrhythmic drugs may worsen such arrhythmias. Dystonic reactions are rapidly abolished by injection of drugs such as benzatropine or diazepam (section 4.8.2, emulsion preferred).

Emergency treatment of poisoning

Stimulants

Amphetamines These cause wakefulness, excessive activity, paranoia, hallucinations, and hypertension followed by exhaustion, convulsions, hyperthermia, and coma. The early stages can be controlled by diazepam or lorazepam; advice should be sought from a poisons information centre (p. 32) on the management of hypertension. Later, tepid sponging, anticonvulsants, and artificial respiration may be needed.

Cocaine Cocaine stimulates the central nervous system, causing agitation, dilated pupils, tachycardia, hypertension, hallucinations, hyperthermia, hypertonia, and hyperreflexia; cardiac effects include chest pain, myocardial infarction, and arrhythmias.

Initial treatment of cocaine poisoning involves intravenous administration of diazepam to control agitation and cooling measures for hyperthermia (see p. 33); hypertension and cardiac effects require specific treatment and expert advice should be sought.

Ecstasy Ecstasy (methylenedioxymethamfetamine, MDMA) may cause severe reactions, even at doses that were previously tolerated. The most serious effects are delirium, coma, convulsions, ventricular arrhythmias, hyperpyrexia, rhabdomyolysis, acute renal failure, acute hepatitis, disseminated intravascular coagulation, adult respiratory distress syndrome, hyperreflexia, hypotension and intracerebral haemorrhage; hyponatraemia has also been associated with ecstasy use and syndrome of inappropriate antidiuretic hormone secretion (SIADH) can occur.

Treatment of methylenedioxymethamfetamine poisoning is supportive, with diazepam to control severe agitation or persistent convulsions and close monitoring including ECG. Self-induced water intoxication should be considered in patients with ecstasy poisoning.

'Liquid ecstasy' is a term used for sodium oxybate (gamma-hydroxybutyrate, GHB), which is a sedative.

Theophylline

Theophylline and related drugs are often prescribed as modified-release formulations and toxicity may therefore be delayed. They cause vomiting (which may be severe and intractable), agitation, restlessness, dilated pupils, sinus tachycardia, and hyperglycaemia. More serious effects are haematemesis, convulsions, and supraventricular and ventricular arrhythmias. Profound hypokalaemia may develop rapidly.

Repeated doses of activated charcoal can be used to eliminate theophylline even if more than 1 hour has lapsed after ingestion and especially if a modified-release preparation has been taken (see also under Active Elimination Techniques). Hypokalaemia is corrected by intravenous infusion of potassium chloride in 0.9% sodium chloride and may be so severe as to require high doses under ECG monitoring. Convulsions should be controlled by intravenous administration of diazepam (emulsion preferred). Sedation with lorazepam or diazepam (emulsion preferred) may be necessary in agitated children.

Provided the child does **not** suffer from asthma, a short-acting beta-blocker (section 2.4) may be administered intravenously to reverse severe tachycardia, hypokalaemia, and hyperglycaemia.

Other poisons

Consult either a poisons information centre day and night or TOXBASE, see p. 32.

The **poisons information centres** (Tel: 0870 600 6266) will provide specialist advice on all aspects of poisoning day and night

Cyanides

Cyanide antidotes include dicobalt edetate, given alone, and sodium nitrite followed by sodium thiosulphate. These antidotes are held for emergency use in hospitals as well as in centres where cyanide poisoning is a risk such as factories and laboratories. The use of sodium nitrite with sodium thiosulphate is preferred over the use of dicobalt edetate because dicobalt edetate itself is toxic and is associated with anaphylactic reactions. Hydroxocobalamin is an alternative antidote but its use should ideally be discussed with a poisons information centre; the usual dose is hydroxocobalamin 70 mg/kg by intravenous infusion (repeated once or twice according to severity). *Cyanokit®*, which provides hydroxocobalamin 2.5 g/bottle, is available but it is not licensed for use in the UK.

DICOBALT EDETATE

Cautions owing to toxicity to be used only for definite cyanide poisoning when patient tending to lose, or has lost, consciousness; **not** to be used as a precautionary measure

Side-effects hypotension, tachycardia, and vomiting; anaphylactic reactions including facial and laryngeal oedema and cardiac abnormalities

Indication and dose

Acute poisoning with cyanides
- By intravenous injection
  Consult a poisons information centre

[1]**Dicobalt Edetate** (Cambridge) PoM
Injection, dicobalt edetate 15 mg/mL, net price 20-mL (300-mg) amp = £10.58

1. PoM restriction does not apply where administration is for saving life in emergency

SODIUM NITRITE

Side-effects flushing and headache due to vasodilatation

Indication and dose

Poisoning with cyanides (used in conjunction with sodium thiosulphate) See under preparation below

[1]**Sodium Nitrite** PoM
Injection, sodium nitrite 3% (30 mg/mL) in water for injections

Dose
- **By intravenous injection over 5–20 minutes**
  Child 1 month–18 years 4–10 mg/kg max. 300 mg (0.13–0.33 mL/kg, max. 10 mL, of 3% solution) followed by sodium thiosulphate injection 400 mg/kg, max. 12.5 g (0.8 mL/kg, max. 25 mL, of 50% solution) over 10 minutes

Available as a manufactured special; contact Martindale, or regional hospital manufacturing unit

1. PoM restriction does not apply where administration is for saving life in emergency

SODIUM THIOSULPHATE

Indication and dose

Poisoning with cyanides (used in conjunction with sodium nitrite)
see above under Sodium Nitrite

[1]**Sodium Thiosulphate** PoM
Injection, sodium thiosulphate 50% (500 mg/mL) in water for injections
Available as a manufactured special; contact Martindale, or regional hospital manufacturing unit

1. PoM restriction does not apply where administration is for saving life in emergency

Ethylene glycol and methanol

Ethanol (by mouth or by intravenous infusion) is used for the treatment of ethylene glycol or methanol (methyl alcohol) poisoning. Fomepizole (*Antizol®*, available from specialist importing companies) has also been used for the treatment of ethylene glycol or methanol poisoning. Advice on the treatment of ethylene glycol or methanol poisoning should be obtained from a poisons information centre.

Heavy metals

Heavy metal antidotes include dimercaprol, penicillamine, and sodium calcium edetate. Other antidotes for heavy metal poisoning include succimer (DMSA) and unithiol (DMPS) [both unlicensed]; their use may be valuable in certain cases and the advice of a poisons information centre should be sought.

DIMERCAPROL
(BAL)

Cautions hypertension, pregnancy and breast-feeding; **interactions:** Appendix 1 (dimercaprol)

Renal impairment discontinue or use with extreme caution if impairment develops during treatment

Contra-indications not indicated for iron, cadmium, or selenium poisoning; severe hepatic impairment (unless due to arsenic poisoning)

Side-effects hypertension, tachycardia, malaise, nausea, vomiting, salivation, lacrimation, sweating, burning sensation (mouth, throat, and eyes), feeling of constriction of throat and chest, headache, muscle spasm, abdominal pain, tingling of extremities; pyrexia; local pain and abscess at injection site

Licensed use licensed for use in children (age range not specified by manufacturer)

Indication and dose

Poisoning by antimony, arsenic, bismuth, gold, mercury, possibly thallium; adjunct (with sodium calcium edetate) in lead poisoning
- **By intramuscular injection**

  Child 1 month–18 years 2.5–3 mg/kg every 4 hours for 2 days, 2–4 times on the third day, then 1–2 times daily for 10 days or until recovery

Dimercaprol (Sovereign) PoM

Injection, dimercaprol 50 mg/mL. Net price 2-mL amp = £42.73

Note Contains arachis (peanut) oil as solvent

PENICILLAMINE

Cautions see section 9.8.1

Contra-indications see section 9.8.1

Side-effects see section 9.8.1

Licensed use licensed for use in children (age range not specified by manufacturer)

Indication and dose

Lead poisoning
- **By mouth**

  Child 1 month–18 years 20 mg/kg daily in divided doses before food until urinary lead is stabilised at less than 500 micrograms/day

Preparations

Section 9.8.1

SODIUM CALCIUM EDETATE
(Sodium Calciumedetate)

Cautions renal impairment

Side-effects nausea, diarrhoea, abdominal pain, pain at site of injection, thrombophlebitis if given too rapidly, renal damage particularly in overdosage; hypotension, lacrimation, myalgia, nasal congestion, sneezing, malaise, thirst, fever, chills, headache also reported

Licensed use licensed for use in children (age range not specified by manufacturer)

Indication and dose

Poisoning by heavy metals, especially lead
- **By intravenous infusion**

  Child 1 month–18 years up to 40 mg/kg twice daily for up to 5 days, repeated if necessary after 48 hours

Administration for *intravenous infusion*, dilute to a concentration of not more 30 mg/mL with Glucose 5% *or* Sodium Chloride 0.9%; give over at least 1 hour

Ledclair® (Durbin) PoM

Injection, sodium calcium edetate 200 mg/mL, net price 5-mL amp = £7.29

Noxious gases

Carbon monoxide Carbon monoxide poisoning is usually due to inhalation of smoke, car exhaust, or fumes caused by blocked flues or incomplete combustion of fuel gases in confined spaces. Its toxic effects are entirely due to hypoxia.

Immediate treatment of carbon monoxide poisoning is essential. The child should be moved to fresh air, the airway cleared, and **oxygen** 100% administered as soon as available. Artificial respiration should be given as necessary and continued until adequate spontaneous breathing starts, or stopped only after persistent and efficient treatment of cardiac arrest has failed. The child should be admitted to hospital because complications may arise after a delay of hours or days. Cerebral oedema should be anticipated in severe poisoning and is treated with an intravenous infusion of mannitol (section 2.2.5). Referral for hyperbaric oxygen treatment should be discussed with the poisons information services if the patient is or has been unconscious, or has psychiatric or neurological features other than a headache or has myocardial ischaemia or an arrhythmia, or has a blood carboxyhaemoglobin concentration of more than 20%, or is pregnant.

Sulphur dioxide, chlorine, phosgene, ammonia All of these gases can cause upper respiratory tract and conjunctival irritation. Pulmonary oedema, with severe breathlessness and cyanosis may develop suddenly up to 36 hours after exposure. Death may occur. Children are kept under observation and those who develop pulmonary oedema are given oxygen. Assisted ventilation may be necessary in the most serious cases.

CS Spray

CS spray, which is used for riot control, irritates the eyes (hence 'tear gas') and the respiratory tract; symptoms normally settle spontaneously within 15 minutes. If symptoms persist, the patient should be removed to a well-ventilated area, and the exposed skin washed with soap and water after removal of contaminated clothing. Contact lenses should be removed and rigid ones washed (soft ones should be discarded). Eye symptoms should be treated by irrigating the eyes with physiological saline (or water if saline not available) and advice sought from an ophthalmologist. Patients with features of severe poisoning, particularly respiratory complications, should be admitted to hospital for symptomatic treatment.

Nerve agents

Treatment of nerve agent poisoning is similar to organophosphorus insecticide poisoning (see below), but advice must be sought from a poisons information centre. The risk of cross-contamination is significant; adequate decontamination and protective clothing for healthcare personnel are essential. In emergencies involving the release of nerve agents, kits ('NAAS pods') which contain **pralidoxime mesilate** may be obtained through the Ambulance Service from the National Blood Service (or the Welsh Blood Service in South Wales or designated hospital pharmacies in Northern Ireland and Scotland—see TOXBASE for list of designated centres). If the child does not respond to atropine and pralidoxime it may be appropriate to use **obidoxime**, but advice should be sought from a poisons information centre. In the very rare circumstances where the nerve agent is tabun (GA), obidoxime will also be supplied as part of the pod.

> The **poisons information centres** (Tel: 0870 600 6266) will provide specialist advice on all aspects of poisoning day and night

Pesticides

Paraquat Concentrated liquid paraquat preparations (e.g. *Gramoxone*®), available to farmers and horticulturists, contain 10–20% paraquat and are extremely toxic. Granular preparations, for garden use, contain only 2.5% paraquat and have caused few deaths.

Paraquat has local and systemic effects. Splashes in the eyes irritate and ulcerate the cornea and conjunctiva. Copious washing of the eye should aid healing but it may be a long process. Skin irritation, blistering, and ulceration can occur from prolonged contact both with the concentrated and dilute forms. Inhalation of spray, mist, or dust containing paraquat may cause nose bleeding and sore throat but not systemic toxicity.

Ingestion of concentrated paraquat solutions is followed by nausea, vomiting, and diarrhoea. Painful ulceration of the tongue, lips, and fauces may appear after 36 to 48 hours together with renal failure. Some days later there may be dyspnoea with pulmonary fibrosis due to proliferative alveolitis and bronchiolitis.

Treatment should be started immediately. The single most useful measure is oral administration of **activated charcoal**. Vomiting may preclude the use of activated charcoal and an anti-emetic may be required. Gastric lavage is of doubtful value. Intravenous fluids and analgesics are given as necessary. Oxygen therapy should be avoided in the early stages of management since this may exacerbate damage to the lungs, but oxygen may be required in the late stages to palliate symptoms. Measures to enhance elimination of absorbed paraquat are probably valueless but should be discussed with the poisons information centres who will also give guidance on predicting the likely outcome from plasma concentrations. Paraquat absorption can be confirmed by a simple qualitative urine test.

Organophosphorus insecticides Organophosphorus insecticides are usually supplied as powders or dissolved in organic solvents. All are absorbed through the bronchi and intact skin as well as through the gut and inhibit cholinesterase activity thereby prolonging and intensifying the effects of acetylcholine. Toxicity between different compounds varies considerably, and onset may be delayed after skin exposure.

Anxiety, restlessness, dizziness, headache, miosis, nausea, hypersalivation, vomiting, abdominal colic, diarrhoea, bradycardia, and sweating are common features of organophosphorus poisoning. Muscle weakness and fasciculation may develop and progress to generalised flaccid paralysis including the ocular and respiratory muscles. Convulsions, coma, pulmonary oedema with copious bronchial secretions, hypoxia, and arrhythmias occur in severe cases. Hyperglycaemia and glycosuria without ketonuria may also be present.

Further absorption of the organophosphorus insecticide should be prevented by moving the child to fresh air, removing soiled clothing, and washing contaminated skin. In severe poisoning it is vital to ensure a clear airway, frequent removal of bronchial secretions, and adequate ventilation and oxygenation; gastric lavage may be considered provided that the airway is protected. **Atropine** will reverse the muscarinic effects of acetylcholine and is given in a dose of 20 micrograms/kg (max. 2 mg) as atropine sulphate (intramuscularly or intravenously according to the severity of poisoning) every 5 to 10 minutes until the skin becomes flushed and dry, the pupils dilate, and tachycardia develops.

Pralidoxime mesilate (P2S), a cholinesterase reactivator, is used as an adjunct to atropine in moderate or severe poisoning. It improves muscle tone within 30 minutes of administration. Repeated doses are required; an intravenous infusion is required in severe cases. Pralidoxime mesilate may be obtained from designated centres, the names of which are held by the poisons information centres (see p. 32).

PRALIDOXIME MESILATE

(P2S)

Cautions renal impairment, myasthenia gravis

Contra-indications poisoning due to carbamates and to organophosphorus compounds without anticholinesterase activity

Side-effects drowsiness, dizziness, disturbances of vision, nausea, tachycardia, headache, hyperventilation, and muscular weakness

Licensed use licensed for use in children (age range not specified by manufacturer)

Indication and dose

Adjunct to atropine in the treatment of poisoning by organophosphorus insecticide or nerve agent

- By slow intravenous injection (diluted to 10–15 mL with water for injections) over 5–10 minutes

Child initially 30 mg/kg then either 30 mg/kg every 4 hours *or by intravenous infusion*, 8–10 mg/kg/hour; usual max. 12 g in 24 hours

Note Pralidoxime mesilate doses may differ from those in product literature

PRALIDOXIME MESILATE (*continued*)

[1]**Pralidoxime Mesilate** PoM

Injection, pralidoxime mesilate 200 mg/mL

Available as 5-mL amps (from designated centres for organophosphorus insecticide poisoning or from the National Blood Service and the Welsh Blood Service for nerve agent poisoning—see TOXBASE for list of designated centres)

1. PoM restriction does not apply where administration is for saving life in emergency

The **poisons information centres** (Tel: 0870 600 6266) will provide specialist advice on all aspects of poisoning day and night

Snake bites and animal stings

Snake bites Envenoming from snake bite is uncommon in the UK. Many exotic snakes are kept, some illegally, but the only indigenous venomous snake is the adder (*Vipera berus*). The bite may cause local and systemic effects. Local effects include pain, swelling, bruising, and tender enlargement of regional lymph nodes. Systemic effects include early anaphylactoid symptoms (transient hypotension with syncope, angioedema, urticaria, abdominal colic, diarrhoea, and vomiting), with later persistent or recurrent hypotension, ECG abnormalities, spontaneous systemic bleeding, coagulopathy, adult respiratory distress syndrome, and acute renal failure. Fatal envenoming is rare but the potential for severe envenoming must not be underestimated.

Early anaphylactoid symptoms should be treated with **adrenaline (epinephrine)** (section 3.4.3). Indications for antivenom treatment include systemic envenoming, especially hypotension (see above), ECG abnormalities, vomiting, haemostatic abnormalities, and marked local envenoming such that after bites on the hand or foot, swelling extends beyond the wrist or ankle within 4 hours of the bite. The contents of one vial (10 mL) of **European viper venom antiserum** (available from Farillon) is given *by intravenous injection* over 10–15 minutes or *by intravenous infusion* over 30 minutes after diluting in sodium chloride intravenous infusion 0.9% (use 5 mL diluent/kg body-weight). The **same dose** should be used for **adults** and **children**. The dose can be repeated in 1–2 hours if symptoms of **systemic envenoming** persist. Adrenaline (epinephrine) injection must be immediately to hand for treatment of anaphylactic reactions to the antivenom (for the management of anaphylaxis see section 3.4.3).

Antivenom is available for certain foreign snakes, spiders and scorpions. For information on identification, management, and supply, telephone:

Oxford	(01865) 220 968 *or* (01865) 221 332 *or* (01865) 741 166
Liverpool	(0151) 708 9393
Liverpool (Royal Liverpool University Hospital) (emergency supply only)	(0151) 706 2000
London (emergency supply only)	(020) 7771 5394

Insect stings Stings from ants, wasps, hornets, and bees cause local pain and swelling but seldom cause severe direct toxicity unless many stings are inflicted at the same time. If the sting is in the mouth or on the tongue local swelling may threaten the upper airway. The stings from these insects are usually treated by cleaning the area. Bee stings should be removed as quickly as possible. Anaphylactic reactions require immediate treatment with intramuscular **adrenaline (epinephrine)**; self-administered (or administered by a carer) intramuscular adrenaline (e.g. *EpiPen*®) is the best first-aid treatment for children with severe hypersensitivity. An inhaled bronchodilator should be used for asthmatic reactions. For the management of anaphylaxis, see section 3.4.3. A short course of an **oral antihistamine** or a **topical corticosteroid** may help to reduce inflammation and relieve itching.

Marine stings The severe pain of weeverfish (*Trachinus vipera*) stings can be relieved by immersing the stung area in uncomfortably hot, but not scalding, water (not more than 45° C). Children stung by jellyfish and Portuguese man-o'-war around the UK coast should be removed from the sea as soon as possible. Adherent tentacles should be lifted off carefully (wearing gloves or using tweezers) or washed off with seawater. Alcoholic solutions including suntan lotions should **not** be applied because they may cause further discharge of stinging hairs. Ice packs will reduce pain and a slurry of baking soda (sodium bicarbonate), but not vinegar, may be useful for treating stings from UK species.

1 Gastro-intestinal system

This chapter includes advice on the drug management of the following:

antibiotic-associated colitis, p. 68
constipation, p. 75
Crohn's disease, p. 66
food allergy, p. 75
Helicobacter pylori infection, p. 58
irritable bowel syndrome, p. 67
malabsorption syndromes, p. 68
NSAID-associated ulcers, p. 59
ulcerative colitis, p. 66

1.1 Dyspepsia and gastro-oesophageal reflux disease

Dyspepsia

Dyspepsia covers pain, fullness, early satiety, bloating, and nausea. It can occur with gastric and duodenal ulceration (section 1.3), gastro-oesophageal reflux disease, gastritis, and upper gastro-intestinal motility disorders, but most commonly it is of uncertain origin.

A compound alginate preparation (section 1.1.2) may provide relief from dyspepsia; persistent dyspepsia requires investigation. Treatment with a H_2-receptor antagonist (section 1.3.1) or a proton pump inhibitor (section 1.3.5) should be initiated only on the advice of a hospital specialist.

Helicobacter pylori may be present in children with dyspepsia. *H. pylori* eradication therapy (section 1.3) should be considered for persistent dyspepsia if it is ulcer-like. However, there is no evidence that children with functional (investigated, non-ulcer) dyspepsia benefit symptomatically from *H. pylori* eradication.

Gastro-oesophageal reflux disease

Gastro-oesophageal reflux disease includes non-erosive gastro-oesophageal reflux and erosive oesophagitis. Uncomplicated gastro-oesophageal reflux is common in infancy and most symptoms, such as intermittent vomiting or repeated, effortless regurgitation, resolve without treatment between 12 and 18 months of age. Older children with gastro-oesophageal reflux disease may have heartburn, acid regurgitation and dysphagia. Oesophageal inflammation (oesophagitis), ulceration or stricture formation may develop in early childhood; gastro-oesophageal reflux disease may also be associated with chronic respiratory disorders including asthma.

Management of gastro-oesophageal reflux disease

- *Neonates and infants*: provide parental reassurance; increase the frequency and decrease the volume of feeds; use a suitable compound alginate preparation (section 1.1.2) or use a feed thickener or pre-thickened formula feeds (Appendix 2) on the advice of a dietitian
- *Older children* should be advised about life-style changes such as weight reduction if obese, and the avoidance of alcohol and smoking; treat with an alginate-containing antacid
- On the advice of a specialist paediatrician, a **histamine H_2-receptor antagonist** (section 1.3.1) or a **proton pump inhibitor** (section 1.3.5) may be added.

H_2-receptor antagonists (section 1.3.1) relieve symptoms of gastro-oesophageal reflux disease, promote mucosal healing and permit reduction in antacid consumption.

Proton pump inhibitors (section 1.3.5) may be used in infants and children for the treatment of moderate, non-erosive oesophagitis that is unresponsive to an H_2-receptor antagonist. Endoscopically confirmed *erosive*, *ulcerative*, or *stricturing* disease in children is usually treated with a proton pump inhibitor. Reassessment is necessary if symptoms persist despite 4–6 weeks of treatment; long-term use of an H_2-receptor antagonist or proton pump inhibitor should not be undertaken without full assessment of the underlying condition.

Motility stimulants (section 1.2), such as domperidone or erythromycin may improve gastro-oesophageal sphincter contraction and accelerate gastric emptying. Evidence for the long-term efficacy of motility stimulants in the management of gastro-oesophageal reflux in children is unconvincing.

For advice on specialised formula feeds, see section 9.4.2

1.1.1 Antacids and simeticone

Antacids (usually containing aluminium or magnesium compounds) are suitable for short-term relief of intermittent symptoms of *ulcer dyspepsia* and *non-erosive gastro-oesophageal reflux* (see above) in children; they are also used in functional (non-ulcer) dyspepsia, but the evidence of benefit is uncertain.

Aluminium- and **magnesium-containing** antacids, being relatively insoluble in water, are long-acting if retained in the stomach. Magnesium-containing antacids tend to be laxative whereas aluminium-containing antacids may be constipating; antacids containing both magnesium and aluminium may reduce these colonic side-effects. Aluminium-containing antacids should not be used in children with renal impairment, or in neonates and infants because accumulation may lead to increased plasma-aluminium concentrations.

Complexes such as **hydrotalcite** confer no special advantage.

Calcium-containing antacids can induce rebound acid secretion; with modest doses the clinical significance of this is doubtful, but prolonged high doses also cause hypercalcaemia and alkalosis.

Simeticone (activated dimeticone) is used to treat infantile colic, but the evidence of benefit is uncertain. Simeticone is added to an antacid as an antifoaming agent to relieve flatulence; such preparations may also be useful for the relief of hiccup in palliative care (see Prescribing in Palliative Care, p. 26).

Alginates act as mucosal protectants in gastro-oesophageal reflux disease (section 1.1.2) The amount of additional ingredient or antacid in individual preparations varies widely, as does their sodium content, so that preparations may not be freely interchangeable.

Interactions Antacids should preferably not be taken at the same time as other drugs since they may impair absorption. Antacids may also damage enteric coatings designed to prevent dissolution in the stomach. See also **Appendix 1** (antacids, calcium salts).

> Low Na^+
> The words low Na^+ added after some preparations indicate a sodium content of less than 1 mmol per tablet or 10-mL dose.

Aluminium- and magnesium-containing antacids

ALUMINIUM HYDROXIDE

Cautions see notes above; **interactions:** Appendix 1 (antacids)

Renal impairment risk of aluminium accumulation in severe impairment

Pregnancy use with caution especially in first trimester

Contra-indications hypophosphataemia; neonates; porphyria (section 9.8.2)

Side-effects see notes above

Indication and dose

Dyspepsia for dose see under preparation

Hyperphosphataemia section 9.5.2.2

Co-magaldrox

Co-magaldrox is a mixture of aluminium hydroxide and magnesium hydroxide; the proportions are expressed in the form *x*/*y* where *x* and *y* are the strengths in milligrams per unit dose of magnesium hydroxide and aluminium hydroxide respectively

Maalox® (Sanofi-Aventis)

Suspension, sugar-free, co-magaldrox 195/220 (magnesium hydroxide 195 mg, dried aluminium hydroxide 220 mg/5 mL (low Na^+)). Net price 500 mL = £2.59

Dose

- **By mouth**
  Child 14–18 years 10–20 mL 20–60 minutes after meals and at bedtime

Mucogel® (Forest)

Suspension, sugar-free, co-magaldrox 195/220 (magnesium hydroxide 195 mg, dried aluminium hydroxide 220 mg/5 mL (low Na^+)). Net price 500 mL = £1.71

Dose

- **By mouth**
  Child 12–18 years 10–20 mL 3 times daily, 20–60 minutes after meals, and at bedtime when required

MAGNESIUM TRISILICATE

Cautions heart failure, hypertension; metabolic or respiratory alkalosis, hypermagnesaemia; **interactions:** Appendix 1 (antacids)

Renal impairment increased risk of toxicity in moderate impairment—avoid or reduce dose

Pregnancy use with caution especially in first trimester; avoid antacid preparations containing high sodium content

Contra-indications severe renal failure; hypophosphataemia

Side-effects see notes above; silica-based renal stones reported on long-term treatment

Indication and dose

Dyspepsia for dose see under preparation

Magnesium Trisilicate Mixture, BP (Magnesium Trisilicate Oral Suspension)
Oral suspension, 5% each of magnesium trisilicate, light magnesium carbonate, and sodium bicarbonate in a suitable vehicle with a peppermint flavour. Contains about 6 mmol Na^+/10 mL

Dose

- By mouth
  Child 5–12 years 5–10 mL with water 3 times daily
  Child 12–18 years 10–20 mL with water 3 times daily

Aluminium-magnesium complexes

HYDROTALCITE

Aluminium magnesium carbonate hydroxide hydrate

Cautions see notes above; **interactions:** Appendix 1 (antacids)

Side-effects see notes above

Indication and dose

Dyspepsia for dose see under preparation

Hydrotalcite (Peckforton)
Suspension, hydrotalcite 500 mg/5 mL (low Na^+). Net price 500-mL pack = £1.96

Note The brand name *Altacite*® [NHS] is used for hydrotalcite suspension; for *Altacite Plus*® suspension, see below

Dose

- By mouth
  Child 6–12 years 5 mL 3 times daily between meals and at bedtime
  Child 12–18 years 10 mL 3 times daily between meals and at bedtime

Antacid preparations containing simeticone

Altacite Plus® (Peckforton)
Suspension, sugar-free, co-simalcite 125/500 (simeticone 125 mg, hydrotalcite 500 mg)/5 mL (low Na^+). Net price 500 mL = £1.96

Dose

- By mouth
  Child 8–12 years 5 mL 3 times daily between meals and at bedtime when required
  Child 12–18 years 10 mL 3 times daily between meals and at bedtime when required

Asilone® (Thornton & Ross)
Suspension, sugar-free, dried aluminium hydroxide 420 mg, simeticone 135 mg, light magnesium oxide 70 mg/5 mL (low Na^+). Net price 500 mL = £1.95

Dose

- By mouth
  Child 12–18 years 5–10 mL after meals and at bedtime or when required up to 4 times daily

Maalox Plus® (Sanofi-Aventis)
Suspension, sugar-free, dried aluminium hydroxide 220 mg, simeticone 25 mg, magnesium hydroxide 195 mg/5 mL (low Na^+). Net price 500 mL = £2.59

Dose

- By mouth
  Child 2–5 years 5 mL 3 times daily
  Child 5–12 years 5–10 mL 3–4 times daily
  Child 12–18 years 5–10 mL 4 times daily, after meals and at bedtime when required

Simeticone alone

SIMETICONE

Activated dimeticone

Indication and dose

Colic, gripes, wind pain for dose see under individual preparations

Dentinox® (DDD) ◢
Colic drops (= emulsion), simeticone 21 mg/2.5-mL dose. Net price 100 mL = £1.73

Dose

- By mouth
  Neonate 2.5 mL with or after each feed (max. 6 doses in 24 hours); may be added to bottle feed
  Child 1 month–2 years 2.5 mL with or after each feed (max. 6 doses in 24 hours); may be added to bottle feed

Note The brand name *Dentinox*® is also used for other preparations including teething gel

1 Gastro-intestinal system

SIMETICONE (*continued*)

Infacol® (Forest)
Liquid, sugar-free, simeticone 40 mg/mL (low Na^+). Net price 50 mL = £2.03 Counselling, use of dropper

Dose
- By mouth
  Neonate 0.5–1 mL before feeds
  Child 1 month–2 years 0.5–1 mL before feeds

1.1.2 Compound alginate preparations

Alginate-containing antacids form a 'raft' that floats on the surface of the stomach contents to reduce reflux and protect the oesophageal mucosa; they are used in the management of mild symptoms of dyspepsia and gastro-oesophageal reflux disease (section 1.1).

Preparations containing aluminium should not be used in children with renal impairment, neonates or infants (section 1.1.1).

Compound alginate preparations

Acidex® (Pinewood)
Liquid, sugar-free, sodium alginate 250 mg, sodium bicarbonate 133.5 mg, calcium carbonate 80 mg/5 mL. Contains about 3 mmol Na^+/5 mL, net price 500 mL (aniseed- or peppermint-flavour) = £1.70

Dose
- By mouth
  Child 6–12 years 5–10 mL after meals and at bedtime
  Child 12–18 years 10–20 mL after meals and at bedtime

Algicon® (Sanofi-Aventis)
Suspension, yellow, aluminium hydroxide-magnesium carbonate co-gel 140 mg, magnesium alginate 250 mg, magnesium carbonate 175 mg, potassium bicarbonate 50 mg/5 mL (low Na^+). Net price 500 mL (lemon-flavoured) = £3.07

Dose
- By mouth
  Child 12–18 years 10–20 mL 4 times daily (after meals and at bedtime)

Gastrocote® (Thornton & Ross)
Tablets, alginic acid 200 mg, dried aluminium hydroxide 80 mg, magnesium trisilicate 40 mg, sodium bicarbonate 70 mg. Contains about 1 mmol Na^+/tablet. Net price 100-tab pack = £3.51
Cautions diabetes mellitus (high sugar content)

Dose
- By mouth
  Child 6–18 years 1–2 tablets chewed 4 times daily (after meals and at bedtime)

Liquid, sugar-free, peach-coloured, dried aluminium hydroxide 80 mg, magnesium trisilicate 40 mg, sodium alginate 220 mg, sodium bicarbonate 70 mg/5 mL. Contains 1.8 mmol Na^+/5 mL. Net price 500 mL = £2.67

Dose
- By mouth
  Child 6–18 years 5–15 mL 4 times daily (after meals and at bedtime)

Gaviscon® Advance (R&C)
Tablets, sugar-free, sodium alginate 500 mg, potassium bicarbonate 100 mg. Contains 2.25mmol Na^+, 1 mmol K^+/tablet. Net price 60–tab pack (peppermint-flavour) = £3.24
Excipients: include aspartame (section 9.4.1)

Dose
- By mouth
  Child 6–12 years 1 tablet to be chewed after meals and at bedtime (under medical advice only)
  Child 12–18 years 1–2 tablets to be chewed after meals and at bedtime

Suspension, sugar-free, sodium alginate 500 mg, potassium bicarbonate 100 mg/5 mL. Contains 2.3 mmol Na^+, 1 mmol K^+/5 mL. Net price 500 mL (aniseed- or peppermint-flavour) = £5.40

Dose
- By mouth
  Child 2–12 years 2.5–5 mL after meals and at bedtime (under medical advice only)
  Child 12–18 years 5–10 mL after meals and at bedtime

Gaviscon® Infant (R&C)
Oral powder, sugar-free, sodium alginate 225 mg, magnesium alginate 87.5 mg, with colloidal silica and mannitol/dose (half dual-sachet). Contains 0.92 mmol Na^+/dose. Net price 15 dual-sachets (30 doses) = £2.46

Dose
- By mouth
  Neonate body-weight under 4.5 kg 1 dose (half dual-sachet) mixed with feeds (or water, for breast-fed infants) when required (max. 6 times in 24 hours)
  Neonate body-weight over 4.5 kg 2 doses (1 dual-sachet) mixed with feeds (or water, for breast-fed infants) when required (max. 6 times in 24 hours)
  Child 1 month–2 years 2 doses (1 dual-sachet) mixed with feeds (or water, for breast-fed infants) when required (max. 6 times in 24 hours)

Note Not to be used in preterm neonates, or where excessive water loss likely (e.g. fever, diarrhoea, vomiting, high room temperature), or if intestinal obstruction. Not to be used with other preparations containing thickening agents

Safe Practice Each half of the dual-sachet is identified as 'one dose'. To avoid errors prescribe as 'dual-sachet' with directions in terms of 'dose'

Peptac® (IVAX)
Suspension, sugar-free, sodium bicarbonate 133.5 mg, sodium alginate 250 mg, calcium carbonate 80 mg/5 mL. Contains 3.1 mmol Na^+/5mL. Net price 500 mL (aniseed- or peppermint-flavoured) = £2.16

Dose

Child 6–12 years 5–10 mL 4 times daily after meals and at bedtime

Child 12–18 years 10–20 mL 4 times daily. after meals and at bedtime

Rennie® Duo (Roche Consumer Health)
Suspension, sugar-free, calcium carbonate 600 mg, magnesium carbonate 70 mg, sodium alginate 150 mg/5 mL. Contains 2.6 mmol Na^+/5 mL. Net price 500 mL (mint flavour) = £2.67

Dose

- **By mouth**
  Child 12–18 years 10 mL after meals and at bedtime; an additional 10 mL may be taken between doses for heartburn if necessary, max. 80 mL daily

Excipients: include propylene glycol

Topal® (Fabre)
Tablets, alginic acid 200 mg, dried aluminium hydroxide 30 mg, light magnesium carbonate 40 mg with lactose 220 mg, sucrose 880 mg, sodium bicarbonate 40 mg (low Na^+). Net price 42-tab pack = £1.67

Cautions diabetes mellitus (high sugar content)

Dose

- **By mouth**
  Child 12–18 years 1–3 tablets chewed 4 times daily (after meals and at bedtime)

1.2 Antispasmodics and other drugs altering gut motility

Drugs in this section include antimuscarinic compounds and drugs believed to be direct relaxants of intestinal smooth muscle. The smooth muscle relaxant properties of antimuscarinic and other antispasmodic drugs may be useful in *irritable bowel syndrome.*

The dopamine-receptor antagonist **domperidone** stimulates transit in the gut.

Antimuscarinics

Antimuscarinics (formerly termed 'anticholinergics') reduce intestinal motility. They are occasionally used for the management of *irritable bowel syndrome* but the evidence of their value has not been established and response varies. Other indications of antimuscarinic drugs include asthma and airways disease (section 3.1.2), motion sickness (section 4.6), urinary frequency and enuresis (section 7.4.2), mydriasis and cycloplegia (section 11.5), premedication (section 15.1.3), palliative care (p. 26), and as an antidote to organophosphorus poisoning (p. 46).

Antimuscarinics that are used for gastro-intestinal smooth muscle spasm include the tertiary amine **dicycloverine hydrochloride** (dicyclomine hydrochloride) and the quaternary ammonium compounds **propantheline bromide** and **hyoscine butylbromide**. The quaternary ammonium compounds are less lipid soluble than atropine and so are less likely to cross the blood-brain barrier; they are also less well absorbed.

Dicycloverine hydrochloride may also have some direct action on smooth muscle. Hyoscine butylbromide is advocated as a gastro-intestinal antispasmodic, but it is poorly absorbed; the injection is useful in endoscopy and radiology.

Cautions Antimuscarinics should be used with caution in children (especially children with Down's Syndrome) due to increased risk of side-effects; they should also be used with caution in hypertension, conditions characterised by tachycardia (including hyperthyroidism, cardiac insufficiency, cardiac surgery), pyrexia, pregnancy and breast-feeding. Antimuscarinics are not used in children with gastro-oesophageal reflux disease, diarrhoea or ulcerative colitis. **Interactions:** Appendix 1 (antimuscarinics).

Contra-indications Antimuscarinics are contra-indicated in angle-closure glaucoma, myasthenia gravis (but may be used to decrease muscarinic side-effects of anticholinesterases—section 10.2.1), paralytic ileus, and pyloric stenosis.

Side-effects Side-effects of antimuscarinics include constipation, transient bradycardia (followed by tachycardia, palpitations and arrhythmias), reduced bronchial secretions, urinary urgency and retention, dilatation of the pupils with loss of accommodation, photophobia, dry mouth, flushing and dryness of the skin. Side-effects that occur occasionally include nausea, vomiting, and giddiness.

DICYCLOVERINE HYDROCHLORIDE

(Dicyclomine hydrochloride)

Cautions see notes above

Contra-indications see notes above; child under 6 months

Side-effects see notes above

Indication and dose

Symptomatic relief of gastro-intestinal disorders characterised by smooth muscle spasm
- By mouth
  Child 6 months–2 years 5–10 mg 3–4 times daily 15 minutes before feeds
  Child 2–12 years 10 mg 3 times daily
  Child 12–18 years 10–20 mg 3 times daily

[1]**Merbentyl®** (Sanofi-Aventis) PoM
Tablets, dicycloverine hydrochloride 10 mg, net price 20 = £1.01; 20 mg (*Merbentyl 20®*), 84-tab pack = £8.47

Syrup, dicycloverine hydrochloride 10 mg/5 mL, net price 120 mL = £1.84

1. Dicycloverine hydrochloride can be sold to the public provided that max. single dose is 10 mg and max. daily dose is 60 mg

Compound preparations

Kolanticon® (Peckforton)
Gel, sugar-free, dicycloverine hydrochloride 2.5 mg, dried aluminium hydroxide 200 mg, light magnesium oxide 100 mg, simeticone 20 mg/5 mL, net price 200 mL = £1.69, 500 mL = £1.85

Dose

Child 12–18 years 10–20 mL every 4 hours when required

HYOSCINE BUTYLBROMIDE

Cautions see notes above; also intestinal and urinary outlet obstruction

Pregnancy manufacturer advises use only if potential benefit outweighs risk

Breast-feeding amount too small to be harmful

Contra-indications see notes above; avoid in porphyria (section 9.8.2)

Side-effects see notes above; also, *rarely* hypotension, dyspnoea in patients with history of bronchial asthma or allergy

Licensed use *tablets* not licensed for use in children under 6 years; *injection* not licensed for use in children (age range not specified by manufacturer)

Indication and dose

Symptomatic relief of gastro-intestinal or genito-urinary disorders characterised by smooth muscle spasm
- By mouth
  Child 6–12 years 10 mg 3 times daily
  Child 12–18 years 20 mg 3 times daily
- By intramuscular or intravenous injection
  Child 1 month–4 years 300–500 micrograms/kg (max. 5 mg) 3–4 times daily
  Child 5–12 years 5–10 mg 3–4 times daily
  Child 12–18 years 10–20 mg 3–4 times daily

Excessive respiratory secretions and bowel colic in palliative care (see also, p. 26)
- By mouth
  Child 1 month–2 years 300–500 micrograms/kg (max. 5 mg) 3–4 times daily
  Child 2–5 years 5 mg 3–4 times daily
  Child 5–12 years 10 mg 3–4 times daily
  Child 12–18 years 10–20 mg 3–4 times daily

Acute spasm, spasm in diagnostic procedures
- By intramuscular or intravenous injection
  Child 2–6 years 5 mg repeated after 30 minutes if necessary (may be repeated more frequently in endoscopy), max. 15 mg daily
  Child 6–12 years 5–10 mg repeated after 30 minutes if necessary (may be repeated more frequently in endoscopy), max. 30 mg daily
  Child 12–18 years 20 mg repeated after 30 minutes if necessary (may be repeated more frequently in endoscopy), max. 80 mg daily

Administration for *intravenous injection*, may be diluted with Glucose 5% *or* Sodium Chloride 0.9%; give over at least 1 minute.
For administration *by mouth*, injection solution may be used; content of ampoule may be stored in a refrigerator for up to 24 hours after opening

Buscopan® (Boehringer Ingelheim) PoM
[1]Tablets, coated, hyoscine butylbromide 10 mg. Net price 56-tab pack = £2.59

Injection, hyoscine butylbromide 20 mg/mL. Net price 1-mL amp = 20p

1. Hyoscine butylbromide can be sold to the public provided single dose does not exceed 20 mg, daily dose does not exceed 80 mg, and pack does not contain a total of more than 240 mg

PROPANTHELINE BROMIDE

Cautions see notes above

Pregnancy manufacturer advises avoid

Breast-feeding may suppress lactation

Contra-indications see notes above

Side-effects see notes above

Licensed use *tablets* not licensed for use in children under 12 years

Indication and dose

Symptomatic relief of gastro-intestinal disorders characterised by smooth muscle spasm
- By mouth

  Child 1 month–12 years 300 micrograms/kg (max. 15 mg) 3–4 times daily at least one hour before food

  Child 12–18 years 15 mg 3 times daily at least one hour before meals and 30 mg at night (max. 120 mg daily)

Pro-Banthine® (Concord) PoM

Tablets, pink, s/c, propantheline bromide 15 mg, net price 112-tab pack = £15.32. Label: 23

Extemporaneous formulations available see Extemporaneous Preparations, p. 8

Other antispasmodics

Alverine, **mebeverine**, and **peppermint oil** are believed to be direct relaxants of intestinal smooth muscle and may relieve pain in *irritable bowel syndrome* and primary dysmenorrhoea. They have no serious adverse effects; peppermint oil occasionally causes heartburn.

ALVERINE CITRATE

Cautions

Pregnancy caution

Breast-feeding little information available—manufacturer advises avoid

Contra-indications paralytic ileus; when combined with sterculia, intestinal obstruction, faecal impaction, colonic atony

Side-effects nausea, headache, pruritus, rash and dizziness

Indication and dose

Adjunct in gastro-intestinal disorders characterised by smooth muscle spasm, dysmenorrhoea
- By mouth

  Child 12–18 years 60–120 mg up to 3 times daily

Spasmonal® (Norgine)

Capsules, alverine citrate 60 mg (blue/grey), net price 100-cap pack = £11.95; 120 mg (*Spasmonal® Forte*, blue/grey), 60-cap pack = £13.80

MEBEVERINE HYDROCHLORIDE

Cautions avoid in porphyria (section 9.8.2.)

Pregnancy not known to be harmful—manufacturers advise caution

Breast-feeding amount too small to be harmful

Contra-indications paralytic ileus

Side-effects *rarely* allergic reactions (including rash, urticaria, angioedema)

Licensed use *tablets and liquid* not licensed for use in children under 10 years; *granules* not licensed for use in children under 12 years; *modified release capsules* not licensed for use in children (age range not specified by manufacturers)

Indication and dose

Adjunct in gastro-intestinal disorders characterised by smooth muscle spasm
- By mouth

  Child 3–4 years 25 mg 3 times daily, preferably 20 minutes before meals

  Child 4–8 years 50 mg 3 times daily, preferably 20 minutes before meals

  Child 8–10 years 100 mg 3 times daily, preferably 20 minutes before meals

  Child 10–18 years 135–150 mg 3 times daily, preferably 20 minutes before meals

[1]**Mebeverine Hydrochloride** (Non-proprietary) PoM

Tablets, mebeverine hydrochloride 135 mg, net price 20 = £1.34

Oral suspension, mebeverine hydrochloride (as mebeverine embonate) 50 mg/5 mL. Contains Na^+ 0.87 mmol/5 mL. Net price 300 mL = £107.00

1. Mebeverine hydrochloride can be sold to the public for symptomatic relief of irritable bowel syndrome in children over 10 years, provided that max. single dose is 135 mg and max. daily dose is 405 mg;

Colofac® (Solvay) PoM

Tablets, s/c, mebeverine hydrochloride 135 mg. Net price 20 = £1.50

1 Gastro-intestinal system

MEBEVERINE HYDROCHLORIDE (*continued*)

Modified release

Colofac® MR (Solvay) PoM
Capsules, m/r, mebeverine hydrochloride 200 mg, net price 60-cap pack = £6.67. Label: 25

Dose

Irritable bowel syndrome
- By mouth
  Child 12–18 years 1 capsule twice daily preferably 20 minutes before food

Compound preparations

[1]**Fybogel® Mebeverine** (R&C) PoM
Granules, buff, effervescent, ispaghula husk 3.5 g, mebeverine hydrochloride 135 mg/sachet. Contains 7 mmol K^+/sachet (caution in renal impairment). Net price 60 sachets = £15.00. Label: 13, 22, counselling, see below

Dose

Irritable bowel syndrome
- By mouth
  Child 12–18 years 1 sachet in water, morning and evening 30 minutes before food; an additional sachet may also be taken before the midday meal if necessary

Counselling Preparations that swell in contact with liquid should always be carefully swallowed with water and should not be taken immediately before going to bed

1. 10-sachet pack can be sold to the public for use in children over 12 years

PEPPERMINT OIL

Cautions sensitivity to menthol

Breast-feeding significant levels of menthol in breast milk unlikely

Side-effects heartburn, perianal irritation; *rarely*, allergic reactions (including rash, headache, bradycardia, muscle tremor, ataxia)

Local irritation Capsules should not be broken or chewed because peppermint oil may irritate mouth or oesophagus

Indication and dose

Relief of abdominal colic and distension, particularly in irritable bowel syndrome
- By mouth
  Child 15–18 years 1–2 capsules, swallowed whole with water, 3 times daily for up to 3 months if necessary

Colpermin® (Pharmacia)
Capsules, e/c, light blue/dark blue, blue band, peppermint oil 0.2 mL. Net price 100-cap pack = £12.05. Label: 5, 25
Excipients: include arachis (peanut) oil

Motility stimulants

Domperidone and **metoclopramide** (section 4.6) are dopamine antagonists which stimulate gastric emptying and small intestinal transit, and enhance the strength of oesophageal sphincter contraction. Metoclopramide and occasionally domperidone may induce an acute dystonic reaction—for further details of this and other side-effects, see section 4.6.

A low dose of **erythromycin** stimulates gastro-intestinal motility and may be used on the advice of a paediatric gastroenterologist to promote tolerance of enteral feeds; erythromycin may be less effective as a prokinetic drug in preterm neonates than in older children.

DOMPERIDONE

Cautions see under Domperidone (section 4.6)

Side-effects see under Domperidone (section 4.6)

Licensed use not licensed for use in gastro-intestinal stasis

Indication and dose

Gastro-intestinal stasis
- By mouth
  Neonate 100–300 micrograms/kg 4–6 times daily before feeds
  Child 1 month–12 years 200–400 micrograms/kg (max. 20 mg) 3–4 times daily before food
  Child 12–18 years 10–20 mg, 3–4 times daily before food

Nausea and vomiting section 4.6

Preparations

For Preparations see section 4.6

ERYTHROMYCIN

Cautions see section 5.1.5; **interactions:** Appendix 1 (macrolides)

Side-effects see section 5.1.5

Licensed use not licensed for use in gastro-intestinal stasis

Indication and dose

Gastro-intestinal stasis
- By mouth

Neonate 3 mg/kg 4 times daily

Child 1 month–18 years 3 mg/kg 4 times daily

Preparations

For Preparations see section 5.1.5

1.3 Ulcer-healing drugs

Peptic ulceration commonly involves the stomach, duodenum, and lower oesophagus; after gastric surgery it involves the gastro-enterostomy stoma.

Healing can be promoted by general measures, stopping smoking and taking antacids and by antisecretory drug treatment, but relapse is common when treatment ceases. Nearly all duodenal ulcers and most gastric ulcers not associated with NSAIDs are caused by *Helicobacter pylori*.

The management of *H. pylori* infection and of NSAID-associated ulcers is discussed below.

Helicobacter pylori infection

Long-term healing of gastric and duodenal ulcers can be achieved rapidly by eradicating *Helicobacter pylori*; it is recommended that the presence of *H. pylori* is confirmed before starting eradication treatment. If possible the antibacterial sensitivity of the organism should be established at the time of endoscopy and biopsy. Acid inhibition combined with antibacterial treatment is highly effective in the eradication of *H. pylori*; reinfection is rare. Antibiotic-induced colitis is an uncommon risk.

Treatment to eradicate *H. pylori* infection in children should be initiated under specialist supervision. One-week triple-therapy regimens that comprise omeprazole, amoxicillin, and either clarithromycin or metronidazole are recommended. There is normally no need to continue antisecretory treatment (with a proton pump inhibitor or H_2-receptor antagonist) unless the ulcer is complicated by haemorrhage or perforation. Resistance to clarithromycin or to metronidazole is much more common than to amoxicillin and can develop during treatment. A regimen containing amoxicillin and clarithromycin is therefore recommended for initial therapy and one containing amoxicillin and metronidazole for eradication failure. Lansoprazole may be considered if omeprazole is unsuitable. Treatment failure usually indicates antibacterial resistance or poor compliance.

Two-week triple-therapy regimens offer the possibility of higher eradication rates compared to one-week regimens, but adverse effects are common and poor compliance is likely to offset any possible gain.

Two-week dual-therapy regimens using a proton pump inhibitor and a single antibacterial produce low rates of *H. pylori* eradication and are **not** recommended.

There is insufficient evidence to support eradication therapy in children infected with *H. pylori* who continue to take NSAIDs.

Recommended regimens for *Helicobacter pylori* eradication

Eradication therapy	Age range	Oral dose (to be used in combination with omeprazole, section 1.3.5)
Amoxicillin	1–6 years	250 mg twice daily (with clarithromycin) 125 mg 3 times daily (with metronidazole)
	6–12 years	500 mg twice daily (with clarithromycin) 250 mg 3 times daily (with metronidazole)
	12–18 years	1 g twice daily (with clarithromycin) 500 mg 3 times daily (with metronidazole)
Clarithromycin	1–2 years	62.5 mg twice daily (with metronidazole or amoxicillin)
	2–6 years	125 mg twice daily (with metronidazole or amoxicillin)
	6–9 years	187.5 mg twice daily (with metronidazole or amoxicillin)
	9–12 years	250 mg twice daily (with metronidazole or amoxicillin)
	12–18 years	500 mg twice daily (with metronidazole or amoxicillin)
Metronidazole	1–6 years	100 mg twice daily (with clarithromycin) 100 mg 3 times daily (with amoxicillin)
	6–12 years	200 mg twice daily (with clarithromycin) 200 mg 3 times daily (with amoxicillin)
	12–18 years	400 mg twice daily (with clarithromycin) 400 mg 3 times daily (with amoxicillin)

Test for *Helicobacter pylori*

^{13}C-Urea breath test kits are available for confirming the presence of gastro-duodenal infection with *Helicobacter pylori*. The test involves collection of breath samples before and after ingestion of an oral solution of ^{13}C-urea; the samples are sent for analysis by an appropriate laboratory. The test should not be performed within 4 weeks of treatment with an antibacterial or within 2 weeks of treatment with an antisecretory drug. A specific ^{13}C-Urea breath test kit for children is available (*Helicobacter Test INFAI for children of the age 3–11®*). However the appropriateness of testing for *H. pylori* infection in children has not been established. Breath, saliva, faecal, and urine tests for *H. pylori* are frequently unreliable in children; the most accurate method of diagnosis is endoscopy with biopsy.

Helicobacter Test INFAI for children of the age 3-11® (Infai) PoM
Oral powder, ^{13}C-urea 45 mg, net price 1 kit (including 4 breath sample containers, straws) = £19.20 (spectrometric analysis included)

Helicobacter Test INFAI® (Infai) PoM
Oral powder, ^{13}C-urea 75 mg, net price 1 kit (including 4 breath-sample containers, straws) = £19.20 (spectrometric analysis included); 1 kit (including 2 breath bags) = £14.20 (spectroscopic analysis not included); 50-test set = £855.00 (spectrometric analysis included)

NSAID-associated ulcers

Gastro-intestinal bleeding and ulceration can occur with NSAID use (section 10.1.1). Wherever possible, NSAIDs should be **withdrawn** if an ulcer occurs.

Ulcer-healing drugs are not licensed for the prevention or treatment of NSAID-associated gastric and duodenal ulcers in children. However, in those at risk of ulceration a proton pump inhibitor (section 1.3.5) or an H_2-receptor antagonist such as ranitidine may be considered for protection against NSAID-associated gastric and duodenal ulcers.

NSAID use and *H. pylori* infection are independent risk factors for gastro-intestinal bleeding and ulceration. In children already on an NSAID, eradication of *H. pylori* is not recommended because it is unlikely to reduce the risk of NSAID-induced bleeding or ulceration. However, in children about to start long-term NSAID treatment who are *H. pylori* positive and have dyspepsia or a history of gastric or duodenal ulcer, eradication of *H. pylori* may reduce the overall risk of ulceration.

If the *NSAID can be discontinued* in a child who has developed an ulcer, a proton pump inhibitor usually produces the most rapid healing, alternatively the ulcer can be treated with an H_2-receptor antagonist.

If *NSAID treatment needs to continue*, the ulcer is treated with a proton pump inhibitor (section 1.3.5).

1.3.1 H_2-receptor antagonists

H_2-receptor antagonists heal *gastric and duodenal ulcers* by reducing gastric acid output as a result of histamine H_2-receptor blockade; they can also be expected to relieve *dyspepsia* and *gastro-oesophageal reflux disease* (section 1.1). High doses of H_2-receptor antagonists have been used in *Zollinger–Ellison syndrome*, but a proton pump inhibitor may be preferred.

Maintenance treatment with low doses has largely been replaced in *Helicobacter pylori* positive children by eradication regimens (section 1.3).

H_2-receptor antagonist therapy can promote healing of *NSAID-associated ulcers* (section 1.3).

Treatment has not been shown to be beneficial in haematemesis and melaena, but prophylactic use reduces the frequency of bleeding from *gastroduodenal erosions in hepatic coma*, and possibly in other conditions requiring intensive care. Treatment also reduces the risk of *acid aspiration* in obstetric patients at delivery (Mendelson's syndrome).

H_2-receptor antagonists are also used to reduce the degradation of pancreatic enzyme supplements (section 1.9.4) in children with cystic fibrosis.

Side-effects Side-effects of the H_2-receptor antagonists include diarrhoea and other gastro-intestinal disturbances, altered liver function tests (rarely liver damage), headache, dizziness, rash, and tiredness. Rare side-effects include acute pancreatitis, bradycardia, AV block, confusion, depression, and hallucinations particularly in the very ill, hypersensitivity reactions (including fever, arthralgia, myalgia, anaphylaxis), blood disorders (including agranulocytosis, leucopenia, pancytopenia, thrombocytopenia), and skin reactions (including erythema multiforme and toxic epidermal necrolysis). There have been occasional reports of gynaecomastia and impotence.

Interactions Cimetidine retards oxidative hepatic drug metabolism by binding to microsomal cytochrome P450. It should be avoided in patients stabilised on warfarin, phenytoin, and theophylline (or aminophylline), but other interactions (see **Appendix** 1, Histamine H_2-antagonists) may be of less clinical relevance. Ranitidine does not share the drug metabolism inhibitory properties of cimetidine.

CIMETIDINE

Cautions preferably avoid intravenous injection (use intravenous infusion) particularly in high dosage and in cardiovascular impairment (risk of arrhythmias); **interactions:** Appendix 1 (histamine H_2-antagonists) and notes above

Hepatic impairment increased risk of confusion—reduce dose

Renal impairment use 75% of normal dose if creatinine clearance 15–30 mL/minute/1.73m^2; use 50% of normal dose if creatinine clearance less than 15 mL/minute/1.73m^2

Pregnancy manufacturer advises avoid unless essential

Breast-feeding significant amount present in milk—not known to be harmful but manufacturer advises avoid

Side-effects see notes above; also alopecia; *very rarely* tachycardia, interstitial nephritis

Licensed use not licensed for use in children under 1 year

Indication and dose

Reflux oesophagitis, benign gastric and duodenal ulceration, Zollinger-Ellison syndrome, other conditions where gastric acid reduction is beneficial see notes above and section 1.9.4

- **By mouth**

Neonate 5 mg/kg 4 times daily (half dose may be adequate for prophylaxis)

Child 1 month–12 years 5–10 mg/kg (max. 400 mg) 4 times daily

Child 12–18 years 400 mg 2–4 times daily

- **By slow intravenous injection or infusion**

Neonate 5 mg/kg every 6 hours

Child 1 month–12 years 5–10 mg/kg (max. 400 mg) every 6 hours

Child 12–18 years 200–400 mg every 6 hours

Administration For *intravenous injection*, dilute to a concentration not exceeding 10 mg/mL with

Sodium Chloride 0.9%, give over at least 10 minutes; for *intermittent intravenous infusion* dilute with Glucose 5% *or* Sodium Chloride 0.9%

[1]**Cimetidine** (Non-proprietary) PoM

Tablets, cimetidine 200 mg, net price 60-tab pack = £1.98; 400 mg, 60-tab pack = £2.32; 800 mg, 30-tab pack = £2.87

Brands include *Acitak®*, *Peptimax®*

Oral solution, cimetidine 200 mg/5 mL, net price 300 mL = £14.25

1. Cimetidine can be sold to the public for children over 16 years (provided packs do not contain more than 2 weeks' supply) for the short-term symptomatic relief of heartburn, dyspepsia, and hyperacidity (max. single dose 200 mg, max. daily dose 800 mg), and for the prophylactic management of nocturnal heartburn (single night-time dose 100 mg)

Dyspamet® (Goldshield) PoM

Suspension, sugar-free, cimetidine 200 mg/5 mL. Contains sorbitol 2.79 g/5 mL. Net price 600 mL = £24.08

Tagamet® (GlaxoSmithKline) PoM

Injection, cimetidine 100 mg/mL. Net price 2-mL amp = 33p

Tagamet® (Chemidex) PoM

Tablets, all green, f/c, cimetidine 200 mg, net price 120-tab pack = £19.58; 400 mg, 60-tab pack = £22.62; 800 mg, 30-tab pack = £22.62

Syrup, orange, cimetidine 200 mg/5 mL. Net price 600 mL = £28.49

Excipients: include propylene glycol

RANITIDINE

Cautions avoid in porphyria (section 9.8.2); **interactions:** Appendix 1 (histamine H_2-antagonists) and notes above

Renal impairment use half normal dose in severe impairment

Pregnancy manufacturer advises avoid unless essential, but not known to be harmful

Breast-feeding significant amount present in milk, but not known to be harmful

Side-effects see notes above; also *rarely* tachycardia, agitation, visual disturbances, alopecia; *very rarely* interstitial nephritis

Licensed use *oral* preparations licensed for treatment of peptic ulcer in children (age range not specified by manufacturer); *injection* not licensed for use in children (age range not specified by manufacturer)

Indication and dose

Reflux oesophagitis, benign gastric and duodenal ulceration, Zollinger-Ellison syndrome, other conditions where gastric acid reduction is beneficial (see notes above and section 1.9.4)

- **By mouth**

Neonate 2 mg/kg 3 times daily but absorption unreliable; max. 3 mg/kg 3 times daily

Child 1–6 months 1 mg/kg 3 times daily; max. 3 mg/kg 3 times daily

Child 6 months–12 years 2–4 mg/kg (max. 150 mg) twice daily

Child 12–18 years 150 mg twice daily

Note In fat malabsorption syndrome, give 1–2 hours before food to enhance effects of pancreatic enzyme replacement

- **By slow intravenous injection**

Neonate 0.5–1 mg/kg every 6–8 hours

Child 1 month–18 years 1 mg/kg (max. 50 mg) every 6–8 hours (may be given as an intermittent infusion at a rate of 25 mg/hour)

- **By continuous intravenous infusion**

Neonate 30–60 micrograms/kg/hour (max. 3 mg/kg daily)

Child 1 month–18 years 125–250 micrograms/kg/hour

Administration For *slow intravenous injection* dilute to a concentration of 2.5 mg/mL with Glucose 5%, Sodium Chloride 0.9%, *or* Compound Sodium Lactate. Give over at least 3 minutes. For *continuous intravenous infusion*, further dilution is required.

[1]**Ranitidine** (Non-proprietary) PoM

Tablets, ranitidine (as hydrochloride) 150 mg, net price 60-tab pack = £1.86; 300 mg, 30-tab pack = £1.86

Brands include *Ranitic®*, *Rantec®*

Effervescent tablets, ranitidine (as hydrochloride) 150 mg, net price 60-tab pack = £20.20; 300 mg, 30-tab pack = £20.14. Label: 13

Excipients: may include sodium (check with supplier)

Oral solution, ranitidine (as hydrochloride) 75 mg/5 mL, net price 300 mL = £22.32

1. Ranitidine can be sold to the public for children over 16 years (provided packs do not contain more than 2 weeks' supply) for the short-term symptomatic relief of heartburn, dyspepsia, and hyperacidity, and for the prevention of these symptoms when associated with consumption of food or drink (max. single dose 75 mg, max. daily dose 300 mg)

Zantac® (GSK) PoM

Tablets, f/c, ranitidine (as hydrochloride) 150 mg, net price 60-tab pack = £1.30; 300 mg, 30-tab pack = £1.30

Effervescent tablets, pale yellow, ranitidine (as hydrochloride) 150 mg (contains 14.3 mmol Na^+/tablet), net price 60-tab pack = £25.94; 300 mg (contains 20.8 mmol Na^+/tablet), 30-tab pack = £25.51. Label: 13

Excipients: include aspartame (section 9.4.1)

Syrup, sugar-free, ranitidine (as hydrochloride) 75 mg/5 mL. Net price 300 mL = £20.76

Excipients: include alcohol 8%

Injection, ranitidine (as hydrochloride) 25 mg/mL. Net price 2-mL amp = 60p

1.3.2 Selective antimuscarinics

Classification not used in BNF for Children

1.3.3 Chelates and complexes

Sucralfate is a complex of aluminium hydroxide and sulphated sucrose that appears to act by protecting the mucosa from acid-pepsin attack; it has minimal antacid properties. Sucralfate is not licensed for use in children but is used to prevent stress ulceration in children receiving intensive care. It should be used with caution in this situation (**important**: reports of bezoar formation, see CSM advice below)

SUCRALFATE

Cautions administration of sucralfate and enteral feeds should be separated by 1 hour; **interactions:** Appendix 1 (sucralfate)

Renal impairment manufacturer advises caution in severe renal impairment—aluminium is absorbed and may accumulate

Breast-feeding amount probably too small to be harmful

Bezoar formation Following reports of bezoar formation associated with sucralfate, the **CSM** has advised caution in seriously ill patients, especially those receiving concomitant enteral feeds or those with predisposing conditions such as delayed gastric emptying

Side-effects constipation, diarrhoea, nausea, indigestion, gastric discomfort, dry mouth, rash, hypersensitivity reactions, back pain, dizziness, headache, vertigo and drowsiness, bezoar formation (see above)

Licensed use not licensed for use in children under 15 years

Indication and dose

Duodenal and gastric ulcer, prophylaxis of stress ulceration in child under intensive care

- **By mouth**

  Child 1 month–2 years 250 mg 4–6 times daily

  Child 2–12 years 500 mg 4–6 times daily

  Child 12–18 years 1 g 4–6 times daily

Administration for administration *by mouth*, sucralfate should be given 1 hour before meals, see also Cautions, above; *oral suspension* blocks fine-bore feeding tubes; crushed *tablets* may be dispersed in water.

Antepsin® (Chugai) PoM

Tablets, scored, sucralfate 1 g, net price 50-tab pack = £4.37. Label: 5

Counselling tablets may be dispersed in water

Suspension, sucralfate, 1 g/5 mL, net price 250 mL (aniseed- and caramel-flavoured) = £4.37. Label: 5

1.3.4 Prostaglandin analogues

Classification not used in BNF for Children

1.3.5 Proton pump inhibitors

The proton pump inhibitors **omeprazole** and **lansoprazole** inhibit gastric acid by blocking the hydrogen-potassium adenosine triphosphatase enzyme system (the 'proton pump') of the gastric parietal cell. Omeprazole is currently only licensed in children for the treatment of *gastro-oesophageal reflux disease* with severe symptoms. Lansoprazole is not licensed for use in children, but may be considered when treatment with the available formulations of omeprazole is unsuitable. Proton pump inhibitors are effective short-term treatments for *gastric and duodenal ulcers*; they are also used in combination with antibacterials for the eradication of *Helicobacter pylori* (see p. 59 for specific regimens). An initial short course of a proton pump inhibitor is the treatment of choice in *gastro-oesophageal reflux disease* with severe symptoms; children with endoscopically confirmed *erosive*, *ulcerative*, or *stricturing oesophagitis* usually need to be maintained on a proton pump inhibitor (section 1.1).

Proton pump inhibitors are also used in the prevention and treatment of NSAID-associated ulcers (see p. 59 and guidance issued by NICE, below). In children who need to continue NSAID treatment after an ulcer has healed, the dose of proton pump inhibitor should normally not be reduced because asymptomatic ulcer deterioration may occur.

Proton pump inhibitors are effective in the treatment of the *Zollinger-Ellison syndrome* (including cases resistant to other treatment). They are also used to reduce the degradation of pancreatic enzyme supplements (section 1.9.4) in children with cystic fibrosis.

Side-effects Side-effects of the proton pump inhibitors include gastro-intestinal disturbances (including nausea, vomiting, abdominal pain, flatulence, diarrhoea, constipation), headache, and dizziness. Less frequent side-effects include dry mouth, insomnia, drowsiness, malaise, blurred vision, rash, and pruritus. Other side-effects reported rarely or very rarely include taste disturbance, liver dysfunction, peripheral oedema, hypersensitivity reactions (including urticaria, angioedema, bronchospasm, anaphylaxis), photosensitivity, fever, sweating, depression, interstitial nephritis, blood disorders (including leucopenia, leucocytosis, pancytopenia, thrombocytopenia), arthralgia, myalgia and skin reactions (including Stevens-Johnson syndrome, toxic epidermal necrolysis, bullous eruption). Proton pump inhibitors, by decreasing gastric acidity, may increase the risk of gastro-intestinal infections.

NICE advice (proton pump inhibitors)
NICE has provided guidance (July 2000) on the use of proton pump inhibitors for the following indications:

- Gastro-oesophageal reflux disease—use only for severe symptoms (reduce dose when symptoms abate) and in disease complicated by stricture, ulceration, or haemorrhage (full dose should be maintained);
- NSAID-associated ulceration in patients who need to continue NSAID treatment—on healing of the ulcer a lower dose of proton pump inhibitor may be used [but see notes above].

LANSOPRAZOLE

Cautions interactions: Appendix 1 (proton pump inhibitors)

Hepatic impairment may accumulate in severe impairment

Pregnancy manufacturer advises avoid

Breast-feeding present in milk in *animal* studies—manufacturer advises avoid

Side-effects see notes above; also reported, alopecia, paraesthesia, bruising, purpura, petechiae, fatigue, vertigo, hallucinations, confusion; *rarely* gynaecomastia, impotence

Licensed use not licensed for use in children

Indication and dose

Gastro-oesophageal reflux disease, acid-related dyspepsia, treatment of duodenal and benign gastric ulcer including those complicating NSAID therapy

- By mouth

Child body-weight under 30 kg 0.5–1 mg/kg (max. 15 mg) once daily in the morning

Child body-weight over 30 kg 15–30 mg once daily in the morning

Administration for administration through an *enteral feeding tube, Zoton FasTab®* should be divided if necessary before mixing with water; *Zoton® Suspension* is not suitable for administration through feeding tubes.

Zoton® (Wyeth) PoM

FasTab® (= orodispersible tablet), lansoprazole 15 mg, net price 28-tab pack = £10.86; 30 mg, 7-tab pack = £4.98, 14-tab pack = £9.94, 28-tab pack = £19.88. Label: 5, counselling, administration

Excipients: include aspartame (section 9.4.1)

Counselling Tablets should be placed on the tongue, allowed to disperse and swallowed, or may be swallowed whole with a glass of water; tablets should not be crushed or chewed.

Suspension, pink, powder for reconstitution, lansoprazole 30 mg/sachet (strawberry flavour), net price 28-sachet pack = £33.97. Label: 5, 13

OMEPRAZOLE

Cautions interactions: Appendix 1 (proton pump inhibitors)

Hepatic impairment no more than 700 micrograms/kg (max. 20 mg) once daily

Pregnancy not known to be harmful

Breast-feeding present in milk but not known to be harmful

Side-effects see notes above; also reported, paraesthesia, vertigo, alopecia, gynaecomastia, *rarely* impotence, stomatitis, encephalopathy in severe liver disease; hyponatraemia; reversible confusion, agitation, and hallucinations in the severely ill; visual impairment reported with high-dose injection

Licensed use *capsules* and *tablets*, not licensed for use in children except for severe ulcerating reflux oesophagitis; not licensed for use in children under 1 year; *preparations for injection*, not licensed for use in children under 12 years

Indication and dose

Gastro-oesophageal reflux disease, acid-related dyspepsia, treatment of duodenal and benign gastric ulcers including those complicating NSAID therapy, prophylaxis of acid aspiration, Zollinger-Ellison syndrome

- By mouth

Neonate 700 micrograms/kg once daily, increased if necessary after 7–14 days to 1.4 mg/kg; some neonates may require up to 2.8 mg/kg once daily

Child 1 month–2 years 700 micrograms/kg once daily, increased if necessary to 3 mg/kg (max. 20 mg) once daily

Child body-weight 10–20 kg 10 mg once daily increased if necessary to 20 mg once daily (in severe ulcerating reflux oesophagitis, max. 12 weeks at higher dose)

OMEPRAZOLE (*continued*)

Child body-weight over 20 kg 20 mg once daily increased if necessary to 40 mg once daily (in severe ulcerating reflux oesophagitis, max. 12 weeks at higher dose)

- **By intravenous injection over 5 minutes *or* by intravenous infusion**

  Child 1 month–12 years initially 500 micrograms/kg (max. 20 mg) once daily, increased to 2 mg/kg (max. 40 mg) once daily if necessary

  Child 12–18 years 40 mg once daily

Helicobacter pylori eradication (in combination with antibacterials see p. 59)

- **By mouth**

  Child 1–12 years 1–2 mg/kg (max. 40 mg) once daily

  Child 12–18 years 40 mg once daily

Administration for administration *by mouth*, swallow whole, *or* disperse *Losec MUPS®* tablets in water, *or* mix capsule contents or *Losec MUPS®* tablets with fruit juice or yoghurt.

For administration through an *enteral feeding tube*, use *Losec MUPS®* or the contents of a capsule containing omeprazole dispersed in a large volume of water, or in 10 mL Sodium Bicarbonate 8.4% (1 mmol Na^+/mL) (allow to stand for 10 minutes before administration).

For *intermittent intravenous infusion*, dilute reconstituted solution to a concentration of 400 micrograms/mL with Glucose 5% *or* Sodium Chloride 0.9%; give over 20–30 minutes

Omeprazole (Non-proprietary) PoM

Capsules, enclosing e/c granules, omeprazole 10 mg, net price 28-cap pack = £5.81; 20 mg, 28-cap pack = £9.67; 40 mg, 7-cap pack = £5.77. Label: 5, counselling, administration

Tablets, e/c, omeprazole 10 mg, net price 28-tab pack = £8.60; 20 mg, 28-tab pack = £19.42; 40 mg, 7-tab pack = £9.77. Label: 25

Losec® (AstraZeneca) PoM

MUPS® (multiple-unit pellet system = dispersible tablets), f/c, omeprazole 10 mg (light pink), net price 28-tab pack = £19.34; 20 mg (pink), 28-tab pack = £29.22; 40 mg (red-brown), 7-tab pack = £14.61. Counselling, administration

Capsules, enclosing e/c granules, omeprazole 10 mg (pink), net price 28-cap pack = £19.34; 20 mg (pink/brown), 28-cap pack = £29.22; 40 mg (brown), 7-cap pack = £14.61. Counselling, administration

Intravenous infusion, powder for reconstitution, omeprazole (as sodium salt), net price 40-mg vial = £5.21

Injection, powder for reconstitution, omeprazole (as sodium salt), net price 40-mg vial (with solvent) = £5.21

1.3.6 Other ulcer-healing drugs

Classification not used in BNF for Children

1.4 Acute diarrhoea

The priority in acute diarrhoea, as in gastro-enteritis, is the prevention or reversal of fluid and electrolyte depletion—this is particularly important in infants. For details of **oral rehydration preparations**, see section 9.2.1.2. Severe dehydration requires immediate admission to hospital and urgent replacement of fluid and electrolytes.

Antimotility drugs (section 1.4.2) relieve symptoms of diarrhoea. They are used in the management of uncomplicated acute diarrhoea in adults, but are **not** recommended for use in children under 12 years. Fluid and electrolyte replacement (section 9.2.1.2) are of prime importance in the treatment of acute diarrhoea.

Antispasmodics (section 1.2) are occasionally of value in treating abdominal cramp associated with diarrhoea but they should **not** be used for primary treatment. Antispasmodics and antiemetics should be **avoided** in young children with gastro-enteritis since they are rarely effective and have troublesome side-effects.

Antibacterial drugs are generally unnecessary in simple gastro-enteritis because the complaint usually resolves quickly without such treatment, and infective diarrhoeas in the UK often have a viral cause. Systemic bacterial infection does, however, need appropriate systemic treatment; for drugs used in campylobacter enteritis, shigellosis, and salmonellosis, see p. 283

Colestyramine (cholestyramine, section 1.9.2) binds unabsorbed bile salts and provides symptomatic relief of diarrhoea following ileal disease or resection.

1.4.1 Adsorbents and bulk-forming drugs

Adsorbents such as kaolin are **not** recommended for *acute diarrhoeas*. Bulk-forming drugs, such as ispaghula, methylcellulose, and sterculia (section 1.6.1) are rarely effective in controlling faecal consistency in ileostomy and colostomy.

1.4.2 Antimotility drugs

Antimotility drugs have a role in the management of uncomplicated *acute diarrhoea* in adults but not in children under 12 years; see also section 1.4. However, in the case of dehydration, fluid and electrolyte replacement (section 9.2.1.2) are of primary importance.

For comments on their role in *chronic diarrhoeas* see section 1.5.

CODEINE PHOSPHATE

Cautions see section 4.7.2; tolerance and dependence may occur with prolonged use; **interactions**: Appendix 1 (opioid analgesics)

Contra-indications see section 4.7.2; also conditions where inhibition of peristalsis should be avoided, where abdominal distension develops, or in acute diarrhoeal conditions such as acute ulcerative colitis or antibiotic-associated colitis

Side-effects see section 4.7.2

Indication and dose

Diarrhoea (but see notes above)
- By mouth
  Child 12–18 years 30 mg (range 15–60 mg) 3–4 times daily

Pain section 4.7.2

Codeine Phosphate (Non-proprietary) PoM

Tablets, codeine phosphate 15 mg, net price 28 = £1.46; 30 mg, 28 = £1.67; 60 mg, 28 = £2.61. Label: 2

Note Travellers needing to take codeine phosphate tablets abroad may require a doctor's letter explaining why they are necessary.

CO-PHENOTROPE

A mixture of diphenoxylate hydrochloride and atropine sulphate in the mass proportions 100 parts to 1 part respectively

Cautions see under Codeine Phosphate; also young children are particularly susceptible to **overdosage** and symptoms may be delayed and observation is needed for at least 48 hours after ingestion; presence of subclinical doses of atropine may give rise to atropine side-effects in susceptible individuals or in overdosage; **interactions**: Appendix 1 (opioid analgesics)

Pregnancy may depress neonatal respiration; withdrawal effects in neonates of dependent mothers; gastric stasis and risk of inhalation pneumonia in mother during labour

Breast-feeding may be present in milk

Contra-indications see under Codeine Phosphate; jaundice

Side-effects see under Codeine Phosphate, section 4.7.2

Licensed use not licensed for use in children under 4 years

Indication and dose

Chronic mild ulcerative colitis, control of faecal consistency after colostomy or ileostomy, adjunct to rehydration in acute diarrhoea (but see notes above)
- By mouth
  Child 2–4 years half tablet 3 times daily
  Child 4–9 years 1 tablet 3 times daily
  Child 9–12 years 1 tablet 4 times daily
  Child 12–16 years 2 tablets 3 times daily
  Child 16–18 years initially 4 tablets then 2 tablets 4 times daily

Administration for administration *by mouth* tablets may be crushed

[1]**Lomotil®** (Goldshield) PoM

Tablets, co-phenotrope 2.5/0.025 (diphenoxylate hydrochloride 2.5 mg, atropine sulphate 25 micrograms), net price 20 = £1.63

1. Co-phenotrope 2.5/0.025 can be sold to the public for children over 16 years (provided packs do not contain more than 20 tablets) as an adjunct to rehydration in acute diarrhoea (max. daily dose 10 tablets)

LOPERAMIDE HYDROCHLORIDE

Cautions see notes above; **interactions**: Appendix 1 (loperamide)

Hepatic impairment risk of accumulation—manufacturer advises avoid

Pregnancy manufacturer advises avoid—no information available

Breast-feeding amount probably too small to be harmful

Contra-indications conditions where inhibition of peristalsis should be avoided, where abdominal distension develops, or in conditions such as active ulcerative colitis or antibiotic-associated colitis

Side-effects abdominal cramps, dizziness, drowsiness, and skin reactions including urticaria;

LOPERAMIDE HYDROCHLORIDE (*continued*)

paralytic ileus and abdominal bloating also reported

Licensed use *capsules* not licensed for use in children under 8 years; *syrup* not licensed for use in children under 4 years; not licensed for use in children for chronic diarrhoea

Indication and dose

Chronic diarrhoea
- **By mouth**

Child 1 month–1 year 100–200 micrograms/kg twice daily, 30 minutes before feeds; up to 2 mg/kg daily in divided doses occasionally required

Child 1–12 years 100–200 micrograms/kg (max. 2mg) 3–4 times daily; up to 1.25 mg/kg daily in divided doses may be required (max. 16 mg daily)

Child 12–18 years 2–4 mg 2–4 times daily (max. 16 mg daily)

Acute diarrhoea (but see notes above)
- **By mouth**

Child 4–8 years 1 mg 3–4 times daily for *up to 3 days only*

Child 8–12 years 2 mg 4 times daily for up to 5 days

Child 12–18 years initially 4 mg, then 2 mg after each loose stool for up to 5 days (usual dose 6–8 mg daily; max. 16 mg daily)

[1]**Loperamide** (Non-proprietary) PoM

Capsules, loperamide hydrochloride 2 mg, net price 30-cap pack = £1.09

Tablets, loperamide hydrochloride 2 mg, net price 30-tab pack = £2.15

Brands include *Norimode*®

1. Loperamide can be sold to the public, for use in children over 12 years, provided it is licensed and labelled for the treatment of acute diarrhoea

[1]**Imodium**® (Janssen-Cilag) PoM

Capsules, green/grey, loperamide hydrochloride 2 mg. Net price 30-cap pack = £1.16

Syrup, red, sugar-free, loperamide hydrochloride 1 mg/5 mL. Net price 100 mL = £1.00

1. Loperamide can be sold to the public, for use in children over 12 years, provided it is licensed and labelled for the treatment of acute diarrhoea

Compound preparations

Imodium® Plus (J&J MSD)

Tablets (chewable), scored, loperamide hydrochloride 2 mg, simeticone 125 mg, net price 6-tab pack = £1.97, 12-tab pack = £3.40, 18-tab pack = £4.54. Label: 24

Caplets (= tablets), loperamide hydrochloride 2 mg, simeticone 125 mg, net price 6-tab pack = £2.14, 12-tab pack = £3.40

Dose

Acute diarrhoea with abdominal colic

Child 12–18 years initially 1 tablet or caplet then 1 tablet or caplet after each loose stool; max. 4 tablets or caplets daily for up to 2 days

1.5 Chronic bowel disorders

Individual symptoms of chronic bowel disorders need specific treatment including dietary manipulation as well as drug treatment and the maintenance of a liberal fluid intake.

Inflammatory bowel disease

Chronic inflammatory bowel diseases include *ulcerative colitis* and *Crohn's disease.* The treatment of inflammatory bowel disease in children should be initiated and supervised by a paediatric gastroenterologist. Effective management requires drug therapy, attention to nutrition, and in severe or chronic active disease, surgery.

Aminosalicylates (balsalazide, mesalazine, olsalazine, and sulfasalazine), and **corticosteroids** (hydrocortisone, budesonide, and prednisolone) form the basis of drug treatment.

Treatment of acute ulcerative colitis and Crohn's disease Acute mild to moderate disease affecting the rectum (proctitis) or the recto-sigmoid (distal colitis) is treated initially with local application of a corticosteroid or an aminosalicylate; foam preparations and suppositories are useful for children who have difficulty retaining liquid enemas.

Diffuse inflammatory bowel disease or disease that does not respond to local therapy requires oral treatment; mild disease affecting the colon may be treated with an aminosalicylate alone but refractory or moderate disease usually requires adjunctive use of an oral corticosteroid (section 6.3.2) such as **prednisolone** for 4–8 weeks. Modified-release **budesonide** is rarely used for children with Crohn's disease affecting the ileum and the ascending colon; it causes fewer systemic side-effects than oral prednisolone but may be less effective.

Active Crohn's disease affecting the small intestine may be treated with **enteral nutrition** (Appendix 2) for 6–8 weeks. Alternatively, an oral corticosteroid may be used but at the expense of side-effects; the dose of the corticosteroid is reduced gradually over 8–10 weeks.

Severe inflammatory bowel disease calls for hospital admission and treatment with an intravenous corticosteroid (section 6.3); other therapy may include intravenous fluid and electrolyte replacement, blood transfusion, and possibly parenteral nutrition and antibiotics. Children with ulcerative colitis that fails to respond adequately to these measures may benefit from a short course of ciclosporin. Children with unresponsive or chronically active Crohn's disease may benefit from azathioprine, mercaptopurine, or once-weekly methotrexate.

Infliximab is used in specialist centres for children with severe active Crohn's disease whose condition has not responded adequately to treatment with a corticosteroid and a conventional immunosuppressant or who are intolerant of them. Infliximab is also used for the management of refractory fistulating Crohn's disease. The benefits of treatment with infliximab appear to be short-lived (6–8 weeks).

Crohn's disease of the mouth or of the perineum is more common in children than in adults and it is difficult to treat; elimination diets and the use of a topical corticosteroid (section 13.4) may be beneficial, but a systemic corticosteroid (section 6.3.2) and occasionally azathioprine may be required in severe cases.

> NICE guidance (infliximab for Crohn's disease)
> NICE has recommended (April 2002) that infliximab is used only for the treatment of severe active Crohn's disease (with or without fistulae) when treatment with immunomodulating drugs and corticosteroids has failed or is not tolerated and when surgery is inappropriate. Treatment may be repeated if the condition responded to the initial course but relapsed subsequently. Infliximab should be prescribed only by a gastroenterologist.

Metronidazole may be beneficial for the treatment of active Crohn's disease with colonic and perianal involvement, possibly through its antibacterial activity. Metronidazole is usually given for a month but no longer than 3 months because of concerns about developing peripheral neuropathy. **Ciprofloxacin** may be used as an alternative to metronidazole or the two may be used together but the combination is less well tolerated. Other antibacterials should be given if specifically indicated (e.g. sepsis associated with fistulas and perianal disease) and for managing bacterial overgrowth in the small bowel.

Maintenance of remission of acute ulcerative colitis and Crohn's disease

Aminosalicylates are of great value in the maintenance of remission of ulcerative colitis. They are of less value in the maintenance of remission of Crohn's disease; an oral formulation of mesalazine is available for the long-term management of ileal disease. Corticosteroids are **not** suitable for maintenance treatment because of side-effects. In resistant or frequently relapsing cases either **azathioprine** or **mercaptopurine** may be helpful. Once-weekly methotrexate (section 10.1.3) is tried in Crohn's disease if azathioprine or mercaptopurine cannot be used. **Infliximab** p. 74 may be used for maintenance therapy in Crohn's disease.

Adjunctive treatment of inflammatory bowel disease Due attention should be paid to diet; high-fibre or low-residue diets should be used as appropriate.

Antimotility drugs such as codeine phosphate and loperamide, and antispasmodic drugs may precipitate paralytic ileus and megacolon in active ulcerative colitis; treatment of the inflammation is more logical. Laxatives may be required in proctitis. Diarrhoea resulting from the loss of bile-salt absorption (e.g. in terminal ileal disease or bowel resection) may improve with **colestyramine** (section 1.9.2), which binds bile salts.

Irritable bowel syndrome

Irritable bowel syndrome can present with pain, constipation, or diarrhoea. In some children there may be important psychological aggravating factors which respond to reassurance. A laxative (section 1.6) may be needed to relieve constipation. Antimotility drugs such as loperamide (section 1.4.2) may relieve diarrhoea and antispasmodic drugs (section 1.2) may relieve pain. Opioids with a central action such as codeine are better avoided because of the risk of dependence.

Antibiotic-associated colitis

Antibiotic-associated colitis (pseudomembranous colitis) is caused by colonisation of the colon with *Clostridium difficile* which may follow antibacterial therapy. It is usually of acute onset, but may run a chronic course; it is a particular hazard of clindamycin but few antibacterials are free of this side-effect. Oral **vancomycin** (section 5.1.7) or **metronidazole** (section 5.1.11) are used as specific treatment; vancomycin may be preferred for very sick patients.

Malabsorption syndromes

Individual conditions need specific management and also general nutritional consideration. Coeliac disease (gluten enteropathy) usually needs a gluten-free diet (Appendix 2) and pancreatic insufficiency needs pancreatin supplements (section 1.9.4).

For further information on specialised feeds (ACBS), see Appendix 2.

Aminosalicylates

Sulfasalazine is a combination of 5-aminosalicylic acid ('5-ASA') and sulfapyridine; sulfapyridine acts only as a carrier to the colonic site of action but still causes side-effects. In the newer aminosalicylates, **mesalazine** (5-aminosalicylic acid), **balsalazide** (a prodrug of 5-aminosalicylic acid) and **olsalazine** (a dimer of 5-aminosalicylic acid which cleaves in the lower bowel), the sulphonamide-related side-effects of sulfasalazine are avoided, but 5-aminosalicylic acid alone can still cause side-effects including blood disorders (see recommendation below) and lupoid phenomenon also seen with sulfasalazine.

Cautions Blood disorders can occur with aminosalicylates (see recommendation below).

Blood disorders

Children receiving aminosalicylates and their carers should be advised to report any unexplained bleeding, bruising, purpura, sore throat, fever or malaise that occurs during treatment. A blood count should be performed and the drug stopped immediately if there is suspicion of a blood dyscrasia.

Contra-indications Aminosalicylates should be avoided in salicylate hypersensitivity.

Side-effects Side-effects of the aminosalicylates include diarrhoea, nausea, vomiting, abdominal pain, exacerbation of symptoms of colitis, headache, hypersensitivity reactions (including rash and urticaria); side-effects that occur rarely include acute pancreatitis, hepatitis, myocarditis, pericarditis, lung disorders (including eosinophilia and fibrosing alveolitis), peripheral neuropathy, blood disorders (including agranulocytosis, aplastic anaemia, leucopenia, methaemoglobinaemia, neutropenia, and thrombocytopenia—see also recommendation above), renal dysfunction (interstitial nephritis, nephrotic syndrome), myalgia, arthralgia, skin reactions (including lupus erythematosus-like syndrome, Stevens-Johnson syndrome), alopecia.

BALSALAZIDE SODIUM

Cautions see notes above; also history of asthma; test renal function initially and periodically thereafter (risk of serious renal toxicity); **interactions:** Appendix 1 (aminosalicylates)

Blood disorders see recommendation above

Renal impairment manufacturer advises avoid in moderate to severe impairment

Pregnancy manufacturer advises avoid

Breast-feeding manufacturer advises avoid

Contra-indications see notes above

Hepatic impairment avoid in severe impairment

Side-effects see notes above; also cholelithiasis

Licensed use not licensed for use in children under 18 years

Indication and dose

Treatment of mild to moderate ulcerative colitis and maintenance of remission

- By mouth

Child 12–18 years acute attack, 2.25 g 3 times daily until remission occurs or for up to max. 12 weeks; maintenance, 1.5 g twice daily, adjusted according to response (max. 3 g twice daily)

BALSALAZIDE SODIUM (*continued*)

Colazide® (Shire) PoM
Capsules, beige, balsalazide sodium 750 mg. Net price 130-cap pack = £39.00. Label: 21, 25, counselling, blood disorder symptoms (see recommendation above)

MESALAZINE

Cautions see notes above; with *oral* preparations, test renal function initially and every 3 months for first year then every 6 months for next 4 years and annually thereafter (risk of serious renal toxicity); **interactions:** Appendix 1 (aminosalicylates)

Blood disorders see recommendation above

Renal impairment use with caution in moderate impairment; manufacturers advise avoid in severe impairment

Pregnancy negligible quantity crosses placenta

Breast-feeding diarrhoea reported but manufacturers advise negligible amounts detected in breast milk

Contra-indications see notes above; blood clotting abnormalities

Hepatic impairment avoid in severe impairment

Side-effects see notes above

Licensed use *Asacol®* (all preparations) *Pentasa® enemas, Salofalk® tablets, suppositories, rectal enema,* no dose recommendations for children (age range not specified by manufacturer); *Salofalk® granules* not licensed for use in children under 6 years; *Ipocol®*, *Mesren MR®*, *Pentasa® granules, Salofalk® rectal foam,* not licensed for use in children under 12 years; *Pentasa® SR tablets* and *suppositories* not licensed for use in children under 15 years

Indication and dose

Treatment of mild to moderate ulcerative colitis and maintenance of remission for dose see under preparations below

Note The delivery characteristics of enteric-coated mesalazine preparations may vary; these preparations should not be considered interchangeable

Asacol® (Procter & Gamble Pharm.) PoM
Foam enema, mesalazine 1 g/metered application, net price 14-application cannister with disposable applicators and plastic bags = £37.82. Counselling, blood disorder symptoms (see recommendation above)

Dose

Acute attack affecting the rectosigmoid region
- **By rectum**
  Child 12–18 years 1 metered application (mesalazine 1 g) into the rectum daily for 4–6 weeks

Acute attack affecting the descending colon
- **By rectum**
  Child 12–18 years 2 metered applications (mesalazine 2 g) once daily for 4–6 weeks

Suppositories, mesalazine 250 mg, net price 20-suppos pack = £6.83; 500 mg, 10-suppos pack = £6.83. Counselling, blood disorder symptoms (see recommendation above)

Dose

Treatment and maintenance of remission of ulcerative colitis affecting the rectosigmoid region
- **By rectum**
  Child 12–18 years 1–2 suppositories of 250 mg 3 times daily (max. 1.5 g daily), with last dose at bedtime

Asacol® MR (Procter & Gamble Pharm.) PoM
Tablets, red, e/c, mesalazine 400 mg, net price 90-tab pack = £31.22, 120-tab pack = £41.62. Label: 5, 25, counselling, blood disorder symptoms (see recommendation above)

Dose

Acute attack
- **By mouth**
  Child 12–18 years 2 tablets 3 times daily

Maintenance of remission of ulcerative colitis and Crohn's ileo-colitis
- **By mouth**
  Child 12–18 years 1–2 tablets 2–3 times daily

Note Preparations that lower stool pH (e.g. lactulose) may prevent release of mesalazine

Ipocol® (Sandoz) PoM
Tablets, e/c, mesalazine 400 mg, net price 120-tab pack = £35.20. Label: 5, 25, counselling, blood disorder symptoms (see recommendation above)

Dose

Acute attack
- **By mouth**
  Child 12–18 years 2 tablets 3 times daily

Maintenance of remission
- **By mouth**
  Child 12–18 years 1–2 tablets 3 times daily

Note Preparations that lower stool pH (e.g. lactulose) may prevent release of mesalazine

Mesren MR® (IVAX) PoM
Tablets, red-brown, e/c, mesalazine 400 mg, net price 90-tab pack = £20.29, 120-tab pack = £27.05. Label: 5, 25, counselling, blood disorder symptoms (see recommendation above)

Dose

Acute attack
- **By mouth**
  Child 12–18 years 2 tablets 3 times daily

Maintenance of remission
- **By mouth**
  Child 12–18 years 1–2 tablets 3 times daily

Note Preparations that lower stool pH (e.g. lactulose) may prevent release of mesalazine

MESALAZINE (*continued*)

Pentasa® (Ferring) PoM

Slow release tablets, m/r, scored, mesalazine 500 mg (grey), net price 100-tab pack = £25.48. Counselling, administration (see dose), blood disorder symptoms (see recommendation above)

Dose

Acute attack
- By mouth
  Child 5–15 years 15–20 mg/kg (max. 1 g) 3 times daily
  Child 15–18 years 1–2 g twice daily; total daily dose may alternatively be given in 3 divided doses

Maintenance of remission
- By mouth
  Child 5–15 years 10 mg/kg (max. 500 mg) 2–3 times daily
  Child 15–18 years 500 mg 3 times daily; total daily dose may alternatively be given in 2 divided doses

Administration tablets may be halved, quartered, or dispersed in water, but should not be chewed

Prolonged release granules, m/r, pale brown, mesalazine 1 g/sachet, net price 50-sachet pack = £30.02. Counselling, administration (see dose), blood disorder symptoms (see recommendation above)

Dose

Acute attack
- By mouth
  Child 5–12 years 15–20 mg/kg (max. 1 g) 3 times daily
  Child 12–18 years 1–2 g twice daily; total daily dose may alternatively be given in 3–4 divided doses

Maintenance of remission
- By mouth
  Child 5–12 years 10 mg/kg (max. 500 mg) 2–3 times daily
  Child 12–18 years 500 mg–1 g twice daily

Administration contents of one sachet should be weighed and divided immediately before use; discard any remaining granules. Granules should be placed on tongue and washed down with water or orange juice without chewing

Retention enema, mesalazine 1 g in 100-mL pack. Net price 7 enemas = £18.09. Counselling, blood disorder symptoms (see recommendation above)

Dose

Acute attack affecting the rectosigmoid region
- By rectum
  Child 12–18 years 1 enema at bedtime

Suppositories, mesalazine 1 g. Net price 28-suppos pack = £41.55. Counselling, blood disorder symptoms (see recommendation above)

Dose

Acute attack, ulcerative proctitis
- By rectum
  Child 12–18 years 1 suppository daily for 2–4 weeks

Maintenance, ulcerative proctitis
- By rectum
  Child 12–18 years 1 suppository daily

Salofalk® (Dr Falk) PoM

Tablets, e/c, yellow, mesalazine 250 mg. Net price 100-tab pack = £17.40. Label: 5, 25, counselling, blood disorder symptoms (see recommendation above)

Dose

Acute attack
- By mouth
  Child 12–18 years 2 tablets 3 times daily

Maintenance of remission
- By mouth
  Child 12–18 years 1–2 tablets 2–3 times daily

Granules, m/r, grey, mesalazine 500 mg/sachet, net price 100-sachet pack = £29.30/sachet, 50-sachet pack = £29.30. Counselling, administration (see dose), blood disorder symptoms (see recommendation above)

Excipients: include aspartame (section 9.4.1)

Dose

Acute attack
- By mouth
  Child 6–12 years 10–15 mg/kg (max.1 g) 3 times daily
  Child 12–18 years 0.5 –1 g 3 times daily

Maintenance of remission
- By mouth
  Child 6–12 years 7.5–15 mg/kg (max. 500 mg) twice daily (*or* **child body-weight under 40 kg** 250 mg 3 times daily)
  Child 12–18 years 500 mg 3 times daily

Administration Granules should be placed on tongue and washed down with water without chewing

Note Preparations that lower stool pH (e.g. lactulose) may prevent release of mesalazine

Suppositories, mesalazine 500 mg. Net price 30-suppos pack = £15.90 Counselling, blood disorder symptoms (see recommendation above)

Dose

Acute attack
- By rectum
  Child 12–18 years 1–2 suppositories 2–3 times daily adjusted according to response

Enema, mesalazine 2 g in 59-mL pack. Net price 7 enemas = £31.20 Counselling, blood disorder symptoms (see recommendation above)

Dose

Acute attack *or* maintenance
- By rectum
  Child 12–18 years 1 enema once daily at bedtime

Rectal foam, mesalazine 1 g/metered application, net price 14-application cannister with disposable applicators and plastic bags = £31.10. Counselling, blood disorder symptoms (see recommendation above)

Dose

Mild ulcerative colitis affecting sigmoid colon and rectum
- By rectum
  Child 12–18 years 2 metered applications (mesalazine 2 g) into the rectum at bedtime increased if necessary to 2 metered applications (mesalazine 2 g) twice daily

OLSALAZINE SODIUM

Cautions see notes above; **interactions:** Appendix 1 (aminosalicylates)

Blood disorders see recommendation above

Renal impairment use with caution in moderate impairment; manufacturer advises avoid in severe impairment

Pregnancy manufacturer advises avoid unless potential benefit outweighs risk

Breast-feeding manufacturer advises avoid

Contra-indications see notes above

Side-effects see notes above; also watery diarrhoea

Licensed use not licensed for use in children

Indication and dose

Treatment of acute attack of mild ulcerative colitis
- By mouth

Child 2–18 years 500 mg twice daily after food increased if necessary over 1 week to max. 1 g 3 times daily

Maintenance of remission of mild ulcerative colitis
- By mouth

Child 2–18 years 250–500 mg twice daily after food

Administration Capsules can be opened and contents sprinkled on food

Dipentum® (Celltech) PoM

Capsules, brown, olsalazine sodium 250 mg. Net price 112-cap pack = £20.57. Label: 21, counselling, blood disorder symptoms (see recommendation above)

Tablets, yellow, scored, olsalazine sodium 500 mg. Net price 60-tab pack = £22.04. Label: 21, counselling, blood disorder symptoms (see recommendation above)

SULFASALAZINE
(Sulphasalazine)

Cautions see notes above; also history of allergy; hepatic impairment; G6PD deficiency (section 9.1.5); slow acetylator status; risk of haematological and hepatic toxicity (differential white cell, red cell and platelet counts initially and at monthly intervals for first 3 months, liver function tests at monthly intervals for first 3 months); kidney function tests at regular intervals; upper gastro-intestinal side-effects common with doses over 4 g daily; porphyria (section 9.8.2); **interactions:** Appendix 1 (aminosalicylates)

Blood disorders see recommendation above

Renal impairment in moderate impairment risk of toxicity including crystalluria—ensure high fluid intake; avoid in severe impairment

Pregnancy theoretical risk of neonatal haemolysis in third trimester; adequate folate supplements should be given to mother

Breast-feeding small amount in milk (1 report of bloody diarrhoea and rashes); theoretical risk of neonatal haemolysis especially in G6PD-deficient infants

Contra-indications see notes above; also sulphonamide hypersensitivity; child under 2 years of age

Side-effects see notes above; also loss of appetite; fever; blood disorders (including Heinz body anaemia, megaloblastic anaemia); hypersensitivity reactions (including exfoliative dermatitis, epidermal necrolysis, pruritus, photosensitisation, anaphylaxis, serum sickness); ocular complications (including periorbital oedema); stomatitis, parotitis; ataxia, aseptic meningitis, vertigo, tinnitus, insomnia, depression, hallucinations; kidney reactions (including proteinuria, crystalluria, haematuria); oligospermia; urine may be coloured orange; some soft contact lenses may be stained

Indication and dose

Treatment of acute attack of mild to moderate and severe ulcerative colitis, active Crohn's disease
- By mouth

Child 2–12 years 10–15 mg/kg (max. 1 g) 4–6 times daily until remission occurs; increased to max. 60 mg/kg daily in divided doses, if necessary

Child 12–18 years 1–2 g 4 times daily until remission occurs

Maintenance of remission of mild to moderate and severe ulcerative colitis
- By mouth

Child 2–12 years 5–7.5 mg/kg (max. 500 mg) 4 times daily

Child 12–18 years 0.5–1 g 4 times daily

Treatment of mild to moderate or severe ulcerative colitis and maintenance of remission, active Crohn's disease
- By rectum as suppositories

Child 5–8 years 500 mg twice daily

Child 8–12 years 500 mg in the morning and 1 g at night

Child 12–18 years 1 g twice daily

- By rectum as rectal enema, retained for at least 1 hour

Child 2–7 years 1–1.5 g at night

Child 7–12 years 1.5–2.25 g at night

Child 12–18 years 3 g at night

Juvenile idiopathic arthritis section 10.1.3

SULFASALAZINE (*continued*)

Sulfasalazine (Non-proprietary) PoM

Tablets, sulfasalazine 500 mg. Net price 112 = £10.71. Label: 14, counselling, blood disorder symptoms (see recommendation above), contact lenses may be stained

Tablets, e/c, sulfasalazine 500 mg. Net price 112-tab pack = £8.43. Label: 5, 14, 25, counselling, blood disorder symptoms (see recommendation above), contact lenses may be stained

Brands include *Sulazine EC*®

Salazopyrin® (Pharmacia) PoM

Tablets, yellow, scored, sulfasalazine 500 mg. Net price 112-tab pack = £6.97. Label: 14, counselling, blood disorder symptoms (see recommendation above), contact lenses may be stained

EN-Tabs® (= tablets e/c), yellow, f/c, sulfasalazine 500 mg. Net price 112-tab pack = £8.43. Label: 5, 14, 25, counselling, blood disorder symptoms (see recommendation above), contact lenses may be stained

Suspension, yellow, sulfasalazine 250 mg/5 mL. Net price 500 mL = £18.84. Label: 14, counselling, blood disorder symptoms (see recommendation above), contact lenses may be stained

Suppositories, yellow, sulfasalazine 500 mg. Net price 10 = £3.30. Label: 14, counselling, blood disorder symptoms (see recommendation above), contact lenses may be stained

Retention enema, sulfasalazine 3 g in 100-mL single-dose disposable packs fitted with a nozzle. Net price 7× 100 mL = £11.87. Label: 14, counselling, blood disorder symptoms (see recommendation above), contact lenses may be stained

Corticosteroids

BUDESONIDE

Cautions see section 6.3.2

Hepatic impairment plasma-budesonide concentration may increase

Pregnancy risk of intra-uterine growth restriction on prolonged or repeated treatment (see also CSM advice, section 6.3.2)

Breast-feeding amount too small to be harmful

Contra-indications see section 6.3.2

Side-effects see section 6.3.2

Licensed use *Budenofalk*® not licensed for use in children

Indication and dose

See under preparations, below

Administration Capsules can be opened and the contents mixed with apple or orange juice

Budenofalk® (Dr Falk) PoM

Capsules, pink, enclosing e/c pellets, budesonide 3 mg, net price 100-cap pack = £76.70. Label: 5, 10, steroid card, 22, 25

Dose

Mild to moderate Crohn's disease affecting ileum or ascending colon, chronic diarrhoea due to collagenous colitis
- **By mouth**
  Child 12–18 years 3 mg 3 times daily for up to 8 weeks; reduce dose for the last 2 weeks of treatment. See also section 6.3.2

Entocort® (AstraZeneca) PoM

CR Capsules, grey/pink, enclosing e/c, m/r granules, budesonide 3 mg, net price 100-cap pack = £99.00. Label: 5, 10, steroid card, 22, 25

Note Dispense in original container (contains desiccant)

Dose

Mild to moderate Crohn's disease affecting the ileum or ascending colon
- **By mouth**
  Child 12–18 years 9 mg once daily in the morning before breakfast for up to 8 weeks; reduce dose for the last 2–4 weeks of treatment. See also section 6.3.2

Enema, budesonide 2 mg/100 mL when dispersible tablet reconstituted in isotonic saline vehicle, net price pack of 7 dispersible tablets and bottles of vehicle = £33.00

Dose

Ulcerative colitis involving rectal and recto-sigmoid disease
- **By rectum**
  Child 12–18 years 1 enema at bedtime for 4 weeks

HYDROCORTISONE

Cautions see section 6.3.2; systemic absorption may occur; prolonged use should be avoided

Pregnancy see Budesonide, above

Breast-feeding see Budesonide, above

Contra-indications use of enemas and rectal foams in obstruction, bowel perforation, and extensive fistulas; untreated infection

Side-effects see section 6.3.2; local irritation

Indication and dose

See under preparations, below

Colifoam® (Meda) PoM

Foam in aerosol pack, hydrocortisone acetate 10%, net price 14-application cannister with applicator = £8.21

Dose

Ulcerative colitis, proctitis, proctosigmoiditis
- **By rectum**
  Child 2–18 years initially 1 metered application (125 mg hydrocortisone acetate) inserted into the rectum once or twice daily for 2–3 weeks, then once on alternate days

PREDNISOLONE

Cautions see under Hydrocortisone and section 6.3.2

Contra-indications see under Hydrocortisone and section 6.3.2

Side-effects see under Hydrocortisone and section 6.3.2

Licensed use *Predfoam®, Predsol® retention enema* not licensed for use in children (age range not specified by manufacturer)

Indication and dose

Ulcerative colitis, Crohn's disease see also under preparations, below

- By mouth

  Child 2–18 years 1–2 mg/kg daily (max. 40 mg) in single or divided doses until remission occurs, followed by reducing doses

- By rectum

  See under preparations

Other indications section 6.3.2

Oral preparations

Section 6.3.2

Rectal preparations

Predenema® (Forest) PoM

Retention enema, prednisolone 20 mg (as sodium metasulphobenzoate) in 100-mL single-dose disposable pack. Net price 1 (standard tube) = 71p, 1 (long tube) = £1.21

Dose

Ulcerative colitis

- By rectum

  Child 12–18 years initially 1 enema at bedtime for 2–4 weeks, continued if good response

Predfoam® (Forest) PoM

Foam in aerosol pack, prednisolone 20 mg (as metasulphobenzoate sodium)/metered application, net price 14-application cannister with disposable applicators = £6.32

Dose

Proctitis and distal ulcerative colitis

- By rectum

  Child 12–18 years 1 metered application (20 mg prednisolone) inserted into the rectum once or twice daily for 2 weeks, continued for further 2 weeks if good response

Predsol® (Celltech) PoM

Suppositories, prednisolone 5 mg (as sodium phosphate). Net price 10 = £1.40

Dose

Proctitis and rectal complications of Crohn's disease

- By rectum

  Child 2–18 years 1 suppository inserted night and morning after a bowel movement

Other immunosuppressants

Azathioprine and **mercaptopurine** are used to induce remission in unresponsive or chronically active Crohn's disease, and they may also be helpful for retaining remission in frequently relapsing inflammatory bowel disease. Response to azathioprine may not become apparent for several months.

Ciclosporin (cyclosporin) is a potent immunosuppressant and it is markedly nephrotoxic. In children with severe ulcerative colitis unresponsive to other treatment, ciclosporin may reduce the need for urgent colorectal surgery.

AZATHIOPRINE

Cautions see section 8.2.1; **interactions:** Appendix 1 (azathioprine)

Contra-indications see section 8.2.1

Side-effects see section 8.2.1

Licensed use not licensed for use in ulcerative colitis or Crohn's disease

Indication and dose

Severe ulcerative colitis and Crohn's disease

- By mouth

  Child 2–18 years initially 2 mg/kg (if necessary up to 3 mg/kg) once daily, then reduced according to response to lowest effective dose; total daily dose may alternatively be given in 2 divided doses

Transplantation rejection and auto-immune conditions section 8.2.1

Preparations

Section 8.2.1

CICLOSPORIN

Cautions see section 8.2.2; **interactions:** Appendix 1 (ciclosporin)

Contra-indications see section 8.2.2

Side-effects see section 8.2.2

Licensed use not licensed for use in ulcerative colitis

CICLOSPORIN (*continued*)

Indication and dose

Refractory ulcerative colitis
- By mouth

  Child 2–18 years initially 2 mg/kg twice daily then adjusted according to blood-ciclosporin concentration and response; max. 5 mg/kg twice daily

  Important For advice on counselling and conversion between preparations, see section 8.2.2
- By intravenous infusion

  Child 2–18 years initially 100–200 micrograms/kg daily, then adjusted according to blood-ciclosporin concentration and response

Nephrotic syndrome section 8.2.2

Transplantation rejection and auto-immune conditions section 8.2.2

Atopic dermatitis and psoriasis section 13.5.3

Administration for *intermittent intravenous infusion*, dilute to a concentration of 0.5–2.5 mg/mL with Glucose 5% *or* Sodium Chloride 0.9% and give over 2–6 hours; not to be used with PVC equipment

Preparations
section 8.2.2

MERCAPTOPURINE

Cautions see section 8.1.3; see also Azathioprine, section 8.2.1

Contra-indications see section 8.1.3

Side-effects see section 8.1.3

Licensed use not licensed for use in severe ulcerative colitis and Crohn's disease; for other indications, see section 8.1.3

Indication and dose

Severe ulcerative colitis and Crohn's disease
- By mouth

  Child 2–18 years 1–1.5 mg/kg once daily (initial max. 50 mg; may be increased to 75 mg once daily)

Acute leukaemias section 8.1.3

Preparations
section 8.1.3

1 Gastro-intestinal system

Cytokine inhibitors

Infliximab is a monoclonal antibody which inhibits the pro-inflammatory cytokine, tumour necrosis factor α. It should be administered under specialist supervision where adequate resuscitation facilities are available and is used in the treatment of severe refractory or fistulating Crohn's disease in children. Infliximab should be used only when treatment with other immunomodulating drugs has failed or is not tolerated and for children in whom surgery is inappropriate.

INFLIXIMAB

Cautions hepatic impairment; renal impairment; monitor for infections before, during, and for 6 months after treatment (see also Tuberculosis below); heart failure (discontinue if symptoms develop or worsen; avoid in moderate or severe heart failure); demyelinating CNS disorders (risk of exacerbation); **interactions**: Appendix 1 (infliximab)

Tuberculosis Children should be evaluated for tuberculosis before treatment. Active tuberculosis should be treated with standard treatment (section 5.1.9) for at least 2 months before starting infliximab. Children who have previously received adequate treatment for tuberculosis can start infliximab but should be monitored every 3 months for possible recurrence. In those without active tuberculosis but who were previously not treated adequately, chemo-prophylaxis should ideally be completed before starting infliximab. Children and their carers should be advised to seek medical attention if symptoms suggestive of tuberculosis (e.g. persistent cough, weight loss, and fever) develop

Hypersensitivity reactions Hypersensitivity reactions (including fever, chest pain, hypotension, hypertension, dyspnoea, pruritus, urticaria, serum sickness-like reactions, angioedema, anaphylaxis) reported during or within 1–2 hours after infusion (risk greatest during first or second infusion or in children who discontinue other immunosuppressants). All children should be observed carefully for 1–2 hours after infusion and resuscitation equipment should be available for immediate use. Prophylactic antipyretics, antihistamines, or hydrocortisone may be administered. Readministration not recommended after infliximab-free interval of more than 16 weeks—risk of delayed hypersensitivity reactions. Children and carers should be advised to keep Alert card with them at all times and seek medical advice if symptoms of delayed hypersensitivity develop

Contra-indications severe infections (see also under cautions)

Pregnancy avoid; manufacturer advises adequate contraception during and for at least 6 months after last dose

Breast-feeding avoid; manufacturer advises avoid for at least 6 months after last dose

Side-effects see under Cytokine Inhibitors (section 10.1.3) and Cautions above; also dyspepsia, diarrhoea, constipation, hepatitis, cholecystitis, diverticulitis, gastro-intestinal haemorrhage, flushing, bradycardia, arrhythmias, palpitation, syncope, vasospasm, peripheral ischaemia,

INFLIXIMAB (*continued*)

ecchymosis, haematoma, interstitial pneumonitis or fibrosis, fatigue, anxiety, drowsiness, dizziness, insomnia, confusion, agitation, amnesia, seizures, demyelinating disorders, vaginitis, myalgia, arthralgia, endophthalmitis, rash, sweating, hyperkeratosis, skin pigmentation, alopecia

Licensed use not licensed for use in children

Indication and dose

Severe active Crohn's disease
- **By intravenous infusion**

  Child 2–18 years initially 5 mg/kg, then if the condition responds within 2 weeks of initial dose, either 5 mg/kg 2 weeks and 6 weeks after initial dose, then 5 mg/kg every 8 weeks *or* after initial dose, further dose of 5 mg/kg if signs and symptoms recur

Fistulating Crohn's disease
- **By intravenous infusion**

  Child 2–18 years initially 5 mg/kg, then 5 mg/kg 2 weeks and 6 weeks after initial dose, then if condition has responded, consult literature for guidance on further doses

Administration for *intravenous infusion* reconstitute each 100-mg vial of powder with 10 mL Water for Injections; to dissolve, gently swirl vial without shaking; allow to stand for 5 minutes; dilute required dose with Sodium Chloride 0.9% to a final volume of 250 mL and give through a low protein-binding filter (1.2 micron or less) over at least 2 hours; start infusion within 3 hours of reconstitution

Remicade (Schering-Plough) ▼ PoM

Intravenous infusion, powder for reconstitution, infliximab, net price 100-mg vial = £451.20. Label: 10, alert card, counselling, tuberculosis and hypersensitivity reactions

Food allergy

Allergy with classical symptoms of vomiting, colic and diarrhoea caused by specific foods such as cow's milk should be managed by strict avoidance. The condition should be distinguished from symptoms of occasional food intolerance in children with irritable bowel syndrome. **Sodium cromoglicate** (sodium cromoglycate) may be helpful as an adjunct to dietary avoidance.

SODIUM CROMOGLICATE
(Sodium cromoglycate)

Side-effects occasional nausea, rashes, and joint pain

Indication and dose

Food allergy (in conjunction with dietary restriction)
- **By mouth**

  Child 2–14 years 100 mg 4 times daily before meals, dose may be increased after 2–3 weeks to a max. 40 mg/kg daily and then reduced according to response

  Child 14–18 years 200 mg 4 times daily before meals, dose may be increased after 2–3 weeks to max. 40 mg/kg daily and then reduced according to response

Asthma section 3.3

Allergic conjunctivitis section 11.4.2

Allergic rhinitis section 12.2.1

Administration capsules may be swallowed whole or the contents dissolved in hot water and diluted with cold water before taking

Nalcrom® (Sanofi-Aventis) PoM

Capsules, sodium cromoglicate 100 mg. Net price 100-cap pack = £63.32. Label: 22, counselling, administration

1.6 Laxatives

Before prescribing laxatives it is important to be sure that the child *is* constipated and that the constipation is *not* secondary to an underlying undiagnosed complaint.

The use of laxatives in children should be discouraged unless prescribed by a doctor or other prescribers with special expertise in the management of gastrointestinal disorders in children. Delays of greater than 3 days between stools may increase the likelihood of pain on passing hard stools leading to anal fissure, anal spasm and eventually to a learned response to avoid defaecation.

In infants, increased intake of fluids, particularly fruit juice containing sorbitol (e.g. prune, pear, or apple), may be sufficient to soften the stool. In infants under 1 year with mild constipation, **lactulose** (section 1.6.4) can be used to soften the stool; glycerol suppositories may be used to clear faecal impaction. The infant should be referred to a hospital paediatric specialist if these measures fail.

In children over 1 year with infrequent bowel motion or hard stools, if increased fluid and fibre intake is insufficient, an osmotic laxative containing **macrogols** or **lactulose** (section 1.6.4) can be used. If there is evidence of minor faecal retention, the addition of a **stimulant laxative** (section 1.6.2) may overcome withholding but may lead to colic or, in the presence of faecal impaction in the rectum, an increase of faecal overflow.

Long-term regular use of laxatives is essential to maintain well-formed stools and prevent recurrence of faecal impaction; intermittent use may provoke relapses. For children with chronic constipation, it may be necessary to exceed the licensed doses of some laxatives.

In children with faecal impaction, an oral preparation containing **macrogols** (section 1.6.4) can be used to clear faecal mass and to establish and maintain soft well-formed stools. Rectal administration of laxatives may be effective but the use of this route is frequently distressing for the child and may lead to a persistence of withholding. Referral to hospital may be needed unless the child evacuates the impacted mass spontaneously. Enemas may be administered under heavy sedation in hospital or alternatively a **bowel cleansing solution** (section 1.6.5) may be tried. In severe cases or where the child is afraid, a manual evacuation under anaesthetic may be appropriate.

Pregnancy If dietary and lifestyle changes fail to control constipation in pregnancy, moderate doses of poorly absorbed laxatives may be used. A bulk-forming laxative should be tried first. An osmotic laxative, such as lactulose, can also be used. Bisacodyl or senna may be suitable, if a stimulant effect is necessary.

Laxatives are also of value in *drug-induced constipation* (see Prescribing in Palliative Care, p. 26), in *distal intestinal obstruction syndrome* in children with cystic fibrosis, for the expulsion of *parasites* after anthelmintic treatment, and to clear the alimentary tract before *surgery and radiological procedures* (section 1.6.5).

The laxatives that follow have been divided into 5 main groups (sections 1.6.1–1.6.5). This simple classification disguises the fact that some laxatives have a complex action.

1.6.1 Bulk-forming laxatives

Bulk-forming laxatives are of value if the diet is deficient in fibre. They relieve constipation by increasing faecal mass which stimulates peristalsis; children and their carers should be advised that the full effect may take some days to develop.

During treatment with bulk-forming laxatives, adequate fluid intake must be maintained to avoid intestinal obstruction. Proprietary preparations containing a bulking agent such as ispaghula husk are often difficult to administer to children; unprocessed wheat **bran**, taken with food or fruit juice, is a most effective bulk-forming preparation. Finely ground bran, though more palatable, has poorer water-retaining properties, but can be taken as bran bread or biscuits in appropriately increased quantities. Oat bran is also used.

Bulk-forming laxatives may be used in the management of children with *haemorrhoids, anal fissure,* and *irritable bowel syndrome.*

ISPAGHULA HUSK

Cautions adequate fluid intake should be maintained to avoid intestinal obstruction

Contra-indications difficulty in swallowing, intestinal obstruction, colonic atony, faecal impaction

Side-effects flatulence and abdominal distension (especially during the first few days of treatment), gastro-intestinal obstruction or impaction; hypersensitivity reported

Licensed use not licensed for use in children under 6 years (unless on specialist practitioner advice)

Indication and dose

See under preparations

Counselling Preparations that swell in contact with liquid should always be carefully swallowed with water and should not be taken immediately before going to bed

ISPAGHULA HUSK (*continued*)

Fibrelief® (Manx)
Granules, sugar- and gluten-free, ispaghula husk 3.5 g/sachet (natural or orange flavour), net price 10 sachets = £1.23, 30 sachets = £2.07. Label: 13, counselling, , see above
Excipients: include aspartame (section 9.4.1)

Dose

Constipation
- **By mouth**
  Child 12–18 years 1–6 sachets daily in water in 1–3 divided doses

Fybogel® (R&C)
Granules, buff, effervescent, sugar- and gluten-free, ispaghula husk 3.5 g/sachet (low Na^+), net price 30 sachets (plain, lemon, or orange flavour) = £2.12, 150 g (orange flavour) = £3.44. Label: 13, counselling, see above
Excipients: include aspartame 16 mg/sachet (see section 9.4.1)

Dose

Constipation
- **By mouth**
  Child 2–12 years ½–1 level 5-mL spoonful in water twice daily preferably after meals
  Child 12–18 years 1 sachet *or* 2 level 5-mL spoonfuls in water twice daily preferably after meals

Isogel® (Chefaro UK)
Granules, brown, sugar- and gluten-free, ispaghula husk 90%. Net price 200 g = £2.67. Label: 13, counselling, see above

Dose

Constipation
- **By mouth**
  Child 2–12 years 1 level 5-mL spoonful in water once or twice daily, preferably at mealtimes
  Child 12–18 years 2 level 5-mL spoonfuls in water once or twice daily, preferably at mealtimes

Ispagel Orange® (LPC)
Granules, beige, effervescent, sugar- and gluten-free, ispaghula husk 3.5 g/sachet, net price 30 sachets = £2.10. Label: 13, counselling, see above
Excipients: include aspartame (section 9.4.1)

Dose

Constipation
- **By mouth**
  Child 2–12 years ½–1 level 5-mL spoonful in water twice daily preferably after meals
  Child 12–18 years 1 sachet (or 2 level 5-mL) spoonfuls in water twice daily preferably after meals

Regulan® (Procter & Gamble)
Powder, beige, sugar- and gluten-free, ispaghula husk 3.4 g/5.85-g sachet (orange or lemon/lime flavour). Net price 30 sachets = £2.12. Label: 13, counselling, see above
Excipients: include aspartame (section 9.4.1)

Dose

Constipation
- **By mouth**
  Child 2–12 years ½–1 level 5-mL spoonful in water 1–3 times daily
  Child 12–18 years 1 sachet in 150 mL water 1–3 times daily

METHYLCELLULOSE

Cautions see under Ispaghula Husk

Contra-indications see under Ispaghula Husk; also infective bowel disease

Side-effects see under Ispaghula Husk

Licensed use no age limit specified by manufacturer

Indication and dose

See under preparation below

Counselling Preparations that swell in contact with liquid should always be carefully swallowed with water and should not be taken immediately before going to bed

Celevac® (Shire)
Tablets, pink, scored, methylcellulose '450' 500 mg. Net price 112-tab pack = £2.69. Counselling, see above and dose

Dose

Constipation, diarrhoea (see notes above)
- **By mouth**
  Child 7–12 years 2 tablets twice daily
  Child 12–18 years 3–6 tablets twice daily.

Administration In constipation the dose should be taken with at least 300 mL liquid. In diarrhoea, ileostomy, and colostomy control, minimise liquid intake for 30 minutes before and after dose

Extemporaneous formulations available see Extemporaneous Preparations, p. 8

STERCULIA

Cautions see under Ispaghula Husk

Contra-indications see under Ispaghula Husk

Side-effects see under Ispaghula Husk

Indication and dose

Constipation for dose see under preparation

Counselling Preparations that swell in contact with liquid should always be carefully swallowed with water and should not be taken immediately before going to bed

STERCULIA (continued)

Normacol® (Norgine)
Granules, coated, gluten-free, sterculia 62%. Net price 500 g = £6.18; 60 × 7-g sachets = £5.19. Label: 25, 27, counselling, see above

Dose

- **By mouth**
  Child 6–12 years ½–1 heaped 5-mL spoonful, or the contents of ½–1 sachet, washed down without chewing with plenty of liquid once or twice daily after meals
  Child 12–18 years 1–2 heaped 5-mL spoonfuls, or the contents of 1–2 sachets, washed down without chewing with plenty of liquid once or twice daily after meals

Administration May be mixed with soft food (e.g. yoghurt) before swallowing, followed by plenty of liquid.

Normacol Plus® (Norgine)
Granules, brown, coated, gluten-free, sterculia 62%, frangula (standardised) 8%. Net price 500 g = £6.60; 60 × 7 g sachets = £5.56. Label: 25, 27, counselling, see above

Dose

- **By mouth**
  Child 6–18 years 1–2 heaped 5-mL spoonfuls or the contents of 1–2 sachets washed down without chewing with plenty of liquid once or twice daily after meals

1.6.2 Stimulant laxatives

Stimulant laxatives include **bisacodyl**, **sodium picosulphate** and members of the **anthraquinone** group, **senna** and **dantron** (danthron). The indications for dantron are limited (see below) by its potential carcinogenicity (based on *rodent* carcinogenicity studies) and evidence of genotoxicity. Powerful stimulants such as **cascara** (an anthraquinone) and **castor oil** are obsolete. **Docusate sodium** probably acts both as a stimulant and as a softening agent.

Stimulant laxatives increase intestinal motility and often cause abdominal cramp; they should be avoided in intestinal obstruction. Stools should be softened by increasing dietary fibre and liquid or with an osmotic laxative (section 1.6.4) before giving a stimulant laxative. In chronic constipation, especially where withholding of stool occurs, additional doses of a stimulant laxative may be required. Long-term use of stimulant laxatives is sometimes necessary (see section 1.6), but excessive use can cause diarrhoea and related effects such as hypokalaemia.

Glycerol suppositories act as a lubricant and as a rectal stimulant by virtue of the mildly irritant action of glycerol.

BISACODYL

Cautions prolonged use (risk of electrolyte imbalance)

Contra-indications ileus, intestinal obstruction, acute abdominal conditions, acute inflammatory bowel disease, severe dehydration

Side-effects abdominal cramps; *suppositories* local irritation

Indication and dose

Constipation (tablets act in 10–12 hours; suppositories act in 20–60 minutes)

- **By mouth**
  Child 4–10 years 5 mg at night
  Child 10–18 years 5–10 mg at night; increased if necessary (max. 20 mg)
- **By rectum (suppository)**
  Child 2–10 years 5 mg in the morning
  Child 10–18 years 10 mg in the morning

Bowel clearance before radiological procedures and surgery

- **By mouth and by rectum**
  Child 4–10 years *by mouth*, 5 mg at bedtime for 2 days before procedure and, if necessary, *by rectum*, 5 mg suppository 1 hour before procedure
  Child 10–18 years *by mouth*, 10 mg at bedtime for 2 days before procedure and, if necessary, *by rectum*, 10 mg suppository 1 hour before procedure

Bisacodyl (Non-proprietary)
Tablets, e/c, bisacodyl 5 mg. Net price 20 = 43p. Label: 5, 25

Suppositories, bisacodyl 10 mg. Net price 12 = 77p

Paediatric suppositories, bisacodyl 5 mg. Net price 5 = 94p

Note The brand name *Dulco-lax®* (NHS) (Boehringer Ingelheim) is used for bisacodyl tablets, net price 10-tab pack = 74p; suppositories (10 mg), 10 = £1.57; paediatric suppositories (5 mg), 5 = 94p
The brand names *Dulco-lax® Liquid* and *Dulco-lax Perles®* are used for sodium picosulfate preparations

DANTRON

(Danthron)

Cautions avoid prolonged contact with skin (as in incontinent patients)—risk of irritation and excoriation; *rodent* studies indicate potential carcinogenic risk

Pregnancy manufacturer advises avoid

Breast-feeding *rodent* studies indicate potential carcinogenic risk

Contra-indications see Bisacodyl above

Side-effects urine may be coloured red

Indication and dose

Constipation in terminally ill children for dose see under preparations

With poloxamer '188' (as co-danthramer)

Note Co-danthramer suspension 5 mL = one co-danthramer capsule, **but** strong co-danthramer suspension 5 mL = two strong co-danthramer capsules

Co-danthramer (Non-proprietary) PoM

Capsules, co-danthramer 25/200 (dantron 25 mg, poloxamer '188' 200 mg). Net price 60-cap pack = £12.86. Label: 14, (urine red)

Dose

- **By mouth**

  Child 6–12 years 1 capsule at night (restricted indications, see notes above)

  Child 12–18 years 1–2 capsules at night (restricted indications, see notes above)

Strong capsules, co-danthramer 37.5/500 (dantron 37.5 mg, poloxamer '188' 500 mg). Net price 60-cap pack = £15.55. Label: 14, (urine red)

Dose

- **By mouth**

  Child 12–18 years 1–2 capsules at night (restricted indications, see notes above)

Suspension, co-danthramer 25/200 in 5 mL (dantron 25 mg, poloxamer '188' 200 mg/5 mL). Net price 300 mL = £11.27, 1 litre = £37.57. Label: 14, (urine red)

Brands include *Codalax*® NHS, *Danlax*®

Dose

- **By mouth**

  Child 2–12 years 2.5–5 mL at night (restricted indications, see notes above)

  Child 12–18 years 5–10 mL at night (restricted indications, see notes above)

Strong suspension, co-danthramer 75/1000 in 5 mL (dantron 75 mg, poloxamer '188' 1 g/5 mL). Net price 300 mL = £30.13. Label: 14, (urine red)

Brands include *Codalax Forte*® NHS

Dose

- **By mouth**

  Child 12–18 years 5 mL at night (restricted indications, see notes above)

With docusate sodium (as co-danthrusate)

Co-danthrusate (Non-proprietary) PoM

Capsules, co-danthrusate 50/60 (dantron 50 mg, docusate sodium 60 mg). Net price 63-cap pack = £13.46. Label: 14, (urine red)

Brands include *Capsuvac*®, *Normax*® NHS

Dose

- **By mouth**

  Child 6–12 years 1 capsule at night (restricted indications, see notes above)

  Child 12–18 years 1–3 capsules at night (restricted indications, see notes above)

Suspension, yellow, co-danthrusate 50/60 (dantron 50 mg, docusate sodium 60 mg/5 mL). Net price 200 mL = £8.75. Label: 14, (urine red)

Brands include *Normax*®

Dose

- **By mouth**

  Child 6–12 years 5 mL at night (restricted indications, see notes above)

  Child 12–18 years 5–15 mL at night (restricted indications, see notes above)

DOCUSATE SODIUM

(Dioctyl sodium sulphosuccinate)

Cautions see notes above; do not give with liquid paraffin

Pregnancy not known to be harmful—manufacturer advises caution

Breast-feeding present in milk following oral administration—manufacturer advises caution

Contra-indications for *rectal preparations*, haemorrhoids or anal fissure

Side-effects see notes above

Licensed use *adult oral solution and capsules* not licensed for use in children under 12 years

Indication and dose

Constipation

- **By mouth**

  Child 6 months–2 years 12.5 mg 3 times daily (use paediatric oral solution)

  Child 2–12 years 12.5–25 mg 3 times daily (use paediatric oral solution)

  Child 12–18 years up to 500 mg daily in divided doses

Note Oral preparations act within 1–2 days; response to rectal administration usually occurs within 20 minutes; recommended doses may be exceeded on specialist advice

Adjunct in abdominal radiological procedures

Child 12–18 years 400 mg with barium meal

Administration for administration *by mouth*, solution may be mixed with milk or squash

Dioctyl® (Schwarz)

Capsules, yellow/white, docusate sodium 100 mg, net price 30-cap pack = £2.40, 100-cap pack = £8.00

Docusol® (Typharm)

Adult oral solution, sugar-free, docusate sodium 50 mg/5 mL, net price 300 mL = £2.48

Paediatric oral solution, sugar-free, docusate sodium 12.5 mg/5 mL, net price 300 mL = £1.63

DOCUSATE SODIUM (*continued*)

Rectal preparations

Norgalax Micro-enema® (Norgine)
Enema, docusate sodium 120 mg in 10-g single-dose disposable packs. Net price 10-g unit = 60p

Dose
- By rectum
  Child 12–18 years 1 enema as a single dose

GLYCEROL
(Glycerin)

Indication and dose

Constipation
- By rectum
  Child 1 month–1 year 1 g suppository as required
  Child 1–12 years 2 g suppository as required
  Child 12–18 years 4 g suppository as required

Glycerol Suppositories, BP
(Glycerin Suppositories)
Suppositories, gelatin 140 mg, glycerol 700 mg, purified water to 1 g. Net price 12 = 81p (infant, 1-g mould), 82p (child, 2-g mould), 76p (adult, 4-g mould)
Administration Moisten with water before insertion

SENNA

Cautions see notes above
Pregnancy see notes above
Breast-feeding not known to be harmful
Contra-indications see notes above
Side-effects see notes above
Licensed use *syrup* not licensed for use in children under 2 years

Indication and dose

Constipation for dose see under preparations

Note Onset of action 8–12 hours; initial dose should be low; recommended doses may be exceeded on specialist advice

Senna (Non-proprietary)
Tablets, total sennosides (calculated as sennoside B) 7.5 mg. Net price 20 = 65p
Brands include *Senokot®* (NHS)

Dose
- By mouth
  Child 6–12 years 1–2 tablets at night (or in the morning if preferred)
  Child 12–18 years 2–4 tablets at night (or in the morning if preferred)

Manevac® (Galen)
Granules, coated, senna fruit 12.4%, ispaghula 54.2%, net price 400 g = £7.45. Label: 25, 27, counselling, see below

Dose
- By mouth
  Child 5–12 years 1 level 5-mL spoonful once daily
  Child 12–18 years 1–2 level 5-mL spoonfuls after evening meal and, if necessary, before breakfast or every 6 hours in resistant cases for 1–3 days

Administration granules can be taken mixed with a cold or warm drink *or* be sprinkled on food
Counselling Preparations that swell in contact with liquid should always be carefully swallowed with water and should not be taken immediately before going to bed

Senokot® (R&C)
Tablets (NHS), see above

Granules, brown, total sennosides (calculated as sennoside B) 15 mg/5 mL or 5.5 mg/g (one 5-mL spoonful = 2.7 g). Net price 100 g = £3.10

Dose
- By mouth
  Child 6–12 years 2.5–5 mL at night or in the morning
  Child 12–18 years 5–10 mL usually at bedtime

Syrup, sugar-free, brown, total sennosides (calculated as sennoside B) 7.5 mg/5 mL. Net price 500 mL = £2.69

Dose
- By mouth
  Child 1 month–2 years 0.5 mL/kg (max. 2.5 mL) once daily
  Child 2–6 years 2.5–5 mL once daily in the morning
  Child 6–12 years 5–10 mL once daily at night *or* in the morning
  Child 12–18 years 10–20 mL once daily, usually at bedtime

SODIUM PICOSULFATE
(Sodium picosulphate)

Cautions see notes above; active inflammatory bowel disease (avoid if fulminant)
Breast-feeding not known to be present in milk but manufacturer advises avoid
Contra-indications see notes above; severe dehydration
Side-effects see notes above
Licensed use *elixir*, licensed for use in children (age range not specified by manufacturer; *Perles®* not licensed for use in children under 4 years

SODIUM PICOSULFATE (*continued*)

Indication and dose

Constipation
- By mouth

Child 1 month–4 years 250 micrograms/kg (max. 5 mg) at night

Child 4–10 years 2.5–5 mg at night

Child 10–18 years 5–10 mg at night

Note onset of action 6–12 hours; recommended doses may be exceeded on specialist advice

Bowel evacuation before abdominal radiological and endoscopic procedures on the colon, and surgery section 1.6.5

Sodium Picosulfate (Non-proprietary)
Elixir, sodium picosulfate 5 mg/5 mL, net price 100 mL = £1.85
Note The brand names *Laxoberal*® NHS and *Dulco-lax*® *Liquid* (both Boehringer Ingelheim) are used for sodium picosulfate elixir 5 mg/5 mL

Dulco-lax® (Boehringer Ingelheim)
Perles® (= capsules), sodium picosulfate 2.5 mg, net price 20-cap pack = £1.93, 50-cap pack = £2.73
Note The brand name *Dulco-lax*® is also used for bisacodyl tablets and suppositories

Bowel cleansing solutions
Section 1.6.5

1.6.3 Faecal softeners

Enemas containing **arachis oil** (ground-nut oil, peanut oil) lubricate and soften impacted faeces and promote a bowel movement.

Liquid paraffin, the classical lubricant, has disadvantages (see below) and should be used **only** on the advice of a specialist practitioner. Liquid paraffin is not recommended for use in children with difficulty swallowing or impaired neurodevelopment.

Bulk laxatives (section 1.6.1) and non-ionic surfactant 'wetting' agents e.g. docusate sodium (section 1.6.2) also have softening properties. Such drugs are useful for oral administration in the management of anal fissure; glycerol suppositories (section 1.6.2) are useful for rectal use.

ARACHIS OIL

Cautions intestinal obstruction; hypersensitivity to soya

Contra-indications inflammatory bowel disease, hypersensitivity to arachis oil or peanuts

Licensed use licensed for use in children (age range not specified by manufacturer

Indication and dose

Impacted faeces
- By rectum

Child 3–7 years 45–65 mL as required

Child 7–12 years 65–100 mL as required

Child 12–18 years 100–130 mL as required

Administration warm enema in warm water before use

Fletchers' Arachis Oil Retention Enema® (Forest)
Enema, arachis (peanut) oil in 130-mL single-dose disposable packs. Net price 130 mL = 96p

LIQUID PARAFFIN

Cautions avoid prolonged use

Contra-indications abdominal pain, nausea or vomiting; children under 3 years

Side-effects anal seepage of paraffin and consequent anal irritation after prolonged use, granulomatous reactions caused by absorption of small quantities of liquid paraffin (especially from the emulsion), lipoid pneumonia

Licensed use no licensed preparation available

Indication and dose

Refractory constipation (specialist use only) for dose see under preparation

Liquid Paraffin Oral Emulsion, BP (Non-proprietary)
Oral emulsion, liquid paraffin 5 mL, vanillin 5 mg, chloroform 0.025 mL, benzoic acid solution 0.2 mL, methylcellulose-20 200 mg, saccharin sodium 500 micrograms, water to 10 mL, net price 500-mL = £3.00

Dose
- By mouth

Child 3–12 years 0.5–1 mL/kg (max. 30 mL) once daily

Child 12–18 years 10–30 mL once daily

Counselling Should not be taken immediately before going to bed

Liquid Paraffin Light BP (Non-proprietary)
Liquid, liquid paraffin light, net price 500-mL = £2.40

Dose
- By mouth

Child 3–18 years 0.5–1 mL/kg (up to max. 45 mL) once daily

Administration Mix liquid paraffin with ice-cream or yoghurt to improve palatability. Take after the evening meal, but not immediately before going to bed.

1.6.4 Osmotic laxatives

Osmotic laxatives increase the amount of water in the large bowel, either by drawing fluid from the body into the bowel or by retaining the fluid they were administered with.

Lactulose is a semi-synthetic disaccharide which is not absorbed from the gastro-intestinal tract. It produces an osmotic diarrhoea of low faecal pH, and discourages the proliferation of ammonia-producing organisms. It is therefore useful in the treatment of *hepatic encephalopathy*.

Macrogols are inert polymers of ethylene glycol which sequester fluid in the bowel; giving fluid with macrogols may reduce the dehydrating effect sometimes seen with osmotic laxatives. Macrogols are an effective non-traumatic means of evacuation in children with faecal impaction and can be used in the long-term management of chronic constipation.

Saline purgatives such as **magnesium hydroxide** are commonly abused but are satisfactory for occasional use; adequate fluid intake should be maintained. **Magnesium salts** are useful where rapid bowel evacuation is required. **Sodium salts** should be avoided as they may give rise to sodium and water retention in susceptible individuals. **Phosphate enemas** are useful in bowel clearance before radiology, endoscopy, and surgery. Enemas containing **phosphate** or **sodium citrate**, and oral **bowel cleansing solutions** (section 1.6.5) should only be used on the advice of a specialist practitioner.

LACTULOSE

Cautions lactose intolerance

Contra-indications galactosaemia, intestinal obstruction

Side-effects flatulence, cramps, and abdominal discomfort

Indication and dose

Constipation (may take up to 48 hours to act)
- By mouth

Child 1 month–1 year 2.5 mL twice daily, adjusted according to response

Child 1–5 years 5 mL twice daily, adjusted according to response

Child 5–10 years 10 mL twice daily, adjusted according to response

Child 10–18 years initially 15 mL twice daily, adjusted according to response

Hepatic encephalopathy
- By mouth

Child 12–18 years 30–50 mL 3 times daily; adjust dose to produce 2–3 soft stools per day

Lactulose (Non-proprietary)

Solution, lactulose 3.1–3.7 g/5 mL with other ketoses. Net price 500-mL pack = £2.44

Brands include *Duphalac*® (NHS), *Lactugal*®, *Regulose*®

MACROGOLS
(Polyethylene glycols)

Cautions discontinue if symptoms of fluid and electrolyte disturbance

Pregnancy manufacturer advises use only if essential—no information available

Breast-feeding no information available, but absorption from gastro-intestinal tract negligible

Contra-indications intestinal perforation or obstruction, paralytic ileus, severe inflammatory conditions of the intestinal tract (such as Crohn's disease, ulcerative colitis, and toxic megacolon)

Side-effects abdominal distension and pain, nausea

Licensed use *Movicol® Paediatric Plain* not licensed for use in faecal impaction in children under 5 years, or for chronic constipation in children under 2 years

Indication and dose

See under preparations below

Idrolax® (Schwarz)

Oral powder, macrogol '4000' (polyethylene glycol '4000') 10 g/sachet, net price 20-sachet pack (orange-grapefruit flavour) = £4.84. Label: 13

Dose

Constipation
- By mouth

Child 8–18 years 1–2 sachets preferably as a single dose in the morning for max. 3 months

Administration Mix content of each sachet in a glass (approx. 250 mL) of water

Movicol® (Norgine)

Oral powder, macrogol '3350' (polyethylene glycol '3350') 13.125 g, sodium bicarbonate 178.5 mg, sodium chloride 350.7 mg, potassium chloride 46.6 mg/sachet, net price 20-sachet pack (lime and lemon flavour) = £4.63, 30-sachet pack = £6.95. Label: 13

MACROGOLS (*continued*)

Cautions patients with cardiovascular impairment should not take more than 2 sachets in any 1 hour

Dose

Chronic constipation
- By mouth

  Child 12–18 years 1–3 sachets daily in divided doses usually for up to 2 weeks; maintenance, 1–2 sachets daily

  Administration Mix content of each sachet in half a glass (approx. 125 mL) of water

Faecal impaction
- By mouth

  Child 12–18 years 8 sachets daily, usually for max. 3 days

  Administration Mix contents of 8 sachets in 1 litre water. After reconstitution the solution should be kept in a refrigerator and discarded if unused after 6 hours

Movicol®-Half (Norgine)
Oral powder, macrogol '3350' (polyethylene glycol '3350') 6.563 g, sodium bicarbonate 89.3 mg, sodium chloride 175.4 mg, potassium chloride 23.3 mg/sachet, net price 20-sachet pack (lime and lemon flavour) = £2.78, 30-sachet pack = £4.17. Label: 13

Cautions patients with impaired cardiovascular function should not take more than 4 sachets in any 1 hour

Dose

Chronic constipation
- By mouth

  Child 12–18 years 2–6 sachets daily in divided doses usually for up to 2 weeks; maintenance, 2–4 sachets daily

  Administration Mix content of each sachet dissolved in quarter of a glass (approx. 60–65 mL) of water

Faecal impaction
- By mouth

  Child 12–18 years 16 sachets daily, usually for max. 3 days

  Administration Mix contents of 16 sachets in 1 litre of water. After reconstitution the solution should be kept in a refrigerator and discarded if unused after 6 hours

Movicol® Paediatric Plain (Norgine) PoM
Oral powder, macrogol '3350' (polyethylene glycol '3350') 6.563 g, sodium bicarbonate 89.3 mg, sodium chloride 175.4 mg, potassium chloride 25.1 mg/sachet, net price 30-sachet pack = £4.63. Label: 13

Contra-indications cardiovascular impairment, renal impairment—no information available

Dose

Chronic constipation, prevention of faecal impaction
- By mouth

  Child 1–6 years 1 sachet daily; adjust dose to produce regular soft stools (max. 4 sachets daily)

  Child 6–12 years 2 sachets daily; adjust dose to produce regular soft stools (max. 4 sachets daily)

  Administration Mix content of each sachet in quarter of a glass (approx. 60–65 mL) of water

Faecal impaction
- By mouth

  Child 1–5 years (treat until impaction resolves or for max. 7 days) 2 sachets on first day, then 4 sachets daily for 2 days, then 6 sachets daily for 2 days, then 8 sachets daily for 2 days

  Child 5–12 years (treat until impaction resolves or for max. 7 days) 4 sachets on first day, then increased in steps of 2 sachets daily to max. 12 sachets daily

  Administration Mix each sachet in quarter of a glass (approx. 60–65 mL) of water; total daily dose to be taken over a 12-hour period

MAGNESIUM SALTS

Cautions see also notes above; **interactions:** Appendix 1 (antacids)

Hepatic impairment avoid in hepatic coma if risk of renal impairment

Renal impairment avoid or reduce dose in moderate impairment; risk of magnesium accumulation

Contra-indications acute gastro-intestinal conditions

Side-effects colic

Indication and dose

Constipation see under preparations below

Magnesium hydroxide

Magnesium Hydroxide Mixture, BP
Aqueous suspension containing about 8% hydrated magnesium oxide. Do not store in cold place

Dose
- By mouth

  Child 3–12 years 5–10 mL at bedtime

  Child 12–18 years 25–50 mL when required

Bowel cleansing solutions

Section 1.6.5

PHOSPHATES (RECTAL)

Cautions see also notes above; impaired renal function, heart disease, pre-existing electrolyte disturbances

Contra-indications acute gastro-intestinal conditions

Side-effects local irritation

Indication and dose

Constipation, bowel evacuation before abdominal radiological procedures, endoscopy, and surgery
for dose see under preparations

Carbalax® (Forest)
Suppositories, sodium acid phosphate (anhydrous) 1.3 g, sodium bicarbonate 1.08 g, net price 12 = £2.01

Dose
- By rectum

  Child 12–18 years 1 suppository, inserted 30 minutes before evacuation required; moisten with water before use

PHOSPHATES (RECTAL) (*continued*)

Fleet® Ready-to-use Enema (De Witt)
Enema, sodium acid phosphate 21.4 g, sodium phosphate 9.4 g/118 mL. Net price single-dose pack (standard tube) = 46p

Dose

- **By rectum**
  Child 3–7 years 40–60 mL once daily
  Child 7–12 years 60–90 mL once daily
  Child 12–18 years 90–118 mL once daily

Fletchers' Phosphate Enema® (Forest)
Enema, sodium acid phosphate 12.8 g, sodium phosphate 10.24 g, purified water, freshly boiled and cooled, to 128 mL (corresponds to Phosphates Enema Formula B). Net price 128 mL with standard tube = 41p, with long rectal tube = 57p

Dose

- **By rectum**
  Child 3–7 years 45–65 mL once daily
  Child 7–12 years 65–100 mL once daily
  Child 12–18 years 100–128 mL once daily

SODIUM CITRATE (RECTAL)

Cautions see notes above

Contra-indications acute gastro-intestinal conditions

Indication and dose

Constipation for dose see under preparations

Micolette Micro-enema® (Pinewood)
Enema, sodium citrate 450 mg, sodium lauryl sulphoacetate 45 mg, glycerol 625 mg, together with citric acid, potassium sorbate, and sorbitol in a viscous solution, in 5-mL single-dose disposable packs with nozzle. Net price 5 mL = 31p

Dose

- **By rectum**
  Child 3–18 years 5–10 mL as a single dose

Micralax Micro-enema® (Celltech)
Enema, sodium citrate 450 mg, sodium alkylsulphoacetate 45 mg, sorbic acid 5 mg, together with glycerol and sorbitol in a viscous solution in 5-mL single-dose disposable packs with nozzle. Net price 5 mL = 41p

Dose

- **By rectum**
  Child 3–18 years 5 mL as a single dose

Relaxit Micro-enema® (Crawford)
Enema, sodium citrate 450 mg, sodium lauryl sulphate 75 mg, sorbic acid 5 mg, together with glycerol and sorbitol in a viscous solution in 5-mL single-dose disposable packs with nozzle. Net price 5 mL = 32p

Dose

- **By rectum**
  Child 1 month–18 years 5 mL as a single dose (insert only half nozzle length in child under 3 years)

1.6.5 Bowel cleansing solutions

Bowel cleansing solutions are used before colonic surgery, colonoscopy, or radiological examination to ensure the bowel is free of solid contents. They are **not** treatments for constipation.

Gastrografin® is an **amidotrizoate** radiological contrast medium with high osmolality; it is used in the treatment of meconium ileus in neonates and in the management of distal intestinal obstruction syndrome in children with cystic fibrosis.

BOWEL CLEANSING SOLUTIONS

Cautions recent gastro-intestinal surgery; heart disease; inflammatory bowel disease; reflux oesophagitis; impaired gag reflex; administer solution via nasogastric tube in semi-conscious or unconscious patients

Renal impairment avoid in severe impairment (risk of hypermagnesaemia with *Citramag®* and *Picolax®*)

Pregnancy no evidence of harm in *animal* studies; manufacturer advises caution especially in first trimester

Breast-feeding not excreted in breast milk

Contra-indications gastro-intestinal obstruction, gastric retention, gastro-intestinal ulceration, perforated bowel, congestive cardiac failure; toxic colitis, toxic megacolon or ileus

Side-effects nausea and bloating; *less frequently* abdominal cramps (usually transient—reduced by taking more slowly); vomiting

Licensed use *Klean-Prep®* not licensed for use in children

Indication and dose

Clearance of bowel prior to radiological examination, colonoscopy, or surgery for dose, see under preparations

Citramag® (Sanochemia)
Powder, effervescent, magnesium carbonate 11.57 g, anhydrous citric acid 17.79 g/sachet, net price 10-sachet pack (lemon and lime flavour) = £14.90. Label: 10, patient information leaflet, 13, counselling, see below

Dose

- **By mouth**
  Child 5–10 years on day before procedure, one-third of a sachet at 8 a.m. and one-third of a sachet between 2 and 4 p.m.

1 Gastro-intestinal system

BOWEL CLEANSING SOLUTIONS (*continued*)

Child 10–18 years on day before procedure, ½–1 sachet at 8 a.m. and ½–1 sachet between 2 and 4 p.m.

Counselling The patient information leaflet advises that hot water (200 mL) is needed to make the solution and provides guidance on the timing and procedure for reconstitution; it also mentions need for high fluid, low residue diet beforehand (according to hospital advice), and explains that only clear fluids can be taken after *Citramag*® until procedure completed

Fleet Phospho-soda® (De Witt)

Oral solution, sugar-free, sodium dihydrogen phosphate dihydrate 24.4 g, disodium phosphate dodecahydrate 10.8 g/45 mL. Net price 2 × 45-mL bottles = £4.79. Label: 10, patient information leaflet, counselling

Dose

- **By mouth**

Child 15–18 years 45 mL diluted with half a glass (120 mL) of cold water, followed by one full glass (240 mL) of cold water

Timing of doses is dependent on the time of the procedure

For morning procedure, first dose should be taken at 7 a.m. and second at 7 p.m. on day before the procedure

For afternoon procedure, first dose should be taken at 7 p.m. on day before and second dose at 7 a.m. on day of the procedure

Solid food must not be taken during dosing period; clear liquids or water should be substituted for meals

Klean-Prep® (Norgine)

Oral powder, macrogol '3350' (polyethylene glycol '3350') 59 g, anhydrous sodium sulphate 5.685 g, sodium bicarbonate 1.685 g, sodium chloride 1.465 g, potassium chloride 743 mg/sachet, net price 4 sachets = £8.56. Label: 10, patient information leaflet, counselling

Excipients: include aspartame (section 9.4.1)

Note Allergic reactions reported

Dose

Clearance of bowel prior to radiological examination, colonoscopy or surgery

- **By mouth**

Child 12–18 years a glass (approx. 250 mL) of reconstituted solution every 10–15 minutes, or by nasogastric tube 20–30 mL/minute, until 4 litres have been consumed or watery stools are free of solid matter. The solution from all 4 sachets should be drunk within 4–6 hours (250 mL drunk rapidly every 10–15 minutes)

Alternatively total volume for administration given in 2 divided doses, first dose taken on the evening before examination and second dose on the morning of the examination

Distal intestinal obstruction syndrome

- **By mouth, nasogastric or gastrostomy tube**

Child 1–18 years 10 mL/kg/hour for 30 minutes, then 20 mL/kg/hour for 30 minutes, then increase to 25 mL/kg/hour if tolerated; max. 100 mL/kg (or 4 litres) over 4 hours; repeat 4-hour treatment if necessary.

Administration Each sachet should be made up to 1 litre with water; flavouring such as clear fruit cordials may be added if required; to facilitate gastric emptying domperidone (section 1.2) may be given 30 minutes before starting. After reconstitution the solution should be kept in a refrigerator and discarded if unused after 24 hours.

Picolax® (Ferring)

Oral powder, sugar-free, sodium picosulfate 10 mg/sachet, with magnesium citrate, net price 2-sachet pack = £3.53. Label: 10, patient information leaflet, 13, counselling, see below

Dose

- **By mouth**

Child 1–2 years ¼ sachet in the morning and ¼ sachet in the afternoon

Child 2–4 years ½ sachet in the morning and ½ sachet in the afternoon

Child 4–9 years 1 sachet in the morning and ½ sachet in the afternoon

Child 9–18 years 1 sachet in the morning and 1 sachet in the afternoon

Administration morning dose to be taken before 8 a.m and afternoon dose to be taken between 2 and 4 p.m. on day preceding procedure

Note Acts within 3 hours of first dose. Low residue diet recommended for 2 days before procedure and copious intake of water or other clear fluids recommended during treatment

Counselling. Children and carers should be warned that heat is generated on addition to water; for this reason the powder should be added initially to 30 mL (2 tablespoonfuls) of water; after 5 minutes (when reaction complete) the solution should be further diluted to 150 mL (approx. half a glass)

AMIDOTRIZOATES

Diatrizoates

Cautions asthma or history of allergy, latent hyperthyroidism, dehydration and electrolyte disturbance (correct first); in children with oesophageal fistulae (aspiration may lead to pulmonary oedema); benign nodular goitre

Contra-indications hypersensitivity to iodine, hyperthyroidism

Side-effects diarrhoea; *rarely* nausea, vomiting, urticaria

Licensed use not licensed for use in distal intestinal obstruction syndrome

Indication and dose

Uncomplicated meconium ileus

- **By rectum**

Neonate 15–30 mL as a single dose

Distal intestinal obstruction syndrome

- **By mouth or by rectum**

Child 1 month–2 years 15–30 mL as a single dose

Child body-weight 15–25 kg 50 mL as a single dose

Child body-weight over 25 kg 100 mL as a single dose

Administration Intravenous prehydration is essential in neonates and infants. Fluid intake should be encouraged for 3 hours after administration. *By mouth*, for child bodyweight under 25 kg, dilute *Gastrografin*® with 3 times its volume of water or fruit juice; for child bodyweight over 25 kg, dilute *Gastrografin*® with twice its volume of water or fruit juice. *By rectum*, administration

AMIDOTRIZOATES (*continued*)

must be carried out slowly under radiological supervision to ensure required site is reached. For child under 5 years, dilute *Gastrografin*® with 5 times its volume of water; for child over 5 years dilute *Gastrografin*® with 4 times its volume of water. Administer using a large syringe and soft rubber catheter (No.8 French); the buttocks may be taped tightly together to minimise leakage, but a balloon catheter should not be used.

Radiological investigations dose to be recommended by radiologist

Gastrografin® (Schering Health)
Solution, sodium amidotrizoate 100 mg, meglumine amidotrizoate 600 mg/mL, net price 100-mL bottle = £14.16
Excipients: include disodium edetate

1.7 Local preparations for anal and rectal disorders

In children with perianal soreness or pruritus ani, good toilet hygiene is essential; the use of alcohol-free 'wet-wipes' after each bowel motion, regular bathing and the avoidance of local irritants such as bath additives is recommended. Excoriated skin is best treated with a protective barrier emollient 9section 13.2.2); in children over 1 month, **hydrocortisone** ointment or cream (section 13.4) or a compound rectal preparation (section 1.7.2) may be used for a short period of time, up to a maximum of 7 days.

Pruritus ani caused by threadworm infection requires treatment with an anthelmintic (section 5.5.1). Topical application of **white soft paraffin** or other bland emollient (section 13.2.1) may reduce anal irritation caused by threadworms.

Perianal erythema caused by streptococcal infection should be treated initially with an oral antibacterial such as **phenoxymethylpenicillin** (section 5.1.1.1) or **erythromycin** (section 5.1.5), while awaiting results of culture and sensitivity testing.

Perianal candidiasis (thrush) requires treatment with oral **nystatin** (section 5.2) and another antifungal preparation applied topically (section 13.10.2). For treatment of vulvovaginal candidiasis, see section 7.2.2.

Proctitis associated with inflammatory bowel disease in children is treated with corticosteroids and aminosalicylates (section 1.5).

For the management of anal fissures, see section section 1.7.4.

1.7.1 Soothing anal and rectal preparations

Haemorrhoids in children are rare, but may occur in infants with portal hypertension. Soothing rectal preparations containing mild astringents such as bismuth subgallate, zinc oxide, and hammamelis may provide symptomatic relief, but proprietary preparations which also contain lubricants, vasoconstrictors, or mild antiseptics may cause further perianal irritation.

Local anaesthetics may be used to relieve pain in children with anal fissures or pruritus ani, but local anaesthetics are absorbed through the rectal mucosa and may cause sensitisation of the anal skin. Excessive use of local anaesthetics may result in systemic effects, see section 15.2. Preparations containing local anaesthetics should be used for no longer than 2–3 days.

Lidocaine (lignocaine) ointment (section 15.2) may be applied before defaecation to relieve pain associated with anal fissure, but local anaesthetics can cause stinging initially and this may aggravate the child's fear of pain.

Other local anaesthetics such as tetracaine (amethocaine), cinchocaine, and pramocaine (pramoxine) may be included in rectal preparations, but these are more irritant than lidocaine.

Corticosteroids are often combined with local anaesthetics and soothing agents in topical preparations for haemorrhoids and proctitis. Topical preparations containing corticosteroids (section 1.7.2) should not be used long-term or if infection (such as herpes simplex) is present. For further information on the use of topical corticosteroids, see section 13.4.

1.7.2 Compound anal and rectal preparations with corticosteroids

Anugesic-HC® (Pfizer) PoM

Cream, benzyl benzoate 1.2%, bismuth oxide 0.875%, hydrocortisone acetate 0.5%, Peru balsam 1.85%, pramocaine hydrochloride 1%, zinc oxide 12.35%. Net price 30 g (with rectal nozzle) = £3.71

Dose

Haemorrhoids, pruritus ani
- By rectum
  Child 12–18 years apply night and morning and after a bowel movement; do not use for longer than 7 days

Suppositories, buff, benzyl benzoate 33 mg, bismuth oxide 24 mg, bismuth subgallate 59 mg, hydrocortisone acetate 5 mg, Peru balsam 49 mg, pramocaine hydrochloride 27 mg, zinc oxide 296 mg, net price 12 = £2.69

Dose

Haemorrhoids, pruritus ani
- By rectum
  Child 12–18 years insert 1 suppository night and morning and after a bowel movement; do not use for longer than 7 days

Anusol-HC® (Pfizer Consumer) PoM

Ointment, benzyl benzoate 1.25%, bismuth oxide 0.875%, bismuth subgallate 2.25%, hydrocortisone acetate 0.25%, Peru balsam 1.875%, zinc oxide 10.75%. Net price 30 g (with rectal nozzle) = £3.50

Dose

Haemorrhoids, pruritus ani
- By rectum
  Child 12–18 years apply night and morning and after a bowel movement; do not use for longer than 7 days

Suppositories, benzyl benzoate 33 mg, bismuth oxide 24 mg, bismuth subgallate 59 mg, hydrocortisone acetate 10 mg, Peru balsam 49 mg, zinc oxide 296 mg. Net price 12 = £2.46

Dose

Haemorrhoids, pruritus ani
- By rectum
  Child 12–18 years insert 1 suppository night and morning and after a bowel movement; do not use for longer than 7 days

Perinal® (Dermal)

Spray application, hydrocortisone 0.2%, lidocaine hydrochloride 1%. Net price 30-mL pack = £6.39

Dose

Haemorrhoids, pruritus ani
- By rectum
  Child 2–18 years spray once over the affected area up to 3 times daily; do not use for longer than 1–2 weeks (child under 14 years, on medical advice only)

Proctofoam HC® (Meda) PoM

Foam in aerosol pack, hydrocortisone acetate 1%, pramocaine hydrochloride 1%. Net price 21.2-g pack (approx. 40 applications) with applicator = £5.06

Dose

Pain and irritation associated with local, non-infected anal or perianal conditions
- By rectum
  Child 12–18 years 1 applicatorful (4–6 mg hydrocortisone acetate, 4–6 mg pramocaine hydrochloride) by rectum 2–3 times daily and after a bowel movement (max. 4 times daily); do not use for longer than 7 days

Proctosedyl® (Aventis Pharma) PoM

Ointment, cinchocaine (dibucaine) hydrochloride 0.5%, hydrocortisone 0.5%. Net price 30 g = £7.83 (with cannula)

Dose

Haemorrhoids, pruritus ani
- By rectum
  Child 1 month–18 years apply morning and night and after a bowel movement, externally or by rectum; do not use for longer than 7 days

Suppositories, cinchocaine (dibucaine) hydrochloride 5 mg, hydrocortisone 5 mg. Net price 12 = £3.53

Dose

Haemorrhoids, pruritus ani
- By rectum
  Child 12–18 years insert 1 suppository night and morning and after a bowel movement; do not use for longer than 7 days

Scheriproct® (Schering Health) PoM

Ointment, cinchocaine (dibucaine) hydrochloride 0.5%, prednisolone hexanoate 0.19%. Net price 30 g = £3.00

Dose

Haemorrhoids, pruritus ani
- By rectum
  Child 1 month–18 years apply twice daily for 5–7 days (3–4 times daily on 1st day if necessary), then once daily for a few days after symptoms have cleared

Suppositories, cinchocaine (dibucaine) hydrochloride 1 mg, prednisolone hexanoate 1.3 mg. Net price 12 = £1.41

Dose

Haemorrhoids, pruritus ani
- By rectum
  Child 12–18 years insert 1 suppository daily after a bowel movement, for 5–7 days (in severe cases initially 2–3 times daily)

Ultraproct® (Meadow) PoM

Ointment, cinchocaine (dibucaine) hydrochloride 0.5%, fluocortolone caproate 0.095%, fluocortolone pivalate 0.092%, net price 30 g (with rectal nozzle) = £4.57

Dose

Haemorrhoids, pruritus ani
Child 1 month–18 years apply twice daily for 5–7 days (3–4 times daily on 1st day if necessary), then once daily for a few days after symptoms have cleared

Suppositories, cinchocaine (dibucaine) hydrochloride 1 mg, fluocortolone caproate 630 micrograms, fluocortolone pivalate 610 micrograms, net price 12 = £2.15

Dose

Haemorrhoids, pruritus ani
- By rectum
  Child 12–18 years insert 1 suppository daily after a bowel movement, for 5–7 days (in severe cases initially 2–3 times daily) then 1 suppository every other day for 1 week

Uniroid-HC® (Chemidex) PoM
Ointment, cinchocaine (dibucaine) hydrochloride 0.5%, hydrocortisone 0.5%. Net price 30 g (with applicator) = £4.23

Dose

Haemorrhoids, pruritus ani
- **By rectum**
  Child 1 month–18 years apply twice daily and after a bowel movement, externally or by rectum; do not use for longer than 7 days (child under 12 years, on medical advice only)

Suppositories, cinchocaine (dibucaine) hydrochloride 5 mg, hydrocortisone 5 mg. Net price 12 = £1.91

Dose

Haemorrhoids, pruritus ani
- **By rectum**
  Child 12–18 years insert 1 suppository twice daily and after a bowel movement; do not use for longer than 7 days

Xyloproct® (AstraZeneca) PoM
Ointment (water-miscible), aluminium acetate 3.5%, hydrocortisone acetate 0.275%, lidocaine 5%, zinc oxide 18%, net price 20 g (with applicator) = £2.26

Dose

Haemorrhoids, pruritus ani
- **By rectum**
  Child 1 month–18 years apply several times daily; short-term use only

Gastro-intestinal system 1

1.7.3 Rectal sclerosants

Classification not used in BNF for Children.

1.7.4 Management of anal fissures

The management of anal fissures includes stool softening (section 1.6) and the short-term use of a topical preparation containing a local anaesthetic (section 1.7.1). Children with chronic anal fissures should be referred to a hospital specialist for assessment and treatment with a topical nitrate, or for surgery. Topical **glyceryl trinitrate**, 0.05% or 0.1% ointment, may be used in children to relax the anal sphincter, relieve pain and aid healing of anal fissures. Excessive application of topical nitrates causes side-effects such as headache, flushing, dizziness, and postural hypotension.

Diltiazem 2% ointment has also been used to treat chronic anal fissures resistant to topical nitrates.

Ointments containing glyceryl trinitrate in a range of strengths or diltiazem 2% are available as manufactured specials (see Special-order Manufacturers, p. 861).

1.8 Stoma and enteral feeding tubes

Stoma

Prescribing for children with stoma calls for special care. The following is a brief account of some of the main points to be borne in mind.

When a solid-dose formulation such as a capsule or a tablet is given the contents of the ostomy bag should be checked for any remnants; response to treatment should be carefully monitored because of the possibility of incomplete absorption. *Enteric-coated* and *modified-release* preparations are **unsuitable**, particularly in children with an ileostomy, as there may not be sufficient release of the active ingredient.

Laxatives Enemas and washouts should be used in children with stoma only under specialist supervision; they should **not** be prescribed for those with an ileostomy as they may cause rapid and severe loss of water and electrolytes.

Children with colostomy may suffer from constipation and whenever possible it should be treated by increasing fluid intake or dietary fibre. If a laxative (section 1.6) is required, it should generally be used for short periods only.

Antidiarrhoeals **Loperamide**, **codeine phosphate**, and **co-phenotrope** (section 1.4.2) are effective for controlling excessive stool losses. Bulk-forming drugs (section 1.6.1) may be tried but it is often difficult to adjust the dose appropriately.

Antibacterials should **not** be given for an episode of acute diarrhoea.

Antacids The tendency to diarrhoea from magnesium salts or constipation from aluminium salts may be increased in children with stoma.

Diuretics Diuretics should be used with caution in children with an ileostomy because they may become excessively dehydrated and potassium depletion may easily occur. It is usually advisable to use a **potassium-sparing** diuretic (section 2.2.3).

Digoxin Children with stoma are particularly susceptible to hypokalaemia. This predisposes children on digoxin to digoxin toxicity; potassium supplements (section 9.2.1.1) or a potassium-sparing diuretic (section 2.2.3) may be advisable.

Analgesics Opioid analgesics (section 4.7.2) may cause troublesome constipation in children with colostomy. When a non-opioid analgesic is required **paracetamol** is usually suitable; anti-inflammatory analgesics may cause gastric irritation and bleeding.

Iron preparations Iron supplements may cause loose stools and sore skin at the stoma site. If this is troublesome and if iron is definitely indicated a parenteral iron preparation (section 9.1.1.2) should be used. Modified-release iron preparations should be **avoided**.

Care of stoma Children and carers are usually given advice about the use of *cleansing agents, protective creams, lotions, deodorants*, or *sealants* whilst in hospital, either by the surgeon or by a stoma-care nurse. Voluntary organisations offer help and support to patients with stoma.

Enteral feeding tubes

Care is required in choosing an appropriate formulation of a drug for administration through a nasogastric narrow-bore feeding tube or through a percutaneous endoscopic gastrostomy (PEG) or jejunostomy tube. Liquid preparations (or soluble tablets) are preferred; injection solutions may also be suitable for administration through an enteral tube.

If a solid formulation of a medicine needs to be given, it should be given as a suspension of particles fine enough to pass through the tube. It is possible to crush many immediate-release tablets but enteric-coated or modified-release preparations should **not** be crushed.

Enteral feeds may affect the absorption of drugs and it is therefore important to consider the timing of drug administration in relation to feeds. If more than one drug needs to be given, they should be given separately and the tube should be flushed with water after each drug has been given.

Clearing blockages Carbonated (sugar-free) drinks may be marginally more effective than water in unblocking feeding tubes, but mildly acidic liquids (such as pineapple juice or cola-based drinks) can coagulate protein in feeds, causing further blockage. If these measures fail to clear the enteral feeding tube, an alkaline solution containing pancreatic enzymes may be introduced into the tube (followed after at least 5 minutes by water). Specific products designed to break up blockages caused by formula feeds are also available.

1.9 Drugs affecting intestinal secretions

1.9.1 Drugs affecting biliary composition and flow

Bile acids (**ursodeoxycholic** and **chenodeoxycholic acid**) may be used as dietary supplements in children with inborn errors of bile acid synthesis. Ursodeoxycholic acid is used to improve the flow of bile in children with cholestatic conditions such as familial intrahepatic cholestasis, biliary atresia in infants, cystic-fibrosis-related liver disease, and cholestasis caused by total parenteral nutrition or following liver transplantation. Ursodeoxycholic acid may also relieve the severe itching associated with cholestasis.

In primary biliary cirrhosis and primary sclerosing cholangitis, ursodeoxycholic acid is used to lower liver enzyme and serum-bilirubin concentrations.

Ursodeoxycholic acid is used in the treatment of intrahepatic cholestasis in pregnancy.

Smith-Lemli-Opitz syndrome Chenodeoxycholic and ursodeoxycholic acid have been used with cholesterol in children with Smith-Lemli-Opitz syndrome. Chenodeoxycholic acid is also used in combination with cholic acid to treat bile acid synthesis defects but cholic acid is difficult to obtain. Chenodeoxycholic acid and cholesterol are available from specialist importing companies, see p. 848.

URSODEOXYCHOLIC ACID

Cautions interactions: Appendix 1 (ursodeoxycholic acid)

Hepatic impairment avoid in chronic liver disease (but used in primary biliary cirrhosis)

Pregnancy no evidence of harm but manufacturer advises avoid

Breast-feeding not known to be harmful but manufacturer advises avoid

Contra-indications radio-opaque stones; non-functioning gall bladder (in patients with radiolucent gallstones)

Side-effects *rarely*, diarrhoea

Licensed use *Ursofalk®*, not licensed for use in improvement of hepatic metabolism of essential fatty acids or cholestasis associated with total parenteral nutrition; *all other preparations*, not licensed for use in any condition other than dissolution of gallstones

Indication and dose

Cholestasis in biliary atresia
- By mouth

Neonate 15 mg/kg once daily, adjust dose and frequency according to response, up to a max. 30 mg/kg daily

Child 1 month–2 years 15 mg/kg once daily, adjust dose and frequency according to response, up to a max. 30 mg/kg daily

Improvement of hepatic metabolism of essential fatty acids and bile flow, in children with cystic fibrosis
- By mouth

Child 1 month–18 years 10–15 mg/kg twice daily; total daily dose may alternatively be given in 3 divided doses

Cholestasis associated with total parenteral nutrition
- By mouth

Neonate 10mg/kg 3 times daily

Child 1 month–18 years 10 mg/kg 3 times daily

Primary biliary cirrhosis
- By mouth

Child 1 month–18 years 5–10 mg/kg 2–3 times daily, adjusted according to response, max. 45 mg/kg daily

Ursodeoxycholic Acid (Non-proprietary) PoM

Tablets, ursodeoxycholic acid 150 mg, net price 60-tab pack = £18.51. Label: 21

Capsules, ursodeoxycholic acid 250 mg, net price 60-cap pack = £35.11. Label: 21

Destolit® (Norgine) PoM

Tablets, scored, ursodeoxycholic acid 150 mg, net price 60-tab pack = £18.39. Label: 21

Urdox® (CP) PoM

Tablets, f/c, ursodeoxycholic acid 300 mg, net price 60-tab pack = £30.24. Label: 21

Ursofalk® (Provalis) PoM

Capsules, ursodeoxycholic acid 250 mg, net price 60-cap pack = £31.10, 100-cap pack = £32.85. Label: 21

Suspension, sugar-free, ursodeoxycholic acid 250 mg/5 mL, net price 250 mL = £28.50. Label: 21

Ursogal® (Galen) PoM

Tablets, scored, ursodeoxycholic acid 150 mg, net price 60-tab pack = £17.05. Label: 21

Capsules, ursodeoxycholic acid 250 mg, net price 60-cap pack = £30.50. Label: 21

Other preparations for bile synthesis defects

CHENODEOXYCHOLIC ACID

Cautions see under Ursodeoxycholic Acid

Pregnancy avoid—fetotoxicity reported in *animal* studies

Contra-indications see under Ursodeoxycholic Acid

Side-effects see under Ursodeoxycholic Acid

Licensed use not licensed

CHENODEOXYCHOLIC ACID (*continued*)

Indication and dose

Cerebrotendinous xanthomatosis
- By mouth

Neonate 5 mg/kg 3 times daily

Child 1 month–18 years 5 mg/kg 3 times daily

Defective synthesis of bile acid
- By mouth

Neonate initially 5 mg/kg 3 times daily, reduced to 2.5 mg/kg 3 times daily

Child 1 month–18 years initially 5 mg/kg 3 times daily, reduced to 2.5 mg/kg 3 times daily

Smith-Lemli-Opitz syndrome see notes above
- By mouth

Neonate 7 mg/kg once daily or in divided doses

Child 1 month–18 years 7 mg/kg once daily or in divided doses

Administration for administration *by mouth*, add the contents of a 250-mg capsule to 25 mL of sodium bicarbonate solution 8.4% (1 mmol/mL) to produce a suspension containing chenodeoxycholic acid 10 mg/mL; use immediately after preparation, discard any remaining suspension

Chenofalk (Non-proprietary) PoM
Capsules, chenodeoxycholic acid 250mg
Available from specialist importing companies, see p. 848

CHOLESTEROL

Cautions consult product literature

Contra-indications consult product literature

Licensed use not licensed

Indication and dose

Smith-Lemli-Opitz syndrome
- By mouth

Neonate 5–10 mg/kg 3–4 times daily

Child 1 month–18 years 5–10 mg/kg 3–4 times daily (doses up to 15 mg/kg 4 times daily have been used)

Administration cholesterol powder can be mixed with a vegetable oil before administration

Cholesterol Powder (Non-proprietary)
Available from specialist importing companies, see p. 848

1.9.2 Bile acid sequestrants

Colestyramine (cholestyramine) is an anion-exchange resin that forms an insoluble complex with bile acids in the gastro-intestinal tract; it is used to relieve diarrhoea associated with surgical procedures such as ileal resection, or following radiation therapy. Colestyramine is also used in the treatment of familial hypercholesterolaemia (see section 2.12), and to relieve pruritus in children with partial biliary obstruction, (for treatment of pruritus, see section 3.4.1). Colestyramine is not absorbed from the gastro-intestinal tract, but will interfere with the absorption of a number of drugs, so timing of administration is important.

COLESTYRAMINE
(Cholestyramine)

Cautions see section 2.12

Contra-indications see section 2.12

Side-effects see section 2.12

Licensed use not licensed for use in children under 6 years

Indication and dose

Pruritus associated with partial biliary obstruction and primary biliary cirrhosis, diarrhoea associated with Crohn's disease, ileal resection, vagotomy, diabetic vagal neuropathy, and radiation
- By mouth

Child 1 month–1 year 1 g once daily, mixed with water (or other suitable liquid) adjusted according to response; total daily dose may alternatively be given in 2–4 divided doses (max. 9 g daily)

Child 1–6 years 2 g once daily, mixed with water (or other suitable liquid) adjusted according to response; total daily dose may alternatively be given in 2–4 divided doses (max. 18 g daily)

Child 6–12 years 4 g once daily, mixed with water (or other suitable liquid) adjusted according to response; total daily dose may alternatively be given in 2–4 divided doses (max. 24 g daily)

Child 12–18 years 4–8 g once daily, mixed with water (or other suitable liquid) adjusted according to response; total daily dose may alternatively be given in 2–4 divided doses (max. 36 g daily)

Counselling Other drugs should be taken at least 1 hour before or 4–6 hours after colestyramine to reduce possible interference with absorption

Note For treatment of diarrhoea induced by bile acid malabsorption, if no response within 3 days an alternative therapy should be initiated

Hypercholesterolaemia section 2.12

Preparations
Section 2.12

1.9.3 Aprotinin

Classification not used in BNF for Children.

1.9.4 Pancreatin

Pancreatin containing a mixture of protease, lipase and amylase in varying proportions aids the digestion of starch, fat, and protein. Supplements of pancreatin are given by mouth to compensate for reduced or absent exocrine secretion in cystic fibrosis, and following pancreatectomy, total gastrectomy, or chronic pancreatitis.

The dose of pancreatin is adjusted according to size, number, and consistency of stools, and the nutritional status of the child; extra allowance may be needed if snacks are taken between meals. Daily dose should not exceed 10 000 lipase units per kg body-weight per day, (**important**: see CSM advice on Higher-strength preparations below).

Pancreatin preparations

Preparation	Protease units	Amylase units	Lipase units
Creon® 10 000 capsule, e/c granules	600	8000	10 000
Creon® Micro e/c granules (per 100 mg)	200	3600	5000
Nutrizym 10® capsule, e/c granules	500	9000	10 000
Pancrease® capsule, e/c granules	330	2900	5000
Pancrex V® capsule, powder	430	9000	8000
Pancrex V '125'® capsule, powder	160	3300	2950
Pancrex V® e/c tablet	110	1700	1900
Pancrex V® Forte e/c tablet	330	5000	5600

Higher-strength pancreatin preparations *Pancrease HL®* and *Nutrizym 22®* have been associated with the development of large bowel strictures (fibrosing colonopathy) in children with cystic fibrosis aged between 2 and 13 years. The **CSM** (1995) has recommended the following:

- *Pancrease HL®*, *Nutrizym 22®* should not be used in children under 16 years with cystic fibrosis;
- the total dose of pancreatic enzyme supplements used in patients with cystic fibrosis should not usually exceed 10 000 units of lipase per kg body-weight daily;
- if a patient on any pancreatin preparation develops new abdominal symptoms (or any change in existing abdominal symptoms) the patient should be reviewed to exclude the possibility of colonic damage.

Possible risk factors are gender (boys at greater risk than girls), more severe cystic fibrosis, and concomitant use of laxatives. The peak age for developing fibrosing colonopathy is between 2 and 8 years.

Higher-strength pancreatin preparations

Preparation	Protease units	Amylase units	Lipase units
Creon® 25 000 capsule, e/c granules	1000	18 000	25 000
Creon® 40 000 capsule, e/c granules	1600	25 000	40 000
Nutrizym 22® capsule, e/c granules	1100	19 800	22 000
Pancrease HL® capsule, e/c granules	1250	22 500	25 000
Pancrex® granules (per gram)	300	4000	5000
Pancrex V® powder (per gram)	1400	30 000	25 000

Pancreatin is inactivated by gastric acid therefore pancreatin preparations are best taken with food (or immediately before or after food). In children with cystic fibrosis with persistent fat malabsorption despite optimal use of enzyme replacement, an **H_2-receptor antagonist** (section 1.3.1), or a **proton pump inhibitor** (section 1.3.5) may improve fat digestion and absorption. Enteric-coated preparations are designed to deliver a higher enzyme concentration in the duodenum (provided the capsule contents are swallowed whole without chewing). If the capsules are opened the enteric-coated granules should be mixed with milk, slightly acidic soft food or liquid such as apple juice, and then swallowed

1 Gastro-intestinal system

immediately without chewing. Any left-over food or liquid containing pancreatin should be discarded. Since pancreatin is also inactivated by heat, excessive heat should be avoided if preparations are mixed with liquids or food.

Pancreatin can irritate the perioral skin and buccal mucosa if retained in the mouth, and excessive doses can cause perianal irritation. Hypersensitivity reactions may occur particularly if the powder is handled.

PANCREATIN

Note The pancreatin preparations which follow are all of porcine origin

Cautions see CSM advice above; hyperuricaemia and hyperuricosuria have been associated with very high doses; **interactions:** Appendix 1 (pancreatin)

Side-effects nausea, vomiting, abdominal discomfort; skin and mucosal irritation (see notes above)

Indication and dose

Pancreatic insufficiency for dose see individual preparations, below

Creon® 10 000 (Solvay)

Capsules, brown/clear, enclosing buff-coloured e/c granules of pancreatin, providing: protease 600 units, lipase 10 000 units, amylase 8000 units. Net price 100-cap pack = £16.66. Counselling, see dose

Dose

- By mouth

  Child 1 month–18 years 1–2 capsules with meals either taken whole or contents mixed with fluid or soft food (then swallowed immediately without chewing), see notes above

Creon® Micro (Solvay)

Gastro-resistant granules, brown, pancreatin, providing: protease 2000 units, lipase 50 000 units, amylase 36 000 units/g, net price 20 g = £31.50. Counselling, see dose

Dose

- By mouth

  Neonate initially 100 mg before each feed; granules can be mixed with a small amount of breast milk or formula feed and administered immediately (manufacturer recommends mixing with a small amount of apple juice before administration)

  Child 1 month–18 years initially 100 mg before each feed or meal; granules can be mixed with a small amount of milk or soft food and administered immediately (manufacturer recommends mixing with acidic liquid or pureed fruit before administration); see notes above

  Note 100 mg granules = one measured scoopful (scoop supplied with product). Granules should not be chewed before swallowing.

Nutrizym 10® (Merck)

Capsules, red/yellow, enclosing e/c minitablets of pancreatin providing minimum of: protease 500 units, lipase 10 000 units, amylase 9000 units. Net price 100 = £14.47. Counselling, see dose

Dose

- By mouth

  Child 1 month–18 years 1–2 capsules with meals and 1 capsule with snacks, swallowed whole or contents taken with water or sprinkled on soft food (then swallowed immediately without chewing, see notes above); higher doses may be required according to response

Pancrease® (Janssen-Cilag)

Capsules, enclosing e/c beads of pancrelipase USP, providing minimum of: protease 330 units, lipase 5000 units, amylase 2900 units. Net price 100 = £16.22. Counselling, see dose

Dose

- By mouth

  Child 1 month–18 years 1–2 (occasionally 3) capsules during each meal and 1 capsule with snacks swallowed whole or contents sprinkled on slightly acidic liquid or soft food (then swallowed immediately without chewing); higher doses may be required according to response

Pancrex® (Paines & Byrne)

Granules, pancreatin, providing minimum of: protease 300 units, lipase 5000 units, amylase 4000 units/g. Net price 300 g = £20.39. Label: 25, counselling, see dose

Excipients: include lactose (7 g per 10 g dose)

Dose

- By mouth

  Child 2–18 years 5–10 g just before meals washed down or mixed with milk or water

Pancrex V® (Paines & Byrne)

Capsules, pancreatin, providing minimum of: protease 430 units, lipase 8000 units, amylase 9000 units. Net price 300-cap pack = £15.80. Counselling, see dose

Dose

- By mouth

  Child 1 month–1 year contents of 1–2 capsules mixed with feeds

  Child 1–18 years 2–6 capsules with meals, swallowed whole or sprinkled on food

Capsules '125', pancreatin, providing minimum of: protease 160 units, lipase 2950 units, amylase 3300 units. Net price 300-cap pack = £9.72. Counselling, see dose

Dose

- By mouth

  Neonate contents of 1–2 capsules in each feed (or mix with feed and give by spoon)

Tablets, e/c, pancreatin, providing minimum of: protease 110 units, lipase 1900 units, amylase 1700 units. Net price 300-tab pack = £4.51. Label: 5, 25, counselling, see dose

Dose

- By mouth

  Child 2–18 years 5–15 tablets before meals

Tablets forte, e/c, pancreatin, providing minimum of: protease 330 units, lipase 5600 units, amylase 5000 units. Net price 300-tab pack = £13.74. Label: 5, 25, counselling, see dose

Dose

- By mouth

  Child 2–18 years 6–10 tablets before meals

PANCREATIN (*continued*)

Powder, pancreatin, providing minimum of: protease 1400 units, lipase 25 000 units, amylase 30 000 units/g. Net price 300 g = £24.28. Counselling, see dose

Dose

- By mouth

Neonate 250–500 mg with each feed

Child 1 month–18 years 0.5–2 g with meals, washed down or mixed with milk or water

Higher-strength preparations

See **CSM** warning above

Counselling It is important to ensure adequate hydration at all times in children receiving higher-strength pancreatin preparations.

Creon® 25 000 (Solvay) PoM

Capsules, orange/clear, enclosing brown-coloured e/c pellets of pancreatin, providing: protease (total) 1000 units, lipase 25 000 units, amylase 18 000 units, net price 100-cap pack = £30.03. Counselling, see above and under dose

Dose

- By mouth

Child 2–18 years initially 1 capsule with meals either taken whole or contents mixed with fluid or soft food (then swallowed immediately without chewing), see notes above

Creon® 40 000 (Solvay) PoM

Capsules, brown/clear, enclosing brown-coloured e/c granules of pancreatin, providing: protease (total) 1600 units, lipase 40 000 units, amylase 25 000 units, net price 100-cap pack = £60.00. Counselling, see above and under dose

Dose

- By mouth

Child 2–18 years initially 1–2 capsules with meals either taken whole or contents mixed with fluid or soft food (then swallowed immediately without chewing), see notes above

Nutrizym 22® (Merck) PoM

Capsules, red/yellow, enclosing e/c minitablets of pancreatin, providing minimum of: protease 1100 units, lipase 22 000 units, amylase 19 800 units. Net price 100-cap pack = £33.33. Counselling, see above and under dose

Dose

- By mouth

Child 15–18 years 1–2 capsules with meals and 1 capsule with snacks, swallowed whole or contents taken with water or sprinkled on soft food (then swallowed immediately without chewing), see notes above

Pancrease HL® (Janssen-Cilag) PoM

Capsules, enclosing light brown e/c minitablets of pancreatin, providing minimum of: protease 1250 units, lipase 25 000 units, amylase 22 500 units. Net price 100 = £34.37. Counselling, see above and under dose

Dose

- By mouth

Child 15–18 years 1–2 capsules during each meal and 1 capsule with snacks swallowed whole or contents sprinkled on slightly acidic liquid or soft food (then swallowed immediately without chewing), see notes above

2 Cardiovascular system

2.1 Positive inotropic drugs

Positive inotropic drugs increase the force of contraction of the myocardium. Drugs which produce inotropic effects include cardiac glycosides, phosphodiesterase inhibitors, and some sympathomimetics (section 2.7.1).

2.1.1 Cardiac glycosides

The cardiac glycoside digoxin increases the force of myocardial contraction and reduces conductivity within the atrioventricular (AV) node.

Digoxin is most useful in the treatment of supraventricular tachycardias, especially for controlling ventricular response in persistent atrial fibrillation (section 2.3.1). Digoxin has a limited role in children with chronic heart failure; for reference to the role of digoxin in heart failure, see section 2.2.

For management of atrial fibrillation the maintenance dose of digoxin can usually be determined by the lowest acceptable ventricular rate at rest.

Digoxin is now rarely used for rapid control of heart rate (see section 2.3.1), even with intravenous administration, response may take many hours; persistence of tachycardia is therefore not an indication for exceeding the recommended dose. The intramuscular route is **not** recommended.

Unwanted effects depend both on the concentration of digoxin in the plasma and on the sensitivity of the conducting system or of the myocardium, which is often increased in heart disease. It may sometimes be difficult to distinguish between toxic effects and clinical deterioration because the symptoms of both are similar. Also, the plasma-digoxin concentration alone cannot indicate toxicity reliably but the likelihood of toxicity increases progressively through the range 1.5 to 3 micrograms/litre for digoxin. Renal function is very important in determining digoxin dosage.

Care should be taken to avoid hypokalaemia if a diuretic is used with a cardiac glycoside because hypokalaemia predisposes the child to digitalis toxicity. Hypokalaemia is managed by giving a potassium-sparing diuretic or, if necessary, potassium supplements (or foods rich in potassium).

Toxicity can often be managed by discontinuing digoxin and correcting hypokalaemia if appropriate; serious manifestations require urgent specialist management. **Digoxin-specific antibody fragments** are available for reversal of life-threatening overdosage (see below).

DIGOXIN

Cautions sick sinus syndrome; thyroid disease; hypoxia; avoid hypokalaemia or hypomagnesaemia (risk of digitalis toxicity); avoid rapid intravenous administration (nausea and risk of arrhythmias); **interactions:** Appendix 1 (cardiac glycosides)

Renal impairment reduce dose; toxicity increased by electrolyte disturbances, adjust dose according to plasma-digoxin concentration

Pregnancy may need dosage adjustment

Breast-feeding amount too small to be harmful

Contra-indications intermittent complete heart block, second degree AV block; supraventricular arrhythmias caused by Wolff-Parkinson-White syndrome; ventricular tachycardia or fibrillation; hypertrophic obstructive cardiomyopathy (unless concomitant atrial fibrillation and heart failure — but with caution)

Side-effects usually associated with excessive dosage, include: anorexia, nausea, vomiting, diarrhoea, abdominal pain; visual disturbances, headache, fatigue, drowsiness, confusion, delirium, hallucinations, depression; arrhythmias, heart block; rarely rash, intestinal ischaemia; gynaecomastia on long-term use; thrombocytopenia reported; see also notes above

Pharmacokinetics For plasma-digoxin concentration assay, blood should ideally be taken at least 6 hours after a dose; plasma-digoxin concentration should be maintained in the range 0.8–2 micrograms/litre (see also notes above)

DIGOXIN (*continued*)

Licensed use heart failure, supraventricular arrhythmias

Indication and dose

Supraventricular arrhythmias and chronic heart failure (see also notes above) consult product literature for details

- By mouth

Neonate under 1.5 kg initially 25 micrograms/kg daily in 3 divided doses for 24 hours then 4–6 micrograms/kg daily in 1–2 divided doses

Neonate 1.5–2.5 kg initially 30 micrograms/kg daily in 3 divided doses for 24 hours then 4–6 micrograms/kg daily in 1–2 divided doses

Neonate over 2.5 kg initially 45 micrograms/kg daily in 3 divided doses for 24 hours then 10 micrograms/kg daily in 1–2 divided doses

Child 1 month–2 years initially 45 micrograms/kg daily in 3 divided doses for 24 hours then 10 micrograms/kg daily in 1–2 divided doses

Child 2–5 years initially 35 micrograms/kg daily in 3 divided doses for 24 hours then 10 micrograms/kg daily in 1–2 divided doses

Child 5–10 years initially 25 micrograms/kg daily (max. 750 micrograms daily) in 3 divided doses for 24 hours then 6 micrograms/kg daily (max. 250 micrograms daily) in 1–2 divided doses

Child 10–18 years initially 0.75–1.5 mg daily in 3 divided doses for 24 hours then 62.5–750 micrograms daily in 1–2 divided doses

- By intravenous infusion (but rarely necessary)

Neonate under 1.5 kg initially 20 micrograms/kg daily in 3 divided doses for 24 hours then 4–6 micrograms/kg daily in 1–2 divided doses

Neonate 1.5–2.5 kg initially 30 micrograms/kg daily in 3 divided doses for 24 hours then 4–6 micrograms/kg daily in 1–2 divided doses

Neonate over 2.5 kg initially 35 micrograms/kg daily in 3 divided doses for 24 hours then 10 micrograms/kg daily in 1–2 divided doses

Child 1 month–2 years initially 35 micrograms/kg daily in 3 divided doses for 24 hours then 10 micrograms/kg daily in 1–2 divided doses

Child 2–5 years initially 35 micrograms/kg daily in 3 divided doses for 24 hours then 10 micrograms/kg daily in 1–2 divided doses

Child 5–10 years initially 25 micrograms/kg daily (max. 500 micrograms daily) in 3 divided doses for 24 hours then 6 micrograms/kg daily (max. 250 micrograms daily) in 1–2 divided doses

Child 10–18 years initially 0.5–1 mg daily in 3 divided doses for 24 hours then 62.5–750 micrograms daily in 1–2 divided doses

Less urgent digitalisation

- By mouth

Rapid digitalisation may not always be required.

Child 10–18 years 250–500 micrograms daily (higher dose may be divided) for 5–7 days followed by maintenance dose

Note The above doses may need to be reduced if digoxin (or another cardiac glycoside) has been given in the preceding 2 weeks. When switching from intravenous to oral route may need to increase dose by 20–30% to maintain the same plasma digoxin concentration. Plasma monitoring may be required when changing formulation to take account of varying bioavailabilities. For plasma concentration monitoring, blood should ideally be taken at least 6 hours after a dose

Administration For *intravenous infusion*, dilute with sodium chloride 0.9% intravenous infusion *or* glucose 5% to a max. concentration of 50 micrograms/mL; loading doses should be given over 30–60 minutes and maintenance dose over 10–20 minutes.

For *oral* administration, oral solution must **not** be diluted

Digoxin (Non-proprietary) PoM

Tablets, digoxin 62.5 micrograms, net price 20 = 58p; 125 micrograms, 20 = 43p; 250 micrograms, 20 = 43p

Injection, digoxin 250 micrograms/mL, net price 2-mL amp = 70p

Excipients: include alcohol, propylene glycol (see excipients)

Available from Antigen

Paediatric injection, digoxin 100 micrograms/mL

Available as a manufactured special

Lanoxin® (GSK) PoM

Tablets, digoxin 125 micrograms, net price 20 = 32p; 250 micrograms (scored), 20 = 32p

Injection, digoxin 250 micrograms/mL. Net price 2-mL amp = 66p

Lanoxin-PG® (GSK) PoM

Tablets, blue, digoxin 62.5 micrograms. Net price 20 = 32p

Elixir, yellow, digoxin 50 micrograms/mL. Do not dilute, measure with pipette. Net price 60 mL = £5.35. Counselling, use of pipette

2 Cardiovascular system

Digoxin-specific antibody

Digoxin-specific antibody fragments are indicated for the treatment of known or strongly suspected digoxin or digitoxin overdosage, where measures beyond the withdrawal of the cardiac glycoside and correction of any electrolyte abnormality are felt to be necessary (see also notes above).

Digibind® (GSK) PoM

Injection, powder for preparation of infusion, digoxin-specific antibody fragments (F(ab)) 38 mg. Net price per vial = £93.97 (hosp. and poisons centres only)

Dose

Consult product literature or Poisons Information Centre

2.1.2 Phosphodiesterase inhibitors

Enoximone and **milrinone** are selective phosphodiesterase inhibitors which exert most of their effect on the myocardium. They possess positive inotropic and vasodilator activity and are useful in infants and children with low cardiac output especially after cardiac surgery. Phosphodiesterase inhibitors should be limited to short-term use because long-term oral administration has been associated with increased mortality in adults with congestive heart failure.

ENOXIMONE

Cautions heart failure associated with hypertrophic cardiomyopathy, stenotic or obstructive valvular disease or other outlet obstruction; monitor blood pressure, heart rate, ECG, central venous pressure, fluid and electrolyte status, renal function, platelet count, hepatic enzymes; avoid extravasation

Hepatic impairment dose reduction may be required in hepatic impairment

Renal impairment consider dose reduction in renal impairment

Pregnancy manufacturer advises use only if potential benefit outweighs risk

Breast-feeding manufacturer advises caution—no information available

Side-effects ectopic beats; less frequently ventricular tachycardia or supraventricular arrhythmias (more likely in children with pre-existing arrhythmias); hypotension; also headache, insomnia, nausea and vomiting, diarrhoea; occasionally, chills, oliguria, fever, urinary retention; upper and lower limb pain

Licensed use not licensed for use in children

Indication and dose

Congestive heart failure, low cardiac output following cardiac surgery

- **By intravenous injection and continuous intravenous infusion**

Neonate initial loading dose of 500 micrograms/kg *by slow intravenous injection*, followed by 5–20 micrograms/kg/minute *by continuous intravenous infusion* over 24 hours adjusted according to response; max 24 mg/kg over 24 hours

Child 1 month–18 years initial loading dose of 500 micrograms/kg *by slow intravenous injection*, followed by 5–20 micrograms/kg/minute *by continuous intravenous infusion* over 24 hours adjusted according to response; max. 24 mg/kg over 24 hours

Administration For *intravenous* administration dilute to concentration of 2.5mg/mL with sodium chloride 0.9% intravenous infusion *or* water for injections; the initial loading dose should be given by slow intravenous injection over at least 15 minutes

Perfan® (Myogen) PoM

Injection, enoximone 5 mg/mL. For dilution before use. Net price 20-mL amp = £15.02

Excipients: include alcohol, propylene glycol

Note Plastic apparatus should be used; crystal formation if glass used

MILRINONE

Cautions see under Enoximone; also correct hypokalaemia, monitor renal function

Renal impairment reduce dose in renal impairment; monitor response

Pregnancy manufacturer advises use only if potential benefit outweighs risk

Breast-feeding manufacturer advises caution—no information available

Side-effects see under Enoximone; also chest pain, tremor, bronchospasm, anaphylaxis, thrombocytopenia and rash reported

Licensed use not licensed for use in children

Indication and dose

Congestive heart failure, low cardiac output following cardiac surgery, shock

- **By intravenous infusion**

Neonate initially 50–75 micrograms/kg over 30–60 minutes (reduce or omit initial dose if at risk of hypotension) then 30–45 micrograms/kg/hour by continuous intravenous infusion for 2–3 days (usually for 12 hours after cardiac surgery)

Child 1 month–18 years initially 50–75 micrograms/kg over 30–60 minutes (reduce or omit initial dose if at risk of hypotension) then 30–45 micrograms/kg/hour by continuous intravenous infusion for 2–3 days (usually for 12 hours after cardiac surgery)

Administration For *intravenous infusion* dilute with glucose 5% *or* sodium chloride 0.9% *or* sodium chloride and glucose intravenous infusion to a concentration of 200 micrograms/mL, (higher concentrations of 400 micrograms/mL have been used)

Primacor® (Sanofi-Synthelabo) PoM

Injection, milrinone (as lactate) 1 mg/mL. For dilution before use. Net price 10-mL amp = £16.61

2.2 Diuretics

Diuretics are used for a variety of conditions in children including pulmonary oedema (caused by conditions such as respiratory distress syndrome and bronchopulmonary dysplasia), congestive heart failure, and hypertension. Hypertension in children is often resistant to therapy and may require the use of several drugs in combination (see section 2.5). Maintenance of fluid and electrolyte balance can be difficult in children on diuretics, particularly neonates whose renal function may be immature.

Thiazides (section 2.2.1) are often used in combination with loop diuretics or spironolactone in the management of pulmonary oedema and, in lower doses, for hypertension associated with cardiac disease.

Loop diuretics (section 2.2.2) are used more frequently than thiazide diuretics. They are used for pulmonary oedema, congestive heart failure, and hypertension in cardiac or renal disease.

Aminophylline infusion has been used with intravenous furosemide to relieve fluid overload in critically ill children.

Heart failure Heart failure is less common in children than in adults; it may occur as a result of congenital heart disease (e.g. septal defects), dilated cardiomyopathy, myocarditis, or cardiac surgery.

Acute heart failure may occur after cardiac surgery or as a complication in severe acute infections with or without myocarditis. Therapy consists of volume loading, vasodilator or inotropic drugs.

Chronic heart failure is initially treated with a **loop diuretic** (section 2.2.2), usually furosemide supplemented with spironolactone or potassium.

If diuresis with furosemide is insufficient, the addition of metolazone or a thiazide diuretic (section 2.2.1) may be considered. With metolazone, the resulting diuresis may be profound and care is needed to avoid potentially dangerous electrolyte disturbance.

If diuretics are insufficient an ACE inhibitor or digoxin may be used. **ACE inhibitors** (section 2.5.5.1) are used for the treatment of all grades of heart failure in adults and may also be useful for children with heart failure.

Some beta-blockers improve outcome in adults with heart failure, but data on beta-blockers in children are limited. **Carvedilol** (section 2.4) has vasodilatory properties and therefore (like ACE inhibitors) also lowers afterload.

In children receiving specialist cardiology care, the selective phosphodiesterase inhibitor **enoximone** is sometimes used by mouth for its inotropic and vasodilator effects. **Spironolactone** (section 2.2.3) is usually used as a potassium-sparing drug with a loop diuretic; in adults low doses of spironolactone are effective in the treatment of heart failure. Careful monitoring of serum potassium is necessary if spironolactone is used in combination with an ACE inhibitor.

Potassium loss Hypokalaemia may occur with both thiazide and loop diuretics. The risk of hypokalaemia depends on the duration of action as well as the potency and is thus greater with thiazides than with an equipotent dose of a loop diuretic.

Hypokalaemia is particularly dangerous in children being treated with cardiac glycosides. In hepatic failure hypokalaemia caused by diuretics can precipitate encephalopathy.

The use of potassium-sparing diuretics (section 2.2.3) avoids the need to take potassium supplements.

2.2.1 Thiazides and related diuretics

Thiazides and related compounds are moderately potent diuretics; they inhibit sodium reabsorption at the beginning of the distal convoluted tubule. They are usually administered early in the day so that the diuresis does not interfere with sleep.

In the management of *hypertension* a low dose of a thiazide produces a maximal or near-maximal blood pressure lowering effect, with very little biochemical disturbance. Higher doses cause more marked changes in plasma potassium, sodium, uric acid, glucose, and lipids, with little advantage in blood pressure control. For reference to the use of thiazides in chronic heart failure see section 2.2.

Bendroflumethiazide is licensed for use in children; **chlorothiazide** is also used.

Metolazone is particularly effective when combined with a loop diuretic (even in renal failure) and is most effective when given 30–60 minutes before furosemide; profound diuresis may occur and the child should therefore be monitored carefully.

BENDROFLUMETHIAZIDE

(Bendrofluazide)

Cautions electrolytes may need to be monitored with high doses or in renal impairment, aggravates diabetes and gout; may exacerbate systemic lupus erythematosus; **interactions:** Appendix 1 (diuretics)

Pregnancy not used to treat hypertension in pregnancy; may cause neonatal thrombocytopenia

Breast-feeding amount too small to be harmful; large doses may suppress lactation

Contra-indications refractory hypokalaemia, hyponatraemia, hypercalcaemia; symptomatic hyperuricaemia; Addison's disease

Hepatic impairment avoid in severe liver disease; hypokalaemia may precipitate coma (potassium-sparing diuretics can prevent)

Renal impairment avoid if creatinine clearance less than 30 mL/minute/1.73m^2—ineffective

Side-effects postural hypotension and mild gastro-intestinal effects; impotence (reversible on withdrawal of treatment); hypokalaemia (see also notes above), hypomagnesaemia, hyponatraemia, hypercalcaemia, hypochloraemic alkalosis, hyperuricaemia, gout, hyperglycaemia, and altered plasma lipid concentration; less commonly rashes, photosensitivity; blood disorders (including neutropenia and thrombocytopenia—when given in late pregnancy neonatal thrombocytopenia has been reported); pancreatitis, intrahepatic cholestasis, and hypersensitivity reactions (including pneumonitis, pulmonary oedema, severe skin reactions) also reported

Indication and dose

Oedema and hypertension
- By mouth

Child 1 month–2 years 50–100 micrograms/kg daily adjusted according to response

Child 2–12 years initially 50–400 micrograms/kg daily (max. 10 mg daily) then 50–100 micrograms/kg daily adjusted according to response

Child 12–18 years initially 5–10 mg daily or on alternate days (2.5 mg in hypertension) as a single morning dose, adjusted according to response

Bendroflumethiazide (Non-proprietary) PoM

Tablets, bendroflumethiazide 2.5 mg, net price 20 = 83p; 5 mg, 20 = 59p

Brands include *Aprinox®*, *Neo-NaClex®*

Extemporaneous formulations available see Extemporaneous Preparations, p. 8

CHLOROTHIAZIDE

Cautions see under Bendroflumethiazide; neonate (theoretical risk of kernicterus if very jaundiced); **interactions**: Appendix 1 (diuretics)

Pregnancy see under Bendroflumethiazide

Breast-feeding see under Bendroflumethiazide

Contra-indications see under Bendroflumethiazide

Hepatic impairment avoid in severe liver disease; hypokalaemia may precipitate coma (potassium-sparing diuretics can prevent)

Renal impairment avoid if creatinine clearance less than 30 mL/minute/1.73 m^2—ineffective

Side-effects see under Bendroflumethiazide

Licensed use Not licensed

Indication and dose

Heart failure, hypertension
- By mouth

Neonate 10–20 mg/kg twice daily

Child 1–6 months 10–20 mg/kg twice daily

Child 6 months–12 years 10 mg/kg twice daily (max. 1 g daily)

Child 12–18 years 0.25–1 g once daily *or* 125–500 mg twice daily

Chronic hypoglycaemia section 6.1.4

Diabetes insipidus section 6.5.2

Preparations

Chlorothiazide oral suspension 250 mg/5 mL is available from specialist manufacturers and specialist importing companies

METOLAZONE

Cautions see under Bendroflumethiazide; also profound diuresis on concomitant administration with furosemide (monitor child carefully); porphyria (section 9.8.2)

Renal impairment remains effective in moderate impairment but risk of excessive diuresis

Pregnancy see under Bendroflumethiazide

Breast-feeding see under Bendroflumethiazide

Contra-indications see under Bendroflumethiazide

Hepatic impairment see under Bendroflumethiazide

Side-effects see under Bendroflumethiazide

Licensed use Not licensed for use in children

Indication and dose

Oedema resistant to loop diuretics; adjunct to loop diuretics to induce diuresis
- By mouth

Child 1 month–12 years 100–200 micrograms/kg once or twice a day

Child 12–18 years 5–10 mg once daily in the morning, increased to 5–10 mg twice daily in resistant oedema; max. 80 mg daily

Administration Tablets may be crushed and mixed with water immediately before use

Metenix 5® (Borg) PoM
Tablets, blue, metolazone 5 mg. Net price 100-tab pack = £20.37

Extemporaneous formulations available see Extemporaneous Preparations, p. 8

2.2.2 Loop diuretics

Loop diuretics inhibit reabsorption of sodium, potassium and chloride from the ascending limb of the loop of Henlé in the renal tubule and are powerful diuretics. Hypokalaemia may develop, and care is needed to avoid hypotension.

Furosemide (frusemide) and **bumetanide** are similar in activity; the diuresis associated with these drugs is dose related. In children with impaired renal function very large doses may occasionally be needed; in such doses both drugs can cause deafness and bumetanide can cause myalgia. Furosemide is extensively used in children. It may be used for pulmonary oedema (e.g. in respiratory distress syndrome and bronchopulmonary dysplasia), congestive heart failure, and hypertension due to cardiac or renal disease. Furosemide may occasionally cause ototoxicity but the risk can be reduced by giving large oral doses in 2 or more divided doses. Long-term use of furosemide in neonates may lead to nephrocalcinosis due to increased urinary calcium loss; a thiazide may be of value in this case.

FUROSEMIDE

(Frusemide)

Cautions hypotension; correct hypovolaemia before using in oliguria; precomatose states associated with liver cirrhosis; some liquid preparations contain alcohol, caution especially in neonates; **interactions:** Appendix 1 (diuretics)

Hepatic impairment hypokalaemia may precipitate coma (use potassium-sparing diuretic to prevent this)

Renal impairment in moderate impairment, may need high doses; deafness may follow rapid intravenous injection

Pregnancy not to be used to treat hypertension in pregnancy

Breast-feeding amount too small to be harmful

Contra-indications renal failure with anuria

Side-effects hyponatraemia, hypokalaemia (see also section 2.2), and hypomagnesaemia, hypochloraemic alkalosis, increased calcium excretion and nephrocalcinosis (especially in neonates with prolonged use), hypotension; less commonly nausea, gastro-intestinal disturbances, hyperuricaemia and gout; hyperglycaemia (less common than with thiazides); rarely rashes, photosensitivity and bone marrow depression (withdraw treatment), pancreatitis (with large parenteral doses), tinnitus and deafness (usually with large parenteral doses and rapid administration and in renal impairment)

Licensed use Not licensed for use in children for hypertension

Indication and dose

Oedema and hypertension
- By mouth

Neonate 0.5–2 mg/kg every 12–24 hours (every 24 hours if postmenstrual age under 31 weeks)

Child 1 month–12 years 0.5–2 mg/kg 2–3 times a day (every 24 hours if postmenstrual age under 31 weeks); higher doses may be required in resistant oedema; max. 12 mg/kg daily, not to exceed 80 mg daily

Child 12–18 years 20–40 mg daily, increased in resistant oedema to 80 mg daily or more

- By slow intravenous injection

Neonate 0.5–1 mg/kg every 12–24 hours (every 24 hours if post-menstrual age under 31 weeks)

Child 1 month–12 years 0.5–1 mg/kg (max. 4 mg/kg) repeated every 8 hours as necessary

FUROSEMIDE (*continued*)

Child 12–18 years 20–40 mg repeated every 8 hours as necessary; higher doses may be required in resistant cases

- **By continuous intravenous infusion**

Child 1 month–18 years 0.1–2 mg/kg/hour (following cardiac surgery, initially 100 micrograms/kg/hour, doubled every 2 hours until urine output exceeds 1 mL/kg/hour)

Oliguria
- **By mouth**

Child 12–18 years initially 250 mg daily; if necessary, dose increased in steps of 250 mg given every 4–6 hours; max. single dose 2 g (rarely used)

- **By intravenous infusion**

Child 1 month–12 years 2–5 mg/kg up to 4 times daily (max. 1 g daily)

Child 12–18 years initially 250 mg over 1 hour (rate not exceeding 4 mg/minute), increase to 500 mg over 2 hours if satisfactory urine output not obtained, then give a further 1 g over 4 hours if no satisfactory response within subsequent hour, if no response obtained dialysis probably required; effective dose (up to 1 g) can be repeated every 24 hours

Administration For administration *by mouth* tablets may be crushed and mixed with water *or* injection solution diluted and given by mouth; for *intravenous injection* give over 5–10 minutes at a usual rate of 100 micrograms/kg/minute (not exceeding 500 micrograms/kg/minute), max. 4 mg/minute; for *intravenous infusion* dilute with sodium chloride 0.9% intravenous infusion to a concentration of 1–2 mg/mL—glucose solutions unsuitable (infusion pH must be above 5.5)

Furosemide (Non-proprietary) PoM

Tablets, furosemide 20 mg, net price 28 = 93p; 40 mg, 28-tab pack = £1.05; 500 mg, 28 = £7.72
Brands include *Froop®*, *Rusyde®*

Oral solution, sugar-free, furosemide, net price 20 mg/5 mL, 150 mL = £12.07; 40 mg/5 mL, 150 mL = £15.58; 50 mg/5 mL, 150 mL = £16.84
Brands include *Frusol®* (contains alcohol 10%)

Injection, furosemide 10 mg/mL, net price 2-mL amp = 55p; 5-mL amp = 66p

Lasix® (Sanofi-Aventis) PoM

Injection, furosemide 10 mg/mL, net price 2-mL amp = 78p
Note Large-volume furosemide injections also available; brands include *Minijet®*

BUMETANIDE

Cautions see under Furosemide

Hepatic impairment hypokalaemia may precipitate coma (use potassium-sparing diuretic to prevent this)

Renal impairment may need high doses in moderate impairment

Pregnancy not to be used for treating hypertension in pregnancy

Breast-feeding manufacturer advises avoid if possible—no information available

Contra-indications see under Furosemide

Side-effects see under Furosemide; also myalgia

Licensed use Not licensed for use in children under 12 years

Indication and dose

Oedema
- **By mouth**

Child 1 month–12 years 15–50 micrograms/kg 1–4 times daily (max. single dose 2 mg); do not exceed 5 mg daily

Child 12–18 years 1 mg in the morning, repeated after 6–8 hours if necessary; severe cases up to 5 mg daily

- **By intravenous injection**

Child 12–18 years 1–2 mg, repeated after 20 minutes if necessary

- **By intravenous infusion over 30–60 minutes**

Child 1 month–12 years 25–50 micrograms/kg

Child 12–18 years 1–5 mg

Administration For *intravenous infusion*, dilute with glucose 5% intravenous infusion *or* sodium chloride 0.9% intravenous infusion to a concentration of 24 micrograms/mL

Bumetanide (Non-proprietary) PoM

Tablets, bumetanide 1 mg, net price 28-tab pack = £1.71; 5 mg, 28-tab pack = £11.14

Liquid, bumetanide 1 mg/5 mL, net price 150 mL = £15.22
Available from Leo

Injection, bumetanide 500 micrograms/mL, net price 4-mL amp = £1.79

Burinex® (Leo) PoM

Tablets, both scored, bumetanide 1 mg, net price 28-tab pack = £1.52; 5 mg, 28 = £9.67

Extemporaneous formulations available see Extemporaneous Preparations, p. 8

2.2.3 Potassium-sparing diuretics and aldosterone antagonists

Spironolactone is the most commonly used potassium-sparing diuretic in children; it is an aldosterone antagonist and enhances potassium retention and sodium excretion in the distal tubule. Spironolactone is combined with other diuretics to reduce urinary potassium loss. It is also used in the long-term management of Bartter's syndrome and high doses can help to control ascites in babies with chronic neonatal hepatitis. The clinical value of spironolactone in the management of pulmonary oedema in preterm neonates with chronic lung disease is uncertain.

Amiloride on its own is a weak diuretic. It causes retention of potassium and is therefore used as an alternative to giving potassium supplements with thiazide or loop diuretics (see section 2.2.4 for compound preparations with thiazides or loop diuretics).

A potassium-sparing diuretic such as spironolactone or amiloride may also be used in the management of amphotericin-induced hypokalaemia.

Potassium supplements must **not** be given with potassium-sparing diuretics. It is also important to bear in mind that administration of a potassium-sparing diuretic to a child receiving an ACE inhibitor or an angiotensin-II receptor antagonist (section 2.5.5) can cause severe hyperkalaemia.

AMILORIDE HYDROCHLORIDE

Cautions diabetes mellitus; **interactions:** Appendix 1 (diuretics)

Renal impairment monitor plasma-potassium concentration (high risk of hyperkalaemia in renal impairment)

Pregnancy not to be used for treating hypertension in pregnancy

Breast-feeding manufacturer advises avoid—no information available

Contra-indications hyperkalaemia, renal failure

Side-effects include gastro-intestinal disturbances, dry mouth, rashes, confusion, postural hypotension, hyperkalaemia, hyponatraemia

Licensed use Not licensed for use in children

Indication and dose

Adjunct to thiazide and loop diuretics in oedema (where potassium conservation desirable)

- **By mouth**

Neonate 100–200 micrograms/kg twice daily

Child 1 month–12 years 100–200 micrograms/kg twice daily; max. 20 mg daily

Child 12–18 years 5–10 mg twice daily

Amiloride (Non-proprietary) PoM

Tablets, amiloride hydrochloride 5 mg, net price 28 = £1.46

Oral solution, sugar-free, amiloride hydrochloride 5 mg/5 mL, net price 150 mL = £37.35

Brands include *Amilamont®*

Compound preparations with thiazide or loop diuretics

See section 2.2.4

Aldosterone antagonists

SPIRONOLACTONE

Cautions potential metabolic products carcinogenic in *rodents*; monitor electrolytes (discontinue if hyperkalaemia); porphyria (section 9.8.2); **interactions:** Appendix 1 (diuretics)

Renal impairment in mild impairment monitor plasma-potassium concentration; avoid in moderate to severe impairment

Pregnancy feminisation of male fetus in *animal* studies

Breast-feeding metabolites present in milk but unlikely to be harmful; manufacturer advises avoid

Contra-indications hyperkalaemia, hyponatraemia; Addison's disease

Side-effects gastro-intestinal disturbances; impotence, gynaecomastia; menstrual irregularities; lethargy, headache, confusion; rashes; hyperkalaemia (discontinue); hyponatraemia; hepatotoxicity, osteomalacia, and blood disorders reported

Licensed use Not licensed for reduction of hypokalaemia induced by diuretics or amphotericin

Indication and dose

Diuresis in congestive cardiac failure, ascites and oedema, reduction of hypokalaemia induced by diuretics or amphotericin

- **By mouth**

Neonate 1–2 mg/kg daily in 1–2 divided doses; up to 7 mg/kg daily in resistant ascites

Child 1 month–12 years 1–3 mg/kg daily in 1–2 divided doses; up to 9 mg/kg daily in resistant ascites

Child 12–18 years 50–100 mg daily in 1–2 divided doses; up to 9 mg/kg daily (max. 400 mg daily) in resistant ascites

SPIRONOLACTONE (*continued*)

Spironolactone (Non-proprietary) PoM
Tablets, spironolactone 25 mg, net price 28 = £3.02; 50 mg, 28 = £4.22; 100 mg, 28 = £4.51
Brands include *Spirospare®*

Oral suspensions, sugar-free, spironolactone 5 mg/5 mL, 10 mg/5 mL, 25 mg/5 mL, 50 mg/5 mL and 100 mg/5 mL
Available from Rosemont as a manufactured special

Aldactone® (Searle) PoM
Tablets, all f/c, spironolactone 25 mg (buff), net price 100-tab pack = £8.89; 50 mg (off-white), 100-tab pack = £17.78; 100 mg (buff), 28-tab pack = £9.96

2.2.4 Potassium-sparing diuretics with other diuretics

Although it is preferable to prescribe diuretics separately in children, the use of fixed combinations may be justified if compliance is a problem. The most commonly used preparations are listed below (but they may not be licensed for use in children—consult product literature), for other preparations see the BNF. For **interactions**, see Appendix 1 (diuretics).

Amiloride with thiazides

Co-amilozide (Non-proprietary) PoM
Tablets, co-amilozide 2.5/25 (amiloride hydrochloride 2.5 mg, hydrochlorothiazide 25 mg), net price 28-tab pack = £1.85
Brands include *Moduret 25®*

Amiloride with loop diuretics

Co-amilofruse (Non-proprietary) PoM
Tablets, co-amilofruse 2.5/20 (amiloride hydrochloride 2.5 mg, furosemide 20 mg). Net price 28-tab pack = £2.01, 56-tab pack = £2.64
Brands include *Frumil LS®*

Tablets, co-amilofruse 5/40 (amiloride hydrochloride 5 mg, furosemide 40 mg). Net price 28-tab pack = £1.47
Brands include *Froop-Co®*, *Fru-Co®*, *Frumil®*, *Lasoride®*

2.2.5 Osmotic diuretics

Osmotic diuretics are rarely used in heart failure as they may acutely expand the blood volume. **Mannitol** has a valuable role in preventing or minimising the damage caused by acute cerebral oedema, usually following cerebral trauma, and in reducing raised intracranial pressure. Mannitol is also used to reduce raised intra-ocular pressure (section 11.6).

MANNITOL

Cautions extravasation causes inflammation and thrombophlebitis, monitor fluid and electrolyte balance, serum osmolality, and renal function

Contra-indications congestive cardiac failure, pulmonary oedema, intracranial bleeding after head injury, dehydration

Side-effects chills, fever

Indication and dose

Cerebral oedema, raised intra-ocular pressure
- By intravenous infusion over 30 minutes

Neonate 0.5–1 g/kg (2.5–5 mL/kg of 20% solution) repeated if necessary 1–2 times after 4–8 hours

Child 1 month–18 years 0.5–1.5 g/kg (2.5–7.5 mL/kg of 20% solution) repeated if necessary 1–2 times after 4–8 hours

Peripheral oedema and ascites
- By intravenous infusion over 2–6 hours

Child 1 month–18 years 1–2 g/kg

Administration Examine infusion for crystals; if crystals present, dissolve by warming infusion fluid (allow to cool to body temperature before administration); use 5-micron in-line filter

Mannitol (Baxter) PoM
Intravenous infusion, mannitol 10% and 20%

2.2.6 Mercurial diuretics

Classification not used in BNF for Children.

2.2.7 Carbonic anhydrase inhibitors

The carbonic anhydrase inhibitor **acetazolamide** is a weak diuretic although it is little used for its diuretic effect. Acetazolamide and eye drops of dorzolamide and brinzolamide inhibit the formation of aqueous humour and are used in glaucoma (section 11.6). In children, acetazolamide is also used in the treatment of epilepsy (section 4.8.1), and raised intracranial pressure (section 11.6).

2.2.8 Diuretics with potassium

Diuretics and potassium supplements should be prescribed separately for children.

2.3 Anti-arrhythmic drugs

2.3.1 Management of arrhythmias

Management of an arrhythmia requires precise diagnosis of the type of arrhythmia; electrocardiography and referral to a paediatric cardiologist is essential; underlying causes such as heart failure require appropriate treatment.

Arrhythmias may be broadly divided into bradycardias, supraventricular tachycardias, and ventricular arrhythmias.

Bradycardia Adrenaline (epinephrine) is useful in the treatment of symptomatic bradycardia in an infant or child.

Supraventricular tachycardias

In supraventricular tachycardia adenosine is given by rapid intravenous injection. If necessary, injections are repeated every 2 minutes and the dose is increased with each injection. If adenosine is ineffective, intravenous amiodarone, flecainide, or a beta-blocker (such as esmolol, see section 2.4) may be tried; verapamil may also be considered in children over 1 year. Atenolol and sotalol (section 2.4) are used for the prophylaxis of paroxysmal supraventricular tachycardias.

The use of d.c. shock and vagal stimulation also have a role in the treatment of supraventricular tachycardia.

Wolff-Parkinson-White syndrome Amiodarone, flecainide, or a beta-blocker are used to prevent recurrence of supraventricular tachycardia in infants and young children with Wolff-Parkinson-White syndrome.

Atrial flutter In atrial flutter without structural heart defects, sinus rhythm is established with d.c. shock and drug treatment is usually not necessary. Amiodarone is used in atrial flutter when structural heart defects are present or after heart surgery. Sotalol (section 2.4) may also be considered.

Atrial fibrillation In atrial fibrillation, d.c. shock is used to restore sinus rhythm; beta-blockers, together with digoxin, may be useful for ventricular rate control especially in children with thyrotoxicosis.

Ectopic tachycardia Intravenous amiodarone is used in conjunction with body cooling and synchronised pacing in *postoperative* junctional ectopic tachycardia. Oral amiodarone or flecainide are used in *congenital* junctional ectopic tachycardia.

Amiodarone, flecainide, or a beta-blocker are used in atrial ectopic tachycardia; amiodarone is preferred in those with poor ventricular function.

Ventricular tachycardia and ventricular fibrillation

Pulseless ventricular tachycardia or ventricular fibrillation requires resuscitation, see Paediatric Advanced Life Support algorithm (inside back cover). Amiodarone is used in resuscitation for pulseless ventricular tachycardia or ventricular fibrillation unresponsive to d.c. shock; lidocaine may be used as an alternative to amiodarone.

Amiodarone is also used in a haemodynamically stable child where drug treatment is required; lidocaine may be used as an alternative to amiodarone.

Torsades de pointes Intravenous magnesium sulphate injection (section 9.5.1.3) may be used to treat torsades de pointes (dose recommendations vary—consult local guidelines). Anti-arrhythmics (including lidocaine) may further prolong the QT interval, thus worsening the condition.

2.3.2 Drugs for arrhythmias

Anti-arrhythmic drugs can be classified clinically as those acting on supraventricular arrhythmias (adenosine, digoxin, and verapamil), those acting on both supraventricular and ventricular arrhythmias (amiodarone, beta-blockers, disopyramide, flecainide, procainamide, and quinidine), and those acting on ventricular arrhythmias (lidocaine (lignocaine)). For the treatment of bradycardia see section 2.3.1.

Anti-arrhythmic drugs can also be classified according to their effects on the electrical behaviour of myocardial cells during activity (the Vaughan Williams classification) although this classification is of less clinical significance:

> Class Ia, b, c: membrane stabilising drugs (e.g. quinidine, lidocaine, flecainide respectively)
>
> Class II: beta-blockers
>
> Class III: amiodarone and sotalol (also Class II)
>
> Class IV: calcium-channel blockers (includes verapamil but not dihydropyridines)

Cautions The negative inotropic effects of anti-arrhythmic drugs tend to be additive. Therefore special care should be taken if two or more are used, especially if myocardial function is impaired. Most or all drugs that are effective in countering arrhythmias can also provoke them in some circumstances; moreover, hypokalaemia enhances the arrhythmogenic (pro-arrhythmic) effect of many drugs.

Adenosine is the treatment of choice for terminating supraventricular tachycardias, including those associated with Wolff-Parkinson-White syndrome. It is also used in the diagnosis of supraventricular arrhythmias. It is not negatively inotropic and does not cause significant hypotension; it may be used safely in children with impaired cardiac function or post-operative arrhythmias. The injection should be administered by rapid intravenous injection into a central or large peripheral vein.

Amiodarone is useful in the management of both supraventricular and ventricular tachyarrhythmias. It may be given by intravenous infusion and by mouth and causes little or no myocardial depression. Unlike oral amiodarone, intravenous amiodarone acts relatively rapidly. Intravenous amiodarone is also used in cardiopulmonary resuscitation for ventricular fibrillation or pulseless ventricular tachycardia unresponsive to d.c. shock (see algorithm, inside back cover).

Amiodarone has a very long half-life (extending to several weeks) and only needs to be given once daily (but high doses may cause nausea unless divided). Many weeks or months may be required to achieve steady-state plasma-amiodarone concentration; this is particularly important when drug interactions are likely (see also Appendix 1).

Most patients taking amiodarone develop corneal microdeposits (reversible on withdrawal of treatment); these rarely interfere with vision, but drivers may be dazzled by headlights at night. However, if vision is impaired or if optic neuritis or optic neuropathy occur, amiodarone must be stopped to prevent blindness and expert advice sought. Because of the possibility of phototoxic reactions, children and carers should be advised to shield the child's skin from light during treatment and for several months after discontinuing amiodarone; a wide-spectrum sunscreen (section 13.8.1) should be used to protect against both long ultraviolet and visible light.

Amiodarone contains iodine and can cause disorders of thyroid function; both hypothyroidism and hyperthyroidism may occur. Clinical assessment alone is unreliable, and laboratory tests should be performed before treatment and every 6 months. Thyroxine (T4) may be raised in the absence of hyperthyroidism; therefore tri-iodothyronine (T3), T4, and thyroid-stimulating hormone (thyrotrophin, TSH) should all be measured. A raised T3 and T4 with a very low or undetectable TSH concentration suggests the development of thyrotoxicosis. The thyrotoxicosis may be very refractory, and amiodarone should usually be withdrawn at least temporarily to help achieve control; treatment with carbimazole may be required. Hypothyroidism can be treated with replacement therapy without withdrawing amiodarone if it is essential; careful supervision is required.

Pneumonitis should always be suspected if new or progressive shortness of breath or cough develops in a patient taking amiodarone. Fresh neurological symptoms should raise the possibility of peripheral neuropathy. Amiodarone is also associated with hepatotoxicity (see under amiodarone below).

Beta-blockers act as anti-arrhythmic drugs principally by attenuating the effects of the sympathetic system on automaticity and conductivity within the heart, for details see section 2.4. For special reference to the role of **sotalol** in ventricular arrhythmias, see section 2.4.

Oral administration of **digoxin** (section 2.1.1) slows the ventricular rate in atrial fibrillation and in atrial flutter. However, intravenous infusion of digoxin is rarely effective for rapid control of ventricular rate.

Flecainide is useful in the treatment of resistant re-entry supraventricular tachycardia, ventricular tachycardia, ventricular ectopic beats, arrhythmias associated with Wolff-Parkinson-White syndrome, and paroxysmal atrial fibrillation. Flecainide crosses the placenta and can be used to control fetal supraventricular arrhythmias.

Lidocaine (lignocaine) is used as an alternative to amiodarone in cardiopulmonary resuscitation in children with ventricular fibrillation or pulseless ventricular tachycardia unresponsive to d.c. shock. Doses may need to be reduced in children with persistently poor cardiac output and hepatic or renal failure (see under lidocaine, below).

Verapamil (section 2.6.2) may cause severe haemodynamic compromise (refractory hypotension and cardiac arrest) when used for the acute treatment of arrhythmias in neonates and infants; it is contra-indicated in children under 1 year. It is also contra-indicated in those with congestive heart failure, Wolff-Parkinson-White syndrome and in most receiving concomitant beta-blockers. It may be useful in older children with supraventricular tachycardia.

ADENOSINE

Cautions atrial fibrillation or flutter with accessory pathway (conduction down anomalous pathway may increase); asthma; ECG monitoring should be carried out and resuscitation facilities should be available during administration; **interactions:** Appendix 1 (adenosine)

Pregnancy no evidence of harm

Breast-feeding no information available—unlikely to be present in milk owing to short half-life

Contra-indications second- or third-degree AV block and sick sinus syndrome (unless pacemaker fitted)

Side-effects include transient facial flush, chest pain, dyspnoea, bronchospasm, choking sensation, nausea, light-headedness; severe bradycardia reported (requiring temporary pacing); ECG may show transient rhythm disturbances

Licensed use not licensed for use in children

Indication and dose

Arrhythmias (see also section 2.3.1 and see algorithm inside back cover), Diagnosis of arrhythmias

- By intravenous injection

Neonates 150 micrograms/kg; if necessary repeat injection every 2 minutes increasing dose by 50 micrograms/kg until tachycardia terminated or max. single dose of 300 micrograms/kg given

Child 1 month–1 year 150 micrograms/kg; if necessary repeat injection every 2 minutes increasing the dose by 50 micrograms/kg until tachycardia terminated or max. single dose of 300 micrograms/kg given

Child 1–12 years 100 micrograms/kg; if necessary repeat injection every 2 minutes increasing dose by 50 micrograms/kg until tachycardia terminated or max. single dose of 500 micrograms/kg given

Child 12–18 years initially 3 mg; if necessary followed by 6 mg after 1–2 minutes, and then by 12 mg after a further 1–2 minutes

Note In some children over 12 years 3-mg dose ineffective and higher initial dose sometimes used; however, those with *heart transplant* are **very sensitive** to the effects of adenosine, and should **not** receive higher initial doses. In children receiving dipyridamole reduce dose to a quarter of usual dose of adenosine

Administration By *rapid intravenous injection* over 2 seconds into central or large peripheral vein followed by rapid sodium chloride 0.9% flush. Injection solution may be diluted with sodium chloride 0.9% intravenous infusion if required.

Adenocor® (Sanofi-Synthelabo) PoM
Injection, adenosine 3 mg/mL in physiological saline. Net price 2-mL vial = £4.45 (hosp. only)

Note Intravenous infusion of adenosine (*Adenoscan®*, Sanofi Winthrop) may be used in conjunction with radionuclide myocardial perfusion imaging in patients who cannot exercise adequately or for whom exercise is inappropriate—consult product literature

AMIODARONE HYDROCHLORIDE

Cautions liver-function and thyroid-function tests required before treatment and then every 6 months (see notes above for tests of thyroid function); hypokalaemia (measure serum-potassium concentration before treatment); pulmonary function tests and chest x-ray required before treatment; heart failure; severe bradycardia and conduction disturbances in excessive dosage; intravenous use may cause moderate and transient fall in blood pressure (circulatory collapse precipitated by rapid administration or overdosage) or severe hepato-cellular toxicity (monitor transaminases closely); porphyria (section 9.8.2); avoid benzyl alcohol containing injections in neonates (see Excipients p. 3); **interactions:** Appendix 1 (amiodarone)

Contra-indications sinus bradycardia, sino-atrial heart block; unless pacemaker fitted avoid in severe conduction disturbances or sinus node disease; thyroid dysfunction; iodine sensitivity; avoid *intravenous use* in severe respiratory failure, circulatory collapse (except in cardiac arrest), severe arterial hypotension; avoid bolus injection in congestive heart failure or cardiomyopathy;

Pregnancy possible risk of neonatal goitre if amiodarone used in second or third trimester; use only if no alternative

Breast-feeding avoid; significant amount present in milk theoretical risk of neonatal thyroid dysfunction

Side-effects nausea, vomiting, taste disturbances, raised serum transaminases (may require dose reduction or withdrawal if accompanied by acute liver disorders), jaundice; bradycardia (see Cautions); pulmonary toxicity (including pneumonitis and fibrosis); tremor, sleep disorders; hypothyroidism, hyperthyroidism; reversible corneal microdeposits (sometimes with night glare); phototoxicity, persistent slate-grey skin discoloration (see also notes above); *less commonly* onset or worsening of arrhythmia, conduction disturbances (see Cautions), peripheral neuropathy and myopathy (usually reversible on withdrawal); *very rarely* chronic liver disease including cirrhosis, sinus arrest, bronchospasm (in patients with severe respiratory failure), ataxia, benign intracranial hypertension, headache, vertigo, epididymo-orchitis, impotence, haemolytic or aplastic anaemia, thrombocytopenia, rash (including exfoliative dermatitis), hypersensitivity including vasculitis, alopecia, impaired vision due to optic neuritis or optic neuropathy (including blindness), anaphylaxis on rapid injection, also hypotension, respiratory distress syndrome, sweating, and hot flushes

Licensed use Not licensed for use in children under 3 years

Indication and dose

Supraventricular and ventricular arrhythmias see notes above (initiated in hospital or under specialist supervision)

- **By mouth**

Neonate initially 5–10 mg/kg twice daily for 7–10 days, then reduced to maintenance dose of 5–10 mg/kg once daily

Child 1 month–12 years initially 5–10 mg/kg (max. 200 mg) twice daily for 7–10 days, then reduced to maintenance dose of 5–10 mg/kg once daily (max. 200 mg daily)

Child 12–18 years 200 mg 3 times daily for 1 week then 200 mg twice daily for 1 week then usually 200 mg daily adjusted according to response

Administration For *oral* administration tablets may be crushed and dispersed in water; injection solution should **not** be given orally (irritant)

- **By intravenous infusion**

Neonate initially 5 mg/kg over 30 minutes then 5 mg/kg over 30 minutes every 12–24 hours

Child 1 month–18 years initially 5–10 mg/kg over 20 minutes–2 hours then *by continuous infusion* 300 micrograms/kg/hour, increased according to response to max. 1.5 mg/kg/hour; do not exceed 1.2 g in 24 hours

Administration Intravenous administration via central venous catheter preferred; ECG monitoring and resuscitation facilities necessary. For *intravenous infusion* dilute with glucose 5% to a concentration of not less than 600 micrograms/mL; incompatible with sodium chloride infusion; avoid equipment containing the plasticizer di-2-ethylhexphthalate (DEHP)

Ventricular fibrillation or pulseless ventricular tachycardia (see also section 2.3.1)

- **By intravenous injection**

Neonate 5 mg/kg over at least 3 minutes

Child 1 month–18 years 5 mg/kg (max. 300 mg) over at least 3 minutes

Amiodarone (Non-proprietary) PoM

Tablets, amiodarone hydrochloride 100 mg, net price 28-tab pack = £1.97; 200 mg, 28-tab pack = £2.42. Label: 11

Brands include *Amyben®*

Injection, amiodarone hydrochloride 30 mg/mL, net price 10-mL prefilled syringe = £10.25

Excipients: may include benzyl alcohol (avoid in neonates, see Excipients, p. 3)

Sterile concentrate, amiodarone hydrochloride 50 mg/mL, net price 3-mL amp = £1.33, 6-mL amp = £2.86. For dilution and use as an infusion

Excipients: may include benzyl alcohol (avoid in neonates, see Excipients, p. 3)

Extemporaneous formulations available see Extemporaneous Preparations, p. 8

Cordarone X® (Sanofi-Synthelabo) PoM

Tablets, both scored, amiodarone hydrochloride 100 mg, net price 28-tab pack = £4.45; 200 mg, 28-tab pack = £7.27. Label: 11

Sterile concentrate, amiodarone hydrochloride 50 mg/mL. Net price 3-mL amp = £1.33. For dilution and use as an infusion

Excipients: include benzyl alcohol (avoid in neonates, see Excipients, p. 3)

FLECAINIDE ACETATE

Cautions patients with pacemakers (especially those who may be pacemaker dependent because stimulation threshold may rise appreciably); avoid in sinus node dysfunction, atrial conduction defects, second-degree or greater AV block, bundle branch block or distal block unless pacing rescue available; atrial fibrillation following heart surgery; **interactions:** Appendix 1 (flecainide)

Hepatic impairment avoid or reduce dose in severe impairment; monitor plasma concentration (see pharmacokinetics below)

Renal impairment reduce dose by 25–50% if creatinine clearance less than 35 mL/minute/ $1.73m^2$ and monitor plasma-flecainide concentration

Pregnancy not known to be harmful in humans—used in pregnancy to treat maternal and fetal arrhythmias in specialist centres; toxicity reported in *animal* studies

Breast-feeding significant amount present in milk but not known to be harmful

Contra-indications heart failure; long-standing atrial fibrillation where conversion to sinus rhythm not attempted; haemodynamically significant valvular heart disease

Side-effects nausea, vomiting; pro-arrhythmic effects; dyspnoea; visual disturbances; less commonly gastro-intestinal disturbances, jaundice, hepatic dysfunction, AV block, heart failure, myocardial infarction, hypotension, pneumonitis, hallucinations, depression, convulsions, peripheral neuropathy, paraesthesia, ataxia, dyskinesia, hypoaesthesia, tinnitus, vertigo, reduction in red blood cells, in white blood cells and in platelets, corneal deposits, rashes, alopecia, sweating, urticaria, photosensitivity, increased antinuclear antibodies

Pharmacokinetics plasma-flecainide concentration for optimal response 200–800 micrograms/litre; blood sample should be taken immediately before next dose

Licensed use Not licensed for use in children under 12 years

Indication and dose

Resistant re-entry tachycardia, ventricular ectopics or ventricular tachycardia, arrhythmias associated with Wolff-Parkinson-White syndrome, paroxysmal atrial fibrillation

- **By mouth**

Neonate 2 mg/kg 2–3 times daily adjusted according to response and plasma-flecainide concentration

Child 1 month–12 years 2 mg/kg 2–3 times daily adjusted according to response and plasma-flecainide concentration (max. 8 mg/kg/day or 300 mg daily)

Child 12–18 years initially 50–100 mg twice daily (max. 300 mg daily)

Administration Liquid has a local anaesthetic effect and should be given at least 30 minutes before or after food. Milk, infant formula, and dairy products may reduce absorption of flecainide—separate doses from feeds. Do not store liquid in refrigerator as precipitation occurs.

- **By slow intravenous injection or intravenous infusion**

Neonate 1–2 mg/kg over 10–30 minutes; if necessary followed by continuous infusion at a rate of 100–250 micrograms/kg/hour until arrhythmia controlled; if continued for more than 24 hours monitor plasma concentration; transfer to *oral* treatment as above

Child 1 month–12 years 2 mg/kg over 10–30 minutes; if necessary followed by continuous infusion at a rate of 100–250 micrograms/kg/hour until arrhythmia controlled (max. cumulative dose 600 mg in 24 hours); if continued for more than 24 hours monitor plasma concentration; transfer to *oral* treatment as above

Child 12–18 years 2 mg/kg (max. 150 mg) over 10–30 minutes; if necessary followed by continuous infusion at a rate of 1.5 mg/kg/hour for 1 hour, then reduced to 100–250 micrograms/kg/hour until arrhythmia controlled (max. cumulative dose 600 mg in first 24 hours) monitor plasma concentration if continued for more than 24 hours; transfer to *oral* treatment as above

Administration ECG monitoring and resuscitation facilities should always be available. Administer initial dose over 30 minutes in children with sustained ventricular tachycardia or cardiac failure.
Dilute injection using glucose 5% intravenous infusion; concentrations of more than 300micrograms/mL are unstable in chloride containing solutions

Flecainide (Non-proprietary) PoM

Tablets, flecainide acetate 50 mg, net price 60-tab pack = £11.90; 100 mg, 60-tab pack = £15.43

Liquid, available on a named-patient basis (Penn Pharmaceuticals)

Tambocor® (3M) PoM

Tablets, flecainide acetate 50 mg, net price 60-tab pack = £14.46; 100 mg (scored), 60-tab pack = £20.66

Injection, flecainide acetate 10 mg/mL. Net price 15-mL amp = £4.40

LIDOCAINE HYDROCHLORIDE

(Lignocaine hydrochloride)

Cautions lower doses in congestive cardiac failure, in hepatic failure, and following cardiac surgery; ECG monitoring should be carried out and resuscitation facilities should be available; **interactions:** Appendix 1 (lidocaine)

Hepatic impairment manufacturer advises caution—increased risk of side-effects

Renal impairment caution in severe renal impairment

Pregnancy crosses the placenta but not known to be harmful in animal studies—use if benefit outweighs risk

Breast-feeding amount too small to be harmful

2 Cardiovascular system

LIDOCAINE HYDROCHLORIDE (*continued*)

Contra-indications sino-atrial disorders, all grades of atrioventricular block, severe myocardial depression; porphyria (see section 9.8.2)

Side-effects dizziness, paraesthesia, or drowsiness (particularly if injection too rapid); other CNS effects include confusion, respiratory depression and convulsions; hypotension and bradycardia (may lead to cardiac arrest); hypersensitivity reported

Licensed use not licensed for use in children under 12 years

Indication and dose

Ventricular arrhythmias, pulseless ventricular tachycardia or ventricular fibrillation

- **By intravenous or intraosseous injection, and intravenous infusion**

Neonate 0.5–1 mg/kg by injection followed by infusion of 0.6–3 mg/kg/hour; if infusion not immediately available following initial injection, injection of 0.5–1 mg/kg may be repeated at intervals of not less than 5 minutes (to max. total dose 3 mg/kg)

Child 1 month–12 years 0.5–1 mg/kg by injection followed by infusion of 0.6–3 mg/kg/hour; if infusion not immediately available following initial injection, injection of 0.5–1 mg/kg may be repeated at intervals of not less than 5 minutes (to max. total dose 3 mg/kg)

Child 12–18 years 50–100 mg by injection followed by infusion of 120 mg over 30 minutes *then* 240 mg over 2 hours *then* 60 mg/hour; reduce dose further if infusion continued beyond 24 hours; if infusion not immediately available following initial injection, injection of 50–100 mg may be repeated at intervals of not less than 5 minutes (to max. 300 mg in 1 hour)

Administration For *intravenous infusion* dilute with glucose 5% intravenous infusion or sodium chloride 0.9%

For use as a local anaesthetic see section 15.2

Lidocaine (Non-proprietary) PoM

Injection 2%, lidocaine hydrochloride 20 mg/mL, net price 2-mL amp = 28p; 5-mL amp = 25p; 10-mL amp = 60p; 20-mL amp = 61p

Available from Braun

Infusion, lidocaine hydrochloride 0.1% (1 mg/mL) and 0.2% (2 mg/mL) in glucose intravenous infusion 5%. 500-mL containers

Available from Baxter

Minijet® Lignocaine (Celltech) PoM

Injection, lidocaine hydrochloride 1% (10 mg/mL), net price 10-mL disposable syringe = £4.40; 2% (20 mg/mL), 5-mL disposable syringe = £4.30

2.4 Beta-adrenoceptor blocking drugs

Beta-adrenoceptor blocking drugs (beta-blockers) block the beta-adrenoreceptors in the heart, peripheral vasculature, bronchi, pancreas, and liver.

Many beta-blockers are available but experience in children is limited to the use of only a few.

Differences between beta-blockers may affect choice. The water-soluble beta-blockers, atenolol and sotalol, are less likely to enter the brain and may therefore cause less sleep disturbance and nightmares. Water-soluble beta-blockers are excreted by the kidneys and dosage reduction is often necessary in renal impairment.

Some beta-blockers, such as atenolol, have an intrinsically longer duration of action and need to be given only once daily. Carvedilol and labetalol are beta-blockers which have, in addition, an arteriolar vasodilating action and thus lower peripheral resistance. Although carvedilol and labetalol possess both alpha- and beta-blocking properties, these drugs have no important advantages over other beta-blockers in the treatment of hypertension.

Beta-blockers slow the heart and can depress the myocardium; they are contra-indicated in children with second- or third-degree heart block. Sotalol may prolong the QT interval, and it occasionally causes life-threatening ventricular arrhythmias (**important**: particular care is required to avoid hypokalaemia in children taking sotalol).

Beta-blockers may precipitate asthma and they should be **avoided** in children with a history of asthma or bronchospasm; if there is no alternative, a cardioselective beta-blocker may be used with extreme caution under specialist supervision. Atenolol and metoprolol have less effect on the $beta_2$ (bronchial) receptors and are, therefore, relatively *cardioselective*, but they are **not** *cardiospecific*. They have a lesser effect on airways resistance but are **not** free of this side-effect.

Beta-blockers are also associated with fatigue, coldness of the extremities, and sleep disturbances with nightmares (may be less common with the water-soluble beta-blockers, see above).

Beta-blockers are not contra-indicated in diabetes; however, they can lead to a small deterioration of glucose tolerance and interfere with metabolic and autonomic responses to hypoglycaemia. The cardioselective beta-blockers (e.g. atenolol and metoprolol) may be preferable in diabetes but beta-blockers should be avoided altogether in those with frequent episodes of hypoglycaemia.

Hypertension Beta-blockers are effective for reducing blood pressure (section 2.5), but their mode of action is not understood; they reduce cardiac output, alter baroceptor reflex sensitivity, and block peripheral adrenoceptors. Some beta-blockers depress plasma renin secretion. It is possible that a central effect may also explain their mode of action. Blood pressure can usually be controlled with relatively few side-effects. In general the dose of beta-blocker does not have to be high.

Labetalol may be given intravenously for *hypertensive emergencies* in children (section 2.5); however, care is needed to avoid dangerous hypotension or beta-blockade, particularly in neonates. **Esmolol** is also used intravenously for the treatment of hypertension particularly in the peri-operative period.

Beta-blockers can be used to control the pulse rate in children with *phaeochromocytoma* (section 2.5.4). However, they should never be used alone as beta-blockade without concurrent alpha-blockade may lead to a hypertensive crisis; phenoxybenzamine should always be used together with the beta-blocker.

Arrhythmias In arrhythmias (section 2.3), beta-blockers act principally by attenuating the effects of the sympathetic system on automaticity and conductivity within the heart. They may be used in conjunction with digoxin to control the ventricular rate in *atrial fibrillation*, especially in children with thyrotoxicosis. Beta-blockers are also useful in the management of *supraventricular tachycardias* and *ventricular tachycardias*.

Esmolol is a relatively cardioselective beta-blocker with a very short duration of action, used intravenously for the short-term treatment of supraventricular arrhythmias and sinus tachycardia, particularly in the peri-operative period.

Sotalol is a non-cardioselective beta-blocker with additional class III anti-arrhythmic activity. Atenolol and sotalol suppress ventricular ectopic beats and non-sustained ventricular tachycardia (section 2.3.1). However, the pro-arrhythmic effects of sotalol, particularly in children with sick sinus syndrome, may prolong the QT interval and induce torsades de pointes.

Heart failure Beta-blockers may produce benefit in heart failure by blocking sympathetic activity and the addition of a beta-blocker such as **carvedilol** to other treatment for heart failure may be beneficial. Treatment should be initiated by those experienced in the management of heart failure (see section 2.2 for details on heart failure).

Thyrotoxicosis Beta-blockers are used in the management of *thyrotoxicosis* including neonatal thyrotoxicosis; **propranolol** can reverse clinical symptoms within 4 days. Beta-blockers are also used for the pre-operative preparation for thyroidectomy; the thyroid gland is rendered less vascular, thus facilitating surgery (section 6.2.2).

Other uses In Tetralogy of Fallot, esmolol or propranolol may be given intravenously in the initial management of *cyanotic spells*; propranolol is given by mouth for preventing cyanotic spells. If a severe cyanotic spell in a child with congenital heart disease persists despite optimal use of 100% oxygen, propranolol is given by intravenous infusion (for dose, see below). If cyanosis is still present after 10 minutes, sodium bicarbonate intravenous infusion is given in a dose of 1 mmol/kg to correct acidosis (or dose calculated according to arterial blood gas results); sodium bicarbonate 4.2% intravenous infusion is appropriate for a child under 1 year and sodium bicarbonate 8.4% intravenous infusion in children over 1 year. If blood-glucose concentration is less than 3 mmol/litre, glucose 10% intravenous infusion is given in a dose of 2 mL/kg (glucose 200 mg/kg) over 10 minutes, followed by morphine in a dose of 100 micrograms/kg by intravenous or intramuscular injection.

Beta-blockers are also used in the *prophylaxis of migraine* (section 4.7.4.2). Betaxolol, carteolol, levobunolol, and timolol are used topically in *glaucoma* (section 11.6).

PROPRANOLOL HYDROCHLORIDE

Cautions avoid abrupt withdrawal; first-degree AV block; portal hypertension (risk of deterioration in liver function); diabetes; history of obstructive airways disease (introduce cautiously and monitor lung function—see also Bronchospasm below); myasthenia gravis; history of hypersensitivity—may increase sensitivity to allergens and result in more serious hypersensitivity response, also may reduce response to adrenaline (epinephrine); see also notes above; **interactions:** Appendix 1 (beta-blockers), **important:** verapamil interaction, see also p. 136

Hepatic impairment reduce oral dose in liver disease

Renal impairment start with smaller dose in severe impairment; may reduce renal blood flow and adversely affect renal function in severe renal impairment

Pregnancy may cause intra-uterine growth restriction, neonatal hypoglycaemia, and bradycardia; risk greater in severe hypertension

Breast-feeding present in milk but amount probably too small to be harmful; monitor infant for symptoms of beta-blockade

Contra-indications asthma (**important:** see Bronchospasm below), uncontrolled heart failure, marked bradycardia, hypotension, sick sinus syndrome, second- or third- degree AV block, cardiogenic shock, metabolic acidosis, severe peripheral arterial disease; phaeochromocytoma (apart from specific use with alpha-blockers, see also notes above)

Bronchospasm The CSM has advised that beta-blockers, including those considered to be cardioselective, should not be given to patients with a history of asthma or bronchospasm. However, in rare situations where there is no alternative a cardioselective beta-blocker is given to these patients with extreme caution and under specialist supervision

Side-effects bradycardia, heart failure, hypotension, conduction disorders, bronchospasm, peripheral vasoconstriction (including exacerbation of intermittent claudication and Raynaud's phenomenon), gastro-intestinal disturbances, fatigue, sleep disturbances; rare reports of rashes and dry eyes (reversible on withdrawal), sexual dysfunction, and exacerbation of psoriasis; see also notes above; **overdosage:** see Emergency Treatment of Poisoning, p. 40

Licensed use Not licensed for treatment of hypertension in children

Indication and dose

Arrhythmias
- By mouth

Neonate 250–500 micrograms/kg 3 times daily, adjusted according to response

Child 1 month–12 years 250–500 micrograms/kg 3–4 times daily, adjusted according to response; max. 1 mg/kg 4 times daily, total daily dose not to exceed 160 mg daily

Child 12–18 years 10–40 mg 3–4 times daily, adjusted according to response

- By slow intravenous injection, with ECG monitoring

Neonate 20–50 micrograms/kg repeated if necessary every 6-8 hours

Child 1 month–12 years 25–50 micrograms/kg repeated every 6–8 hours if necessary

Child 12–18 years 1 mg over 1 minute; if necessary repeat at 2-minute intervals; max. 10 mg (5 mg in anaesthesia)

Hypertension
- By mouth

Neonate initially, 250 micrograms/kg 3 times daily, increased if necessary to max. 2 mg/kg 3 times daily

Child 1 month–12 years 0.25–1 mg/kg 3 times daily, increased in weekly intervals to max. 5 mg/kg daily

Child 12–18 years initially 80 mg twice daily; increased at weekly intervals as required; maintenance 160–320 mg daily; slow-release preparations may be used for once daily administration

Tetralogy of Fallot
- By mouth

Neonate 0.25–1 mg/kg 2–3 times daily, max. 2 mg/kg 3 times daily

Child 1 month–12 years 0.25–1 mg/kg 3–4 times daily, max. 5 mg/kg daily

- By slow intravenous injection with ECG monitoring

Neonate initially 15–20 micrograms/kg (max. 100 micrograms/kg), repeated every 12 hours if necessary

Child 1 month–12 years initially 15–20 micrograms/kg (max. 100 micrograms/kg), repeated every 6–8 hours if necessary; higher doses rarely necessary

Migraine prophylaxis
- By mouth

Child 2–12 years 200–500 micrograms/kg 3 times daily; max. 4 mg/kg daily, usual dose 10–20 mg 2–3 times daily

Child 12–18 years 20–40 mg 2–3 times daily; maintenance 80–160 mg daily

Administration Give by slow intravenous injection over at least 3–5 minutes. Rate of administration should not exceed 1 mg/minute. May be diluted with sodium chloride 0.9% or glucose 5% intravenous infusion. Incompatible with bicarbonate.

Note Excessive bradycardia can be countered with intravenous injection of atropine sulphate; for **overdosage** see Emergency Treatment of Poisoning, p. 40

Propranolol (Non-proprietary) PoM

Tablets, propranolol hydrochloride 10 mg, net price 28 = £1.25; 40 mg, 28 = £1.18; 80 mg, 56 = £1.76; 160 mg, 56 = £2.76. Label: 8

Brands include *Angilol®*

2 Cardiovascular system

PROPRANOLOL HYDROCHLORIDE (*continued*)

Oral solution, propranolol hydrochloride 5 mg/ 5 mL, net price 150 mL = £12.50; 10 mg/5 mL, 150 mL = £16.45; 50 mg/5 mL, 150 mL = £19.98
Brands include *Syprol®*

Inderal® (AstraZeneca) PoM
Injection, propranolol hydrochloride 1 mg/mL, net price 1-mL amp = 21p

Modified release
Note For use in older children only

Half-Inderal LA® (AstraZeneca) PoM
Capsules, m/r, lavender/pink, propranolol hydrochloride 80 mg. Net price 28-cap pack = £5.40. Label: 8, 25
Note Modified-release capsules containing propranolol hydrochloride 80 mg also available; brands include *Bedranol SR®*, *Half Beta Prograne®*

ATENOLOL

Cautions see under Propranolol Hydrochloride

Renal impairment initially use 50% of usual dose if creatinine clearance 10–35 mL/minute/1.73m²; initially use 30–50% of usual dose if creatinine clearance less than 10 mL/minute/1.73m²

Pregnancy may cause intra-uterine growth restriction, neonatal hypoglycaemia, and bradycardia; risk greater in severe hypertension

Breast-feeding present in milk in greater amounts than some other beta-blockers; possible toxicity due to beta-blockade—monitor infant and use with caution

Contra-indications see under Propranolol Hydrochloride

Side-effects see under Propranolol Hydrochloride

Licensed use not licensed for use in children

Indication and dose

Hypertension, arrhythmias
- By mouth

Neonate 0.5–2 mg/kg once daily; may be given twice daily if necessary

Child 1 month–12 years 0.5–2 mg/kg once daily; may be given twice daily if necessary (max. 100 mg daily)

Child 12–18 years 50 mg daily (higher doses rarely necessary for hypertension); max. 100 mg daily

Atenolol (Non-proprietary) PoM
Tablets, atenolol 25 mg, net price 28-tab pack = £1.12; 50 mg, 28-tab pack = 84p; 100 mg, 28-tab pack = £1.20. Label: 8
Brands include *Atenix®*

Tenormin® (AstraZeneca) PoM
'25' tablets, f/c, atenolol 25 mg. Net price 28-tab pack = £4.41. Label: 8

LS tablets, orange, f/c, scored, atenolol 50 mg. Net price 28-tab pack = £5.11. Label: 8

Tablets, orange, f/c, scored, atenolol 100 mg. Net price 28-tab pack = £6.50. Label: 8

Syrup, sugar-free, atenolol 25 mg/5mL. Net price 300 mL = £8.55. Label: 8

CARVEDILOL

Cautions see under Propranolol Hydrochloride; before increasing dose ensure renal function and heart failure not deteriorating; severe heart failure, avoid in acute or decompensated heart failure requiring intravenous inotropes

Pregnancy see under Propranolol Hydrochloride; also lack of experience in human pregnancy limits any assessment of fetal risk

Breast-feeding present in milk in *animal* studies but amount probably too small to be harmful; monitor infant for symptoms of alpha- and beta-blockade

Contra-indications see under Propranolol Hydrochloride; severe chronic heart failure

Hepatic impairment avoid

Side-effects postural hypotension, dizziness, headache, fatigue, gastro-intestinal disturbances, bradycardia; occasionally diminished peripheral circulation, peripheral oedema and painful extremities, dry mouth, dry eyes, eye irritation or disturbed vision, impotence, disturbances of micturition, influenza-like symptoms; rarely angina, AV block, exacerbation of intermittent claudication or Raynaud's phenomenon; allergic skin reactions, exacerbation of psoriasis, nasal stuffiness, wheezing, depressed mood, sleep disturbances, paraesthesia, heart failure, changes in liver enzymes, thrombocytopenia, leucopenia also reported

Licensed use Not licensed for use in children under 18 years

Indication and dose

Adjunct in heart failure (limited information available)
- By mouth

Child 2–18 years initially 50 micrograms/kg (max. 3.125 mg) twice daily, double dose at intervals of at least 2 weeks up to 350 micrograms/kg (max. 25 mg) twice daily

Carvedilol (Non-proprietary) PoM
Tablets, carvedilol 3.125 mg, net price 28-tab pack = £6.67; 6.25 mg, 28-tab pack = £7.71; 12.5 mg, 28-tab pack = £8.69; 25 mg, 28-tab pack = £10.56. Label: 8

Eucardic® (Roche) PoM
Tablets, all scored, carvedilol 3.125 mg (pink), net price 28-tab pack = £7.57; 6.25 mg (yellow), 28-tab pack = £8.41; 12.5 mg (peach), 28-tab pack = £9.35; 25 mg, 28-tab pack = £11.68. Label: 8

ESMOLOL HYDROCHLORIDE

Cautions see under Propranolol Hydrochloride

Renal impairment manufacturer advises caution

Contra-indications see under Propranolol Hydrochloride

Side-effects see under Propranolol Hydrochloride; infusion causes venous irritation and thrombophlebitis

Licensed use not licensed for use in children

Indication and dose

Arrhythmias, hypertensive emergencies (see also notes above and section 2.5)

- **By intravenous administration**

Child 1 month–18 years initially by intravenous injection over 1 minute 500 micrograms/kg then by intravenous infusion 50 micrograms/kg/minute for 4 minutes (rate reduced if low blood pressure or low heart rate); if inadequate response, repeat loading dose and increase maintenance infusion by 50 microgram/kg/minute increments; repeat until effective or max. infusion of 200 micrograms/kg/minute reached; doses over 300 micrograms/kg/minute not recommended

Tetralogy of Fallot

- **By intravenous administration**

Neonate initially by intravenous injection over 1–2 minutes 600 micrograms/kg then if necessary by intravenous infusion 300–900 micrograms/kg/minute

Administration Dilute injection solution (with Glucose 5% *or* Sodium Chloride 0.9%) to a concentration of 10 mg/mL (20 mg/mL if fluid restricted) and give through central line; incompatible with bicarbonate

Brevibloc® (Baxter) PoM

Injection, esmolol hydrochloride 10 mg/mL, net price 10-mL vial = £7.79, 250-mL infusion bag = £81.54

Injection concentrate, esmolol hydrochloride 250 mg/mL (for dilution before infusion), 10-mL amp = £79.08

LABETALOL HYDROCHLORIDE

Cautions see under Propranolol Hydrochloride; interferes with laboratory tests for catecholamines; liver damage (see below)

Liver damage Severe hepatocellular damage reported after both short-term and long-term treatment. Appropriate laboratory testing needed at first symptom of liver dysfunction and if laboratory evidence of damage (or if jaundice) labetalol should be stopped and not restarted

Pregnancy use in treatment of maternal hypertension does not pose risk, except possibly in first trimester, monitor neonate for signs of alpha- and beta-blockade

Breast-feeding present in milk but amount probably too small to be harmful—monitor infant for possible symptoms of alpha- and beta-blockade

Contra-indications see under Propranolol Hydrochloride

Side-effects postural hypotension (avoid upright position during and for 3 hours after intravenous administration), tiredness, weakness, headache, rashes, scalp tingling, difficulty in micturition, epigastric pain, nausea, vomiting; liver damage (see above); rarely lichenoid rash

Licensed use not licensed for use in children

Indication and dose

Hypertensive emergencies see also section 2.5

- **By intravenous infusion**

Neonate 500 micrograms/kg/hour adjusted at intervals of at least 15 minutes according to response; max. 4 mg/kg/hour

Child 1 month–12 years initially 0.5–1 mg/kg/hour adjusted at intervals of at least 15 minutes according to response; max. 3 mg/kg/hour

Child 12–18 years 30–120 mg/hour adjusted at intervals of at least 15 minutes according to response

Note Consult local guidelines. In hypertensive encephalopathy reduce blood pressure to normotensive level over 24–48 hours (more rapid reduction may lead to cerebral infarction, blindness, and death). If child fitting, reduce blood pressure rapidly, but not to normal levels

Hypertension

- **By mouth**

Child 1 month–12 years 1–2 mg/kg 3–4 times a day

Child 12–18 years initially 50–100 mg twice daily increased if required at intervals of 3–14 days to usual dose of 200–400 mg twice daily (3–4 divided doses if higher); max. 2.4 g daily

Administration Injection may be given orally with squash or juice

- **By intravenous injection**

Child 1 month–12 years 250–500 micrograms/kg as a single dose; max. 20 mg

Child 12–18 years 50 mg over at least 1 minute, repeated after 5 minutes if necessary; max. total dose 200 mg

Note Excessive bradycardia can be countered with intravenous injection of atropine sulphate; for **overdosage** see p. 40

Administration for *intravenous infusion*, dilute to a concentration of 1 mg/mL in Glucose 5% *or* Sodium Chloride and Glucose 5%; if fluid restricted may be given undiluted, preferably through a central venous catheter. Measure systolic pressure at least every 15 minutes

LABETALOL HYDROCHLORIDE (*continued*)

Labetalol Hydrochloride (Non-proprietary) PoM
Tablets, all f/c, labetalol hydrochloride 100 mg, net price 56 = £6.87; 200 mg, 56 = £10.01; 400 mg, 56 = £15.60. Label: 8, 21

Trandate® (Celltech) PoM
Tablets, all orange, f/c, labetalol hydrochloride 50 mg, net price 56-tab pack = £3.79; 100 mg, 56-tab pack = £4.17; 200 mg, 56-tab pack = £6.77; 400 mg, 56-tab pack = £9.42. Label: 8, 21
Injection, labetalol hydrochloride 5 mg/mL. Net price 20-mL amp = £2.12

Extemporaneous formulations available see Extemporaneous Preparations, p. 8

METOPROLOL TARTRATE

Cautions see under Propranolol Hydrochloride

Hepatic impairment reduce dose

Pregnancy see under Propranolol Hydrochloride

Breast-feeding present in milk but amount probably too small to be harmful—monitor infant for possible symptoms of beta-blockade

Contra-indications see under Propranolol Hydrochloride

Side-effects see under Propranolol Hydrochloride

Licensed use Not licensed for use in children

Indication and dose

Hypertension
- **By mouth**

Child 1 month–12 years initially 1 mg/kg twice daily, increase if necessary to max. 8 mg/kg daily in 2–4 divided doses

Child 12–18 years initially 100 mg daily increased if necessary to 200 mg daily in 1–2 divided doses; max. 400 mg daily (but high doses rarely necessary)

Arrhythmias
- **By mouth**

Child 12–18 years usually 50 mg 2–3 times daily; up to 300 mg daily in divided doses if necessary

Metoprolol Tartrate (Non-proprietary) PoM
Tablets, metoprolol tartrate 50 mg, net price 28 = £1.57; 100 mg, 28 = £2.52. Label: 8

Betaloc® (AstraZeneca) PoM
Tablets, both scored, metoprolol tartrate 50 mg, net price 100-tab pack = £3.30; 100 mg, 100-tab pack = £6.13. Label: 8

Lopresor® (Novartis) PoM
Tablets, both f/c, scored, metoprolol tartrate 50 mg (pink), net price 56-tab pack = £2.57; 100 mg (blue), 56-tab pack = £6.68. Label: 8

Extemporaneous formulations available see Extemporaneous Preparations, p. 8

SOTALOL HYDROCHLORIDE

Cautions see under Propranolol Hydrochloride; correct hypokalaemia, hypomagnesaemia, or other electrolyte disturbances; severe or prolonged diarrhoea; reduce dose or discontinue if corrected QT interval exceeds 550 msec; **interactions:** Appendix 1 (beta-blockers), **important:** verapamil interaction see also p. 136

Renal impairment halve initial dose if creatinine clearance 30–60 mL/minute/1.73m^2; use one-quarter normal dose if creatinine clearance 10–30 mL/minute/1.73m^2; avoid if creatinine clearance less than 10 mL/minute/1.73m^2

Pregnancy see under Propranolol Hydrochloride

Breast-feeding present in milk; possible toxicity due to beta-blockade—monitor infant

CSM advice The use of sotalol should be limited to the treatment of ventricular arrhythmias or prophylaxis of supraventricular arrhythmias (see above). It should no longer be used for angina, hypertension, thyrotoxicosis or for secondary prevention after myocardial infarction; when stopping sotalol for these indications, the dose should be reduced gradually

Contra-indications see under Propranolol Hydrochloride; congenital or acquired long QT syndrome; torsades de pointes

Side-effects see under Propranolol Hydrochloride; arrhythmogenic (pro-arrhythmic) effect (torsades de pointes—increased risk in females)

Licensed use Not licensed for use in children

Indication and dose

Atrial flutter, life-threatening ventricular tachyarrhythmia and supraventricular arrhythmias, ventricular arrhythmias initiated under specialist supervision and ECG monitoring and measurement of corrected QT interval
- **By mouth**

Neonate initially 1 mg/kg twice daily, increased as necessary every 3–4 days to max. 4 mg/kg twice daily

Child 1 month–12 years initially 1 mg/kg twice daily, increased as necessary every 2–3 days to max. 4 mg/kg twice daily (max. 80 mg twice daily)

Child 12–18 years initially 80 mg once daily *or* 40 mg twice daily, increased gradually at intervals of 2–3 days to usual dose 80–160 mg twice daily; higher doses of 480–640 mg daily for life-threatening ventricular arrhythmias under specialist supervision

Administration tablets may be crushed and dispersed in water

Note Excessive bradycardia can be countered with intravenous injection of atropine sulphate; for **overdosage** see Emergency Treatment of Poisoning, p. 40

SOTALOL HYDROCHLORIDE (*continued*)

Sotalol (Non-proprietary) PoM
Tablets, sotalol hydrochloride 40 mg, net price 56 = £2.22; 80 mg, 56-tab pack = £3.29; 160 mg, 28-tab pack = £6.06. Label: 8

Beta-Cardone® (Celltech) PoM
Tablets, all scored, sotalol hydrochloride 40 mg (green), net price 56-tab pack = £1.34; 80 mg (pink), 56-tab pack = £1.99; 200 mg, 28-tab pack = £2.50. Label: 8

Sotacor® (Bristol-Myers Squibb) PoM
Tablets, both scored, sotalol hydrochloride 80 mg, net price 28-tab pack = £3.25; 160 mg, 28-tab pack = £6.41. Label: 8

Injection, sotalol hydrochloride 10 mg/mL. Net price 4-mL amp = £1.76

Extemporaneous formulations available see Extemporaneous Preparations, p. 8

2.5 Hypertension

Hypertension in children and adolescents can have substantial effect on long-term health. Possible causes of hypertension (e.g. congenital heart disease, renal disease and endocrine disorders) and the presence of any complications (e.g. left ventricular hypertrophy) should be established. Treatment should take account of contributory factors and any factors that increase the risk of cardiovascular complications.

Serious hypertension is rare in *neonates* but it can present with signs of congestive heart failure; the cause is often renal and can follow embolic arterial damage.

Children (or their parents or carers) should be given advice on lifestyle changes to reduce blood pressure or cardiovascular risk; these include weight reduction (in obese children), reduction of dietary salt, reduction of total and saturated fat, increasing exercise, increasing fruit and vegetable intake, and smoking cessation (in children who smoke).

Indications for antihypertensive therapy in children include symptomatic hypertension, secondary hypertension, hypertensive target-organ damage, diabetes mellitus, persistent hypertension despite lifestyle measures (see above), and pulmonary hypertension (section 2.5.1.2). The effect of antihypertensive treatment on growth and development is not known; treatment should be started only if benefits are clear.

Antihypertensive therapy should be initiated with a single drug at the lowest recommended dose; the dose can be increased until the target blood pressure is achieved. Once the highest recommended dose is reached, or sooner if the patient begins to experience side-effects, a second drug may be added if blood pressure is not controlled. If more than one drug is required, these should be given as separate products because there is little paediatric experience in using fixed-dose combination products.

Acceptable drug classes for use in children with hypertension include ACE inhibitors (section 2.5.5.1), alpha-blockers (section 2.5.4), beta-blockers (section 2.4), calcium-channel blockers (section 2.6.2), and diuretics (section 2.2). There is limited information on the use of angiotensin II-receptor antagonists in children. Diuretics and beta-blockers have a long history of safety and efficacy in children. The newer classes of antihypertensive drugs, including ACE inhibitors and calcium-channel blockers have been shown to be safe and effective in short-term studies in children. Refractory hypertension may require additional treatment with agents such as minoxidil (section 2.5.1.1) or clonidine (section 2.5.2).

Other measures to reduce cardiovascular risk **Aspirin** (section 2.9) may be used to reduce the risk of cardiovascular events; however, concerns about an increased risk of bleeding and Reye's syndrome need to be considered.

A **statin** can be of benefit in older children who have a high risk of cardiovascular disease and have hypercholesterolaemia (see section 2.12).

Hypertension in diabetes Hypertension can occur in type 2 (non-insulin-dependent) diabetes and treatment prevents both macrovascular and microvascular complications. ACE inhibitors (section 2.5.5.1) may be considered in children with diabetes and microalbuminaemia or proteinuric renal disease (see also section 6.1.5).

Hypertension in renal disease ACE inhibitors may be considered in children with micro-albuminuria or proteinuric renal disease (see also section 6.1.5). High doses of loop diuretics may be required. Specific cautions apply to the use of ACE inhibitors in renal impairment, see section 2.5.5.1, but ACE inhibitors may be effective. Dihydropyridine calcium-channel blockers may be added.

Hypertension in pregnancy High blood pressure in pregnancy may usually be due to pre-existing essential hypertension or to pre-eclampsia. Methyldopa (section 2.5.2) is safe in pregnancy. Beta-blockers are effective and safe in the third trimester. Modified-release preparations of nifedipine [unlicensed] are also used for hypertension in pregnancy. Intravenous administration of labetalol (section 2.4) can be used to control hypertensive crises; alternatively hydralazine (section 2.5.1.1) may be used by the intravenous route.

Hypertensive emergencies Hypertensive emergencies in children may be accompanied by signs of hypertensive encephalopathy, including seizures. Controlled reduction in blood pressure over 72–96 hours is essential; very rapid reduction can reduce perfusion leading to organ damage. It may be necessary to infuse fluids particularly during the first 12 hours to expand plasma volume should the blood pressure drop too rapidly. Once blood pressure is controlled oral therapy should be started.

Controlled reduction of blood pressure is achieved by intravenous infusions of **labetalol** (section 2.4) or **sodium nitroprusside** (section 2.5.1.1). Esmolol (section 2.4) is useful for short-term use and has a short duration of action. **Nicardipine** (section 2.6.2) may be administered as a continuous intravenous infusion but it is not licensed for this use. In less severe cases, **nifedipine** capsules (section 2.6.2) can be used.

In resistant cases, **diazoxide** (section 2.5.1.1) is given intravenously, but it can cause sudden hypotension. Other antihypertensive drugs which may be given intravenously include hydralazine (section 2.5.1.1) and clonidine (section 2.5.2).

Hypertension in acute nephritis occurs as a result of sodium and water retention; it should be treated with sodium and fluid restriction, and with furosemide (section 2.2.2); antihypertensive drugs may be added if necessary.

For advice on short-term management of hypertensive episodes in phaeochromocytoma, see under Phaeochromocytoma, section 2.5.4.

2.5.1 Vasodilator antihypertensive drugs and pulmonary hypertension

2.5.1.1 Vasodilator antihypertensives

Vasodilator antihypertensives are potent drugs, especially when used in combination with a beta-blocker and a thiazide. **Important**: for a warning on the hazards of a very rapid fall in blood pressure, see Hypertensive Emergencies section 2.5.

Sodium nitroprusside is given by intravenous infusion to control severe hypertensive crisis when parenteral treatment is necessary. At low doses it reduces systemic vascular resistance and increases cardiac output; at high doses it can produce profound systemic hypotension—continuous blood pressure monitoring is therefore essential. Sodium nitroprusside may also be used to control paradoxical hypertension after surgery for coarctation of the aorta.

Diazoxide has also been used by intravenous injection in hypertensive emergencies; however it is not first-line therapy.

Hydralazine given by mouth is a useful adjunct to other antihypertensives, but when used alone causes tachycardia and fluid retention. Side-effects can be few if the dose is kept low, but systemic lupus erythematosus should be suspected if there is unexplained weight loss, arthritis, or any other unexplained ill health.

Minoxidil should be reserved for the treatment of severe hypertension resistant to other drugs. Vasodilatation is accompanied by increased cardiac output and tachycardia and children develop fluid retention. For this reason the addition of a beta-blocker and a diuretic (usually furosemide, in high dosage) are mandatory. Hypertrichosis is troublesome and renders this drug unsuitable for females.

Prazosin and doxazosin (section 2.5.4) have alpha-blocking and vasodilator properties.

DIAZOXIDE

Cautions interactions: Appendix 1 (diazoxide)

Renal impairment reduce dose in severe renal impairment

Contra-indications

Pregnancy prolonged use may produce alopecia, hypertrichosis, and impaired glucose tolerance in neonate; inhibits uterine activity during labour

Breast-feeding manufacturer advises avoid—no information available

Side-effects tachycardia, hypotension, hyperglycaemia, sodium and water retention; *rarely* cardiomegaly, hyperosmolar non-ketotic coma, leucopenia, thrombocytopenia, and hirsuitism

Licensed use intractable hypoglycaemia (section 6.1.4)

Indication and dose

Hypertensive emergencies initiated on specialist advice

- **By intravenous injection**

Child 1 month–18 years 1–3 mg/kg (max. 150 mg) as a single dose, repeat dose after 5–15 minutes until blood pressure controlled; max. 4 doses in 24 hours

Administration intravenous injection over 30 seconds. Do not dilute

Resistant hypertension

- **By mouth**

Neonate initially 1.7 mg/kg 3 times daily, adjusted according to response; usual max. 15 mg/kg daily

Child 1 month–18 years initially 1.7 mg/kg 3 times daily, adjusted according to response; usual max. 15 mg/kg daily

Intractable hypoglycaemia section 6.1.4

Eudemine® (Goldshield) PoM

Injection, diazoxide 15 mg/mL. Net price 20-mL amp = £30.00

Tablets, section 6.1.4

Extemporaneous formulations available see Extemporaneous Preparations, p. 8

HYDRALAZINE HYDROCHLORIDE

Cautions cerebrovascular disease; occasionally blood pressure reduction too rapid even with low parenteral doses; manufacturer advises test for antinuclear factor and for proteinuria every 6 months and check acetylator status before increasing dose, but evidence of clinical value unsatisfactory; **interactions**: Appendix 1 (hydralazine)

Hepatic impairment reduce dose

Renal impairment reduce dose if creatinine clearance less than 30 mL/minute/1.73m^2

Pregnancy manufacturer advises avoid before third trimester; no reports of serious harm following use in third trimester

Breast-feeding present in milk but not known to be harmful; monitor infant

Contra-indications idiopathic systemic lupus erythematosus, severe tachycardia, high output heart failure, myocardial insufficiency due to mechanical obstruction, cor pulmonale; porphyria (section 9.8.2)

Side-effects tachycardia, palpitation, flushing, hypotension, fluid retention, gastro-intestinal disturbances; headache, dizziness; systemic lupus erythematosus-like syndrome after long-term therapy (especially in slow acetylator individuals); rarely rashes, fever, peripheral neuritis, polyneuritis, paraesthesia, arthralgia, myalgia, increased lacrimation, nasal congestion, dyspnoea, agitation, anxiety, anorexia; blood disorders (including leucopenia, thrombocytopenia, haemolytic anaemia), abnormal liver function, jaundice, raised plasma creatinine, proteinuria and haematuria reported

Licensed use not licensed for use in children

Indication and dose

Hypertension

- **By mouth**

Neonate 250–500 micrograms/kg every 8–12 hours increased as necessary to max. 2–3 mg/kg every 8 hours

Child 1 month–12 years 250–500 micrograms/kg every 8–12 hours increased as necessary to max. 7.5 mg/kg daily (not exceeding 200 mg daily)

Child 12–18 years 25 mg twice daily, increased to usual max. 50–100 mg twice daily

- **By slow intravenous injection**

Neonate 100–500 micrograms/kg repeated every 4–6 hours as necessary; max 3 mg/kg daily

2 Cardiovascular system

HYDRALAZINE HYDROCHLORIDE (*continued*)

Child 1 month–12 years 100–500 micrograms/kg repeated every 4–6 hours as necessary; max 3 mg/kg daily (not exceeding 60 mg daily)

Child 12–18 years 5–10 mg repeated every 4–6 hours as necessary

- **By continuous intravenous infusion (preferred route in cardiac patients)**

Neonate 12.5–50 micrograms/kg/hour

Child 1 month–12 years 12.5–50 micrograms/kg/hour; max. 3 mg/kg daily

Child 12–18 years initially 3–9 mg/hour; max. 3 mg/kg daily

Administration For *intravenous injection* initially reconstitute 20 mg with 1 mL water for injections, then dilute to a concentration of 0.5–1 mg/mL with sodium chloride 0.9% intravenous infusion and administer over 5–20 minutes. For administration *by mouth* diluted injection may be given orally. For *continuous intravenous infusion* initially reconstitute 20 mg with 1 mL water for injections, then dilute with sodium chloride 0.9% or Ringer's solution. Incompatible with glucose intravenous infusion

Hydralazine (Non-proprietary) PoM

Tablets, hydralazine hydrochloride 25 mg, net price 20 = 86p; 50 mg, 20 = £1.37

Apresoline® (Sovereign) PoM

Tablets, yellow, s/c, hydralazine hydrochloride 25 mg, net price 84-tab pack = £2.50

Excipients: include gluten

Injection, powder for reconstitution, hydralazine hydrochloride. Net price 20-mg amp = £1.64

Extemporaneous formulations available see Extemporaneous Preparations, p. 8

MINOXIDIL

Cautions see notes above; porphyria (section 9.8.2); **interactions:** Appendix 1 (minoxidil)

Renal impairment reduce dose if creatinine clearance less than 50 mL/minute/1.73m² and titrate according to response

Pregnancy neonatal hirsutism reported

Breast-feeding present in milk but not known to be harmful

Contra-indications phaeochromocytoma

Side-effects sodium and water retention; weight gain, peripheral oedema, tachycardia, hypertrichosis; reversible rise in creatinine and blood urea nitrogen; occasionally, gastro-intestinal disturbances, breast tenderness, rashes

Indication and dose

Severe hypertension

- By mouth

Child 1 month–12 years initially 200 microgram/kg daily in 1–2 divided doses, increased in steps of 100–200 micrograms/kg daily every 3 days; max. 1 mg/kg daily

Child 12–18 years initially 5 mg daily in 1–2 divided doses increased in steps of 5–10 mg every 3 or more days; max. 100 mg daily (seldom necessary to exceed 50 mg daily)

Loniten® (Pharmacia) PoM

Tablets, all scored, minoxidil 2.5 mg, net price 60-tab pack = £8.88; 5 mg, 60-tab pack = £15.83; 10 mg, 60-tab pack = £30.68

Extemporaneous formulations available see Extemporaneous Preparations, p. 8

SODIUM NITROPRUSSIDE

Cautions hypothyroidism, hyponatraemia, impaired cerebral circulation, hypothermia; monitor blood pressure and blood-cyanide concentration, and if treatment exceeds 3 days also blood-thiocyanate concentration; avoid sudden withdrawal—terminate infusion over 15–30 minutes; **interactions:** Appendix 1 (nitroprusside)

Hepatic impairment avoid in severe liver impairment

Renal impairment avoid prolonged use if creatinine clearance less than 20 mL/minute/1.73m²

Pregnancy potential for accumulation of cyanide in fetus—avoid prolonged use

Breast-feeding manufacturer advises caution—no information available

Contra-indications severe vitamin B_{12} deficiency; Leber's optic atrophy; compensatory hypertension

Side-effects associated with over rapid reduction in blood pressure (reduce infusion rate): headache, dizziness, nausea, retching, abdominal pain, perspiration, palpitation, apprehension, retrosternal discomfort; occasionally reduced platelet count, acute transient phlebitis

Cyanide Side-effects caused by excessive plasma concentration of the cyanide metabolite include tachycardia, sweating, hyperventilation, arrhythmias, marked metabolic acidosis (discontinue and give antidote, see p. 43)

Licensed use not licensed for use in children

Indication and dose

Hypertensive emergencies

- **By continuous infusion**

Neonate 500 nanograms/kg/minute then increased in steps of 200 nanograms/kg/minute as necessary to max. 8 micrograms/kg/minute (max. 4 micrograms/kg/minute if used for longer than 24 hours)

SODIUM NITROPRUSSIDE (*continued*)

Child 1 month–18 years 500 nanograms/kg/minute then increased in steps of 200 nanograms/kg/minute as necessary to max. 8 micrograms/kg/minute (max. 4 micrograms/kg/minute if used for longer than 24 hours)

Administration For *continuous intravenous infusion* reconstitute 50 mg with 2–3 mL glucose 5% intravenous infusion then dilute immediately with glucose 5% to a concentration of 50–200 micrograms/mL (max. 1 mg/mL if fluid restricted); infuse *via* infusion device to allow precise control; protect infusion from light

Sodium Nitroprusside (Mayne) PoM
Intravenous infusion, powder for reconstitution, sodium nitroprusside 10 mg/mL. For dilution and use as an infusion, net price 5-mL vial = £6.64

2.5.1.2 Pulmonary hypertension

Only pulmonary *arterial* hypertension is currently suitable for drug treatment. Pulmonary arterial hypertension includes persistent pulmonary hypertension of the newborn, primary pulmonary hypertension in children, and pulmonary hypertension related to congenital heart disease and cardiac surgery.

Some types of pulmonary hypertension are treated with vasodilator antihypertensive therapy and oxygen. Diuretics (section 2.2) may also have a role in children with right-sided heart failure.

Initial treatment of *persistent pulmonary hypertension of the newborn* involves the administration of **nitric oxide**; **epoprostenol** may be used until nitric oxide is available. Oral sildenafil may be helpful in less severe cases. Epoprostenol and sildenafil can cause profound systemic hypotension. In rare circumstances either **tolazoline** or **magnesium sulphate** may be given by intravenous infusion when nitric oxide and epoprostenol have failed.

Treatment of *primary pulmonary hypertension* is determined by acute vasodilator testing; drugs used for treatment include calcium-channel blockers (usually **nifedipine**, section 2.6.2), long-term intravenous **epoprostenol**, nebulised **iloprost**, **bosentan**, or **sildenafil**. Anticoagulation (usually with warfarin) may also be required to prevent secondary thrombosis.

Inhaled nitric oxide is a potent and selective pulmonary vasodilator. It acts on cyclic gaunosine monophosphate (cGMP) resulting in smooth muscle relaxation. Inhaled nitric oxide is used in the treatment of persistent pulmonary hypertension of the newborn, and may also be useful in other forms of arterial pulmonary hypertension. Dependency can occur with high doses and prolonged use; to avoid rebound pulmonary hypertension the drug should be withdrawn gradually, often with the aid of sildenafil.

Excess nitric oxide can cause methaemoglobinaemia; therefore, methaemoglobin concentration should be measured regularly, particularly in neonates.

Nitric oxide increases the risk of haemorrhage by inhibiting platelet aggregation, but it does not usually cause bleeding.

Epoprostenol (prostacyclin) is a prostaglandin and a potent vasodilator. It is used in the treatment of persistent pulmonary hypertension of the newborn, primary pulmonary hypertension, and in the acute phase following cardiac surgery. It is given by continuous 24-hour intravenous infusion.

Epoprostenol is a powerful inhibitor of platelet aggregation and there is a possible risk of haemorrhage. It is sometimes used as an antiplatelet in renal dialysis either alone or with heparin (see section 2.8.1). It can also cause serious systemic hypotension and, if withdrawn suddenly, can cause pulmonary hypertensive crisis.

Children on prolonged treatment can become tolerant to epoprostenol, and therefore require an increase in dose.

Iloprost is a synthetic analogue of epoprostenol and is efficacious when nebulised in adults with pulmonary arterial hypertension, but experience in children is limited. It is more stable than epoprostenol and has a longer half-life.

Bosentan is a dual endothelin antagonist used orally in the treatment of primary pulmonary hypertension. The concentration of endothelin, a potent vasoconstrictor, is raised in sustained pulmonary hypertension.

Sildenafil, a vasodilator developed for the treatment of erectile dysfunction, is also used for pulmonary arterial hypertension. It is used either alone or as an adjunct to other drugs and has relatively few side-effects.

Sildenafil is a selective phosphodiesterase type-5 inhibitor. Inhibition of this enzyme in the lungs enhances the vasodilatory effects of nitric oxide and promotes relaxation of vascular smooth muscle.

Sildenafil has also been used in pulmonary hypertension for weaning children off inhaled nitric oxide following cardiac surgery, and less successfully in primary pulmonary hypertension.

Tolazoline is now rarely used to correct pulmonary artery vasospasm in pulmonary hypertension of the newborn as better alternatives are available (see above). Tolazoline is an alpha-blocker and produces both pulmonary and systemic vasodilation.

BOSENTAN

Cautions not to be initiated if systemic systolic blood pressure is below 85 mmHg; monitor liver function before and during treatment (reduce dose or suspend treatment if liver enzymes raised significantly)—discontinue if symptoms of liver impairment (see Contra-indications below); monitor haemoglobin, withdraw treatment gradually; **interactions**: Appendix 1 (bosentan)

Contra-indications

Hepatic impairment avoid in moderate and severe hepatic impairment

Pregnancy avoid (teratogenic in *animal* studies); effective contraception required during and for at least 3 months after administration; monthly pregnancy tests advised

Note Bosentan possibly interacts with progestogen; alternative contraceptive recommended

Breast-feeding manufacturer advises avoid—no information available

Side-effects dyspepsia, flushing, hypotension, palpitations, fatigue, oedema, anaemia, pruritus, nasopharyngitis

Licensed use not licensed for use in children under 12 years

Indication and dose

Primary pulmonary arterial hypertension
- By mouth

Child 3–18 years and body-weight 10–20 kg initially 31.25 mg once daily increased after 4 weeks to 31.25 mg twice daily

Child 3–18 years and body-weight 20–40 kg initially 31.25 mg twice daily increased after 4 weeks to 62.5 mg twice daily

Child 12–18 years and body-weight over 40 kg initially 62.5 mg twice daily increased after 4 weeks to 125 mg twice daily; max. 250 mg twice daily

Administration Tablets may be cut, or dissolved in water or non-acidic liquid. Solution is stable at room-temperature (max. 25°C) for 24 hours

Tracleer® (Actelion) ▼ PoM

Tablets, f/c, orange, bosentan (as monohydrate) 62.5 mg, net price 56-tab pack = £1541.00; 125 mg, 56-tab pack = £1541.00

EPOPROSTENOL

Cautions anticoagulant monitoring required when given with heparin; haemorrhagic diathesis; avoid abrupt withdrawal (see notes above); monitor blood pressure

Pregnancy manufacturer advises use with caution—no information available

Contra-indications severe left ventricular dysfunction; pulmonary veno-occlusive disease

Side-effects see notes above; gastro-intestinal disturbances, hypotension, bradycardia, tachycardia, pallor, flushing, sweating with higher doses; headache; lassitude, anxiety, agitation; dry mouth, jaw pain, chest pain; also reported, hyperglycaemia and injection-site reactions

Licensed use not licensed for use in children

Indication and dose

Persistent pulmonary hypertension of the newborn
- By continuous intravenous infusion

Neonate initially 2 nanograms/kg/minute adjusted according to response; usual max. 20 nanograms/kg/minute (rarely up to 40 nanograms/kg/minute)

Primary pulmonary hypertension
- By continuous intravenous infusion

Child 1 month–18 years initially 2 nanograms/kg/minute increased as necessary to 40 nanograms/kg/minute

Administration Reconstitute using the solvent provided (pH 10.5) to make a concentrate; filter the concentrate using the filter provided; the concentrate can be administered via a central vein, alternatively it may be diluted further with the glycine buffer provided *or* with not more than 6 times the volume of sodium chloride 0.9% intravenous infusion; solution stable for 12 hours at room temperature, although some units use for 24 hours and allow for loss of potency; solution stable for 24 hours if prepared in glycine buffer only and administered via an ambulatory cold pouch system (to maintain solution at 2–8°C)

Flolan® (GSK) PoM

Infusion, powder for reconstitution, epoprostenol (as sodium salt). Net price 500-microgram vial (with diluent) = £64.57; 1.5-mg vial (with diluent) = £130.07

ILOPROST

Cautions unstable pulmonary hypertension with advanced right heart failure; hypotension (do not initiate if systolic blood pressure below 85 mmHg); **interactions:** Appendix 1 (iloprost)

Hepatic impairment dose may need to be halved in liver cirrhosis—initially 2.5 micrograms at intervals of at least 3 hours (max. 6 times daily), adjusted according to response

Contra-indications decompensated cardiac failure (unless under medical supervision); severe arrhythmias; congenital or acquired valvular defects of the myocardium; pulmonary veno-occlusive disease; conditions which increase risk of haemorrhage

Pregnancy manufacturer advises avoid (toxicity in *animal* studies); effective contraception must be used during treatment

Breast-feeding manufacturer advises avoid—no information available

Side-effects vasodilatation, hypotension, syncope, cough, headache, trismus

Licensed use not licensed for use in children

Indication and dose

Primary pulmonary hypertension
- By inhalation of nebulised solution

  Child 8–18 years 2.5–5 micrograms 6–9 times daily, adjusted according to response

Raynaud's syndrome section 2.6.4.1

Ventavis (Schering Health) ▼ PoM
Nebuliser solution, iloprost (as trometamol) 10 micrograms/mL, net price 30 × 2 mL (20 microgram) unit-dose vials = £425.00; 100 × 2-mL = £1415.08; 300 × 2-mL = £4243.88. For use with *Prodose®* NHS nebuliser (available on loan from Schering)

SILDENAFIL

Cautions other cardiovascular disease, predisposition to prolonged erection (e.g. in sickle-cell disease, multiple myeloma, or leukaemia); bleeding disorders or active peptic ulceration; ocular disorders; initiate cautiously if child also on epoprostenol, iloprost, bosentan or nitric oxide; withdraw treatment gradually; **interactions:** Appendix 1 (sildenafil)

Hepatic impairment use half initial dose; manufacturer advises avoid in severe hepatic impairment

Renal impairment use half initial dose if creatinine clearance less than 30 mL/minute/1.73m^2

Contra-indications children receiving nitrates; manufacturer contra-indicates sildenafil in hypotension and hereditary degenerative retinal disorders

Side-effects dyspepsia; flushing; headache, dizziness; penile erection; visual disturbances, raised intra-ocular pressure; nasal congestion; *rarely* vomiting, serious cardiovascular disorders, priapism, painful red eyes, and hypersensitivity reactions (including rash)

Licensed use not licensed for use in children

Indication and dose

Pulmonary hypertension after cardiac surgery, weaning from nitric oxide, primary pulmonary hypertension, persistent pulmonary hypertension of the newborn
- By mouth

  Neonate initially 250–500 micrograms/kg every 4–8 hours, adjusted according to response; max. 2 mg/kg every 4 hours; start with lower dose and frequency especially if used with other vasodilators (see Cautions above); withdraw gradually

  Child 1 month– 18 years initially 250–500 micrograms/kg every 4–8 hours, adjusted according to response; max. 2 mg/kg every 4 hours; start with lower dose and frequency especially if used with other vasodilators (see Cautions above)

Administration tablet may be dissolved in water or blackcurrant drink and given by mouth or through a nasogastric tube

Viagra® (Pfizer) PoM NHS
Tablets, all blue, f/c, sildenafil (as citrate), 25 mg, net price 4-tab pack = £16.59, 8-tab pack = £33.19; 50 mg, 4-tab pack = £19.34, 8-tab pack = £38.67; 100 mg, 4-tab pack = £23.50, 8-tab pack = £46.99

Revatio® (Pfizer) ▼ PoM
Tablets, f/c, sildenafil (as citrate), 20 mg, net price 90-tab pack = £373.50

Extemporaneous formulations available see Extemporaneous Preparations, p. 8

TOLAZOLINE

Cautions mitral stenosis; cardiotoxic accumulation may occur with continuous infusion, particularly in renal impairment—monitor blood pressure regularly for sustained systemic hypotension; **interactions:** Appendix 1 (alpha-blockers)

Renal impairment accumulates in renal impairment; risk of cardiotoxicity; lower doses may be necessary

Contra-indications peptic ulcer disease

Side-effects nausea, vomiting, diarrhoea, epigastric pain; flushing, tachycardia, cardiac arrhyth-

TOLAZOLINE (*continued*)

mias; headache, shivering, sweating; oliguria, metabolic alkalosis, haematuria, blood dyscrasias (including thrombocytopenia); blotchy skin; at high doses severe hypotension, marked hypertension, renal failure, and haemorrhage reported

Licensed use not licensed for use in children

Indication and dose

Correction of pulmonary vasospasm in neonates
- By intravenous injection and continuous intravenous infusion (maintenance)

Neonate initially 1 mg/kg *by intravenous injection* over 2–5 minutes, followed if necessary *by continuous intravenous infusion* of 200 micrograms/kg/hour with careful blood pressure monitoring; doses above 300 micrograms/kg/hour associated with cardiotoxicity and renal failure

- By endotracheal administration

Neonate 200 micrograms/kg

Administration For *continuous intravenous infusion* dilute with glucose 5% *or* sodium chloride 0.9% intravenous infusion. Prepare a fresh solution every 24 hours.

For *endotracheal administration* dilute with 0.5–1 mL of sodium chloride 0.9% solution for injection

Tolazoline (Non-proprietary)
Injection, tolazoline 25 mg/mL
Available as a manufactured special

MAGNESIUM SULPHATE

Cautions see section 9.5.1.3

Side-effects see section 9.5.1.3

Licensed use see section 9.5.1.3

Indication and dose

Persistent pulmonary hypertension of the newborn
- By intravenous infusion

Neonate initially 200 mg/kg over 20–30 minutes; if response occurs, then by continuous intravenous infusion of 20–75 mg/kg/hour to maintain plasma-magnesium concentration between 3.5–5.5 mmol/litre), given for up to 5 days

Neonatal hypocalcaemia see section 9.5.1.3

Hypomagnesaemia see section 9.5.1.3

Administration For *intravenous infusion* dilute with glucose 5% *or* sodium chloride 0.9% intravenous infusion to a max. concentration of 100 mg/mL (200 mg/mL if fluid restricted)

Magnesium Sulphate (Non-proprietary) PoM
Injection, magnesium sulphate 50% (Mg^{2+} approx. 2 mmol/mL), net price 2-mL (1-g) amp= £2.88, 5-mL (2.5-g) amp = £2.39, 10-mL (5-g) amp = £3.20; prefilled 10-mL (5-g) syringe = £4.72

2.5.2 Centrally acting antihypertensive drugs

Methyldopa, a centrally acting antihypertensive, is of little value in the management of refractory sustained hypertension in infants and children. On prolonged use it is associated with fluid retention (which may be alleviated by concomitant use of diuretics).

Methyldopa is effective for the management of hypertension in pregnancy.

Clonidine is also a centrally acting antihypertensive but has the disadvantage that sudden withdrawal may cause a hypertensive crisis. Clonidine is also used under specialist supervision for pain management, sedation, and opioid withdrawal, attention deficit hyperactivity disorder, and Tourette syndrome.

CLONIDINE HYDROCHLORIDE 

Cautions must be withdrawn gradually to avoid hypertensive crisis; Raynaud's syndrome or other occlusive peripheral vascular disease; history of depression; avoid in porphyria (section 9.8.2); **interactions:** Appendix 1 (clonidine)

Skilled tasks Drowsiness may affect performance of skilled tasks (e.g. driving); effects of alcohol may be enhanced

Pregnancy may lower fetal heart rate, but risk to fetus should be balanced against risk of uncontrolled maternal hypertension; avoid intravenous injection

Breast-feeding present in milk—manufacturer advises avoid

Side-effects dry mouth, sedation, depression, fluid retention, bradycardia, Raynaud's phenomenon, headache, dizziness, euphoria, nocturnal unrest, rash, nausea, constipation, rarely impotence

Licensed use not licensed for use in children

Indication and dose

Severe hypertension
- By mouth

Child 2–18 years initially 0.5–1 microgram/kg 3 times daily, increased gradually if necessary; max. 25 micrograms/kg daily in divided doses (not exceeding 1.2 mg daily)

CLONIDINE HYDROCHLORIDE (*continued*)

- By slow intravenous injection
  Child 2–18 years 2–6 micrograms/kg (max. 300 micrograms) as a single dose

Administration For *intravenous injection* give over 10–15 minutes; compatible with sodium chloride 0.9% *or* glucose 5% intravenous infusion.

For administration *by mouth* tablets may be crushed and dissolved in water

Catapres® (Boehringer Ingelheim) PoM
Tablets, both scored, clonidine hydrochloride 100 micrograms, net price 100-tab pack = £5.60; 300 micrograms, 100-tab pack = £13.04. Label: 3, 8

Injection, clonidine hydrochloride 150 micrograms/mL. Net price 1-mL amp = 29p

Extemporaneous formulations available see Extemporaneous Preparations, p. 8

METHYLDOPA

Cautions withdraw treatment gradually; blood counts and liver-function tests advised; history of depression; positive direct Coombs' test in up to 20% of patients (may affect blood cross-matching); interference with laboratory tests; **interactions:** Appendix 1 (methyldopa)

Skilled tasks Drowsiness may affect performance of skilled tasks (e.g. driving); effects of alcohol may be enhanced

Hepatic impairment manufacturer advises caution in history of liver disease; avoid in active liver disease

Renal impairment if creatinine clearance less than 20 mL/minute/1.73m^2, start with small dose; increased sensitivity to hypotensive and sedative effect

Pregnancy not known to be harmful

Breast-feeding amount too small to be harmful

Contra-indications depression, active liver disease, phaeochromocytoma; porphyria (section 9.8.2)

Side-effects gastro-intestinal disturbances, dry mouth, stomatitis, sialadenitis; bradycardia, postural hypotension, oedema; sedation, headache, dizziness, asthenia, myalgia, arthralgia, paraesthesia, nightmares, mild psychosis, depression, impaired mental acuity, parkinsonism, Bell's palsy; abnormal liver function tests, hepatitis, jaundice; pancreatitis; haemolytic anaemia; bone-marrow depression, leucopenia, thrombocytopenia, eosinophilia; hypersensitivity reactions including lupus erythematosus-like syndrome, drug fever, myocarditis, pericarditis; rashes (including toxic epidermal necrolysis); nasal congestion, failure of ejaculation, impotence, decreased libido, gynaecomastia, hyperprolactinaemia, amenorrhoea

Indication and dose

Refractory hypertension (but see notes above)
- By mouth
  Child 1 month–12 years initially 2.5 mg/kg 3 times daily, increased as necessary at intervals of at least 2 days to max. 65 mg/kg daily (not exceeding 3 g daily)

  Child 12–18 years initially 250 mg 2–3 times daily increased as necessary at intervals of at least 2 days to max. 3 g daily

Methyldopa (Non-proprietary) PoM
Tablets, coated, methyldopa (anhydrous) 125 mg, net price 56 tab pack = £2.87; 250 mg, 56 tab pack = £2.69; 500 mg, 56 tab pack = £4.25. Label: 3, 8

Aldomet® (MSD) PoM
Tablets, all yellow, f/c, methyldopa (anhydrous) 250 mg, net price 60 = £1.88; 500 mg, 30 = £1.90. Label: 3, 8

Extemporaneous formulations available see Extemporaneous Preparations, p. 8

2.5.3 Adrenergic neurone blocking drugs

Adrenergic neurone blocking drugs prevent the release of noradrenaline from postganglionic adrenergic neurones. These drugs do not control supine blood pressure and may cause postural hypotension. For this reason they have largely fallen from use in adults and are rarely used in children.

2.5.4 Alpha-adrenoceptor blocking drugs

Doxazosin and **prazosin** have post-synaptic alpha-blocking and vasodilator properties and rarely cause tachycardia. They may, however, reduce blood pressure rapidly after the first dose and should be introduced with caution.

Alpha-blockers may be used with other antihypertensive drugs in the treatment of hypertension.

DOXAZOSIN

Cautions care with initial dose (postural hypotension); susceptibility to heart failure; **interactions:** Appendix 1 (alpha-blockers)

Hepatic impairment no information available—manufacturer advises caution

Pregnancy no evidence of teratogenicity, manufacturer advises use only when potential benefit outweighs risk

Breast-feeding accumulates in milk in *animal* studies—manufacturer advises avoid

DOXAZOSIN (*continued*)

Side-effects postural hypotension; dizziness, vertigo, headache, fatigue, asthenia, oedema, somnolence, nausea, rhinitis; less frequently abdominal discomfort, diarrhoea, vomiting, agitation, tremor, rash, pruritus; rarely blurred vision, epistaxis, haematuria, thrombocytopenia, purpura, leucopenia, hepatitis, jaundice, cholestasis, and urinary incontinence; isolated cases of priapism and impotence reported

Licensed use not licensed for use in children

Indication and dose

Hypertension (see notes above)

- By mouth

Child 6–12 years 500 micrograms once daily, increased at 1-week intervals to 2–4 mg daily

Child 12–18 years 1 mg daily, increased after 1–2 weeks to 2 mg once daily, and thereafter to 4 mg once daily if necessary; usual max. 4 mg daily (rarely up to 16 mg daily may be required)

Doxazosin (Non-proprietary) PoM

Tablets, doxazosin (as mesilate) 1 mg, net price 28-tab pack = £1.64; 2 mg, 28-tab pack = £2.04; 4 mg, 28-tab pack = £4.23

Brands include *Doxadura®*

Cardura® (Pfizer) PoM

Tablets, doxazosin (as mesilate) 1 mg, net price 28-tab pack = £10.56; 2 mg, 28-tab pack = £14.08

Extemporaneous formulations available see Extemporaneous Preparations, p. 8

Modified-release

Cardura® XL (Pfizer) PoM

Tablets, m/r, doxazosin (as mesilate) 4 mg, net price 28-tab pack = £6.33; 8 mg, 28-tab pack = £12.67. Label: 25

PRAZOSIN

Cautions first dose may cause collapse due to hypotension (therefore should be taken on retiring to bed); **interactions:** Appendix 1 (alpha-blockers)

Hepatic impairment start with low doses and adjust according to response

Renal impairment if creatinine clearance less than 20 mL/minute/1.73m^2 start with low doses; increase with caution

Pregnancy no evidence of teratogenicity; manufacturer advises use only when potential benefit outweighs risk

Breast-feeding present in milk; manufacturer advises use with caution

Contra-indications not recommended for congestive heart failure due to mechanical obstruction (e.g. aortic stenosis)

Side-effects postural hypotension, drowsiness, weakness, dizziness, headache, lack of energy, nausea, palpitations; urinary frequency, incontinence and priapism reported

Licensed use not licensed for use in children under 12 years

Indication and dose

Hypertension (see notes above)

- By mouth

Child 1 month–12 years 10–15 micrograms/kg 2–4 times daily (initial dose at bedtime) increased gradually to max. 500 micrograms/kg daily in divided doses (not exceeding 20 mg daily)

Child 12–18 years 500 micrograms 2–3 times daily (initial dose at bedtime), increased after 3–7 days to 1 mg 2–3 times daily; further increased gradually if necessary to max. 20 mg daily in divided doses

Congestive heart failure (but rarely used, see section 2.2)

- By mouth

Child 1 month–12 years 5 micrograms/kg twice daily (initial dose at bedtime), increased gradually to max. 100 micrograms/kg daily in divided doses

Child 12–18 years 500 micrograms 2–4 times daily (initial dose at bedtime), increasing to 4 mg daily in divided doses; maintenance 4–20 mg daily in divided doses

Administration For *oral* administration tablets may be dispersed in water

Prazosin (Non-proprietary) PoM

Tablets, prazosin (as hydrochloride) 500 micrograms, net price 56-tab pack = £2.51; 1 mg, 56-tab pack = £3.23; 2 mg, 56-tab pack = £4.39; 5 mg, 56-tab pack = £8.75. Label: 3, counselling, , initial dose

Hypovase® (Pfizer) PoM

Tablets, prazosin (as hydrochloride) 500 micrograms, net price 56-tab pack = £2.51; 1 mg (orange, scored), 56-tab pack = £3.23; 2 mg (scored), 56-tab pack = £4.39. Label: 3, counselling, initial dose

Phaeochromocytoma

Long-term management of phaeochromocytoma involves surgery. However, surgery should not take place until there is adequate blockade of both alpha- and beta-adrenoceptors. Alpha-blockers are used in the short-term management of hypertensive episodes in phaeochromocytoma. Once alpha blockade is established, tachycardia can be controlled by the cautious addition of a beta-blocker (section 2.4); a cardioselective beta-blocker is preferred.

Phenoxybenzamine, a powerful alpha-blocker, is effective in the management of phaeochromocytoma but it has many side-effects. Phenoxybenzamine has also been used to treat severe shock in the presence of adequate circulating blood volume, and to lower systemic vascular resistance after cardiac surgery.

Phentolamine is a short-acting alpha-blocker used mainly during surgery of phaeochromocytoma; its use for the diagnosis of phaeochromocytoma has been superseded by measurement of catecholamines in blood and urine. It has also been used in children with paroxysmal hypertension.

PHENOXYBENZAMINE HYDROCHLORIDE

Cautions congestive heart failure; severe heart disease (see also Contra-indications); cerebrovascular disease (avoid if history of cerebrovascular accident); carcinogenic in *animals*; avoid in porphyria (section 9.8.2); avoid infusion in hypovolaemia; avoid extravasation (irritant to tissues); avoid contact with skin (risk of contact sensitisation)

Renal impairment use with caution

Pregnancy hypotension in newborn may occur—use with caution

Breast-feeding may be present in milk

Contra-indications history of cerebrovascular accident

Side-effects postural hypotension with dizziness and marked compensatory tachycardia, lassitude, nasal congestion, miosis, inhibition of ejaculation; rarely gastro-intestinal disturbances; decreased sweating and dry mouth after intravenous infusion; idiosyncratic profound hypotension within few minutes of starting infusion

Licensed use not licensed for use in children

Indication and dose

Hypertension in phaeochromocytoma
- **By mouth**
  Child 1 month–18 years 0.5–1 mg/kg twice daily adjusted according to response
- **By intravenous infusion**
  Child 1 month–18 years 0.5–1 mg/kg daily adjusted according to response; occasionally up to 2 mg/kg daily may be required; do not repeat dose within 24 hours

Severe shock following cardiac surgery
- **By intravenous infusion**
  Child 1 month–18 years initially 1 mg/kg then if necessary 500 micrograms/kg every 8–12 hours adjusted according to response

Administration for administration *by mouth*, capsules may be opened

For *intravenous infusion*, dilute with Sodium Chloride 0.9% and give over at least 2 hours; max. 4 hours between dilution and completion of infusion

Phenoxybenzamine (Goldshield) PoM
Injection concentrate, phenoxybenzamine hydrochloride 50 mg/mL. To be diluted before use. Net price 3 × 2-mL amp = £94.88 (hosp. only)

Dibenyline® (Goldshield) PoM
Capsules, red/white, phenoxybenzamine hydrochloride 10 mg. Net price 30-cap pack = £10.84

PHENTOLAMINE MESILATE

Cautions monitor blood pressure (avoid in hypotension), heart rate; renal impairment; gastritis, peptic ulcer; **interactions**: Appendix 1 (alpha-blockers)

Asthma Presence of sulphites in ampoules may (especially in patients with asthma) lead to hypersensitivity (with bronchospasm and shock)

Pregnancy use with caution; may cause marked decrease in maternal blood pressure with resulting fetal anoxia

Breast-feeding no information available—manufacturer advises avoid

Contra-indications hypotension; history of cardiac muscle damage; coronary insufficiency, or evidence of coronary artery disease

Side-effects postural hypotension, tachycardia, dizziness, flushing; nausea and vomiting, diarrhoea, nasal congestion; also acute or prolonged hypotension, chest pain, arrhythmias

Indication and dose

Hypertension during surgery for phaeochromocytoma
- **By intravenous injection over 3–5 minutes**
  Child 1 month–12 years 50–100 micrograms/kg (max. 5 mg) 1–2 hours before surgery, repeated if necessary
  Child 12–18 years 2–5 mg 1–2 hours before surgery, repeated if necessary

Diagnosis of phaeochromocytoma consult product literature (but see notes above)

Rogitine® (Alliance) PoM
Injection, phentolamine mesilate 10 mg/mL. Net price 1-mL amp = £1.66

2.5.5 Drugs affecting the renin-angiotensin system

2.5.5.1 Angiotensin-converting enzyme inhibitors

Angiotensin-converting enzyme inhibitors (ACE inhibitors) inhibit the conversion of angiotensin I to angiotensin II. The main indications of ACE inhibitors in children are shown below. In infants and young children with heart failure, captopril is often considered first.

Initiation under specialist supervision Treatment with ACE inhibitors should be initiated under specialist supervision and with careful clinical monitoring in children.

Heart failure ACE inhibitors have a valuable role in all grades of heart failure, usually combined with a loop diuretic (section 2.2). Potassium supplements and potassium-sparing diuretics should be discontinued before introducing an ACE inhibitor because of the risk of hyperkalaemia. In adults, a low dose of spironolactone may be beneficial in severe heart failure and can be used with an ACE inhibitor provided serum potassium is monitored carefully. Profound first-dose hypotension may occur when ACE inhibitors are introduced to children with heart failure who are already taking a high dose of a loop diuretic (see Cautions below). Temporary withdrawal of the loop diuretic reduces the risk, but may cause severe rebound pulmonary oedema.

Hypertension ACE inhibitors may be considered for hypertension when thiazides and beta-blockers are contra-indicated, not tolerated, or fail to control blood pressure; they may be considered for hypertension in insulin-dependent diabetics with nephropathy (see also section 6.1.5). ACE inhibitors may cause very rapid falls of blood pressure in some patients particularly in those receiving diuretic therapy (see Cautions, below); the first dose should preferably be given at bedtime.

Diabetic nephropathy For comment on the role of ACE inhibitors in the management of diabetic nephropathy, see section 6.1.5.

Renal effects In children with severe bilateral renal artery stenosis (or severe stenosis of the artery supplying a single functioning kidney), ACE inhibitors reduce or abolish glomerular filtration and are likely to cause severe and progressive renal failure. They are therefore contra-indicated in children known to have these forms of critical renovascular disease.

ACE inhibitor treatment is unlikely to have an adverse effect on overall renal function in children with severe unilateral renal artery stenosis and a normal contralateral kidney, but glomerular filtration is likely to be reduced (or even abolished) in the affected kidney and the long-term consequences are unknown.

In general, ACE inhibitors are therefore best avoided in those with known or suspected renovascular disease, unless the blood pressure cannot be controlled by other drugs. If they are used in these circumstances renal function needs to be monitored.

ACE inhibitors should also be used with particular caution in children who may have undiagnosed and clinically silent renovascular disease. This includes those with peripheral vascular disease or those with severe generalised atherosclerosis. ACE inhibitors are useful for the management of hypertension and proteinuria in children with nephritis. They are thought to have a beneficial effect by reducing intra-glomerular hypertension and protecting the glomerular capillaries and membrane.

Renal function and electrolytes should be checked before starting ACE inhibitors and monitored during treatment (more frequently if features mentioned above are present).

Concomitant treatment with NSAIDs increases the risk of renal damage, and potassium-sparing diuretics (or potassium-containing salt substitutes) increase the risk of hyperkalaemia.

Cautions ACE inhibitors need to be initiated with care in children receiving diuretics (**important**: see Concomitant diuretics, below); first doses may cause hypotension especially in children taking high doses of diuretics, on a low-sodium diet, on dialysis, dehydrated or with heart failure. Renal function should be monitored before and during treatment, and the dose reduced in renal impairment (see also above and under individual drugs). The risk of agranulocytosis is possibly increased in collagen vascular disease (blood counts recommended). ACE inhibitors should be used with care in children with severe or symptomatic aortic stenosis (risk of hypotension). They should be used with care (or avoided) in those with a history of idiopathic or hereditary angioedema. **Interactions:** Appendix 1 (ACE inhibitors)

Anaphylactoid reactions To prevent anaphylactoid reactions, ACE inhibitors should be avoided during dialysis with high-flux polyacrylonitrile membranes and during low-density lipoprotein apheresis with dextran sulphate; they should also be withheld before desensitisation with wasp or bee venom

Concomitant diuretics ACE inhibitors can cause a very rapid fall in blood pressure in volume-depleted children; treatment should therefore be initiated with very low doses. In some children the diuretic dose may need to be reduced or the diuretic discontinued at least 24 hours beforehand. If high-dose diuretic therapy cannot be stopped, close observation is recommended after administration of the first dose of ACE inhibitor, for at least 2 hours or until the blood pressure has stabilised.

Contra-indications ACE inhibitors are contra-indicated in children with hypersensitivity to ACE inhibitors (including angioedema) and in known or suspected renovascular disease (see also above). ACE inhibitors should not be used in pregnancy; they may adversely affect fetal and neonatal blood pressure control and renal function, and possibly cause skull defects and oligohydramnios; toxicity in *animal* studies has been reported.

Side-effects ACE inhibitors can cause profound hypotension (see Cautions) and renal impairment (see Renal effects above), and a persistent dry cough. They may also cause angioedema (onset may be delayed), rash (which may be associated with pruritus and urticaria), pancreatitis and upper respiratory-tract symptoms such as sinusitis, rhinitis, and sore throat. Gastro-intestinal effects reported with ACE inhibitors include nausea, vomiting, dyspepsia, diarrhoea, constipation, and abdominal pain. Altered liver function tests, cholestatic jaundice and hepatitis have been reported. Blood disorders including thrombocytopenia, leucopenia, neutropenia and haemolytic anaemia have also been reported. Other reported side-effects include headache, dizziness, fatigue, malaise, taste disturbance, paraesthesia, bronchospasm, fever, serositis, vasculitis, myalgia, arthralgia, positive antinuclear antibody, raised erythrocyte sedimentation rate, eosinophilia, leucocytosis and photosensitivity.

Neonates The neonatal response to treatment with ACE inhibitors is very variable, and some neonates develop profound hypotension with even small doses; a test-dose should be used initially and increased cautiously. Adverse effects such as apnoea, seizures, renal failure, and severe unpredictable hypotension are very common in the first month of life and it is therefore recommended that ACE inhibitors are avoided whenever possible, particularly in preterm neonates.

CAPTOPRIL

Cautions see notes above; porphyria (section 9.8.2)

Renal impairment see notes above; start with low dose and adjust according to response

Breast-feeding present in milk—manufacturer advises avoid

Contra-indications see notes above

Pregnancy avoid

Side-effects see notes above; tachycardia, serum sickness, weight loss, stomatitis, maculopapular rash, photosensitivity, flushing and acidosis

Licensed use not licensed for use in children

Indication and dose

Hypertension, heart failure, proteinuria in nephritis or diabetic nephropathy (under specialist supervision)

• **By mouth**

Neonate (caution, see neonatal information above) test dose, 10–50 micrograms/kg (10 micrograms/kg in neonate less than 37 weeks postmenstrual age), monitor blood pressure carefully for 1–2 hours; if tolerated give 10–50 micrograms/kg 2–3 times daily increased as necessary to max. 2 mg/kg daily in divided doses (max. 300 micrograms/kg daily in divided

CAPTOPRIL (*continued*)

doses in neonate less than 37 weeks post menstrual age)

Child 1 month–12 years test dose, 100 micrograms/kg (max. 6.25 mg), monitor blood pressure carefully for 1–2 hours; if tolerated give 100–300 micrograms/kg 2–3 times a day, increased as necessary to max. 6 mg/kg daily in divided doses (max. 4 mg/kg daily in divided doses for child 1 month–1 year)

Child 12–18 years test dose, 100 micrograms/kg *or* 6.25 mg, monitor blood pressure carefully for 1–2 hours; if tolerated give 12.5–25 mg 2–3 times a day, increased as necessary to max. 150 mg daily in divided doses

Administration Administer under close supervision, see notes above. Give test dose whilst child supine. Tablets can be dispersed in water

Captopril (Non-proprietary) PoM
Tablets, captopril 12.5 mg, net price 56-tab pack = £2.14; 25 mg, 56-tab pack = £3.05; 50 mg, 56-tab pack = £3.89
Brands include *Ecopace®*, *Kaplon®*, *Tensopril®*

Note Liquid formulation available from specialist importing companies

Capoten® (Squibb) PoM
Tablets, captopril 12.5 mg (scored), net price 56-tab pack = £9.82; 25 mg, 56-tab pack = £11.19, 84-tab pack = £16.79; 50 mg (scored), 56-tab pack = £19.07, 84-tab pack = £28.60 (also available as *Acepril®*)

Extemporaneous formulations available see Extemporaneous Preparations, p. 8

ENALAPRIL MALEATE

Cautions see notes above

Hepatic impairment monitor closely

Renal impairment not recommended in children if creatinine clearance less than 30 mL/minute/1.73m^2

Breast-feeding amount probably too small to be harmful; see also notes above

Contra-indications see notes above

Pregnancy avoid

Side-effects see notes above; also palpitations, arrhythmias, chest pain, Raynaud's syndrome, syncope, cerebrovascular accident; anorexia, ileus, stomatitis, hepatic failure; dermatological side-effects including erythema multiforme, Stevens-Johnson syndrome, toxic epidermal necrolysis, exfoliative dermatitis and pemphigus; confusion, depression, nervousness, asthenia, drowsiness, insomnia, dream abnormalities, blurred vision, tinnitus, sweating, flushing, impotence, alopecia, dyspnoea, asthma, pulmonary infiltrates and muscle cramps

Licensed use not licensed for use in children for congestive heart failure, proteinuria in nephritis or diabetic nephropathy; not licensed for use in children less than 20 kg for hypertension

Indication and dose

Hypertension, congestive heart failure, proteinuria in nephritis or diabetic nephropathy (under specialist supervision)

- **By mouth**

Neonate (limited information) initially 10 micrograms/kg once daily, monitor blood pressure carefully for 1–2 hours, increased as necessary up to 500 micrograms/kg daily in 1–3 divided doses

Child 1 month–12 years initially 100 micrograms/kg once daily, monitor blood pressure carefully for 1–2 hours, increased as necessary up to max. 1 mg/kg daily in 1–2 divided doses

Child 12–18 years initially 2.5 mg once daily, monitor blood pressure carefully for 1–2 hours, usual maintenance dose 10–20 mg daily in 1–2 divided doses, max. 40 mg daily if body-weight over 50 kg

Administration Tablets may be crushed and suspended in water immediately before use

Enalapril Maleate (Non-proprietary) PoM
Tablets, enalapril maleate 2.5 mg, net price 28-tab pack = 95p; 5 mg, 28-tab pack = £1.28; 10 mg, 28-tab pack = £1.38; 20 mg, 28-tab pack = £1.54
Brands include *Ednyt®*

Innovace® (MSD) PoM
Tablets, enalapril maleate 2.5 mg, net price 28-tab pack = £5.35; 5 mg (scored), 28-tab pack = £7.51; 10 mg (red), 28-tab pack = £10.53; 20 mg (peach), 28-tab pack = £12.51

LISINOPRIL

Cautions see notes above

Renal impairment not recommended in children if creatinine clearance less than 30 mL/minute/1.73m^2

Breast-feeding no information available—manufacturer advises caution

Contra-indications see notes above

Pregnancy avoid

Side-effects see notes above; tachycardia, cerebrovascular accident; dry mouth, blurred vision, confusion, mood changes, asthenia, sweating, impotence and alopecia

Licensed use not licensed for use in children

LISINOPRIL (*continued*)

Indication and dose

Hypertension (under specialist supervision)
Child 6–12 years initially 70 micrograms/kg (max. 5 mg) once daily, increased in intervals of 1–2 weeks to max. 600 micrograms/kg (*or* 40 mg) once daily

Child 12–18 years initially 2.5 mg daily; usual maintenance dose 10–20 mg daily; max. 40 mg daily

Heart failure (adjunct) (under specialist supervision)
Child 12–18 years initially 2.5 mg daily; usual maintenance dose 5–20 mg daily

Lisinopril (Non-proprietary) PoM
Tablets, lisinopril (as dihydrate) 2.5 mg, net price 28-tab pack = £1.17; 5 mg, 28-tab pack = £1.34; 10 mg, 28-tab pack = £1.70; 20 mg, 28-tab pack = £2.22
Note Liquid formulation available as manufactured special

Carace® (Bristol-Myers Squibb) PoM
Tablets, lisinopril 2.5 mg (blue), net price 28-tab pack = £6.79; 5 mg (scored), 28-tab pack = £8.51; 10 mg (yellow, scored), 28-tab pack = £10.51; 20 mg (orange, scored), 28-tab pack = £11.89

Zestril® (AstraZeneca) PoM
Tablets, lisinopril (as dihydrate) 2.5 mg, net price 28-tab pack = £6.26; 5 mg (pink, scored), 28-tab pack = £7.86; 10 mg (pink), 28-tab pack = £9.70; 20 mg (pink), 28-tab pack = £10.97

Extemporaneous formulations available see Extemporaneous Preparations, p. 8

2.5.5.2 Angiotensin-II receptor antagonists

Losartan is a specific angiotensin-II receptor antagonist with many properties similar to those of the ACE inhibitors. However, unlike ACE inhibitors, losartan does not inhibit the breakdown of bradykinin and other kinins, and therefore does not appear to cause the persistent dry cough which commonly complicates ACE inhibitor therapy. It is therefore an alternative for children who have to discontinue an ACE inhibitor because of persistent cough.

Losartan may also be used as an alternative to an ACE inhibitor in the management of hypertension; however, evidence for its use in children is very limited.

Cautions and contraindications Losartan should be used with caution in renal artery stenosis (see also Renal Effects under ACE Inhibitors, section 2.5.5.1). Monitoring of plasma-potassium concentration is advised, particularly in children with renal impairment; lower initial doses may be appropriate in these patients and losartan should be avoided when creatinine clearance falls below 30 mL/minute/1.73 m². Losartan should also be used with caution in aortic or mitral valve stenosis and in obstructive hypertrophic cardiomyopathy. Afro-caribbean children, particularly those with left ventricular hypertrophy, may not benefit from an angiotensin-II receptor antagonist. Angiotensin-II receptor antagonists, like the ACE inhibitors, should be avoided in pregnancy. **Interactions:** Appendix 1 (Angiotensin-II receptor antagonists).

Side-effects Side-effects are usually mild. Symptomatic hypotension including dizziness may occur, particularly in children with intravascular volume depletion (e.g. those taking high-dose diuretics). Hyperkalaemia occurs occasionally; angio-edema has also been reported.

LOSARTAN POTASSIUM

Cautions see notes above

Hepatic impairment consider lower dose

Renal impairment not recommended in children 16 years old or under with creatinine clearance less than 30 mL/minute/1.73m²; child 16–18 years with creatinine clearance less than 20 mL/minute/1.73m², start with 25 mg once daily

Pregnancy see notes above

Breast-feeding manufacturer advises avoid—no information available

Contra-indications see notes above

Side-effects see notes above; diarrhoea, taste disturbance, cough, arthralgia, myalgia, asthenia, fatigue, migraine, vertigo, urticaria, pruritus, rash; *rarely* hepatitis, anaemia (in severe renal disease or following renal transplant), thrombocytopenia, vasculitis (including Henoch-Schönlein purpura)

Licensed use not licensed for use in children

Indication and dose

Hypertension (under specialist supervision)
- By mouth

Child 6–16 years

Body-weight 20–50 kg initially 25 mg once daily; adjusted according to response to max. 50 mg once daily

Body-weight 50 kg and over initially 50 mg once daily adjusted according to response to max. 100 mg once daily

LOSARTAN POTASSIUM (*continued*)

Child 16–18 years initially 50 mg once daily (intravascular volume depletion, initially 25 mg once daily); if necessary increased after several weeks to 100 mg once daily

Cozaar® (MSD) PoM
Tablets, f/c, losartan potassium 25 mg, net price 28-tab pack = £18.09; 50 mg (scored), 28-tab pack = £18.09; 100 mg, 28-tab pack = £24.20

2.6 Nitrates, calcium-channel blockers, and other antianginal drugs

Nitrates and calcium-channel blockers have a vasodilating and, consequently, blood-pressure lowering effect. Vasodilators are known to act in heart failure either by arteriolar dilatation which reduces both peripheral vascular resistance and left ventricular pressure at systole and results in improved cardiac output, *or* venous dilatation which results in dilatation of capacitance vessels, increase of venous pooling, and diminution of venous return to the heart (decreasing left ventricular end-diastolic pressure).

2.6.1 Nitrates

Nitrates are potent coronary vasodilators, but their principal benefit follows from a reduction in venous return which reduces left ventricular work. Unwanted effects such as flushing, headache, and postural hypotension may limit therapy, especially if the child is unusually sensitive to the effects of nitrates or is hypovolaemic.

For the use of glyceryl trinitrate in extravasation, see section 10.3.

Children receiving nitrates continuously throughout the day can develop tolerance (with reduced therapeutic effects). Reduction of blood-nitrate concentrations to low levels for 4 to 8 hours each day usually maintains effectiveness in such patients.

GLYCERYL TRINITRATE

Cautions hypothyroidism, malnutrition, or hypothermia; head trauma, cerebral haemorrhage; hypoxaemia or other ventilation and perfusion abnormalities; metal-containing transdermal systems should be removed before cardioversion or diathermy; avoid abrupt withdrawal; tolerance (see notes above); **interactions:** Appendix 1 (nitrates)

Hepatic impairment caution in severe hepatic impairment

Renal impairment caution in severe renal impairment

Pregnancy not known to be harmful but most manufacturers advise avoid unless potential benefit outweighs risk

Breast-feeding no information available—manufacturers advise use only if potential benefit outweighs risk

Contra-indications hypersensitivity to nitrates; hypotensive conditions and hypovolaemia; hypertrophic obstructive cardiomyopathy, aortic stenosis, cardiac tamponade, constrictive pericarditis, mitral stenosis; marked anaemia, closed-angle glaucoma

Side-effects postural hypotension, tachycardia (but paradoxical bradycardia has occurred); throbbing headache, dizziness, *less commonly* nausea, vomiting, heartburn; flushing

Injection Specific side-effects following injection (particularly if given too rapidly) include severe hypotension, diaphoresis, apprehension, restlessness, muscle twitching, retrosternal discomfort, palpitation, abdominal pain, syncope; prolonged administration has been associated with methaemoglobinaemia

Licensed use not licensed for use in children

Indication and dose

Hypertension during and after cardiac surgery, cardiac failure after cardiac surgery, coronary vasodilation in myocardial ischaemia

- **By continuous intravenous infusion**

Neonate 0.2–0.5 micrograms/kg/minute, dose adjusted according to response; usual dose 1–3 micrograms/kg/minute; max. 10 micrograms/kg/minute

Child 1 month–18 years initially 0.2–0.5 micrograms/kg/minute, dose adjusted according to response, usual dose 1–3 micrograms/kg/minute; max. 10 micrograms/kg/minute (do not exceed 200 micrograms/minute)

Administration For *intravenous infusion* dilute with glucose 5% *or* sodium chloride 0.9% intravenous infusion to max. concentration of 400 micr-

GLYCERYL TRINITRATE (*continued*)

ograms/mL, but concentration of 1 mg/mL has been used via a central venous catheter.
Glass or polyethylene apparatus is preferable; loss of potency will occur if PVC is used

Glyceryl Trinitrate (Non-proprietary) PoM
Injection, glyceryl trinitrate 5 mg/mL. To be diluted before use. Net price 5-mL amp = £6.49; 10-mL amp = £12.98
Excipients: include ethanol, propylene glycol

Nitrocine® (Schwarz) PoM
Injection, glyceryl trinitrate 1 mg/mL. To be diluted before use or given undiluted with syringe pump. Net price 10-mL amp = £7.34; 50-mL bottle = £17.21
Excipients: include propylene glycol

Nitronal® (Merck) PoM
Injection, glyceryl trinitrate 1 mg/mL. To be diluted before use or given undiluted with syringe pump. Net price 5-mL vial = £1.92; 50-mL vial = £15.67

2.6.2 Calcium-channel blockers

Calcium-channel blockers (less correctly called 'calcium-antagonists') interfere with the inward displacement of calcium ions through the slow channels of active cell membranes. They influence the myocardial cells, the cells within the specialised conducting system of the heart, and the cells of vascular smooth muscle. Thus, myocardial contractility may be reduced, the formation and propagation of electrical impulses within the heart may be depressed, and coronary or systemic vascular tone may be diminished.

Calcium-channel blockers differ in their predilection for the various possible sites of action and, therefore, their therapeutic effects are disparate, with much greater variation than those of beta-blockers. There are important differences between verapamil, diltiazem, and the dihydropyridine calcium-channel blockers (amlodipine, nicardipine, nifedipine, and nimodipine). Verapamil and diltiazem should usually be **avoided** in *heart failure* because they may further depress cardiac function and cause clinically significant deterioration.

Verapamil is used for the treatment of *hypertension* and *arrhythmias* (section 2.3.2). However, it is no longer first-line treatment for arrhythmias in children because it has been associated with fatal collapse especially in infants under 1 year; adenosine is now recommended for first-line use.

Verapamil is a highly negatively inotropic calcium channel-blocker and it reduces cardiac output, slows the heart rate, and may impair atrioventricular conduction. It may precipitate heart failure, exacerbate conduction disorders, and cause hypotension at high doses and should **not** be used with beta-blockers (see p. 136). Constipation is the most common side-effect.

Nifedipine relaxes vascular smooth muscle and dilates coronary and peripheral arteries. It has more influence on vessels and less on the myocardium than does verapamil, and unlike verapamil has no anti-arrhythmic activity. It rarely precipitates heart failure because any negative inotropic effect is offset by a reduction in left ventricular work. Short-acting formulations of nifedipine are not recommended for long-term management of hypertension; their use may be associated with large variations in blood pressure and reflex tachycardia. However, they may be used if a modified-release preparation delivering the appropriate dose is not available or if a child is unable to swallow (a liquid preparation may be prepared using capsules). Nifedipine may also be used for the management of angina due to coronary artery disease in Kawasaki disease or progeria and in the management of Raynaud's syndrome.

Nicardipine has similar effects to those of nifedipine and may produce less reduction of myocardial contractility; it is used to treat hypertensive crisis.

Amlodipine also resembles nifedipine and nicardipine in its effects and does not reduce myocardial contractility or produce clinical deterioration in heart failure. It has a longer duration of action and can be given once daily. Nifedipine and amlodipine are used for the treatment of hypertension. Side-effects associated with vasodilatation such as flushing and headache (which become less obtrusive after a few days), and ankle swelling (which may respond only partially to diuretics) are common.

Nimodipine is related to nifedipine but the smooth muscle relaxant effect preferentially acts on cerebral arteries. Its use is confined to prevention of *vascular spasm following aneurysmal subarachnoid haemorrhage.*

Diltiazem is a peripheral vasodilator and also has mild depressor effects on the myocardium. It is used in the treatment of Raynaud's syndrome.

Withdrawal There is some evidence that sudden withdrawal of calcium-channel blockers may be associated with an exacerbation of myocardial ischaemia.

AMLODIPINE

Cautions interactions: Appendix 1 (calcium-channel blockers)

Hepatic impairment half-life prolonged—may need dose reduction

Pregnancy no information available—manufacturer advises avoid, but risk to fetus should be balanced against risk of uncontrolled maternal hypertension

Breast-feeding no information available—manufacturer advises avoid

Contra-indications cardiogenic shock, significant aortic stenosis

Side-effects abdominal pain, nausea; palpitation, flushing, oedema; headache, dizziness, sleep disturbances, fatigue; *less commonly* gastro-intestinal disturbances, dry mouth, taste disturbances, hypotension, syncope, chest pain, dyspnoea, rhinitis, mood changes, tremor, paraesthesia, urinary disturbances, impotence, gynaecomastia, weight changes, myalgia, visual disturbances, tinnitus, pruritus, rashes (including isolated reports of erythema multiforme), alopecia, purpura, and skin discolouration; *very rarely* gastritis, pancreatitis, hepatitis, jaundice, cholestasis, gingival hyperplasia, myocardial infarction, arrhythmias, vasculitis, coughing, hyperglycaemia, thrombocytopenia, angioedema, and urticaria

Licensed use not licensed for use in children

Indication and dose

Hypertension
- **By mouth**

  Child 1 month–12 years initially 100–200 micrograms/kg once daily; if necessary increase at intervals of 1–2 weeks up to 400 micrograms/kg once daily; max. 10 mg once daily

  Child 12–18 years initially 5 mg once daily; if necessary increase at intervals of 1–2 weeks to max. 10 mg once daily

Administration Tablets may be dispersed in water

Note Tablets from various suppliers may contain different salts (e.g. amlodipine besilate, amlodipine maleate, and amlodipine mesilate) but the strength is expressed in terms of amlodipine (base); tablets containing different salts are considered interchangeable

Amlodipine (Non-proprietary) PoM

Tablets, amlodipine (as maleate or as mesilate) 5 mg, net price 28-tab pack = £5.48; 10 mg, 28-tab pack = £7.96

Brands include Amlostin®

Istin® (Pfizer) PoM

Tablets, amlodipine (as besilate) 5 mg. Net price 28-tab pack = £13.04; 10 mg, 28-tab pack = £19.47

Extemporaneous formulations available see Extemporaneous Preparations, p. 8

DILTIAZEM HYDROCHLORIDE

Cautions heart failure or significantly impaired left ventricular function, bradycardia (avoid if severe), first degree AV block, or prolonged PR interval; **interactions**: Appendix 1 (calcium-channel blockers)

Hepatic impairment reduce dose

Renal impairment start with smaller dose

Breast-feeding significant amount present in milk—no evidence of harm but avoid unless no safer alternative

Contra-indications severe bradycardia, left ventricular failure with pulmonary congestion, second- or third-degree AV block (unless pacemaker fitted), sick sinus syndrome

Pregnancy avoid

Side-effects bradycardia, sino-atrial block, AV block, palpitation, dizziness, hypotension, malaise, asthenia, headache, hot flushes, gastro-intestinal disturbances, oedema (notably of ankles); rarely rashes (including erythema multiforme and exfoliative dermatitis), photosensitivity; hepatitis, gynaecomastia, gum hyperplasia, extrapyramidal symptoms, depression reported

Licensed use not licensed for use in children

Indication and dose

Raynaud's syndrome
- **By mouth**

  Child 12–18 years 30–60 mg 2–3 times daily

Standard formulations

Note These formulations are licensed as generics and there is no requirement for brand name dispensing. Although their means of formulation has called for the strict designation 'modified-release' their duration of action corresponds to that of tablets requiring administration more frequently

Diltiazem (Non-proprietary) PoM

Tablets, m/r (but see note above), diltiazem hydrochloride 60 mg. Net price 100 = £5.25. Label: 25

Brands include *Optil®*

Tildiem® (Sanofi-Synthelabo) PoM

Tablets, m/r (but see note above), off-white, diltiazem hydrochloride 60 mg. Net price 90-tab pack = £8.28. Label: 25

NICARDIPINE HYDROCHLORIDE

Cautions congestive heart failure or significantly impaired left ventricular function; avoid grapefruit juice (may affect metabolism); **interactions:** Appendix 1 (calcium-channel blockers)

Hepatic impairment reduce dose

Renal impairment start with smaller dose

Pregnancy may inhibit labour; toxicity in *animal* studies; manufacturer advises avoid, but risk to fetus should be balanced against risk of uncontrolled maternal hypertension

Contra-indications cardiogenic shock; advanced aortic stenosis

Breast-feeding no information available—manufacturer advises avoid

Side-effects dizziness, headache, peripheral oedema, flushing, palpitation, nausea; also gastro-intestinal disturbances, drowsiness, insomnia, tinnitus, hypotension, rashes, dyspnoea, paraesthesia, frequency of micturition; thrombocytopenia, depression and impotence reported

Licensed use not licensed for use in children

Indication and dose

Hypertensive crisis
- By continuous intravenous infusion

Neonate initially 500 nanograms/kg/minute, adjusted according to response; usual maintenance of 1–4 micrograms/kg/minute

Child 1 month–18 years initially 500 nanograms/kg/minute, adjusted according to response; usual maintenance of 1–4 micrograms/kg/minute (max. 250 micrograms/minute)

Administration For *intravenous infusion* dilute in glucose 5% *or* sodium chloride 0.9% intravenous infusion to a concentration of 100 micrograms/mL; to minimise peripheral venous irritation, change site of infusion every 12 hours

Cardene IV® PoM
Injection, nicardipine 2.5 mg/mL (10-mL ampoule)
Available from specialist importing companies

NIFEDIPINE

Cautions poor cardiac reserve; heart failure or significantly impaired left ventricular function (heart failure deterioration observed); severe hypotension; diabetes mellitus; avoid grapefruit juice (may affect metabolism); **interactions:** Appendix 1 (calcium-channel blockers)

Hepatic impairment reduce dose in severe liver disease

Pregnancy may inhibit labour; toxicity in *animal* studies; manufacturer advises avoid, but risk to fetus should be balanced against risk of uncontrolled maternal hypertension

Breast-feeding amount too small to be harmful but manufacturer advises avoid

Contra-indications cardiogenic shock; advanced aortic stenosis; porphyria (section 9.8.2)

Side-effects headache, flushing, dizziness, lethargy; tachycardia, palpitation; short-acting preparations may induce an exaggerated fall in blood pressure and reflex tachycardia which may lead to myocardial or cerebrovascular ischaemia; gravitational oedema, rash (erythema multiforme reported), pruritus, urticaria, nausea, constipation or diarrhoea, increased frequency of micturition, eye pain, visual disturbances, gum hyperplasia, asthenia, paraesthesia, myalgia, tremor, impotence, gynaecomastia; depression, telangiectasia, cholestasis, jaundice reported

Licensed use not licensed for use in children

Indication and dose

Hypertensive crisis
- By mouth

Child 1 month–18 years 250–500 micrograms/kg as a single dose

Administration use liquid if 5 or 10 mg dose inappropriate; if liquid unavailable, extract contents of capsule via a syringe and use immediately—cover syringe with foil to protect contents from light

Hypertension
- By mouth

Child 1 month–12 years 200–300 micrograms/kg 3 times daily; max. 3 mg/kg daily *or* 100 mg daily

Child 12–18 years 5–20 mg 3 times daily; max. 100 mg daily

Administration Dose frequency depends on preparation used; modified release tablets may be crushed—this may alter the release profile; crushed tablets should be administered within 30–60 seconds to avoid significant loss of potency of drug

Angina in Kawasaki disease or progeria see cautions above
- By mouth

Child 1 month–18 years 200–300 micrograms/kg 3 times daily *or* if over 12 years 5–20 mg 3 times daily (max. 3 mg/kg/day *or* 100 mg/day)

Administration dose frequency depends on preparation used; use liquid if 5 or 10 mg dose inappropriate; if liquid unavailable, extract contents of capsule via a syringe and use immediately—cover syringe with foil to protect contents from light

Raynaud's syndrome
- By mouth

Child 2–18 years 2.5–10 mg 2–4 times daily; start with low doses at night and increase gradually to avoid postural hypotension

Administration Dose frequency depends on preparation used; modified release tablets may be crushed—this may alter the release profile; crushed tablets should be administered within 30–60 seconds to avoid significant loss of potency of drug

Persistent hyperinsulinaemic hypoglycaemia see also section 6.1.4
- By mouth

Neonates 100–200 micrograms/kg (max. 600 micrograms/kg) 4 times daily

NIFEDIPINE (*continued*)

Nifedipine (Non-proprietary) PoM
Capsules, nifedipine 5 mg, net price 84-cap pack = £3.68; 10 mg, 84-cap pack = £3.72

Dose

Give 3 times daily

Oral liquid, available from specialist importing companies

Adalat® (Bayer) PoM
Capsules, both orange, nifedipine 5 mg, net price 90-cap pack = £6.08; 10 mg, 90-cap pack = £7.74

Dose

Give 3 times daily

Modified release

Note Different versions of modified-release preparations may not have the same clinical effect. To avoid confusion between these different formulations of nifedipine, prescribers should specify the brand to be dispensed. Modified-release formulations may not be suitable for dose titration in hepatic disease

Adalat® LA (Bayer) PoM
LA 20 tablets, m/r, pink, nifedipine 20 mg, net price 28-tab pack = £5.27. Label: 25

LA 30 tablets, m/r, pink, nifedipine 30 mg, net price 28-tab pack = £7.59. Label: 25

LA 60 tablets, m/r, pink, nifedipine 60 mg, net price 28-tab pack = £9.69. Label: 25

Counselling Tablet membrane may pass through gastro-intestinal tract unchanged, but being porous has no effect on efficacy

Cautions dose form not appropriate for use in hepatic impairment or where there is a history of oesophageal or gastro-intestinal obstruction, decreased lumen diameter of the gastro-intestinal tract, or inflammatory bowel disease (including Crohn's disease)

Dose

Give once daily

Adalat® Retard (Bayer) PoM
Retard 10 tablets, m/r, pink, nifedipine 10 mg. Net price 56-tab pack = £8.50. Label: 25

Retard 20 tablets, m/r, pink, nifedipine 20 mg. Net price 56-tab pack = £10.20. Label: 25

Dose

Give twice daily

Adipine® MR (Trinity-Chiesi) PoM
Tablets, m/r, nifedipine 10 mg (apricot), net price 56-tab pack = £5.96; 20 mg (pink), 56-tab pack = £7.43. Label: 21, 25

Dose

Give twice daily

Adipine® XL (Trinity-Chiesi) PoM
Tablets, m/r, both red, nifedipine 30 mg, net price 28-tab pack = £8.95. Label: 25

Dose

Give once daily

Cardilate MR® (IVAX) PoM
Tablets, m/r, nifedipine 10 mg (pink), net price 56-tab pack = £4.97; 20 mg (brown), net price 100-tab pack = £16.62. Label: 25

Dose

Give twice daily

Coracten SR® (Celltech) PoM
Capsules, m/r, nifedipine 10 mg (grey/pink, enclosing yellow pellets), net price 60-cap pack = £4.27; 20 mg (pink/brown, enclosing yellow pellets), 60-cap pack = £5.93. Label: 25

Dose

Give twice daily

Coracten XL® (Celltech) PoM
Capsules, m/r, nifedipine 30 mg (brown), net price 28-cap pack = £5.89; 60 mg (orange), 28-cap pack = £8.84. Label: 25

Dose

Give once daily

Fortipine LA 40® (Goldshield) PoM
Tablets, m/r, red, nifedipine 40 mg, net price 30-tab pack = £8.00. Label: 21, 25

Dose

Give 1–2 times daily

Hypolar® Retard 20 (Sandoz) PoM
Tablets, m/r, red, f/c, nifedipine 20 mg. Net price 56-tab pack = £7.00. Label: 25

Dose

Give twice daily

Nifedipress® MR (Dexcel) PoM
Tablets, m/r, pink, nifedipine 10 mg, net price 56-tab pack = £9.23. Label: 25

Dose

Give twice daily

Nifopress® Retard (Goldshield) PoM
Tablets, m/r, pink, nifedipine 20 mg, net price 112-tab pack = £10.80. Label: 21, 25

Dose

Give twice daily

Slofedipine® (Sterwin) PoM
Tablets, m/r, pink, nifedipine 20 mg, net price 56-tab pack = £10.32. Label: 25

Dose

Give twice daily

Slofedipine XL® (Sterwin) PoM
Tablets, m/r, brown, nifedipine 30 mg, net price 28-tab pack = £9.89; 60 mg, 28-tab pack = £14.71. Label: 25

Cautions dose form not appropriate for use in hepatic impairment or where there is a history of oesophageal or gastro-intestinal obstruction, decreased lumen diameter

NIFEDIPINE (*continued*)

of the gastro-intestinal tract, or inflammatory bowel disease (including Crohn's disease)

Dose

Give once daily

Tensipine MR® (Genus) PoM

Tablets, m/r, both pink, nifedipine 10 mg, net price 56-tab pack = £3.75; 20 mg, 56-tab pack = £5.25. Label: 21, 25

Dose

Give twice daily

NIMODIPINE

Cautions cerebral oedema or severely raised intracranial pressure; hypotension; avoid concomitant administration of nimodipine tablets and infusion, other calcium-channel blockers, or beta-blockers; concomitant nephrotoxic drugs; avoid grapefruit juice (may affect metabolism); **interactions:** Appendix 1 (calcium-channel blockers, alcohol (infusion only))

Hepatic impairment elimination reduced in cirrhosis—monitor blood pressure; reduce oral dose by 50% in children with severe cirrhosis

Renal impairment manufacturer advises monitor renal function closely

Pregnancy manufacturer advises use only if potential benefit outweighs risks

Side-effects hypotension, variation in heart-rate, flushing, headache, gastro-intestinal disorders, nausea, sweating and feeling of warmth; thrombocytopenia and ileus reported

Licensed use not licensed for use in children

Indication and dose

Treatment of vasospasm following subarachnoid haemorrhage under specialist advice only

- **By intravenous infusion**

Child 1 month–12 years initially 15 micrograms/kg/hour (max. 500 micrograms/hour) *or* initially 7.5 micrograms/kg/hour if blood pressure unstable; increase after 2 hours to 30 micrograms/kg/hour (max. 2 mg/hour) if no severe decrease in blood pressure; continue for at least 5 days (max. 14 days)

Child 12–18 years initially 500 micrograms/hour (up to 1 mg/hour if body-weight over 70 kg and blood pressure stable), increase after 2 hours to 1–2 mg/hour if no severe fall in blood pressure; continue for at least 5 days (max. 14 days)

Administration For *intravenous infusion* administer undiluted *via* a Y-piece on a central venous catheter connected to a running infusion of glucose 5% *or* sodium chloride 0.9% intravenous infusion; not to be added to an infusion container; incompatible with polyvinyl chloride giving sets or containers; protect infusion from light

Prevention of vasospasm following subarachnoid haemorrhage

- **By mouth**

Child 1 month–18 years 0.9–1.2 mg/kg (max. 60 mg) 6 times daily, starting within 4 days of haemorrhage and continued for 21 days

Administration Tablets may be crushed or halved but are light sensitive—administer immediately

Nimotop® (Bayer) PoM

Tablets, yellow, f/c, nimodipine 30 mg. Net price 100-tab pack = £38.85

Intravenous infusion, nimodipine 200 micrograms/mL; also contains ethanol 20% and macrogol '400' 17%. Net price 50-mL vial (with polyethylene infusion catheter) = £13.24

Note Polyethylene, polypropylene or glass apparatus should be used; PVC should be avoided

VERAPAMIL HYDROCHLORIDE

Cautions first-degree AV block; patients taking beta-blockers (**important:** see below); avoid grapefruit juice (may affect metabolism); **interactions:** Appendix 1 (calcium-channel blockers)

Verapamil and beta-blockers **Verapamil** injection should not be given to patients recently treated with beta-blockers because of the risk of hypotension and asystole. The suggestion that when verapamil injection has been given first, an interval of 30 minutes before giving a beta-blocker is sufficient has not been confirmed.
It may also be hazardous to give verapamil and a beta-blocker together by mouth (should only be contemplated if myocardial function well preserved).

Hepatic impairment oral dose may need to be reduced

Pregnancy may reduce uterine blood flow with fetal hypoxia; manufacturer advises avoid during first trimester unless absolutely necessary; may inhibit labour

Breast-feeding amount too small to be harmful

Contra-indications hypotension, bradycardia, second- and third-degree AV block, sick sinus syndrome, cardiogenic shock, sino-atrial block; history of heart failure or significantly impaired left ventricular function, even if controlled by therapy; atrial flutter or fibrillation complicating Wolff-Parkinson-White syndrome; porphyria (section 9.8.2)

Side-effects constipation; less commonly nausea, vomiting, flushing, headache, dizziness, fatigue, ankle oedema; rarely allergic reactions (erythema, pruritus, urticaria, angioedema, Stevens-Johnson syndrome); myalgia, arthralgia, paraesthesia, erythromelalgia; increased prolactin concentration; rarely gynaecomastia and gingival hyperplasia after long-term treatment; after intravenous administration or high doses, hypotension, heart failure, bradycardia, heart block, and asystole; hypersensitivity reactions involving reversibly raised liver function tests

VERAPAMIL HYDROCHLORIDE (*continued*)

Licensed use Modified release preparation not licensed for use in children

Indication and dose

Hypertension, prophylaxis of supraventricular arrhythmias under specialist advice only
- By mouth
  Child 1–2 years 20 mg 2–3 times daily
  Child 2–18 years 40–120 mg 2–3 times daily

Treatment of supraventricular arrhythmias
- By intravenous injection over 2–3 minutes (with ECG and blood-pressure monitoring and under specialist advice)
  Child 1–18 years 100–300 micrograms/kg (max. 5 mg) as a single dose, repeated after 30 minutes if necessary

Administration for *intravenous injection* may be diluted with Glucose 5% *or* Sodium Chloride 0.9%; incompatible with solutions of pH greater than 6

Verapamil (Non-proprietary) PoM
Tablets, coated, verapamil hydrochloride 40 mg, net price 20 = 47p; 80 mg, 20 = 56p; 120 mg, 20 = £1.12; 160 mg, 20 = £1.69

Oral solution, verapamil hydrochloride 40 mg/5 mL, net price 150 mL = £36.90
Brands include *Zolvera®*

Cordilox® (IVAX) PoM
Tablets, all yellow, f/c, verapamil hydrochloride 40 mg, net price 84-tab pack = £1.50; 80 mg, 84-tab pack = £2.05; 120 mg, 28-tab pack = £1.15; 160 mg, 56-tab pack = £2.80

Injection, verapamil hydrochloride 2.5 mg/mL, net price 2-mL amp = £1.11

Securon® (Abbott) PoM
Tablets, f/c, verapamil hydrochloride 40 mg, net price 100 = £4.57; 120 mg (scored), 60-tab pack = £6.29

Injection, verapamil hydrochloride 2.5 mg/mL. Net price 2-mL amp = £1.08

Extemporaneous formulations available see Extemporaneous Preparations, p. 8

Modified release

Half Securon SR® (Abbott) PoM
Tablets, m/r, f/c, verapamil hydrochloride 120 mg. Net price 28-tab pack = £7.50. Label: 25

Dose

Give once daily (doses above 240 mg daily, give 2–3 times daily)

Securon SR® (Abbott) PoM
Tablets, m/r, pale green, f/c, scored, verapamil hydrochloride 240 mg. Net price 28-tab pack = £6.29. Label: 25

Dose

Give once daily (doses above 240 mg daily, give 2–3 times daily)

Univer® (Zeneus) PoM
Capsules, m/r, verapamil hydrochloride 120 mg (yellow/dark blue), net price 28-cap pack = £7.51; 180 mg (yellow), 56-cap pack = £18.15; 240 mg (yellow/dark blue), 28-cap pack = £12.24. Label: 25

Dose

Give once daily

Verapress MR® (Dexcel) PoM
Tablets, m/r, pale green, f/c, verapamil hydrochloride 240 mg. Net price 28-tab pack = £9.90. Label: 25

Dose

Give 1–2 times daily

Note Also available as *Cordilox® MR*

Vertab® SR 240 (Trinity-Chiesi) PoM
Tablets, m/r, pale green, f/c, scored, verapamil hydrochloride 240 mg, net price 28-tab pack = £8.63. Label: 25

Dose

Give 1–2 times daily

2.6.3 Other antianginal drugs

Classification not used in BNF for Children

2.6.4 Peripheral vasodilators and related drugs

Raynaud's syndrome consists of recurrent, long-lasting, and episodic vasospasm of the fingers and toes often associated with exposure to cold. Management includes avoidance of exposure to cold and stopping smoking (if appropriate). More severe symptoms may require vasodilator treatment, which is most often successful in primary Raynaud's syndrome. **Nifedipine** and **diltiazem** (section 2.6.2) are useful for reducing the frequency and severity of vasospastic attacks. In very severe cases, where digital infarction is likely, intravenous infusion of the prostacyclin analogue **iloprost** may be helpful.

Vasodilator therapy is not established as being effective for *chilblains* (section 13.14).

ILOPROST

Cautions see section 2.5.1.2

Contra-indications see section 2.5.1.2

Side-effects see section 2.5.1.2

Licensed use not licensed for use in children

Indication and dose

Raynaud's syndrome see notes above

- **By intravenous infusion**

  Child 12–18 years initially 30 nanograms/kg/hour, increased gradually to 60–120 nanograms/kg/hour given over 6 hours daily for 3–5 days

Pulmonary hypertension section 2.5.1.2

Administration For intravenous infusion dilute with glucose 5% intravenous infusion or sodium chloride 0.9% intravenous infusion to a concentration of 200 nanograms/mL; alternatively, may be diluted to a concentration of 2 micrograms/mL and given via syringe driver

Iloprost (Non-proprietary)

Concentrate for infusion, iloprost 100 micrograms/mL (as iloprost trometamol).

For dilution and use as an intravenous infusion

Note available on a named patient basis from Schering Healthcare in 0.5 mL and 1 mL ampoules

2.7 Sympathomimetics

The properties of sympathomimetics vary according to whether they act on alpha or on beta adrenergic receptors. Response to sympathomimetics can also vary considerably in children, particularly neonates. It is important to titrate the dose to the desired effect and to monitor the child closely.

2.7.1 Inotropic sympathomimetics

The cardiac stimulants **dobutamine** and **dopamine** act on $beta_1$ receptors in cardiac muscle and increase contractility with little effect on rate.

Dopamine has a variable, unpredictable, and dose dependent impact on vascular tone. Low dose infusion (2 micrograms/kg/minute) normally causes vasodilatation, but there is little evidence that this is clinically beneficial; moderate doses increase myocardial contractility and cardiac output in older children, but in neonates moderate doses may cause a reduction in cardiac output. High doses cause vasoconstriction and increase vascular resistance, and should therefore be used with caution following cardiac surgery, or where there is co-existing neonatal pulmonary hypertension.

In neonates the response to inotropic sympathomimetics varies considerably, particularly in those born prematurely; careful dose titration and monitoring are necessary.

Isoprenaline injection is available on special order only.

Shock Shock is a medical emergency associated with a high mortality. The underlying causes of shock such as haemorrhage, sepsis or myocardial insufficiency should be corrected. The profound hypotension of shock must be treated promptly to prevent tissue hypoxia and organ failure. Volume replacement is essential to correct the hypovolaemia associated with haemorrhage and sepsis but may be detrimental in cardiogenic shock.

Neonatal septic shock can be complicated by the transition from fetal to neonatal circulation. Treatment to reverse right ventricular failure, by decreasing pulmonary artery pressures, is commonly needed in neonates with fluid-refractory shock and persistent pulmonary hypertension of the newborn (section 2.5.1.2). Rapid administration of fluid in neonates with patent ductus arteriosus may cause left-to-right shunting and congestive heart failure induced by ventricular overload.

The use of sympathomimetic inotropes and vasoconstrictors should preferably be confined to the intensive care setting and undertaken with invasive haemodynamic monitoring.

For advice on the management of anaphylactic shock, see section 3.4.3.

DOBUTAMINE

Cautions severe hypotension complicating cardiogenic shock; **interactions:** Appendix 1 (sympathomimetics)

Pregnancy no information available

Contra-indications marked obstruction of cardiac ejection, such as idiopathic hypertrophic subaortic stenosis

Side-effects tachycardia and marked increase in systolic blood pressure indicate overdosage; phlebitis; *rarely* thrombocytopenia

Licensed use not licensed for use in children

Indication and dose

Inotropic support in low cardiac output states, after cardiac surgery, cardiomyopathies, shock
- By continuous intravenous infusion

Neonate initially 5 micrograms/kg/minute, adjusted according to response to 2–15 micrograms/kg/minute; max. 20 micrograms/kg/minute

Child 1 month–18 years initially 5 micrograms/kg/minute adjusted according to response to 2–20 micrograms/kg/minute; max. 40 micrograms/kg/minute (but increased side-effects)

Administration Intravenous infusion using infusion pump; dilute injection solution with glucose 5% *or* sodium chloride 0.9% to 0.5–1 mg/mL (max. 5 mg/mL in fluid restricted children)—infuse higher concentration solutions through central venous catheter; incompatible with bicarbonate and other strong alkaline solutions.

Dobutamine (Non-proprietary) PoM
Strong sterile solution, dobutamine (as hydrochloride) 12.5 mg/mL. For dilution and use as an intravenous infusion. Net price 20-mL amp = £5.25

DOPAMINE HYDROCHLORIDE

Cautions correct hypovolaemia; **interactions:** Appendix 1 (sympathomimetics)

Pregnancy manufacturer advises use only if potential benefit outweighs risk

Contra-indications tachyarrhythmia, phaeochromocytoma

Side-effects nausea and vomiting, peripheral vasoconstriction, hypotension, hypertension, tachycardia

Licensed use not licensed for use in children

Indication and dose

To correct the haemodynamic imbalance due to acute hypotension, shock, cardiac failure, adjunct following cardiac surgery
- By continuous intravenous infusion

Neonate initially 3 micrograms/kg/minute, adjusted according to response (max. 20 micrograms/kg/minute)

Child 1 month–18 years initially 5 micrograms/kg/minute adjusted according to response (max. 20 micrograms/kg/minute)

Administration For *intravenous administration* dilute injection solution in sodium chloride 0.9% *or* glucose 5% to max. concentration of 3.2 mg/mL. Infuse higher concentrations through central venous catheter using a syringe pump to avoid extravasation and fluid overload. Incompatible with bicarbonate and other alkaline solutions.

Dopamine (Non-proprietary) PoM
Sterile concentrate, dopamine hydrochloride 40 mg/mL, net price 5-mL amp = £3.88; 160 mg/mL, net price 5-mL amp = £14.75. For dilution and use as an intravenous infusion
Intravenous infusion, dopamine hydrochloride 1.6 mg/mL in glucose 5% intravenous infusion, net price 250-mL container (400 mg) = £11.69; 3.2 mg/mL, 250-mL container (800 mg) = £22.93 (both hosp. only)

Select-A-Jet® Dopamine (Celltech) PoM
Strong sterile solution, dopamine hydrochloride 40 mg/mL. Net price 5-mL vial = £4.55; 10-mL vial = £7.32. For dilution and use as an intravenous infusion

2.7.2 Vasoconstrictor sympathomimetics

Vasoconstrictor sympathomimetics raise blood pressure transiently by acting on alpha-adrenergic receptors to constrict peripheral vessels. They are sometimes used as an emergency method of elevating blood pressure where other measures have failed (see also section 2.7.1).

The danger of vasoconstrictors is that although they raise blood pressure they also reduce perfusion of vital organs such as the kidney.

Ephedrine is used to reverse hypotension caused by spinal and epidural anaesthesia.

Metaraminol is used as a vasopressor during cardiopulmonary bypass.

Phenylephrine causes peripheral vasoconstriction and increases arterial pressure.

Ephedrine, metaraminol and phenylephrine are rarely needed in children and should be used under specialist supervision.

Noradrenaline (norepinephrine) is reserved for children with low systemic vascular resistance that is unresponsive to fluid resuscitation following septic shock, spinal shock, and anaphylaxis.

Adrenaline (epinephrine) is mainly used for its inotropic action. Low doses (acting on beta receptors) cause systemic and pulmonary vasodilation, with some increase in heart rate and stroke volume and also an increase in contractility; high doses act predominantly on alpha receptors causing intense systemic vasoconstriction.

EPHEDRINE HYDROCHLORIDE

Cautions hyperthyroidism, diabetes mellitus, hypertension, angle-closure glaucoma, **interactions:** Appendix 1 (sympathomimetics)

Renal impairment avoid in severe impairment; increased CNS toxicity

Pregnancy increased fetal heart rate reported

Contra-indications

Breast-feeding irritability and disturbed sleep reported in breast-fed infants

Side-effects nausea, vomiting, anorexia; tachycardia (sometimes bradycardia), arrhythmias, anginal pain, vasoconstriction with hypertension, vasodilation with hypotension, dizziness and flushing; dyspnoea; headache, anxiety, restlessness, confusion, psychoses, insomnia, tremor; difficulty in micturition, urine retention; sweating, hypersalivation; changes in blood-glucose concentration

Indication and dose

Reversal of hypotension from epidural and spinal anaesthesia

- **By slow intravenous injection of a solution containing ephedrine hydrochloride 3 mg/mL**

  Child 1–12 years 500–750 micrograms/kg *or* 17–25 mg/m² every 3–4 minutes according to response; max. 30 mg during episode

  Child 12–18 years 3–7.5 mg (max. 9 mg) repeated every 3–4 minutes according to response, max. 30 mg during episode

Nasal congestion section 12.2.2

Administration By slow intravenous injection, via central line.

Ephedrine Hydrochloride (Non-proprietary) PoM

Injection, ephedrine hydrochloride 3 mg/mL, net price 10-mL amp = £2.70; 30 mg/mL, net price 1-mL amp = £1.70

METARAMINOL

Cautions see under Noradrenaline; longer duration of action than noradrenaline (norepinephrine), see below; cirrhosis; **interactions:** Appendix 1 (sympathomimetics)

Hypertensive response Metaraminol has a longer duration of action than noradrenaline, and an excessive vasopressor response may cause a prolonged rise in blood pressure

Breast-feeding manufacturer advises caution—no information available

Contra-indications see under Noradrenaline

Pregnancy may reduce placental prefusion—manufacturer advises use only if potential benefit outweighs risk

Side-effects see under Noradrenaline; tachycardia; fatal ventricular arrhythmia reported in Laennec's cirrhosis

Licensed use Not licensed for use in children

Indication and dose

Acute hypotension

- **By intravenous infusion**

  Child 12–18 years 15–100 mg adjusted according to response

Emergency treatment of acute hypotension

- **By intravenous administration**

  Child 12–18 years initially by intravenous injection 0.5–5 mg, then by intravenous infusion 15–100 mg adjusted according to response

Administration For *intravenous infusion* dilute injection solution with glucose 5% *or* sodium chloride 0.9% intravenous infusion to a concentration of 30–200 micrograms/mL and give through a central venous catheter

Metaraminol (Non-proprietary) PoM

Injection, metaraminol 10 mg (as tartrate)/mL. Available from regional hospital manufacturing unit ('special order')

NORADRENALINE/NOREPINEPHRINE

Cautions coronary, mesenteric, or peripheral vascular thrombosis; Prinzmetal's variant angina, hyperthyroidism, diabetes mellitus; hypoxia or hypercapnia; uncorrected hypovolaemia; extravasation at injection site may cause necrosis; **interactions:** Appendix 1 (sympathomimetics)

Contra-indications hypertension (monitor blood pressure and rate of flow frequently)

Pregnancy avoid—may reduce placental perfusion

Side-effects hypertension, headache, bradycardia, arrhythmias, peripheral ischaemia

NORADRENALINE/NOREPINEPHRINE (*continued*)

Licensed use not licensed for use in children

Indication and dose

Acute hypotension (septic shock) or shock secondary to excessive vasodilation (as noradrenaline)

- **By continuous intravenous infusion**

Neonate 20–100 nanograms(base)/kg/minute adjusted according to response; max. 1 microgram(base)/kg/minute

Child 1 month–18 years 20–100 nanograms(base)/kg/minute adjusted according to response; max. 1 microgram(base)/kg/minute

Note 1 mg of noradrenaline acid tartrate is equivalent to 500 micrograms of the base. Dose expressed as the base

Administration dilute (with glucose 5% intravenous infusion *or* sodium chloride and glucose intravenous infusion) to a concentration of noradrenaline (base) up to 40 micrograms/mL and give through central line; incompatible with bicarbonate or alkaline solutions; protect from light (discard if discoloured)

Noradrenaline/Norepinephrine (Abbott) PoM
Injection, noradrenaline acid tartrate 2 mg/mL (equivalent to noradrenaline base 1 mg/mL). For dilution before use. Net price 2-mL amp = £1.01, 4-mL amp = £1.50, 20-mL amp = £6.35
Excipients: may include sodium metabisulphite

PHENYLEPHRINE HYDROCHLORIDE

Cautions see under Noradrenaline; longer duration of action than noradrenaline (norepinephrine), see below; coronary disease

Hypertensive response Phenylephrine has a longer duration of action than noradrenaline, and an excessive vasopressor response may cause a prolonged rise in blood pressure

Contra-indications see under Noradrenaline; severe hyperthyroidism

Pregnancy avoid if possible; malformations reported following use in first trimester; fetal hypoxia and bradycardia reported in late pregnancy and labour

Side-effects see under Noradrenaline; tachycardia or reflex bradycardia

Licensed use not licensed for use in children by intravenous infusion or injection

Indication and dose

Acute hypotension

- **By subcutaneous or intramuscular injection (but intravenous injection preferred, see below)**

Child 1–12 years 100 micrograms/kg every 1–2 hours as needed (max. 5 mg)

Child 12–18 years 2–5 mg, followed if necessary by further doses of 1–10 mg (max. initial dose 5 mg)

- **By slow intravenous injection**

Child 1–12 years 5–20 micrograms/kg (max. 500 micrograms) repeated as necessary after at least 15 minutes

Child 12–18 years 100–500 micrograms repeated as necessary after at least 15 minutes

Administration Dilute with water for injection to a concentration of 1 mg/mL and administer slowly

- **By intravenous infusion**

Child 1–16 years 100–500 nanograms/kg/minute, adjusted according to response

Child 16–18 years initially up to 180 micrograms/minute reduced to 30–60 micrograms/minute according to response

Administration For *intravenous infusion* dilute injection solution with glucose 5% *or* sodium chloride 0.9% intravenous infusion to a concentration of 20 micrograms/ml and administer as a continuous infusion via a central venous catheter using a controlled infusion device.

Phenylephrine (Sovereign) PoM
Injection, phenylephrine hydrochloride 10 mg/mL (1%). Net price 1-mL amp = £5.50

ADRENALINE/EPINEPHRINE

Cautions diabetes mellitus, hyperthyroidism, hypertension, arrhythmias, cerebrovascular disease, avoid extravasation, monitor urine output, limb perfusion (especially at higher doses), central venous pressures and ECG; **interactions:** Appendix 1 (sympathomimetics)

Side-effects nausea, vomiting, sweating, tachycardia, dyspnoea, anxiety, tremor, headache, weakness, dizziness and hyperglycaemia , cold extremities; in overdosage hypertension, arrhythmias, cerebral haemorrhage, pulmonary oedema

Indication and dose

Acute hypotension

- **By continuous intravenous infusion**

Neonate initially 100 nanograms/kg/minute adjusted according to response; higher doses up to 1.5 micrograms/kg/minute have been used in acute hypotension

Child 1 month–18 years initially 100 nanograms/kg/minute adjusted according to response; higher doses up to 1.5 micrograms/kg/minute have been used in acute hypotension

Anaphylaxis section 3.4.3

Administration For *intravenous infusion* dilute injection solution with glucose 5% *or* sodium

ADRENALINE/EPINEPHRINE (*continued*)

chloride 0.9% intravenous infusion and give *via* central venous catheter; incompatible with bicarbonate and alkaline solutions; protect from light

Preparations
Section 3.4.3

2.7.3 Cardiopulmonary resuscitation

The algorithms for cardiopulmonary resuscitation (see inside back cover) reflect the recommendations of the Resuscitation Council (UK); they cover paediatric basic life support, paediatric advanced life support, newborn life support, and adult life support. The guidelines are available at www.resus.org.uk.

Paediatric advanced life support Cardiopulmonary (cardiac) arrest in children is rare and frequently represents the terminal event of progressive shock or respiratory failure.

During cardiopulmonary arrest in children without intravenous access, the intraosseous route is chosen because it provides rapid and effective response; if circulatory access cannot be gained, the endotracheal tube can be used. When the endotracheal route is used ten times the intravenous dose should be used; the drug should be injected quickly down a narrow bore suction catheter beyond the tracheal end of the tube and then flushed in with 1 or 2 mL of sodium chloride 0.9%. The endotracheal route is useful for lipid-soluble drugs, including lidocaine, adrenaline, atropine, and naloxone. Drugs that are not lipid-soluble (e.g. sodium bicarbonate and calcium chloride) should **not** be administered by this route because they will injure the airways.

For the management of acute anaphylaxis see section 3.4.3.

2.8 Anticoagulants and protamine

Although thrombotic episodes are uncommon in childhood, anticoagulants may be required in children with congenital heart disease; in children undergoing haemodialysis; for preventing thrombosis in children requiring chemotherapy and following surgery; and for systemic venous thromboembolism secondary to inherited thrombophilias, systemic lupus erythematosus, or indwelling central venous catheters.

2.8.1 Parenteral anticoagulants

Heparin

Heparin initiates anticoagulation rapidly but has a short duration of action. It is now often referred to as being **standard** or **unfractionated heparin** to distinguish it from the **low molecular weight heparins** (see p. 144), which have a longer duration of action. For children at high risk of bleeding, heparin is more suitable than low molecular weight heparin because its effect can be terminated rapidly by stopping the infusion.

Heparin is used in both the treatment and prophylaxis of thromboembolic disease; however, it is mainly used to prevent further clotting rather than to lyse existing clots—surgery or a thrombolytic drug may be necessary if a thrombus obstructs major vessels.

Treatment For the initial treatment of thrombotic episodes heparin is given as an *intravenous loading dose*, followed by *continuous intravenous infusion* (using an infusion pump) or by *intermittent subcutaneous injection*; the use of *intermittent intravenous injection* is no longer recommended. Alternatively, a low molecular weight heparin may be given for initial treatment. An oral anticoagulant (usually warfarin, section 2.8.2) is started at the same time as the heparin (the heparin needs to be continued for at least 5 days and until the INR has been in the therapeutic range for 2 consecutive days). Laboratory monitoring of coagulation activity, preferably on a daily basis, involves determination of the activated partial prothrombin time (APTT) or of the anti-factor Xa concentration. Local guidelines on recommended APTT for neonates and children should be followed.

Prophylaxis Low-dose heparin by subcutaneous injection is used to prevent thrombotic episodes in 'high-risk' patients; laboratory monitoring of APTT is also required in prophylactic regimens in children. **Aspirin** (section 2.9) and **warfarin** (section 2.8.2) may also be used for prophylaxis.

Extracorporeal circuits Heparin is also used in the maintenance of extracorporeal circuits in *cardiopulmonary bypass* and *haemodialysis.*

Haemorrhage If haemorrhage occurs it is usually sufficient to withdraw heparin, but if rapid reversal of the effects of heparin is required, protamine sulphate (section 2.8.3) is a specific antidote (but only partially reverses the effects of low molecular weight heparins).

HEPARIN

Cautions hypersensitivity to low molecular weight heparins; **interactions:** Appendix 1 (heparin)

Heparin-induced thrombocytopenia Clinically important thrombocytopenia is immune-mediated, and does not usually develop until after 6 to 10 days; it may be complicated by thrombosis. Platelet counts are recommended for patients receiving heparin (including low molecular weight heparins) for longer than 5 days (heparin should be stopped immediately, and not repeated, in those who develop thrombocytopenia or a 50% reduction in platelet count). Children with heparin-induced thrombocytopenia who require continued anticoagulation should preferably be given a heparinoid such as danaparoid

Hyperkalaemia Inhibition of aldosterone secretion by heparin (including low molecular weight heparins) may result in hyperkalaemia; patients with diabetes mellitus, chronic renal failure, acidosis, raised plasma potassium, or those taking potassium-sparing drugs seem to be more susceptible. The risk appears to increase with duration of therapy and the CSM has recommended that plasma potassium should be measured in patients at risk before starting heparin and monitored regularly thereafter, particularly if heparin is to be continued for more than 7 days

Hepatic impairment risk of bleeding increased—possibly reduce dose in severe impairment

Renal impairment risk of bleeding increased—consider reduced dose in severe impairment

Pregnancy no evidence of harm and is the anticoagulant of choice if indicated during pregnancy; maternal osteoporosis reported after prolonged use; increased risk of maternal bleeding

Contra-indications haemophilia and other haemorrhagic disorders, thrombocytopenia (including history of heparin-induced thrombocytopenia), peptic ulcer, recent cerebral haemorrhage, severe hypertension, severe liver disease (including oesophageal varices), after major trauma or recent surgery to eye or nervous system, acute bacterial endocarditis; spinal or epidural anaesthesia with treatment doses of heparin; hypersensitivity to heparin

Side-effects haemorrhage (see notes above), skin necrosis, thrombocytopenia (see Cautions), hyperkalaemia (see Cautions), hypersensitivity reactions (including urticaria, angioedema, and anaphylaxis); osteoporosis after prolonged use (and rarely alopecia)

Licensed use Some preparations licensed for use in children

Indication and dose

Treatment of thrombotic episodes
- **By intravenous administration**

Neonate initially 75 units/kg (50 units/kg if under 35 weeks post-menstrual age) *by intravenous injection*, then *by continuous intravenous infusion* 25 units/kg/hour, adjusted according to APTT

Child 1 month–1 year initially 75 units/kg *by intravenous injection*, then *by continuous intravenous infusion* 25 units/kg/hour, adjusted according to APTT

Child 1–18 years initially 75 units/kg *by intravenous injection*, then *by continuous intravenous infusion* 20 units/kg/hour, adjusted according to APTT

- **By subcutaneous injection**

Child 1 month–18 years 250 units/kg twice daily, adjusted according to APTT

Prophylaxis of thrombotic episodes
- **By subcutaneous injection**

Child 1 month–18 years 100 units/kg (max. 5000 units) twice daily, adjusted according to APTT

Prevention of clotting in extracorporeal circuits consult product literature

Administration For *intravenous infusion* dilute with glucose 5% intravenous infusion *or* sodium chloride 0.9% intravenous infusion

Heparin (Non-proprietary) PoM

Injection, heparin sodium 1000 units/mL, net price 1-mL amp = 19p, 5-mL amp = 85p, 5-mL vial = 47p, 10-mL amp = £1.46, 20-mL amp = £2.40; 5000 units/mL, 1-mL amp = 36p, 5-mL amp = £1.00, 5-mL vial = 92p; 25 000 units/mL, 1-mL amp = £1.01, 5-mL vial = £3.68

Calciparine® (Sanofi-Synthelabo) PoM

Injection (subcutaneous only), heparin calcium 25 000 units/mL. Net price 0.2-mL syringe = 60p; 0.5-mL syringe = £1.46

HEPARIN (*continued*)

Monoparin® (CP) PoM
Injection, heparin sodium (mucous) 1000 units/mL, net price 1-mL amp = 19p; 5-mL amp = 52p; 10-mL amp = 69p; 20-mL amp = £1.24; 5000 units/mL, 1-mL amp = 36p; 5-mL amp = £1.00; 25 000 units/mL, 0.2-mL amp = 46p, 1-mL amp = £1.01

Monoparin Calcium® (CP) PoM
Injection, heparin calcium 25 000 units/mL. Net price 0.2-mL amp = 48p

Multiparin® (CP) PoM
Injection, heparin sodium (mucous) 1000 units/mL, net price 5-mL vial = 47p; 5000 units/mL, 5-mL vial = 92p; 25 000 units/mL, 5-mL vial = £3.68

Low molecular weight heparins

Dalteparin, **enoxaparin**, and **tinzaparin** are low molecular weight heparins used in children. The duration of action is longer than that of unfractionated heparin; *once-daily subcutaneous* dosage means that they are convenient to use especially in children with poor venous access. The standard prophylactic regimen does not require monitoring in older children and minimal monitoring is required in younger children and neonates.

Some low molecular weight heparins are also used in the treatment of thrombotic episodes.

Haemorrhage See under Heparin.

Hepatic impairment Reduce dose in severe hepatic impairment—risk of bleeding may be increased.

Renal impairment Reduce dose in severe renal impairment—risk of bleeding may be increased; use of unfractionated heparin may be preferable.

Pregnancy Low molecular weight heparins do not cross the placenta.

Breast-feeding Due to the relatively high molecular weight of these drugs and inactivation in the gastro-intestinal tract, passage into milk and subsequent risk to the nursing infant are likely to be negligible; however manufacturers advise avoid

DALTEPARIN SODIUM

Cautions see under Heparin; antithrombotic effect monitored by assessing anti-Factor Xa activity—blood should be taken 3–4 hours after a dose

Hepatic impairment see notes above

Renal impairment see notes above

Pregnancy see notes above

Breast-feeding see notes above

Contra-indications see under Heparin

Side-effects see under Heparin

Licensed use Not licensed for use in children

Indication and dose

Treatment of thrombotic episodes
- **By subcutaneous injection**

Neonate 100 units/kg twice daily

Child 1 month–12 years 100 units/kg twice daily

Child 12–18 years 200 units/kg (max. 18 000 units) once daily, if increased risk of bleeding reduced to 100 units/kg twice daily

Prophylaxis of thrombotic episodes
- **By subcutaneous injection**

Neonate 100 units/kg once daily

Child 1 month–12 years 100 units/kg once daily

Child 12–18 years 2500–5000 units once daily

Fragmin® (Pharmacia) PoM
Injection (single-dose syringe), dalteparin sodium 12 500 units/mL, net price 0.2-mL (2500-unit) syringe = £1.86; 25 000 units/mL, 0.2-mL (5000-unit) syringe = £2.82, 0.3-mL (7500-unit) syringe = £4.23, 0.4-mL (10 000-unit) syringe = £5.65, 0.5-mL (12 500-unit) syringe = £7.06, 0.6-mL (15 000-unit) syringe = £8.47, 0.72-mL (18 000-unit) syringe = £10.16

Injection, dalteparin sodium 2500 units/mL (for subcutaneous or intravenous use), net price 4-mL (10 000-unit) amp = £5.12; 10 000-units/mL (for subcutaneous or intravenous use), 1-mL (10 000-unit) amp = £5.12; 25 000 units/mL (for subcutaneous use only), 4-mL (100 000-unit) vial = £48.66

Injection (graduated syringe), dalteparin sodium 10 000 units/mL, net price 1-mL (10 000-unit) syringe = £5.65

ENOXAPARIN SODIUM

Cautions see under Heparin

Hepatic impairment see notes above

Renal impairment see notes above

Pregnancy see notes above

Breast-feeding see notes above

Contra-indications see under Heparin

2 Cardiovascular system

ENOXAPARIN SODIUM (*continued*)

Side-effects see under Heparin

Licensed use Not licensed for use in children

Indication and dose

Treatment of thrombotic episodes
• By subcutaneous injection
Neonate 1.5–2 mg/kg twice daily
Child 1–2 months 1.5 mg/kg twice daily
Child 2 months–18 years 1 mg/kg twice daily

Prophylaxis of thrombotic episodes
• By subcutaneous injection
Neonate 750 micrograms/kg twice daily
Child 1–2 months 750 micrograms/kg twice daily
Child 2 months–18 years 500 micrograms/kg (max. 40 mg) twice daily

Clexane® (Rhône-Poulenc Rorer) PoM
Injection, enoxaparin sodium 100 mg/mL, net price 0.2-mL (20-mg, 2000-units) syringe = £3.15, 0.4-mL (40-mg, 4000-units) syringe = £4.20, 0.6-mL (60-mg, 6000-units) syringe = £4.75, 0.8-mL (80-mg, 8000-units) syringe = £5.40, 1-mL (100-mg, 10 000-units) syringe = £6.69; 150 mg/mL (*Clexane® Forte*), 0.8-mL (120-mg, 12 000-units) syringe = £9.77, 1-mL (150-mg, 15 000-units) syringe = £11.10

TINZAPARIN SODIUM

Cautions see under Heparin

Hepatic impairment see notes above

Renal impairment see notes above; also anti-Factor Xa activity must be monitored on a daily basis

Pregnancy see notes above

Breast-feeding see notes above

Contra-indications see under Heparin

Side-effects see under Heparin

Licensed use Not licensed for use in children

Indication and dose

Treatment of thrombotic episodes
• By subcutaneous injection
Child 1 month–18 years 175 units/kg once daily for at least 6 days

Prophylaxis of thrombotic episodes
Child 1 month–18 years 50 units/kg once daily

Innohep® (Leo) PoM
Injection, tinzaparin sodium 10 000 units/mL, net price 2500-unit (0.25-mL) syringe = £2.13, 3500-unit (0.35-mL) syringe = £2.98, 4500-unit (0.45-mL) syringe = £3.83, 20 000-unit (2-mL) vial = £11.36

Injection, tinzaparin sodium 20 000 units/mL, net price 0.5-mL (10 000-unit) syringe = £9.65, 0.7-mL (14 000-unit) syringe = £13.51, 0.9-mL (18 000-unit) syringe = £17.37, 2-mL (40 000-unit) vial = £36.77

Asthma Presence of sulphites in formulation may (especially in children with asthma) lead to hypersensitivity (with bronchospasm and shock)

Heparinoids

Danaparoid is a heparinoid that has a role in children who develop thrombocytopenia in association with heparin, providing they have no evidence of cross-reactivity.

DANAPAROID SODIUM

Cautions recent bleeding or risk of bleeding; antibodies to heparins (risk of antibody-induced thrombocytopenia)

Hepatic impairment use with caution in moderate impairment (increased risk of bleeding); avoid in severe impairment unless no alternative

Renal impairment increased risk of bleeding in moderate impairment (monitor anti-Factor Xa activity); avoid in severe impairment unless no alternative

Pregnancy limited information available but not known to be harmful—manufacturer advises avoid

Breast-feeding amount probably too small to be harmful but manufacturer advises avoid

Contra-indications haemophilia and other haemorrhagic disorders, thrombocytopenia (unless patient has heparin-induced thrombocytopenia), recent cerebral haemorrhage, severe hypertension, active peptic ulcer (unless this is the reason for operation), diabetic retinopathy, acute bacterial endocarditis, spinal or epidural anaesthesia with treatment doses of danaparoid

Side-effects haemorrhage; hypersensitivity reactions (including rash)

Licensed use not licensed for use in children

Indication and dose

Thromboembolic disease in children with history of heparin-induced thrombocytopenia
• By intravenous administration
Neonate initially 30 units/kg *by intravenous injection* then *by continuous intravenous infusion* 1.2–2 units/kg/hour adjusted according to coagulation activity
Child 1 month–16 years initially 30 units/kg (max. 1250 units if bodyweight under 55 kg, 2500 units if over 55 kg) *by intravenous injection* then *by continuous intravenous infusion* 1.2–2 units/kg/hour adjusted according to coagulation activity

DANAPAROID SODIUM (*continued*)

Child 16–18 years initially 2500 units (1250 units if bodyweight under 55 kg, 3750 units if over 90 kg) *by intravenous injection* then *by continuous intravenous infusion* 400 units/hour for 2 hours, *then* 300 units/hour for 2 hours, *then* 200 units/hour for 5 days adjusted according to coagulation activity

Administration for *intravenous infusion*, dilute with Glucose 5% *or* Sodium Chloride 0.9%

Orgaran® (Organon) PoM
Injection, danaparoid sodium 1250 units/mL, net price 0.6-mL amp (750 units) = £29.80

Heparin flushes

For maintaining patency of peripheral venous catheters, sodium chloride 0.9% injection is as effective as heparin flushes. However, heparin flushes do have a role in maintaining patency of arterial catheters and implanted central venous access devices.

Heparin Sodium (Non-proprietary) PoM
Solution, heparin sodium 10 units/mL, net price 5-mL amp = 25p; 100 units/mL, 2-mL amp = 28p

Canusal® (CP) PoM
Solution, heparin sodium 100 units/mL. Net price 2-mL amp = 28p

Hepsal® (CP) PoM
Solution, heparin sodium 10 units/mL. Net price 5-mL amp = 25p

Epoprostenol

Epoprostenol (prostacyclin) can be given to inhibit platelet aggregation during renal dialysis either alone or with heparin. For its use in pulmonary hypertension, see section 2.5.1.2. It is a potent vasodilator and therefore its side-effects include flushing, headache, and hypotension.

2.8.2 Oral anticoagulants

Oral anticoagulants antagonise the effects of vitamin K and take at least 48 to 72 hours for the anticoagulant effect to develop fully; if an immediate effect is required, heparin must be given concomitantly.

Uses Warfarin is the drug of choice for the treatment of systemic thromboembolism in children (not neonates) after initial heparinisation. It may also be used occasionally for the treatment of intravascular or intracardiac thrombi. Warfarin is used prophylactically in those with chronic atrial fibrillation, dilated cardiomyopathy, certain forms of reconstructive heart surgery, mechanical prosthetic heart valves, and some forms of hereditary thrombophilia (e.g. homozygous protein C deficiency).

Dose Whenever possible, the base-line prothrombin time should be determined but the initial dose should not be delayed whilst awaiting the result.

An induction dose[1] is usually given over 3 days (see under Warfarin Sodium below). The subsequent maintenance dose depends on the prothrombin time, reported as INR (international normalised ratio) and should be taken at the same time each day. The following indications and target INRs[2] for **adults** take into account recommendations of the British Society for Haematology[3];

- INR 2.5 for treatment of deep-vein thrombosis and pulmonary embolism (or for recurrence in patients no longer receiving warfarin), atrial fibrillation, cardioversion, dilated cardiomyopathy, mural thrombus following myocardial infarction, and rheumatic mitral valve disease;

1. Induction dose may need to be altered if base-line prothrombin time prolonged, if liver-function tests abnormal, or if patient in cardiac failure, on parenteral feeding, less than average body weight, or receiving other drugs known to potentiate oral anticoagulants.
2. An INR which is within 0.5 units of the target value is generally satisfactory; larger deviations require dosage adjustment. Target values (rather than ranges) are now recommended.
3. Guidelines on Oral Anticoagulation: third edition. *Br J Haematol* 1998; **101**: 374–87

- INR 3.5 for recurrent deep-vein thrombosis and pulmonary embolism (in patients currently receiving warfarin with INR above 2) and mechanical prosthetic heart valves.

Monitoring It is essential that the INR be determined daily or on alternate days in early days of treatment, *then* at longer intervals (depending on response[1]) *then* up to every 12 weeks.

Haemorrhage The main adverse effect of all oral anticoagulants is haemorrhage. Checking the INR and omitting doses when appropriate is essential; if the anticoagulant is stopped but not reversed, the INR should be measured 2–3 days later to ensure that it is falling. The following recommendations are based on the result of the INR and whether there is major or minor bleeding; the recommendations (which take into account the recommendations of the British Society for Haematology) apply to **adults** taking warfarin:

- Major bleeding—stop warfarin; give phytomenadione (vitamin K_1) 5–10 mg by slow intravenous injection; give prothrombin complex concentrate (factors II, VII, IX and X) 30–50 units/kg *or* (if no concentrate available) fresh frozen plasma 15 mL/kg
- INR > 8.0, no bleeding or minor bleeding—stop warfarin, restart when INR < 5.0; if there are other risk factors for bleeding give phytomenadione (vitamin K_1) 500 micrograms by slow intravenous injection or 5 mg by mouth (for partial reversal of anticoagulation give smaller oral doses of phytomenadione e.g. 0.5–2.5 mg using the intravenous preparation orally); repeat dose of phytomenadione if INR still too high after 24 hours
- INR 6.0–8.0, no bleeding or minor bleeding—stop warfarin, restart when INR < 5.0
- INR < 6.0 but more than 0.5 units above target value—reduce dose or stop warfarin, restart when INR < 5.0
- Unexpected bleeding at therapeutic levels—always investigate possibility of underlying cause e.g. unsuspected renal or gastro-intestinal tract pathology

Pregnancy Oral anticoagulants are teratogenic and should not be given in the first trimester of pregnancy. Adolescents at risk of pregnancy should be warned of this danger since stopping warfarin before the sixth week of gestation largely avoids the risk of fetal abnormality. Oral anticoagulants cross the placenta with risk of placental or fetal haemorrhage, especially during the last few weeks of pregnancy and at delivery. Therefore, if at all possible, oral anticoagulants should be avoided in pregnancy, especially in the first and third trimesters. Difficult decisions may have to be made, particularly in those with prosthetic heart valves or with a history of recurrent venous thrombosis, pulmonary embolism, or atrial fibrillation.

Babies of mothers taking warfarin at the time of delivery need to be offered immediate prophylaxis with at least 100 micrograms/kg of intramuscular phytomenadione (vitamin K_1), see section 9.6.6.

Dietary differences Infant formula is supplemented with vitamin K, which makes formula-fed infants resistant to warfarin; they may therefore need higher doses. In contrast breast milk contains low concentrations of vitamin K making breast-fed infants more sensitive to warfarin.

Treatment booklets Anticoagulant treatment booklets should be issued to children or their carers, and are available for distribution to local healthcare professionals from Health Authorities and also from:

England and Wales:
Astron
The Causeway
Oldham Broadway
Business Park
Chadderton
Oldham OL9 9XD
(0161) 683 2376

Scotland:
Banner Business Supplies
20 South Gyle Crescent
Edinburgh EH12 9EB
(0131) 479 3279

Northern Ireland:
Central Services Agency
25 Adelaide St
Belfast BT2 8FH
(028) 9053 5652

1. Change in child's clinical condition, particularly associated with liver disease, intercurrent illness, or drug administration, necessitates more frequent testing. See also **interactions**, Appendix 1 (warfarin). Major changes in diet (especially involving salads and vegetables) and in alcohol consumption may also affect warfarin control.

These booklets include advice for children or their carers on anticoagulant treatment.

WARFARIN SODIUM

Cautions recent surgery; **interactions**: Appendix 1 (warfarin)

Hepatic impairment avoid in severe impairment, especially if prothrombin time already prolonged

Renal impairment avoid in severe impairment

Breast-feeding not excreted in breast milk; no evidence of harm

Contra-indications peptic ulcer, severe hypertension, bacterial endocarditis

Pregnancy see notes above

Side-effects haemorrhage—see notes above; other side-effects reported include hypersensitivity, rash, alopecia, diarrhoea, unexplained drop in haematocrit, 'purple toes', skin necrosis, jaundice, hepatic dysfunction; also nausea, vomiting, and pancreatitis

Licensed use Not licensed for use in children

Indication and dose

Treatment and prophylaxis of thrombotic episodes

- By mouth

Neonate (under specialist advice) 200 micrograms/kg as a single dose on first day, reduced to 100 micrograms/kg once daily for following 2 days (but if INR still below 1.5 use 200 micrograms/kg once daily, or if INR above 3 use 50 micrograms/kg once daily, if INR above 3.5 omit dose); then adjusted according to INR, usual maintenance 100–300 micrograms/kg once daily (may need up to 400 micrograms/kg once daily especially if bottle fed—see notes above)

Child 1 month–18 years 200 micrograms/kg (max. 10 mg) as a single dose on first day, reduced to 100 micrograms/kg (max. 5 mg) once daily for following 2 days (but if INR still below 1.5 use 200 micrograms/kg (max. 10 mg) once daily, or if INR above 3 use 50 micrograms/kg (max. 2.5 mg) once daily, or if INR above 3.5 omit dose); then adjusted according to INR, usual maintenance 100–300 micrograms/kg once daily (may need up to 400 micrograms/kg once daily especially if bottle fed—see notes above)

Note Induction dose may need to be altered according to condition, concomitant interacting drugs, and if baseline INR above 1.3.

Warfarin (Non-proprietary) PoM

Tablets, warfarin sodium 0.5 mg (white), net price 28-tab pack = £1.00; 1 mg (brown), 28 = 90p; 3 mg (blue), 28 = £1.34; 5 mg (pink), 28 = £1.53. Label: 10, anticoagulant card

Brands include *Marevan®*

Extemporaneous formulations available see Extemporaneous Preparations, p. 8

2.8.3 Protamine sulphate

Although protamine sulphate is used to counteract overdosage with heparin, if used in excess it has an anticoagulant effect.

PROTAMINE SULPHATE
(Protamine Sulfate)

Cautions see above; also if increased risk of allergic reaction to protamine (includes previous treatment with protamine or protamine insulin, allergy to fish, and adolescent males who are infertile)

Side-effects nausea, vomiting, lassitude, flushing, hypotension, bradycardia, dyspnoea; hypersensitivity reactions (including angioedema, anaphylaxis) reported

Indication and dose

Heparin overdose

- **By intravenous injection (at rate not exceeding 5 mg/minute)**

Child 1 month–18 years *to neutralise each 100 units of unfractionated heparin*, 1 mg if less than 30 minutes lapsed since overdose, 500–750 micrograms if 30–60 minutes lapsed, 375–500 micrograms if 60–120 minutes lapsed, 250–375 micrograms if over 120 minutes lapsed; max. 50 mg

Administration May be diluted if necessary with sodium chloride 0.9% intravenous infusion

Protamine Sulphate (Non-proprietary) PoM

Injection, protamine sulphate 10 mg/mL, net price 5-mL amp = £1.14, 10-mL amp = £3.96

Prosulf® (CP) PoM

Injection, protamine sulphate 10 mg/mL. Net price 5-mL amp = 96p (glass), £1.20 (polypropylene)

2.9 Antiplatelet drugs

Antiplatelet drugs decrease platelet aggregation and may inhibit thrombus formation in the arterial circulation, where anticoagulants have little effect.

Aspirin has limited use in children because it has been associated with Reye's syndrome. The CSM has advised that aspirin-containing preparations should not be given to children and adolescents under 16 years, unless specifically indicated, e.g. for Kawasaki syndrome (see below), for prophylaxis of clot formation after cardiac surgery, or for prophylaxis of stroke in children at high risk.

Dipyridamole is also used as an antiplatelet drug to prevent clot formation after cardiac surgery and may be used with specialist advice for treatment of persistent coronary artery aneurysms in Kawasaki syndrome.

Kawasaki syndrome A high initial dose of aspirin reduces pyrexia in Kawasaki syndrome; a single dose of intravenous normal immunoglobulin (p. 701) and continuation of aspirin at a lower dose can reduce the risk of developing coronary artery abnormalities.

ASPIRIN (antiplatelet)
(Acetylsalicylic Acid)

Cautions asthma; uncontrolled hypertension; previous peptic ulceration (but manufacturer's package insert may advise avoidance of low-dose aspirin in history of peptic ulceration); **interactions:** Appendix 1 (aspirin)

Hepatic impairment avoid in severe impairment—increased risk of gastro-intestinal bleeding

Renal impairment avoid in severe impairment—sodium and water retention, deterioration in renal function, and increased risk of gastro-intestinal bleeding

Pregnancy use with caution during third trimester; impaired platelet function and risk of haemorrhage; delayed onset and increased duration of labour with increased blood loss; avoid analgesic doses if possible in last few weeks (low doses probably not harmful); with high doses, closure of fetal ductus arteriosus *in utero* and possibly persistent pulmonary hypertension of newborn; kernicterus in jaundiced neonates

Contra-indications for use other than as an antiplatelet in children under 16 years (risk of Reye's syndrome); active peptic ulceration; haemophilia and other bleeding disorders

Breast-feeding avoid—possible risk of Reye's syndrome; regular use of high doses could impair platelet function and produce hypoprothrombinaemia in infant if neonatal vitamin K stores low

Side-effects bronchospasm; gastro-intestinal haemorrhage (occasionally major), also other haemorrhage (e.g. subconjunctival)

Licensed use Not licensed for use in children under 16 years

Indication and dose

Antiplatelet, prevention of thrombus formation after cardiac surgery
- By mouth

Neonate 5 mg/kg once daily

Child 1 month–18 years 1–5 mg/kg (usual max. 75 mg) once daily

Kawasaki syndrome
- By mouth

Neonate initially 8 mg/kg 4 times daily for 2 weeks *or* until afebrile, followed by 5 mg/kg once daily for 6–8 weeks; if no evidence of coronary lesions after 8 weeks, discontinue treatment or seek expert advice

Child 1 month–12 years initially 7.5–12.5 mg/kg 4 times daily for 2 weeks or until afebrile, then 2–5 mg/kg once daily for 6–8 weeks; if no evidence of coronary lesions after 8 weeks, discontinue treatment or seek expert advice

Aspirin (Non-proprietary) PoM
Dispersible tablets, aspirin 75 mg, net price 20 = 22p; 300 mg, 20 = 21p. Label: 13, 21, 32

Tablets, e/c, aspirin 75 mg, net price 56-tab pack = £1.39; 300 mg, 100-tab pack = £4.89. Label: 5, 25, 32
Brands include *Gencardia*®, *Micropirin*®

Suppositories, available from specialist manufacturers

Angettes 75® (Bristol-Myers Squibb)
Tablets, aspirin 75 mg. Net price 28-tab pack = 94p. Label: 32

Caprin® (Sinclair) PoM
Tablets, e/c, pink, aspirin 75 mg, net price 28-tab pack = £1.55, 56-tab pack = £3.08, 100-tab pack = £5.24; 300 mg, 100-tab pack = £4.89. Label: 5, 25, 32

Nu-Seals® **Aspirin** (Alliance) PoM
Tablets, e/c, aspirin 75 mg, net price 56-tab pack = £2.60; 300 mg, 100-tab pack = £3.46. Label: 5, 25, 32

DIPYRIDAMOLE

Cautions aortic stenosis, heart failure; may exacerbate migraine; hypotension; myasthenia gravis (risk of exacerbation); **interactions:** Appendix 1 (dipyridamole)

Pregnancy not known to be harmful

Breast-feeding small amount present in milk—manufacturer advises caution

Side-effects gastro-intestinal effects, dizziness, myalgia, throbbing headache, hypotension, hot flushes and tachycardia; hypersensitivity reactions such as rash, urticaria, severe bronchospasm and angioedema; increased bleeding during or after surgery; thrombocytopenia reported

Licensed use Not licensed for use in children

DIPYRIDAMOLE (*continued*)

Indication and dose

Prevention of thrombus formation after cardiac surgery
- By mouth

Child 1 month–12 years 2.5 mg/kg twice daily

Child 12–18 years 100–200 mg 3 times daily

Kawasaki syndrome
- By mouth

Child 1 month–12 years 1 mg/kg 3 times daily

Administration Injection solution can be given orally

Dipyridamole (Non-proprietary) PoM

Tablets, coated, dipyridamole 25 mg, net price 20 = 37p; 100 mg, 20 = £1.06; 84 = £4.48. Label: 22

Oral suspension, dipyridamole 50 mg/5 ml, net price 150 mL = £34.00

Persantin® (Boehringer Ingelheim) PoM

Tablets, both s/c, dipyridamole 25 mg (orange), net price 84-tab pack = £1.57; 100 mg, 84-tab pack = £4.38. Label: 22

Injection, dipyridamole 5 mg/mL. Net price 2-mL amp = 11p

2.10 Myocardial infarction and fibrinolysis

2.10.1 Management of myocardial infarction

Classification not used in BNF for Children.

2.10.2 Fibrinolytic drugs

Fibrinolytic drugs act as thrombolytics by activating plasminogen to form plasmin, which degrades fibrin and so breaks up thrombi.

Alteplase, **streptokinase**, and **urokinase** are used in children to dissolve intravascular thrombi and unblock occluded shunts and catheters. Treatment should be started as soon as possible after a clot has formed and discontinued once a pulse in the affected limb is detected, or the shunt or catheter unblocked.

The safety and efficacy of treatment remains uncertain, especially in neonates. A fibrinolytic drug is probably only appropriate where arterial occlusion threatens ischaemic damage; an anticoagulant may stop the clot getting bigger. Alteplase is the preferred fibrinolytic in children and neonates; there is less risk of adverse effects including allergic reactions.

Cautions Risk of bleeding including that from venepuncture or invasive procedures, external chest compression, pregnancy (see individual drugs), abdominal aneurysm or conditions in which thrombolysis might give rise to embolic complications such as enlarged left atrium with atrial fibrillation (risk of dissolution of clot and subsequent embolisation), diabetic retinopathy (very small risk of retinal bleeding), recent or concurrent anticoagulant therapy.

Contra-indications Recent haemorrhage, trauma, or surgery (including dental extraction), coagulation defects, bleeding diatheses, aortic dissection, coma, history of cerebrovascular disease especially recent events or with any residual disability, recent symptoms of possible peptic ulceration, heavy vaginal bleeding, severe hypertension, active pulmonary disease with cavitation, acute pancreatitis, severe liver disease, oesophageal varices; also in the case of streptokinase, previous allergic reactions to streptokinase.

Prolonged persistence of antibodies to streptokinase may reduce the effectiveness of subsequent treatment; therefore, streptokinase should not be used again beyond 4 days of first administration. Streptokinase should also be avoided in children who have had streptococcal infection in the last 12 months. Antibodies may also appear after topical use of streptokinase on wounds.

Side-effects Side-effects of thrombolytics are mainly bleeding, nausea and vomiting. Hypotension may also occur and can usually be controlled by elevating the patient's legs, or by reducing the rate of infusion or stopping it temporarily. Back pain has been reported. Bleeding is usually limited to the site of injection, but intracerebral haemorrhage or bleeding from other sites may occur. Serious bleeding calls for discontinuation of the thrombolytic and may require administration of coagulation factors and antifibrinolytic drugs (aprotinin or tranexamic acid). Streptokinase may cause allergic reactions (including rash, flushing and uveitis) and anaphylaxis has been reported (for details of management see Allergic Emergencies, section 3.4.3). Guillain-Barré syndrome has been reported rarely after streptokinase treatment.

ALTEPLASE

(rt-PA, tissue-type plasminogen activator)

Cautions see notes above; in children who have had an *acute stroke*, monitor for intracranial haemorrhage and monitor blood pressure

Hepatic impairment avoid in severe impairment

Renal impairment risk of hyperkalaemia in moderate or severe impairment

Pregnancy no evidence of teratogenicity; possibility of premature separation of placenta in first 18 weeks; theoretical possibility of fetal haemorrhage throughout pregnancy; avoid postpartum use—maternal haemorrhage

Contra-indications see notes above; in children who have had an *acute stroke*, convulsion accompanying stroke, severe stroke, history of stroke in children with diabetes, stroke in last 3 months, hypoglycaemia, hyperglycaemia

Side-effects see notes above; also risk of cerebral bleeding increased in acute stroke

Licensed use Not licensed for use in children

Indication and dose

Intravascular thrombosis doses may vary—consult local guidelines

- **By intravenous infusion**

Neonate 100–500 micrograms/kg/hour for 3–6 hours; use ultrasound assessment to monitor effect before considering a second course of treatment

Child 1 month–18 years 100–500 micrograms/kg/hour for 3–6 hours; max. 100 mg total daily dose; use ultrasound assessment to monitor effect before considering a second course of treatment

Administration Can be given by intravenous infusion. Dissolve in water for injections to a concentration of 1 mg/mL and infuse intravenously; alternatively dilute further in sodium chloride 0.9% to a concentration of not less than 200 micrograms/mL; not to be diluted in glucose solution

Occluded arteriovenous shunts, catheters, and indwelling central lines

- **By injection direct into catheter or central line**

Child 1 month–18 years using 1 mg/mL solution, instill up to 2 mL according to type of catheter or central line; aspirate lysate after 4 hours; flush with sodium chloride 0.9% injection

Actilyse® (Boehringer Ingelheim) PoM

Injection, powder for reconstitution, alteplase 10 mg (5.8 million units)/vial, net price per vial (with diluent) = £135.00; 20 mg (11.6 million units)/vial (with diluent and transfer device) = £180.00; 50 mg (29 million units)/vial (with diluent, transfer device, and infusion bag) = £300.00

STREPTOKINASE

Cautions see notes above

Hepatic impairment avoid in severe hepatic impairment

Pregnancy possibility of premature separation of placenta in first 18 weeks; theoretical possibility of fetal haemorrhage throughout pregnancy; risk of maternal haemorrhage on post-partum use

Contra-indications see notes above

Side-effects see notes above

Licensed use Licensed for use in children for intravascular dissolution of thrombi and emboli

Indication and dose

Intravascular thrombosis

- **By intravenous infusion**

Child 1 month–12 years initially 2500–4000 units/kg over 30 minutes, followed by *continuous intravenous infusion* of 500–1000 units/kg/hour for up to 3 days until reperfusion occurs

Child 12–18 years initially 250 000 units over 30 minutes, followed by *continuous intravenous infusion* of 100 000 units/hour for up to 3 days until reperfusion occurs

Administration May be diluted with glucose 5% or sodium chloride 0.9% intravenous infusion after reconstitution. Monitor fibrinogen concentration closely; if fibrinogen concentration less than 1g/litre, stop streptokinase infusion and start heparin; restart streptokinase once fibrinogen concentration reaches 1g/litre

Topical use see section 13.11.7

Streptokinase (Non-proprietary) PoM

Injection, powder for reconstitution, streptokinase, net price 100 000-unit vial = £10.00; 250 000-unit vial = £14.33; 750 000-unit vial = £38.20; 1.5 million-unit vial = £81.18

Streptase® (ZLB Behring) PoM

Injection, powder for reconstitution, streptokinase, net price 250 000-unit vial = £17.11; 750 000-unit vial = £44.86; 1.5 million-unit vial = £89.72 (hosp. only)

UROKINASE

Cautions see notes above

Hepatic impairment avoid in severe hepatic impairment

Pregnancy possibility of premature separation of placenta; theoretical possibility of fetal haemorrhage throughout pregnancy; risk of maternal haemorrhage on post-partum use

Contra-indications see notes above

Side-effects see notes above

Licensed use Urokinase not licensed

Indication and dose

Intravascular thrombosis

- **By intravenous injection and infusion**

Neonate 5000 units/kg/hour *by intravenous infusion*, adjusted according to response

Child 1 month–18 years 4400 units/kg as a single dose *by intravenous injection* in 15 mL diluent, followed by 4400 units/kg/hour *by intravenous infusion* for 12 hours, adjusted according to response

Administration May be diluted, after reconstitution, with sodium chloride 0.9% intravenous infusion or glucose 5% intravenous infusion

Occluded arteriovenous shunts, catheters, and indwelling central lines

- **By injection directly into catheter or central line**

Neonate 5000–10 000 units in sodium chloride 0.9% to fill catheter dead-space; leave for 2–4 hours then aspirate the lysate; flush with heparinised saline

Child 1 month–18 years 5000–10 000 units in sodium chloride 0.9% to fill catheter dead-space; leave for 2–4 hours then aspirate the lysate; flush with heparinised saline

Urokinase

Injection, powder for reconstitution, urokinase, available as 10 000-unit vial; 50 000-unit vial; 100 000-unit vial; 250 000-unit vial (named patient supply)

2.11 Antifibrinolytic drugs and haemostatics

Fibrin dissolution can be impaired by the administration of **tranexamic acid**, which inhibits fibrinolysis. It may be useful to prevent bleeding (e.g. in prostatectomy and dental extraction in haemophilia) and can be particularly useful in menorrhagia. Tranexamic acid may also be used in hereditary angioedema, epistaxis and in thrombolytic overdose.

Desmopressin (section 6.5.2) is used in the management of mild to moderate haemophilia.

Aprotinin is a proteolytic enzyme inhibitor acting on plasmin and kallidinogenase (kallikrein). It is used for children at high risk of major blood loss during and after open heart surgery with extracorporeal circulation and for patients in whom optimal blood conservation during open heart surgery is an absolute priority; it is also indicated for the treatment of life-threatening haemorrhage due to hyperplasminaemia (occasionally observed during the mobilisation and dissection of malignant tumours, in acute promyelocytic leukaemia, and following thrombolytic therapy). Aprotinin is also used in liver transplantation [unlicensed].

APROTININ

Cautions

Pregnancy manufacturer advises use only if potential benefit outweighs risk; possibly reduced fibrinolytic activity in newborn

Side-effects occasionally hypersensitivity reactions and localised thrombophlebitis

Licensed use Licensed for hyperplasminaemia in children

Indication and dose

Prevention of blood loss in open heart surgery with extracorporeal membrane oxygenation

- **By intravenous administration and introduction to extracorporeal circuit**

Child 1 month–18 years consult local guidelines for test dose and peri-operative doses

Hyperplasminaemia

- **By slow intravenous injection or by intravenous infusion**

Child 1 month–18 years consult local guidelines; suggested test dose 200 units/kg then after 10 minutes 10 000 units/kg over 20 minutes then by *continuous intravenous infusion* 3000 units/kg/hour until bleeding controlled

Trasylol® (Bayer) PoM

Injection, aprotinin 10 000 kallikrein inactivator units/mL. Net price 50-mL vial = £20.53

Note A non-proprietary aprotinin injection containing 10 000 kallikrein inactivator units/mL is also available

TRANEXAMIC ACID

Cautions massive haematuria (avoid if risk of ureteric obstruction); not for use in disseminated intravascular coagulation; regular eye examinations and liver function tests in long-term treatment of hereditary angioedema

Note Requirement for regular eye examinations during long-term treatment is based on unsatisfactory evidence

Renal impairment reduce dose in mild to moderate renal impairment; avoid in severe renal impairment

Pregnancy no evidence of teratogenicity in *animal* studies; manufacturer advises use only if potential benefit outweighs risk—crosses the placenta

Breast-feeding small amount present in milk—antifibrinolytic effect in infant unlikely

Contra-indications thromboembolic disease

Side-effects nausea, vomiting, diarrhoea (reduce dose); disturbances in colour vision (discontinue) and thromboembolic events reported rarely; giddiness on rapid intravenous injection

Licensed use Licensed for inhibition of fibrinolysis

Indication and dose

Inhibition of fibrinolysis, hereditary angioedema (section 3.4.3)

- **By mouth**

  Child 1 month–18 years 15–25 mg/kg (max. 1.5 g) 2–3 times daily

- **By intravenous injection over at least 10 minutes**

  Child 1 month–18 years 10 mg/kg (max 1 g) 2–3 times daily

- **By continuous intravenous infusion**

  Child 1 month–18 years 45 mg/kg over 24 hours

Administration Dilute with glucose 5% *or* sodium chloride 0.9% intravenous infusion

Prevention of excessive bleeding after dental procedures (e.g. in haemophilia)

- **By intravenous injection (pre-operatively) and by mouth (post-operatively)**

  Child 6–18 years 10 mg/kg (max 1.5 g) *by intravenous injection* pre-operatively, followed by 15–25 mg/kg(max. 1.5 g) 2–3 times daily *by mouth* for up to 8 days

- **Mouthwash**

  Child 6–18 years 5–10% solution may be used

  Note Mouthwash available only as extemporaneously prepared preparation

Menorrhagia

- **By mouth**

  Child 12–18 years 1 g 3–4 times daily for up to 4 days; max. 4 g daily (initiate when menstruation has started)

Tranexamic acid (Non-proprietary) PoM

Tablets, tranexamic acid 500 mg, net price 60-tab pack = £12.28

Cyklokapron® (Meda) PoM

Tablets, f/c, scored, tranexamic acid 500 mg. Net price 60-tab pack = £14.30

Injection, tranexamic acid 100 mg/mL. Net price 5-mL amp = £1.55

Blood products

Classification not used in BNF for Children

2.12 Lipid-regulating drugs

Atherosclerosis begins in childhood and raised serum-cholesterol in children is associated with cardiovascular disease in adulthood. Lowering the cholesterol, without hindering growth and development in children and adolescents, should reduce the risk of cardiovascular disease in later life.

The risk factors for developing cardiovascular disease include raised serum cholesterol concentration, smoking, hypertension, male sex, and a family history of cardiovascular disease. In children with heterozygous familial hypercholesterolaemia, the family history of cardiovascular disease is most important when considering initiation of a lipid-regulating drug. Homozygous familial hypercholesterolaemia is rare and requires specialist management.

Secondary causes of hypercholesterolaemia should be addressed, these include diet, diabetes mellitus, hypothyroidism (see below), nephrotic syndrome, obstructive biliary disease, glycogen storage disease, and drugs such as corticosteroids.

Treatment Dietary intervention is the mainstay of treatment of hypercholesterolaemia in children. The aim is to reduce the risk of atherosclerosis whilst ensuring adequate growth and development. Advice should also be given on lifestyle measures (e.g. increased exercise, and if appropriate, stopping smoking). Blood pressure should also be reduced if required (section 2.5).

When 6–12 months of dietary intervention alone has failed, drug therapy is indicated in children over 6 years who are at high risk of developing cardiovascular disease. Dietary therapy and lifestyle measures should continue even if lipid-regulating drugs have been introduced.

Lipid-regulating drugs are considered if dietary intervention fails to reduce total serum-cholesterol adequately; experience of their use in children is limited and they should be initiated on specialist advice.

Statins (**atorvastatin**, **pravastatin**, and **simvastatin**) are generally well tolerated and are considered to be the drugs of first choice. Alternatively, **anion-exchange resins** are used but tolerability and compliance with these drugs is poor.

Evidence for the use of a **fibrate** (**bezafibrate** or **fenofibrate**) in children is limited; fibrates should be considered only if dietary intervention and treatment with a statin and an anion-exchange resin is unsuccessful.

In hypertriglyceridaemia which cannot be controlled by very strict diet, omega-3 fatty acid compounds may be helpful.

Hypothyroidism Children with hypothyroidism should receive adequate thyroid replacement therapy before their requirement for lipid-regulating treatment is assessed because correction of hypothyroidism itself may resolve the lipid abnormality. Untreated hypothyroidism increases the risk of myositis with lipid-regulating drugs.

CSM advice (muscle effects). The CSM has advised that rhabdomyolysis associated with lipid-regulating drugs such as the fibrates and statins appears to be rare (approx. 1 case in every 100 000 treatment years) but may be increased in those with renal impairment and possibly in those with hypothyroidism (see also notes above). Concomitant treatment with drugs that increase plasma-statin concentration increase the risk of muscle toxicity; concomitant treatment with a fibrate and a statin may also be associated with an increased risk of serious muscle toxicity.

Anion-exchange resins

Colestyramine (cholestyramine) and **colestipol** are anion-exchange resins used in the management of hypercholesterolaemia. They act by binding bile acids, preventing their reabsorption; this promotes hepatic conversion of cholesterol into bile acids; the resultant increased LDL-receptor activity of liver cells increases the clearance of LDL-cholesterol. Thus both compounds effectively reduce LDL-cholesterol but can aggravate hypertriglyceridaemia.

Cautions Anion-exchange resins interfere with the absorption of fat-soluble vitamins; supplements of vitamins A, D and K may be required when treatment is prolonged. **Interactions:** Appendix 1 (colestyramine and colestipol).

Side-effects As colestyramine and colestipol are not absorbed, gastro-intestinal side-effects predominate. Constipation is common, but diarrhoea has occurred, as have nausea, vomiting, and gastro-intestinal discomfort. Hypertriglyceridaemia may be aggravated. An increased bleeding tendency has been reported due to hypoprothrombinaemia associated with vitamin K deficiency.

Counselling Other drugs should be taken at least 1 hour before or 4–6 hours after colestyramine or colestipol to reduce possible interference with absorption.

COLESTYRAMINE
(Cholestyramine)

Cautions see notes above

Hepatic impairment interferes with absorption of fat-soluble vitamins and may aggravate malabsorption in primary biliary cirrhosis; likely to be ineffective in complete biliary obstruction

Contra-indications complete biliary obstruction (not likely to be effective)

Side-effects see notes above; hyperchloraemic acidosis reported on prolonged use

Licensed use licensed in children over 6 years to reduce cholesterol; see also section 1.9.2

COLESTYRAMINE (*continued*)

Indication and dose

Familial hypercholesterolaemia
- By mouth

Child 6–12 years initially 4 g once daily increased to 4 g up to 3 times daily according to response

Child 12–18 years initially 4 g once daily increased to 4–8 g up to 4 times daily according to response; max. 36 g daily in up to 4 divided doses

Cholestatic pruritus section 1.9.2

Diarrhoea section 1.9.2

Administration Mix with water, fruit juice, skimmed milk, thin soup, or pulped fruit; total daily dose may be given as a single dose if tolerated

Colestyramine (Non-proprietary) PoM
Powder, colestyramine (anhydrous) 4 g/sachet, net price 60-sachet pack = £19.23. Label: 13, counselling, avoid other drugs at same time (see notes above)
Excipients: include aspartame (section 9.4.1)

Questran® (Bristol-Myers Squibb) PoM
Powder, colestyramine (anhydrous) 4 g/sachet. Net price 50-sachet pack = £17.55. Label: 13, counselling, avoid other drugs at same time (see notes above)
Excipients: include sucrose 3.79g/sachet

Questran Light® (Bristol-Myers Squibb) PoM
Powder, sugar-free, colestyramine (anhydrous) 4 g/sachet, net price 50-sachet pack = £18.43. Label: 13, counselling, avoid other drugs at same time (see notes above)
Excipients: include aspartame (section 9.4.1)

COLESTIPOL HYDROCHLORIDE

Cautions see notes above

Side-effects see notes above

Licensed use not licensed for use in children

Indication and dose

Familial hypercholesterolaemia
- By mouth

Child 12–18 years initially 5 g once daily increased if necessary at intervals of 1 month to max. of 30 g daily in 1–2 divided doses

Administration Mix with water, fruit juice, skimmed milk, thin soup, or pulped fruit; total daily dose may be given as a single dose if tolerated

Colestid® (Pharmacia) PoM
Granules, yellow, colestipol hydrochloride 5 g/sachet. Net price 30 sachets = £15.05. Label: 13, counselling, avoid other drugs at same time (see notes above)

Colestid Orange, granules, yellow/orange, colestipol hydrochloride 5 g/sachet, with aspartame. Net price 30 sachets = £15.05. Label: 13, counselling, avoid other drugs at same time (see notes above)

Ezetimibe

Ezetimibe inhibits the intestinal absorption of cholesterol. It is given in combination with a statin or alone if a statin is inappropriate.

EZETIMIBE

Cautions interactions: Appendix 1 (ezetimibe)

Hepatic impairment avoid in moderate and severe impairment—may accumulate

Pregnancy manufacturer advises use only if potential benefit outweighs risk—no information available

Contra-indications

Breast-feeding present in milk in *animal* studies—manufacturer advises avoid

Side-effects gastro-intestinal disturbances; headache, fatigue; myalgia; *rarely* hypersensitivity reactions including rash and angioedema, hepatitis; *very rarely* pancreatitis, cholelithiasis, thrombocytopenia, raised creatine kinase, myopathy, and rhabdomyolysis

Indication and dose

Adjunct to dietary measures and statin in primary hypercholesterolaemia and homozygous familial hypercholesterolaemia (statin omitted in primary hypercholesterolaemia if inappropriate or not tolerated) adjunct to dietary measures in homozygous sitosterolaemia

Child 10–18 years 10 mg once daily

Ezetrol® (MSD, Schering-Plough) ▼ PoM
Tablets, ezetimibe 10 mg, net price 28-tab pack = £26.31

Fibrates

Bezafibrate and **fenofibrate** act mainly by decreasing serum triglycerides; they have variable effects on LDL-cholesterol. Fibrates may reduce the risk of coronary heart disease in those with low HDL-cholesterol or with raised triglycerides.

Fibrates can cause a myositis-like syndrome, especially in children with impaired renal function. Also, combination of a fibrate with a statin increases the risk of muscle effects (especially rhabdomyolysis) and should be used with caution (see CSM advice on p. 154).

There is limited evidence to support their use in children.

BEZAFIBRATE

Cautions correct hypothyroidism before initiating treatment (see Lipid-regulating Drugs, p. 154); see under Myotoxicity below; **interactions:** Appendix 1 (fibrates)

Myotoxicity Special care needed in patients with renal disease, as progressive increases in serum creatinine concentration or failure to follow dosage guidelines may result in myotoxicity (rhabdomyolysis); discontinue if myotoxicity suspected or creatine kinase concentration increases significantly

Hepatic impairment avoid in severe impairment

Renal impairment reduce dose if creatinine clearance 15–60 mL/minute/1.73 m^2; avoid if creatinine clearance less than 15 mL/minute/ 1.73 m^2; see also Myotoxicity below

Contra-indications hypoalbuminaemia, primary biliary cirrhosis, gall bladder disease, nephrotic syndrome

Pregnancy embryotoxicity in *animal* studies—manufacturers advise avoid

Breast-feeding manufacturer advises avoid—no information available

Side-effects gastro-intestinal disturbances; rash, pruritus, *less commonly* headache, fatigue, dizziness, insomnia; *rarely* gallstones, hepatomegaly, cholestasis, hypoglycaemia, impotence, anaemia, leucopenia, thrombocytopenia, increased risk of bleeding, alopecia, photosensitivity reactions, raised serum creatinine (unrelated to renal impairment) and myotoxicity (with myasthenia or myalgia)—special risk in renal impairment (see Cautions)

Licensed use Not licensed for use in children

Indication and dose

Hyperlipidaemia including familial hypercholesterolaemia (on specialist advice only)

- By mouth

  Child 10–18 years 200 mg once daily adjusted according to response to max. 200 mg 3 times daily

Bezafibrate (Non-proprietary) PoM

Tablets, bezafibrate 200 mg, net price 100-tab pack = £9.81. Label: 21

Bezalip® (Roche) PoM

Tablets, f/c, bezafibrate 200 mg. Net price 100-tab pack = £9.15. Label: 21

FENOFIBRATE

Cautions see under Bezafibrate; liver function tests recommended every 3 months for first year (discontinue treatment if significantly raised)

Hepatic impairment avoid in severe impairment

Renal impairment reduce dose if creatinine clearance less than 60 mL/minute/1.73m^2; avoid if creatinine clearance less than 10 mL/minute/ 1.73m^2

Contra-indications gall bladder disease; photosensitivity to ketoprofen

Pregnancy embryotoxicity in animal studies—manufacturer advises avoid

Breast-feeding manufacturer advises avoid—no information available

Side-effects see under Bezafibrate; also *very rarely* hepatitis, pancreatitis, and interstitial pneumopathies

Licensed use *Lipantil® Micro 67* is licensed for use in children with hypercholesterolaemia

Indication and dose

Hyperlipidaemias including familial hypercholesterolaemia (on specialist advice only)

- By mouth

  Child 4–15 years 1 capsule/20 kg body-weight daily

  Child 15–18 years initially 3 capsules daily in divided doses; usual range 2-4 capsules daily

Lipantil® (Fournier) PoM

Lipantil® Micro 67 capsules, yellow, fenofibrate (micronised) 67 mg, net price 90-cap pack = £23.30. Label: 21

Statins

The statins (**atorvastatin**, **pravastatin**, and **simvastatin**) competitively inhibit 3-hydroxy-3-methylglutaryl coenzyme A (HMG CoA) reductase, an enzyme involved in cholesterol synthesis, especially in the liver. They are more effective than other classes of drugs in lowering LDL-cholesterol but less effective than the fibrates in reducing triglycerides. Statins also increase concentrations of HDL-cholesterol.

Statins reduce, all atherosclerotic cardiovascular disease events, and total mortality in adults.

Cautions Statins should be used with caution in those with a history of liver disease or with a high alcohol intake (use should be avoided in active liver disease). Hypothyroidism should be managed adequately before starting treatment with a statin (see Hypothyroidism, section 2.12). Liver-function tests should be carried out before and within 1–3 months of starting treatment and thereafter at intervals of 6 months for 1 year, unless indicated sooner by signs or symptoms suggestive of hepatotoxicity. Treatment should be discontinued if serum transaminase concentration rises to, and persists at, 3 times the upper limit of the reference range. Statins should be used with caution in those with risk factors for myopathy or rhabdomyolysis; children or their carers should be advised to report unexplained muscle pain (see Muscle Effects below). Statins should be avoided in porphyria (section 9.8.2) but rosuvastatin is thought to be safe.

Contra-indications Statins are contra-indicated in active liver disease (or persistently abnormal liver function tests), in pregnancy (adequate contraception required during treatment and for 1 month afterwards), and breast-feeding.

Side-effects Reversible myositis is a rare but significant side-effect of the statins (see also Muscle Effects, p. 154 and below). The statins also cause headache, altered liver-function tests (rarely, hepatitis), paraesthesia, and gastro-intestinal effects including abdominal pain, flatulence, diarrhoea, nausea, and vomiting. Rash and hypersensitivity reactions (including angioedema and anaphylaxis) have been reported rarely.

Muscle effects Myalgia, myositis and myopathy have been reported with the statins; if myopathy is suspected and creatine kinase is markedly elevated (more than 5 times upper limit of normal), treatment should be discontinued; in children at high risk of muscle effects, a statin should not be started if creatine kinase is elevated. There is an increased incidence of myopathy if the statins are given with a fibrate (see also CSM advice p. 154), with lipid-lowering doses of nicotinic acid, or with immunosuppressants such as ciclosporin; close monitoring of liver function and, if symptomatic, of creatine kinase is required in patients receiving these drugs. Rhabdomyolysis with acute renal impairment secondary to myoglobinuria has also been reported.

Counselling Advise children or their carers to report promptly unexplained muscle pain, tenderness, or weakness.

ATORVASTATIN

Cautions see notes above

Hepatic impairment avoid in active liver disease or unexplained persistent elevations in serum transaminases

Contra-indications see notes above

Pregnancy avoid—congenital anomalies reported; decreased synthesis of cholesterol possibly affects fetal development

Breast-feeding manufacturer advises avoid—no information available

Side-effects see notes above; also chest pain, angina; insomnia, dizziness, hypoaesthesia, arthralgia; back pain; *less commonly* anorexia, malaise, weight gain, amnesia, impotence, thrombocytopenia, tinnitus, and alopecia; *rarely* pancreatitis, peripheral neuropathy, and peripheral oedema; *very rarely* cholestatic jaundice, hypoglycaemia, and Stevens-Johnson syndrome

Indication and dose

Hyperlipidaemia including familial hypercholesterolaemia

- **By mouth**

Child 10–17 years initially 10 mg once daily, increased if necessary, at intervals of at least 4 weeks to usual max. 20 mg once daily

Child 17–18 years initially 10 mg once daily, increased if necessary, at intervals of at least 4 weeks to max. 80 mg once daily

Lipitor® (Parke-Davis) PoM
Tablets, all f/c, atorvastatin (as calcium trihydrate) 10 mg, net price 28-tab pack = £18.03; 20 mg, 28-tab pack = £24.64; 40 mg 28-tab pack = £28.21; 80 mg, 28-tab pack = £28.21. Counselling, muscle effects, see notes above

PRAVASTATIN SODIUM

Cautions see notes above

Hepatic impairment avoid in active liver disease or unexplained persistent elevations in serum transaminases

Renal impairment start with lower doses in moderate to severe renal impairment

Contra-indications see notes above

Pregnancy avoid—congenital anomalies reported; decreased synthesis of cholesterol possibly affects fetal development

Breast-feeding small amounts present in breast milk—manufacturer advises avoid

Side-effects see notes above; *less commonly* fatigue, dizziness, sleep disturbances, abnormal urination (including dysuria, nocturia, and frequency), sexual dysfunction, visual disturbances, alopecia; *very rarely* pancreatitis, jaundice, fulminant hepatic necrosis, peripheral neuropathy, lupus erythematosus-like syndrome

Licensed use licensed in children over 8 years for familial hypercholesterolaemia

2 Cardiovascular system

PRAVASTATIN SODIUM (*continued*)

Indication and dose

Hyperlipidaemia including familial hypercholesterolaemia
- By mouth

Child 8–14 years 10 mg once daily at night, adjusted at intervals of not less than 4 weeks to max. 20 mg once daily at night

Child 14–18 years 10 mg once daily at night, adjusted at intervals of not less than 4 weeks to max. 40 mg once daily at night

Pravastatin (Non-proprietary) PoM
Tablets, pravastatin sodium 10 mg, net price 28-tab pack = £3.41; 20 mg, 28-tab pack = £4.22; 40 mg, 28-tab pack = £4.59
Counselling muscle effects, see notes above

Lipostat® (Squibb) PoM
Tablets, all yellow, pravastatin sodium 10 mg, net price 28-tab pack = £15.05; 20 mg, 28-tab pack = £27.61; 40 mg, 28-tab pack = £27.61. Counselling, muscle effects, see notes above

SIMVASTATIN

Cautions see notes above

Hepatic impairment avoid in active liver disease or unexplained persistent elevations in serum transaminases

Renal impairment doses above 5 mg daily (10 mg daily in children over 10 years) should be used with caution if creatinine clearance less than 30 mL/minute/1.73 m²

Contra-indications see notes above

Pregnancy avoid—congenital anomalies reported; decreased synthesis of cholesterol possibly affects fetal development

Breast-feeding manufacturer advises avoid—no information available

Side-effects see notes above; also alopecia, anaemia, dizziness, peripheral neuropathy, asthenia, hepatitis, jaundice, pancreatitis

Licensed use not licensed for use in children

Indication and dose

Hyperlipidaemia including familial hypercholesterolaemia
- By mouth

Child 5–10 years initially 5 mg at night increased, if necessary, at intervals of at least 4 weeks to max. 20 mg at night

Child 10–18 years initially 10 mg at night increased, if necessary, at intervals of at least 4 weeks to max. 40 mg at night

Note Reduced dose required with concomitant ciclosporin, danazol, fibrates, amiodarone, diltiazem, or verapamil—seek specialist advice

Simvastatin (Non-proprietary) PoM
Tablets, simvastatin 10 mg, net price 28-tab pack = £1.65, 20 mg, 28-tab pack = £1.48; 40 mg, 28-tab pack = £3.57; 80 mg, 28-tab pack = £20.29. Counselling, muscle effects, see notes above
Brands include *Simvador®*, *Simzal®*

Zocor® (MSD) PoM
Tablets, all f/c, simvastatin 10 mg (peach), net price 28-tab pack = £18.03; 20 mg (tan), 28-tab pack = £29.69; 40 mg (red), 28-tab pack = £29.69; 80 mg (red), 28-tab pack = £29.69. Counselling, muscle effects, see notes above

2.13 Local sclerosants

Classification not used in BNF for Children.

2.14 Drugs affecting the ductus arteriosus

Closure of the ductus arteriosus

Patent ductus arteriosus is a frequent problem in premature neonates with respiratory distress syndrome. Substantial left-to-right shunting through the ductus arteriosus may increase the risk of intraventricular haemorrhage, necrotising enterocolitis, bronchopulmonary dysplasia, and possibly death.

Indometacin or ibuprofen may be used to close the ductus arteriosus. **Indometacin** has been used for many years and is effective but it reduces cerebral blood flow, and causes a transient fall in renal and gastro-intestinal blood flow. **Ibuprofen** may also be used; it has little effect on renal function (there may be a small reduction in sodium excretion) when used in doses for closure of the ductus arteriosus; gastro-intestinal problems are uncommon.

If drug treatment fails to close the ductus arteriosus, surgery may be indicated.

IBUPROFEN

Cautions may mask symptoms of infection; monitor for bleeding; monitor gastro-intestinal function; allergic disorders; **interactions:** Appendix 1 (NSAIDs)

Hepatic impairment avoid in severe liver disease

Renal impairment causes sodium and water retention; use lowest effective dose and monitor renal function; avoid if possible in moderate to severe renal impairment

Contra-indications life-threatening infection; active bleeding especially intracranial or gastro-intestinal; thrombocytopenia or coagulation defects; marked unconjugated hyperbilirubinaemia; known or suspected necrotising enterocolitis; pulmonary hypertension

Side-effects necrotising enterocolitis, intestinal perforation; intraventricular haemorrhage; ischaemic brain injury; bronchopulmonary dysplasia, pulmonary haemorrhage; thrombocytopenia, neutropenia, oliguria, haematuria, fluid retention, hyponatraemia; *less commonly* gastro-intestinal haemorrhage; hypoxaemia

Licensed use Orphan licence for the injection for closure of ductus arteriosus in premature neonates less than 34 weeks gestational age

Indication and dose

Closure of ductus arteriosus
- **By slow intravenous injection**

Neonate initially 10 mg/kg as a single dose followed at 24-hour intervals by 2 doses of 5 mg/kg; course may be repeated after 48 hours if necessary

Mild to moderate pain, pain and inflammation of soft tissue injuries and rheumatic disease, pyrexia section 10.1.1

Administration By slow intravenous injection over 15 minutes, preferably undiluted. May be diluted, with Glucose 5% or Sodium Chloride 0.9%

Pedea® (Orphan Europe) PoM
Intravenous solution, ibuprofen 5 mg/mL, 2-mL amp

INDOMETACIN

Cautions see notes above; also may mask symptoms of infection; may reduce urine output by 50% or more (monitor carefully—see also under Anuria or Oliguria, below) and precipitate renal impairment especially if extracellular volume depleted, heart failure, sepsis, or concomitant use of nephrotoxic drugs; may induce hyponatraemia; inhibition of platelet aggregation (monitor for bleeding); **interactions:** Appendix 1 (NSAIDs)

Anuria or oliguria If anuria or marked oliguria (urinary output less than 0.6 mL/kg/hour), delay further doses until renal function returns to normal

Hepatic impairment can cause fluid retention; avoid in severe hepatic impairment

Renal impairment causes sodium and water retention; use lowest effective dose and monitor renal function; avoid if possible in moderate to severe renal impairment; see also Cautions and Anuria and oliguria above

Contra-indications untreated infection, bleeding (especially with active intracranial haemorrhage or gastro-intestinal bleeding); thrombocytopenia, coagulation defects, necrotising enterocolitis

Side-effects haemorrhagic, renal, gastro-intestinal (including necrotising enterocolitis), metabolic, and coagulation disorders; pulmonary hypertension, intracranial bleeding, fluid retention, and exacerbation of infection

Indication and dose

Closure of ductus arteriosus
- **By intravenous infusion over 20–30 minutes**

Neonate under 48 hours initially 200 micrograms/kg as a single dose followed by (if urine output adequate) 2 doses of 100 micrograms/kg at intervals of 12–24 hours; course may be repeated after 48 hours if necessary

Neonate 2–7 days initially 200 micrograms/kg as a single dose followed by (if urine output adequate) 2 doses of 200 micrograms/kg at intervals of 12–24 hours; course may be repeated after 48 hours if necessary

Neonate over 7 days initially 200 micrograms/kg as a single dose followed by (if urine output adequate) 2 doses of 250 micrograms/kg at intervals of 12–24 hours; course may be repeated after 48 hours if necessary

Note In some units *by intravenous infusion* initially 100 micrograms/kg (200 micrograms/kg if symptomatic) then 100 micrograms/kg every 24 hours for 5 further doses

Pain and inflammation in rheumatic disease section 10.1.1

Administration For *intravenous infusion* dilute each vial with 1–2 mL sodium chloride 0.9% *or* water for injections (not glucose and no preservatives)

Indocid PDA® (MSD) PoM
Injection, powder for reconstitution, indometacin (as sodium trihydrate). Net price 3 × 1-mg vials = £22.50 (hosp. only)

2 Cardiovascular system

Maintenance of patency

In the newborn with duct-dependent congenital heart disease it is often necessary to maintain the patency of the ductus arteriosus whilst awaiting surgery.

Alprostadil (prostaglandin E1) and **dinoprostone** (prostaglandin E2) are potent vasodilators that are effective for maintaining the patency of the ductus arteriosus. They are usually given by continuous intravenous infusion, but oral dosing of dinoprostone is still used in some centres.

During the infusion of a prostaglandin, the newborn requires careful monitoring of heart rate, blood pressure, respiratory rate, and core body temperature. In the event of complications such as apnoea, profound bradycardia, or severe hypotension, the infusion should be temporarily stopped and the complication dealt with; the infusion should be recommenced at a lower dose. Recurrent or prolonged apnoea may require ventilatory support in order for the prostaglandin infusion to continue.

ALPROSTADIL

Cautions see notes above; also history of haemorrhage; avoid in hyaline membrane disease; monitor arterial pressure, respiratory rate, heart rate, temperature, and venous blood pressure in arm and leg; facilities for intubation and ventilation must be immediately available; **interactions:** Appendix 1 (alprostadil)

Side-effects apnoea (particularly in neonates under 2 kg), flushing, bradycardia, hypotension, tachycardia, cardiac arrest, oedema, diarrhoea, fever, convulsions, disseminated intravascular coagulation, hypokalaemia; cortical proliferation of long bones, weakening of the wall of the ductus arteriosus and pulmonary artery may follow prolonged use; gastric-outlet obstruction reported

Indication and dose

Maintaining patency of the ductus arteriosus
- By continuous intravenous infusion

Neonate initially 50–100 nanograms/kg/minute then decreased to lowest effective dose (but lower dose such as 10 nanograms/kg/minute may be effective and safer; dinoprostone is an alternative)

Administration Dilute with glucose 5% *or* sodium chloride 0.9%; add directly to the infusion solution avoiding contact with the walls of plastic containers

Prostin VR® (Pharmacia) PoM
Intravenous solution, alprostadil 500 micrograms/mL in alcohol. For dilution and use as an infusion. Net price 1-mL amp = £75.19 (hosp.only)

DINOPROSTONE

Cautions see notes above; also history of haemorrhage; avoid in hyaline membrane disease; monitor arterial oxygenation, heart rate, temperature, and blood pressure in arm and leg; facilities for intubation and ventilation must be immediately available; **interactions:** Appendix 1 (prostaglandins)

Contra-indications

Hepatic impairment manufacturer advises avoid in hepatic impairment

Renal impairment manufacturer advises avoid in renal impairment

Side-effects nausea, vomiting, diarrhoea; flushing, bradycardia, hypotension, cardiac arrest; respiratory depression and apnoea, particularly with high doses and in low birth-weight neonates, bronchospasm; pyrexia and raised white blood cell count, shivering; local reactions, erythema; if used for longer than 5 days, gastric outlet obstruction, cortical hyperostosis; may be associated with necrotising enterocolitis

Licensed use not licensed for use in children

Indication and dose

Maintaining patency of ductus arteriosus
- By continuous intravenous infusion

Neonate initially 5–10 nanograms/kg/minute, increased as necessary in 5 nanogram/kg/minute increments to 20 nanograms/kg/minute
Note Doses up to 100 nanograms/kg/minute have been used but are associated with increased side-effects
Administration Dilute to a concentration of 1 microgram/mL with glucose 5% or sodium chloride 0.9% intravenous infusion

- By mouth

Neonate 20–25 micrograms/kg every 1–2 hours doubled if necessary; if treatment continues for more than 1 week gradually reduce the dose

Administration Injection solution can be given orally; dilute with water

Prostin E2 (Pharmacia) PoM
Intravenous solution, for dilution and use as an infusion, dinoprostone 1 mg/mL, net price 0.75-mL amp = £8.52; 10 mg/mL, 0.5-mL amp = £18.40 (both hosp. only)

Extemporaneous formulations available see Extemporaneous Preparations, p. 8

3 Respiratory system

This chapter includes advice on the drug management of the following:

acute asthma, p. 163
anaphylaxis, p. 189
angioedema, p. 190
chronic asthma, p. 165
croup, p. 164

3.1 Bronchodilators

3.1.1 Adrenoceptor agonists
3.1.2 Antimuscarinic bronchodilators
3.1.3 Theophylline
3.1.4 Compound bronchodilator preparations
3.1.5 Peak flow meters, inhaler devices and nebulisers

Asthma

Drugs used in the management of asthma include beta$_2$ agonists (section 3.1.1), antimuscarinic bronchodilators (section 3.1.2), theophylline (section 3.1.3), corticosteroids (section 3.2), cromoglicate and nedocromil (section 3.3.1), and leukotriene receptor antagonists (section 3.3.2).

For a table outlining the management of chronic asthma see p. 165.

3 Respiratory system

Administration of drugs for asthma

Inhalation This route delivers the drug directly to the airways; the dose is smaller than that for the drug given by mouth and side-effects are reduced. A *pressurised metered-dose* inhaler is commonly used to administer drugs in asthma; a spacer device must be used with a pressurised metered-dose inhaler to improve drug delivery in children under 5 years. A *dry-powder inhaler* may be used for children over 5 years, and a *breath-actuated inhaler* may be more suitable for children over 7 years (see section 3.1.5).

Solutions for nebulisation for use in acute severe asthma are administered over 5–10 minutes from a nebuliser, usually driven by oxygen in hospital. Electric compressors are best suited to domiciliary use.

Oral Systemic side-effects occur more frequently when a drug is given orally rather than by inhalation. Oral corticosteroids, theophylline, and leukotriene receptor antagonists are sometimes required for the management of asthma. Oral administration of a beta$_2$ agonist is generally not recommended for children, but may be necessary in infants and young children unable to use an inhaler device.

Parenteral Drugs such as beta$_2$ agonists, corticosteroids, and aminophylline may be given by injection in acute severe asthma when drug administration by nebulisation is inadequate or inappropriate; in these circumstances the child should generally be treated in a high-dependency or intensive care unit.

Pregnancy and breast-feeding

Women with asthma should be closely monitored during pregnancy. Well-controlled asthma has no important effects on pregnancy, labour, or on the fetus. Drugs for asthma should preferably be administered by inhalation to minimise fetal drug exposure.

Severe exacerbations of asthma can have an adverse effect on pregnancy and should be treated promptly with conventional therapy, including oral or parenteral administration of a corticosteroid and nebulisation of a beta$_2$ agonist; prednisolone is the preferred corticosteroid for oral administration since very little of the drug reaches the fetus. Oxygen should be given immediately to maintain arterial oxygen saturation above 95% and prevent maternal and fetal hypoxia.

Inhaled drugs, theophylline, and prednisolone can be taken as normal during breast-feeding.

Assessment of asthma severity[1]

Each episode of acute asthma requiring emergency consultation should be treated as being *severe* until proven otherwise; failure of the child to respond adequately to treatment for acute asthma *at any time* requires immediate referral to hospital.

It is essential to assess the severity of the child's condition accurately bearing in mind that clinical signs may correlate poorly with severity of airways obstruction; some children with acute severe asthma do not appear distressed. Lung-function measurements cannot be used as a guide to management in children under 5 years.

Child (all ages) **Mild:** cough and wheeze without distress, cyanosis, or increased respiration rate; able to speak normally between breaths

Child under 2 years **Moderate:** oxygen saturation $\geq 92\%$, audible wheezing, using accessory muscles of breathing, still feeding

Severe: oxygen saturation $< 92\%$, cyanosis, marked respiratory distress, too breathless to feed

Child 2–5 years **Moderate:** oxygen saturation $\geq 92\%$, no clinical features of severe asthma

1. Advice on the management of acute asthma is based on the recommendations of the British Thoracic Society and Scottish Intercollegiate Guidelines Network (updated November 2005)

Severe: oxygen saturation < 92%, too breathless to talk or eat, heart rate > 130 beats/minute, respiratory rate > 50 breaths/minute, use of accessory muscles of breathing

Life-threatening: oxygen saturation < 92%; silent chest, poor respiratory effort, agitation or altered consciousness, cyanosis

Child 5–18 years **Moderate:** oxygen saturation ≥ 92%, peak flow ≥ 50% best or predicted, no clinical features of severe asthma
Severe: oxygen saturation < 92%, peak flow < 50% best or predicted, too breathless to talk, heart rate > 120 beats/minute, respiratory rate > 30 breaths/minute, use of accessory muscles of breathing
Life-threatening: oxygen saturation < 92%, peak flow < 33% best or predicted, silent chest, poor respiratory effort, altered consciousness, cyanosis

Management of acute asthma[1]

> Important
> Failure to respond adequately **at any time** requires immediate referral to hospital

Child under 2 years

Acute mild to moderate exacerbation of asthma Administer a **short-acting beta$_2$ agonist** using a pressurised metered-dose inhaler with a spacer device and close-fitting facemask. Give 1 puff every 15–30 seconds up to a maximum of 10 puffs; repeat dose after 20–30 minutes if necessary.

If response is poor or if a relapse occurs within 3–4 hours, send child **immediately** to hospital for assessment and further treatment.

Children under 18 months often respond poorly to bronchodilators; nebulised beta$_2$ agonists have been associated with mild paradoxical bronchospasm and transient worsening of oxygen saturation; response to prednisolone may also be poor in this age group.

Severe or life-threatening exacerbation of asthma Send **immediately** to hospital. Administer oxygen using a close-fitting face mask or nasal prongs to achieve oxygen saturation above 92%.

Treat with inhaled **short-acting beta$_2$ agonist** as above, or with salbutamol 2.5 mg or terbutaline 5 mg as a nebulised solution. Repeat dose every 20–30 minutes if necessary, then reduce frequency according to response. If response is poor, add nebulised **ipratropium bromide** 125–250 micrograms every 20–30 minutes for the first 2 hours, reduce dose frequency as condition improves. Give oral **prednisolone** 1–2 mg/kg (max. 40 mg) once daily for 3–5 days or, if oral administration is not possible, use intravenous **hydrocortisone** (preferably as sodium succinate; for doses see p. 429). If necessary, transfer the child to a paediatric intensive care unit for treatment with a parenteral **short-acting beta$_2$ agonist** (section 3.1.1.1) or parenteral **aminophylline** (section 3.1.3).

Child 2–18 years

Acute mild to moderate exacerbation of asthma Administer a **short-acting beta$_2$ agonist** using a pressurised metered-dose inhaler with a spacer device; for a child under 5 years use a close-fitting facemask with the spacer. Give 1 puff every 15–30 seconds, up to a maximum of 10 puffs. Repeat treatment after 20–30 minutes if necessary.

In all cases, give oral **prednisolone** 1–2 mg/kg once daily (max. 20 mg daily for child under 5 years; for child 5–18 years, max. 40 mg daily) for 3–5 days.

If response is poor or a relapse occurs within 3–4 hours, send child **immediately** to hospital for assessment and further treatment.

Acute severe or life-threatening exacerbation of asthma Send **immediately** to hospital. Administer oxygen using a close-fitting face mask or nasal prongs to achieve oxygen saturation above 92%.

1. Advice on the management of acute asthma is based on the recommendations of the British Thoracic Society and Scottish Intercollegiate Guidelines Network (updated November 2005)

3 Respiratory system

Treat with an inhaled **short-acting beta$_2$ agonist** (as above) or with nebulised salbutamol 2.5 mg or terbutaline 5 mg (nebulised doses may be doubled for child over 5 years); repeat dose every 20–30 minutes if necessary.

If symptoms do not improve, add nebulised **ipratropium bromide** 250 micrograms—in severe exacerbations administer every 20–30 minutes over the first 2 hours then reduce frequency on improvement.

Give oral **prednisolone**, 1–2 mg/kg once daily for 3–5 days—or if oral administration not possible use intravenous **hydrocortisone** (preferably as sodium succinate; for doses see p. 429).

If the condition does not respond or is life-threatening, transfer the child to an intensive care unit and treat with parenteral bronchodilators including salbutamol (section 3.1.1.1) and aminophylline (section 3.1.3). Children with severe asthma may be helped by intravenous infusion of **magnesium sulphate** 40 mg/kg (max. 2 g) over 20 minutes (section 9.5.1.3), but evidence of benefit is limited.

Croup

Mild croup is largely self-limiting, but treatment with a single dose of **dexamethasone** 150 micrograms/kg by mouth is of benefit.

Severe croup (or mild croup that might cause complications) calls for hospital admission—a single dose of either dexamethasone 150 micrograms/kg or prednisolone 1–2 mg/kg, which may be administered by mouth before transfer to hospital. In hospital, dexamethasone 150 micrograms/kg (by mouth or by injection) or budesonide 2 mg by nebulisation (section 3.2) will often reduce symptoms; the dose may be repeated after 12 hours if necessary.

For severe croup not effectively controlled with corticosteroid treatment, nebulised **adrenaline** (section 3.4.3) solution 1 in 1000 (1 mg/mL) may be given with close clinical monitoring in a dose of 400 micrograms/kg (max. 5 mg) repeated after 30 minutes if necessary (the dose may be diluted with sterile sodium chloride 0.9% solution). The effects of nebulised adrenaline last 2–3 hours; the child needs to be carefully monitored for recurrence of the obstruction.

3.1.1 Adrenoceptor agonists (Sympathomimetics)

The selective beta$_2$ agonists (selective beta$_2$-adrenoceptor agonists, selective beta$_2$ stimulants) such as salbutamol or terbutaline are the safest and most effective short-acting beta$_2$ agonists for the treatment of asthma. Less selective beta$_2$ agonists, such as orciprenaline, are no longer recommended for the treatment of asthma.

Adrenaline (epinephrine), which has both alpha- and beta-adrenoceptor agonist properties, is used in the emergency management of allergic and anaphylactic reactions (section 3.4.3); it is also used as a nebuliser solution to treat severe croup.

3.1.1.1 Selective beta$_2$ agonists

Selective beta$_2$ agonists produce bronchodilation. A short-acting beta$_2$ agonist is used for immediate relief of asthma symptoms while a long-acting beta$_2$ agonist is generally used in addition to an inhaled corticosteroid in children requiring prophylactic treatment.

Short-acting beta$_2$ agonists Mild to moderate symptoms of asthma respond rapidly to the inhalation of a selective short-acting beta$_2$ agonist such as **salbutamol** or **terbutaline**. If beta$_2$ agonist inhalation is needed more often than once daily, prophylactic treatment should be considered, using a stepped approach as outlined in the Management of Chronic Asthma table, p. 165; regular treatment with a short-acting beta$_2$ agonist provides no clinical benefit.

A short-acting beta$_2$ agonist inhaled immediately before exertion reduces *exercise-induced asthma*; however, frequent exercise-induced asthma probably reflects poor overall control and calls for reassessment of asthma treatment.

MANAGEMENT OF CHRONIC ASTHMA

Start at **step most appropriate** to initial severity

Children 5–18 years

Step 1: occasional relief bronchodilators

Inhaled short-acting $beta_2$ agonist as required (up to once daily)

NOTE Check compliance and inhaler technique; move to step 2 if needed 3 times a week or more, or if night-time symptoms more than once a week or if exacerbation in the last 2 years requiring systemic corticosteroid or nebulised bronchodilator

Step 2: regular inhaled preventer therapy

Inhaled short-acting $beta_2$ agonist as required

plus

Regular standard-dose[1] inhaled corticosteroid (alternatives[2] are considerably less effective)

Step 3: inhaled corticosteroids + long-acting inhaled $beta_2$ agonist

Inhaled short-acting $beta_2$ agonist as required

plus

Regular standard-dose[1] inhaled corticosteroid

plus

Regular inhaled long-acting $beta_2$ agonist (salmeterol *or* formoterol (eformoterol)) but discontinue long-acting $beta_2$ agonist in the absence of response

If asthma not controlled

Increase dose of inhaled corticosteroid to upper end of standard-dose[1]

If asthma still not controlled

Add one of
- Leukotriene receptor antagonist
- Modified-release oral theophylline
- Modified-release oral $beta_2$ agonist

Step 4: high-dose inhaled corticosteroids + regular bronchodilators

Inhaled short-acting $beta_2$ agonist as required

with

Regular high-dose[3] inhaled corticosteroid

plus

Inhaled long-acting $beta_2$ agonist

plus

A 6-week sequential therapeutic trial of one or more of
- Leukotriene receptor antagonist
- Modified-release oral theophylline
- Modified-release oral $beta_2$ agonist

Step 5: regular corticosteroid tablets

Refer child to respiratory paediatrician

Inhaled short-acting $beta_2$ agonist as required

with

Regular high-dose[3] inhaled corticosteroid

and

one or more long-acting bronchodilators (see step 4)

plus

Regular prednisolone tablets (as single daily dose)

NOTE In addition to regular prednisolone, continue high-dose inhaled corticosteroid (in exceptional cases may exceed licensed doses)

Stepping down

Review treatment every 3 months; if control achieved stepwise reduction may be possible; use lowest possible dose of corticosteroid; reduce dose of *inhaled* corticosteroid slowly (consider reduction every 3 months, decreasing dose by up to 50% each time) to the lowest dose which controls asthma

Children under 5 years[4]

Step 1: occasional relief bronchodilators

Short-acting $beta_2$ agonist as required (not more than once daily)

NOTE Preferably by inhalation (less effective and more side-effects when given as tablets or syrup); check compliance, technique and that inhaler device is appropriate
Move to step 2 if needed 3 times a week or more, or if night-time symptoms more than once a week, or if exacerbation in last 2 years

Step 2: regular preventer therapy

Inhaled short-acting $beta_2$ agonist as required

plus

Either regular standard-dose[1] inhaled corticosteroid
Or (if inhaled corticosteroid cannot be used) leukotriene receptor antagonist or theophylline

Step 3: add-on therapy

Children 2–5 years:

Inhaled short-acting $beta_2$ agonist as required

plus

Regular standard-dose[1] inhaled corticosteroid

plus

Leukotriene receptor antagonist

Children under 2 years:

Refer child to respiratory paediatrician

Step 4: persistent poor control

Refer child to respiratory paediatrician

Stepping down

Regularly review need for treatment

1. **Standard doses** of inhaled corticosteroids (metered-dose inhaler used with large-volume spacer)
   Beclometasone dipropionate or **budesonide**:
   Child under 2 years 50–100 micrograms twice daily; Child 2–5 years 100–200 micrograms twice daily; Child 5–12 years 100–200 micrograms twice daily; Child 12–18 years 100–400 micrograms twice daily.
   Fluticasone:
   Child under 5 years 50–100 micrograms twice daily; Child 5–12 years 50–100 micrograms twice daily; Child 12–18 years 50–200 micrograms twice daily.
   Mometasone furoate (given through dry powder inhaler):
   Child 12–18 years 200 micrograms twice daily.
2. Alternatives to inhaled corticosteroid are leukotriene receptor antagonists, theophylline, inhaled nedocromil (in child 5–18 years), or inhaled cromoglicate (in child 12–18 years)
3. **High doses** of inhaled corticosteroids (metered-dose inhaler used with large-volume spacer)
   Beclometasone dipropionate or **budesonide**:
   Child under 2 years up to 200 micrograms twice daily; Child 2–5 years up to 400 micrograms twice daily; Child 5–12 years up to 400 micrograms twice daily; Child 12–18 years 0.4–1 mg twice daily.
   Fluticasone:
   Child under 5 years 100–200 micrograms twice daily; Child 5–12 years 100–200 micrograms twice daily; Child 12–18 years 200–500 micrograms twice daily.
   Mometasone furoate (given through dry powder inhaler):
   Child 12–18 years up to 400 micrograms twice daily.
4. Lung-function measurements cannot be used to guide management in those under 5 years

Advice on the management of chronic asthma is based on the recommendations of the British Thoracic Society and Scottish Intercollegiate Guidelines Network (updated November 2005)

Long-acting beta$_2$ agonists **Formoterol** (eformoterol) and **salmeterol** are longer-acting beta$_2$ agonists which are administered by inhalation. Added to regular inhaled corticosteroid treatment, they have a role in the long-term control of chronic asthma (see Management of Chronic Asthma table, p. 165) and they can be useful in nocturnal asthma. Salmeterol should not be used for the relief of an asthma attack; it has a slower onset of action than salbutamol or terbutaline. Formoterol is licensed for short-term symptom relief and for the prevention of exercise-induced bronchospasm; its speed of onset of action is similar to that of salbutamol.

When used without an inhaled corticosteroid, salmeterol has been associated with rare life-threatening attacks of asthma and high doses of formoterol (e.g. 24 micrograms twice daily) may be associated with an increase in severe exacerbation of asthma. Therefore, a long-acting beta$_2$ agonist should be *added* to existing corticosteroid treatment and should not replace it; the long-acting beta$_2$ agonist should be discontinued in the absence of a clinical response. Lower doses of a long-acting beta$_2$ agonist are effective for most children and should be tried first.

Management of Chronic Asthma, see p. 165
Management of Acute Asthma, see p. 163
For guidance on the use of inhalers and spacer devices see section 3.1.5

Inhalation A *pressurised metered-dose inhaler* is an effective method of drug administration in mild to moderate chronic asthma; to deliver the drug effectively particularly in children under 12 years, a spacer device should be used (see also NICE guidance, section 3.1.5). When a pressurised metered-dose inhaler with a spacer is unsuitable or inconvenient, a *dry-powder inhaler* or *breath-actuated inhaler* may be used instead if the child is able to use the device effectively. At recommended inhaled doses the duration of action of salbutamol and terbutaline is about 3 to 5 hours and for salmeterol and formoterol is about 12 hours. The **dose**, the frequency, and the maximum number of inhalations in 24 hours of the beta$_2$ agonist should be **stated explicitly** to the child and the child's carer. High doses of beta$_2$ agonists can be dangerous in some children (see Cautions, below). Excessive use is usually an indication of **inadequately controlled** asthma and should be managed with a prophylactic drug such as an inhaled corticosteroid. The child and the child's carer should be advised to seek medical advice when the prescribed dose of beta$_2$ agonist fails to provide the usual degree of symptomatic relief because this usually indicates a worsening of the asthma and the child may require alternative medication (see Management of Chronic Asthma, p. 165).

Children and their carers should be advised to follow manufacturers' instructions on the care and cleansing of inhaler devices.

CFC-free inhalers Chlorofluorocarbon (CFC) propellants in pressurised metered-dose inhalers are being replaced by hydrofluoroalkane (HFA) propellants. Carers and children receiving CFC-free inhalers should be reassured about the efficacy of the new inhalers and counselled that the aerosol may feel and taste different to their previous CFC-based inhaler; any difficulty with the new inhaler should be discussed with the doctor or pharmacist.

Nebuliser (or respirator) solutions of salbutamol and terbutaline are used for the treatment of acute asthma both in hospital and in general practice. Children with a severe attack of asthma should have oxygen if possible during nebulisation since beta$_2$ agonists can increase arterial hypoxaemia. See also guidelines in section 3.1.5.

Oral Oral preparations of beta$_2$ agonists may be used for children if an inhaler device cannot be used but inhaled beta$_2$ agonists are more effective and have fewer side-effects. A modified-release formulation of salbutamol may be of value in nocturnal asthma as an alternative to modified-release theophylline preparations (section 3.1.3), but an inhaled long-acting beta$_2$ agonist is preferable.

Parenteral Beta$_2$ agonists may be given intravenously in children with severe or life-threatening acute asthma. Chronic asthma unresponsive to stepwise treatment (see Management of Chronic Asthma, p. 165) may benefit from continuous subcutaneous infusion of a beta$_2$ agonist but this should be used only under the supervision of a respiratory specialist; the evidence of benefit is uncertain and it may be difficult to withdraw such treatment once started.

Cautions Beta$_2$ agonists should be used with caution in diabetes—monitor blood glucose (risk of ketoacidosis, especially when a beta$_2$ agonist is given intravenously). Beta$_2$ agonists should also be used with caution in hyperthyroidism, cardiovascular disease, arrhythmias, susceptibility to QT-interval prolongation, and hypertension. If high doses of beta$_2$ agonists are needed during pregnancy they should be given by inhalation because a parenteral beta$_2$ agonist can affect the myometrium and possibly cause cardiac problems; see also Pregnancy and Breast-feeding, section 3.1. **Interactions:** Appendix 1 (sympathomimetics, beta$_2$).

Hypokalaemia The CSM has advised that potentially serious hypokalaemia may result from beta$_2$ agonist therapy. Particular caution is required in severe asthma, because this effect may be potentiated by concomitant treatment with theophylline and its derivatives, corticosteroids, and diuretics, and by hypoxia. Plasma-potassium concentration should therefore be monitored in severe asthma.

Side-effects Side-effects of the beta$_2$ agonists include fine tremor (particularly in the hands), nervous tension, headache, peripheral dilatation and palpitations. Other side-effects include tachycardia and arrhythmias and disturbances of sleep and behaviour in children. Muscle cramps and hypersensitivity reactions including paradoxical bronchospasm, urticaria, and angioedema have also been reported. Beta$_2$ agonists are associated with hypokalaemia after high doses (for CSM advice see under Cautions). Pain may occur on intramuscular injection.

SALBUTAMOL

Cautions see notes above

Side-effects see notes above

Licensed use not licensed for use in renal hyperkalaemia; *syrup* not licensed for use in children under 2 years; *modified-release tablets* not licensed for use in children under 3 years; *injection* not licensed for use in children

Indication and dose

Acute asthma

- **By aerosol or nebulised solution inhalation**
  see Management of Acute Asthma, section 3.1

- **By intravenous injection over 5 minutes**
  Child 1 month–2 years 5 micrograms/kg as a single dose

  Child 2–18 years 15 micrograms/kg (max. 250 micrograms) as a single dose

- **By continuous intravenous infusion**
  Child 1 month–18 years 60–300 micrograms/kg/hour, dose adjusted according to response and heart rate (doses above 120 micrograms/kg/hour with close monitoring)

Exacerbations of reversible airways obstruction (including nocturnal asthma) and prevention of exercise-induced bronchospasm, see Management of Chronic Asthma, p. 165

- **By aerosol inhalation**
  Child 1 month–18 years 100–200 micrograms (1–2 puffs) up to 4 times daily (for occasional use only)

- **By inhalation of powder**
  Child 5–12 years 200 micrograms up to 4 times daily (for occasional use only)

  Child 12–18 years 200–400 micrograms up to 4 times daily (for occasional use only)

  Note Bioavailability appears to be lower, so recommended doses for dry powder inhalers are twice those in a metered-dose aerosol inhaler; for *Ventolin Accuhaler*® dose see under preparation

- **By mouth (but not recommended)**
  Child 1 month–2 years 100 micrograms/kg (max. 2 mg) 3–4 times daily

  Child 2–6 years 1–2 mg 3–4 times daily

  Child 6–12 years 2 mg 3–4 times daily

  Child 12–18 years 4 mg (sensitive patients initially 2 mg) 3–4 times daily; max. single dose 8 mg (but unlikely to provide extra benefit or to be tolerated)

Severe hyperkalaemia (section 9.2.1.1)

- **By intravenous injection over 5 minutes**
  Neonate 4 micrograms/kg as a single dose; repeat if necessary

  Child 1 month–18 years 4 micrograms/kg as a single dose; repeat if necessary

- **By inhalation of nebulised solution (but intravenous injection preferred)**
  Neonate 2.5–5 mg as a single dose; repeat if necessary

  Child 1 month–18 years 2.5–5 mg as a single dose; repeat if necessary

Administration for *continuous intravenous infusion*, dilute to a concentration of 10 micrograms/mL with Glucose 5% *or* Sodium Chloride 0.9%; if fluid-restricted, may be given undiluted through central venous catheter.

For *nebulisation*, dilute nebuliser solution with a suitable volume of sterile Sodium Chloride 0.9% solution according to nebuliser type and duration of administration; salbutamol and ipratropium bromide solutions are compatible and may be mixed for nebulisation.

Oral

Salbutamol (Non-proprietary) PoM

Tablets, salbutamol (as sulphate) 2 mg, net price 28-tab pack = £1.92; 4 mg, 28-tab pack = £2.23

Oral solution, salbutamol (as sulphate) 2 mg/5 mL, net price 150 mL = £1.37

Brands include *Salapin*® (sugar-free)

3 Respiratory system

SALBUTAMOL (*continued*)

Ventmax® SR (Trinity) PoM
Capsules, m/r, salbutamol (as sulphate) 4 mg (green/grey), net price 56-cap pack = £8.57; 8 mg (white), 56-cap pack = £10.28. Label: 25

Dose

Chronic asthma (but see notes above)
- **By mouth**
  Child 3–12 years 4 mg twice daily
  Child 12–18 years 8 mg twice daily

Ventolin® (A&H) PoM
Syrup, sugar-free, salbutamol (as sulphate) 2 mg/5 mL, net price 150 mL = 60p

Volmax® (A&H) PoM
Tablets, m/r, salbutamol (as sulphate) 4 mg, net price 56-tab pack = £9.81; 8 mg, 56-tab pack = £11.77. Label: 25

Dose

Chronic Asthma (but see notes above)
- **By mouth**
  Child 3–12 years 4 mg twice daily
  Child 12–18 years 8 mg twice daily

Parenteral

Ventolin® (A&H) PoM
Injection, salbutamol (as sulphate) 500 micrograms/mL, net price 1-mL amp = 40p

Solution for intravenous infusion, salbutamol (as sulphate) 1 mg/mL. Dilute before use. Net price 5-mL amp = £2.58

Inhalation

Counselling Advise children and carers not to exceed prescribed dose and to follow manufacturer's directions; if a previously effective dose of inhaled salbutamol fails to provide at least 3 hours relief, a doctor's advice should be obtained as soon as possible.
Patients receiving CFC-free inhalers should be reassured about their efficacy and counselled that aerosol may feel and taste different (see notes above)

Salbutamol (Non-proprietary) PoM
Aerosol inhalation, salbutamol 100 micrograms/metered inhalation, net price 200-dose unit = £2.91. Counselling, dose
Excipients: include CFC propellants

Aerosol inhalation, salbutamol (as sulphate) 100 micrograms/metered inhalation, net price 200-dose unit = £2.99. Counselling, dose, change to CFC-free inhaler
Excipients: include HFA-134a (a non-CFC propellant), alcohol
Brands include *Salamol®*
Note Can be supplied against a generic prescription but if CFC-free not specified will be reimbursed at price for CFC-containing inhaler

Dry powder for inhalation, salbutamol 100 micrograms/metered inhalation, net price 200-dose unit = £3.46; 200 micrograms/metered inhalation, 100-dose unit = £5.05, 200-dose unit = £6.92. Counselling, dose
Brands include *Easyhaler® Salbutamol, Pulvinal® Salbutamol*

Inhalation powder, *hard capsule* (for use with *Cyclohaler®* device), salbutamol 200 micrograms, net price 120-cap pack = £4.78; 400 micrograms, 120-cap pack = £8.08
Brands include *Salbutamol Cyclocaps®*

Nebuliser solution, salbutamol (as sulphate) 1 mg/mL, net price 20 × 2.5 mL (2.5 mg) = £1.99; 2 mg/mL, 20 × 2.5 mL (5 mg) = £3.98. May be diluted with sterile sodium chloride 0.9%
Brands include *Salamol Steri-Neb®*

Airomir® (IVAX) PoM
Aerosol inhalation, salbutamol (as sulphate) 100 micrograms/metered inhalation, net price 200-dose unit = £1.97. Counselling, dose, change to CFC-free inhaler
Excipients: include HFA-134a (a non-CFC propellant), alcohol
Note Can be supplied against a generic prescription but if 'CFC-free' not specified will be reimbursed at price for CFC-containing inhaler

Autohaler (breath-actuated aerosol inhalation), salbutamol (as sulphate) 100 micrograms/metered inhalation, net price 200-dose unit = £6.02. Counselling, dose, change to CFC-free inhaler
Excipients: include HFA-134a (a non-CFC propellant), alcohol

Asmasal Clickhaler® (Celltech) PoM
Dry powder for inhalation, salbutamol (as sulphate) 95 micrograms/metered inhalation, net price 200-dose unit = £5.88. Counselling, dose

Dose
- **By inhalation of powder**
  Child 5–18 years 1–2 puffs up to 4 times daily (but see Management of Chronic Asthma, p. 165)

Salamol Easi-Breathe® (IVAX) PoM
Aerosol inhalation, salbutamol 100 micrograms/metered inhalation, net price 200-dose breath-actuated unit = £1.58. Counselling, dose
Excipients: include alcohol, HFA-134a (a non-CFC propellant)

Ventodisks® (A&H) PoM
Dry powder for inhalation, disks containing 8 blisters of salbutamol (as sulphate) 200 micrograms/blister, net price 15 disks with *Diskhaler®* device = £6.98, 15-disk refill = £6.45; 400 micrograms/blister, 15 disks with *Diskhaler®* device = £11.83, 15-disk refill = £11.29. Counselling, dose

Ventolin® (A&H) PoM
Accuhaler® (dry powder for inhalation), disk containing 60 blisters of salbutamol (as sulphate) 200 micrograms/blister with *Accuhaler®* device, net price = £5.12. Counselling, dose

Dose
- **By inhalation of powder**
  Child 5–18 years 200 micrograms up to 4 times daily (for occasional use only)

Evohaler® *aerosol inhalation*, salbutamol (as sulphate) 100 micrograms/metered inhalation, net price 200-dose unit = £1.50. Counselling, dose, change to CFC-free inhaler
Excipients: include HFA-134a (a non-CFC propellant)
Note Can be supplied against a generic prescription but if CFC-free not specified will be reimbursed at price for CFC-containing inhaler

Nebules® (for use with nebuliser), salbutamol (as sulphate) 1 mg/mL, net price 20 × 2.5 mL (2.5 mg) = £1.75; 2 mg/mL, 20 × 2.5 mL (5 mg) = £2.95. May be diluted with sterile sodium chloride 0.9%

Respirator solution (for use with a nebuliser or ventilator), salbutamol (as sulphate) 5 mg/mL. Net price 20 mL = £2.27 (hosp. only). May be diluted with sterile sodium chloride 0.9%

TERBUTALINE SULPHATE

Cautions see notes above

Side-effects see notes above

Licensed use *tablets* not licensed for use in children under 7 years; *modified-release tablets* not licensed for use in children under 12 years; *injection* not licensed for use in children under 2 years

Indication and dose

Acute asthma

- **By inhalation of nebulised solution**
  see Management of Acute Asthma section 3.1
- **By subcutaneous, intramuscular, or slow intravenous injection**
  Child 2–18 years 10 micrograms/kg (max. 300 micrograms, child under 15 years; child over 15 years, max. 500 micrograms) every 6 hours if necessary
- **By continuous intravenous infusion**
  Child 1 month–18 years initially 2–4 micrograms/kg as a loading dose, then 1–10 micrograms/kg/hour according to response and heart rate (doses above 10 micrograms/kg/hour with close monitoring)

Exacerbations of reversible airways obstruction (including nocturnal asthma) and prevention of exercise-induced bronchospasm see Management of Chronic Asthma p. 165

- **By inhalation of powder**
  Child 5–18 years 500 micrograms (1 inhalation) up to 4 times daily (for occasional use only)
- **By mouth (but not recommended)**
  Child 1 month–7 years 75 micrograms/kg (max. 2.5 mg) 3 times daily
  Child 7–12 years 2.5 mg 2–3 times daily
  Child 12–18 years initially 2.5 mg 3 times daily, increased if necessary to 5 mg 3 times daily

Administration For *continuous intravenous infusion*, dilute to a concentration of 5 micrograms/mL with Glucose 5% *or* Sodium Chloride 0.9%; if fluid-restricted, dilute to a concentration of 100 micrograms/mL

For *nebulisation*, dilute nebuliser solution with sterile Sodium Chloride 0.9% solution according to nebuliser type and duration of administration; terbutaline and ipratropium bromide solutions are compatible and may be mixed for nebulisation.

Oral and parenteral

Bricanyl® (AstraZeneca) PoM

Tablets, scored, terbutaline sulphate 5 mg. Net price 20 = 82p

Syrup, sugar-free, terbutaline sulphate 1.5 mg/5 mL. Net price 300 mL = £2.60

Injection, terbutaline sulphate 500 micrograms/mL. Net price 1-mL amp = 30p; 5-mL amp = £1.40

Inhalation

Counselling Advise children and carers not to exceed prescribed dose and to follow manufacturer's directions; if a previously effective dose of inhaled terbutaline fails to provide at least 3 hours relief, a doctor's advice should be obtained as soon as possible

Bricanyl® (AstraZeneca) PoM

Turbohaler® (= dry powder inhaler), terbutaline sulphate 500 micrograms/metered inhalation. Net price 100-dose unit = £6.92. Counselling, dose

Respules® (= single-dose units for nebulisation), terbutaline sulphate 2.5 mg/mL. Net price 20 × 2-mL units (5-mg) = £4.04

FORMOTEROL FUMARATE

(Eformoterol fumarate)

Cautions see notes above

Hepatic impairment metabolism possibly reduced in severe cirrhosis

Pregnancy see section 3.1 (manufacturers advise use only if potential benefit outweighs risk)

Breast-feeding amount in milk probably too small to be harmful but manufacturers advise avoid

Side-effects see notes above; oropharyngeal irritation, taste disturbances, rash, insomnia, nausea and pruritus also reported; **important**: potential for paradoxical bronchospasm (calling for discontinuation and alternative therapy)

Indication and dose

Reversible airways obstruction (including nocturnal asthma and prevention of exercise-induced bronchospasm) in patients requiring long-term regular bronchodilator therapy see also Management of Chronic Asthma, p. 165; for dose see preparations below

Counselling Advise children and carers not to exceed prescribed dose, and to follow manufacturer's directions; if a previously effective dose of inhaled formoterol fails to provide adequate relief, a doctor's advice should be obtained as soon as possible

Atimos Modulite® (Trinity-Chiesi) ▼ PoM

Aerosol inhalation, formoterol fumarate 10.1 micrograms/metered inhalation, net price 100-dose unit = £31.28. Counselling, dose

Dose

Chronic Asthma

- **By aerosol inhalation**
  Child 12–18 years 10.1 micrograms twice daily, increased to max. 20.2 micrograms twice daily in more severe airways obstruction

Note Each inhalation of *Atimos Modulite® 12* delivers 10.1 micrograms formoterol fumarate

Foradil® (Novartis) PoM

Dry powder for inhalation, formoterol fumarate 12 micrograms/capsule, net price 60-dose unit (with inhaler device) = £26.57. Counselling, dose

Dose

Chronic asthma

- **By inhalation of powder**
  Child 5–18 years 12 micrograms twice daily, increased to 24 micrograms twice daily in more severe airways obstruction

FORMOTEROL FUMARATE (*continued*)

Oxis® (AstraZeneca) PoM
Turbohaler® (= dry powder inhaler), formoterol fumarate 4.5 micrograms/inhalation, net price 60-dose unit = £24.80; 9 micrograms/inhalation, 60-dose unit = £24.80. Counselling, dose

Dose

Chronic asthma
- **By inhalation of powder**
  Child 6–18 years 9 micrograms 1–2 times daily; occasionally up to 36 micrograms daily may be needed (max. single dose 9 micrograms); reassess treatment if additional doses required on more than 2 days a week

Relief of bronchospasm
- **By inhalation of powder**
  Child 6–18 years 4.5–9 micrograms

Prevention of exercise-induced bronchospasm
- **By inhalation of powder**
  Child 6–18 years 4.5–9 micrograms before exercise

Note Each metered inhalation of *Oxis® 6 Turbohaler®* delivers 4.5 micrograms formoterol fumarate; each metered inhalation of *Oxis® 12 Turbohaler®* delivers 9 micrograms formoterol fumarate

SALMETEROL

Note Not for immediate relief of acute attacks; existing corticosteroid therapy should not be reduced or withdrawn

Cautions see notes above

Side-effects see notes above; **important**: potential for paradoxical bronchospasm (calling for discontinuation and alternative therapy)

Licensed use not licensed for use in children under 4 years

Indication and dose

Reversible airways obstruction (including nocturnal asthma and prevention of exercise-induced bronchospasm) in patients requiring long-term regular bronchodilator therapy see also Management of Chronic Asthma, p. 165
- **By inhalation**
  Child 2–4 years 25 micrograms (1 puff) twice daily
  Child 4–12 years 50 micrograms (2 puffs or 1 blister) twice daily
  Child 12–18 years 50–100 micrograms (2–4 puffs or 1–2 blisters) twice daily
  Counselling Advise children and carers that salmeterol should **not** be used for relief of acute attacks, not to exceed prescribed dose, and to follow manufacturer's directions; if a previously effective dose of inhaled salmeterol fails to provide adequate relief, a doctor's advice should be obtained as soon as possible

Serevent® (A&H) PoM
Accuhaler® (dry powder for inhalation), disk containing 60 blisters of salmeterol (as xinafoate) 50 micrograms/blister with *Accuhaler®* device, net price = £29.26. Counselling, dose

Evohaler® aerosol inhalation, salmeterol (as xinafoate) 25 micrograms/metered inhalation, net price 120-dose unit = £29.26. Counselling, dose, change to CFC-free inhaler
Excipients: include HFA-13Ha (a non-CFC propellant)

Diskhaler® (dry powder for inhalation), disks containing 4 blisters of salmeterol (as xinafoate) 50 micrograms/blister, net price 15 disks with *Diskhaler®* device = £35.79, 15-disk refill = £35.15. Counselling, dose, change to CFC-free inhaler

3.1.1.2 Other adrenoceptor agonists

Adrenaline (epinephrine) injection (1 in 1000) is used in the emergency treatment of acute allergic and anaphylactic reactions (section 3.4.3), in angioedema (section 3.4.3), and in cardiopulmonary resuscitation (section 2.7.3). Adrenaline solution (1 in 1000) is used by nebulisation in the management of severe croup (section 3.1).

3.1.2 Antimuscarinic bronchodilators

Ipratropium by nebulisation may be added to other standard treatment in life-threatening acute asthma or where acute asthma fails to improve with standard therapy (see Management of Acute Asthma, p. 163). Ipratropium can be used to provide short-term relief in chronic asthma, but short-acting beta$_2$ agonists act more quickly and are preferred.

The aerosol inhalation of ipratropium has a maximum effect 30–60 minutes after use; its duration of action is 3 to 6 hours.

IPRATROPIUM BROMIDE

Cautions *first dose* of nebulised solution under medical supervision (risk of paradoxical bronchospasm); risk of glaucoma (see below), bladder outflow obstruction; **interactions**: Appendix 1 (antimuscarinics)
Glaucoma *Acute angle-closure glaucoma* reported with nebulised ipratropium, particularly when given with nebulised salbutamol (and possibly other beta$_2$ agonists); care needed to protect the child's eyes from nebulised drug or from drug powder

Side-effects dry mouth, nausea, tachycardia, atrial fibrillation, headache; *rarely*, constipation, urinary retention

IPRATROPIUM BROMIDE (*continued*)

Indication and dose

Acute asthma
- **By inhalation of nebulised solution**
  See Management of Acute Asthma, section 3.1

Reversible airways obstruction see notes above
- **By aerosol inhalation**
  Neonate 20 micrograms 4 times daily
  Child 1 month–6 years 20 micrograms 3–4 times daily
  Child 6–12 years 20–40 micrograms 3–4 times daily
  Child 12–18 years 20–40 micrograms 3–4 times daily
- **By inhalation of powder**
  Child 12–18 years 40 micrograms 3–4 times daily (dose may be doubled in less responsive condition)

Counselling Advise child and carer not to exceed prescribed dose and to follow manufacturer's directions

Rhinitis section 12.2.2

Ipratropium Bromide (Non-proprietary) PoM
Nebuliser solution, ipratropium bromide 250 micrograms/mL, net price 20 × 1-mL (250-microgram) unit-dose vials = £6.75, 60 × 1-mL = £21.78; 20 × 2-mL (500-microgram) = £7.43, 60 × 2-mL = £26.97

Atrovent® (Boehringer Ingelheim) PoM
Aerocaps® (dry powder for inhalation; for use with *Atrovent Aerohaler®*), green, ipratropium bromide 40 micrograms, net price pack of 100 caps with *Aerohaler®* = £14.53; 100 caps = £10.53. Counselling, dose

Aerosol inhalation ▼, ipratropium bromide 20 micrograms/metered inhalation, net price 200-dose unit = £4.21. Counselling, dose, change to CFC-free inhaler
Excipients: include HFA-134a (a non-CFC propellant), alcohol

Nebuliser solution, isotonic, ipratropium bromide 250 micrograms/mL, net price 20 × 1-mL unit-dose vials = £5.18, 60 × 1-mL vials = £15.55; 20 × 2-mL vials = £6.08, 60 × 2-mL vials = £18.24

Note One *Atrovent Aerocap®* is equivalent to 2 puffs of *Atrovent®* metered aerosol inhalation

Ipratropium Steri-Neb® (IVAX) PoM
Nebuliser solution, isotonic, ipratropium bromide 250 micrograms/mL, net price 20 × 1-mL (250-microgram) unit-dose vials = £8.72; 20 × 2-mL (500-microgram) = £9.94

Respontin® (A&H) PoM
Nebuliser solution, isotonic, ipratropium bromide 250 micrograms/mL, net price 20 × 1-mL (250-microgram) unit-dose vials = £5.07; 20 × 2-mL (500-microgram) = £5.95

3.1.3 Theophylline

Theophylline is a bronchodilator used for asthma, see Management of Chronic Asthma p. 165. It may have an additive effect when used in conjunction with small doses of beta$_2$ agonists; the combination may increase the risk of side-effects, including hypokalaemia (see p. 167).

Theophylline is given by injection as **aminophylline**, a mixture of theophylline with ethylenediamine, which is 20 times more soluble than theophylline alone. Aminophylline injection is rarely needed for severe attacks of asthma (see Management of Acute Asthma, section 3.1). It must be given by **very slow** intravenous injection (over at least 20 minutes) or by intravenous infusion; it is too irritant for intramuscular use. Intravenous aminophylline may be used as a respiratory stimulant in neonates with apnoea, but **caffeine** (section 3.5.1) is usually preferred. Measurement of plasma-theophylline concentration may be helpful and is **essential** if a loading dose of aminophylline is to be given to children who are taking theophylline, because serious side-effects such as convulsions and arrhythmias can occasionally precede other symptoms of toxicity.

Theophylline is metabolised in the liver. Plasma-theophylline concentration is *increased* in heart failure, cirrhosis, viral infections, and by drugs that inhibit its metabolism. The plasma-theophylline concentration is *decreased* in smokers and by drugs that induce liver metabolism. Particular care is required when introducing or withdrawing drugs that interact with theophylline. For other interactions of theophylline see Appendix 1.

Plasma-theophylline concentration In most individuals a plasma-theophylline concentration of 10–20 mg/litre (55–110 micromol/litre) is required for satisfactory bronchodilation, but a lower concentration of 5–15 mg/litre may be effective. Adverse effects can occur within the range 10–20 mg/litre and both the frequency and severity increase if the concentration exceeds 20 mg/litre. In neonates, toxic symptoms sometimes occur when the plasma-theophylline concentration exceeds 14 mg/litre (78 micromol/litre). If theophylline is used in the treatment of *neonatal apnoea*, the usual target range is 8–12 mg/litre (44–67 micromol/litre).

Plasma-theophylline concentration is measured 5 days after starting oral treatment and at least 3 days after any dose adjustment. A blood sample should be taken 1–2 hours after an oral dose (after 4–6 hours in the case of a modified-release preparation). If aminophylline is given intravenously, a blood sample should be taken 4–6 hours after starting treatment; in a child already taking theophylline, plasma-theophylline concentration should be determined before giving the intravenous dose.

THEOPHYLLINE

Cautions cardiac disease, hypertension, hyperthyroidism, peptic ulcer, epilepsy, fever; **CSM** advice on hypokalaemia risk, p. 167; avoid in porphyria (section 9.8.2); **interactions:** Appendix 1 (theophylline) and notes above

Hepatic impairment reduce dose

Pregnancy neonatal irritability and apnoea reported

Breast-feeding present in milk—irritability in infant reported; modified-release preparations preferable

Side-effects tachycardia, palpitations, nausea and other gastro-intestinal disturbances, headache, CNS stimulation, insomnia, arrhythmias, and convulsions especially if given rapidly by intravenous injection; **overdosage:** see Emergency Treatment of Poisoning, p. 42

Licensed use *Slo-Phyllin®* capsules not licensed for use in children under 2 years

Indication and dose

Chronic asthma

see under preparations below and Management of Chronic Asthma p. 165

Note Plasma-theophylline concentration for optimum response 10–20 mg/litre (55–110 micromol/litre); narrow margin between therapeutic and toxic dose, see also notes above

Modified release

Note The rate of absorption from modified-release preparations can vary between different brands. The Council of the Royal Pharmaceutical Society of Great Britain advises pharmacists that if a general practitioner prescribes a modified-release oral theophylline preparation without specifying a brand name, the pharmacist should contact the prescriber and agree the brand to be dispensed. Additionally, it is essential that a child discharged from hospital should be maintained on the brand on which that child was stabilised as an in-patient.

Nuelin SA® (3M)

SA tablets, m/r, theophylline 175 mg. Net price 60-tab pack = £3.19. Label: 21, 25

SA 250 tablets, m/r, scored, theophylline 250 mg. Net price 60-tab pack = £4.46. Label: 21, 25

Dose

Chronic asthma

- By mouth

Child 6–12 years 175 mg every 12 hours

Child 12–18 years 175–350 mg every 12 hours

(SA 250)

Chronic asthma

- By mouth

Child 6–12 years 125–250 mg every 12 hours

Child 12–18 years 250–500 mg every 12 hours

Slo-Phyllin® (Merck)

Capsules, all m/r, theophylline 60 mg (white/clear, enclosing white pellets), net price 56-cap pack = £2.30; 125 mg (brown/clear, enclosing white pellets), 56-cap pack = £2.90; 250 mg (blue/clear, enclosing white pellets), 56-cap pack = £3.62. Label: 25, or counselling, see below

Dose

Chronic asthma

- By mouth

Child 6 months–2 years (body-weight under 10 kg) 12 mg/kg every 12 hours

Child 2–6 years (body-weight over 10 kg) 60–120 mg every 12 hours

Child 6–12 years 125–250 mg every 12 hours

Child 12–18 years 250–500 mg every 12 hours

Administration Contents of the capsule (enteric-coated granules) may be sprinkled on to a spoonful of soft food (e.g. yoghurt) and swallowed without chewing

Uniphyllin Continus® (Napp)

Tablets, m/r, all scored, theophylline 200 mg, net price 56-tab pack = £3.13; 300 mg, 56-tab pack = £4.77; 400 mg, 56-tab pack = £5.65. Label: 25

Dose

Chronic asthma

- By mouth

Child 7–12 years 9 mg/kg every 12 hours; some children with chronic asthma may require 10–16 mg/kg every 12 hours

Child 12–18 years 8 mg/kg (max. 400 mg) every 12 hours

Note May be appropriate to give larger evening or morning dose to achieve optimum therapeutic effect when symptoms most severe; in children whose night or daytime symptoms persist despite other therapy, who are not currently receiving theophylline, total daily requirement may be added as single evening or morning dose

AMINOPHYLLINE

Note Aminophylline is a stable mixture or combination of theophylline and ethylenediamine; the ethylenediamine confers greater solubility in water

Cautions see under Theophylline; also rapid intravenous injection can cause arrhythmias

Side-effects see under Theophylline; also allergy to ethylenediamine can cause urticaria, erythema, and exfoliative dermatitis

Licensed use *Minijet® Aminophylline* not licensed for use in children under 6 months

AMINOPHYLLINE (*continued*)

Indication and dose

Note To avoid excessive dosage in obese children, dose should be calculated on the basis of ideal weight for height

Chronic asthma (see also Management of Chronic Asthma, p. 165)

- **By mouth**

See under preparations below

Severe acute asthma not previously treated with theophylline (with close monitoring; see also Management of Acute Asthma, section 3.1)

- **By intravenous injection over at least 20 minutes**

Child 1 month–18 years 5 mg/kg (max. 500 mg) then by intravenous infusion

Severe acute asthma (with close monitoring; see also Management of Acute Asthma, section 3.1)

- **By intravenous infusion**

Child 1 month–9 years 1 mg/kg/hour adjusted according to plasma-theophylline concentration

Child 9–16 years 800 micrograms/kg/hour adjusted according to plasma-theophylline concentration

Child 16–18 years 500 micrograms/kg/hour adjusted according to plasma-theophylline concentration

Note Plasma-theophylline concentration for optimum response in asthma 10–20 mg/litre (55–110 micromol/litre); narrow margin between therapeutic and toxic dose, see notes on plasma-theophylline concentration above; children taking oral theophylline or aminophylline should not normally receive intravenous aminophylline unless plasma-theophylline concentration is available to guide dosage

Neonatal apnoea (but see notes above)

- **By intravenous injection over 20 minutes**

Neonate initially 6 mg/kg, then 2.5 mg/kg every 12 hours (increased if necessary to 3.5 mg/kg every 12 hours)

Note Plasma-theophylline concentration for optimum response in neonatal apnoea 8–12 mg/litre (44–66 micromol/litre), see also notes above

Administration For *intravenous infusion*, dilute to a concentration of 1 mg/mL with Glucose 5% *or* Sodium Chloride 0.9%

Aminophylline (Non-proprietary) PoM

Injection, aminophylline 25 mg/mL, net price 10-mL amp = 67p

Brands include *Minijet® Aminophylline*

Injection, aminophylline 2 mg/mL, 20-mL amp; 5 mg/mL, 20-mL amp

Available as a manufactured special, see list of Special-order manufacturers

Modified release

Note Advice about modified-release theophylline preparations on p. 172 also applies to modified-release aminophylline preparations

Phyllocontin Continus® (Napp)

Tablets, m/r, yellow, f/c, aminophylline hydrate 225 mg. Net price 56-tab pack = £2.54. Label: 25

Dose

Chronic asthma (see also Management of Chronic Asthma, p. 165)

- **By mouth**

Child 3–12 years initially 6 mg/kg every 12 hours for 1 week then 12 mg/kg every 12 hours; if necessary dose increased up to 20 mg/kg (max. 450 mg) every 12 hours

Child 12–18 years 225 mg every 12 hours for 1 week then 450 mg every 12 hours

Note Brands of modified-release tablets containing aminophylline 225 mg include *Amnivent® 225 SR, Norphyllin® SR*

3.1.4 Compound bronchodilator preparations

In general, children are best treated with single-ingredient preparations, such as a selective beta$_2$ agonist (section 3.1.1.1) or ipratropium bromide (section 3.1.2), so that the dose of each drug can be adjusted. This flexibility is lost with compound bronchodilator preparations.

3.1.5 Peak flow meters, inhaler devices and nebulisers

Peak flow meters

Peak flow meters may be used to assess lung function in children over 5 years with asthma, but symptom monitoring is the most reliable assessment of asthma control.

Standard Range Peak Flow Meter

Conforms to standard EN 13826

MicroPeak®, range 60–800 litres/minute, net price = £6.50, replacement mouthpiece = 38p (Micro Medical)

Mini-Wright®, range 60–800 litres/minute, net price = £6.86, replacement mouthpiece = 38p (Clement Clarke)

Pocketpeak®, range 60–800 litres/minute, net price = £6.53, replacement mouthpiece = 38p (Ferraris)

Vitalograph®, range 50–800 litres/minute, net price = £5.95 (a child's peak flow meter is also available), replacement mouthpiece = 40p (Vitalograph)

Note Readings from new peak flow meters are often lower than those obtained from old Wright-scale peak flow meters and the correct recording chart should be used

Low Range Peak Flow Meter

Compliant to standard EN 13826 except for scale range

Mini-Wright®, range 30–400 litres/minute, net price = £6.90, replacement mouthpiece = 38p (Clement Clarke)

Pocketpeak®, range 50–400 litres/minute, net price = £6.53, replacement mouthpiece = 38p (Ferraris)

Vitalograph®, range 50–400 litres/minute, net price = £5.95, replacement mouthpiece = 40p (Vitalograph)

Note Readings from new peak flow meters are often lower than those obtained from old Wright-scale peak flow meters and the correct recording chart should be used

Drug delivery devices

Inhaler devices A *pressurised metered-dose inhaler* is an effective method of drug administration in mild to moderate chronic asthma; to deliver the drug effectively particularly in children under 12 years, a spacer device should be used (see also NICE guidance, below). When a pressurised metered-dose inhaler with a spacer is unsuitable or inconvenient, a *dry-powder inhaler* or *breath-actuated inhaler* may be used instead if the child is able to use the device effectively.

Breath-actuated inhalers are suitable for use in children over 7 years and *dry powder inhalers* may be useful in children over 5 years, who are unwilling or unable to use a pressurised metered-dose inhaler with a spacer device. On changing from a pressurised metered-dose inhaler to a dry powder inhaler the child may notice a lack of sensation in the mouth and throat previously associated with each actuation; coughing may occur more frequently following use of a dry-powder inhaler. The child or child's carer should be instructed carefully on the use of the inhaler; CFC-free metered-dose inhalers should be cleaned **weekly** according to the manufacturer's instructions. It is important to check that the inhaler is being used correctly; poor inhalation technique may be mistaken for a lack of response to the drug.

NICE guidance (inhaler devices for children with chronic asthma)

The National Institute for Health and Clinical Excellence has advised that the child's needs, ability to develop and maintain effective technique, and likelihood of good compliance should govern the choice of inhaler and spacer device; only then should cost be considered

For children aged under 5 years:

- corticosteroid and bronchodilator therapy should be delivered by pressurised metered-dose inhaler **and** spacer device, with a facemask if necessary;
- if this is not effective, and depending on the child's condition, nebulised therapy may be considered and, in children over 3 years, a dry powder inhaler may also be considered [but see notes above];

For children aged 5–15 years:

- corticosteroid therapy should be routinely delivered by a pressurised metered-dose inhaler **and** spacer device
- children and their carers should be trained in the use of the chosen device; suitability of the device should be reviewed at least annually. Inhaler technique and compliance should be monitored

Spacer devices Spacer devices are particularly useful for infants, for children with poor inhalation technique, or for nocturnal asthma, because the device reduces the need for co-ordination between actuation of a pressurised metered-dose inhaler and inhalation. The spacer device reduces the velocity of the aerosol and subsequent impaction on the oropharynx and allows more time for evaporation of the propellant so that a larger proportion of the particles can be inhaled and deposited in the lungs. Smaller-volume spacers may be more manageable for pre-school children and infants. The spacer device used must be compatible with the prescribed metered-dose inhaler.

Use and care of spacer devices The suitability of the spacer device should be carefully assessed; the opening of the one-way valve is dependent on the child's inspiratory flow. Some devices can be tipped to 45° to open the valve during inhaler actuation and inspiration to assist4 the child. By the age of 3 years, the child can usually be taught to use the spacer device without a mask.

Inhalation from the spacer device should follow the actuation as soon as possible because the drug aerosol is very short-lived. The total dose (which may be more than a single puff) should be administered as single actuations (tidal breathing for 10–20 seconds or 5–6 breaths between each actuation) for children with good inspiratory flow. Larger doses may be necessary for a child with acute bronchospasm; for guidance on the Management of Acute Asthma, see section 3.1.

The device should be cleansed once a month by washing in mild detergent and then allowed to dry in air; the mouthpiece should be wiped clean of detergent before use. More frequent cleaning should be avoided since any electrostatic charge may affect drug delivery. Spacer devices should be replaced every 6–12 months.

Able Spacer® (Clement Clarke)
Spacer device, small-volume device. For use with pressurised (aerosol) inhalers, net price standard device = £4.20; with infant, child or adult mask = £6.86

AeroChamber® Plus (GSK)
Spacer device, medium-volume device. For use with pressurised (aerosol) inhalers, net price standard device (blue) = £4.36, with mask (blue) = £7.27; infant device (orange) with mask = £4.36; child device (yellow) with mask = £7.27

Babyhaler® (A&H) NHS
Spacer device, paediatric use with *Becotide®-50* and *Ventolin®* inhalers. Net price = £11.34

E-Z Spacer® (Vitalograph) NHS
Spacer device, large-volume, collapsible device. For use with pressurised (aerosol) inhalers, price (direct from manufacturer) = £23.00

Haleraid® (A&H)
Device to place over standard inhalers to aid when strength in hands is impaired (e.g. arthritis). Available as *Haleraid®-120* for 120-dose inhalers and *Haleraid®-200* for 200-dose inhalers, net price = 80p

NebuChamber® (AstraZeneca)
Spacer device, for use with *Pulmicort®* aerosol inhalation. Free of charge from manufacturer

Nebuhaler® (AstraZeneca)
Spacer device, large-volume device. For use with *Bricanyl®* and *Pulmicort®* inhalers, net price = £4.28; with paediatric mask = £4.28

PARI Vortex Spacer® (Pari) NHS
Spacer device, small-volume device. For use with a pressurised (aerosol) inhaler, net price with mouthpiece = £6.07; with mask for infant or child = £7.91; with adult mask = £9.97

Pocket Chamber® (Ferraris)
Spacer device, small-volume device. For use with a pressurised (aerosol) inhaler, net price = £4.18; with infant, small, medium, or large mask = £9.75

Spinhaler® (Rhône-Poulenc Rorer)
Inhalation device, for use with *Intal Spincaps®*, net price = £1.92

Volumatic® (A&H)
Spacer inhaler, large-volume device. For use with *Becloforte®*, *Becotide®*, *Flixotide®*, *Seretide®*, *Serevent®*, and *Ventolin®* inhalers, net price = £2.75; with paediatric mask = £2.75

Nebulisers

In England and Wales nebulisers and compressors are not available on the NHS (but they are free of VAT); some nebulisers (but not compressors) are available on form GP10A in Scotland (for details consult Scottish Drug Tariff).

For details of jet nebulisers, home compressors with nebulisers, and compressors, see current BNF.

A nebuliser converts a solution of a drug into an aerosol for inhalation. It is used to deliver higher doses of drug to the airways than is usual with standard inhalers. The main indications for use of a nebuliser are:

- to deliver a beta$_2$ agonist or ipratropium to a child with an *acute exacerbation* of asthma or of airways obstruction;
- to deliver *prophylactic medication* to a child unable to use other conventional devices;
- to deliver an antibacterial (such as colistin, section 5.1.7) or tobramycin (section 5.1.4) to a child with chronic purulent infection (as in cystic fibrosis or bronchiectasis);
- to deliver pentamidine (section 5.4.8) for the prophylaxis and treatment of pneumocystis pneumonia to a child with AIDS.

The proportion of a nebuliser solution that reaches the lungs depends on the type of nebuliser and although it can be as high as 30% it is more frequently close to 10% and sometimes below 10%. The remaining solution is left in the nebuliser as residual volume or it is deposited in the mouthpiece and tubing. The extent to which the nebulised solution is deposited in the airways or alveoli depends on particle size. Particles with a median diameter of 1–5 microns are deposited in the airways and are therefore appropriate for asthma whereas a particle size of 1–2 microns is needed for alveolar deposition of pentamidine to combat pneumocystis infection. The type of nebuliser is therefore chosen according to the deposition required and according to the viscosity of the solution (antibacterial solutions usually being more viscous).

Some jet nebulisers are able to increase drug output during inspiration and hence increase efficiency.

The dose of a bronchodilator given by nebulisation is usually **much higher** than that from an aerosol inhaler.

Nebulised bronchodilators may be given to children with chronic persistent asthma or those with severe acute asthma. In chronic asthma, nebulised bronchodilators should only be used to relieve persistent daily wheeze (see Management of Chronic Asthma table, p. 165). The use of nebulisers in chronic persistent asthma should only be considered:

- after a review of the diagnosis and use of current inhaler devices;
- if the airflow obstruction is significantly reversible by bronchodilators without unacceptable side-effects;
- if the child does not benefit from use of conventional inhaler device, such as pressurised metered-dose inhaler plus spacer;
- if the child is complying with the prescribed dose and frequency of anti-inflammatory treatment including regular use of high-dose inhaled corticosteroid.

When a nebuliser is prescribed, the child or child's carer must:

- have clear instructions from doctor, specialist nurse or pharmacist on the use of the nebuliser (and on peak-flow monitoring—see notes above);
- be instructed not to treat acute attacks without also seeking medical help;
- have regular follow up with doctor or specialist nurse.

Jet nebulisers are more widely used than ultrasonic nebulisers. Most jet nebulisers require an optimum flow rate of 6–8 litres/minute and in hospital can be driven by piped air or oxygen; in acute asthma the nebuliser should be driven by oxygen. Domiciliary oxygen cylinders do not provide an adequate flow rate therefore an electrical compressor is required for domiciliary use.

> Safe practice
> The Department of Health has reminded users of the need to use the correct grade of tubing when connecting a nebuliser to a medical gas supply or compressor.

For a list of available devices see BNF (section 3.1.5).

Nebuliser diluent

Nebulisation may be carried out using an undiluted nebuliser solution or it may require dilution beforehand. The usual diluent is sterile sodium chloride 0.9% (physiological saline).

Sodium Chloride (Non-proprietary) PoM
Nebuliser solution, sodium chloride 0.9%, net price
20 × 2.5 mL = £5.49
Brands include *Saline Steripoule®*, *Saline Steri-Neb®*

3.2 Corticosteroids

Corticosteroids are very effective in *asthma*; they reduce airway inflammation.

Inhalation Inhaled corticosteroids are recommended for prophylactic treatment of asthma when a child needs to use a beta$_2$ agonist more than 3 times a week or if symptoms disturb sleep more than once a week or if the child has suffered exacerbations in the last 2 years requiring a systemic corticosteroid or a nebulised bronchodilator (see Management of Chronic Asthma, p. 165). *Regular use* of inhaled corticosteroids reduces the risk of exacerbation of asthma.

Corticosteroid inhalers must be used regularly for maximum benefit; alleviation of symptoms usually occurs 3 to 7 days after initiation but may take longer. **Beclometasone dipropionate** (beclomethasone dipropionate), **budesonide**, **fluticasone propionate,** and **mometasone furoate** appear to be equally effective. A spacer device should be used for administering inhaled corticosteroids in children under 15 years (see NICE guidance, section 3.1.5); a spacer device is also useful in children over 15 years, particularly if high doses are required.

Doses for CFC-free corticosteroid inhalers may be different from those that contain CFCs.

CFC-free inhalers Chlorofluorocarbon (CFC) propellants in pressurised aerosol inhalers are being replaced by hydrofluoroalkane (HFA) propellants. Carers of children and children receiving CFC-free inhalers should be reassured about the efficacy of the new inhalers and counselled that the aerosol may feel and taste different; any difficulty with the new inhaler should be discussed with the doctor, asthma nurse specialist, or pharmacist.

If the inhaled corticosteroid makes the child cough, the use of an inhaled $beta_2$ agonist beforehand may help.

High doses of inhaled corticosteroids may be prescribed for children who respond only partially to standard doses and long-acting $beta_2$ agonists or other long-acting bronchodilators (see Management of Chronic Asthma, p. 165). High doses should be continued only if there is clear benefit over the lower dose. The recommended maximum dose of an inhaled corticosteroid should not generally be exceeded; however, if higher doses are required they should be initiated and supervised by a respiratory paediatrician. The use of high doses of an inhaled corticosteroid can minimise the requirement for oral corticosteroid.

Cautions of inhaled corticosteroids Caution is required in active or quiescent tuberculosis; systemic therapy may be required during periods of stress, during episodes of infection, or when airways obstruction or mucus prevent drug access to smaller airways. An inhaled corticosteroid may be used during pregnancy and breast-feeding, see p. 162; **interactions:** Appendix 1 (corticosteroids)

Paradoxical bronchospasm The potential for paradoxical bronchospasm (calling for discontinuation and alternative therapy) should be borne in mind—mild bronchospasm may be prevented by inhalation of a short-acting $beta_2$ agonist (or by transfer from an aerosol inhalation to a dry powder inhalation if suitable).

Side-effects of inhaled corticosteroids Inhaled corticosteroids have considerably fewer systemic effects than oral corticosteroids, but adverse effects have been reported.

Higher doses of inhaled corticosteroids have the potential to induce adrenal suppression (section 6.3.2) and children on high doses should be given a 'steroid card'; these children may need corticosteroid cover during an episode of stress (e.g. an operation). Inhaled corticosteroids in children have occasionally been associated with adrenal crisis and coma; excessive doses should be **avoided**.

Bone mineral density may be reduced following long-term inhalation of higher doses of corticosteroids, predisposing patients to osteoporosis (section 6.6). It is therefore sensible to ensure that the dose of an inhaled corticosteroid is no higher than necessary to keep a child's asthma under good control.

Growth retardation associated with oral corticosteroid therapy does not seem to be a significant problem with recommended doses of inhaled corticosteroids; although initial growth velocity may be reduced, there appears to be no effect on eventual adult height. However, the CSM recommends that the height of children receiving prolonged treatment is monitored; if growth is slowed, referral to a paediatrician should be considered.

Hoarseness and candidiasis of the mouth or throat have been reported, usually only with high doses (see also below). Hypersensitivity reactions (including rash and angioedema) have been reported rarely.

Candidiasis Candidiasis can be reduced by using a spacer device (see notes above) and by rinsing the mouth with water (or cleaning the child's teeth) after inhalation of a corticosteroid; candidiasis can be treated with antifungal oral suspension or lozenges (section 12.3.2) while continuing corticosteroid therapy.

Oral An acute attack of asthma should be treated with a short course (3–5 days) of oral corticosteroid, see Management of Acute Asthma, p. 163. The dose can usually be stopped abruptly in a mild exacerbation of asthma (see also Withdrawal of Corticosteroids, section 6.3.2) but it should be reduced gradually in children with poorer asthma control, to reduce the possibility of serious relapse.

In chronic continuing asthma, when the response to other drugs has been inadequate, longer term administration of an oral corticosteroid may be necessary; in such cases high doses of an inhaled corticosteroid should be continued to minimise oral corticosteroid requirements.

An oral corticosteroid should normally be taken as a single dose in the morning to reduce the disturbance to circadian cortisol secretion. Dosage should always be titrated to the lowest dose that controls symptoms.

Parenteral For the use of hydrocortisone injection in the emergency treatment of acute severe asthma, see Management of Acute Asthma, p. 163.

BECLOMETASONE DIPROPIONATE

(Beclomethasone Dipropionate)

Cautions see notes above

Side-effects see notes above

Licensed use *Asmabec Clickhaler®-50* not licensed for use in children under 6 years; *Becodisk®-400*, *Becotide®-200*, *Qvar®*, and *high-dose inhalers* are not licensed for use in children (age range not specified by manufacturers)

Indication and dose

Prophylaxis of asthma

for doses, see Management of Chronic Asthma, p. 165

Important for *Qvar®* see under preparation below

Standard-dose inhalers

Beclometasone (Non-proprietary) PoM

Aerosol inhalation, beclometasone dipropionate 50 micrograms/metered inhalation, net price 200-dose unit = £3.97; 100 micrograms/metered inhalation, 200-dose unit = £8.24; 200 micrograms/metered inhalation, 200-dose unit = £8.14. Label: 8, counselling, dose

Excipients: include CFC propellants

Brands include *Beclazone®*, *Filair®*

Dry powder for inhalation, beclometasone dipropionate 100 micrograms/metered inhalation, net price 100-dose unit = £5.58; 200 micrograms/metered inhalation, 100-dose unit = £10.29, 200-dose unit = £15.60. Label: 8, counselling, dose

Brands include *Pulvinal® Beclometasone Dipropionate, Easyhaler® Beclometasone Dipropionate*

Inhalation powder, hard capsule (for use with *Cyclohaler®* device), beclometasone dipropionate 100 micrograms, net price 120-cap pack = £7.59; 200 micrograms, 120-cap pack = £14.41. Label: 8, counselling, dose

Brands include *Beclometasone Cyclocaps®*

AeroBec® (3M) PoM

AeroBec 50 Autohaler® (breath-actuated aerosol inhalation), beclometasone dipropionate 50 micrograms/metered inhalation, net price 200-dose unit = £4.04. Label: 8, counselling, dose

Excipients: include CFC propellants

AeroBec 100 Autohaler® (breath-actuated aerosol inhalation), beclometasone dipropionate 100 micrograms/metered inhalation, net price 200-dose unit = £7.66. Label: 8, counselling, dose

Excipients: include CFC propellants

Asmabec Clickhaler® (Celltech) PoM

Dry powder for inhalation, beclometasone dipropionate 50 micrograms/metered inhalation, net price 200-dose unit = £6.68; 100 micrograms/metered inhalation, 200-dose unit = £9.81. Label: 8, counselling, dose

Beclazone Easi-Breathe® (IVAX) PoM

Aerosol inhalation, beclometasone dipropionate 50 micrograms/metered inhalation, net price 200-dose breath-actuated unit = £3.26; 100 micrograms/metered inhalation, 200-dose breath-actuated unit = £6.18. Label: 8, counselling, dose

Excipients: include CFC propellants

Becodisks® (A&H) PoM

Dry powder for inhalation, disks containing 8 blisters of beclometasone dipropionate 100 micrograms/blister, net price 15 disks with *Diskhaler®* device = £12.00, 15-disk refill = £11.42; 200 micrograms/blister, 15 disks with *Diskhaler®* device = £22.87, 15-disk refill = £22.28. Label: 8, counselling, dose

Becotide® (A&H) PoM

Becotide®-50 aerosol inhalation, beclometasone dipropionate 50 micrograms/metered inhalation. Net price 200-dose unit = £1.79. Label: 8, counselling, dose

Excipients: include CFC propellants

Becotide®-100 aerosol inhalation, beclometasone dipropionate 100 micrograms/metered inhalation. Net price 200-dose unit = £2.79. Label: 8, counselling, dose

Excipients: include CFC propellants

Becotide®-200 aerosol inhalation, beclometasone dipropionate 200 micrograms/metered inhalation. Net price 200-dose unit = £8.14. Label: 8, counselling, dose, 10, steroid card

Excipients: include CFC propellants

Qvar® (IVAX) PoM

Qvar® 50 aerosol inhalation, beclometasone dipropionate 50 micrograms/metered inhalation, net price 200-dose unit = £7.87. Label: 8, counselling, dose

Excipients: include HFA-134a (a non-CFC propellant), ethanol

Qvar® 100 aerosol inhalation, beclometasone dipropionate 100 micrograms/metered inhalation, net price 200-dose unit = £17.21. Label: 8, counselling, dose, 10, steroid card

Excipients: include HFA-134a (a non-CFC propellant), ethanol

BECLOMETASONE DIPROPIONATE (*continued*)

Qvar 50 Autohaler® (breath-actuated aerosol inhalation), beclometasone dipropionate 50 micrograms/metered inhalation, net price 200-dose unit = £7.87. Label: 8, counselling, dose
Excipients: include HFA-134a (a non-CFC propellant), ethanol

Qvar 100 Autohaler® (breath-actuated aerosol inhalation), beclometasone dipropionate 100 micrograms/metered inhalation, net price 200-dose unit = £17.21. Label: 8, counselling, dose, 10, steroid card
Excipients: include HFA-134a (a non-CFC propellant), ethanol

Qvar Easi-Breathe® (breath-actuated aerosol inhalation), beclometasone dipropionate 50 micrograms/metered inhalation, net price 200-dose = £8.24; 100 micrograms/metered inhalation, 200-dose = £18.02. Label: 8, counselling, dose, 10, steroid card
Excipients: include HFA-134a (a non-CFC propellant), ethanol

Note When transferring a patient from a CFC-containing inhaler (asthma well controlled), initially a 100-microgram metered dose of *Qvar®* should be substituted for:

- 200–250 micrograms of beclometasone dipropionate or budesonide
- 100 micrograms of fluticasone propionate

When transferring a patient from a CFC-containing inhaler (asthma poorly controlled), initially a 100-microgram metered dose of *Qvar®* should be substituted for 100 micrograms of beclometasone dipropionate, budesonide or fluticasone propionate; max. adult dose of *Qvar®* 400 micrograms twice daily

High-dose inhalers

Note High-dose inhalers not licensed for use in children (age range not specified by manufacturers)

Beclometasone (Non-proprietary) PoM
Aerosol inhalation, beclometasone dipropionate 250 micrograms/metered inhalation, net price 200-dose unit = £12.93. Label: 8, counselling, dose, 10, steroid card
Excipients: include CFC propellants
Brands include *Beclazone®*, *Filair Forte®*

Dry powder for inhalation, beclometasone dipropionate 400 micrograms/metered inhalation, net price 100-dose unit = £20.41. Label: 8, counselling, dose, 10, steroid card
Brands include *Pulvinal® Beclometasone Dipropionate*, *Easyhaler® Beclometasone Dipropionate*

Inhalation powder, hard capsule (for use with *Cyclohaler®* device), beclometasone dipropionate 400 micrograms, net price 120-cap pack = £27.38. Label: 8, counselling, dose, 10, steroid card
Brands include *Beclometasone 400 Cyclocaps®*

AeroBec Forte® (3M) PoM
Aerosol inhalation, beclometasone dipropionate 250 micrograms/metered inhalation, net price 200-inhalation breath-actuated unit (*Autohaler®*) = £16.76. Label: 8, counselling, dose, 10, steroid card
Excipients: include CFC propellants

Asmabec Clickhaler® (Celltech) PoM
Dry powder for inhalation, beclometasone dipropionate 250 micrograms/metered inhalation, net price 100-dose unit = £12.31. Label: 8, counselling, dose, 10, steroid card

Beclazone Easi-Breathe® (IVAX) PoM
Aerosol inhalation, beclometasone dipropionate 250 micrograms/metered inhalation, net price 200-dose breath-actuated unit = £13.52. Label: 8, counselling, dose, 10, steroid card
Excipients: include CFC propellants

Becloforte® (A&H) PoM
Aerosol inhalation, beclometasone dipropionate 250 micrograms/metered inhalation. Net price 200-dose unit = £6.99. Label: 8, counselling, dose, 10, steroid card
Excipients: include CFC propellants

Becodisks® (A&H) PoM
Dry powder for inhalation, disks containing 8 blisters of beclometasone dipropionate 400 micrograms/blister, 15 disks with *Diskhaler®* device = £45.14, 15-disk refill = £44.57. Label: 8, counselling, dose, 10, steroid card

Qvar® (IVAX) PoM
See under Standard-dose inhalers above

BUDESONIDE

Cautions see notes above

Side-effects see notes above

Licensed use *Pulmicort® nebuliser solution* not licensed for use in children under 3 months; not licensed for use in bronchopulmonary dysplasia

Indication and dose

Prophylaxis of asthma for doses, see Management of Chronic Asthma, p. 165

Croup
- **By inhalation of nebuliser suspension**
  Child over 1 month 2 mg as single dose or in 2 divided doses separated by 30 minutes; dose may be repeated after 12 hours if necessary

Bronchopulmonary dysplasia
- **By aerosol inhalation**
  Neonate 400 micrograms twice daily
  Child 1–4 months 400 micrograms twice daily

Bronchopulmonary dysplasia with spontaneous respiration
- **By inhalation of nebuliser suspension**
  Neonate 500 micrograms twice daily
  Child 1–4 months 500 micrograms twice daily; for severe symptoms in child body-weight 2.5 kg or over, 1 mg twice daily

Administration For *aerosol inhalation*, use medium-volume spacer (section 3.1.5) attached directly to endotracheal tube; hand-ventilate through spacer, using a bag system; inflate chest 10 times between activations of inhaler

Budesonide (Non-proprietary) PoM
Dry powder for inhalation, budesonide 100 micrograms/metered inhalation, net price 200-dose unit = £9.25; 200 micrograms/metered inhalation

BUDESONIDE (*continued*)

200-dose unit = £18.50; 400 micrograms/metered inhalation 100-dose unit = £18.50. Label: 8, counselling, dose, 10, steroid card
Brands include *Easyhaler® Budesonide*

Inhalation powder, hard capsule (for use with *Cyclohaler®* device), budesonide 200 micrograms, net price 100-cap pack = £15.48; 400 micrograms, 50-cap pack = £15.48. Label: 8, counselling, dose, 10, steroid card
Brands include *Budesonide Cyclocaps®*

Novolizer® (Viatris) ▼ PoM
Dry powder for inhalation, budesonide 200 micrograms, net price refillable inhaler device and 100-dose cartridge = £14.86; 100-dose refill cartridge = £9.59. Label: 8, counselling, dose, 10, steroid card

Pulmicort® (AstraZeneca) PoM
LS aerosol inhalation, budesonide 50 micrograms/metered inhalation, net price 200-dose unit = £7.33. Label: 8, counselling, dose
Excipients: include CFC propellants

Aerosol inhalation, budesonide 200 micrograms/metered inhalation, net price 200-dose unit = £20.90; 100-dose unit = £7.60 (hosp. only; may be difficult to obtain). Label: 8, counselling, dose, 10, steroid card
Excipients: include CFC propellants

Turbohaler® (= dry powder inhaler), budesonide 100 micrograms/metered inhalation, net price 200-dose unit = £18.50; 200 micrograms/metered inhalation, 100-dose unit = £18.50; 400 micrograms/metered inhalation, 50-dose unit = £18.50. Label: 8, counselling, dose, 10, steroid card

Respules® (= single-dose units for nebulisation), budesonide 250 micrograms/mL, net price 20 × 2-mL (500-microgram) unit = £32.00; 500 micrograms/mL, 20 × 2-mL (1-mg) unit = £44.64. May be diluted with sterile sodium chloride 0.9%. Label: 8, counselling, dose,, 10, steroid card

Compound preparations

Symbicort® (AstraZeneca) PoM
Symbicort 100/6 Turbohaler® (= dry powder inhaler), budesonide 80 micrograms, formoterol fumarate 4.5 micrograms/metered inhalation, net price 120-dose unit = £33.00. Label: 8, counselling, dose, 10, steroid card
Note Each metered inhalation of *Symbicort® 100/6* delivers the same quantity of budesonide as a 100-microgram metered inhalation of *Pulmicort Turbohaler®* and of formoterol fumerate as a 4.5-microgram metered inhalation of *Oxis® 6 Turbohaler®*

Dose

Chronic asthma
- **By inhalation of powder**
  Child 6–12 years 2 puffs twice daily reduced to 1 puff once daily if control maintained
  Child 12–18 years 1–2 puffs twice daily reduced to 1 puff once daily if control maintained

Symbicort 200/6 Turbohaler® (= dry powder inhaler), budesonide 160 micrograms, formoterol fumarate 4.5 micrograms/metered inhalation, net price 120-dose unit = £38.00. Label: 8, counselling, dose, 10, steroid card
Note Each metered inhalation of *Symbicort® 200/6* delivers the same quantity of budesonide as a 200-microgram metered inhalation of *Pulmicort Turbohaler®* and of formoterol fumerate as a 4.5-microgram metered inhalation of *Oxis® 6 Turbohaler®*

Dose

Chronic asthma
- **By inhalation of powder**
  Child 12–18 years 1–2 puffs twice daily reduced in well-controlled asthma to 1 puff once daily

Symbicort 400/12 Turbohaler® (= dry powder inhaler), budesonide 320 micrograms, formoterol fumarate 9 micrograms/metered inhalation, net price 60-dose unit = £38.00. Label: 8, counselling, dose, 10, steroid card
Note Each metered inhalation of *Symbicort® 400/12* delivers the same quantity of budesonide as a 400-microgram metered inhalation of *Pulmicort Turbohaler®* and of formoterol fumerate as a 9-microgram metered inhalation of *Oxis® 12 Turbohaler®*

Dose

Chronic asthma
- **By inhalation of powder**
  Child 12–18 years 1 puff twice daily; may be reduced in well-controlled asthma to 1 puff once daily

FLUTICASONE PROPIONATE

Cautions see notes above

Side-effects see notes above

Licensed use *Flixotide Evohaler®* 125 micrograms/metered dose and 250 micrograms/metered dose, *Flixotide Accuhaler®* and *Flixotide Diskhaler®* 250 micrograms/blister and 500 micrograms/blister, *Flixotide Nebules®*, consult product literature; all other *Flixotide®* preparations, *Seretide 100 Accuhaler®*, *Seretide 50 Evohaler®*, not licensed for use in children under 4 years; *Seretide 250 Accuhaler®*, *Seretide 500 Accuhaler®*, *Seretide 125 Evohaler®*, *Seretide 250 Evohaler®*, not licensed for use in children under 12 years

Indication and dose

Prophylaxis of asthma for doses, see Management of Chronic Asthma, p. 165

Flixotide® (A&H) PoM
Accuhaler® (dry powder for inhalation), disk containing 60 blisters of fluticasone propionate 50 micrograms/blister with *Accuhaler®* device, net price = £6.38; 100 micrograms/blister with *Accuhaler®* device = £8.93; 250 micrograms/blister with *Accuhaler®* device = £21.26; 500 micrograms/blister with *Accuhaler®* device = £36.14. Label: 8, counselling, dose; 250- and 500-microgram strengths also label 10, steroid card

Diskhaler® (dry powder for inhalation), fluticasone propionate 50 micrograms/blister, net price 15 disks of 4 blisters with *Diskhaler®* device = £8.17, 15-disk refill = £7.64; 100 micrograms/blister, 15 disks of 4 blisters with *Diskhaler®* device = £12.71, 15-disk refill = £12.18; 250 micrograms/blister, 15 disks of 4 blisters with *Diskhaler®* device = £24.11, 15-disk refill = £23.58; 500 micrograms/blister, 15 disks of 4 blisters with *Diskhaler®* device = £40.05,

FLUTICASONE PROPIONATE (*continued*)

15-disk refill = £39.52. Label: 8, counselling, dose; 250- and 500-microgram strengths also label 10, steroid card

Evohaler® *aerosol inhalation*, fluticasone propionate 50 micrograms/metered inhalation, net price 120-dose unit = £5.44; 125 micrograms/metered inhalation, 120-dose unit = £21.26; 250 micrograms/metered inhalation, 120-dose unit = £36.14. Label: 8, counselling, dose, change to CFC-free inhaler; 250-microgram strength also label 10, steroid card
Excipients: include HFA-134a (a non-CFC propellant)

Nebules® (= single-dose units for nebulisation) fluticasone propionate 250 micrograms/mL, net price 10 × 2-mL (500-microgram) unit = £9.34; 1 mg/mL, 10 × 2-mL (2-mg) unit = £37.35. May be diluted with sterile sodium chloride 0.9%. Label: 8, counselling, dose, 10, steroid card

Dose

Chronic asthma
- **By inhalation of nebuliser suspension**
  Child 4–16 years 1 mg twice daily
  Child 16–18 years 0.5–2 mg twice daily

Compound preparations

Seretide® (A&H) PoM

Seretide 100 Accuhaler® (dry powder for inhalation), disk containing 60 blisters of fluticasone propionate 100 micrograms, salmeterol (as xinafoate) 50 micrograms/blister with *Accuhaler®* device, net price = £31.19. Label: 8, counselling, dose

Dose

Chronic asthma
- **By inhalation of powder**
  Child 4–18 years 1 blister twice daily, reduced to 1 blister once daily if control maintained

Seretide 250 Accuhaler® (dry powder for inhalation), disk containing 60 blisters of fluticasone propionate 250 micrograms, salmeterol (as xinafoate) 50 micrograms/blister with *Accuhaler®* device, net price = £36.65. Label: 8, counselling, dose, 10, steroid card

Dose

Chronic asthma
- **By inhalation of powder**
  Child 12–18 years 1 blister twice daily

Seretide 500 Accuhaler® (dry powder for inhalation), disk containing 60 blisters of fluticasone propionate 500 micrograms, salmeterol (as xinafoate) 50 micrograms/blister with *Accuhaler®* device, net price = £40.92. Label: 8, counselling, dose, 10, steroid card

Dose

Chronic asthma
- **By inhalation of powder**
  Child 12–18 years 1 blister twice daily

Seretide 50 Evohaler® (aerosol inhalation), fluticasone propionate 50 micrograms, salmeterol (as xinafoate) 25 micrograms/metered inhalation, net price 120-dose unit = £19.50. Label: 8, counselling, dose, change to CFC-free inhaler
Excipients: include HFA-134a (a non-CFC propellant)

Dose

Chronic asthma
- **By aerosol inhalation**
  Child 4–18 years 2 puffs twice daily, reduced to 2 puffs once daily if control maintained

Seretide 125 Evohaler® (aerosol inhalation), fluticasone propionate 125 micrograms, salmeterol (as xinafoate) 25 micrograms/metered inhalation, net price 120-dose unit = £39.41. Label: 8, counselling, dose, change to CFC-free inhaler, 10, steroid card
Excipients: include HFA-134a (a non-CFC propellant)

Dose

Chronic asthma
- **By aerosol inhalation**
  Child 12–18 years 2 puffs twice daily

Seretide 250 Evohaler® (aerosol inhalation), fluticasone propionate 250 micrograms, salmeterol (as xinafoate) 25 micrograms/metered inhalation, net price 120-dose unit = £66.98. Label: 8, counselling, dose, change to CFC-free inhaler, 10, steroid card
Excipients: include HFA-134a (a non-CFC propellant)

Dose

Chronic asthma
- **By aerosol inhalation**
  Child 12–18 years 2 puffs twice daily

MOMETASONE FUROATE

Cautions see notes above

Side-effects see notes above; also pharyngitis, headache; *less commonly* palpitation

Indication and dose

Prophylaxis of asthma see also Management of Chronic Asthma, p. 165
- **By inhalation of powder**
  Child 12–18 years 200–400 micrograms as a single dose in the evening or in 2 divided doses; dose increased to 400 micrograms twice daily if necessary

Asmanex® (Schering-Plough) ▼ PoM

Twisthaler (= dry powder inhaler), mometasone furoate 200 micrograms/metered inhalation, net price 30-dose unit = £16.00, 60-dose unit = £24.00; 400 micrograms/metered inhalation, 30-dose unit = £22.20, 60-dose unit = £36.75. Label: 8, counselling, dose, 10, steroid card

3.3 Cromoglicate and related therapy, leukotriene receptor antagonists, and omalizumab

3.3.1 Cromoglicate and related therapy

The mode of action of **sodium cromoglicate** and **nedocromil** is not completely understood; they may be of value as *prophylaxis* in asthma with an allergic basis, but the evidence for benefit of sodium cromoglicate in children is contentious. Prophylaxis with cromoglicate or nedocromil is less effective than with inhaled corticosteroids (see Management of Chronic Asthma, p. 165).

Nedocromil may be of some benefit in the prophylaxis of exercise-induced asthma.

For the use of sodium cromoglicate and nedocromil in allergic conjunctivitis see section 11.4.2; sodium cromoglicate is used also in allergic rhinitis (section 12.2.1) and allergy-related diarrhoea (section 1.5).

SODIUM CROMOGLICATE

(Sodium Cromoglycate)

Side-effects coughing, transient bronchospasm, and throat irritation due to inhalation of powder

Indication and dose

Prophylaxis of asthma (but see notes above)
Counselling Regular use is necessary

- **By aerosol inhalation**
  Child 12–18 years 10 mg (2 puffs) 4 times daily, increased in severe cases or during periods of risk to 6–8 times daily; additional doses may also be taken before exercise; maintenance 5 mg (1 puff) 4 times daily

- **By inhalation of powder (*Spincaps*®)**
  Child 12–18 years 20 mg 4 times daily, increased in severe cases to 8 times daily; additional doses may also be taken before exercise

- **By inhalation of nebulised solution**
  Child 12–18 years 20 mg 4 times daily, increased in severe cases to 6 times daily

Food allergy section 1.5

Allergic conjunctivitis section 11.4.2

Allergic rhinitis section 12.2.1

Sodium Cromoglicate (Non-proprietary) PoM
Aerosol inhalation, sodium cromoglicate 5 mg/metered inhalation. Net price 112-dose unit = £5.92. Label: 8
Excipients: include CFC propellants
Brands include *Cromogen*®

Cromogen Easi-Breathe® (IVAX) PoM
Aerosol inhalation, sodium cromoglicate 5 mg/metered inhalation. Net price 112-dose breath-actuated unit = £13.91. Label: 8
Excipients: include CFC propellants

Intal® (Rhône-Poulenc Rorer) PoM
Aerosol inhalation, sodium cromoglicate 5 mg/metered inhalation. Net price 112-dose unit with large volume spacer inhaler (*Fisonair*®) = £20.52. Label: 8
Excipients: include CFC propellants

Spincaps®, yellow/clear, sodium cromoglicate 20 mg. Net price 112-cap pack = £15.44. Label: 8

Spinhaler insufflator® (for use with *Intal Spincaps*). Net price = £1.92

NEDOCROMIL SODIUM

Side-effects see under Sodium Cromoglicate; also headache, nausea, vomiting, dyspepsia and abdominal pain; bitter taste (masked by mint flavour)

Licensed use not licensed for use in children under 6 years

Indication and dose

Prophylaxis of asthma (but see notes above)
Counselling Regular use is necessary

- **By aerosol inhalation**
  Child 5–18 years 4 mg (2 puffs) 4 times daily, when control achieved may be possible to reduce to twice daily

Allergic conjunctivitis section 11.4.2

Tilade CFC-free inhaler® (Sanofi-Aventis) ▼ PoM
Aerosol inhalation, mint-flavoured, nedocromil sodium 2 mg/metered inhalation. Net price 112-dose unit = £39.94. Label: 8, counselling, change to CFC-free inhaler
Excipients: include HFA-227 (a non-CFC propellant)

3.3.2 Leukotriene receptor antagonists and omalizumab

The leukotriene receptor antagonists, **montelukast** and **zafirlukast**, block the effects of cysteinyl leukotrienes in the airways; they may be used with an inhaled corticosteroid (see Management of Chronic Asthma, p. 165) but adequate control is not always achieved. Montelukast has not been shown to be more effective than a standard dose of inhaled corticosteroid but the two drugs appear to have an additive effect. The leukotriene receptor antagonists may be of benefit in exercise-induced asthma and in those with concomitant rhinitis but they are less effective in children with severe asthma who are also receiving high doses of other drugs.

Churg-Strauss syndrome Churg-Strauss syndrome has occurred very rarely in association with the use of leukotriene receptor antagonists; in many of the reported cases the reaction followed the reduction or withdrawal of oral corticosteroid therapy. The CSM has advised that prescribers should be alert to the development of eosinophilia, vasculitic rash, worsening pulmonary symptoms, cardiac complications, or peripheral neuropathy.

MONTELUKAST

Cautions interactions: Appendix 1 (leukotriene antagonists)

Pregnancy manufacturer advises avoid unless essential

Breast-feeding manufacturer advises avoid unless essential

Side-effects abdominal pain, thirst; hyperkinesia (in young children), headache; *very rarely* dry mouth, diarrhoea, dyspepsia, nausea, vomiting, hepatic disorders, palpitation, oedema, increased bleeding, Churg-Strauss syndrome (sec notes above), asthenia, dizziness, hallucinations, paraesthesia, hypoaesthesia, sleep disturbances, abnormal dreams, agitation, aggression, seizures, arthralgia, myalgia, pruritus, and rash

Indication and dose

Prophylaxis of asthma see notes above and Management of Chronic Asthma, p. 165

- By mouth

Child 6 months–6 years 4 mg once daily in the evening

Child 6–15 years 5 mg once daily in the evening

Child 15–18 years 10 mg once daily in the evening

Singulair® (MSD) PoM

Chewable tablets, pink, cherry-flavoured, montelukast (as sodium salt) 4 mg, net price 28-tab pack = £25.69; 5 mg, 28-tab pack = £25.69. Label: 24

Excipients: include aspartame equivalent to phenylalanine 674 micrograms/4-mg tablet and 842 micrograms/5-mg tablet (section 9.4.1)

Granules, montelukast (as sodium salt) 4 mg, net price 28-sachet pack = £25.69. Counselling, administration

Counselling Granules may be swallowed whole or mixed with cold food (but not fluid) and taken immediately

Tablets, beige, f/c, montelukast (as sodium salt) 10 mg, net price 28-tab pack = £26.97

ZAFIRLUKAST

Cautions interactions: Appendix 1 (leukotriene antagonists)

Hepatic disorders Children or their carers should be told how to recognise development of liver disorder and advised to seek medical attention if symptoms or signs such as persistent nausea, vomiting, malaise or jaundice develop

Renal impairment manufacturer advises caution in moderate to severe impairment

Pregnancy manufacturer advises use only if potential benefit outweighs risk

Contra-indications hepatic impairment

Breast-feeding present in milk—manufacturer advises avoid

Side-effects gastro-intestinal disturbances; headache; *rarely* bleeding disorders, hypersensitivity reactions including angioedema and skin reactions, arthralgia, myalgia, hepatitis, hyperbilirubinaemia, thrombocytopenia; *very rarely* Churg-Strauss syndrome (see notes above), agranulocytosis

Indication and dose

Prophylaxis of asthma see notes above and Management of Chronic Asthma, p. 165

- By mouth

Child 12–18 years 20 mg twice daily

Accolate® (AstraZeneca) PoM

Tablets, f/c, zafirlukast 20 mg, net price 56-tab pack = £28.26. Label: 23

Omalizumab

Omalizumab is a monoclonal antibody that binds to immunoglobulin E (IgE). It is licensed for use as additional therapy in children over 12 years with proven IgE-mediated sensitivity to inhaled allergens, whose severe persistent allergic asthma cannot be controlled adequately with high-dose inhaled corticosteroid together with a long-acting beta$_2$ agonist. Omalizumab should be initiated by physicians experienced in the treatment of severe persistent asthma.

OMALIZUMAB

Cautions autoimmune disease; susceptibility to helminth infections—discontinue if infection does not respond to anthelmintic

Hepatic impairment manufacturer advises caution—no information available

Renal impairment manufacturer advises caution—no information available

Pregnancy manufacturer advises avoid unless essential; no evidence of teratogenicity in *animal* studies

Contra-indications

Breast-feeding manufacturer advises avoid—present in milk in *animal* studies

Side-effects headache; injection-site reactions; *less commonly* nausea, diarrhoea, dyspepsia, postural hypotension, flushing, pharyngitis, cough, fatigue, dizziness, drowsiness, paraesthesia, weight gain, influenza-like symptoms, rash, pruritus, and photosensitivity

Indication and dose

Prophylaxis of severe persistent allergic asthma (see notes above)

- **By subcutaneous injection**

  Child over 12 years according to immunoglobulin E concentration and body-weight, consult product literature

Xolair® (Novartis) ▼ PoM

Injection, powder for reconstitution, omalizumab, net price 150-mg vial = £256.15 (with solvent)

Excipients: include sucrose 108 mg/vial

3.4 Antihistamines, immunotherapy, and allergic emergencies

3.4.1 Antihistamines

Antihistamines (histamine H$_1$-antagonists) are classified as *sedating* or *non-sedating*, according to their relative potential for CNS depression. Antihistamines differ in their duration of action, incidence of drowsiness, and antimuscarinic effects; the response to an antihistamine may vary from child to child (see below, Side-effects). Either a sedating or a non-sedating antihistamine may be used to treat an acute allergic reaction; for conditions with more persistent symptoms, a non-sedating antihistamine should be used regularly.

An oral antihistamine may be used to prevent urticaria, and for the treatment of acute urticarial rashes, pruritus, insect bites, and stings. Antihistamines are also used in the management of nausea and vomiting (section 4.6), of migraine (section 4.7.4.1), and the adjunctive management of anaphylaxis and angioedema (section 3.4.3).

Oral antihistamines are also used in the treatment of nasal allergies, particularly seasonal allergic rhinitis (hay fever), and may be of some value in vasomotor rhinitis; rhinorrhoea and sneezing is reduced, but antihistamines are usually less effective for nasal congestion. Antihistamines are used topically to treat allergic reactions in the eye (section 11.4.2) and in the nose (section 12.2.1). Topical application of antihistamines to the skin is not recommended (section 13.3).

Sedating antihistamines are occasionally useful when insomnia is associated with urticaria and pruritus (section 4.1.1). Most of the sedating antihistamines are relatively short acting, but promethazine may be effective up to 12 hours. **Alimemazine** (trimeprazine) and **promethazine** have a more sedative effect than **chlorphenamine** (chlorpheniramine) and **cyclizine** (section 4.6). Chlorphenamine is used as an adjunct to adrenaline (epinephrine) in the emergency treatment of anaphylaxis and angioedema (section 3.4.3).

The *non-sedating* antihistamine **cetirizine** is safe and effective in children; it causes less sedation and psychomotor impairment than the sedating antihistamines. Other non-sedating antihistamines that are used in children include **desloratadine** (an active metabolite of loratadine), **fexofenadine** (an active metabolite of terfenadine), **levocetirizine** (an isomer of cetirizine), **loratadine**, and **mizolastine**. Most non-sedating antihistamines are long-acting (usually 12–24 hours). There is little evidence that desloratadine or levocetirizine confer any additional benefit—they should be reserved for children who cannot tolerate other therapies.

Cautions and contra-indications Antihistamines should be used with caution in hepatic impairment (see below), and the dose may need to be reduced in renal impairment (see under individual drugs for details); also, use with caution in children with epilepsy. Most antihistamines should be avoided in porphyria, but some (e.g. chlorphenamine and cetirizine) are thought to be safe (see section 9.8.2). Sedating antihistamines should not be given to children under 2 years, except on specialist advice, because the safety of such use has not been established. Sedating antihistamines have significant antimuscarinic activity—they should **not** be used in neonates and should be used with caution in children with urinary retention, glaucoma, or pyloroduodenal obstruction. **Interactions:** see Appendix 1 (antihistamines).

Hepatic impairment Sedating antihistamines should be avoided in children with severe liver disease—increased risk of coma.

Pregnancy and breast-feeding No evidence of teratogenicity associated with the use of antihistamines, except for hydroxyzine and loratadine where embryotoxicity has been reported with high doses in *animal* studies. However, manufacturers of some antihistamines advise avoiding use during pregnancy. The use of sedating antihistamines in the latter part of the third trimester may cause adverse effects in neonates. Significant amounts of some antihistamines are present in breast milk; although not known to be harmful, manufacturers advise avoiding use in mothers who are breast-feeding.

Side-effects Drowsiness is a significant side-effect with most of the older antihistamines although paradoxical stimulation may occur rarely in children, especially with high doses. Drowsiness may diminish after a few days of treatment and is considerably less of a problem with the newer antihistamines (see also notes above). Side-effects that are more common with the older antihistamines include headache, psychomotor impairment, and antimuscarinic effects such as urinary retention, dry mouth, blurred vision, and gastro-intestinal disturbances. Other rare side-effects of antihistamines include hypotension, extrapyramidal effects, dizziness, confusion, depression, sleep disturbances, tremor, convulsions, palpitation, arrhythmias, hypersensitivity reactions (including bronchospasm, angioedema, anaphylaxis, rashes, and photosensitivity reactions), blood disorders, and liver dysfunction.

Non-sedating antihistamines

Skilled tasks Although drowsiness is rare, children and their carers should be advised that it can occur and may affect performance of skilled tasks (e.g. cycling or driving); alcohol should be avoided.

CETIRIZINE HYDROCHLORIDE

Cautions see notes above

Renal impairment creatinine clearance less than 20 mL/minute/1.73 m², reduce dose by half

Contra-indications see notes above

Side-effects see notes above

Licensed use not licensed for use in children under 6 years except for use in children 2–6 years for treatment of seasonal allergic rhinitis

Indication and dose

Symptomatic relief of allergy such as hay fever, chronic idiopathic urticaria, atopic dermatitis
- **By mouth**

Child 1–2 years 250 micrograms/kg twice daily

Child 2–6 years 5 mg daily in 1–2 divided doses

Child 6–18 years 10 mg daily in 1–2 divided doses

Cetirizine (Non-proprietary)

Tablets, cetirizine hydrochloride 10 mg, net price 30-tab pack = £1.46. Counselling, skilled tasks

Oral solution, cetirizine hydrochloride 5 mg/5 mL, net price 200 mL = £8.39. Counselling, skilled tasks

DESLORATADINE

Note Desloratadine is a metabolite of loratadine

Cautions see notes above

Contra-indications see notes above; also hypersensitivity to loratadine

Side-effects see notes above; *rarely* myalgia

Indication and dose

Symptomatic relief of allergy such as hay fever, chronic idiopathic urticaria
- By mouth

Child 1–6 years 1.25 mg once daily

Child 6–12 years 2.5 mg once daily

Child 12–18 years 5 mg once daily

Neoclarityn® (Schering-Plough) PoM

Tablets, blue, f/c, desloratadine 5 mg, net price 30-tab pack = £7.04. Counselling, skilled tasks

Syrup, desloratadine 2.5 mg/5 mL, net price 100 mL (bubblegum-flavour) = £7.04. Counselling, skilled tasks

FEXOFENADINE HYDROCHLORIDE

Note Fexofenadine is a metabolite of terfenadine

Cautions see notes above

Contra-indications see notes above

Side-effects see notes above

Indication and dose

Symptomatic relief of seasonal allergic rhinitis
- By mouth

Child 6–12 years 30 mg twice daily

Child 12–18 years 120 mg once daily

Symptomatic relief of chronic idiopathic urticaria
- By mouth

Child 12–18 years 180 mg once daily

Telfast® (Aventis Pharma) PoM

Tablets, f/c, peach, fexofenadine hydrochloride 30 mg, net price 60-tab pack = £5.68; 120 mg, 30-tab pack = £6.23; 180 mg, 30-tab pack = £7.89. Counselling, skilled tasks

LEVOCETIRIZINE HYDROCHLORIDE

Note Levocetirizine is an isomer of cetirizine

Cautions see notes above

Renal impairment creatinine clearance 30–50 mL/minute/1.73 m², reduce dose frequency to alternate days; creatinine clearance 10–30 mL/minute/1.73 m², reduce dose frequency to every 3 days; creatinine clearance less than 10 mL/minute/1.73 m², avoid

Contra-indications see notes above

Side-effects see notes above

Indication and dose

Symptomatic relief of allergy such as hay fever, urticaria
- By mouth

Child 6–18 years 5 mg once daily

Xyzal® (UCB Pharma) ▼ PoM

Tablets, f/c, levocetirizine hydrochloride 5 mg, net price 30-tab pack = £7.45. Counselling, skilled tasks

LORATADINE

Cautions see notes above

Contra-indications see notes above

Side-effects see notes above

Indication and dose

Symptomatic relief of allergy such as hay fever, chronic idiopathic urticaria
- By mouth

Child 2–6 years 5 mg once daily

Child 6–18 years 10 mg once daily

Loratadine (Non-proprietary)

Tablets, loratadine 10 mg, net price 30-tab pack = £1.73

Syrup, loratadine 5 mg/5 mL, net price 100 mL = £7.57. Counselling, skilled tasks

MIZOLASTINE

Cautions see notes above

Contra-indications see notes above; also susceptibility to QT-interval prolongation (including cardiac disease and hypokalaemia)

Hepatic impairment manufacturer recommends avoid in significant hepatic impairment

Side-effects see notes above; also may cause weight gain

Indication and dose

Symptomatic relief of allergy such as hay fever, urticaria
- By mouth

Child 12–18 years 10 mg once daily

MIZOLASTINE (*continued*)

Mizollen® (Schwarz) PoM
Tablets, m/r, f/c, scored, mizolastine 10 mg, net price 30-tab pack = £5.77. Label: 25, Counselling, skilled tasks

Sedating antihistamines

Skilled tasks Drowsiness may affect performance of skilled tasks (e.g. cycling or driving); sedating effects enhanced by alcohol.

ALIMEMAZINE TARTRATE
(Trimeprazine tartrate)

Cautions see notes above

Renal impairment creatinine clearance less than 20 mL/minute/1.73 m², use with caution; manufacturer advises avoid in severe impairment

Contra-indications see notes above

Side-effects see notes above

Licensed use not licensed for use in children under 2 years

Indication and dose

Urticaria, pruritus
- By mouth

Child 6 months–2 years 250 micrograms/kg (max. 2.5 mg) 3–4 times daily—specialist use only

Child 2–5 years 2.5 mg 3–4 times daily

Child 5–12 years 5 mg 3–4 times daily

Child 12–18 years 10 mg 2–3 times daily, in severe cases max. 100 mg daily

Premedication section 15.1.4
- By mouth

Child 2–7 years up to 2 mg/kg (max. 60 mg) 1–2 hours before operation

Vallergan® (Castlemead) PoM
Tablets, blue, f/c, alimemazine tartrate 10 mg, net price 28-tab pack = £3.01. Label: 2

Syrup, straw-coloured, alimemazine tartrate 7.5 mg /5 mL, net price 100 mL = £3.44. Label: 2

Syrup forte, alimemazine tartrate 30 mg/5 mL, net price 100 mL = £5.32. Label: 2

CHLORPHENAMINE MALEATE
(Chlorpheniramine maleate)

Cautions see notes above

Contra-indications see notes above

Side-effects see notes above; also exfoliative dermatitis and tinnitus reported; injections may cause transient hypotension or CNS stimulation and may be irritant

Licensed use *syrup* not licensed for use in children under 1 year; *tablets* not licensed for use in children under 6 years; *injection* not licensed for use in neonates

Indication and dose

Symptomatic relief of allergy such as hay fever, urticaria
- By mouth

Child 1 month–2 years 1 mg twice daily

Child 2–6 years 1 mg every 4–6 hours, max. 6 mg daily

Child 6–12 years 2 mg every 4–6 hours, max. 12 mg daily

Child 12–18 years 4 mg every 4–6 hours, max. 24 mg daily

Symptomatic relief of allergy, emergency treatment of anaphylactic reactions (section 3.4.3)
- By subcutaneous, intramuscular or intravenous injection

Child 1 month–1 year 250 micrograms/kg (max. 2.5 mg), repeated if required up to 4 times in 24 hours

Child 1–6 years 2.5–5 mg, repeated if required up to 4 times in 24 hours

Child 6–12 years 5–10 mg, repeated if required up to 4 times in 24 hours

Child 12–18 years 10–20 mg,, repeated if required up to 4 times in 24 hours (max. 40 mg in 24 hours)

Note Intravenous route recommended for anaphylaxis; subcutaneous and intramuscular injections rarely act quicker than oral administration

Administration for *intravenous injection*, give over 1 minute; if small dose required, dilute with Sodium Chloride 0.9%

Chlorphenamine (Non-proprietary)
Tablets, chlorphenamine maleate 4 mg, net price 28 = 1.02p. Label: 2

Dental prescribing on NHS Chlorphenamine tablets may be prescribed

Oral solution, chlorphenamine maleate 2 mg/5 mL, net price 150 mL = £2.28. Label: 2

Injection PoM[1], chlorphenamine maleate 10 mg/mL, net price 1-mL amp = £1.62

1. PoM restriction does not apply where administration is for saving life in emergency

Piriton® (GSK Consumer Healthcare)
Tablets, yellow, scored, chlorphenamine maleate 4 mg, net price 20 = 19p. Label: 2

Syrup, chlorphenamine maleate 2 mg/5 mL, net price 150 mL = £2.28. Label: 2

HYDROXYZINE HYDROCHLORIDE

Cautions see notes above

Renal impairment use half normal dose

Contra-indications see notes above

Side-effects see notes above

Indication and dose

Pruritus
- By mouth

Child 1–6 years initially 1 mg/kg (or 5–15 mg) at night, increased if necessary to 2.5 mg/kg (or 50 mg) daily in 3–4 divided doses

Child 6–12 years initially 1 mg/kg (or 15–25 mg) at night, increased if necessary to 2 mg/kg (or 50–100 mg) daily in 3–4 divided doses

Child 12–18 years initially 25 mg at night, increased if necessary to 100 mg daily in 3–4 divided doses (max. 300 mg daily in severe cases)

Atarax® (Pfizer) PoM

Tablets, both s/c, hydroxyzine hydrochloride 10 mg (orange), net price 84-tab pack = £1.82; 25 mg (green), 28-tab pack = £1.22. Label: 2

Ucerax® (UCB Pharma) PoM

Tablets NHS, f/c, scored, hydroxyzine hydrochloride 25 mg, net price 25-tab pack = 85p. Label: 2

Syrup, hydroxyzine hydrochloride 10 mg/5 mL. Net price 200-mL pack = £1.78. Label: 2

PROMETHAZINE HYDROCHLORIDE

Cautions see notes above

Contra-indications see notes above; child under 2 years (risk of respiratory depression)

Side-effects see notes above; intramuscular injection may be painful

Indication and dose

Symptomatic relief of allergy such as hayfever, insomnia associated with urticaria and pruritus
- By mouth

Child 2–5 years 5 mg twice daily *or* 5–15 mg at night

Child 5–10 years 5–10 mg twice daily *or* 10–25 mg at night

Child 10–18 years 10–20 mg 2–3 times daily *or* 25 mg at night increased to 25 mg twice daily if necessary

Sedation section 4.1.1

Motion sickness section 4.6

Phenergan® (Rhône-Poulenc Rorer)

Tablets, both blue, f/c, promethazine hydrochloride 10 mg, net price 56-tab pack = £1.71; 25 mg, 56-tab pack = £2.55. Label: 2

Dental prescribing on NHS May be prescribed as Promethazine Hydrochloride Tablets 10 mg or 25 mg

Elixir, sugar-free, golden, promethazine hydrochloride 5 mg/5 mL. Net price 100 mL = £1.49. Label: 2

Dental prescribing on NHS May be prescribed as Promethazine Hydrochloride Oral Solution 5 mg/5 mL

Injection PoM[1], promethazine hydrochloride 25 mg/mL. Net price 1-mL amp = 58p

1. PoM restriction does not apply where administration is for saving life in emergency

3.4.2 Allergen immunotherapy

Immunotherapy using allergen vaccines containing house dust mite, animal dander (cat or dog), or extracts of grass and tree pollen can improve symptoms of asthma and allergic rhino-conjunctivitis in children. A vaccine containing extracts of wasp and bee venom is used to reduce the risk of severe anaphylaxis and systemic reactions in children with hypersensitivity to wasp and bee stings. Children requiring immunotherapy must be referred to a hospital specialist for accurate allergy diagnosis, assessment, and treatment.

CSM advice. After re-examination of the efficacy and safety of desensitising vaccines, the CSM has concluded that they should only be used for the following indications:

- Seasonal allergic hay fever (which has not responded to anti-allergy drugs) caused by pollens, using licensed products only—patients with *asthma* should not be treated with desensitising vaccines as they are more likely to develop severe adverse reactions.
- Hypersensitivity to wasp and bee venoms—since reactions can be life-threatening, *asthma* is not an absolute contra-indication.

Desensitising vaccines should be avoided in pregnant women, in children under 5 years, and in those taking beta-blockers (adrenaline will be ineffective if a hypersensitivity reaction occurs), or ACE inhibitors (risk of severe anaphylactoid reactions).

3 Respiratory system

Hypersensitivity reactions to immunotherapy (especially to wasp and bee venom extracts) can be life-threatening; bronchospasm usually develops within 1 hour and anaphylaxis within 30 minutes of injection. Therefore the child needs to be monitored for at least 1 hour after injection. If symptoms or signs of hypersensitivity develop (e.g. rash, urticaria, bronchospasm, faintness), **even when mild**, the child should be observed until these have **resolved completely**.

For details of the management of anaphylactic shock, see section 3.4.3.

Each set of allergen extracts usually contains vials for the administration of graded amounts of allergen. Maintenance sets containing vials at the highest strength are also available. Product literature must be consulted for details of allergens, vial strengths, and administration.

BEE AND WASP ALLERGEN EXTRACTS

Cautions see notes above including CSM advice and consult product literature

CSM advice. The CSM has advised that facilities for cardiopulmonary resuscitation must be immediately available and patients monitored closely for 1 hour after each injection, for full details see above.

Contra-indications see notes above and consult product literature

Side-effects consult product literature

Indication and dose

Hypersensitivity to wasp or bee venom (see notes above)

- **By subcutaneous injection**

For dose, consult product literature

Pharmalgen® (ALK-Abelló) PoM

Bee venom extract (*Apis mellifera*) or wasp venom extract (*Vespula* spp.). Net price initial treatment set = £59.77 (bee), £73.28 (wasp); maintenance treatment set = £69.54 (bee), £89.45 (wasp)

GRASS AND TREE POLLEN EXTRACTS

Cautions see notes above including CSM advice and consult product literature

CSM advice. The CSM has advised that facilities for cardiopulmonary resuscitation must be immediately available and patients must be monitored closely for 1 hour after each injection, for full details see above.

Contra-indications see notes above and consult product literature

Side-effects consult product literature

Indication and dose

Treatment of seasonal allergic hay fever due to grass or tree pollen in patients who have failed to respond to anti-allergy drugs (see notes above)

- **By subcutaneous injection**

For dose, consult product literature

Pollinex® (Allergy) PoM

Grasses and rye or tree pollen extract, net price initial treatment set (3 vials) and extension course treatment (1 vial) = £320.00

3.4.3 Allergic emergencies

Adrenaline (epinephrine) provides physiological reversal of the immediate symptoms (such as laryngeal oedema, bronchospasm, and hypotension) associated with hypersensitivity reactions such as *anaphylaxis* and *angioedema*.

Anaphylaxis

Anaphylactic shock requires prompt energetic treatment of *laryngeal oedema*, *bronchospasm*, and *hypotension*. Atopic individuals are particularly susceptible. Insect stings are a recognised risk (in particular wasp and bee stings). Certain foods, including eggs, fish, cow's milk protein, peanuts, and tree nuts may also precipitate anaphylaxis. Medicinal products particularly associated with anaphylaxis include blood products, vaccines, allergen immunotherapy preparations, antibacterials, aspirin and other NSAIDs, heparin, and neuromuscular blocking drugs. In the case of drugs, anaphylaxis is more likely after parenteral administration; resuscitation facilities must always be available when giving injections associated with special risk. Refined arachis (peanut) oil, which may be present in some medicinal products, is unlikely to cause an allergic reaction—nevertheless it is wise to check the full formula of preparations which may contain allergenic fats or oils.

Treatment of anaphylaxis
First-line treatment includes:

- securing the airway, restoration of blood pressure (laying the child flat, raising the feet);
- administering **adrenaline** (epinephrine) by **intramuscular** injection (for doses see Intramuscular Adrenaline below); the dose should be repeated if necessary at 5-minute intervals according to blood pressure, pulse, and respiratory function [important: *for intravenous route using dilute solution* (Adrenaline 1 in 10 000), see Intravenous Adrenaline p. 191];
- administering **oxygen**;
- administering an antihistamine, such as **chlorphenamine** (chlorpheniramine), by slow intravenous injection (section 3.4.1), as adjunctive treatment given after adrenaline injection and the antihistamine continued orally for 24 to 48 hours to prevent relapse.

Continuing deterioration requires further treatment including intravenous fluids (section 9.2.2). A nebulised beta$_2$ agonist (**salbutamol** or **terbutaline**) or intravenous aminophylline (section 3.1.3) may be required in a child with severe bronchoconstriction (especially if the child is asthmatic), see Management of Acute Asthma, p. 163. In addition to oxygen, assisted respiration and possibly emergency tracheotomy may be necessary.

An intravenous corticosteroid (section 6.3.2) such as **hydrocortisone** (as sodium succinate) is of secondary value in the initial management of anaphylactic shock because the onset of action is delayed for several hours, but should be given to prevent further deterioration in severely affected children.

When a child is so ill that there is doubt as to the adequacy of the circulation, the initial injection of adrenaline may need to be given as a *dilute solution by the intravenous route*, or by the intraosseous route if venous access is difficult—for details of cautions, dose and strength, see under Intravenous Adrenaline (Epinephrine), p. 191.

Some children with severe allergy to insect stings or foods are encouraged to carry prefilled adrenaline syringes for *self-administration* during periods of risk.

Angioedema

Angioedema is dangerous if *laryngeal oedema* is present. In this circumstance adrenaline (epinephrine) injection and oxygen should be given as described under Anaphylaxis (see above); antihistamines and corticosteroids should also be given (see again above). Tracheal intubation may be necessary. In some children with laryngeal oedema, adrenaline 1 in 1000 (1 mg/mL) solution may be given by nebuliser. However, nebulised adrenaline cannot be relied upon for a systemic effect—intramuscular adrenaline should be used.

Hereditary angioedema The administration of C_1 esterase inhibitor (in fresh frozen plasma or in partially purified form) may terminate acute attacks of *hereditary angioedema*, but is not practical for long-term prophylaxis. **Tranexamic acid** (section 2.11) is used for long-term or short-term prophylaxis of hereditary angioedema; short-term prophylaxis is started several days before planned procedures which may trigger an acute attack of hereditary angioedema (e.g. dental work) and continued for 2–5 days afterwards. Danazol [unlicensed indication, see BNF section 6.7.2] is best avoided in children because of its androgenic effects but it can be used for short-term prophylaxis of hereditary angioedema.

Intramuscular adrenaline (epinephrine)

The *intramuscular route* is the *first choice route* for the administration of adrenaline in the management of anaphylactic shock. Adrenaline has a rapid onset of action after intramuscular administration and in the shocked patient its absorption from the intramuscular site is faster and more reliable than from the subcutaneous site. The intravenous route should be reserved for extreme emergency when there is doubt about the adequacy of the circulation; for details of cautions, dose and strength see under Intravenous Adrenaline (Epinephrine), below.

Carers of children or the child with severe allergy should ideally be instructed in the self-administration of adrenaline by intramuscular injection (for details see under Self-administration of Adrenaline (Epinephrine), below).

Prompt injection of adrenaline is of paramount importance. The following adrenaline doses are based on the revised recommendations of the Project Team of the Resuscitation Council (UK).

Dose of intramuscular injection of adrenaline (epinephrine) for anaphylactic shock

Age	Dose	Volume of adrenaline **1 in 1000** (1 mg/mL)
Under 6 months	50 micrograms	0.05 mL[1]
6 months–6 years	120 micrograms	0.12 mL[1]
6–12 years	250 micrograms	0.25 mL
12–18 years	500 micrograms	0.5 mL

These doses may be repeated several times if necessary at 5-minute intervals according to blood pressure, pulse and respiratory function.
Subcutaneous injection **not** generally recommended.

1. Use suitable syringe for measuring small volume

Intravenous adrenaline (epinephrine)

Where the child is severely ill and there is real doubt about adequacy of the circulation and absorption from the intramuscular injection site, adrenaline may be given by **slow** *intravenous injection* (for dose see Adrenaline/Epinephrine below). Great vigilance is needed to ensure that the *correct strength* is used; anaphylactic shock kits need to make a *very clear distinction* between the 1 in 10 000 strength and the 1 in 1000 strength. It is also important that, where intramuscular injection might still succeed, time should not be wasted seeking intravenous access.

For reference to the use of the intravenous route for *acute hypotension*, see section 2.7.2.

Self-administration of adrenaline (epinephrine)

Children at considerable risk of anaphylaxis need to carry (or have available) adrenaline at all times and the child, or child's carers, need to be *instructed in advance* how to inject it. Packs for self-administration need to be **clearly labelled with instructions** on how to administer adrenaline (intramuscularly, preferably at the midpoint of the outer thigh, through light clothing if necessary). It is important to ensure that an adequate supply is provided to treat symptoms until medical assistance is available.

Adrenaline for administration by intramuscular injection is available in pre-assembled syringes (e.g. *Anapen*® or *EpiPen*®) fitted with a needle suitable for very rapid administration (if necessary by a bystander). A syringe delivering 300 micrograms of adrenaline is recommended for a child over 30 kg. A syringe delivering 150 micrograms of adrenaline is recommended for a child 15–30 kg, but on the basis of a dose of 10 micrograms/kg, 300 micrograms may be more appropriate for some children.

Other products for the immediate treatment of anaphylaxis are available but are not licensed. *Ana-Guard*® is a prefilled syringe that delivers two 300-microgram doses of adrenaline *by subcutaneous or intramuscular injection*; it can be adjusted to administer smaller doses. *Ana-Kit*® includes a prefilled adrenaline syringe, chewable tablets of chlorphenamine maleate (chlorpheniramine maleate) 2 mg, 2 sterile pads impregnated with 70% isopropyl alcohol, and a tourniquet. *Ana-Guard*® and *Ana-Kit*® are available from specialist importing companies (see Special-orders manufacturers).

ADRENALINE/EPINEPHRINE

Cautions hyperthyroidism, diabetes mellitus, heart disease, hypertension, arrhythmias, cerebrovascular disease, angle-closure glaucoma, second stage of labour

Interactions Severe anaphylaxis in children on non-cardioselective beta-blockers may not respond to adrenaline injection calling for intravenous injection of salbutamol (see section 3.1.1.1); furthermore, adrenaline may cause severe hypertension in those receiving beta-blockers. Children on tricyclic antidepressants are considerably more susceptible to arrhythmias, calling for a much reduced dose of adrenaline. Other **interactions**, see Appendix 1 (sympathomimetics).

Side-effects anxiety, tremor, tachycardia, arrhythmias, headache, cold extremities; also hypertension (risk of cerebral haemorrhage) and pulmonary oedema (on excessive dosage or extreme sensitivity); nausea, vomiting, sweating, weakness, dizziness and hyperglycaemia also reported

Indication and dose

Emergency treatment of acute anaphylaxis, angioedema
- **By intramuscular injection (preferably midpoint in anterolateral thigh) (or by subcutaneous injection) of 1 in 1000 (1 mg/mL) solution**

See notes and table above

Acute anaphylaxis when there is doubt as to the adequacy of the circulation
- **By slow intravenous injection of 1 in 10 000 (100 micrograms/mL) solution (extreme caution)**

Neonate 10 micrograms/kg (0.1 mL/kg of the dilute 1 in 10 000 adrenaline injection), given over several minutes, stopping when response obtained

Child 1 month–12 years 10 micrograms/kg (0.1 mL/kg of the dilute 1 in 10 000 adrenaline injection), given over several minutes, stopping when response obtained

Child 12–18 years 500 micrograms (5 mL of the dilute 1 in 10 000 adrenaline injection given at a rate of 100 micrograms/minute, stopping when response obtained

Safe Practice Intravenous route should be used with **extreme care**, see notes above

Croup (section 3.1)
- **By inhalation of nebulised solution of adrenaline 1 in 1000 (1 mg/mL)**

Child 1 month–12 years 400 micrograms/kg (max. 5 mg), repeated after 30 minutes if necessary

Administration For nebulisation, dilute adrenaline 1 in 1000 solution with sterile sodium chloride 0.9% solution

Acute hypotension, low cardiac output section 2.7.2

Cardiopulmonary resuscitation section 2.7.3

Intramuscular or subcutaneous

[1]**Adrenaline/Epinephrine 1 in 1000** (Non-proprietary) PoM

Injection, adrenaline (as acid tartrate) 1 mg/mL, net price 0.5-mL amp = 51p; 1-mL amp = 42p

Excipients: include sulphites

1. PoM restriction does not apply to adrenaline injection 1 mg/mL where administration is for saving life in emergency

[1]**Minijet® Adrenaline** (Celltech) PoM

Injection, adrenaline (as hydrochloride) 1 in 1000 (1 mg/mL). Net price 1 mL (with 25 gauge × 0.25 inch needle for subcutaneous injection) = £8.11, 1 mL (with 21 gauge × 1.5 inch needle for intramuscular injection) = £5.00 (both disposable syringes)

Excipients: include sulphites

1. PoM restriction does not apply to adrenaline injection 1 mg/mL where administration is for saving life in emergency

Intravenous

Extreme caution, see notes above

Adrenaline/Epinephrine 1 in 10 000, Dilute (Non-proprietary) PoM

Injection, adrenaline (as acid tartrate) 100 micrograms/mL, 10-mL amp, 1-mL and 10-mL prefilled syringe

Excipients: include sulphites

Brands include *Minijet® Adrenaline*

Intramuscular injection for self-administration

Anapen® (Celltech) PoM

[1]Anapen® 0.3 mg solution for injection (delivering a single dose of adrenaline 300 micrograms), adrenaline 1 mg/mL (1 in 1000), net price 1.05-mL auto-injector device = £30.67

Excipients: include sulphites

Note 0.75 mL of the solution remains in the auto-injector device after use

Dose

Acute anaphylaxis
- **By intramuscular injection**

Child over 30 kg 300 micrograms repeated after 10–15 minutes as necessary

Anapen® Junior 0.15 mg solution for injection (delivering a single dose of adrenaline 150 micrograms), adrenaline 500 micrograms/mL (1 in 2000), net price 1.05-mL auto-injector device = £30.67

Excipients: include sulphites

Note 0.75 mL of the solution remains in the auto-injector device after use

Dose

Acute anaphylaxis
- **By intramuscular injection**

Child 15–30 kg 150 micrograms (but on the basis of a dose of 10 micrograms/kg, 300 micrograms may be more appropriate for some children) repeated after 10–15 minutes as necessary

1. PoM restriction does not apply to adrenaline injection 1 mg/mL where administration is for saving life in emergency

ADRENALINE/EPINEPHRINE (*continued*)

EpiPen® (ALK-Abelló) PoM

[1]EpiPen® Auto-injector 0.3 mg (delivering a single dose of adrenaline 300 micrograms), adrenaline 1 mg/mL (1 in 1000), net price 2-mL auto-injector = £28.05

Excipients: include sulphites

Note 1.7 mL of the solution remains in the *Auto-injector* after use

Dose

Acute anaphylaxis
- **By intramuscular injection**
  CHILD over 30 kg 300 micrograms repeated after 15 minutes as necessary

Epipen® Jr Auto-injector 0.15 mg (delivering a single dose of adrenaline 150 micrograms), adrenaline 500 micrograms/mL (1 in 2000), net price 2-mL auto-injector = £28.05

Excipients: include sulphites

Note 1.7 mL of the solution remains in the *Auto-injector* after use

Dose

Acute anaphylaxis
- **By intramuscular injection**
  CHILD 15–30 kg 150 micrograms (but on the basis of a dose of 10 micrograms/kg, 300 micrograms may be more appropriate for some children) repeated after 15 minutes as necessary

1. PoM restriction does not apply to adrenaline injection 1 mg/mL where administration is for saving life in emergency

3.5 Respiratory stimulants and pulmonary surfactants

3.5.1 Respiratory stimulants

Respiratory stimulants (analeptic drugs) such as caffeine citrate and doxapram, should only be given under **expert supervision** in hospital; it is important to rule out any underlying disorder, such as seizures, hypoglycaemia, or infection, causing respiratory exhaustion before starting treatment with a respiratory stimulant.

Caffeine (as caffeine citrate) is used in preference to theophylline in the treatment of idiopathic apnoea in preterm neonates, and it may also be used to improve trigger ventilation, or assist extubation in ventilated infants. Caffeine has fewer adverse effects and a longer half-life than theophylline in neonates. It is well absorbed when given orally; intravenous treatment is rarely necessary. Plasma-caffeine concentration should be measured if the child has previously been treated with theophylline. The therapeutic range for plasma-caffeine concentration is usually 10–20 mg/litre (50–100 micromol/litre) but a concentration of 25–35 mg/litre (130–180 micromol/litre) may be required.

Doxapram may be given by continuous intravenous infusion or by mouth for preterm neonates and infants who continue to have troublesome apnoea despite treatment with caffeine. When given by continuous intravenous infusion, blood pressure monitoring and frequent measurement of arterial blood gas and pH are necessary to ensure correct dosage.

CAFFEINE CITRATE

Cautions see under Theophylline (section 3.1.3)

Side-effects physical signs of withdrawal including irritability, lethargy; headache, tachycardia (early sign of toxicity), raised serum glucose concentration

Licensed use no licensed product available

Indication and dose

Neonatal apnoea; adjunct to extubation in preterm infants
- **By mouth or by intravenous injection**
  Neonate initially 20 mg/kg, then 5 mg/kg once daily starting 24 hours after initial dose (some neonates may require 10 mg/kg); neonate over 44 weeks postmenstrual age may require 10 mg/kg twice daily

Note Dose expressed as caffeine *citrate*

Safe medication practice When prescribing, always state dose in terms of caffeine *citrate*

Caffeine *citrate* 2 mg = caffeine base 1 mg

Preparations

Caffeine citrate oral liquid and injection are available from specialist manufacturers, see list of manufacturers, p. 861

3 Respiratory system

DOXAPRAM HYDROCHLORIDE

Cautions impaired cardiac reserve; risk of QT interval prolongation; **interactions:** Appendix 1 (doxapram)

Contra-indications severe hypertension, thyrotoxicosis, epilepsy, physical obstruction of respiratory tract

Side-effects perineal warmth, dizziness, sweating, moderate increase in blood pressure and heart rate; hyperexcitability; high doses may cause convulsions; oral dose may cause slowed gastric emptying

Licensed use not licensed for use in children

Indication and dose

Neonatal apnoea (see notes above)

- **By intravenous infusion**

Neonate initially 2.5 mg/kg over 5–10 minutes, then by *continuous intravenous infusion* 300 microgram/kg/hour adjusted according to response, up to max. 1.5 mg/kg/hour

- **By mouth (after initial intravenous dose)**

Neonate 6 mg/kg 4 times daily

Administration for *intravenous infusion,* dilute injection solution (20 mg/mL) to a concentration of 1 mg/mL with Glucose 5% *or* Sodium Chloride 0.9%.

For administration *by mouth,* dilute doxapram injection solution with Glucose 5% if necessary

Dopram® (Anpharm) PoM

Injection, doxapram hydrochloride 20 mg/mL. Net price 5-mL amp = £2.24

Intravenous infusion, doxapram hydrochloride 2 mg/mL in glucose 5%. Net price 500-mL bottle = £21.33

3.5.2 Pulmonary surfactants

Pulmonary surfactants derived from animal lungs, **beractant** and **poractant alfa** are used to prevent and treat respiratory distress syndrome (hyaline membrane disease) in preterm neonates. Prophylactic use of a pulmonary surfactant may reduce the need for mechanical ventilation and is more effective than 'rescue treatment' in preterm neonates of 29 weeks or less post-menstrual age.

Pulmonary surfactants may also be of benefit in neonates with meconium aspiration syndrome or intrapartum streptococcal infection.

Pulmonary immaturity with surfactant deficit is the commonest reason for respiratory failure in the neonate, especially in those of less than 30 weeks post-menstrual age. Betamethasone (section 6.3.2) given to the mother (at least 12 hours but preferably 48 hours) before delivery substantially enhances pulmonary maturity in the neonate.

Cautions Continuous monitoring is required to avoid hyperoxaemia (due to rapid improvement in arterial oxygen concentration).

Side-effects Pulmonary haemorrhage, especially in more preterm neonates, has been rarely associated with therapy; obstruction of the endotracheal tube by mucous secretions has also been reported.

BERACTANT

Cautions see notes above

Side-effects see notes above

Licensed use licensed for use in respiratory distress syndrome in newborn premature infants, birth-weight over 700 g, and as prophylaxis in neonates less than 32 weeks post-menstrual age

Indication and dose

Treatment of respiratory distress syndrome in preterm neonate; prophylaxis of respiratory distress syndrome in preterm neonate

- **By endotracheal tube**

Neonate phospholipid 100 mg/kg equivalent to a volume of 4 mL/kg, preferably within 8 hours of birth; may be repeated within 48 hours at intervals of at least 6 hours for up to 4 doses

Survanta® (Abbott) PoM

Suspension, beractant (bovine lung extract) providing phospholipid 25 mg/mL, with lipids and proteins, net price 8-mL vial = £306.43

PORACTANT ALFA

Cautions see notes above

Side-effects see notes above

Licensed use licensed for use in respiratory distress syndrome in newborn premature infants, birth-weight over 700 g, and as prophylaxis in neonates 24–32 weeks post-menstrual age

Indication and dose

Treatment of respiratory distress syndrome or hyaline membrane disease in preterm neonate; prophylaxis of respiratory distress syndrome in preterm neonate

- **By endotracheal tube**

Neonate *treatment*, 100–200 mg/kg; further doses of 100 mg/kg may be repeated 12 hours later and after further 12 hours if still intubated; max. total dose 300–400 mg/kg; *prophylaxis*, 100–200 mg/kg soon after birth (preferably within 15 minutes); further doses of 100 mg/kg may be repeated 6–12 hours later and after further 12 hours if still intubated; max. total dose 300–400 mg/kg

Curosurf® (Trinity) PoM

Suspension, poractant alfa (porcine lung phospholipid fraction) 80 mg/mL, net price 1.5-mL vial = £382.00; 3-mL vial = £764.00

3.6 Oxygen

Oxygen should be regarded as a drug. It is used to increase alveolar oxygen tension and decrease the work of breathing. The concentration depends on the condition being treated; administration of an inappropriate concentration of oxygen may have serious or even fatal consequences. High concentrations of oxygen can cause pulmonary epithelial damage (bronchopulmonary dysplasia), convulsions, and retinal damage, especially in preterm neonates.

For neonates and infants with breathing difficulties, *high concentration oxygen therapy* is usually given in an incubator or by nasal cannula if the concentration of oxygen required is less than 50%; a humidified headbox must be used for concentration of oxygen greater than 60%.

In severe acute asthma, the arterial carbon dioxide (P_aCO_2) is usually subnormal but as asthma deteriorates it may rise steeply. These patients usually require a high concentration (40–60%) of oxygen and if the arterial carbon dioxide (P_aCO_2) remains high despite treatment, intermittent positive pressure ventilation needs to be considered urgently. Where facilities for blood gas measurements are not immediately available, for example while transferring the patient to hospital, 35% to 50% oxygen delivered through a conventional mask is recommended. Oxygen saturation of at least 92% should be maintained.

In children with chronic pulmonary conditions, *low concentration oxygen therapy* (controlled oxygen therapy) 24–28% may be used to provide enough oxygen to improve hypoxaemia and maintain target blood-oxygen saturation of at least 92%.

Domiciliary oxygen Oxygen should only be prescribed for use in the home after careful evaluation in hospital by a respiratory care specialist. Children and their carers should be **advised of the fire risks** when oxygen is being administered from a cylinder or an oxygen concentrator.

Long-term oxygen therapy

The aim of long-term oxygen therapy is to maintain oxygen saturation of at least 92%. Children (especially those with chronic neonatal lung disease) often require supplemental oxygen, either for 24-hours a day or during periods of sleep; many children are eventually weaned off long-term oxygen therapy as their condition improves. Oxygen delivered from a cylinder should be passed through a humidifier if used for long periods.

3 Respiratory system

Oxygen concentrators are more economical than oxygen cylinders when oxygen is required for long periods. Portable oxygen cylinders will be required for ambulatory use in addition to an oxygen concentrator for children requiring continuous long-term oxygen therapy. The Royal College of Physicians has produced guidelines for oxygen therapy (*Domiciliary oxygen therapy services: Clinical guidelines and advice for prescribers; June 1999*).

Short-burst oxygen therapy

Oxygen is occasionally prescribed for short-burst (intermittent) use for episodes of breathlessness, for example in children who are at risk of nocturnal hypoxaemia.

Ambulatory oxygen therapy

Ambulatory oxygen is prescribed for children on long-term oxygen therapy who need to be away from home on a regular basis. Ambulatory oxygen therapy is not recommended for children and adolescents who smoke.

Oxygen therapy equipment

Under the NHS oxygen may be supplied as **oxygen cylinders**. Oxygen flow can be adjusted by means of an oxygen flow meter.

Oxygen concentrators are more economical for patients requiring oxygen for long periods, and in England and Wales can be ordered on the NHS on a regional tendering basis (see below). A concentrator is recommended for a patient requiring oxygen for more than 8 hours a day (or 21 cylinders per month). Exceptionally, if a higher concentration of oxygen is required the output of 2 oxygen concentrators can be combined using a 'Y' connection.

A nasal cannula is usually preferred for long-term oxygen therapy form an oxygen concentrator. It can, however, produce dermatitis and mucosal drying in sensitive individuals.

Giving oxygen by nasal cannula allows the patient to talk and eat but the concentration is not controlled and the method may not be appropriate for acute respiratory failure. When given through a nasal cannula at a rate of 1–2 litres/minute the inspiratory oxygen concentration is usually low, but it varies with ventilation and can be high if the patient is underventilating.

Arrangements for supplying oxygen

The following services may be ordered in England and Wales:

- emergency oxygen;
- short-burst (intermittent) oxygen therapy;
- long-term oxygen therapy;
- ambulatory oxygen.

The type of oxygen service (or combination of services) should be ordered on a Home Oxygen Order Form (HOOF); the amount of oxygen required (hours per day) and flow rate should be specified. The supplier will determine the appropriate equipment to be provided. Special needs or preferences should be specified on the HOOF.

The clinician should obtain the patient's consent to pass on the patient's details to the supplier and the fire brigade. The supplier will contact the patient to make arrangements for delivery, installation, and maintenance of the equipment. The supplier will also train the patient to use the equipment.

The clinician should send order forms to the supplier by facsimile (see below); a copy of the HOOF should be sent to the Primary Care Trust or Local Health

Board. The supplier will continue to provide the service until a revised order is received, or until notified that the patient no longer requires the home oxygen service.

Region	Supplier
Eastern	BOC Medical *to order:* Tel: 0800 136 603 Fax: 0800 169 9989
South East London Kent, Surrey and Sussex South West London Thames Valley, Hampshire and Isle of Wight	Allied Respiratory *to order:* Tel: 0500 823 773 Fax: 0800 781 4610
North West Yorkshire and Humberside East Midlands West Midlands North London South West Wales	Air Products *to order:* Tel: 0800 373 580 Fax: 0800 214 709
North East	Linde Gas UK *to order:* Tel: 0808 202 0999 Fax: 0191 497 4340

In **Scotland** refer the patient for assessment by a respiratory consultant If the need for a concentrator is confirmed the consultant will arrange for the provision of a concentrator through the Common Services Agency. In **Northern Ireland** oxygen concentrators and cylinders should be prescribed on form HS21; oxygen concentrators are supplied by a local contractor. In **Scotland** and **Northern Ireland** prescriptions for oxygen cylinders and accessories can be dispensed by pharmacies contracted to provide domiciliary oxygen services.

3.7 Mucolytics

Mucolytics, such as **carbocisteine** and **mecysteine**, are used to facilitate mucociliary clearance and expectoration by reducing sputum viscosity but evidence of efficacy is limited.

Dornase alfa is a genetically engineered version of a naturally occurring human enzyme which cleaves extracellular deoxyribonucleic acid (DNA); it is used to reduce sputum viscosity in children with cystic fibrosis. Dornase alfa is administered by inhalation using a jet nebuliser (section 3.1.5), usually once daily at least 1 hour before physiotherapy; however, alternate-day therapy may be as effective as daily treatment. Not all children benefit from treatment with dornase alfa; improvement occurs within 2 weeks, but in more severely affected children a trial of 6–12 weeks may be required.

Hypertonic sodium chloride (3–7%) solution inhaled twice daily may improve mucociliary clearance in children with cystic fibrosis.

Mesna (*Mistabron*®, available from specialist importing companies) is used in some children with cystic fibrosis when other mucolytics have failed to reduce sputum viscosity; 3–6 mL of a 20% solution is nebulised twice daily.

Acetylcysteine has been used to treat meconium ileus in neonates and distal intestinal obstruction syndrome in children with cystic fibrosis, but evidence of efficacy is lacking. *Gastrografin*® (section 1.6.5), or a bowel cleansing preparation containing macrogols (section 1.6.5), is usually more effective. Acetylcysteine may be used as a mucolytic to prevent further obstruction.

DORNASE ALFA

Phosphorylated glycosylated recombinant human deoxyribonuclease 1 (rhDNase)

Cautions

Pregnancy no evidence of teratogenicity; manufacturer advises use only if potential benefit outweighs risk

Breast-feeding amount probably too small to be harmful—manufacturer advises caution

Side-effects pharyngitis, voice changes, chest pain; occasionally laryngitis, rashes, urticaria, conjunctivitis

DORNASE ALFA (*continued*)

Indication and dose

Management of cystic fibrosis patients with a forced vital capacity (FVC) of greater than 40% of predicted to improve pulmonary function

- **By inhalation of nebulised solution (by jet nebuliser)**

  Child 5–18 years 2500 units (2.5 mg) once daily

Pulmozyme® (Roche) PoM
Nebuliser solution, dornase alfa 1000 units (1 mg)/mL. Net price 2.5-mL (2500 units) vial = £18.52
Note For use undiluted with jet nebulisers only; ultrasonic nebulisers are unsuitable

ACETYLCYSTEINE

Cautions history of peptic ulceration; asthma

Side-effects hypersensitivity-like reactions including rashes and anaphylaxis

Licensed use not licensed for use in meconium ileus or for distal intestinal obstructive syndrome in children with cystic fibrosis

Indication and dose

Meconium ileus (but see notes above)

- **By mouth**

  Neonate 200–400 mg up to 3 times daily if necessary

Treatment of distal intestinal obstructive syndrome (but see notes above)

- **By mouth**

  Child 1 month–2 years 0.4–3 g as a single dose

  Child 2–7 years 2–3 g as a single dose

  Child 7–18 years 4–6 g as a single dose

Prevention of distal intestinal obstruction syndrome

- **By mouth**

  Child 1 month–2 years 100–200 mg 3 times daily

  Child 2–12 years 200 mg 3 times daily

  Child 12–18 years 200–400 mg 3 times daily

Administration For *oral* administration, use oral granules, *or* dilute injection solution (200 mg/mL) to a concentration of 50 mg/mL; orange or blackcurrant juice or cola drink may be used as a diluent to mask the bitter taste

Acetylcysteine (Non-proprietary) PoM
Oral granules, acetylcysteine 100 mg/sachet; 200 mg/sachet. Label: 13
Available from specialist importing companies

Parvolex® (Celltech) PoM
Injection, acetylcysteine 200 mg/mL, net price 10-mL amp = £2.65

CARBOCISTEINE

Cautions history of peptic ulceration
Pregnancy manufacturer advises avoid in first trimester

Contra-indications active peptic ulceration

Side-effects *rarely* gastro-intestinal bleeding and rashes

Indication and dose

Reduction of sputum viscocity

- **By mouth**

  Child 2–6 years 62.5–125 mg 4 times daily

  Child 6–12 years 250 mg 3 times daily

  Child 12–18 years initially 750 mg 3 times daily, then 1.5 g daily in divided doses

Carbocisteine (Beacon) PoM
Capsules, carbocisteine 375 mg. Net price 120-cap pack = £16.68
Brands include *Mucodyne®*

Oral liquid, carbocisteine 125 mg/5 mL, net price 300 mL = £4.57; 250 mg/5 mL, 300 mL = £5.84
Brands include *Mucodyne® Paediatric* 125 mg/5 mL (cherry- and raspberry-flavoured) and *Mucodyne®* 250 mg/5 mL (cinnamon- and rum-flavoured)

MECYSTEINE HYDROCHLORIDE
(Methyl Cysteine Hydrochloride)

Cautions history of peptic ulceration

Side-effects nausea, heartburn

Indication and dose

Reduction of sputum viscosity

- **By mouth**

  Child 5–12 years 100 mg 3 times daily

  Child 12–18 years 200 mg 4 times daily for 2 days, then 200 mg 3 times daily for 6 weeks, then 200 mg twice daily

Visclair® (Sinclair)
Tablets, yellow, s/c, e/c, mecysteine hydrochloride 100 mg. Net price 20 = £3.66. Label: 5, 22, 25

3.8 Aromatic inhalations

Inhalations containing volatile substances such as eucalyptus oil are traditionally used to relieve congestion and ease breathing. Although the vapour may contain little of the additive it encourages deliberate inspiration of warm moist air which is often comforting. Boiling water should not be used for inhalations owing to the risk of scalding.

Strong aromatic decongestants (applied as rubs or to pillows) are not recommended for infants under the age of 3 months. **Sodium chloride 0.9%** solution given as nasal drops can be used to liquefy mucous secretions and relieve nasal congestion in infants and young children.

Benzoin Tincture, Compound, BP (Friars' Balsam)
Tincture, balsamic acids approx. 4.5%. Label: 15

Dose

Nasal congestion
- **By inhalation**
  Add one teaspoonful to a pint of hot, **not** boiling, water and inhale the vapour

Menthol and Eucalyptus Inhalation, BP 1980
Inhalation, racementhol or levomenthol 2 g, eucalyptus oil 10 mL, light magnesium carbonate 7 g, water to 100 mL

Dose

Nasal congestion
- **By inhalation**
  Add one teaspoonful to a pint of hot, **not** boiling, water and inhale the vapour

Dental prescribing on the NHS May be prescribed as Menthol and Eucalyptus Inhalation BP, 1980

Karvol® (Crookes) NHS

Inhalation capsules, levomenthol 35.55 mg, with chlorobutanol, pine oils, terpineol, and thymol, net price 10-cap pack = £2.25; 20-cap pack = £4.06

Inhalation solution, levomenthol 7.9%, with chlorobutanol, pine oils, terpineol, and thymol, net price 12-mL dropper bottle = £1.90

Dose

Nasal congestion
- **By inhalation**
  Express into handkerchief or add to a pint of hot, **not** boiling, water the contents of 1 capsule or 6 drops of solution; avoid in infants under 3 months

3.9 Cough preparations

3.9.1 Cough suppressants

Cough may be a symptom of an underlying disorder e.g. asthma (section 3.1) or gastro-oesophageal reflux disease (section 1.1), which should be addressed before prescribing cough suppressants. Cough may also result from bronchiectasis including that associated with cystic fibrosis; cough may also have a significant habit component. There is little evidence of any significant benefit from the use of cough suppressants in children with acute cough in ambulatory settings. Cough suppressants may cause sputum retention and this may be harmful in children with bronchiectasis.

Codeine is constipating and can cause dependence; **dextromethorphan** and **pholcodine** have fewer side-effects. The use of cough suppressants containing codeine or similar opioid analgesics is not generally recommended in children and should be avoided altogether in those under 1 year.

Sedating antihistamines are used as the cough suppressant component of many compound cough preparations on sale to the public; all tend to cause drowsiness which may reflect their main mode of action.

PHOLCODINE

Cautions may cause sputum retention

Contra-indications

Hepatic impairment avoid or reduce dose—may precipitate coma

Pregnancy avoid in third trimester, respiratory depression and withdrawal effects in neonate

Side-effects nausea, sputum retention, constipation

PHOLCODINE (*continued*)

Indication and dose

Dry or painful cough (but not generally recommended for children, see notes above)

- **By mouth**
  Child 3 months–1 year 1 mg 3 times daily
  Child 1–5 years 2 mg 3 times daily
  Child 5–12 years 2–5 mg 3–4 times daily
  Child 12–18 years 5–10 mg 3–4 times daily

Pholcodine Linctus, BP
Linctus (= oral solution), pholcodine 5 mg/5 mL in a suitable flavoured vehicle, containing citric acid monohydrate 1%. Net price 100 mL = 24p
Brands include *Pavacol-D®* (sugar-free), *Galenphol®* (sugar-free)

Pholcodine Linctus, Strong, BP
Linctus (= oral solution), pholcodine 10 mg/5 mL in a suitable flavoured vehicle, containing citric acid monohydrate 2%. Net price 100 mL = 33p
Brands include *Galenphol®*

Galenphol® (Thornton & Ross)
Paediatric linctus (= oral solution), orange, sugar-free, pholcodine 2 mg/5 mL. Net price 90-mL pack = £1.11

3.9.2 Expectorant and demulcent cough preparations

Expectorants are claimed to promote expulsion of bronchial secretions but there is no evidence that any drug can specifically facilitate expectoration.

Simple linctus and other demulcent cough preparations containing soothing substances, such as syrup or glycerol, may temporarily relieve a dry irritating cough. These preparations have the advantage of being harmless and inexpensive and sugar-free versions are available.

Compound cough preparations for children are on sale to the public; the rationale for some is dubious.

Simple Linctus, BP
Linctus (= oral solution), citric acid monohydrate 2.5% in a suitable vehicle with an anise flavour. Net price 100 mL = 32p
A sugar-free version is also available

Dose

Cough
- **By mouth**
  Child 12–18 years 5 mL 3–4 times daily

Simple Linctus, Paediatric, BP
Linctus (= oral solution), citric acid monohydrate 0.625% in a suitable vehicle with an anise flavour. Net price 100 mL = 17p
A sugar-free version is also available

Dose

Cough
- **By mouth**
  Child 1 month–12 years 5–10 mL 3–4 times daily

3.10 Systemic nasal decongestants

Nasal congestion in children due to allergic or vasomotor rhinitis should be treated with oral antihistamines (section 3.4.1) or topical nasal preparations containing corticosteroids (section 12.2.1) or topical decongestants (section 12.2.2).

There is little evidence to support the use of systemic decongestants in children.

Pseudoephedrine has few sympathomimetic effects, and is commonly combined with other ingredients (including antihistamines) in preparations intended for the relief of cough and cold symptoms.

PSEUDOEPHEDRINE HYDROCHLORIDE

Cautions hypertension, heart disease, diabetes, hyperthyroidism, raised intra-ocular pressure; **interactions**: Appendix 1 (sympathomimetics)

Hepatic impairment caution in severe hepatic impairment

Renal impairment avoid in severe renal impairment; increased CNS toxicity

Pregnancy not known to be harmful

Breast-feeding amount too small to be harmful

Contra-indications treatment with MAOI within previous 2 weeks

Side-effects tachycardia, anxiety, restlessness, insomnia; *rarely* hallucinations, rash; urinary retention also reported

PSEUDOEPHEDRINE HYDROCHLORIDE (*continued*)

Indication and dose

Congestion of mucous membranes of upper respiratory tract
- By mouth

  Child 2–6 years 15 mg 3–4 times daily

  Child 6–12 years 30 mg 3–4 times daily

  Child 12–18 years 60 mg 3–4 times daily

Galpseud® (Thornton & Ross)

Tablets, pseudoephedrine hydrochloride 60 mg. Net price 20 = 91p

Linctus, orange, sugar-free, pseudoephedrine hydrochloride 30 mg/5 mL. Net price 100 mL = 69p

Sudafed® (Warner Lambert)

Tablets, red, f/c, pseudoephedrine hydrochloride 60 mg. Net price 24 = £2.12

Elixir, red, pseudoephedrine hydrochloride 30 mg/5 mL. Net price 100 mL = £1.48

4 Central nervous system

4.1 Hypnotics and anxiolytics

Most anxiolytics ('sedatives') will induce sleep when given at night and most hypnotics will sedate when given during the day. Hypnotics and anxiolytics should be reserved for short courses to alleviate acute conditions after causal factors have been established.

The role of drug therapy in the management of anxiety disorders in children and adolescents is uncertain; drug therapy should be initiated only by specialists after psychosocial interventions have failed. Benzodiazepines and tricyclic antidepressants have been used but adverse effects may be problematic.

Skilled tasks Hypnotics and anxiolytics may impair judgement and increase reaction time, and so affect ability to drive or perform skilled tasks; they increase the effects of alcohol. Moreover the hangover effects of a night dose may impair performance on the following day.

CSM advice

1. Benzodiazepines are indicated for the short-term relief (two to four weeks only) of anxiety that is severe, disabling or subjecting the individual to unacceptable distress, occurring alone or in association with insomnia or short-term psychosomatic, organic or psychotic illness.
2. The use of benzodiazepines to treat short-term 'mild' anxiety is inappropriate and unsuitable.
3. Benzodiazepines should be used to treat insomnia only when it is severe, disabling, or subjecting the individual to extreme distress.

4.1.1 Hypnotics

The prescribing of hypnotics to children, except for occasional use such as for night terrors and somnambulism (sleep-walking), is not justified. There is a risk of habituation with prolonged use and problems settling children at night should be managed psychologically.

Melatonin is a pineal hormone which may affect sleep pattern. Clinical experience suggests that it may be of value for treating sleep disorders in children with conditions such as visual impairment, cerebral palsy, attention deficit hyperactivity disorder, and autism; it is also sometimes used before EEG investigations. Melatonin appears to have few short-term adverse effects but it has been associated with seizures; little is known about its long-term effects. It should preferably be avoided in endocrine disorders. Melatonin is not licensed because efficacy is unproven, and is available from several sources and in a variety of formulations.

The dose of melatonin has also not been established but an initial dose of 2–3 mg (given 30–60 minutes before bedtime) has been used; in the absence of improvement after 1–2 weeks, the dose is increased to 4–6 mg at night. The maximum dose is generally accepted to be 10 mg but higher doses have been used.

Treatment with melatonin should be initiated and supervised by a specialist and the need for continuing melatonin should be reviewed regularly.

Dental procedures Some anxious children may benefit from the use of a hypnotic for 1 to 3 nights before the dental appointment. Hypnotics do not relieve pain, and if pain interferes with sleep an appropriate analgesic should be given.

Chloral and derivatives

Chloral hydrate and derivatives were formerly popular hypnotics for children. **Triclofos** causes fewer gastro-intestinal disturbances than chloral hydrate.

Chloral hydrate and triclofos are now mainly used for sedation during diagnostic procedures (section 15.1.4) and in intensive care units. These drugs accumulate on prolonged use and they should be avoided in severe renal or hepatic impairment.

CHLORAL HYDRATE

Cautions respiratory disease, history of drug or alcohol abuse, marked personality disorder; reduce dose in debilitated; avoid prolonged use (and abrupt withdrawal thereafter); avoid contact with skin and mucous membranes; **interactions**: Appendix 1 (anxiolytics and hypnotics)

Hepatic impairment reduce dose in mild to moderate hepatic impairment; avoid in severe impairment

Skilled tasks Drowsiness may persist the next day and affect performance of skilled tasks (e.g. driving); effects of alcohol enhanced

Contra-indications cardiac disease, gastritis, (see also notes above), porphyria (section 9.8.2)

Renal impairment avoid in severe impairment

Side-effects gastric irritation (nausea and vomiting reported), abdominal distention and flatulence; also ataxia, confusion, rashes, headache, lightheadedness, ketonuria, excitement, nightmares, delirium (especially on abrupt withdrawal); dependence (may be associated with gastritis and renal damage) on prolonged use

Licensed use not licensed for use in children for sedation for painless procedures or for long-term sedation; rectal route not licensed

4 Central nervous system

CHLORAL HYDRATE (*continued*)

Indication and dose

Night sedation
- By mouth or by rectum (if oral route not available)

Neonate 30–50 mg/kg at bedtime

Child 1 month–12 years 30–50 mg/kg (max. 1 g) at night

Child 12–18 years 0.5–1 g at night

Sedation for painless procedures
- By mouth or by rectum (if oral route not available)

Neonate 25–50 mg/kg 45–60 minutes before procedure; doses up to 100 mg/kg may be used with respiratory monitoring

Child 1 month–12 years 30–50 mg/kg (max. 1 g) 45–60 minutes before procedure; higher doses up to 100 mg/kg (max. 2 g) may be used but respiratory monitoring is required

Child 12–18 years 1–2 g 45–60 minutes before procedure

Long-term sedation
- By mouth or by rectum (if oral route not available)

Neonate 20–30 mg/kg 3–4 times daily; up to 50 mg/kg 4 times daily has been used but risk of accumulation

Child 1 month–12 years 20–50 mg/kg (max. 1 g) 3–4 times daily; up to 50 mg/kg 4 times daily has been used but risk of accumulation

Administration for administration *by mouth* dilute liquid with plenty of water or juice to mask unpleasant taste.

For administration *by rectum* use oral solution

Chloral Mixture, BP 2000 PoM
(Chloral Oral Solution)
Mixture, chloral hydrate 500 mg/5 mL in a suitable vehicle. Extemporaneous and manufactured special preparations available, see guidance on Unlicensed Medicines

Chloral Elixir, Paediatric, BP 2000 PoM
(Chloral Oral Solution, Paediatric)
Elixir, chloral hydrate 200 mg/5mL (4%) in a suitable vehicle with a black currant flavour. Extemporaneous and manufactured special preparations available, see guidance on Unlicensed Medicines

Cloral betaine

Welldorm® (Alphashow) PoM
Tablets, blue-purple, f/c, cloral betaine 707 mg (≡ chloral hydrate 414 mg). Net price 30-tab pack = £2.43. Label: 19, 27

Dose

Short-term treatment of insomnia
- By mouth

Child 12–18 years 1–2 tablets with water or milk at bedtime, max. 5 tablets (chloral hydrate 2 g) daily

Elixir, red, chloral hydrate 143.3 mg/5 mL. Net price 150-mL pack = £2.05. Label: 19, 27

Dose

Short-term treatment of insomnia
- By mouth

Neonate 1–1.75 mL/kg (chloral hydrate 30–50 mg/kg) with water or milk at bedtime

Child 1 month–12 years 1–1.75 mL/kg (chloral hydrate 30–50 mg/kg) with water or milk at bedtime; max. 35 mL (chloral hydrate 1 g) daily

Child 12–18 years 15–45 mL (chloral hydrate 0.4–1.3 g) with water or milk at bedtime; max. 70 mL (chloral hydrate 2 g) daily

TRICLOFOS SODIUM

Cautions see Chloral Hydrate

Contra-indications see Chloral Hydrate

Side-effects see Chloral Hydrate but less gastric irritation

Licensed use not licensed as sedation for painless procedures

Indication and dose

Night sedation
- By mouth

Child 1 month–1 year 25–30 mg/kg at night

Child 1–5 years 250–500 mg at night

Child 6–12 years 0.5–1 g at night

Child 12–18 years 1–2 g at night

Sedation for painless procedures
- By mouth

Child 1 month–18 years 30–50 mg/kg (max. 2 g) 45–60 minutes before procedure; higher doses up to 100 mg/kg (max. 2 g) may be used but respiratory monitoring is required

Triclofos Oral Solution, BP PoM
(Triclofos Elixir)
Oral solution, triclofos sodium 500 mg/5 mL. Net price 300 mL = £27.83. Label: 19

Antihistamines

Some **antihistamines** (section 3.4.1) such as diphenhydramine and promethazine are used for occasional insomnia in adults; their prolonged duration of action may often lead to drowsiness the following day. The sedative effect of antihistamines may diminish after a few days of continued treatment; antihistamines are associated with headache, psychomotor impairment and antimuscarinic effects.

The use of antihistamines as hypnotics in children is not usually justified.

PROMETHAZINE HYDROCHLORIDE

Cautions section 3.4.1

Contra-indications section 3.4.1

Side-effects section 3.4.1

Indication and dose

Night sedation and insomnia (short-term use)
- By mouth

Child under 2 years not recommended

Child 2–10 years 20–25 mg at bedtime

Child 10–18 years 25 mg at bedtime increased to 50 mg if necessary

Allergy, urticaria, premedication section 3.4.1

Nausea and vertigo section 4.6

Preparations
Section 3.4.1

4.1.2 Anxiolytics

Anxiolytic treatment should be used in children only to relieve acute anxiety (and related insomnia) caused by fear (e.g. before surgery, section 15.1.4.1).

Anxiolytic treatment should be limited to the lowest possible dose for the shortest possible time (see CSM advice, section 4.1).

Benzodiazepines

DIAZEPAM

Cautions respiratory disease, muscle weakness and myasthenia gravis, history of drug or alcohol abuse, marked personality disorder; avoid prolonged use (and abrupt withdrawal thereafter); special precautions for intravenous injection (section 4.8.2); when given parenterally, close observation required until full recovery from sedation; porphyria (section 9.8.2); **interactions**: Appendix 1 (anxiolytics and hypnotics)

Hepatic impairment reduce dose as may precipitate coma; avoid in severe impairment

Renal impairment start with small doses; increased cerebral sensitivity

Pregnancy avoid regular use (risk of neonatal withdrawal symptoms); use only if clear indication such as seizure control (high doses during late pregnancy or labour may cause neonatal hyperthermia, hypotonia, and respiratory depression)

Breast-feeding avoid if possible—present in milk

Skilled tasks Drowsiness may affect performance of skilled tasks (e.g. driving); effects of alcohol enhanced

Contra-indications respiratory depression; marked neuromuscular respiratory weakness including unstable myasthenia gravis; acute pulmonary insufficiency; sleep apnoea syndrome; severe hepatic impairment; not for chronic psychosis; should not be used alone in depression or in anxiety with depression; avoid injections containing benzyl alcohol in neonates (see under preparations below)

Side-effects drowsiness and lightheadedness the next day; confusion and ataxia; amnesia; dependence; paradoxical increase in aggression (see also section 4.1); muscle weakness; *occasionally:* headache, vertigo, hypotension, salivation changes, gastro-intestinal disturbances, visual disturbances, dysarthria, tremor, changes in libido, incontinence, urinary retention; blood disorders and jaundice reported; skin reactions; on intravenous injection, pain, thrombophlebitis, and rarely apnoea; **overdosage:** see Emergency Treatment of Poisoning, p. 40

Indication and dose

Night terrors and somnambulism
- By mouth

Child 12–18 years 1–5 mg at bedtime

Status epilepticus section 4.8.2

Febrile convulsions section 4.8.3

Muscle spasm section 10.2.2

Peri-operative use section 15.1.4.1

Diazepam (Non-proprietary) PoM

Tablets, diazepam 2 mg, net price 20 = 65p; 5 mg, 20 = 68p; 10 mg, 20 = 95p. Label: 2 or 19
Brands include *Rimapam®* NHS, *Tensium®* NHS

Oral solution, diazepam 2 mg/5 mL, net price 100 mL = £1.75. Label: 2 or 19
Brands include *Dialar®* NHS

Strong oral solution, diazepam 5 mg/5 mL, net price 100-mL pack = £6.38. Label: 2 or 19 NHS
Brands include *Dialar®* NHS

Dental prescribing on NHS Diazepam Tablets or Diazepam Oral Solution 2 mg/5 mL may be prescribed

Rectal solution and parenteral preparations
Section 4.8.2

Buspirone

Buspirone is thought to act at specific serotonin ($5HT_{1A}$) receptors; safety and efficacy in children have yet to be determined.

4.1.3 Barbiturates

Classification not used in BNF for Children.

4.2 Drugs used in psychoses and related disorders

Advice of Royal College of Psychiatrists on doses above BNF for Children upper limit. Unless otherwise stated, doses in the BNF for Children are licensed doses—any higher dose is therefore **unlicensed** (for an explanation of the significance of this, see p. 2).

1. Consider alternative approaches including adjuvant therapy.
2. Bear in mind risk factors, including obesity.
3. Consider potential for drug interactions—see **interactions:** Appendix 1 (antipsychotics).
4. Carry out ECG to exclude untoward abnormalities such as prolonged QT interval; repeat ECG periodically and reduce dose if prolonged QT interval or other adverse abnormality develops.
5. Increase dose slowly and not more often than once weekly.
6. Carry out regular pulse, blood pressure, and temperature checks; ensure that patient maintains adequate fluid intake.
7. Consider high-dose therapy to be for limited period and review regularly; abandon if no improvement after 3 months (return to standard dosage).

Important: When prescribing an antipsychotic for administration on an emergency basis, the intramuscular dose should be **lower** than the corresponding oral dose (owing to absence of first-pass effect), particularly if the child is very active (increased blood flow to muscle considerably increases the rate of absorption). The prescription should specify the dose for **each route** and should **not** imply that the same dose can be given by mouth or by intramuscular injection. The dose of antipsychotic for emergency use should be reviewed at least **daily**.

4.2.1 Antipsychotic drugs

There is little information on the efficacy and safety of antipsychotic drugs in children and adolescents and much of the information available has been extrapolated from adult data. It is not possible to make recommendations for drug treatment of psychoses, Gilles de la Tourette syndrome and autism; treatment of these conditions should be managed only by an appropriate specialist.

Antipsychotic drugs are also known as 'neuroleptics' and (misleadingly) as 'major tranquillisers'. Antipsychotic drugs generally tranquillise without impairing consciousness and without causing paradoxical excitement but they should not be regarded merely as tranquillisers. For conditions such as schizophrenia the tranquillising effect is of secondary importance.

In the short term they are used to calm disturbed children whatever the underlying psychopathology, which may be schizophrenia, brain damage, mania, toxic delirium, or agitated depression. Antipsychotic drugs are used to alleviate severe anxiety but this too should be a short-term measure.

Schizophrenia Antipsychotic drugs relieve florid psychotic symptoms such as thought disorder, hallucinations, and delusions, and prevent relapse. Although they are usually less effective in apathetic withdrawn children, they sometimes appear to have an activating influence. Children with acute schizophrenia generally respond better than those with chronic symptoms.

Long-term treatment of a child with a definite diagnosis of schizophrenia may be necessary even after the first episode of illness in order to prevent the manifest illness from becoming chronic. Withdrawal of drug treatment requires careful surveillance because children who appear well on medication may suffer a disastrous relapse if treatment is withdrawn inappropriately. In addition the need for continuation of treatment may not become immediately evident because relapse is often delayed for several weeks after cessation of treatment.

Antipsychotic drugs are considered to act by interfering with dopaminergic transmission in the brain by blocking dopamine D_2 receptors, which may give rise to the extrapyramidal effects described below, and also to hyperprolactinaemia. Antipsychotic drugs may also affect cholinergic, alpha-adrenergic, histaminergic, and serotonergic receptors.

Choice of drug is influenced by the potential for side-effects and is often guided by individual circumstances e.g. the psychological effects of potential weight gain. The drugs most commonly used in children are haloperidol, risperidone, and olanzapine.

Cautions and contra-indications Antipsychotics should be used with **caution** in children with hepatic impairment (can precipitate coma), renal impairment (start with small dose; increased cerebral sensitivity), cardiovascular disease, epilepsy (and conditions predisposing to epilepsy), depression, myasthenia gravis, or a personal or family history of angle-closure glaucoma (avoid chlorpromazine, pericyazine and prochlorperazine in these conditions). Caution is also required in severe respiratory disease and in children with a history of jaundice or who have blood dyscrasias (perform blood counts if unexplained infection or fever develops). As photosensitisation may occur with higher dosages, children should avoid direct sunlight.

Antipsychotic drugs may be **contra-indicated** in comatose states, CNS depression, and phaeochromocytoma. Most antipsychotics are best avoided during pregnancy unless essential; extrapyramidal effects may occur in neonates. Although the amount present in breast milk is probably too small to be harmful, *animal* studies indicate possible adverse effects of these drugs on developing nervous system and therefore it is advisable to discontinue breast-feeding during treatment; **interactions:** Appendix 1 (antipsychotics)

Skilled tasks Drowsiness may affect performance of skilled tasks (e.g. driving or operating machinery), especially at start of treatment; effects of alcohol are enhanced

Withdrawal Withdrawal of antipsychotic drugs after long-term therapy should always be gradual and closely monitored to avoid the risk of acute withdrawal syndromes or rapid relapse.

Side-effects Extrapyramidal symptoms are the most troublesome. They occur most frequently with the piperazine phenothiazines (fluphenazine, perphenazine, prochlorperazine, and trifluoperazine), the butyrophenones (benperidol and haloperidol), and the depot preparations. They are easy to recognise but cannot be predicted accurately because they depend on the dose, the type of drug, and on individual susceptibility.

Extrapyramidal symptoms consist of:

- *parkinsonian symptoms* (including tremor), which may appear gradually (but less commonly than in adults) ;
- *dystonia* (abnormal face and body movements) and *dyskinesia*, which appear after only a few doses;
- *akathisia* (restlessness), which characteristically occurs after large initial doses and may resemble an exacerbation of the condition being treated; and
- *tardive dyskinesia* (rhythmic, involuntary movements of tongue, face, and jaw), which usually develops on long-term therapy or with high dosage, but it may develop on short-term treatment with low doses—short-lived tardive dyskinesia may occur after withdrawal of the drug.

Parkinsonian symptoms remit if the drug is withdrawn and may be suppressed by the administration of **antimuscarinic** drugs (section 4.9.2). However, routine administration of such drugs is not justified because not all children are affected and because they may unmask or worsen tardive dyskinesia.

Tardive dyskinesia is of particular concern because it may be irreversible on withdrawing therapy and treatment is usually ineffective. However, some manufacturers suggest that drug withdrawal at the earliest signs of tardive dyskinesia (fine vermicular movements of the tongue) may halt its full development. Tardive dyskinesia may occur and treatment must be carefully and regularly reviewed.

Hypotension and interference with temperature regulation are dose-related side-effects.

Neuroleptic malignant syndrome (hyperthermia, fluctuating level of consciousness, muscular rigidity, and autonomic dysfunction with pallor, tachycardia, labile blood pressure, sweating, and urinary incontinence) is a rare but potentially fatal side-effect of some antipsychotic drugs. Discontinuation of the antipsychotic is essential because there is no proven effective treatment, but cooling, bromocriptine, and dantrolene have been used. The syndrome, which usually lasts for 5–7 days after drug discontinuation, may be unduly prolonged if depot preparations have been used.

Other side-effects include: drowsiness; apathy; agitation, excitement and insomnia; convulsions; dizziness; headache; confusion; gastro-intestinal disturbances; nasal congestion; antimuscarinic symptoms (such as dry mouth, constipation, difficulty with micturition, and blurred vision); cardiovascular symptoms (such as hypotension, tachycardia, and arrhythmias); ECG changes (cases of sudden death have occurred); endocrine effects such as menstrual disturbances, galactorrhoea, gynaecomastia, impotence, and weight gain; blood dyscrasias (such as agranulocytosis and leucopenia), photosensitisation, contact sensitisation and rashes, and jaundice (including cholestatic); corneal and lens opacities, and purplish pigmentation of the skin, cornea, conjunctiva, and retina.

Overdosage: for poisoning with phenothiazines and related compounds, see Emergency Treatment of Poisoning, p. 41.

Classification of antipsychotics The **phenothiazine** derivatives can be divided into 3 main groups.

Group 1: chlorpromazine, levomepromazine (methotrimeprazine), and promazine, generally characterised by pronounced sedative effects and moderate antimuscarinic and extrapyramidal side-effects.

Group 2: pericyazine and pipotiazine, generally characterised by moderate sedative effects, marked antimuscarinic effects, but fewer extrapyramidal side-effects than groups 1 or 3.

Group 3: fluphenazine, perphenazine, prochlorperazine, and trifluoperazine, generally characterised by fewer sedative effects, fewer antimuscarinic effects, but more pronounced extrapyramidal side-effects than groups 1 and 2.

Drugs of other chemical groups tend to resemble the phenothiazines of *group 3*. They include the **butyrophenones** (benperidol and haloperidol); **diphenylbutylpiperidines** (pimozide); **thioxanthenes** (flupentixol and zuclopenthixol); and the **substituted benzamides** (sulpiride).

For details of the newer antipsychotic drugs amisulpride, clozapine, olanzapine, quetiapine, and risperidone, see under Atypical Antipsychotics, p. 212.

Choice As indicated above, the various drugs differ somewhat in predominant actions and side-effects. Selection is influenced by the degree of sedation required and the child's susceptibility to extrapyramidal side-effects. However, the differences between antipsychotic drugs are less important than the great variability in response; moreover, tolerance to secondary effects such as sedation usually develops. The atypical antipsychotics may be appropriate if extrapyramidal side-effects are a particular concern (see under Atypical Antipsychotics, below). **Clozapine** is used for schizophrenia when other antipsychotics are ineffective or not tolerated.

Prescribing of more than one antipsychotic at the same time is **not** recommended; it may constitute a hazard and there is no significant evidence that side-effects are minimised.

Chlorpromazine is still widely used despite the wide range of adverse effects associated with it. It has a marked sedating effect and is useful for treating violent children without causing stupor.

Pimozide (see CSM advice p. 211) is less sedating than chlorpromazine.

Sulpiride in high doses controls florid positive symptoms, but in lower doses it has an alerting effect on children with apathetic withdrawn schizophrenia.

Haloperidol and **trifluoperazine** are also of value but their use is limited by the high incidence of extrapyramidal symptoms. Haloperidol may be preferred for the rapid control of hyperactive psychotic states; it causes less hypotension than chlorpromazine.

Other uses Nausea and vomiting (section 4.6), choreas, motor tics, and intractable hiccup (see under Chlorpromazine Hydrochloride and under Haloperidol).

Equivalent doses of oral antipsychotics

These equivalences are intended **only** as an approximate guide; individual dosage instructions should **also** be checked; children should be carefully monitored after **any** change in medication

Antipsychotic drug	Daily dose
Chlorpromazine	100 mg
Clozapine	50 mg
Haloperidol	2–3 mg
Pimozide	2 mg
Risperidone	0.5–1 mg
Sulpiride	200 mg
Trifluoperazine	5 mg

Important. These equivalences must **not** be extrapolated beyond the max. dose for the drug. Higher doses require careful titration in specialist units and the equivalences shown here may not be appropriate

Dosage
After an initial period of stabilisation, the long half-life of antipsychotic drugs allows the total daily oral dose to be given as a single dose in most children. For the advice of The Royal College of Psychiatrists on doses above the BNF for Children upper limit, see p. 206.

CHLORPROMAZINE HYDROCHLORIDE

Warning Owing to the risk of contact sensitisation, pharmacists, nurses, and other health workers should avoid direct contact with chlorpromazine; tablets should not be crushed and solutions should be handled with care

Cautions see notes above; also children should remain supine and the blood pressure monitored for 30 minutes after intramuscular injection

Contra-indications see notes above

Side-effects see notes above; also intramuscular injection may be painful, cause hypotension and tachycardia, and give rise to nodule formation

Indication and dose

Childhood schizophrenia and other psychoses
- **By mouth**

Child 1–6 years 500 micrograms/kg every 4–6 hours adjusted according to response (max. 40 mg daily)

Child 6-12 years 10 mg 3 times daily, adjusted according to response (max. 75 mg daily)

Child 12–18 years 25 mg 3 times daily (*or* 75 mg at night), adjusted according to response, to usual maintenance dose of 75–300 mg daily (but up to 1 g daily may be required)

Relief of acute symptoms of psychoses but see also Cautions and Side-effects
- **By deep intramuscular injection**

Child 1–6 years 500 micrograms/kg every 6–8 hours (max. 40 mg daily)

Child 6–12 years 500 micrograms/kg every 6–8 hours (max. 75 mg daily)

Child 12–18 years 25–50 mg every 6–8 hours

Induction of hypothermia (to prevent shivering)
- **By deep intramuscular injection**

Child 1–12 years initially 0.5–1 mg/kg, followed by maintenance 500 micrograms/kg every 4–6 hours

Child 12–18 years 25–50 mg every 6–8 hours

Neonatal abstinence syndrome see also section 4.10
- **By mouth**

Neonate initially 0.5–1 mg/kg 3–4 times daily, adjusted according to response (max. 6 mg/kg daily); reduce dose by max. 2 mg/kg daily every third day when stable, consult local guidelines

Chlorpromazine (Non-proprietary) PoM
Tablets, coated, chlorpromazine hydrochloride 10 mg, net price 56-tab pack = 66p; 25 mg, 28-tab pack = £1.94; 50 mg, 28-tab pack = £1.71; 100 mg, 28-tab pack = £2.03. Label: 2, 11
Brands include *Chloractil*®

Oral solution, chlorpromazine hydrochloride 25 mg/5 mL, net price 150 mL = £1.35, 100 mg/5 mL, 150 mL = £3.57. Label: 2, 11

Injection, chlorpromazine hydrochloride 25 mg/mL, net price 1-mL amp = 60p; 2-mL amp = 63p

Largactil® (Hawgreen) PoM
Tablets, all off-white, f/c, chlorpromazine hydrochloride 10 mg. Net price 56-tab pack = 66p; 25 mg, 56-tab pack = 91p; 50 mg, 56-tab pack = £1.91; 100 mg, 56-tab pack = £3.54. Label: 2, 11

Syrup, brown, chlorpromazine hydrochloride 25 mg/5 mL. Net price 100-mL pack = £1.03. Label: 2, 11

CHLORPROMAZINE HYDROCHLORIDE (*continued*)

Suspension forte, orange, sugar-free, chlorpromazine hydrochloride 100 mg (as embonate)/5 mL. Net price 100-mL pack = £2.38. Label: 2, 11

Injection, chlorpromazine hydrochloride 25 mg/mL. Net price 2-mL amp = 63p

HALOPERIDOL

Cautions see notes above; also subarachnoid haemorrhage and metabolic disturbances such as hypokalaemia, hypocalcaemia, or hypomagnesaemia

Contra-indications see notes above

Side-effects see notes above, but less sedating and fewer antimuscarinic or hypotensive symptoms; pigmentation and photosensitivity reactions rare; extrapyramidal symptoms, particularly dystonic reactions and akathisia especially in thyrotoxic patients; rarely weight loss; hypoglycaemia; inappropriate antidiuretic hormone secretion

Licensed use not licensed for use in children for nausea and vomiting in palliative care

Indication and dose

Motor tics (including Gilles de la Tourette syndrome), schizophrenia and other psychoses, mania, short-term adjunctive management of psychomotor agitation, excitement and violent or dangerously impulsive behaviour

- **By mouth**

  Child 2–12 years initially 12.5–25 micrograms/kg twice daily, adjusted according to response to max. 10 mg daily

  Child 12–18 years initially 0.5–3 mg 2–3 times daily *or* 3–5 mg 2–3 times daily in severely affected or resistant disease; in resistant schizophrenia up to 30 mg daily may be needed; adjusted according to response to lowest effective maintenance dose (as low as 5–10 mg daily)

Nausea and vomiting in palliative care

- **By mouth**

  Child 12–18 years 1.5 mg once daily at night, increased to 1.5 mg twice daily if necessary; max. 5 mg twice daily

- **By continuous intravenous or subcutaneous infusion**

  Child 1 month–12 years 25–85 micrograms/kg over 24 hours

  Child 12–18 years 1.5–5 mg over 24 hours

Haloperidol (Non-proprietary) PoM

Tablets, haloperidol 500 micrograms, net price 28-tab pack = 91p; 1.5 mg, 20 = £1.65; 5 mg, 20 = £4.00; 10 mg, 20 = £4.23; 20 mg, 20 = £7.47. Label: 2

Dozic® (Rosemont) PoM

Oral liquid, sugar-free, haloperidol 1 mg/mL. Net price 100-mL pack = £6.86. Label: 2

Haldol® (Janssen-Cilag) PoM

Tablets, both scored, haloperidol 5 mg (blue), net price 20 = £1.56; 10 mg (yellow), 20 = £3.05. Label: 2

Oral liquid, sugar-free, haloperidol 2 mg/mL. Net price 100-mL pack (with pipette) = £4.83. Label: 2

Injection, haloperidol 5 mg/mL. Net price 1-mL amp = 31p

Depot injection (haloperidol decanoate): section 4.2.2

Serenace® (IVAX) PoM

Capsules, green, haloperidol 500 micrograms, net price 30-cap pack = 98p. Label: 2

Tablets, haloperidol 1.5 mg, net price 30-tab pack = £1.73; 5 mg (pink), 30-tab pack = £4.90; 10 mg (pale pink), 30-tab pack = £8.81. Label: 2

Oral liquid, sugar-free, haloperidol 2 mg/mL, net price 500-mL pack = £43.83. Label: 2

LEVOMEPROMAZINE
(Methotrimeprazine)

Cautions see notes above; children receiving large initial doses should remain supine

Contra-indications see notes above

Side-effects see notes above; occasionally raised erythrocyte sedimentation rate occurs

Indication and dose

Restlessness and confusion in palliative care

- **By continuous subcutaneous infusion**

  Child 1–12 years 0.35–3 mg/kg over 24 hours

  Child 12–18 years 12.5–200 mg over 24 hours

Nausea and vomiting in palliative care

- **By continuous intravenous or subcutaneous infusion**

  Child 1 month–12 years 100–400 micrograms/kg over 24 hours

  Child 12–18 years 5–25 mg over 24 hours

Administration for administration by *subcutaneous infusion* dilute with a suitable volume of Sodium Chloride 0.9%

Nozinan® (Link) PoM

Tablets, scored, levomepromazine maleate 25 mg, net price 84-tab pack = £20.26. Label: 2

Injection, levomepromazine hydrochloride 25 mg/mL, net price 1-mL amp = £2.01

4 Central nervous system

PERICYAZINE

(Periciazine)

Cautions see notes above

Contra-indications see notes above

Side-effects see notes above; more sedating; hypotension common when treatment initiated; respiratory depression

Licensed use tablets not licensed for use in children

Indication and dose

Schizophrenia, psychoses (severe mental or behavioural disorders only)
- By mouth

Child 1–12 years initially 500 micrograms daily for 10-kg child, increased by 1 mg for each additional 5 kg to max. total daily dose of 10 mg; dose may be gradually increased according to response but maintenance should not exceed twice initial dose

Child 12–18 years initially 25 mg 3 times daily increased at weekly intervals by steps of 25 mg according to response; usual max. 100 mg 3 times daily; total daily dose may alternatively be given in 2 divided doses

Neulactil® (JHC) PoM

Tablets, all yellow, scored, pericyazine 2.5 mg, net price 84-tab pack = £7.15; 10 mg, 84-tab pack = £9.33. Label: 2

Syrup forte, brown, pericyazine 10 mg/5 mL. Net price 100-mL pack = £9.57. Label: 2

PERPHENAZINE

Cautions see notes above

Contra-indications see notes above

Side-effects see notes above; less sedating; extrapyramidal symptoms, especially dystonia, more frequent, particularly at high dosage; rarely systemic lupus erythematosus

Indication and dose

Schizophrenia and other psychoses, mania, short-term adjunctive management of anxiety, severe psychomotor agitation, excitement, violent or dangerously impulsive behaviour
- By mouth

Child 14–18 years initially 4 mg 3 times daily adjusted according to the response; max. 24 mg daily

Fentazin® (Goldshield) PoM

Tablets, both s/c, perphenazine 2 mg, net price 20 = £3.73; 4 mg, 20 = £4.39. Label: 2

PIMOZIDE

Cautions see notes above

CSM warning Following reports of sudden unexplained death, the CSM recommends ECG before treatment. The CSM also recommends that patients on pimozide should have an annual ECG (if the QT interval is prolonged, treatment should be reviewed and either withdrawn or dose reduced under close supervision) and that pimozide should **not** be given with other antipsychotic drugs (including depot preparations), tricyclic antidepressants or other drugs which prolong the QT interval, such as certain antimalarials, anti-arrhythmic drugs and certain antihistamines and should **not** be given with drugs which cause electrolyte disturbances (especially diuretics)

Contra-indications see notes above; history of arrhythmias or congenital QT prolongation

Side-effects see notes above; less sedating; serious arrhythmias reported; glycosuria and, rarely, hyponatraemia reported

Licensed use not licensed for use in children under 12 years

Indication and dose

Schizophrenia
- By mouth

Child 12–18 years initially 1 mg daily, increased according to response in steps of 2–4 mg at intervals of not less than 1 week; usual dose range 2–20 mg daily

Gilles de la Tourette syndrome
- By mouth

Child 2–12 years 1–4 mg daily

Child 12–18 years 2–10 mg daily

Orap® (Janssen-Cilag) PoM

Tablets, scored, green, pimozide 4 mg, net price 20 = £5.83. Label: 2

SULPIRIDE

Cautions see notes above; also excited, agitated, or aggressive children (even low doses may aggravate symptoms)

Contra-indications see notes above; also porphyria (section 9.8.2)

Side-effects see notes above; also hepatitis

Indication and dose

Schizophrenia, Gilles de la Tourette syndrome
- By mouth

Child 14–18 years 200–400 mg twice daily; max. 800 mg daily in predominantly negative symptoms, dose increased to max. 2.4 g daily in mainly positive symptoms

SULPIRIDE (*continued*)

Sulpiride (Non-proprietary) PoM
Tablets, sulpiride 200 mg, net price 30-tab pack = £4.46; 56-tab pack = £4.47; 400 mg, 30-tab pack = £10.81. Label: 2

Dolmatil® (Sanofi-Synthelabo) PoM
Tablets, both scored, sulpiride 200 mg, net price 100-tab pack = £13.85; 400 mg (f/c), 100-tab pack = £36.29. Label: 2

Sulpitil® (Pharmacia) PoM
Tablets, scored, sulpiride 200 mg. Net price 28-tab pack = £4.29; 112-tab pack = £12.85. Label: 2

Sulpor® (Rosemont) PoM
Oral solution, sugar-free, lemon- and aniseed-flavoured, sulpiride 200 mg/5 mL, net price 150 mL = £25.38. Label: 2

TRIFLUOPERAZINE

Cautions see notes above

Contra-indications see notes above

Side-effects see notes above; extrapyramidal symptoms more frequent, especially at doses exceeding 6 mg daily; pancytopenia; thrombocytopenia; hyperpyrexia; anorexia

Indication and dose

Schizophrenia and other psychoses, short-term adjunctive management of psychomotor agitation, excitement and violent or dangerously impulsive behaviour
- By mouth

Child 3–12 years initially 1–2.5 mg twice daily, adjusted according to response

Child 12–18 years initially 5 mg twice daily, *or* 10 mg daily in modified-release form, increased by 5 mg after 1 week, then at intervals of 3 days, according to response

Short-term adjunctive management of severe anxiety
- By mouth

Child 3–6 years up to 500 micrograms twice daily

Child 6–12 years up to 2 mg twice daily

Child 12–18 years 1–2 mg twice daily *or* 2–4 mg daily in modified-release form, increased if necessary to 3 mg twice daily

Anti-emetic section 4.6

Trifluoperazine (Non-proprietary) PoM
Tablets, coated, trifluoperazine (as hydrochloride) 1 mg, net price 20 = 42p; 5 mg, 20 = 46p. Label: 2

Oral solution, trifluoperazine (as hydrochloride) 5 mg/5 mL. Net price 200-mL = £11.07. Label: 2

Stelazine® (Goldshield) PoM
Tablets, both blue, f/c, trifluoperazine (as hydrochloride) 1 mg, net price 20 = 61p; 5 mg, 20 = 87p. Label: 2

Spansules® (= capsules m/r), all clear/yellow, enclosing dark blue, light blue, and white pellets, trifluoperazine (as hydrochloride) 2 mg, net price 60-cap pack = £4.65; 10 mg, 30-cap pack = £2.83; 15 mg, 30-cap pack = £4.27. Label: 2, 25
Note May be difficult to obtain

Syrup, sugar-free, yellow, trifluoperazine (as hydrochloride) 1 mg/5 mL, net price 200-mL pack = £2.95. Label: 2

Oral solution forte, sugar-free, yellow, peach-flavour, trifluoperazine (as hydrochloride) 5 mg/5 mL, net price 200-mL pack = £10.99. Label: 2

Atypical antipsychotics

The 'atypical antipsychotics' **amisulpride**, **clozapine**, **olanzapine**, **quetiapine**, and **risperidone** may be better tolerated than other antipsychotics; extrapyramidal symptoms may be less frequent than with older antipsychotics.

Clozapine, olanzapine, and quetiapine cause little or no elevation of prolactin concentration; when changing from other antipsychotics, a reduction in prolactin may increase fertility.

Clozapine is used for the treatment of schizophrenia only in children unresponsive to, or intolerant of, conventional antipsychotic drugs. It can cause agranulocytosis and its use is restricted to patients registered with a clozapine Patient Monitoring Service (see under Clozapine, below).

Cautions and contra-indications While atypical antipsychotics have not generally been associated with clinically significant prolongation of the QT interval, they should be used with care if prescribed with other drugs that increase the QT interval. Atypical antipsychotics should be used with caution in children with cardiovascular disease, or a history of epilepsy; **interactions:** Appendix 1 (antipsychotics).

Skilled tasks Atypical antipsychotics may affect performance of skilled tasks (e.g. driving); effects of alcohol are enhanced.

Withdrawal Withdrawal of antipsychotic drugs after long-term therapy should always be gradual and closely monitored to avoid the risk of acute withdrawal syndromes or rapid relapse.

Side-effects Side-effects of the atypical antipsychotics include weight gain, dizziness, postural hypotension (especially during initial dose titration) which may be associated with syncope or reflex tachycardia in some patients, extrapyramidal symptoms (usually mild and transient and which respond to dose reduction or to an antimuscarinic drug), and occasionally tardive dyskinesia on long-term administration (discontinue drug on appearance of early signs). Hyperglycaemia and sometimes diabetes can occur, particularly with clozapine and olanzapine; monitoring weight and plasma glucose may identify the development of hyperglycaemia. Neuroleptic malignant syndrome has been reported rarely.

AMISULPRIDE

Cautions see notes above

Renal impairment Halve dose if creatinine clearance 30–60 mL/minute/1.73 m^2; use one-third dose if creatinine clearance 10–30 mL/minute/1.73 m^2; manufacturers advise intermittent treatment with a reduced dose if creatinine clearance less than 10 mL/minute/1.73 m^2

Contra-indications see notes above; phaeochromocytoma, prolactin-dependent tumours

Pregnancy avoid

Breast-feeding avoid

Side-effects see notes above; also insomnia, anxiety, agitation, drowsiness, gastro-intestinal disorders such as constipation, nausea, vomiting, and dry mouth; hyperprolactinaemia; occasionally bradycardia; *rarely* seizures

Indication and dose

Acute psychotic episode
- **By mouth**

Child 15–18 years 200–400 mg twice daily adjusted according to response; max. 1.2 g daily

Predominantly negative symptoms
- **By mouth**

Child 15–18 years 50–300 mg daily

Amisulpride (Non-proprietary) PoM

Tablets, amisulpride 50 mg, net price 60-tab pack = £17.79; 100 mg, 60-tab pack = £35.59; 200 mg, 60-tab pack = £59.49; 400 mg, 60-tab pack = £118.98. Label: 2

Solian® (Sanofi-Synthelabo) PoM

Tablets, amisulpride 50 mg, net price 60-tab pack = £18.36; 100 mg, 60-tab pack = £36.72; 200 mg, 60-tab pack = £61.38, 400 mg, 60-tab pack = £122.76. Label: 2

Solution, 100 mg/mL, net price 60 mL (caramel flavour) = £30.69. Label: 2

CLOZAPINE

Cautions see notes above; monitor leucocyte and differential blood counts (see Agranulocytosis, below); angle-closure glaucoma; taper off other antipsychotics before starting; close medical supervision during initiation (risk of collapse because of hypotension)

Hepatic impairment monitor hepatic function regularly; avoid in symptomatic, or progressive liver disease or hepatic failure

Pregnancy manufacturers advise caution

Withdrawal On planned withdrawal reduce dose over 1–2 weeks to avoid risk of rebound psychosis. If abrupt withdrawal necessary observe child carefully

Agranulocytosis Neutropenia and potentially fatal agranulocytosis reported. Leucocyte and differential blood counts must be normal before starting; monitor counts every week for 18 weeks then at least every 2 weeks and if clozapine continued and blood count stable after 1 year at least every 4 weeks (and 4 weeks after discontinuation); if leucocyte count below 3000/mm^3 or if absolute neutrophil count below 1500/mm^3 discontinue permanently and refer to haematologist. Avoid drugs which depress leucopoiesis; children (or carers) should report immediately symptoms of infection, especially influenza-like illness

Myocarditis and cardiomyopathy Fatal myocarditis (most commonly in first 2 months) and cardiomyopathy reported. The CSM has advised:

- physical examination and medical history before starting clozapine;
- specialist examination if cardiac abnormalities or history of heart disease found—clozapine initiated only in absence of severe heart disease and if benefit outweighs risk;
- persistent tachycardia especially in first 2 months should prompt observation for other indicators for myocarditis or cardiomyopathy;
- if myocarditis or cardiomyopathy suspected clozapine should be stopped and patient evaluated urgently by cardiologist;
- discontinue permanently in clozapine-induced myocarditis or cardiomyopathy

Gastro-intestinal obstruction Reactions resembling gastro-intestinal obstruction reported. Clozapine should be used cautiously with drugs which cause constipation (e.g. antimuscarinic drugs) or in children with history of colonic disease or bowel surgery. Monitor for constipation and prescribe laxative if required

Contra-indications severe cardiac disorders (e.g. myocarditis; see Myocarditis and Cardiomyopathy, above); history of neutropenia or agranulocytosis (see Agranulocytosis, above); bone-marrow disorders; paralytic ileus (see Gastro-intestinal Obstruction, above); alcoholic and

CLOZAPINE (continued)

toxic psychoses; history of circulatory collapse; drug intoxication; coma or severe CNS depression; uncontrolled epilepsy

Renal impairment avoid in severe renal impairment

Breast-feeding avoid

Side-effects see notes above; also constipation (see Gastro-intestinal Obstruction, above), hypersalivation, dry mouth, nausea, vomiting, anorexia; tachycardia, ECG changes, hypertension; drowsiness, headache, tremor, seizures, fatigue, impaired temperature regulation; urinary incontinence and retention; leucopenia, eosinophilia, leucocytosis; blurred vision; sweating; *less commonly* agranulocytosis (**important**: see Agranulocytosis, above); *rarely* dysphagia, hepatitis, cholestatic jaundice, pancreatitis, circulatory collapse, arrhythmia, myocarditis (**important**: see Myocarditis, above), pericarditis, thromboembolism, agitation, confusion, delirium, anaemia; *very rarely* parotid gland enlargement, intestinal obstruction (see Gastro-intestinal Obstruction, above), cardiomyopathy, myocardial infarction, respiratory depression, priapism, interstitial nephritis, thrombocytopenia, thrombocythaemia, hyperlipidaemia, fulminant hepatic necrosis, and skin reactions

Licensed use not licensed for use in children under 16 years

Indication and dose

Schizophrenia in patients unresponsive to, or intolerant of, conventional antipsychotic drugs
- By mouth

Child 12–18 years 12.5 mg once or twice on first day then 25–50 mg on second day then increased gradually (if well tolerated) in steps of 25–50 mg daily over 14–21 days up to 300 mg daily in divided doses (larger dose at night, up to 200 mg daily may be taken as a single dose at bedtime); if necessary may be further increased in steps of 50–100 mg once (preferably) or twice weekly; usual dose 200–450 mg daily (max. 900 mg daily)

Note *Restarting after interval of more than 2 days,* 12.5 mg once or twice on first day (but may be feasible to increase more quickly than on initiation)—extreme caution if previous respiratory or cardiac arrest with initial dosing

Clozaril® (Novartis) PoM

Tablets, both yellow, clozapine 25 mg (scored), net price 28-tab pack = £6.17, 84-tab pack (hosp. only) = £18.49; 100 mg, 28-tab pack = £24.64, 84-tab pack (hosp. only) = £73.92. Label: 2, 10, patient information leaflet

Note Patient, prescriber, and supplying pharmacist must be registered with the Clozaril Patient Monitoring Service—takes several days to do this

Denzapine® (Denfleet) PoM

Tablets, both yellow, scored, clozapine 25 mg, net price 28-tab pack = £6.17, 84-tab pack = £18.49; 100 mg, 28-tab pack = £24.64, 84-tab pack = £73.92. Label: 2, 10, patient information leaflet

Note Patient, prescriber, and supplying pharmacist must be registered with the Denzapine Patient Monitoring Service—takes several days to do this

Zaponex® (IVAX) PoM

Tablets, both yellow, scored, clozapine 25 mg, net price 84-tab pack = £22.17; 100 mg, 84-tab pack = £88.68. Label: 2, 10, patient information leaflet

Note Patient, prescriber, and supplying pharmacist must be registered with the Zaponex Treatment Access System—takes several days to do this

OLANZAPINE

Cautions see notes above; paralytic ileus, diabetes mellitus (risk of exacerbation or ketoacidosis), low leucocyte or neutrophil count, bone-marrow depression, hyper-eosinophilic disorders, myeloproliferative disease

Hepatic impairment initial dose 5mg daily, increased slowly

Renal impairment initial dose 5mg daily, increased slowly

Pregnancy manufacturer advises use only if potential benefit outweighs risk; neonatal lethargy, tremor and hypertonia reported when used in third trimester

Contra-indications angle-closure glaucoma

Breast-feeding avoid

Side-effects see notes above; also mild, transient antimuscarinic effects; drowsiness, speech difficulty, akathisia, asthenia, increased appetite, raised triglyceride concentration, oedema, hyperprolactinaemia (but clinical manifestations rare), occasionally blood dyscrasias, rarely bradycardia, rash, photosensitivity, diabetes mellitus, priapism, hepatitis, pancreatitis

Licensed use not licensed for use in children

Indication and dose

Schizophrenia, combination therapy for mania
- By mouth

Child 12–18 years initially 5–10 mg daily adjusted to usual range of 5–20 mg daily; doses greater than 10 mg daily only after reassessment; max. 20 mg daily

Monotherapy for mania
- By mouth

Child 12–18 years 15 mg daily adjusted to usual range of 5–20 mg daily; doses greater than 15 mg only after reassessment; max. 20 mg daily

Note When one or more factors present that might result in slower metabolism (e.g. female gender, non-smoker) consider lower initial dose and more gradual dose increase

Zyprexa® (Lilly) PoM

Tablets, f/c, olanzapine 2.5 mg, net price 28-tab pack = £33.29; 5 mg, 28-tab pack = £48.78; 7.5 mg, 56-tab pack = £146.34; 10 mg, 28-tab pack = £79.45, 56-tab pack = £158.90; 15 mg (blue), 28-tab pack = £146.34. Label: 2

OLANZAPINE (*continued*)

Orodispersible tablet (*Velotab*®), yellow, olanzapine 5 mg, net price 28-tab pack = £56.10; 10 mg, 28-tab pack = £112.19; 15 mg, 28-tab pack = £168.29; 20 mg, 28-tab pack = £182.74. Label: 2, counselling, administration

Excipients: include aspartame (section 9.4.1)

Counselling *Velotab*® may be placed on the tongue and allowed to dissolve or dispersed in water, orange juice, apple juice, milk, or coffee

QUETIAPINE

Cautions see notes above; cerebrovascular disease

Hepatic impairment manufacturer advises initial dose of 25 mg daily

Renal impairment manufacturer advises initial dose of 25 mg daily

Pregnancy manufacturer advises use only if potential benefit outweighs risk

Contra-indications

Breast-feeding avoid

Side-effects see notes above; also drowsiness, dyspepsia, constipation, dry mouth, mild asthenia, rhinitis, tachycardia; leucopenia, neutropenia and occasionally eosinophilia reported; elevated plasma-triglyceride and cholesterol concentrations, reduced plasma-thyroid hormone concentrations; possible QT interval prolongation; rarely oedema; very rarely priapism

Licensed use not licensed for use in children

Indication and dose

Schizophrenia
- By mouth

Child 12–18 years initially 25 mg twice daily adjusted in steps of 25–50 mg according to response; max. 750 mg daily

Seroquel® (AstraZeneca) PoM

Tablets, f/c, quetiapine (as fumarate) 25 mg (peach), net price 60-tab pack = £28.20; 100 mg (yellow), 60-tab pack = £113.10; 150 mg (pale yellow), 60-tab pack = £113.10; 200 mg (white), 60-tab pack = £113.10; 300 mg (white), 60-tab pack = £170.00. Label: 2

RISPERIDONE

Cautions see notes above

Hepatic impairment initially 500 micrograms twice daily increased in steps of 500 micrograms twice daily to 1-2 mg twice daily

Renal impairment initially 500 micrograms twice daily increased in steps of 500 micrograms twice daily to 1-2 mg twice daily

Pregnancy manufacturer advises use only if potential benefit outweighs risk

Contra-indications

Breast-feeding avoid

Side-effects see notes above; also insomnia, agitation, anxiety, headache; *less commonly* drowsiness, impaired concentration, fatigue, blurred vision, constipation, nausea and vomiting, dyspepsia, abdominal pain, hyperprolactinaemia (with galactorrhoea, menstrual disturbances, amenorrhoea, gynaecomastia), sexual dysfunction, priapism, urinary incontinence, tachycardia, hypertension, oedema, rash, rhinitis; cerebrovascular accidents, neutropenia and thrombocytopenia have been reported; *rarely* seizures, hyponatraemia, abnormal temperature regulation, and epistaxis

Licensed use not licensed for use in children under 15 years

Indication and dose

Acute and chronic psychoses
- By mouth

Child 12–18 years 2 mg in 1–2 divided doses on first day *then* 4 mg in 1–2 divided doses on second day (slower titration appropriate in some children); usual dose range 4–6 mg daily; doses above 10 mg daily only if benefit considered to outweigh risk (max. 16 mg daily)

Risperdal® (Janssen-Cilag) PoM

Tablets, f/c, scored, risperidone 500 micrograms (brown-red), net price 20-tab pack = £7.06; 1 mg (white), 20-tab pack = £11.61, 60-tab pack = £34.84; 2 mg (orange), 60-tab pack = £68.69; 3 mg (yellow), 60-tab pack = £101.01; 4 mg (green), 60-tab pack = £133.34; 6 mg (yellow), 28-tab pack = £94.28. Label: 2

Orodispersible tablets (*Quicklet*®), all pink, risperidone 500 micrograms, net price 28-tab pack = £11.43; 1 mg, 28-tab pack = £18.39; 2 mg, 28-tab pack = £34.66. Label: 2, counselling, administration

Excipients: include aspartame (section 9.4.1)

Counselling Tablets should be placed on the tongue, allowed to dissolve and swallowed

Liquid, risperidone 1 mg/mL, net price 100 mL = £56.12. Label: 2

Note Liquid may be diluted with mineral water, orange juice or black coffee (should be taken immediately)

4.2.2 Antipsychotic depot injections

There is limited information on the use of antipsychotic depot injections in children and use should be restricted to specialist centres.

4.2.3 Antimanic drugs

Drugs are used in mania both to control acute attacks and also to prevent their recurrence.

Benzodiazepines

Use of benzodiazepines (section 4.1) may be helpful in the initial stages of treatment until lithium achieves its full effect; they should not be used for long periods because of the risk of dependence.

Antipsychotic drugs

In an acute attack of mania, treatment with an antipsychotic drug (section 4.2.1) is usually required because it may take a few days for lithium to exert its antimanic effect. Lithium may be given concurrently with the antipsychotic drug, and treatment with the antipsychotic gradually tailed off as lithium becomes effective. Alternatively, lithium therapy may be commenced once the patient's mood has been stabilised with the antipsychotic. The adjunctive use of atypical antipsychotics such as olanzapine (section 4.2.1) and risperidone [unlicensed indication] with either lithium or valproic acid may also be of benefit.

High doses of haloperidol may be hazardous when used with lithium; irreversible toxic encephalopathy has been reported.

Carbamazepine

Carbamazepine (section 4.8.1) may be used for the prophylaxis of bipolar disorder (manic-depressive disorder) in children unresponsive to lithium; it seems to be particularly effective in those with rapid cycling manic-depressive illness (4 or more affective episodes per year).

Valproic acid

Valproic acid (as the semisodium salt) is licensed in adults for the treatment of manic episodes associated with bipolar disorder. It may be useful in children unresponsive to lithium. Sodium valproate (section 4.8.1) has also been used.

Lithium

Lithium salts are used in the prophylaxis and treatment of mania, in the prophylaxis of bipolar disorder (manic-depressive disorder) and in the prophylaxis of recurrent depression (unipolar illness or unipolar depression). Lithium should be used in children only on the advice of a specialist.

The decision to give prophylactic lithium must be based on careful consideration of the likelihood of recurrence in the individual child, and the benefit weighed against the risks. In long-term use lithium has been associated with thyroid disorders and mild cognitive and memory impairment. Long-term treatment should therefore be undertaken only with careful assessment of risk and benefit, and with regular monitoring of thyroid function. The need for continued therapy should be assessed regularly and children should be maintained on lithium after 3–5 years only if benefit persists.

Serum concentrations Lithium salts have a narrow therapeutic/toxic ratio and should not be prescribed unless facilities for monitoring serum-lithium concentrations are available. There seem few if any reasons for preferring one or other of the salts of lithium available. Doses are adjusted to achieve serum-lithium concentration of 0.4–1 mmol/litre on samples taken 12 hours after the preceding dose. It is important to determine the optimum range for each individual child.

Overdosage, usually with serum-lithium concentration of over 1.5 mmol/litre, may be fatal and toxic effects include tremor, ataxia, dysarthria, nystagmus, renal impairment, and convulsions. If these potentially hazardous signs occur, treatment should be stopped, serum-lithium concentrations redetermined, and steps taken to reverse lithium toxicity. In mild cases withdrawal of lithium and administration of generous amounts of sodium and fluid will reverse the toxicity. Serum-lithium concentration in excess of 2 mmol/litre require urgent treatment as indicated under Emergency Treatment of Poisoning, p. 41.

Interactions Lithium toxicity is made worse by sodium depletion, therefore concurrent use of diuretics (particularly thiazides) is hazardous and should be avoided. For other **interactions** with lithium, see Appendix 1 (lithium).

Withdrawal While there is no clear evidence of withdrawal or rebound psychosis, abrupt discontinuation of lithium increases the risk of relapse. If lithium is to be discontinued, the dose should be reduced gradually over a period of a few weeks and children and carers should be warned of possible relapse if discontinued abruptly.

> Lithium cards
> A lithium treatment card available from pharmacies tells children and carers how to take lithium preparations, what to do if a dose is missed, and what side-effects to expect. It also explains why regular blood tests are important and warns that some medicines and illnesses can change serum-lithium concentration.
> Cards may be purchased from the National Pharmacy Association.
> Tel: (01727) 858 687
> sales@npa.co.uk

LITHIUM CARBONATE

Cautions measure serum-lithium concentration regularly (every 3 months on stabilised regimens), measure renal function and thyroid function every 6–12 months on stabilised regimens and advise children and carers to seek attention if symptoms of hypothyroidism develop (females are at greater risk) e.g. lethargy, feeling cold; maintain adequate sodium and fluid intake; test renal function before initiating and if evidence of toxicity, avoid in cardiac disease, and conditions with sodium imbalance such as Addison's disease; reduce dose or discontinue in diarrhoea, vomiting and intercurrent infection (especially if sweating profusely); psoriasis (risk of exacerbation); diuretic treatment, myasthenia gravis; surgery (section 15.1); if possible avoid abrupt withdrawal (see notes above); **interactions:** Appendix 1 (lithium)

Counselling Children should maintain adequate fluid intake and avoid dietary changes which reduce or increase sodium intake

Renal impairment in mild impairment avoid if possible or reduce dose and monitor serum-lithium concentration carefully; avoid in moderate to severe impairment

Pregnancy avoid if possible in first trimester (risk of teratogenicity, including cardiac abnormalities); dose requirements increased in second and third trimesters (but return to normal abruptly on delivery); close monitoring of serum-lithium concentration advised (risk of toxicity in neonate)

Breast-feeding present in milk and risk of toxicity in infant—manufacturer advises avoid

Side-effects gastro-intestinal disturbances, fine tremor, renal impairment (particularly impaired urinary concentration and polyuria), polydipsia, leucocytosis; also weight gain and oedema (may respond to dose reduction); hyperparathyroidism and hypercalcaemia reported; signs of intoxication are blurred vision, increasing gastro-intestinal disturbances (anorexia, vomiting, diarrhoea), muscle weakness, increased CNS disturbances (mild drowsiness and sluggishness increasing to giddiness with ataxia, coarse tremor, lack of co-ordination, dysarthria), and require withdrawal of treatment; with severe overdosage (serum-lithium concentration above 2 mmol/litre) hyperreflexia and hyperextension of limbs, convulsions, toxic psychoses, syncope, renal failure, circulatory failure, coma, and occasionally, death; goitre, raised antidiuretic hormone concentration, hypothyroidism, hypokalaemia, ECG changes, and kidney changes may also occur; see also Emergency Treatment of Poisoning, p. 41

Indication and dose

Treatment and prophylaxis of mania, bipolar disorder, recurrent depression (see also notes above), aggressive or self-mutilating behaviour
- **By mouth**

  see under preparations below, adjusted to achieve a serum-lithium concentration of 0.4–1 mmol/litre 12 hours after a dose on days 4–7 of treatment, then every week until dosage has remained constant for 4 weeks and every 3 months thereafter; doses are initially divided throughout the day, but once daily administration is preferred when serum-lithium concentration stabilised

Note **Preparations vary widely in bioavailability**; changing the preparation requires the same precautions as initiation of treatment

Note Lithium carbonate 200 mg ≡ lithium citrate 509 mg

Camcolit® (Norgine) PoM

Camcolit 250® tablets, f/c, scored, lithium carbonate 250 mg (Li^+ 6.8 mmol), net price 20 = 64p. Label: 10, lithium card, counselling, see above

Camcolit 400® tablets, m/r, f/c, scored, lithium carbonate 400 mg (Li^+ 10.8 mmol), net price 20 = 86p. Label: 10, lithium card, 25, counselling, see above

Dose

Treatment
- **By mouth**

  (serum monitoring, see above)

  Child 12–18 years initially 1–1.5 g daily

Prophylaxis
- **By mouth**

  (serum monitoring, see above)

  Child 12–18 years initially 300–400 mg daily

4 Central nervous system

LITHIUM CARBONATE (*continued*)

Liskonum® (GSK) PoM
Tablets, m/r, f/c, scored, lithium carbonate 450 mg (Li^+ 12.2 mmol), net price 60-tab pack = £2.88. Label: 10, lithium card, 25, counselling, see above

Dose

Treatment
- **By mouth**
(serum monitoring, see above)
Child 12–18 years initially 225–675 mg twice daily

Prophylaxis
- **By mouth**
(serum monitoring, see above)
Child 12–18 years initially 225–450 mg twice daily

LITHIUM CITRATE

Cautions see under Lithium Carbonate and notes above

Counselling Patients should maintain an adequate fluid intake and should avoid dietary changes which might reduce or increase sodium intake; lithium treatment cards are available from pharmacies (see above)

Side-effects see under Lithium Carbonate and notes above

Licensed use not licensed for use in children

Indication and dose

See under Lithium Carbonate and notes above
- **By mouth**
adjust to achieve serum-lithium concentration of 0.4–1 mmol/litre as described under Lithium Carbonate above

Note **Preparations vary widely in bioavailability**; changing the preparation requires the same precautions as initiation of treatment

Note Lithium carbonate 200 mg ≡ lithium citrate 509 mg

Li-Liquid® (Rosemont) PoM
Oral solution, lithium citrate 509 mg/5 mL (Li^+ 5.4 mmol/5 mL), yellow, net price 150-mL pack = £5.79; 1.018 g/5 mL (Li^+ 10.8 mmol/5 mL), orange, 150-mL pack = £11.58. Label: 10, lithium card, counselling, see above

Priadel® (Sanofi-Synthelabo) PoM
Liquid, sugar-free, lithium citrate 520 mg/5 mL (approx. Li^+ 5.4 mmol/5 mL), net price 150-mL pack = £5.84. Label: 10, lithium card, counselling, see above

4.3 Antidepressant drugs

> The safety and efficacy of drugs used in the treatment of depression in children has not been established; long-term safety information is also lacking.
>
> Depression in children should be managed by an appropriate specialist and treatment should involve psychological therapy.

The major classes of antidepressants include the tricyclics and related antidepressants, the selective serotonin re-uptake inhibitors (SSRIs), and the monoamine oxidase inhibitors (MAOIs).

Choice of antidepressant should be based on the individual child's requirements, including the presence of concomitant disease, existing therapy, suicide risk, and previous response to antidepressant therapy.

Compared to older **tricyclics** (e.g. amitriptyline), the **tricyclic-related drugs** (e.g. trazodone) have a lower incidence of antimuscarinic side-effects, such as dry mouth and constipation. The tricyclic-related drugs may also be associated with a lower risk of cardiotoxicity in overdosage, but some have additional side-effects (for further details see section 4.3.1).

The **selective serotonin re-uptake inhibitors** (SSRIs) have fewer antimuscarinic side-effects than the older tricyclics and they are also less cardiotoxic in overdosage. The SSRIs do, however, have characteristic side-effects of their own; gastro-intestinal side-effects such as nausea and vomiting are common and bleeding disorders have been reported.

St John's wort (*Hypericum perforatum*) is a popular unlicensed herbal remedy for treating mild depression in adults. In the absence of adequate evidence of safety or efficacy in children, St John's wort should not be used for the treatment of depression in children. It interacts with a number of conventional drugs, see Appendix 1 (St John's wort).

> **Hyponatraemia and antidepressant therapy.** Hyponatraemia (possibly due to inappropriate secretion of antidiuretic hormone) has been associated with all types of antidepressants; however, it has been reported more frequently with SSRIs than with other antidepressants. The CSM has advised that hyponatraemia should be considered in all patients who develop drowsiness, confusion, or convulsions while taking an antidepressant.

Withdrawal Gastro-intestinal symptoms of nausea, vomiting, and anorexia, accompanied by headache, giddiness, 'chills', and insomnia, and sometimes by hypomania, panic-anxiety, and extreme motor restlessness may occur if an antidepressant is stopped suddenly after regular administration for 8 weeks or more. The dose should preferably be reduced gradually over about 4 weeks, or longer if withdrawal symptoms emerge (6 months in children who have been on long-term maintenance treatment). SSRIs have been associated with a specific withdrawal syndrome (section 4.3.3).

Anxiety Management of *acute anxiety* in children with drug treatment is contentious (section 4.1.2). For *chronic anxiety* (of longer than 4 weeks' duration), it may be appropriate to use an antidepressant before a benzodiazepine.

4.3.1 Tricyclic antidepressant drugs

> The safety and efficacy of tricyclic antidepressant drugs in the treatment of depression in children has not been established. Treatment should be managed by an appropriate specialist and should involve psychological therapy.

For reference to the role of some tricyclic antidepressants in some forms of *neuralgia*, see section 4.7.3, and in *nocturnal enuresis* in children, see section 7.4.2.

Dosage It is important to use doses that are sufficiently high for effective treatment but not so high as to cause toxic effects. Low doses should be used for initial treatment.

In most children the long half-life of tricyclic antidepressant drugs allows **once-daily** administration, usually at night; the use of modified-release preparations is therefore unnecessary.

Choice Tricyclic antidepressant drugs can be roughly divided into those with additional sedative properties and those without. Those with **sedative** properties include amitriptyline. Those with **less sedative** properties include amoxapine, imipramine and nortriptyline. Tricyclic antidepressants should generally be avoided for the treatment of depression in children (see above).

Imipramine and **amitriptyline** have more marked antimuscarinic and cardiac side-effects than some other tricyclic or related antidepressants; this may be important in some children. **Amoxapine** is related to the antipsychotic loxapine and its side-effects include tardive dyskinesia.

Side-effects *Arrhythmias* and *heart block* occasionally follow the use of tricyclic antidepressants, particularly amitriptyline, and may be a factor in the sudden death of children with cardiac disease. They are also sometimes associated with *convulsions* (and should be prescribed with special caution in epilepsy as they lower the convulsive threshold). *Hepatic* and *haematological* reactions may occur and have been particularly associated with mianserin.

Other side-effects of tricyclic antidepressants include *drowsiness, dry mouth, blurred vision, constipation,* and *urinary retention* (all attributed to antimuscarinic activity), and sweating. The child should be encouraged to persist with treatment as some tolerance to these side-effects seems to develop. They are reduced if low doses are given initially and then gradually increased, but this must be balanced against the need to obtain a full therapeutic effect as soon as possible.

Neuroleptic malignant syndrome (section 4.2.1) may, very rarely, arise in the course of antidepressant treatment.

Overdosage Limited quantities of tricyclic antidepressants should be prescribed at any one time because their cardiovascular effects are dangerous in overdosage. In particular, overdosage with **amitriptyline** is associated with a relatively high rate of fatality. For advice on overdosage see Emergency Treatment of Poisoning, p. 39

Withdrawal If possible tricyclic antidepressants should be withdrawn slowly (see also section 4.3).

Tricyclic antidepressants

AMITRIPTYLINE HYDROCHLORIDE

Cautions cardiac disease (particularly with arrhythmias, see Contra-indications below), history of epilepsy, thyroid disease, phaeochromocytoma, history of mania, psychoses (may aggravate psychotic symptoms), angle-closure glaucoma, history of urinary retention, concurrent electroconvulsive therapy; if possible avoid abrupt withdrawal; anaesthesia (increased risk of arrhythmias and hypotension, see surgery section 15.1); porphyria (section 9.8.2); see section 7.4.2 for additional nocturnal enuresis warnings; **interactions:** Appendix 1 (antidepressants, tricyclic)

Skilled tasks Drowsiness may affect performance of skilled tasks (e.g. driving); effects of alcohol enhanced

Hepatic impairment sedative effects increased; avoid in severe hepatic impairment

Pregnancy manufacturer advises use only if potential benefit outweighs risk

Breast-feeding amount too small to be harmful but manufacturer advises avoid

Contra-indications arrhythmias (particularly heart block), not indicated in manic phase, severe liver disease

Side-effects dry mouth, sedation, blurred vision (disturbance of accommodation, increased intra-ocular pressure), constipation, nausea, difficulty with micturition; cardiovascular side-effects (such as ECG changes, arrhythmias, postural hypotension, tachycardia, syncope, particularly with high doses); sweating, tremor, rashes and hypersensitivity reactions (including urticaria, photosensitivity), behavioural disturbances, hypomania or mania, confusion or delirium, headache, interference with sexual function, blood—glucose changes; increased appetite and weight gain (occasionally weight loss); endocrine side-effects such as testicular enlargement, gynaecomastia, galactorrhoea; also convulsions (see also Cautions), movement disorders and dyskinesias, dysarthria, paraesthesia, taste disturbances, tinnitus, fever, agranulocytosis, leucopenia, eosinophilia, purpura, thrombocytopenia, hyponatraemia (may be due to inappropriate antidiuretic hormone secretion) see CSM advice, p. 219, abnormal liver function tests (jaundice); for a general outline of side-effects see also notes above; **overdosage:** see Emergency Treatment of Poisoning, p. 39 (high rate of fatality—see Overdosage above)

Licensed use not licensed for use in neuropathic pain

Indication and dose

Depression (but see notes above)

• **By mouth**

Child 16–18 years 10–25 mg 3 times daily (total daily dose may alternatively be given as a single dose at bedtime) increased gradually as necessary to 150–200 mg daily

Nocturnal enuresis

• **By mouth**

Child 6–11 years 10–20 mg at night

Child 11–18 years 25–50 mg at night

Note Max. period of treatment (including gradual withdrawal) 3 months—full physical examination before further course, see also section 7.4.2

Neuropathic pain in palliative care

• **By mouth**

Child 2–12 years initially 200–500 micrograms/kg (max. 25 mg) once daily at night, increased if necessary; max. 1 mg/kg twice daily on specialist advice

Child 12–18 years initially 10–25 mg once daily at night, increased gradually if necessary to usual dose 75 mg at night; higher doses on specialist advice

Amitriptyline (Non-proprietary) PoM

Tablets, coated, amitriptyline hydrochloride 10 mg, net price 20 = 71p; 25 mg, 20 = 73p; 50 mg, 20 = 97p. Label: 2

Oral solution, amitriptyline hydrochloride 25 mg/5 mL, net price 200 mL = £16.53; 50 mg/5 mL, 200 mL = £18.00. Label: 2

AMOXAPINE

Cautions see under Amitriptyline Hydrochloride

Contra-indications see under Amitriptyline Hydrochloride

Side-effects see under Amitriptyline Hydrochloride; tardive dyskinesia reported; menstrual irregularities, breast enlargement

Indication and dose

Depressive illness (but see notes above)

- By mouth

Child 16–18 years initially 50 mg 2–3 times daily increased as necessary to max. 100 mg 3 times daily; total daily dose may alternatively be given as a single dose at bedtime

Asendis® (Goldshield) PoM

Tablets, amoxapine 50 mg (orange, scored), net price 84-tab pack = £16.78; 100 mg (blue, scored), 56-tab pack = £18.65. Label: 2

IMIPRAMINE HYDROCHLORIDE

Cautions see under Amitriptyline Hydrochloride

Pregnancy tachycardia, irritability, and muscle spasms reported in neonates when used in third trimester

Contra-indications see under Amitriptyline Hydrochloride

Side-effects see under Amitriptyline Hydrochloride, but less sedating

Licensed use not licensed for use for attention deficit hyperactivity disorder

Indication and dose

Nocturnal enuresis

- By mouth

Child 6–8 years 25 mg at bedtime

Child 8–11 years 25–50 mg at bedtime

Child 11–18 years 50–75 mg at bedtime

Note Max. period of treatment (including gradual withdrawal) 3 months—full physical examination before further course, see also section 7.4.2

Attention deficit hyperactivity disorder (under specialist supervision)

- By mouth

Child 6–18 years 10–30 mg twice daily

Imipramine (Non-proprietary) PoM

Tablets, coated, imipramine hydrochloride 10 mg, net price 20 = 61p; 25 mg, 20 = 72p. Label: 2

NORTRIPTYLINE

Cautions see under Amitriptyline Hydrochloride; manufacturer advises plasma-nortriptyline concentration monitoring if dose above 100 mg daily, but evidence of practical value uncertain

Contra-indications see under Amitriptyline Hydrochloride

Side-effects see under Amitriptyline Hydrochloride, but less sedating

Indication and dose

Depression (but see notes above)

- By mouth

Child 12–18 years low dose initially increased as necessary to 30–50 mg daily in divided doses *or* as a single dose (max. 150 mg daily)

Nocturnal enuresis

- By mouth

Child 6–8 years 10 mg at night

Child 8–11 years 10–20 mg at night

Child 11–18 years 25–35 mg at night

Note Max. period of treatment (including gradual withdrawal) 3 months—full physical examination and ECG before further course, see also section 7.4.2

Allegron® (King) PoM

Tablets, nortriptyline (as hydrochloride) 10 mg, net price 20 = £2.48; 25 mg (orange, scored), 20 = £4.90. Label: 2

4.3.2 Monoamine-oxidase inhibitors (MAOIs)

Classification not used in *BNF for Children*

4.3.3 Selective serotonin re-uptake inhibitors

Citalopram, **escitalopram**, **fluoxetine**, **fluvoxamine**, **paroxetine**, and **sertraline** selectively inhibit the re-uptake of serotonin (5-hydroxytryptamine, 5-HT); they are termed selective serotonin re-uptake inhibitors (SSRIs).

CSM advice (depressive illness in children and adolescents)
The CSM has advised that the balance of risks and benefits for the treatment of depressive illness in individuals under 18 years is considered unfavourable for the SSRIs **citalopram**, **escitalopram**, **paroxetine**, and **sertraline**, and for **mirtazapine** and **venlafaxine**. Clinical trials have failed to show efficacy and have shown an increase in harmful outcomes. However, it is recognised that specialists may sometimes decide to use these drugs in response to individual clinical need; children and adolescents should be monitored carefully for suicidal behaviour, self-harm or hostility, particularly at the beginning of treatment. Only **fluoxetine** has been shown in clinical trials to be effective for treating depressive illness in children and adolescents. However, it is possible that, in common with the other SSRIs, it is associated with a small risk of self-harm and suicidal thoughts. Overall, the balance of risks and benefits for fluoxetine in the treatment of depressive illness in individuals under 18 years is considered favourable, but children and adolescents must be carefully monitored as above.

Cautions SSRIs should be used with caution in children with epilepsy (avoid if poorly controlled, discontinue if convulsions develop), cardiac disease, diabetes mellitus, angle-closure glaucoma, history of mania or bleeding disorders (especially gastro-intestinal bleeding), and if used together with other drugs that increase the risk of bleeding. They should also be used with caution in those receiving concurrent electroconvulsive therapy (prolonged seizures reported with fluoxetine). SSRIs may also impair performance of skilled tasks (e.g. driving). **Interactions:** Appendix 1 (antidepressants, SSRI).

Withdrawal Gastro-intestinal disturbances, headache, anxiety, dizziness, paraesthesia, sleep disturbances, fatigue, influenza-like symptoms, and sweating are the most common features of abrupt withdrawal of an SSRI or marked reduction of the dose; the dose should be tapered over a few weeks to avoid these effects.

Contra-indications SSRIs should not be used if the child enters a manic phase.

Side-effects SSRIs are less sedating and have fewer antimuscarinic and cardiotoxic effects than tricyclic antidepressants (section 4.3). Side-effects of the SSRIs include gastro-intestinal effects (dose-related and fairly common—include nausea, vomiting, dyspepsia, abdominal pain, diarrhoea, constipation), anorexia with weight loss (increased appetite and weight gain also reported) and hypersensitivity reactions including rash (consider discontinuation—may be sign of impending serious systemic reaction, possibly associated with vasculitis), urticaria, angioedema, anaphylaxis, arthralgia, myalgia and photosensitivity; other side-effects include dry mouth, nervousness, anxiety, headache, insomnia, tremor, dizziness, asthenia, hallucinations, drowsiness, convulsions (see Cautions above), galactorrhoea, sexual dysfunction, urinary retention, sweating, hypomania or mania (see Cautions above), movement disorders and dyskinesias, visual disturbances, hyponatraemia (may be due to inappropriate antidiuretic hormone secretion—see CSM warning, section 4.3), and bleeding disorders including ecchymoses and purpura. Suicidal ideation, self harm, and hostility have been linked with SSRIs, see CSM advice above.

CITALOPRAM

Cautions see notes above

Hepatic impairment use doses at lower end of range

Renal impairment no information available in moderate to severe renal impairment

Pregnancy manufacturers advise use only if potential benefit outweighs risk; risk of neonatal withdrawal

Breast-feeding present in milk—manufacturer advises avoid

Contra-indications see notes above

Side-effects see notes above; also palpitation, tachycardia, postural hypotension, coughing, yawning, confusion, impaired concentration, malaise, amnesia, migraine, paraesthesia, abnormal dreams, taste disturbance, increased salivation, rhinitis, tinnitus, polyuria, micturition disorders, euphoria

Licensed use not licensed for use in children

CITALOPRAM (*continued*)

Indication and dose

Major depression
- **By mouth**

Child 12–18 years initially 10 mg once daily, increased if necessary to 20 mg once daily over 2–4 weeks; max. 60 mg once daily

Note 8 mg (4 drops) *Cipramil®* oral drops may be considered to be equivalent in therapeutic effect to 10-mg citalopram tablet

Citalopram (Non-proprietary) PoM

Tablets, citalopram (as hydrobromide) 10 mg, net price 28-tab pack = £2.80; 20 mg, 28-tab pack = £3.02; 40 mg, 28-tab pack = £5.04. Counselling, driving

Cipramil® (Lundbeck) PoM

Tablets, f/c, citalopram (as hydrobromide) 10 mg, net price 28-tab pack = £8.97; 20 mg (scored), 28-tab pack = £14.91; 40 mg, 28-tab pack = £25.20. Counselling, driving

Oral drops, sugar-free, citalopram (as hydrochloride) 40 mg/mL, net price 15 mL = £20.16. Counselling, driving, administration
Excipients: include alcohol

Dose

Major depression
- **By mouth**

Child 12–18 years 8 mg once daily increased if necessary to 16 mg once daily over 2–4 weeks; max. 48 mg once daily

Note 8 mg (4 drops) *Cipramil®* oral drops may be considered to be equivalent in therapeutic effect to 10-mg citalopram tablet.

Mix with water, orange juice, or apple juice before taking

FLUOXETINE

Cautions see notes above

Hepatic impairment reduce dose; avoid in severe hepatic impairment

Renal impairment mild to moderate impairment reduce dose to alternate days; severe impairment, avoid

Pregnancy manufacturer advises use only if potential benefit outweighs risk (no evidence of teratogenicity)

Breast-feeding present in breast milk, manufacturer advises avoid

Contra-indications see notes above

Side-effects see notes above; also vasodilatation, postural hypotension, pharyngitis, dyspnoea, chills, taste disturbances, sleep disturbances, euphoria, confusion, yawning, impaired concentration, changes in blood sugar, alopecia, urinary frequency; *rarely* pulmonary inflammation and fibrosis; *very rarely* hepatitis, toxic epidermal necrolysis, and neuroleptic malignant syndrome-like event

Licensed use not licensed for use in children

Indication and dose

Major depression
- **By mouth**

Child 12–18 years 10 mg once daily increased after 3 weeks if necessary, max. 20 mg once daily (exceptionally, up to 40 mg once daily)

Long duration of action Consider the long half-life of fluoxetine when adjusting dosage (or in overdosage)

Fluoxetine (Non-proprietary) PoM

Capsules, fluoxetine (as hydrochloride) 20 mg, net price 30-cap pack = £1.38; 60 mg, 30-cap pack = £47.61. Counselling, driving
Brands include *Oxactin®*

Liquid, fluoxetine (as hydrochloride) 20 mg/5 mL, net price 70 mL = £10.12. Counselling, driving

Prozac® (Lilly) PoM

Capsules, fluoxetine (as hydrochloride) 20 mg (green/yellow), net price 30-cap pack = £14.21; 60 mg (yellow), 30-cap pack = £47.61. Counselling, driving

Liquid, fluoxetine (as hydrochloride) 20 mg/5 mL, net price 70 mL = £13.26. Counselling, driving

FLUVOXAMINE MALEATE

Cautions see notes above

Hepatic impairment reduce dose

Renal impairment start with smaller dose in moderate renal impairment

Pregnancy manufacturers advise use only if potential benefit outweighs risk; risk of neonatal withdrawal

Breast-feeding present in milk—manufacturer advises avoid

CSM advice The CSM has advised that concomitant use of fluvoxamine and theophylline or aminophylline should usually be avoided; see also **interactions:** Appendix 1 (antidepressants, SSRIs)

Contra-indications see notes above

Side-effects see notes above; palpitation, tachycardia (may also cause bradycardia); *rarely* postural hypotension, confusion, ataxia, paraesthesia, malaise, taste disturbance, neuroleptic malignant syndrome-like event, abnormal liver function tests, usually symptomatic (discontinue treatment)

Indication and dose

Obsessive-compulsive disorder
- **By mouth**

Child 8–18 years initially 25 mg daily increased if necessary in steps of 25 mg every 4–7 days according to response (total daily doses above 50 mg in 2 divided doses); max. 100 mg twice daily

Note If no improvement in obsessive-compulsive disorder within 10 weeks, treatment should be reconsidered

FLUVOXAMINE MALEATE (*continued*)

Fluvoxamine (Non-proprietary) PoM
Tablets, fluvoxamine maleate 50 mg, net price 60-tab pack = £9.17; 100 mg, 30-tab pack = £9.65. Counselling, driving

Faverin® (Solvay) PoM
Tablets, f/c, scored, fluvoxamine maleate 50 mg, net price 60-tab pack = £17.10; 100 mg, 30-tab pack = £17.10. Counselling, driving

SERTRALINE

Cautions see notes above; renal impairment

Hepatic impairment reduce dose in mild or moderate hepatic impairment; avoid in severe impairment

Pregnancy manufacturers advise use only if potential benefit outweighs risk; risk of neonatal withdrawal

Breast-feeding present in milk but not known to be harmful in short-term use

Contra-indications see notes above

Side-effects see notes above; tachycardia, postural hypotension, confusion, amnesia, aggressive behaviour, psychosis, pancreatitis, hepatitis, jaundice, liver failure, menstrual irregularities, paraesthesia; thrombocytopenia also reported (causal relationship not established)

Licensed use not licensed for use in children for depression

Indication and dose

Obsessive-compulsive disorder
- By mouth

Child 6–12 years initially 25 mg daily increased to 50 mg daily after 1 week, further increased if necessary in steps of 50 mg at intervals of at least 1 week; max. 200 mg daily

Child 12–18 years initially 50 mg daily increased if necessary in steps of 50 mg over several weeks; usual range 50–200 mg daily

Major depression
- By mouth

Child 12–18 years initially 50 mg once daily increased if necessary in steps of 50 mg daily at intervals of at least a week; max. 200 mg once daily

Sertraline (Non-proprietary) PoM
Tablets, sertraline (as hydrochloride) 50 mg, net price 28-tab pack = £17.82; 100 mg, 28-tab pack = £29.16. Counselling, driving

Lustral® (Pfizer) PoM
Tablets, both f/c, sertraline (as hydrochloride) 50 mg (scored), net price 28-tab pack = £17.82; 100 mg, 28-tab pack = £29.16. Counselling, driving

Central nervous system 4

4.3.4 Other antidepressant drugs

Classification not used in *BNF for Children*.

4.4 CNS stimulants and other drugs for attention deficit hyperactivity disorder

Methylphenidate is used for the management of *attention deficit hyperactivity disorder* (ADHD) in children and adolescents as part of a comprehensive treatment programme. Growth is not generally affected but it is advisable to monitor growth during treatment. Modified-release methylphenidate preparations are given once daily, avoiding the need for a dose to be given during school hours.

Dexamfetamine (dexamphetamine) is an alternative in children who do not respond to methylphenidate.

Atomoxetine, a selective noradrenaline reuptake inhibitor, is licensed for the management of attention deficit hyperactivity disorder in children. The long-term safety of atomoxetine has not yet been established.

A tricyclic antidepressant such as **imipramine** (section 4.3.1) is sometimes used in the treatment of ADHD; it should not be prescribed concomitantly with a CNS stimulant.

Drug treatment of attention deficit hyperactivity disorder should be initiated by a specialist in ADHD but may be continued by general practitioners, under a shared-care arrangement. Treatment often needs to be continued into adolescence, and may need to be continued into adulthood.

ATOMOXETINE

Cautions cardiovascular disease including hypertension, tachycardia, and postural hypotension; monitor growth; QT-interval prolongation (avoid concomitant administration of drugs that prolong QT-interval); history of seizures; **interactions**: Appendix 1 (atomoxetine)

Hepatic disorders Following rare reports of hepatic disorders, the CSM has advised that children and carers should be advised of the risk and be told how to recognise symptoms; prompt medical attention should be sought in case of abdominal pain, unexplained nausea, malaise, darkening of the urine or jaundice

Suicidal ideation Following reports of suicidal thoughts and behaviour, CSM has advised that patients and their carers should be informed about the risk and told to report clinical worsening, suicidal thoughts or behaviour, irritability, agitation, or depression

Hepatic impairment see hepatic disorders above; also halve dose in moderate liver disease; quarter dose in severe liver disease

Pregnancy no information available; manufacturer advises avoid unless potential benefit outweighs risk

Breast-feeding manufacturer advises avoid—present in milk in *animal* studies

Side-effects anorexia, dry mouth, nausea, vomiting, abdominal pain, constipation, dyspepsia, flatulence; palpitation, tachycardia, increased blood pressure, postural hypotension, hot flushes; sleep disturbance, dizziness, headache, fatigue, lethargy, depression, anxiety, irritability, tremor, rigors; urinary retention, prostatitis, sexual dysfunction, menstrual disturbances; mydriasis, conjunctivitis; dermatitis, pruritus, rash, sweating; *less commonly* cold extremities; *very rarely* hepatic disorders (see Hepatic Disorders above), seizures, and suicidal ideation

Indication and dose

Attention deficit hyperactivity disorder (initiated by a specialist physician experienced in managing the condition)

• By mouth

Child over 6 years (body-weight under 70 kg) initially 500 micrograms/kg daily for 7 days then increased according to response to usual maintenance dose 1.2 mg/kg daily (higher dose unlikely to be beneficial)

Child (body-weight over 70 kg) initially 40 mg daily for 7 days then increased according to response to usual maintenance dose 80 mg daily; max. 100 mg daily

Note Total daily dose may be given *either* as a single dose in the morning *or* in 2 divided doses with last dose no later than early evening

Strattera (Lilly) ▼ PoM

Capsules, atomoxetine (as hydrochloride) 10 mg (white), net price 7-cap pack = £13.65, 28-cap pack = £54.60; 18 mg (gold/white), 7-cap pack = £13.65, 28-cap pack = £54.60; 25 mg (blue/white), 7-cap pack = £13.65, 28-cap pack = £54.60; 40 mg (blue), 7-cap pack = £13.65, 28-cap pack = £54.60; 60 mg (blue/gold), 28-cap pack = £54.60. Label: 3

DEXAMFETAMINE SULPHATE

(Dexamphetamine sulphate)

Cautions mild hypertension (contra-indicated if moderate or severe)—monitor blood pressure; history of epilepsy (discontinue if convulsions occur); tics and Tourette syndrome (use with caution)—discontinue if tics occur; monitor growth (see also below); psychotic children—may exacerbate behavioural disturbances and thought disorder; avoid abrupt withdrawal; data on safety and efficacy of long-term use not complete; porphyria (see section 9.8.2); **interactions:** Appendix 1 (sympathomimetics)

Growth restriction Monitor height and weight as growth restriction may occur during prolonged therapy (drug-free periods may allow catch-up in growth but withdraw slowly to avoid inducing depression or renewed hyperactivity).

Contra-indications cardiovascular disease including moderate to severe hypertension, hyperexcitability or agitated states, hyperthyroidism, history of drug or alcohol abuse, glaucoma

Skilled tasks May affect performance of skilled tasks (e.g. driving); effects of alcohol unpredictable

Pregnancy manufacturer advises avoid (retrospective evidence of uncertain significance suggesting possible embryotoxicity)

Breast-feeding significant amount in milk—avoid

Side-effects insomnia, restlessness, irritability and excitability, nervousness, night terrors, euphoria, tremor, dizziness, headache; convulsions (see also Cautions); dependence and tolerance, sometimes psychosis; anorexia, gastro-intestinal symptoms, growth retardation (see also under Cautions); dry mouth, sweating, tachycardia (and anginal pain), palpitation, increased blood pressure; visual disturbances; cardiomyopathy reported with chronic use; central stimulants have provoked choreoathetoid movements, tics and Tourette syndrome in predisposed individuals (see also Cautions above); **overdosage:** see Emergency Treatment of Poisoning, p. 42

Indication and dose

Hyperkinesia initiated by specialist physician experienced in managing the condition

• By mouth

Child 4–6 years initially 2.5 mg once daily, increased if necessary by 2.5 mg at intervals of 1 week according to response; usual max. 20 mg daily

Child 6–18 years initially 5–10 mg once daily, increased if necessary by 5 mg at intervals of 1 week according to response; usual max. 20 mg daily, up to 40 mg may occasionally be required

Administration tablets can be halved

Dexedrine® (Celltech) CD

Tablets, scored, dexamfetamine sulphate 5 mg. Net price 28-tab pack = £3.00. Counselling, driving

4 Central nervous system

METHYLPHENIDATE HYDROCHLORIDE

Cautions monitor growth (if prolonged treatment), blood pressure and full blood count; history of drug or alcohol dependence; psychosis; epilepsy (discontinue if increased seizure frequency); avoid abrupt withdrawal; **interactions:** Appendix 1 (sympathomimetics)

Pregnancy limited experience—manufacturer advises avoid unless potential benefit outweighs risk; toxicity in *animals*

Contra-indications anxiety or agitation; tics or a family history of Tourette syndrome; hyperthyroidism, cardiac arrhythmias, glaucoma

Breast-feeding no information available—manufacturer advises avoid

Side-effects abdominal pain, nausea, vomiting, dry mouth; tachycardia, palpitation, arrhythmias, changes in blood pressure; insomnia, nervousness, anorexia, headache, drowsiness, dizziness, movement disorders; arthralgia; rash, pruritus, alopecia; *rarely* cerebral arteritis, angina, hyperactivity, convulsions, psychosis, tics including Tourette syndrome, neuroleptic malignant syndrome, tolerance and dependence, growth restriction, reduced weight gain, blood disorders including leucopenia and thrombocytopenia, muscle cramps, visual disturbances, exfoliative dermatitis, erythema multiforme

Licensed use not licensed for use in children under 6 years

Indication and dose

Attention deficit hyperactivity disorder (initiated by specialist physician experienced in managing the condition)

- **By mouth**

  Child 4–6 years 2.5 mg twice daily increased if necessary (max. 1.4 mg/kg daily); discontinue if no response after 1 month, suspend every 1–2 years to assess child's condition

  Child over 6 years initially 5 mg 1–2 times daily, increased if necessary at weekly intervals by 5–10 mg daily to max. 60 mg daily in divided doses; discontinue if no response after 1 month, suspend every 1–2 years to assess child's condition

  Evening dose If effect wears off in evening (with rebound hyperactivity) a dose at bedtime may be appropriate (establish need with trial bedtime dose)

Administration *Equasym®* and *Ritalin®* tablets may be halved

Methylphenidate Hydrochloride (Non-proprietary) CD

Tablets, methylphenidate hydrochloride 5 mg, net price 30-tab pack = £2.78; 10 mg, 30-tab pack = £5.17; 20 mg, 30-tab pack = £9.98

Brands include *Equasym®*

Ritalin® (Novartis) CD

Tablets, scored, methylphenidate hydrochloride 10 mg, net price 30-tab pack = £5.57

Modified release

Concerta® XL (Janssen-Cilag) CD

Tablets, m/r, methylphenidate hydrochloride 18 mg (yellow), net price 30-tab pack = £27.00; 36 mg (white), 30-tab pack = £36.75. Label: 25

Counselling Tablet membrane may pass through gastro-intestinal tract unchanged

Cautions dose form not appropriate for use in dysphagia or where gastro-intestinal lumen restricted

Dose

- **By mouth**

  Child 6–18 years initially 18 mg once daily (in the morning), increased if necessary in weekly steps of 18 mg according to response, max. 54 mg once daily; discontinue if no response after 1 month; suspend every 1–2 years to assess condition

  Note Total daily dose of 15 mg of standard-release formulation is considered equivalent to *Concerta® XL* 18 mg once daily

Equasym XL® (UCB Pharma) CD

Capsules, m/r, methylphenidate hydrochloride 10 mg (white/green), net price 30-cap pack = £25.00; 20 mg (white/blue), 30-cap pack = £30.00; 30 mg (white/brown), 30-cap pack = £35.00. Label: 25

Dose

- **By mouth**

  Child 6–18 years initially 10 mg once daily in the morning before breakfast, increased gradually if necessary to max. 60 mg daily; discontinue if no response after 1 month; suspend every 1–2 years to assess condition

4.5 Drugs used in the treatment of obesity

Classification not used in *BNF for Children*.

4.6 Drugs used in nausea and vertigo

Anti-emetics should be prescribed only when the cause of vomiting is known because otherwise they may delay diagnosis. Anti-emetics are unnecessary and sometimes harmful when the cause can be treated, such as in diabetic ketoacidosis, or in digoxin or antiepileptic overdose.

If anti-emetic drug treatment is indicated, the drug is chosen according to the aetiology of vomiting.

Antihistamines are effective against nausea and vomiting resulting from many underlying conditions. There is no evidence that any one antihistamine is superior to another but their duration of action and incidence of adverse effects (drowsiness and antimuscarinic effects) differ.

The **phenothiazines** are dopamine antagonists and act centrally by blocking the chemoreceptor trigger zone. They may be considered for the prophylaxis and treatment of nausea and vomiting associated with diffuse neoplastic disease, radiation sickness, and the emesis caused by drugs such as opioids, general anaesthetics, and cytotoxics. **Prochlorperazine**, **perphenazine**, and **trifluoperazine** are less sedating than **chlorpromazine**; severe dystonic reactions sometimes occur with phenothiazines (see below). Other antipsychotic drugs including **haloperidol** and **levomepromazine** (**methotrimeprazine**) (section 4.2.1) are also used for the relief of nausea in palliative care (see p. 27 and p. 28). Some phenothiazines are available as rectal suppositories, which can be useful in children with persistent vomiting or with severe nausea; for children over 12 years prochlorperazine can also be administered as a buccal tablet which is placed between the upper lip and the gum.

Metoclopramide is an effective anti-emetic and its activity closely resembles that of the phenothiazines. Metoclopramide also acts directly on the gastro-intestinal tract and it may be superior to the phenothiazines for emesis associated with gastroduodenal, hepatic, and biliary disease. In postoperative nausea and vomiting, metoclopramide has limited efficacy. For the role of metoclopramide in cytotoxic-induced nausea and vomiting see section 8.1.

> Acute dystonic reactions
> Phenothiazines and metoclopramide can all induce acute dystonic reactions such as facial and skeletal muscle spasms and oculogyric crises; children (especially girls, young women, and those under 10 kg) are particularly susceptible. With metoclopramide, dystonic effects usually occur shortly after starting treatment and subside within 24 hours of stopping it. An antimuscarinic drug such as procyclidine (section 4.9.2) is used to abort dystonic attacks.

Domperidone acts at the chemoreceptor trigger zone; it has the advantage over metoclopramide and the phenothiazines of being less likely to cause central effects such as sedation and dystonic reactions because it does not readily cross the blood-brain barrier. For the role of domperidone in cytotoxic-induced nausea and vomiting see section 8.1. Domperidone is also used to treat vomiting due to emergency hormonal contraception (BNF section 7.3.1).

Granisetron, **ondansetron**, and **tropisetron** are specific $5HT_3$ antagonists which block $5HT_3$ receptors in the gastro-intestinal tract and in the CNS. They are of value in the management of nausea and vomiting in children receiving cytotoxics and in postoperative nausea and vomiting.

Nabilone is a synthetic cannabinoid with anti-emetic properties. It may be used for nausea and vomiting caused by cytotoxic chemotherapy that is unresponsive to conventional anti-emetics. Side-effects such as drowsiness and dizziness occur frequently with standard doses.

Dexamethasone (section 6.3.2) has anti-emetic effects. For the role of dexamethasone in cytotoxic-induced nausea and vomiting see section 8.1.

Vomiting of pregnancy

Nausea in the first trimester of pregnancy is generally mild and does not require drug therapy. On rare occasions if vomiting is severe, short-term treatment with an antihistamine, such as **promethazine**, may be required. **Prochlorperazine** or **metoclopramide** may be considered as second-line treatments. If symptoms do not settle in 24 to 48 hours then specialist opinion should be sought. Hyperemesis gravidarum is a more serious condition, which requires intravenous fluid and electrolyte replacement and sometimes nutritional support. Supplementation with thiamine must be considered in order to reduce the risk of Wernicke's encephalopathy.

Postoperative nausea and vomiting

The incidence of postoperative nausea and vomiting depends on many factors including the anaesthetic used, and the type and duration of surgery. The aim is to prevent postoperative nausea and vomiting from occurring. Drugs used include some **phenothiazines** (e.g. prochlorperazine), **metoclopramide**, **$5HT_3$ antagonists**, **antihistamines** (such as cyclizine), and **dexamethasone**. A combination of two anti-emetic drugs acting at different sites may be needed in resistant post-operative nausea and vomiting.

Opioid induced nausea and vomiting

Cyclizine, ondansetron, and prochlorperazine are used to relieve opioid-induced nausea and vomiting; ondansetron has the advantage of not producing sedation.

Motion sickness

Anti-emetics should be given to prevent motion sickness rather than after nausea or vomiting develop. The most effective drug for the prevention of motion sickness is **hyoscine hydrobromide**. For children over 10 years old, a transdermal hyoscine patch provides prolonged activity but it needs to be applied several hours before travelling. The sedating antihistamines are slightly less effective against motion sickness, but are generally better tolerated than hyoscine. If a sedative effect is desired **promethazine** is useful, but generally a slightly less sedating antihistamine such as **cyclizine** or **cinnarizine** is preferred. The $5HT_3$ antagonists, domperidone, metoclopramide, and the phenothiazines (except the antihistamine phenothiazine promethazine) are **ineffective** in motion sickness.

Other vestibular disorders

Management of vestibular diseases is aimed at treating the underlying cause as well as treating symptoms of the balance disturbance and associated nausea and vomiting.

Antihistamines (such as cinnarizine), and **phenothiazines** (such as prochlorperazine) are effective for prophylaxis and treatment of nausea and vertigo resulting from vestibular disorders; however, when nausea and vertigo are associated with middle ear surgery, treatment can be difficult.

Cytotoxic chemotherapy

For the management of nausea and vomiting induced by cytotoxic chemotherapy, see section 8.1.

Palliative care

For the management of nausea and vomiting in palliative care, see p. 27 and p. 28.

Migraine

For the management of nausea and vomiting associated with migraine, see p. 251

Antihistamines

CINNARIZINE

Cautions see section 3.4.1

Hepatic impairment sedation inappropriate in severe liver disease—avoid

Contra-indications see section 3.4.1

Side-effects see section 3.4.1; also *rarely* weight gain, sweating, lichen planus, and lupus-like skin reactions

Indication and dose

Relief of symptoms of vestibular disorders
- By mouth

Child 5–12 years 15 mg 3 times daily

Child 12–18 years 30 mg 3 times daily

Motion sickness
- By mouth

Child 5–12 years 15 mg 2 hours before travel then 7.5 mg every 8 hours during journey if necessary

Child 12–18 years 30 mg 2 hours before travel then 15 mg every 8 hours during journey if necessary

Cinnarizine (Non-proprietary)

Tablets, cinnarizine 15 mg, net price 84-tab pack = £7.43. Label: 2

Brands include *Cinazière*®

Stugeron® (Janssen-Cilag)

Tablets, scored, cinnarizine 15 mg, net price 15-tab pack = £1.48, 100-tab pack = £3.56. Label: 2

4 Central nervous system

CYCLIZINE

Cautions see section 3.4.1; severe heart failure; may counteract haemodynamic benefits of opioids; **interactions:** Appendix 1 (antihistamines)

Hepatic impairment sedation inappropriate in severe liver disease—avoid

Skilled tasks Drowsiness may affect performance of skilled tasks (e.g. driving); effects of alcohol enhanced

Contra-indications see section 3.4.1

Side-effects see section 3.4.1

Licensed use tablets not licensed for use in children under 6 years; injection not licensed for use in children

Indication and dose

Nausea and vomiting of known cause; nausea and vomiting associated with vestibular disorders

- **By mouth or by intravenous injection**

Child 1 month–6 years 0.5–1 mg/kg up to 3 times daily; max. single dose 25 mg

Child 6–18 years 0.5–1 mg/kg up to 3 times daily; max. single dose 50 mg

- **By rectum**

Child 2–6 years 12.5 mg up to 3 times daily

Child 6–12 years 25 mg up to 3 times daily

Child 12 years–18 years 50 mg up to 3 times daily

Valoid® (Amdipharm)

Tablets, scored, cyclizine hydrochloride 50 mg. Net price 20 = £1.44. Label: 2

Injection (PoM), cyclizine lactate 50 mg/mL. Net price 1-mL amp = 70p

Cyclizine (Non-proprietary)

Suppositories, 12.5 mg, 25 mg, 50 mg, 100 mg. Available on a named patient basis as manufactured special

MECLOZINE HYDROCHLORIDE

Cautions see section 3.4.1; **interactions:** Appendix 1 (antihistamines)

Hepatic impairment sedation inappropriate in severe liver disease—avoid

Skilled tasks Drowsiness may affect performance of skilled tasks (e.g. driving); effects of alcohol enhanced

Contra-indications see section 3.4.1

Side-effects see section 3.4.1

Indication and dose

Prevention and treatment of motion sickness

- **By mouth**

Child 2–6 years 6.25 mg as a single dose one hour before travel

Child 6–12 years 12.5 mg as a single dose one hour before travel

Child 12–18 years 25 mg as a single dose one hour before travel

Preparations

A proprietary brand of meclozine hydrochloride tablets 12.5 mg (*Sea-legs®*) is on sale to the public for motion sickness

PROMETHAZINE HYDROCHLORIDE

Cautions see section 3.4.1

Contra-indications see section 3.4.1

Side-effects see section 3.4.1 but more sedating

Indication and dose

Motion sickness prevention

- **By mouth**

Child 2–5 years 5 mg at bedtime on night before travel, repeat following morning if necessary

Child 5–10 years 10 mg at bedtime on night before travel, repeat following morning if necessary

Child 10–18 years 20–25 mg at bedtime on night before travel, repeat following morning if necessary

Preparations

Section 3.4.1

PROMETHAZINE TEOCLATE

Cautions see section 3.4.1

Contra-indications see section 3.4.1

Side-effects see section 3.4.1

Indication and dose

Nausea, vomiting, labyrinthine disorders

- **By mouth**

Child 5–10 years 12.5–37.5 mg daily

Child 10–18 years 25–75 mg daily (max. 100 mg)

Motion sickness prevention

- **By mouth**

Child 5–10 years 12.5 mg at bedtime on night before travel *or* 12.5 mg 1–2 hours before travel

Child 10–18 years 25 mg at bedtime on night before travel *or* 25 mg 1–2 hours before travel

PROMETHAZINE TEOCLATE (*continued*)

Severe vomiting in pregnancy
- By mouth

25 mg at bedtime increased if necessary to max. 100 mg daily (but see also Vomiting of Pregnancy in notes above)

Avomine® (Manx)
Tablets, scored, promethazine teoclate 25 mg. Net price 10-tab pack = £1.13; 28-tab pack = £3.13. Label: 2

Phenothiazines and related drugs

CHLORPROMAZINE HYDROCHLORIDE

Cautions see Chlorpromazine Hydrochloride, section 4.2.1

Contra-indications see Chlorpromazine Hydrochloride, section 4.2.1

Side-effects see Chlorpromazine Hydrochloride, section 4.2.1

Indication and dose

Nausea and vomiting of terminal illness (where other drugs are unsuitable)
- By mouth

Child 1–12 years 500 micrograms/kg every 4–6 hours (1–5 years, max. 40 mg daily, 6–12 years max. 75 mg daily)

Child 12–18 years 10–25 mg every 4–6 hours
- By deep intramuscular injection

Child 1–12 years 500 micrograms/kg every 6–8 hours (1–5 years, max. 40 mg daily, 6–12 years max. 75 mg daily)

Child 12–18 years initially 25 mg then 25–50 mg every 3–4 hours until vomiting stops

Preparations
Section 4.2.1

PERPHENAZINE

Cautions see Perphenazine, section 4.2.1

Contra-indications see Perphenazine, section 4.2.1

Side-effects see Perphenazine, section 4.2.1; extrapyramidal symptoms

Indication and dose

Severe nausea and vomiting unresponsive to other anti-emetics
- By mouth

Child 14–18 years 4 mg 3 times daily, adjusted according to response, max. 24 mg daily

Preparations
Section 4.2.1

PROCHLORPERAZINE

Cautions see notes above and section 4.2.1; hypotension more likely after intramuscular injection

Contra-indications see notes above and section 4.2.1

Side-effects see notes above and section 4.2.1; extrapyramidal symptoms, particularly dystonias, more frequent; respiratory depression may occur in susceptible patients

Licensed use injection not licensed for use in children; suppositories not licensed for use in children under 12 years

Indication and dose

Prevention and treatment of nausea and vomiting
- By mouth

Child 1–5 years and over 10 kg 1.25–2.5 mg, repeated if necessary up to 3 times daily

Child 5–12 years 2.5–5 mg, repeated if necessary up to 3 times daily

Child 12–18 years 5–10 mg, repeated if necessary up to 3 times daily
- By rectum

Child 1–5 years and over 10 kg 2.5 mg, repeated if necessary up to 3 times daily

Child 5–12 years 5–10 mg, repeated if necessary up to 3 times daily

Child 12–18 years 12.5–25 mg, repeated if necessary up to 3 times daily
- By intramuscular injection

Child 2–5 years, 1.25–2.5 mg, repeated if necessary up to 3 times daily

Child 5–12 years 5–6.25 mg, repeated if necessary up to 3 times daily

Child 12–18 years 12.5 mg, repeated if necessary up to 3 times daily

Note Doses are expressed as prochlorperazine maleate or mesilate; 1 mg prochlorperazine maleate ≡ 1 mg prochlorperazine mesilate

Prochlorperazine (Non-proprietary) PoM
Tablets, prochlorperazine maleate 5 mg, net price 20 = 98p. Label: 2
Brands include *Prozière®*

4 Central nervous system

PROCHLORPERAZINE (*continued*)

Stemetil® (Castlemead) PoM
Tablets, prochlorperazine maleate 5 mg (off-white), net price 84-tab pack = £6.18; 25 mg (scored), 56-tab pack = £10.91. Label: 2

Syrup, straw-coloured, prochlorperazine mesilate 5 mg/5 mL. Net price 100-mL pack = £3.48. Label: 2

Eff (= effervescent granules), sugar-free, prochlorperazine mesilate 5 mg/sachet. Net price 21-sachet pack = £6.46. Label: 2, 13
Excipients: include aspartame (section 9.4.1)

Injection, prochlorperazine mesilate 12.5 mg/mL. Net price 1-mL amp = 56p

Suppositories, prochlorperazine maleate (as prochlorperazine), 5 mg, net price 10 = £8.74; 25 mg, 10 = £11.46. Label: 2

Buccal preparation

Buccastem® (R&C) PoM
Tablets (buccal), pale yellow, prochlorperazine maleate 3 mg. Net price 5 × 10-tab pack = £5.75. Label: 2, counselling, administration, see under Dose below

Dose

- By mouth
  Child 12–18 years 1–2 tablets twice daily; tablets are placed high between upper lip and gum and left to dissolve

TRIFLUOPERAZINE

Cautions see Trifluoperazine section 4.2.1

Contra-indications see Trifluoperazine section 4.2.1

Side-effects see Trifluoperazine section 4.2.1; extrapyramidal symptoms

Indication and dose

Severe nausea and vomiting unresponsive to other anti-emetics
- **By mouth**
  Child 3–5 years up to 500 micrograms twice daily
  Child 6–12 years up to 2 mg twice daily
  Child 12–18 years 1–2 mg twice daily; max. 3 mg twice daily

Preparations

Section 4.2.1

Domperidone and metoclopramide

DOMPERIDONE

Cautions not recommended for routine prophylaxis of post-operative vomiting or for chronic administration; **interactions:** Appendix 1 (domperidone)

Renal impairment manufacturer advises reduce dose in renal impairment

Pregnancy manufacturer advises avoid

Breast-feeding amount probably too small to be harmful

Contra-indications

Hepatic impairment avoid

Side-effects rarely gastro-intestinal disturbances (including cramps), raised prolactin concentrations, extrapyramidal effects and rashes reported

Indication and dose

Nausea and vomiting
- **By mouth**
  Child over 2 years
  Body-weight up to 35 kg 250–500 micrograms/kg 3–4 times daily; max. 2.4 mg/kg in 24 hours
  Body-weight 35 kg and over 10–20 mg 3–4 times daily, max. 80 mg daily
- **By rectum**
  Child over 2 years
  Body-weight 15–35 kg 30 mg twice daily
  Body-weight over 35 kg 60 mg twice daily

Gastro-intestinal stasis section 1.2

Domperidone (Non-proprietary) PoM
Tablets, 10 mg (as maleate), net price 30-tab pack = £2.47; 100-tab pack = £4.55

Motilium® (Winthrop) PoM
Tablets, f/c, domperidone 10 mg (as maleate). Net price 30-tab pack = £2.35; 100-tab pack = £7.84

Suspension, sugar-free, domperidone 5 mg/5 mL. Net price 200-mL pack = £1.80

Suppositories domperidone 30 mg. Net price 10 = £2.65

METOCLOPRAMIDE HYDROCHLORIDE

Cautions may mask underlying disorders such as cerebral irritation; epilepsy; porphyria (section 9.8.2); **interactions**: Appendix 1 (metoclopramide)

Hepatic impairment reduce dose

Renal impairment avoid or use small dose; increased risk of extrapyramidal reactions in severe impairment

Pregnancy not known to be harmful but manufacturer advises use only when compelling reasons

Contra-indications gastro-intestinal obstruction, perforation or haemorrhage; 3–4 days after gastro-intestinal surgery; phaeochromocytoma

Breast-feeding small amount present in milk; manufacturer advises avoid large single doses

Side-effects extrapyramidal effects (see p. 227), hyperprolactinaemia, occasionally tardive dyskinesia on prolonged administration; also reported, drowsiness, restlessness, diarrhoea, depression, neuroleptic malignant syndrome, rashes, pruritus, oedema; cardiac conduction abnormalities reported following intravenous administration; rarely methaemoglobinaemia (more severe in G6PD deficiency)

Licensed use not licensed for use in neonates

Indication and dose

Severe intractable vomiting of known cause, vomiting associated with radiotherapy and cytotoxics, aid to gastro-intestinal intubation, as a prokinetic in neonates

- By mouth, or by intramuscular injection or by intravenous injection over 1–2 minutes

Neonate 100 micrograms/kg every 6–8 hours (by mouth or by intravenous injection only)

Child 1 month–1 year and body-weight up to 10 kg 100 micrograms/kg (max. 1 mg) twice daily

Child 1–3 years and body-weight 10–14 kg 1 mg 2–3 times daily

Child 3–5 years and body-weight 15–19 kg 2 mg 2–3 times daily

Child 5–9 years and body-weight 20–29 kg 2.5 mg 3 times daily

Child 9–18 years and body-weight 30–60 kg 5 mg 3 times daily

Child 15–18 years and body-weight over 60 kg 10 mg 3 times daily

Note Daily dose of metoclopramide should not normally exceed 500 micrograms/kg

Pre-medication in diagnostic procedures

- By mouth as a single dose 5–10 minutes before examination

Child 1 month–3 years and body-weight up to 14 kg 100 micrograms/kg, max. 1 mg

Child 3–5 years and body-weight 15–19 kg 2 mg

Child 5–9 years and body-weight 20–29 kg 2.5 mg

Child 9–15 years and body-weight 30–60 kg 5 mg

Child 15–18 years and body-weight over 60 kg 10 mg

Metoclopramide (Non-proprietary) PoM

Tablets, metoclopramide hydrochloride 10 mg, net price 28-tab pack = 87p

Oral solution, metoclopramide hydrochloride 5 mg/5 mL, net price 100-mL pack = £2.55

Note Sugar-free versions are available and can be ordered by specifying 'sugar-free' on the prescription

Injection, metoclopramide hydrochloride 5 mg/mL, net price 2-mL amp = 26p

Maxolon® (Shire) PoM

Tablets, scored, metoclopramide hydrochloride 10 mg, net price 84-tab pack = £5.24

Syrup, sugar-free, metoclopramide hydrochloride 5 mg/5 mL. Net price 200-mL pack = £3.83

Paediatric liquid, sugar-free, metoclopramide hydrochloride 1 mg/mL. Net price 15-mL pack with pipette = £1.51. Counselling, use of pipette

Injection, metoclopramide hydrochloride 5 mg/mL. Net price 2-mL amp = 27p

Compound preparations (for migraine)

Section 4.7.4.1

$5HT_3$ antagonists

GRANISETRON

Cautions

Pregnancy manufacturer advises use only when compelling reasons—no information available

Breast-feeding manufacturer advises avoid—no information available

Side-effects constipation, headache, rash; hypersensitivity reactions reported

Licensed use tablets not licensed for use in children under 12 years; sterile solution not licensed for use in children under 2 years

Indication and dose

Treatment and prevention of nausea and vomiting induced by cytotoxic chemotherapy or radiotherapy

- By mouth

Child 1 month–12 years 20 micrograms/kg (max. 1 mg) within 1 hour before start of treatment, then 20 micrograms/kg (max. 1 mg) twice daily for up to 5 days during treatment

GRANISETRON (*continued*)

Child 12–18 years 1–2 mg within 1 hour before start of treatment, then 1 mg twice daily during treatment (total daily dose may alternatively be given as a single dose); when intravenous infusion also used, max. combined total 9 mg in 24 hours

- **By intravenous infusion**

Child 1 month–12 years prevention, 40 micrograms/kg (max. 3 mg) before start of cytotoxic therapy; treatment, 40 micrograms/kg (max. 3 mg) repeated within 24 hours if necessary (not less than 10 minutes after initial dose)

- **By intravenous injection or by intravenous infusion**

Child 12–18 years prevention, 3 mg before start of cytotoxic therapy (up to 2 additional 3-mg doses may be given within 24 hours); treatment, 3 mg repeated if necessary (doses must not be given less than 10 minutes apart), max. 9 mg in 24 hours

Administration for *intravenous infusion*, dilute 3 mL in 10–30 mL Glucose 5% *or* Sodium Chloride 0.9%, *or* Compound Sodium Lactate; give over 5 minutes

Kytril® (Roche) PoM

Tablets, f/c, granisetron (as hydrochloride) 1 mg, net price 10-tab pack = £65.49; 2 mg, 5-tab pack = £65.49

Sterile solution, granisetron (as hydrochloride) 1 mg/mL, for dilution and use as injection or infusion, net price 1-mL amp = £8.60, 3-mL amp = £25.79

ONDANSETRON

Cautions

Hepatic impairment reduce dose; not more than 8 mg daily in severe liver disease

Pregnancy no information available; manufacturer advises avoid unless potential benefit outweighs risk

Breast-feeding manufacturer advises avoid—no information available

Side-effects constipation; headache, sensation of warmth or flushing, hiccups; occasional alterations in liver enzymes; hypersensitivity reactions reported; occasional transient visual disturbances and dizziness following intravenous administration; involuntary movements, seizures, chest pain, arrhythmias, hypotension and bradycardia also reported; suppositories may cause rectal irritation

Licensed use oral and parenteral preparations not licensed for use in children under 2 years; suppositories not licensed for use in children

Indication and dose

Prevention and treatment of chemotherapy- and radiotherapy-induced nausea and vomiting

- **By slow intravenous injection or by intravenous infusion**

Child 1–12 years 5 mg/m² immediately before chemotherapy (max. single dose 8 mg), then **either** repeat every 8–12 hours during chemotherapy and for at least 24 hours afterwards **or** give by mouth

Child 12–18 years 8 mg immediately before chemotherapy, then **either** repeated every 8–12 hours during chemotherapy and for at least 24 hours afterwards **or** give by mouth

- **By mouth following intravenous administration**

Child 1–12 years 4 mg every 8–12 hours for up to 5 days

Child 12–18 years 8 mg every 8–12 hours for up to 5 days

Treatment and prevention of postoperative nausea and vomiting

- **By intramuscular injection or by slow intravenous injection**

Child 2–12 years 100 micrograms/kg (max. 4 mg), as a single dose before, during, or after induction of anaesthesia

Child 12–18 years 4 mg, as a single dose at induction of anaesthesia

Administration for *slow intravenous injection*, give over 2–5 minutes

For *intravenous infusion*, dilute to a concentration of 320–640 micrograms/mL with Glucose 5% *or* Sodium Chloride 0.9% *or* Ringer's Solution; give over at least 15 minutes

Zofran® (GSK) PoM

Tablets, both yellow, f/c, ondansetron (as hydrochloride) 4 mg, net price 30-tab pack = £107.91; 8 mg, 10-tab pack = £71.94

Oral lyophilisates (*Zofran Melt®*), ondansetron 4 mg, net price 10-tab pack = £35.97; 8 mg, 10-tab pack = £71.94. Counselling, administration

Counselling Tablets should be placed on the tongue, allowed to disperse and swallowed

Excipients: include aspartame (section 9.4.1)

Syrup, sugar-free, ondansetron (as hydrochloride) 4 mg/5 mL. Net price 50-mL pack = £35.97

Injection, ondansetron (as hydrochloride) 2 mg/mL, net price 2-mL amp = £5.99; 4-mL amp = £11.99

Suppositories, ondansetron 16 mg. Net price 5 = £14.39

TROPISETRON

Cautions uncontrolled hypertension (has been aggravated by doses higher than recommended); cardiac conduction disorders; arrhythmias, concomitant administration of drugs that prolong QT interval; **interactions:** Appendix 1 (tropisetron)

Pregnancy manufacturer advises toxicity in *animal* studies

Breast-feeding no information available

Skilled tasks Dizziness or drowsiness may affect performance of skilled tasks (e.g. driving)

Side-effects constipation, diarrhoea, abdominal pain; headache, dizziness, fatigue; hypersensitivity reactions reported (including facial flushing, urticaria, chest tightness, dyspnoea, bronchospasm and hypotension); collapse, syncope, bradycardia, cardiovascular collapse also reported (causal relationship not established)

Indication and dose

Prevention of nausea and vomiting induced by cytotoxic chemotherapy

- **By intravenous injection over at least 1 minute or by intravenous infusion**
  Child 2–18 years 200 micrograms/kg (max. 5 mg) shortly before chemotherapy; then if body-weight less than 25 kg, 200 micrograms/kg daily for 4 days, or if body-weight over 25 kg, (by mouth preferably) 5 mg daily for 5 days
- **By mouth following intravenous administration**
  Child 2–18 years and body-weight over 25 kg 5 mg daily for 5 days

Administration For *intravenous infusion*, dilute to a concentration of 50 micrograms/mL in Glucose 5% *or* Sodium Chloride 0.9%, *or* Ringer's Solution; give by intermittent infusion or via drip tubing

Navoban® (Novartis) PoM
Capsules, white/yellow, tropisetron (as hydrochloride) 5 mg, net price 5-cap pack = £53.86; 50-cap pack = £538.60. Label: 23

Injection, tropisetron (as hydrochloride), 1 mg/mL, net price 2-mL amp = £4.86, 5-mL amp = £12.16

Cannabinoid

NABILONE

Cautions history of psychiatric disorder; hypertension; heart disease; adverse effects on mental state can persist for 48–72 hours after stopping; **interactions:** Appendix 1 (nabilone)

Skilled tasks Drowsiness may affect performance of skilled tasks (e.g. driving); effects of alcohol enhanced

Contra-indications

Hepatic impairment avoid in severe hepatic impairment

Pregnancy manufacturer advises avoid unless essential

Breast-feeding no information available—manufacturer advises avoid

Side-effects drowsiness, vertigo, euphoria, dry mouth, ataxia, visual disturbance, concentration difficulties, sleep disturbance, dysphoria, hypotension, headache and nausea; also confusion, disorientation, hallucinations, psychosis, depression, decreased coordination, tremors, tachycardia, decreased appetite, and abdominal pain

Behavioural effects Children and carers should be made aware of possible changes of mood and other adverse behavioural effects

Licensed use not licensed for use in children

Indication and dose

Nausea and vomiting caused by cytotoxic chemotherapy, unresponsive to conventional antiemetics (under close observation, preferably in hospital setting)

- **By mouth**
  Consult local treatment protocol for details

Nabilone (Cambridge) PoM
Capsules, blue/white, nabilone 1 mg. Net price 20-cap pack = £125.84. Label: 2, counselling, behavioural effects

Hyoscine

HYOSCINE HYDROBROMIDE
(Scopolamine Hydrobromide)

Cautions urinary retention, cardiovascular disease, gastro-intestinal obstruction; porphyria (section 9.8.2); **interactions:** Appendix 1 (antimuscarinics)

Skilled tasks Drowsiness may affect performance of skilled tasks (e.g. driving) and may persist for up to 24 hours or longer after removal of patch; effects of alcohol enhanced

Hepatic impairment manufacturer advises caution

Renal impairment manufacturer advises caution

Pregnancy manufacturer advises use only if potential benefit outweighs risk; injection may depress neonatal respiration

Breast-feeding amount too small to be harmful

Contra-indications closed-angle glaucoma

Side-effects drowsiness, dry mouth, dizziness, blurred vision, difficulty with micturition

4 Central nervous system

☐ **HYOSCINE HYDROBROMIDE (*continued*)**

Licensed use not licensed for use in excessive respiratory secretions

Indication and dose

Motion sickness

- **By mouth**

Child 3–4 years 75 micrograms 20 minutes before start of journey, repeated if necessary; max. 150 micrograms in 24 hours

Child 4–10 years 75–150 micrograms 30 minutes before start of journey, repeated every 6 hours if required; max. 3 doses in 24 hours

Child 10–18 years 150–300 micrograms 30 minutes before start of journey, repeated every 6 hours if required; max. 3 doses in 24 hours

Note Proprietary brands of hyoscine hydrobromide tablets (*Joy-rides®*, *Kwells®*) are on sale to the public for motion sickness

- **By topical application**

Child 10–18 years apply 1 patch (1 mg) to hairless area of skin behind ear 5–6 hours before journey; replace if necessary after 72 hours, siting replacement patch behind the other ear

Premedication

see section 15.1.3

Excessive respiratory secretions

- **By mouth or by sublingual administration**

Child 2–12 years 10 micrograms/kg, max. 300 micrograms 4 times daily

Child 12–18 years 300 micrograms 4 times daily

- **By application of patch to skin**

Child 1 month–3 years 250 micrograms every 72 hours (quarter of a patch)

Child 3–10 years 500 micrograms every 72 hours (half a patch)

Child 10–18 years 1 mg every 72 hours (one patch)

- **By subcutaneous injection, intravenous injection, intravenous infusion, or subcutaneous infusion**

See Prescribing in Palliative Care, p. 26 and p. 28

Administration *patch* applied to hairless area of skin behind ear; if less than whole patch required **either** cut with scissors along full thickness ensuring membrane is not peeled away **or** cover portion to prevent contact with skin

For administration *by mouth*, injection solution may be given orally

Scopoderm TTS® (Novartis Consumer Health) PoM

Patch, self-adhesive, pink, releasing hyoscine approx. 1 mg/72 hours when in contact with skin. Net price 2 = £4.30.Label: 19, counselling, see below

Counselling Explain accompanying instructions to patient and in particular emphasise advice to wash hands after handling and to wash application site after removing, and to use one patch at a time

Note The brand name *Scopoderm®* is used for a hyoscine patch that is available for sale to the public

4.7 Analgesics

The non-opioid drugs (section 4.7.1), paracetamol and ibuprofen (and other NSAIDs), are particularly suitable for pain in musculoskeletal conditions, whereas the opioid analgesics (section 4.7.2) are more suitable for moderate to severe pain, particularly of visceral origin.

Pain in palliative care For advice on pain relief in palliative care see p. 24.

Pain in sickle-cell disease The pain of mild sickle-cell crises is managed with paracetamol, an NSAID, codeine, or dihydrocodeine. Severe crises may require the use of morphine or diamorphine; concomitant use of an NSAID may potentiate analgesia and allow lower doses of the opioid to be used. A mixture of nitrous oxide and oxygen (*Entonox®*, *Equanox®*) may also be used.

Dental and orofacial pain Analgesics should be used judiciously in dental care as a **temporary** measure until the cause of the pain has been dealt with.

Dental pain of inflammatory origin, such as that associated with pulpitis, apical infection, localised osteitis (dry socket) or pericoronitis is usually best managed by treating the infection, providing drainage, restorative procedures, and other local measures. Analgesics provide temporary relief of pain (usually for about 1 to 7 days) until the causative factors have been brought under control. In the case of pulpitis, intra-osseous infection or abscess, reliance on analgesics alone is usually inappropriate.

Similarly the pain and discomfort associated with acute problems of the oral mucosa (e.g. acute herpetic gingivostomatitis, erythema multiforme) may be relieved by **benzydamine** (see p. 602) or topical anaesthetics until the cause of the mucosal disorder has been dealt with. However, where a child is febrile, the antipyretic action of **paracetamol** (see p. 237) or **ibuprofen** (see p. 551) is often helpful.

The *choice* of an analgesic for dental purposes should be based on its suitability for the child. Most dental pain is relieved effectively by non-steroidal anti-inflammatory drugs (NSAIDs) e.g. ibuprofen (section 10.1.1). **Paracetamol** has analgesic and antipyretic effects but no anti-inflammatory effect.

Opioid analgesics (section 4.7.2) such as **dihydrocodeine** act on the central nervous system and are traditionally used for *moderate to severe pain*. However, opioid analgesics are relatively ineffective in dental pain and their side-effects can be unpleasant.

Combining a non-opioid with an opioid analgesic can provide greater relief of pain than a non-opioid analgesic given alone. However, this applies only when an appropriate dose combination is used. Most combination analgesic preparations have not been shown to provide greater relief of pain than an adequate dose of the non-opioid component given alone. Moreover, combination preparations have the disadvantage of an increased number of side-effects.

Any analgesic given before a dental procedure should have a low risk of increasing postoperative bleeding. In the case of pain after the dental procedure, taking an analgesic before the effect of the local anaesthetic has worn off can improve control. Postoperative analgesia with ibuprofen is usually continued for about 24 to 72 hours.

Dysmenorrhoea Paracetamol or a NSAID (section 10.1.1) will generally provide adequate relief of pain from dysmenorrhoea. Alternatively use of a combined hormonal contraceptive in adolescent girls may prevent the pain.

4.7.1 Non-opioid analgesics

Paracetamol has analgesic and antipyretic properties but no demonstrable anti-inflammatory activity. It does not cause respiratory depression and is less irritant to the stomach than the NSAIDs. **Overdosage** with paracetamol is particularly dangerous as it may cause hepatic damage which is sometimes not apparent for 4 to 6 days (see Emergency Treatment of Poisoning, p. 36).

Non-steroidal anti-inflammatory analgesics (NSAIDs, section 10.1.1) are particularly useful for the treatment of children with chronic disease accompanied by pain and inflammation. Some of them are also used in the short-term treatment of mild to moderate pain including transient musculoskeletal pain but paracetamol is now often preferred. They are also suitable for the relief of pain in *dysmenorrhoea* and to treat pain caused by *secondary bone tumours*, many of which produce lysis of bone and release prostaglandins (see Prescribing in Palliative Care, p. 24). Due to an association with Reye's syndrome (section 2.9), **aspirin** should be avoided in children under 16 years except in Kawasaki syndrome or for its antiplatelet action (section 2.9). NSAIDs are also used for peri-operative analgesia (section 15.1.4.2).

Dental and orofacial pain Most dental pain is relieved effectively by NSAIDs (section 10.1.1).

Paracetamol is less irritant to the stomach than NSAIDs. Paracetamol is a suitable analgesic for children; sugar-free versions can be requested by specifying 'sugar-free' on the prescription.

For further information on the management of dental and orofacial pain, see notes above.

Compound analgesic preparations

Compound analgesic preparations that contain a simple analgesic (such as aspirin or paracetamol) with an opioid component reduce the scope for effective titration of the individual components in the management of pain of varying intensity.

Compound analgesic preparations containing paracetamol or aspirin with a *low dose* of an opioid analgesic (e.g. 8 mg of codeine phosphate per compound tablet) may be used in older children but the advantages have not been substantiated. The low dose of the opioid may be enough to cause opioid side-effects (in particular, constipation) and can complicate the treatment of **overdosage** (see p. 38) yet may not provide significant additional relief of pain.

A *full dose* of the opioid component (e.g. 60 mg codeine phosphate) in compound analgesic preparations effectively augments the analgesic activity but is associated with the full range of opioid side-effects (including nausea, vomiting, severe constipation, drowsiness, respiratory depression, and risk of dependence on long-term administration). For details of the **side-effects** of opioid analgesics, see p. 238.

PARACETAMOL

(Acetaminophen)

Cautions alcohol dependence; **interactions:** Appendix 1 (paracetamol)

Hepatic impairment dose-related toxicity—avoid large doses

Renal impairment increase *infusion* dose interval to every 6 hours if creatinine clearance less than 30 mL/minute

Pregnancy not known to be harmful

Breast-feeding amount too small to be harmful

Side-effects side-effects rare, but rashes, blood disorders (including thrombocytopenia, leucopenia, neutropenia) reported; hypotension also reported on infusion; **important:** liver damage (and less frequently renal damage) following **overdosage**, see Emergency Treatment of Poisoning, p. 36

Indication and dose

Pain, pyrexia

• **By mouth**

Neonate 28–32 weeks postmenstrual age 20 mg/kg as a single dose then 10–15 mg/kg every 8–12 hours as necessary; max. 30 mg/kg daily in divided doses

Neonate over 32 weeks postmenstrual age 20 mg/kg as a single dose then 10–15 mg/kg every 6–8 hours as necessary; max. 60 mg/kg daily in divided doses

Child 1–3 months 30–60 mg every 8 hours as necessary; *for severe symptoms* 20 mg/kg as a single dose then 15–20 mg/kg every 6–8 hours; max. 60 mg/kg daily in divided doses

Child 3–12 months 60–120 mg every 4–6 hours (max. 4 doses in 24 hours); *for severe symptoms* 20 mg/kg every 6 hours (max. 90 mg/kg daily in divided doses) for 48 hours (or longer if necessary and if adverse effects ruled out) then 15 mg/kg every 6 hours

Child 1–5 years 120–250 mg every 4–6 hours (max. 4 doses in 24 hours); *for severe symptoms* 20 mg/kg every 6 hours (max. 90 mg/kg daily in divided doses) for 48 hours (or longer if necessary and if adverse effects ruled out) then 15 mg/kg every 6 hours

Child 6–12 years 250–500 mg every 4–6 hours (max. 4 doses in 24 hours); *for severe symptoms* 20 mg/kg (max. 1 g) every 6 hours (max. 90 mg/kg daily in divided doses, not to exceed 4 g) for 48 hours (or longer if necessary and if adverse effects ruled out) then 15 mg/kg every 6 hours; max. 4 g daily

Child 12–18 years 500 mg every 4–6 hours (max. 4 doses in 24 hours); *for severe symptoms* 0.5–1 g every 4–6 hours (max. 4 doses in 24 hours)

• **By rectum**

Neonate 28–32 weeks postmenstrual age 20 mg/kg as a single dose then 15 mg/kg every 12 hours as necessary; max. 30 mg/kg daily in divided doses

Neonate over 32 weeks postmenstrual age 30 mg/kg as a single dose then 20 mg/kg every 8 hours as necessary; max. 60 mg/kg daily in divided doses

Child 1–3 months 30–60 mg every 8 hours as necessary; *for severe symptoms* 30 mg/kg as a single dose then 20 mg/kg every 8 hours; max. 60 mg/kg daily in divided doses

Child 3–12 months 60–125 mg every 4–6 hours as necessary (max. 4 doses in 24 hours); *for severe symptoms* 40 mg/kg as a single dose then 20 mg/kg every 4–6 hours (max. 90 mg/kg daily in divided doses) for 48 hours (or longer if necessary and if adverse effects ruled out) then 15 mg/kg every 6 hours

Child 1–5 years 125–250 mg every 4–6 hours as necessary (max. 4 doses in 24 hours); *for severe symptoms* 40 mg/kg as a single dose then 20 mg/kg every 4–6 hours (max. 90 mg/kg daily in divided doses) for 48 hours (or longer if necessary and if adverse effects ruled out) then 15 mg/kg every 6 hours

Child 5–12 years 250–500 mg every 4–6 hours as necessary (max. 4 doses in 24 hours); *for severe symptoms* 40 mg/kg (max. 1 g) as a single dose then 20 mg/kg every 6 hours (max. 90 mg/kg daily in divided doses) for 48 hours (or longer if necessary and if adverse effects ruled out) then 15 mg/kg every 6 hours

Child 12–18 years 500 mg every 4–6 hours (max. 4 doses in 24 hours); *for severe symptoms* 0.5–1 g every 4–6 hours; max. 4 g daily in divided doses

• **By intravenous infusion over 15 minutes**

Child body-weight 10–50 kg 15 mg/kg every 4–6 hours; max. 60 mg/kg daily

Child body-weight over 50 kg 1 g every 4–6 hours; max. 4 g daily

Post-immunisation pyrexia in infants (see also p. 675)

• **By mouth**

Child 2–3 months 60 mg as a single dose repeated once after 6 hours if necessary

PARACETAMOL (continued)

Paracetamol (Non-proprietary)

Tablets PoM[1], paracetamol 500 mg. Net price 20 = 31p. Label: 29, 30
Brands include *Panadol®* NHS

Soluble Tablets (= Dispersible tablets) PoM[2], paracetamol 500 mg. Net price 60-tab pack = £4.64. Label: 13, 29, 30
Brands include *Panadol Soluble®* NHS

Paediatric Soluble Tablets (= Paediatric dispersible tablets), paracetamol 120 mg. Net price 16-tab pack = 91p. Label: 13, 30
Brands include *Disprol® Soluble Paracetamol* NHS

Oral Suspension 120 mg/5 mL (= Paediatric Mixture), paracetamol 120 mg/5 mL. Net price 100 mL = 42p. Label: 30
Note BP directs that when Paediatric Paracetamol Oral Suspension or Paediatric Paracetamol Mixture is prescribed Paracetamol Oral Suspension 120 mg/5 mL should be dispensed; sugar-free versions can be ordered by specifying 'sugar-free'on the prescription
Brands include *Calpol® Paediatric, Calpol® Paediatric* sugar-free, *Disprol® Paediatric, Medinol® Paediatric* sugar-free, *Paldesic®*, *Panadol®* sugar-free

Oral Suspension 250 mg/5 mL (= Mixture), paracetamol 250 mg/5 mL. Net price 100 mL = 73p. Label: 30
Brands include *Calpol® 6 Plus* NHS, *Medinol® Over 6* NHS, *Paldesic®*

Suppositories, paracetamol 60 mg, net price 10 = £9.96; 125 mg, 10 = £11.50; 250 mg, 10 = £23.00; 500 mg, 10 = £9.90. Label: 30
Brands include *Alvedon®*
Note other strengths available as manufactured specials e.g. 15 mg, 30 mg

Dental prescribing on NHS Paracetamol Tablets, Paracetamol Soluble Tablets 500 mg, and Paracetamol Oral Suspension may be prescribed

Perfalgan® (Bristol-Myers Squibb) ▼ PoM

Intravenous infusion, paracetamol 10 mg/mL, net price 50-mL vial = £1.50, 100-mL vial = £1.50

Co-codamol 8/500

When co-codamol tablets, dispersible (or effervescent) tablets, or capsules are prescribed and **no strength is stated**, tablets, dispersible (or effervescent) tablets, or capsules, respectively, containing codeine phosphate **8 mg** and paracetamol **500 mg** should be dispensed.

[2]**Co-codamol 8/500** (Non-proprietary) PoM

Tablets, co-codamol 8/500 (codeine phosphate 8 mg, paracetamol 500 mg) Net price 20 = 90p. Label: 29, 30
Brands include *Panadeine®* NHS

Dose

Pain, pyrexia
- **By mouth**
  Child 6–12 years ½–1 tablet every 4–6 hours; max. 4 tablets daily
  Child 12–18 years 1–2 tablets every 4–6 hours; max. 8 tablets daily

Effervescent *or* dispersible tablets, co-codamol 8/500 (codeine phosphate 8 mg, paracetamol 500 mg). Net price 20 = £1.48. Label: 13, 29, 30
Brands include *Paracodol®* NHS
Note The Drug Tariff allows tablets of co-codamol labelled 'dispersible' to be dispensed against an order for 'effervescent' and *vice versa*

Dose

Pain, pyrexia
- **By mouth**
  Child 6–12 years ½–1 tablet in water every 4–6 hours; max. 4 tablets daily
  Child 12–18 years 1–2 tablets in water every 4–6 hours; max. 8 tablets daily

Capsules, co-codamol 8/500 (codeine phosphate 8 mg, paracetamol 500 mg). Net price 10-cap pack = £1.10, 20-cap pack = £1.66. Label: 29, 30
Brands include *Paracodol®* NHS

Dose

Pain, pyrexia
- **By mouth**
  Child 12–18 years 1–2 capsules every 4 hours; max. 8 capsules daily

4.7.2 Opioid analgesics

Opioid analgesics are usually used to relieve moderate to severe pain particularly of visceral origin. Repeated administration may cause tolerance, but this is no deterrent in the control of pain in terminal illness, for guidelines see Prescribing in Palliative Care, p. 24. Regular use of a potent opioid may be appropriate for certain cases of chronic non-malignant pain; treatment should be supervised by a specialist and the child should be assessed at regular intervals.

Side-effects Opioid analgesics share many side-effects, although qualitative and quantitative differences exist. The most common include nausea, vomiting, constipation, and drowsiness. Larger doses produce respiratory depression and hypotension. Neonates, particularly if pre-term, may be more susceptible. **Overdose**, see Emergency Treatment of Poisoning, p. 38

Interactions See Appendix 1 (opioid analgesics) (**important:** special hazard with *pethidine and possibly other opioids* and MAOIs).

1. May be sold to the public provided packs contain no more than 32 capsules or tablets; pharmacists can sell multiple packs up to a total quantity of 100 capsules or tablets in justifiable circumstances; for details see *Medicines, Ethics and Practice*, No. 30, London, Pharmaceutical Press, 2006 (and subsequent editions as available)
2. May be sold to the public under certain circumstances; for exemptions see *Medicines, Ethics and Practice*, No. 30, London, Pharmaceutical Press, 2006 (and subsequent editions as available)

Skilled tasks Drowsiness may affect performance of skilled tasks (e.g. driving); effects of alcohol enhanced.

Choice **Morphine** remains the most valuable opioid analgesic for severe pain although it frequently causes nausea and vomiting. It is the standard against which other opioid analgesics are compared. In addition to relief of pain, morphine also confers a state of euphoria and mental detachment.

Morphine is the opioid of choice for the oral treatment of *severe pain in palliative care*. It is given regularly every 4 hours (or every 12 or 24 hours as modified-release preparations). For guidelines on dosage adjustment in palliative care, see p. 24.

Buprenorphine has both opioid agonist and antagonist properties and may precipitate withdrawal symptoms, including pain, in children dependent on other opioids. It has abuse potential and may itself cause dependence. It has a much longer duration of action than morphine and sublingually is an effective analgesic for 6 to 8 hours. Vomiting may be a problem. Unlike most opioid analgesics, the effects of buprenorphine are only partially reversed by naloxone. It is used rarely in children.

Codeine is effective for the relief of mild to moderate pain but is too constipating for long-term use.

Diamorphine (heroin) is a powerful opioid analgesic. It may cause less nausea and hypotension than morphine. In *palliative care* the greater solubility of diamorphine allows effective doses to be injected in smaller volumes and this is important in the emaciated patient.

Dihydrocodeine has an analgesic efficacy similar to that of codeine; doses may be given every 4 hours.

Alfentanil, **fentanyl** and **remifentanil** are used by injection for intra-operative analgesia (section 15.1.4.3).

Methadone is less sedating than morphine and acts for longer periods. In prolonged use, methadone should not be administered more often than twice daily to avoid the risk of accumulation and opioid overdosage. Methadone may be used instead of morphine when excitation (or exacerbation of pain) occurs with morphine. Methadone may also be used to treat children with neonatal abstinence syndrome (section 4.10).

Papaveretum is rarely used; morphine is easier to prescribe and less prone to error with regard to the strength and dose.

Pethidine produces prompt but short-lasting analgesia; it is less constipating than morphine, but even in high doses is a less potent analgesic. It is not suitable for severe continuing pain and is used rarely in children. Pethidine is used for analgesia in labour; however, other opioids, such as morphine or diamorphine, are often preferred for obstetric pain.

Tramadol is used in older children and produces analgesia by two mechanisms: an opioid effect and an enhancement of serotonergic and adrenergic pathways. It has fewer of the typical opioid side-effects (notably, less respiratory depression, less constipation and less addiction potential); psychiatric reactions have been reported.

Dose Doses of opioids may need to be **adjusted individually** according to the degree of analgesia and side-effects; response to opioids varies widely, particularly in the neonatal period. Opioid overdosage can have serious consequences and the dose should be calculated and **checked with care**.

Postoperative analgesia The use of intra-operative opioids affects the prescribing of postoperative analgesics and in many cases delays the need for a postoperative analgesic. A postoperative opioid analgesic should be given with care since it may potentiate any residual respiratory depression (for the treatment of opioid-induced respiratory depression, see section 15.1.7). Non-opioid analgesics are also used for postoperative pain (section 15.1.4.2).

Morphine is used most widely. **Tramadol** is not as effective in severe pain as other opioid analgesics. **Buprenorphine** may antagonise the analgesic effect of previously administered opioids and is generally not recommended. **Pethidine** is metabolised to norpethidine which may accumulate, particularly in neonates and in renal impairment; norpethidine stimulates the central nervous system and may cause convulsions.

Opioids are also given epidurally [unlicensed route] in the postoperative period but are associated with side-effects such as pruritus, urinary retention, nausea and vomiting; respiratory depression can be delayed, particularly with morphine.

For details of patient-controlled analgesia (PCA) and nurse-controlled analgesia (NCA) to relieve postoperative pain, consult hospital protocols. Formulations specifically designed for PCA are available (*Pharma-Ject® Morphine Sulphate*).

Dental and orofacial pain Opioid analgesics are **relatively ineffective** in dental pain. Like other opioids, **dihydrocodeine** often causes nausea and vomiting which limits its value in dental pain; if taken for more than a few doses it is also liable to cause constipation. Dihydrocodeine is not very effective in postoperative dental pain.

For the management of dental and orofacial pain, see p. 235.

Addicts Although caution is necessary, addicts (and ex-addicts) may be treated with analgesics in the same way as other people when there is a real clinical need. Doctors do not require a special licence to prescribe opioid analgesics for addicts for relief of pain due to organic disease or injury.

Dependence and withdrawal Psychological dependence rarely occurs in children when opioids are used for pain relief but tolerance can develop during long-term treatment; they should be withdrawn gradually to avoid abstinence symptoms. For information on the treatment of neonatal abstinence syndrome, see section 4.10.

MORPHINE SALTS

Cautions hypotension, hypothyroidism, asthma (avoid during attack) and decreased respiratory reserve; convulsive disorders, dependence (severe withdrawal symptoms if withdrawn abruptly); use of cough suppressants containing opioid analgesics not generally recommended and should be avoided altogether in those under at least 1 year; neonates and children under 1 year are particularly susceptible to respiratory depression; respiratory monitoring is recommended and respiratory support should be available for non-ventilated children; subcutaneous route not suitable if tissue perfusion impaired or if oedema **interactions:** Appendix 1 (opioid analgesics)

Palliative care In the control of pain in terminal illness these cautions should not necessarily be a deterrent to the use of opioid analgesics

Hepatic impairment may precipitate coma in hepatic impairment—avoid or reduce dose (although many such patients tolerate morphine well)

Renal impairment in moderate to severe impairment reduce dose or avoid, increased and prolonged effect; increased cerebral sensitivity

Pregnancy depresses neonatal respiration; withdrawal effects in neonates of dependent mothers; gastric stasis and risk of inhalation pneumonia in mother during labour

Breast-feeding therapeutic doses unlikely to affect infant; withdrawal symptoms in infants of dependent mothers; breast-feeding not best method of treating dependence in offspring

Contra-indications avoid in acute respiratory depression, acute alcoholism and where risk of paralytic ileus; also avoid in raised intracranial pressure or head injury (affects pupillary responses vital for neurological assessment); avoid injection in phaeochromocytoma (risk of pressor response to histamine release)

Side-effects nausea and vomiting (particularly in initial stages), constipation, and drowsiness; larger doses produce respiratory depression, hypotension, and muscle rigidity; other side-effects include difficulty with micturition, ureteric or biliary spasm, dry mouth, sweating, headache, facial flushing, vertigo, bradycardia, tachycardia, palpitation, postural hypotension, hypothermia, hallucinations, dysphoria, mood changes, dependence, miosis, decreased libido or potency, rashes, urticaria and pruritus; **overdosage:** see Emergency Treatment of Poisoning, p. 38; for reversal of opioid-induced respiratory depression, see section 15.1.7.

Licensed use *Oramorph®* solution not licensed for use in children under 1 year; *Oramorph®* unit dose vials not licensed for use in children under 6 years; *Sevredol®* tablets not licensed for use in children under 3 years; *MST Continus®* preparations licensed to treat children with cancer pain (age-range not specified by manufacturer); *MXL®* capsules not licensed for use in children under 1 year

Indication and dose

Acute pain, postoperative pain

- **By subcutaneous injection or by intramuscular injection**

Neonate 150 micrograms/kg every 6 hours if necessary

Child 1–12 months 200 micrograms/kg every 6 hours if necessary

MORPHINE SALTS (*continued*)

Child 1–5 years 2.5–5 mg every 4 hours if necessary

Child 5–12 years 5–10 mg every 4 hours if necessary

Child 12–18 years 10 mg every 4 hours if necessary

- **By intravenous injection over at least 5 minutes**

Neonate 40–100 micrograms/kg every 6 hours if necessary

Child 1–6 months 100–200 micrograms/kg every 6 hours if necessary

Child 6 months–12 years 100–200 micrograms/kg every 4 hours if necessary

Child 12–18 years 2.5–10 mg every 4 hours if necessary

- **By intravenous injection and infusion**

Premature neonate initially *by intravenous injection* (over at least 5 minutes) 25–50 micrograms/kg then *by continuous intravenous infusion* 5 micrograms/kg/hour adjusted according to response

Neonate initially *by intravenous injection* (over at least 5 minutes) 50–100 micrograms/kg then *by continuous intravenous infusion* 10–20 micrograms/kg/hour adjusted according to response; up to 40 micrograms/kg/hour has been given

Child 1–6 months initially *by intravenous injection* (over at least 5 minutes) 100–200 micrograms/kg then *by continuous intravenous infusion* 10 micrograms/kg/hour adjusted according to response

Child 6 months–12 years initially *by intravenous injection* (over at least 5 minutes) 100–200 micrograms/kg then *by continuous intravenous infusion* 20 micrograms/kg/hour adjusted according to response

Child 12–18 years initially *by intravenous injection* (over at least 5 minutes) 2.5–10 mg then *by continuous intravenous infusion* 20 micrograms/kg/hour adjusted according to response

- **By continuous subcutaneous infusion**

Child 1–3 months 10 micrograms/kg/hour

Child 3 months–18 years 20 micrograms/kg/hour

Chronic pain see also Prescribing in Palliative Care, p. 24.

- **By mouth or by rectum**

Child 1–12 months initially 80 micrograms/kg every 4 hours, adjusted according to response

Child 1–2 years initially 200–400 micrograms/kg every 4 hours, adjusted according to response

Child 2–12 years initially 200–500 micrograms/kg every 4 hours, adjusted according to response

Child 12–18 years initially 10–15 mg every 4 hours, adjusted according to response

- **By subcutaneous or intramuscular injection**

Child 1 month–2 years initially 150–200 micrograms/kg every 4 hours, adjusted according to response

Child 2–12 years initially 200 micrograms/kg every 4 hours, adjusted according to response

Child 12–18 years initially 5–20 mg every 4 hours, adjusted according to response

Neonatal opioid withdrawal under specialist supervision

- **By mouth**

Neonate initially 40 micrograms/kg every 4 hours until symptoms controlled, increase dose if necessary; reduce frequency gradually over 6–10 days, and stop when 40 micrograms/kg once daily achieved; dose may vary, consult local guidelines

Administration for *intravenous infusion*, dilute in Glucose 5% or 10% *or* Sodium Chloride 0.9%

Oral solutions

Note For advice on transfer from oral solutions of morphine to modified-release preparations of morphine, see Prescribing in Palliative Care, p. 24

Morphine Oral Solutions

PoM or CD

Oral solutions of morphine can be prescribed by writing the formula:
Morphine hydrochloride 5 mg
Chloroform water to 5 mL

Note The proportion of morphine hydrochloride may be altered when specified by the prescriber; if above 13 mg per 5 mL the solution becomes **CD**. For sample prescription see Controlled Drugs and Drug Dependence, p. 17. It is usual to adjust the strength so that the dose volume is 5 or 10 mL.

Oramorph® (Boehringer Ingelheim)

Oramorph® oral solution PoM, morphine sulphate 10 mg/5 mL. Net price 100-mL pack = £1.87; 300-mL pack = £5.21; 500-mL pack = £7.86. Label: 2

Oramorph® Unit Dose Vials 10 mg PoM (oral vials), sugar-free, morphine sulphate 10 mg/5-mL vial, net price 20 vials = £2.65. Label: 2

Oramorph® Unit Dose Vials 30 mg CD (oral vials), sugar-free, morphine sulphate 30 mg/5-mL vial, net price 20 vials = £7.44. Label: 2

Oramorph® concentrated oral solution CD, sugar-free, morphine sulphate 100 mg/5 mL. Net price 30-mL pack = £5.24; 120-mL pack = £19.57 (both with calibrated dropper). Label: 2

Oramorph® Unit Dose Vials 100 mg CD (oral vials), sugar-free, morphine sulphate 100 mg/5-mL vial, net price 20 vials = £24.80. Label: 2

Tablets

Sevredol® (Napp) CD

Tablets, f/c, scored, morphine sulphate 10 mg (blue), net price 56-tab pack = £5.61; 20 mg (pink), 56-tab pack = £11.21; 50 mg (pale green), 56-tab pack = £28.02. Label: 2

MORPHINE SALTS (*continued*)

Modified-release oral preparations

MST Continus® (Napp) CD

Tablets, m/r, f/c, morphine sulphate 5 mg (white), net price 60-tab pack = £3.29; 10 mg (brown), 60-tab pack = £5.48; 15 mg (green), 60-tab pack = £9.61; 30 mg (purple), 60-tab pack = £13.17; 60 mg (orange), 60-tab pack = £25.69; 100 mg (grey), 60-tab pack = £40.66; 200 mg (green), 60-tab pack = £81.34. Label: 2, 25

Suspension (= sachet of granules to mix with water), m/r, pink, morphine sulphate 20 mg/sachet, net price 30-sachet pack = £24.58; 30 mg/sachet, 30-sachet pack = £25.54; 60 mg/sachet, 30-sachet pack = £51.09; 100 mg/sachet, 30-sachet pack = £85.15; 200 mg/sachet pack, 30-sachet pack = £170.30. Label: 2, 13

Dose

- **By mouth**

  Every 12 hours, dose adjusted according to daily morphine requirements; for further advice on determining dose, see Prescribing in Palliative Care, p. 24; dosage requirements should be reviewed if the brand is altered

Note Prescriptions must also specify 'tablets' or 'suspension' (i.e. 'MST Continus tablets' or 'MST Continus suspension')

MXL® (Napp) CD

Capsules, m/r, morphine sulphate 30 mg (light blue), net price 28-cap pack = £10.91; 60 mg (brown), 28-cap pack = £14.95; 90 mg (pink), 28-cap pack = £22.04; 120 mg (green), 28-cap pack = £29.15; 150 mg (blue), 28-cap pack = £36.43; 200 mg (red-brown), 28-cap pack = £46.15. Label: 2, counselling, see below

Dose

- **By mouth**

  Every 24 hours, dose adjusted according to daily morphine requirements; for further advice on determining dose, see Prescribing in Palliative Care, p. 24; dosage requirements should be reviewed if the brand is altered

Counselling Swallow whole or open capsule and sprinkle contents on soft food

Note Prescriptions must also specify 'capsules' (i.e. 'MXL capsules')

Suppositories

Morphine (Non-proprietary) CD

Suppositories, morphine hydrochloride or sulphate 10 mg, net price 12 = £7.24; 15 mg, 12 = £7.14; 20 mg, 12 = £8.92; 30 mg, 12 = £10.40. Label: 2

Available from Aurum, Martindale

Note Both the strength of the suppositories and the morphine salt contained in them must be specified by the prescriber

Morphine sulphate 5 mg suppositories available as a manufactured special

Injections

Morphine Sulphate (Non-proprietary) CD

Injection, morphine sulphate 10, 15, 20, and 30 mg/mL, net price 1- and 2-mL amp (all) = 72p–£1.09; 10 mg/mL, 1-mL prefilled syringe = £5.00

Intravenous infusion, morphine sulphate 1 mg/mL, net price 50-mL vial = £5.00; 2 mg/mL, 50-mL vial = £5.10

Minijet® Morphine Sulphate (Celltech) CD

Injection, morphine sulphate 1 mg/mL, net price 10-mL disposable syringe = £7.36

Injection with anti-emetic

Caution **Not recommended** in palliative care, see Nausea and Vomiting, p. 27

Cyclimorph® (Amdipharm) CD

Cyclimorph-10® Injection, morphine tartrate 10 mg, cyclizine tartrate 50 mg/mL. Net price 1-mL amp = £1.34

Dose

Moderate to severe pain (short-term use only)

- **By subcutaneous, intramuscular, or intravenous injection**

  Child 12–18 years 1 mL, repeated not more often than every 4 hours, max. 3 doses in any 24-hour period

Cyclimorph-15® Injection, morphine tartrate 15 mg, cyclizine tartrate 50 mg/mL. Net price 1-mL amp = £1.39

Dose

Moderate to severe pain (short-term use only)

- **By subcutaneous, intramuscular, or intravenous injection**

  Child 12–18 years 1 mL, repeated not more often than every 4 hours, max. 3 doses in any 24-hour period

BUPRENORPHINE

Cautions see under Morphine Salts and notes above; effects only partially reversed by naloxone; **interactions:** Appendix 1 (opioid analgesics)

Hepatic impairment avoid or reduce dose—may precipitate coma

Renal impairment reduce dose or avoid in moderate to severe impairment; increased and prolonged effect; increased cerebral sensitivity

Pregnancy third trimester, depresses neonatal respiration; withdrawal effects in neonates of dependent mothers; gastric stasis and risk of inhalation pneumonia in mother during labour

Breast-feeding amount too small to be harmful; manufacturer advises contra-indicated in the treatment of opioid dependence

Contra-indications see under Morphine Salts and notes above

Side-effects see under Morphine Salts and notes above; can give rise to mild withdrawal symptoms in children who regularly use other opioids; hiccups, dyspnoea; with patches, local reactions such as erythema and pruritus; delayed local allergic reactions with severe inflammation—discontinue treatment

Licensed use sublingual tablets not licensed for use in children under 6 years; injection not licensed for use in children under 6 months

BUPRENORPHINE (*continued*)

Indication and dose

Moderate to severe pain
- **By sublingual administration**

  Child body-weight 16–25 kg 100 micrograms every 6–8 hours

  Child body-weight 25–37.5 kg 100–200 micrograms every 6–8 hours

  Child body-weight 37.5–50 kg 200–300 micrograms every 6–8 hours

  Child body-weight over 50 kg 200–400 micrograms every 6–8 hours

- **By intramuscular or by slow intravenous injection**

  Child 6 months–12 years 3–6 micrograms/kg every 6–8 hours, max. 9 micrograms/kg

  Child 12–18 years 300–600 micrograms every 6–8 hours

Administration tablets may be halved

Temgesic® (Schering-Plough) CD
Tablets (sublingual), buprenorphine (as hydrochloride), 200 micrograms, net price 50-tab pack = £5.33; 400 micrograms, 50-tab pack = £10.66. Label: 2, 26

Injection, buprenorphine (as hydrochloride) 300 micrograms/mL, net price 1-mL amp = 49p

CODEINE PHOSPHATE

Cautions see under Morphine Salts and notes above; avoid intravenous injection (risk of severe hypotension and circulatory collapse); use of cough suppressants containing codeine or similar opioid analgesics not generally recommended and should be avoided altogether in those under 1 year; **interactions:** Appendix 1 (opioid analgesics)

Hepatic impairment avoid or reduce dose—may precipitate coma

Renal impairment in moderate to severe impairment reduce dose or avoid; increased and prolonged effect; increased cerebral sensitivity

Pregnancy third trimester, depresses neonatal respiration; withdrawal effects in neonates of dependent mothers; gastric stasis and risk of inhalation pneumonia in mother during labour

Breast-feeding amount too small to be harmful

Contra-indications see under Morphine Salts and notes above

Side-effects see under Morphine Salts and notes above

Licensed use tablets not licensed for use in children; injection not licensed for use in children under 1 year

Indication and dose

Mild to moderate pain
- **By mouth or by rectum or by subcutaneous injection or by intramuscular injection**

  Neonate 0.5–1 mg/kg every 4–6 hours

  Child 1 month–12 years 0.5–1 mg/kg every 4–6 hours, max. 240 mg daily

  Child 12–18 years 30–60 mg every 4–6 hours, max. 240 mg daily

Cough suppressant section 3.9.1

Codeine Phosphate (Non-proprietary)
Tablets PoM, codeine phosphate 15 mg, net price 28 = £1.46; 30 mg, 28 = £1.67; 60 mg, 28 = £2.61. Label: 2

Note As for schedule 2 controlled drugs, children needing to take codeine phosphate preparations abroad may require a doctor's letter explaining why they are necessary

Syrup PoM, codeine phosphate 25 mg/5 mL. Net price 100 mL = 90p. Label: 2

Injection CD, codeine phosphate 60 mg/mL. Net price 1-mL amp = £2.37

Note Codeine is an ingredient of some compound analgesic preparations, section 4.7.1

DIAMORPHINE HYDROCHLORIDE
(Heroin Hydrochloride)

Cautions see under Morphine Salts and notes above; subcutaneous route not suitable if tissue perfusion impaired or if oedema; **interactions:** Appendix 1 (opioid analgesics)

Hepatic impairment avoid or reduce dose—may precipitate coma

Renal impairment in moderate to severe impairment reduce dose or avoid, increased and prolonged effect; increased cerebral sensitivity

Pregnancy third trimester, depresses neonatal respiration; withdrawal effects in neonates of dependent mothers; gastric stasis and risk of inhalation pneumonia in mother during labour

Breast-feeding therapeutic doses unlikely to affect infant; withdrawal symptoms in infants of dependent mothers; breast-feeding not best method of treating dependence in offspring

Contra-indications see under Morphine Salts and notes above

Side-effects see under Morphine Salts and notes above

Licensed use intranasal route not licensed

Indication and dose

Acute or chronic pain
- **By mouth**

  Child 1 month–12 years 100–200 micrograms/kg (max. 10 mg) every 4 hours as necessary

  Child 12–18 years 5–10 mg every 4 hours as necessary

DIAMORPHINE HYDROCHLORIDE (*continued*)

- **By intravenous administration**

Neonate (ventilated) initially *by intravenous injection* over 30 minutes, 50 micrograms/kg then *by continuous intravenous infusion*, 15 micrograms/kg/hour

Neonate (non-ventilated) *by continuous intravenous infusion* 2.5–7 micrograms/kg/hour

Child 1 month–12 years *by continuous intravenous infusion* 12.5–25 micrograms/kg/hour

- **By intravenous injection**

Child 1–3 months 20 micrograms/kg every 6 hours as necessary

Child 3–6 months 25–50 micrograms/kg every 6 hours as necessary

Child 6–12 months 75 micrograms/kg every 4 hours as necessary

Child 1–12 years 75–100 micrograms/kg every 4 hours as necessary

Child 12–18 years 2.5–5 mg every 4 hours as necessary

- **By continuous subcutaneous infusion**

See Prescribing in Palliative Care, p. 24

- **By subcutaneous or by intramuscular injection**

Child 12–18 years 5 mg every 4 hours as necessary

Acute pain in an emergency setting
- **Intranasally**

Child 3–18 years 100 micrograms/kg

Administration for *intravenous infusion*, dilute in Glucose 5% *or* Sodium Chloride 0.9%; Glucose 5% is preferable

For *intranasal* administration, diamorphine powder should be dissolved in sufficient volume of Water for Injections to provide the requisite dose in 0.2mL of solution; use solution immediately after preparation

Diamorphine (Non-proprietary) CD

Tablets, diamorphine hydrochloride 10 mg. Net price 100-tab pack = £12.30. Label: 2

Injection, powder for reconstitution, diamorphine hydrochloride. Net price 5-mg amp = £1.18, 10-mg amp = £1.36, 30-mg amp = £1.62, 100-mg amp = £4.50, 500-mg amp = £20.68

Extemporaneous formulations available see Extemporaneous Preparations, p. 8

DIHYDROCODEINE TARTRATE

Cautions see under Morphine Salts and notes above; **interactions**: Appendix 1 (opioid analgesics)

Hepatic impairment avoid or reduce dose—may precipitate coma

Renal impairment in moderate to severe impairment reduce dose or avoid; increased and prolonged effect; increased cerebral sensitivity

Pregnancy in third trimester, depresses neonatal respiration—withdrawal effects in neonates of dependent mothers; gastric stasis and risk of inhalation pneumonia in mother during labour

Breast-feeding manufacturer advises use only if potential benefit outweighs risk

Contra-indications see under Morphine Salts and notes above

Side-effects see under Morphine Salts and notes above

Licensed use most preparations not licensed for use in children under 4 years; *DF118 Forte*® and *DHC Continus*® not licensed for use in children under 12 years

Indication and dose

Moderate to severe pain
- **By mouth or by intramuscular injection or by subcutaneous injection**

Child 1–4 years 500 micrograms/kg every 4–6 hours

Child 4–12 years 0.5–1 mg/kg (max. 30 mg) every 4–6 hours

Child 12–18 years 30 mg (max. 50 mg by intramuscular or deep subcutaneous injection) every 4–6 hours

Dihydrocodeine (Non-proprietary)

Tablets PoM, dihydrocodeine tartrate 30 mg. Net price 20 = £1.39. Label: 2, 21

Dental prescribing on NHS Dihydrocodeine Tablets 30 mg may be prescribed

Oral solution PoM, dihydrocodeine tartrate 10 mg/5 mL. Net price 150 mL = £3.08. Label: 2, 21

Injection CD, dihydrocodeine tartrate 50 mg/mL. Net price 1-mL amp = £2.29

DF 118 Forte® (Martindale) PoM

Tablets, dihydrocodeine tartrate 40 mg. Net price 100-tab pack = £11.51. Label: 2, 21

Dose

Severe pain
- **By mouth**

Child 12–18 years 40–80 mg 3 times daily; max. 240 mg daily

Modified release

DHC Continus® (Napp) PoM

Tablets, m/r, dihydrocodeine tartrate 60 mg, net price 56-tab pack = £5.50; 90 mg, 56-tab pack = £8.66; 120 mg, 56-tab pack = £11.57. Label: 2, 25

Dose

Chronic severe pain
- **By mouth**

Child 12–18 years 60–120 mg every 12 hours

Note Dihydrocodeine is an ingredient of some compound analgesic preparations

FENTANYL

Cautions see under Morphine Salts and notes above; **interactions:** Appendix 1 (opioid analgesics)

Fever or external heat Monitor patients using patches for increased side-effects if fever present (increased absorption possible); avoid exposing application site to external heat (may also increase absorption)

Hepatic impairment avoid or reduce dose—may precipitate coma

Renal impairment in moderate to severe impairment reduce dose or avoid; increased and prolonged effect; increased cerebral sensitivity

Pregnancy third trimester, depresses neonatal respiration; withdrawal effects in neonates of dependent mothers; gastric stasis and risk of inhalation pneumonia in mother during labour

Breast-feeding amount too small to be harmful

Contra-indications see under Morphine Salts and notes above

Side-effects see under Morphine Salts and notes above; with patches, local reactions such as rash, erythema and itching reported; muscle rigidity reported following intravenous administration

Licensed use not licensed for use in children

Indication and dose

See under preparations, below; see also section 15.1.4.3

Conversion (from oral morphine to transdermal fentanyl), see Prescribing in Palliative Care, p. 25

Actiq® (Cephalon) CD

Lozenge, (with oromucosal applicator), fentanyl (as citrate) 200 micrograms, net price 3 = £18.58, 30 = £185.80; 400 micrograms, 3 = £18.58, 30 = £185.80; 600 micrograms, 3 = £18.58, 30 = £185.80; 800 micrograms, 3 = £18.58, 30 = £185.80; 1.2 mg, 3 = £18.58, 30 = £185.80; 1.6 mg, 3 = £18.58, 30 = £185.80. Label: 2

Dose

Breakthrough pain

- **By transmucosal application (lozenge with oromucosal applicator)**

  Child 2–18 years (over 10 kg body-weight) 15–20 micrograms/kg as a single dose; max. dose 400 micrograms

  Note If more than 4 episodes of breakthrough pain each day, adjust dose of background analgesic

Premedication analgesia

- **By transmucosal application (lozenge with oromucosal applicator)**

  Child 2–18 years (over 10 kg body-weight) 15–20 micrograms/kg as a single dose; max. 400 micrograms

Durogesic® DTrans® (Janssen-Cilag) CD

Patches, self-adhesive, transparent, fentanyl, '12' patch (releasing approx. 12 micrograms/hour for 72 hours), net price 5 = £19.26; '25' patch (releasing approx. 25 micrograms/hour for 72 hours), 5 = £27.52; '50' patch (releasing approx. 50 micrograms/hour for 72 hours), 5 = £51.40; '75' patch (releasing approx. 75 micrograms/hour for 72 hours), 5 = £71.66; '100' patch (releasing approx. 100 micrograms/hour for 72 hours), 5 = £88.32. Label: 2

Note Prescriptions must also specify 'patches' (i.e. 'Durogesic DTrans patches')

Dose

Chronic pain

- **By transdermal route**

  For children previously stabilised on oral morphine therapy, see Prescribing in Palliative Care, p. 25 for guidance on transferring to transdermal fentanyl

  Dose adjustment When starting, evaluation of the analgesic effect should **not** be made before the system has been worn for **24 hours** (to allow for the gradual increase in plasma-fentanyl concentration)—previous analgesic therapy should be phased out gradually from time of first patch application; if necessary dose should be adjusted at 72-hour intervals in steps of 12–25 micrograms/hour. More than one patch may be used at a time for doses greater than 100 micrograms/hour (but applied at *same time* to avoid confusion)—consider additional or alternative analgesic therapy if dose required exceeds 300 micrograms/hour (**important:** it may take 22 hours or longer for the plasma-fentanyl concentration to decrease by 50%—replacement opioid therapy should be initiated at a low dose, increasing gradually).

  Long duration of action In view of the long duration of action, children who have had severe side-effects should be monitored for up to 24 hours after patch removal

Administration apply to dry, non-irritated, non-irradiated, non-hairy skin on torso or upper arm, removing after 72 hours and siting replacement patch on a different area (avoid using the same area for several days).

Note Prescriptions for fentanyl patches can be written to show the strength in terms of the release rate and it is acceptable to write '*Fentanyl 25 patches*' to prescribe patches that release fentanyl 25 micrograms per hour. The dosage should be expressed in terms of the interval between applying a patch and replacing it with a new one, e.g. '*one patch to be applied every 72 hours*'. The total quantity of patches should be written in words and figures.

HYDROMORPHONE HYDROCHLORIDE

Cautions see Morphine Salts and notes above; **interactions:** Appendix 1 (opioid analgesics)

Hepatic impairment avoid or reduce dose—may precipitate coma

Renal impairment in moderate to severe impairment reduce dose or avoid; increased and prolonged effect; increased cerebral sensitivity

Pregnancy third trimester, depresses neonatal respiration; withdrawal effects in neonates of dependent mothers; gastric stasis and risk of inhalation pneumonia in mother during labour

Breast-feeding manufacturer advises avoid—no information available

Contra-indications see Morphine Salts and notes above

HYDROMORPHONE HYDROCHLORIDE (*continued*)

Side-effects see Morphine Salts and notes above

Indication and dose

Severe pain in cancer
- By mouth

Child 12–18 years 1.3 mg every 4 hours, increased if necessary according to severity of pain

Administration Swallow whole capsule or sprinkle contents on soft food

Palladone® (Napp) CD
Capsules, hydromorphone hydrochloride 1.3 mg (orange/clear), net price 56-cap pack = £8.82; 2.6 mg (red/clear), 56-cap pack = £17.64. Label: 2, counselling, see below

Modified release

Palladone® SR (Napp) CD
Capsules, m/r, hydromorphone hydrochloride 2 mg (yellow/clear), net price 56-cap pack = £20.98; 4 mg (pale blue/clear), 56-cap pack = £28.75; 8 mg (pink/clear), 56-cap pack = £56.08; 16 mg (brown/clear), 56-cap pack = £106.53; 24 mg (dark blue/clear), 56-cap pack = £159.82. Label: 2, counselling, see below

Dose

Severe pain in cancer
- By mouth

Child 12–18 years 4 mg every 12 hours, increased if necessary according to severity of pain

Counselling Swallow whole or open capsule and sprinkle contents on soft food

METHADONE HYDROCHLORIDE

Cautions see under Morphine Salts and notes above; **interactions:** Appendix 1 (opioid analgesics)

Hepatic impairment avoid or reduce dose in liver disease—may precipitate coma

Renal impairment reduce dose or avoid in moderate to severe renal impairment; increased and prolonged effect; increased cerebral sensitivity

Pregnancy third trimester, depresses neonatal respiration; withdrawal effects in neonates of dependent mothers; gastric stasis and risk of inhalation pneumonia in mother during labour

Breast-feeding withdrawal symptoms in infant; breast-feeding permissible during maintenance but dose should be as low as possible and infant monitored to avoid sedation

Contra-indications see under Morphine Salts and notes above

Side-effects see under Morphine Salts and notes above

Licensed use not licensed for use in children

Indication and dose

Neonatal opioid withdrawal dose may vary, consult local guidelines
- By mouth

Neonate initially 100 micrograms/kg increased by 50 micrograms/kg every 6 hours until symptoms are controlled; for maintenance, total daily dose that controls symptoms given in 2 divided doses; to withdraw, reduce dose over 7–10 days

Methadone (Non-proprietary) CD
Oral solution 1 mg/mL, methadone hydrochloride 1 mg/mL, net price 30 mL = 44p, 50 mL = 73p, 100 mL = £1.45, 500 mL = £6.82. Label: 2
Brands include *Metharose®* (sugar-free), *Physeptone* (also as sugar-free)

Safe Practice This preparation is 2½ times the strength of Methadone Linctus; many preparations of this strength are licensed for opioid drug addiction only but some are also licensed for analgesia in severe pain

OXYCODONE HYDROCHLORIDE

Cautions see under Morphine Salts and notes above; avoid in porphyria (section 9.8.2); **interactions:** Appendix 1 (opioid analgesics)

Contra-indications see under Morphine Salts and notes above

Hepatic impairment avoid in moderate to severe impairment

Renal impairment avoid in severe impairment

Breast-feeding present in milk—manufacturer advises avoid

Side-effects see under Morphine Salts and notes above

Licensed use not licensed for use in children

Indication and dose

Moderate to severe pain in palliative care (see also Prescribing in Palliative Care, p. 25)
- By mouth

Child 1 month–12 years initially 200 micrograms/kg (up to 5 mg) every 4–6 hours, dose increased if necessary according to severity of pain

Child 12–18 years initially 5 mg every 4–6 hours, dose increased if necessary according to severity of pain

Oxynorm® (Napp) CD
Capsules, oxycodone hydrochloride 5 mg (orange/beige), net price 56-cap pack = £11.09; 10 mg (white/beige), 56-cap pack = £22.18; 20 mg (pink/beige), 56-cap pack = £44.35. Label: 2

Liquid (= oral solution), sugar-free, oxycodone hydrochloride 5 mg/5 mL, net price 250 mL = £9.43. Label: 2

Concentrate (= concentrated oral solution), sugar-free, oxycodone hydrochloride 10 mg/mL, net price 120 mL = £45.25. Label: 2

OXYCODONE HYDROCHLORIDE (*continued*)

Modified release

OxyContin® (Napp) CD
Tablets, f/c, m/r, oxycodone hydrochloride 5 mg (blue), net price 28-tab pack = £12.16; 10 mg (white), 56-tab pack = £24.30; 20 mg (pink), 56-tab pack = £48.60; 40 mg (yellow), 56-tab pack = £97.22; 80 mg (green), 56-tab pack = £194.44. Label: 2, 25

Dose

Moderate to severe pain in palliative care
- **By mouth**

Child 12–18 years initially, 10 mg every 12 hours, increased if necessary according to severity of pain

PAPAVERETUM

Safe Practice Do **not** confuse with papaverine

A mixture of 253 parts of morphine hydrochloride, 23 parts of papaverine hydrochloride and 20 parts of codeine hydrochloride

The CSM has advised that to avoid confusion the figures of 7.7 mg/mL or 15.4 mg/mL should be used for prescribing purposes

Cautions see Morphine Salts and notes above

Contra-indications see Morphine Salts and notes above

Side-effects see Morphine Salts and notes above

Indication and dose

Premedication, postoperative analgesia, severe chronic pain
- **By subcutaneous or intramuscular injection**

Neonate 115 micrograms/kg repeated every 4 hours if necessary

Child 1–12 months 154 micrograms/kg repeated every 4 hours if necessary

Child 1–6 years 1.93–3.85 mg repeated every 4 hours if necessary

Child 6–12 years 3.85–7.7 mg repeated every 4 hours if necessary

Child 12–18 years 7.7–15.4 mg repeated every 4 hours if necessary

- **By intravenous injection**

Generally 25–50% of the corresponding subcutaneous or intramuscular dose

Papaveretum (Non-proprietary) CD
Injection, papaveretum 15.4 mg/mL (providing the equivalent of 10 mg of anhydrous morphine/mL), net price 1-mL amp = £1.36

PETHIDINE HYDROCHLORIDE

Cautions see under Morphine Salts and notes above; not suitable for severe continuing pain; **interactions:** Appendix 1 (opioid analgesics)

Hepatic impairment avoid or reduce dose—may precipitate coma

Renal impairment reduce dose or avoid in moderate to severe impairment; increased and prolonged effect; increased cerebral sensitivity

Pregnancy third trimester depresses neonatal respiration; withdrawal effects in neonates of dependent mothers; gastric stasis and risk of inhalation pneumonia in mother during labour

Breast-feeding present in milk but not known to be harmful

Contra-indications see under Morphine Salts and notes above

Side-effects see under Morphine Salts and notes above; convulsions reported in **overdosage**

Indication and dose

Moderate to severe acute pain
- **By mouth**

Child 2 months–12 years 0.5–2 mg/kg every 4–6 hours if required

Child 12–18 years 50–100 mg every 4–6 hours if required

Administration Injection solution can be given orally

- **By subcutaneous or by intramuscular injection**

Child 2 months–12 years 0.5–2 mg/kg every 4–6 hours if required

Child 12–18 years 25–100 mg every 4–6 hours if required

- **By intravenous injection**

Neonate 0.5–1 mg/kg every 10–12 hours if required

Child 1 month–2 months 0.5–1 mg/kg every 10–12 hours if required

Child 2 months–12 years 0.5–1 mg/kg every 4–6 hours if required

Child 12–18 years 25–50 mg every 4–6 hours if required

- **By intravenous injection and by continuous intravenous infusion**

Child 1 month–18 years initially 1 mg/kg *by intravenous injection* as a loading dose followed *by continuous intravenous infusion* 100–400 micrograms/kg/hour adjusted according to response

Administration for *intravenous infusion*, dilute with Glucose 5% or Sodium Chloride 0.9% to required volume

For *intravenous injection*, dilute to 5–10 mg/mL with Water for Injections and give over 2–5 minutes

Pethidine (Non-proprietary) CD
Tablets, pethidine hydrochloride 50 mg, net price 20 = £1.97. Label: 2

Dental prescribing on NHS Pethidine Tablets may be prescribed

Injection, pethidine hydrochloride 50 mg/mL, net price 1-mL amp = 53p, 2-mL amp = 56p; 10 mg/mL, 5-mL amp = £2.06, 10-mL amp = £2.18

TRAMADOL HYDROCHLORIDE

Cautions see under Morphine Salts and notes above; history of epilepsy (convulsions reported, usually after rapid intravenous injection); not suitable as substitute in opioid-dependent patients; **interactions:** Appendix 1 (opioid analgesics)

General anaesthesia Not recommended for analgesia during potentially very light planes of general anaesthesia (possibly increased operative recall reported)

Hepatic impairment avoid or reduce dose—may precipitate coma

Renal impairment reduce dose or avoid in moderate to severe impairment; increased and prolonged effect; increased cerebral sensitivity

Pregnancy embryotoxic in *animal studies*—manufacturers advise avoid; third trimester, depress neonatal respiration; withdrawal effects in neonates of dependent mothers; gastric stasis and risk of inhalation pneumonia in mother during labour

Breast-feeding amount probably too small to be harmful, but manufacturer advises avoid

Contra-indications see under Morphine Salts and notes above

Side-effects see under Morphine Salts and notes above; also abdominal discomfort, diarrhoea, hypotension and occasionally hypertension; paraesthesia, anaphylaxis, and confusion reported

Licensed use not licensed for use in children under 12 years

Indication and dose

Moderate to severe pain
- **By mouth**

  Child 12–18 years 50–100 mg not more often than every 4 hours; total of more than 400 mg daily by mouth not usually required

- **By intramuscular injection or by intravenous injection (over 2–3 minutes) or by intravenous infusion**

  Child 12–18 years 50–100 mg every 4–6 hours

Postoperative pain
- **By mouth**

  Child 12–18 years 100 mg initially then 50 mg every 10–20 minutes if necessary during first hour to total max. 250 mg (including initial dose) in first hour, *then* 50–100 mg every 4–6 hours; max. 600 mg daily

Administration for *intravenous infusion*, dilute with Glucose 5% *or* Sodium Chloride 0.9% *or* Compound Sodium Lactate *or* Ringer's Solution

Tramadol Hydrochloride (Non-proprietary) PoM

Capsules, tramadol hydrochloride 50 mg. Net price 30-cap pack = £2.19, 100-cap pack = £4.10. Label: 2

Brands include *Tramake®*

Injection, tramadol hydrochloride 50 mg/mL. Net price 2-mL amp = £1.15

Tramake Insts® (Galen) PoM

Sachets, effervescent powder, sugar-free, lemon-flavoured, tramadol hydrochloride 50 mg (contains Na^+ 9.7 mmol/sachet), net price 60-sachet pack = £8.75; 100 mg (contains Na^+ 14.6 mmol/sachet), 60-sachet pack = £17.00. Label: 2, 13

Excipients: include aspartame (section 9.4.1)

Zamadol® (Viatris) PoM

Capsules, tramadol hydrochloride 50 mg, net price 100-cap pack = £8.00. Label: 2

Orodispersible tablets (*Zamadol Melt®*), tramadol hydrochloride 50 mg, net price 60-tab pack = £7.12, 100-tab pack = £11.88. Label: 2, counselling, administration

Excipients: include aspartame (section 9.4.1)

Counselling *Zamadol Melt®* should be sucked and then swallowed. May also be dispersed in water

Injection, tramadol hydrochloride 50 mg/mL, net price 2-mL amp = £1.10

Zydol® (Grünenthal) PoM

Capsules, green/yellow, tramadol hydrochloride 50 mg, net price 30-cap pack = £3.35, 100-cap pack = £16.91. Label: 2

Soluble tablets, tramadol hydrochloride 50 mg, net price 20-tab pack = £3.05, 100-tab pack = £15.23. Label: 2, 13

Injection, tramadol hydrochloride 50 mg/mL. Net price 2-mL amp = £1.24

Modified release

Dromadol® SR (IVAX) PoM

Tablets, m/r, tramadol hydrochloride 100 mg (white), net price 60-tab pack = £16.00; 150 mg (beige), 60-tab pack = £24.00; 200 mg (orange), 60-tab pack = £32.00. Label: 2, 25

Dose

Moderate to severe pain
- **By mouth**

  Child 12–18 years initially 100 mg twice daily increased if necessary; usual max. 200 mg twice daily

Larapam® SR (Sandoz) PoM

Tablets, m/r, tramadol hydrochloride 100 mg, net price 60-tab pack = £18.25; 150 mg, 60-tab pack = £27.35; 200 mg, 60-tab pack = £36.50. Label: 2, 25

Dose

Moderate to severe pain
- **By mouth**

  Child 12–18 years initially 100 mg twice daily increased if necessary; usual max. 200 mg twice daily

Mabron® (Morningside) PoM

Tablets, m/r, tramadol hydrochloride 100 mg, net price 60-tab pack = £15.00; 150 mg, 60-tab pack = £22.00; 200 mg, 60-tab pack = £30.00. Label: 2, 25

Dose

Moderate to severe pain
- **By mouth**

  Child 12–18 years 100 mg twice daily increased if necessary; usual max. 200 mg twice daily

Zamadol® 24hr (Viatris) PoM

Tablets, all f/c, all m/r, tramadol hydrochloride 150 mg, net price 28-tab pack = £10.70; 200 mg, 28-

TRAMADOL HYDROCHLORIDE (*continued*)

tab pack = £14.26; 300 mg, 28-tab pack = £21.39; 400 mg, 28-tab pack = £28.51. Label: 2, 25

Dose

Moderate to severe pain
- By mouth
  Child 12–18 years initially 150 mg once daily increased if necessary; max. 400 mg once daily

Zamadol® SR (Viatris) PoM
Capsules, m/r, tramadol hydrochloride 50 mg (green), net price 60-cap pack = £7.64; 100 mg, 60-cap pack = £15.28; 150 mg (dark green), 60-cap pack = £22.92; 200 mg (yellow), 60-cap pack = £30.55. Label: 2, 25

Dose

Moderate to severe pain
- By mouth
  Child 12–18 years 50–100 mg twice daily increased if necessary to 150–200 mg twice daily; total of more than 400 mg daily not usually required
  Administration Swallow whole or open capsule and swallow contents immediately without chewing

Zydol SR® (Grünenthal) PoM
Tablets, m/r, f/c, tramadol hydrochloride 100 mg, net price 60-tab pack = £18.26; 150 mg (beige), 60-tab pack = £27.39; 200 mg (orange), 60-tab pack = £36.52. Label: 2, 25

Dose

Moderate to severe pain
- By mouth
  Child 12–18 years 100 mg twice daily increased if necessary to 150–200 mg twice daily; total of more than 400 mg daily not usually required

Zydol XL® (Grünenthal) PoM
Tablets, m/r, f/c, tramadol hydrochloride 150 mg, net price 30-tab pack = £15.22; 200 mg, 30-tab pack = £20.29; 300 mg, 30-tab pack = £30.44; 400 mg, 30-tab pack = £40.59. Label: 2, 25

Dose

Moderate to severe pain
- By mouth
  Child 12–18 years 150 mg daily increased if necessary; more than 400 mg once daily not usually required

With paracetamol

Tramacet (Janssen-Cilag) ▼ PoM
Tablets, f/c, yellow, tramadol hydrochloride 37.5 mg, paracetamol 325 mg, net price 60-tab pack = £10.07. Label: 2, 25, 29, 30

Dose

Moderate to severe pain
- By mouth
  Child 12–18 years 2 tablets not more than every 6 hours; max. 8 tablets daily

4.7.3 Neuropathic pain

Neuropathic pain, which occurs as a result of damage to neural tissue, includes *postherpetic neuralgia, phantom limb pain, complex regional pain syndrome* (reflex sympathetic dystrophy, causalgia) *compression neuropathies, peripheral neuropathies* (e.g. due to diabetes, haematological malignancies, rheumatoid arthritis, alcoholism, drug misuse), *trauma, central pain* (e.g. pain following stroke, spinal cord injury and syringomyelia) and *idiopathic neuropathy*. The pain occurs in an area of sensory deficit and may be described as burning, shooting or scalding and is often accompanied by pain that is evoked by a non-noxious stimulus (allodynia).

Neuropathic pain is generally managed with a tricyclic antidepressant such as amitriptyline (p. 220) or antiepileptic drugs such as carbamazepine (p. 256). Neuropathic pain may respond only partially to opioid analgesics. Nerve blocks, transcutaneous electrical nerve stimulation (TENS) and, in selected cases, central electrical stimulation may help. Many children with chronic neuropathic pain require multidisciplinary management, including physiotherapy and psychological support. A corticosteroid may help to relieve pressure in compression neuropathy and thereby reduce pain.

For the management of neuropathic pain in *palliative care*, see p. 25.

Chronic facial pain Chronic oral and facial pain including persistent idiopathic facial pain (also termed 'atypical facial pain') and temporomandibular dysfunction (previously termed temporomandibular joint pain dysfunction syndrome) may call for prolonged use of analgesics or for other drugs. Tricyclic antidepressants (section 4.3.1) may be useful for facial pain [unlicensed indication], but are not on the Dental Practitioners' List. Long-term prescribing for disorders of this type should follow a full investigation and usually involves specialists. Children on long-term therapy need to be monitored both for progress and for side-effects.

4.7.4 Antimigraine drugs

4.7.4.1 Treatment of the acute migraine attack

Treatment of a migraine attack should be guided by response to previous treatment and the severity of the attacks. A **simple analgesic** such as paracetamol (preferably in a soluble or dispersible form) or an NSAID, usually ibuprofen, is often effective; concomitant **anti-emetic** treatment may be required. If treatment with an analgesic is inadequate, an attack may be treated with a specific anti-migraine compound such as the $5HT_1$ agonist **sumatriptan**. **Ergot alkaloids** are associated with many side-effects and should be avoided.

Frequent and prolonged use of analgesics for migraine (opioid and non-opioid analgesics, $5HT_1$ agonists, and ergotamine) is associated with medication-overuse headache (analgesic-induced headache); therefore, increasing consumption of these medicines needs careful management.

Analgesics

ANALGESICS

Paracetamol
Section 4.7.1

Non-steroidal anti-inflammatory drugs (NSAIDs)
Section 10.1.1

With anti-emetics

Migraleve® (Pfizer Consumer)

Tablets, all f/c, *pink tablets*, buclizine hydrochloride 6.25 mg, paracetamol 500 mg, codeine phosphate 8 mg; *yellow tablets*, paracetamol 500 mg, codeine phosphate 8 mg. Net price 48-tab *Migraleve* PoM (32 pink + 16 yellow) = £5.10; 48 pink (*Migraleve Pink*) = £5.56; 48 yellow (*Migraleve Yellow*) = £4.70. Label: 2, (*Migraleve Pink*), 17, 30

Dose

Treatment of acute migraine attack
- **By mouth**

  Child under 10 years only under close medical supervision

  Child 10–14 years 1 pink tablet at onset of attack, or if it is imminent then 1 yellow tablet every 4 hours if necessary; max. 1 pink and 3 yellow tablets in 24 hours

  Child 14–18 years 2 pink tablets at onset of attack, or if it is imminent, then 2 yellow tablets every 4 hours if necessary; max. in 24 hours 2 pink and 6 yellow

Paramax® (Sanofi-Synthelabo) PoM

Tablets, scored, paracetamol 500 mg, metoclopramide hydrochloride 5 mg. Net price 42-tab pack = £6.69. Label: 17, 30

Sachets, effervescent powder, sugar-free, the contents of 1 sachet = 1 tablet; to be dissolved in ¼ tumblerful of liquid before administration. Net price 42-sachet pack = £8.69. Label: 13, 17, 30

Dose

Treatment of acute migraine attacks
- **By mouth**

  Child 12–18 years 1 at onset of attack then 1 every 4 hours when necessary to max. of 3 in 24 hours (max. dose of metoclopramide 500 micrograms/kg daily)

  Important Metoclopramide can cause **severe extrapyramidal effects** (for further details, see p. 227 and p. 232)

$5HT_1$ agonists

$5HT_1$ agonists are used in the treatment of acute migraine attacks; treatment of children should be initiated by a specialist. The $5HT_1$ agonists ('triptans') act on the 5HT (serotonin) 1B/1D receptors and they are therefore sometimes referred to as $5HT_{1B/1D}$-receptor agonists. A $5HT_1$ agonist may be used during the established headache phase of an attack and is the preferred treatment in those who fail to respond to conventional analgesics.

Sumatriptan is used for migraine in children and it may also be of value in cluster headache (section 4.7.4.3).

SUMATRIPTAN

Cautions pre-existing cardiac disease; history of seizures; $5HT_1$ agonists are recommended as monotherapy and should not be taken concurrently with other therapies for acute migraine; sensitivity to sulphonamides; **interactions:** Appendix 1 ($5HT_1$ agonists)

Skilled tasks Drowsiness may affect performance of skilled tasks (e.g. driving)

Hepatic impairment avoid in severe impairment

Renal impairment caution

Pregnancy limited experience—avoid unless potential benefit outweighs risk

Breast-feeding present in milk but not known to be harmful; withhold breast-feeding for 24 hours

Contra-indications vasospasm; previous cerebrovascular accident or transient ischaemic attack; peripheral vascular disease; moderate and severe hypertension

Side-effects sensations of tingling, heat, heaviness, pressure, or tightness of any part of the body (including throat and chest—discontinue if intense, may be due to coronary vasoconstriction or to anaphylaxis; flushing, dizziness, weakness; nausea and vomiting; drowsiness, transient increase in blood pressure, hypotension, bradycardia or tachycardia, visual disturbances, ischaemic colitis, Raynaud's syndrome, seizures reported; nasal irritation and taste disturbance with nasal spray

Licensed use tablets not licensed for use in children

Indication and dose

Acute migraine attack

- **By mouth**

Child 6–10 years 25 mg as a single dose, repeated once after at least 2 hours if migraine recurs

Child 10–12 years 50 mg as a single dose, repeated once after at least 2 hours if migraine recurs

Child 12–18 years 50–100 mg as a single dose, repeated once after at least 2 hours if migraine recurs

- **Intranasally**

Child 12–18 years 10–20 mg as a single dose, repeated once after at least 2 hours if migraine recurs; max. 40 mg in 24 hours

Note Child not responding to recommended dose should not take second dose for same attack

Imigran® (GSK) PoM

Tablets, f/c, sumatriptan (as succinate) 50 mg, net price 6-tab pack = £27.62, 12-tab pack = £52.48; 100 mg, 6-tab pack = £44.64, 12-tab pack = £89.28. Label: 3, 10, patient information leaflet

Nasal spray, sumatriptan 10 mg/0.1-mL actuation, net price 2 unit-dose spray device = £12.28; 20 mg/ 0.1-mL actuation, 2 unit-dose spray device = £12.28, 6 unit-dose spray device = £36.83. Label: 3, 10, patient information leaflet

Imigran RADIS® (GSK) PoM

Tablets, f/c, sumatriptan (as succinate) 50 mg (pink), net price 6-tab pack = £24.87, 12-tab pack = £49.77; 100 mg (white), 6-tab pack = £44.64, 12-tab pack = £89.28. Label: 3, 10, patient information leaflet

Anti-emetics

Anti-emetics (section 4.6), including **metoclopramide**, **domperidone**, phenothiazines, and antihistamines, relieve the nausea associated with migraine attacks. Anti-emetics may be given by intramuscular injection or rectally if vomiting is a problem. Metoclopramide and domperidone have the added advantage of promoting gastric emptying and normal peristalsis; a single dose should be given at the onset of symptoms (**important**: for warnings relating to extrapyramidal effects of metoclopramide see p. 227 and p. 232).

4.7.4.2 Prophylaxis of migraine

Where migraine attacks are frequent, possible provoking factors such as stress should be sought; combined oral contraceptives may also provoke migraine. Preventive treatment should be considered if migraine attacks interfere with school and social life, particularly for children who:

- suffer at least two attacks a month;
- suffer significant disability despite suitable treatment for migraine attacks;
- cannot take suitable treatment for migraine attacks.

In children it is often possible to stop prophylaxis after a period of treatment.

Propranolol (section 2.4) may be effective in preventing migraine in children but it is contra-indicated in those with asthma. Side-effects such as depression and postural hypotension can further limit its use.

Pizotifen, an antihistamine and serotonin antagonist, taken at night or twice daily, may also be used but its efficacy in children has not been clearly established. Common side-effects include drowsiness and weight gain.

Topiramate (section 4.8.1) is licensed for migraine prophylaxis. Treatment should be supervised by a specialist.

PIZOTIFEN

Cautions urinary retention; angle-closure glaucoma, renal impairment; **interactions:** Appendix 1 (pizotifen)

Skilled tasks Drowsiness may affect performance of skilled tasks (e.g. driving); effects of alcohol enhanced

Pregnancy manufacturer advises avoid unless potential benefit outweighs risk

Breast-feeding amount probably too small to be harmful but manufacturer advises avoid

Side-effects antimuscarinic effects, drowsiness, increased appetite and weight gain; occasionally nausea, dizziness; *rarely* anxiety, aggression and depression; CNS stimulation may occur

Licensed use *Sanomigran®* elixir and 500-microgram tablets not licensed for use in children under 2 years; 1.5 mg-tablets not licensed for use in children

Indication and dose

Prophylaxis of migraine
- By mouth

Child 5–10 years initially 500 micrograms at night increased according to response up to 500 micrograms 3 times daily; max. single dose at night 1 mg; max. 1.5 mg in 24 hours

Child 10–12 years initially 1 mg at night increased according to response up to 500 micrograms 3 times daily; max. single dose at night 1 mg; max. 1.5 mg in 24 hours

Child 12–18 years initially 1.5 mg at night increased according to response to 1.5 mg 3 times daily; max. single dose 3 mg; max. 4.5 mg in 24 hours

Pizotifen (Non-proprietary) PoM

Tablets, pizotifen (as hydrogen malate), 500 micrograms, net price 28-tab pack = £1.96; 1.5 mg, 28-tab pack = £4.34. Label: 2

Sanomigran® (Novartis) PoM

Tablets, both ivory-yellow, s/c, pizotifen (as hydrogen malate), 500 micrograms, net price 60-tab pack = £2.57; 1.5 mg, 28-tab pack = £4.28. Label: 2

Elixir, pizotifen (as hydrogen malate) 250 micrograms/5 mL, net price 300 mL = £4.51. Label: 2

4.7.4.3 Cluster headache

Cluster headache rarely responds to standard analgesics. **Sumatriptan** given by subcutaneous injection is the drug of choice for the *treatment* of cluster headache; treatment should be initiated by a specialist. Alternatively, 100% **oxygen** at a rate of 7–12 litres/minute is useful in aborting an attack.

4.8 Antiepileptics

4.8.1 Control of epilepsy

The decision about when to start treatment with an antiepileptic drug and the choice of medication depend on frequency of seizures, neurological findings, the identification of an epilepsy syndrome, and the wishes of the child and carers. For the majority of children, epilepsy is controlled with a single antiepileptic drug.

The object of treatment is to prevent the occurrence of seizures by maintaining an effective dose of one or more antiepileptic drugs. Careful adjustment of doses is necessary, starting with low doses and increasing gradually until seizures are controlled or there are significant adverse effects. NICE has issued clinical guidance (October 2004) on the diagnosis and management of epilepsies in children and young people.

The frequency of administration is often determined by the plasma half-life, and should be kept as low as possible to encourage better compliance. Most antiepileptics, when used in usual dosage, may be given twice daily. Phenobarbital and sometimes phenytoin, which have long half-lives, may often be given as a daily dose at bedtime. However, with large doses, some antiepileptics may need to be given 3 times daily to avoid adverse effects associated with high peak plasma concentrations. Young children metabolise antiepileptics more rapidly than adults and therefore require more frequent doses and a higher amount per kilogram body-weight.

Combination therapy Therapy with two or more antiepileptic drugs concurrently may be necessary; it should preferably only be used when monotherapy with several alternative drugs has proved ineffective. Combination therapy enhances toxicity and drug interactions may occur between antiepileptics (see below).

Interactions Interactions between antiepileptics are complex and may increase toxicity without a corresponding increase in antiepileptic effect. Interactions are usually caused by *hepatic enzyme induction* or *hepatic enzyme inhibition*; *displacement from protein binding sites* is not usually a problem. These interactions are highly variable and unpredictable.

Significant interactions that occur **between antiepileptics** themselves are as follows:

Note Check under each drug for possible interactions when two or more antiepileptic drugs are used

Carbamazepine
often lowers plasma concentration of *clobazam, clonazepam, lamotrigine, an active metabolite of oxcarbazepine*, and of *phenytoin* (but may also raise phenytoin concentration), *tiagabine, topiramate, and valproate*

sometimes lowers plasma concentration of *ethosuximide, and primidone* (but tendency for corresponding increase in plasma-phenobarbital concentration)

Ethosuximide
sometimes raises plasma concentration of *phenytoin*

Gabapentin
no interactions with gabapentin reported

Lamotrigine
sometimes raises plasma concentration of *an active metabolite of carbamazepine* (but evidence is conflicting)

sometimes raises plasma concentration of *an active metabolite of oxcarbazepine*

Levetiracetam
no interactions with levetiracetam reported

Oxcarbazepine
sometimes lowers plasma concentration of *carbamazepine* (but may raise concentration of *an active metabolite of carbamazepine*)

often lowers plasma concentration of *lamotrigine*

sometimes raises plasma concentration of *phenytoin*

often raises plasma concentration of *phenobarbital*

Phenobarbital *or Primidone*
often lowers plasma concentration of *carbamazepine, clonazepam, lamotrigine, an active metabolite of oxcarbazepine*, and of *phenytoin* (but may also raise phenytoin concentration), *tiagabine, and valproate*

sometimes lowers plasma concentration of *ethosuximide*

Phenytoin
often lowers plasma concentration of *clonazepam, carbamazepine, lamotrigine, an active metabolite of oxcarbazepine*, and of *tiagabine, topiramate, and valproate*

often raises plasma concentration of *phenobarbital*

sometimes lowers plasma concentration of *ethosuximide, and primidone* (by increasing conversion to phenobarbital)

Topiramate
sometimes raises plasma concentration of *phenytoin*

Valproate
sometimes lowers plasma concentration of *an active metabolite of oxcarbazepine*

often raises plasma concentration of *an active metabolite of carbamazepine,* and of *lamotrigine, primidone, phenobarbital, and phenytoin* (but may also lower)

sometimes raises plasma concentration of *ethosuximide, and primidone* (and tendency for significant increase in plasma-phenobarbital concentration)

Vigabatrin
often lowers plasma concentration of *phenytoin*

sometimes lowers plasma concentration of *phenobarbital, and primidone*

For other important interactions see **Appendix** 1; for advice on hormonal contraception and enzyme-inducing drugs (including antiepileptics), see BNF section 7.3.1 and BNF section 7.3.2

Withdrawal Abrupt withdrawal of antiepileptics, particularly the barbiturates and benzodiazepines, should be avoided, as this may precipitate severe rebound seizures. The dose should be reduced in stages and, in the case of the barbiturates, the withdrawal process may take months. The changeover from one antiepileptic drug regimen to another should be made cautiously, withdrawing the first drug only when the new regimen has been largely established.

The decision to withdraw antiepileptics from a seizure-free child, and its timing, depends on individual circumstances such as the type of epilepsy and its cause. Even in children who have been seizure-free for several years, there is a significant risk of seizure recurrence on drug withdrawal.

Drugs should be gradually withdrawn over at least 2–3 months by reducing the daily dose by 10–25% at intervals of 1–2 weeks. Benzodiazepines may need to be withdrawn over 6 months or longer.

In children receiving several antiepileptic drugs, only one drug should be withdrawn at a time.

Monitoring Routine measurement of plasma concentrations of antiepileptic drugs is not usually justified, because the target concentration ranges are arbitrary and often vary between individuals. However, plasma-drug concentrations may be measured in children with worsening seizures, status epilepticus, suspected non-compliance, or suspected toxicity. Similarly, haematological and biochemical monitoring should only be undertaken if clinically indicated.

Driving Older children suffering from epilepsy may drive a motor vehicle provided that they have been seizure-free for one year or, if subject to attacks only while asleep, have established a 3-year period of asleep attacks without awake attacks. Those affected by drowsiness should not drive or operate machinery.

Guidance issued by the Drivers Medical Unit of the Driver and Vehicle Licensing Agency (DVLA) recommends that patients should be advised not to drive during withdrawal of antiepileptic drugs, or for 6 months afterwards.

Pregnancy and breast-feeding During pregnancy, total plasma concentration of antiepileptics (particularly of phenytoin) may fall, particularly in the later stages but the concentration of the unbound drug may remain the same (or even rise). There is an increased risk of teratogenicity associated with the use of antiepileptic drugs (reduced if treatment is limited to a single drug). However, the benefit of antiepileptic treatment usually outweighs the potential teratogenic risk, and treatment should not be stopped during pregnancy without discussing with a specialist (see also under individual drugs). In view of the increased risk of neural tube and other defects associated, in particular, with **carbamazepine**, **oxcarbazepine**, **phenytoin** and **valproate**, women taking antiepileptic drugs who *may become pregnant* should be **informed of the possible consequences**. Those who *wish to become pregnant* should be referred to an appropriate specialist for advice. Young women who become pregnant should be **counselled** and offered **antenatal screening** (including alpha-fetoprotein measurement and a second trimester ultrasound scan).

To counteract the risk of neural tube defects adequate folate supplements are advised for women before and during pregnancy; to prevent recurrence of neural tube defects, women should receive folic acid 5 mg daily (section 9.1.2)—this dose may also be appropriate for women receiving antiepileptic drugs.

In view of the risk of neonatal bleeding associated with carbamazepine, phenobarbital and phenytoin, prophylactic vitamin K_1 (section 9.6.6) is recommended for the mother before delivery as well as for the neonate.

Breast-feeding is acceptable with all antiepileptic drugs, taken in normal doses, with the possible exception of the barbiturates, and also some of the more recently introduced ones, see under individual drugs.

Partial seizures with or without secondary generalisation

Carbamazepine, **lamotrigine**, **sodium valproate** and **topiramate** can be used in monotherapy for secondarily generalised tonic-clonic seizures and for partial (focal) seizures; alternatively, **oxcarbazepine** monotherapy can be used. **Phenobarbital** (phenobarbitone) and **primidone** are also effective but they are more sedating and are not used as first-line drugs.

Where a single drug fails to control the seizures, combination therapy can be tried with the above drugs or with additional drugs, such as gabapentin, levetiracetam, or tiagabine; alternatives include clobazam, clonazepam, and phenytoin.

Generalised seizures

Tonic-clonic seizures (grand mal) The drugs of choice for tonic-clonic seizures are **carbamazepine**, **lamotrigine**, **topiramate**, and **sodium valproate**. For children who have tonic-clonic seizures as part of the syndrome of primary generalised epilepsy, **sodium valproate** is the drug of choice. Second-line drugs include clobazam, levetiracetam, and oxcarbazepine. Other drugs that may be considered include clonazepam and phenytoin; phenobarbital and primidone are also effective but may be more sedating.

Absence seizures (petit mal) **Ethosuximide** and **sodium valproate** are the drugs of choice in simple absence seizures; **lamotrigine** can be used if these are unsuitable. Sodium valproate is also highly effective in treating the tonic-clonic seizures which may co-exist with absence seizures in primary generalised epilepsy. Alternatively, clobazam, clonazepam and topiramate can be used.

Myoclonic seizures Myoclonic seizures (myoclonic jerks) occur in a variety of syndromes, and response to treatment varies considerably. **Sodium valproate** is the drug of choice and **clobazam**, **clonazepam**, **ethosuximide**, **levetiracetam**, **lamotrigine**, or **topiramate** are second-line drugs for treating myoclonic seizures.

Atypical absence, atonic, and tonic seizures *Atypical absence seizures* may be managed with sodium valproate, lamotrigine, or ethosuximide. *Atonic seizures* may respond to sodium valproate, lamotrigine, ethosuximide, or topiramate. *Tonic seizures* may be treated with sodium valproate or topiramate; these seizures may be aggravated by benzodiazepines.

Epilepsy syndromes

Infantile spasms Vigabatrin is the drug of choice for infantile spasms associated with tuberous sclerosis. In spasms of other causes, high doses of corticosteroids such as prednisolone may be more effective. Second-line alternatives include clobazam, clonazepam, sodium valproate, and topiramate; nitrazepam is used but it is sedating. Tetracosactide (section 6.5.1) has also been used.

Lennox-Gastaut syndrome Lamotrigine, sodium valproate, and topiramate are first-line drugs for treating Lennox-Gastaut syndrome. Clobazam, clonazepam, ethosuximide, and levetiracetam are also used.

Landau-Kleffner syndrome Prednisolone, lamotrigine and sodium valproate are commonly used to treat Landau-Kleffner syndrome. Alternatives include clobazam, levetiracetam and topiramate.

Neonatal seizures Seizures can occur before delivery, but they are most common up to 24 hours after birth. Seizures in neonates occur as a result of encephalopathy, biochemical disturbances, inborn errors of metabolism, hypoxic ischaemia, drug withdrawal, severe jaundice (kernicterus), meningitis, or cerebral damage.

Seizures caused by biochemical imbalance and those in neonates with inherited abnormal pyridoxine or biotin metabolism should be corrected by treating the underlying cause. Seizures caused by drug withdrawal following intrauterine exposure are treated with a drug withdrawal regimen.

Phenobarbital may be preferred when there is a risk of seizure recurrence in neonates; phenytoin is an alternative. The benzodiazepines (clonazepam, diazepam, lorazepam, and midazolam) and rectal paraldehyde may be useful in the management of seizures which are likely to be brief with little risk of recurrence.

Carbamazepine and oxcarbazepine

Carbamazepine is a drug of choice for simple and complex partial seizures and for tonic-clonic seizures secondary to a focal discharge. It can exacerbate myoclonic and absence seizures. Carbamazepine has a wider therapeutic index than phenytoin and the relationship between dose and plasma-carbamazepine concentration is linear. It has generally fewer side-effects than phenytoin or the barbiturates, but reversible blurring of vision, dizziness, and unsteadiness are dose-related, and may be dose-limiting. These side-effects may be reduced by altering the timing of medication; use of modified-release tablets also significantly lessens the incidence of dose-related side-effects. It is essential to initiate carbamazepine therapy at a low dose and build this up slowly in small increments every two weeks.

Oxcarbazepine may be used for the treatment of partial seizures with or without secondarily generalised tonic-clonic seizures. Oxcarbazepine induces hepatic enzymes to a lesser extent than carbamazepine.

CARBAMAZEPINE

Cautions cardiac disease (see also Contra-indications), skin reactions (see also Blood, hepatic or skin disorders below and under Side-effects), history of haematological reactions to other drugs; manufacturer recommends blood counts and hepatic and renal function tests (but evidence of practical value unsatisfactory); glaucoma; avoid abrupt withdrawal; **interactions:** see p. 253 and Appendix 1 (carbamazepine)

Hepatic impairment metabolism impaired in advanced liver disease

Renal impairment manufacturer advises caution

Pregnancy see Antiepileptics: pregnancy and breast-feeding, p. 254

Breast-feeding see notes above; amount probably too small to be harmful

Blood, hepatic or skin disorders Children or their carers should be told how to recognise signs of blood, liver, or skin disorders, and advised to seek immediate medical attention if symptoms such as fever, sore throat, rash, mouth ulcers, bruising, or bleeding develop. Leucopenia which is severe, progressive or associated with clinical symptoms requires withdrawal (if necessary under cover of suitable alternative).

Contra-indications AV conduction abnormalities (unless paced); history of bone marrow depression, porphyria (section 9.8.2)

Side-effects nausea and vomiting, dizziness, drowsiness, headache, ataxia, confusion and agitation, visual disturbances (especially diplopia and often associated with peak plasma concentrations); constipation or diarrhoea, anorexia; mild transient generalised erythematous rash may occur in a large number of children (withdraw if worsens or is accompanied by other symptoms); leucopenia and other blood disorders (including thrombocytopenia, agranulocytosis and aplastic anaemia); other side-effects include cholestatic jaundice, hepatitis and acute renal failure, Stevens-Johnson syndrome, toxic epidermal necrolysis, alopecia, thromboembolism, arthralgia, fever, proteinuria, lymph node enlargement, cardiac conduction disturbances (sometimes arrhythmias), dyskinesias, paraesthesia, depression, impotence (and impaired fertility), gynaecomastia, galactorrhoea, aggression, activation of psychosis; photosensitivity, pulmonary hypersensitivity (with dyspnoea and pneumonitis), hyponatraemia, oedema, and disturbances of bone metabolism (with osteomalacia) also reported; suppositories may cause occasional rectal irritation

Pharmacokinetics plasma concentration for optimum response 4–12 mg/litre (20–50 micromol/litre) measured after 1–2 weeks

Licensed use licensed for use in children with generalised tonic-clonic and partial seizures only

Indication and dose

Partial and generalised tonic-clonic seizures, neuropathic pain, some movement disorders (e.g. paroxysmal kinesigenic choreoathetosis), mood stabilisation

- **By mouth**

  Child 1 month–12 years initially 5 mg/kg at night or 2.5 mg/kg twice daily, increased as necessary by 2.5–5 mg/kg every 3–7 days; usual maintenance dose 5 mg/kg 2–3 times daily; doses up to 20 mg/kg daily have been used

  Child 12–18 years initially 100–200 mg 1–2 times daily, increased slowly to usual maintenance of 400–600 mg 2–3 times daily

- **By rectum**

  Child 1 month–18 years use approx. 25% more than the oral dose (max. 250 mg) up to 4 times daily

Administration Oral liquid has been used rectally—should be retained for at least 2 hours (but may have laxative effect)

CARBAMAZEPINE (*continued*)

Carbamazepine (Non-proprietary) PoM
Tablets, carbamazepine 100 mg, net price 20 = £1.42; 200 mg, 20 = £1.70; 400 mg, 20 = £3.47. Label: 3, 8, counselling, blood, hepatic or skin disorder symptoms (see above), driving (see notes above)
Brands include *Epimaz®*
Note Different preparations may vary in bioavailability; to avoid reduced effect or excessive side-effects, it may be prudent to avoid changing the formulation (see also notes above on how side-effects may be reduced)
Dental prescribing on NHS Carbamazepine Tablets may be prescribed

Tegretol® (Novartis) PoM
Tablets, all scored, carbamazepine 100 mg, net price 84-tab pack = £2.43; 200 mg, 84-tab pack = £4.50; 400 mg, 56-tab pack = £5.90. Label: 3, 8, counselling, blood, hepatic or skin disorder symptoms (see above), driving (see notes above)

Chewtabs, orange, carbamazepine 100 mg, net price 56-tab pack = £3.54; 200 mg, 56-tab pack = £6.59. Label: 3, 8, 21, 24, counselling, blood, hepatic or skin disorder symptoms (see above), driving (see notes above)

Liquid, sugar-free, carbamazepine 100 mg/5 mL. Net price 300-mL pack = £6.86. Label: 3, 8, counselling, blood, hepatic or skin disorder symptoms (see above), driving (see notes above)

Suppositories, carbamazepine 125 mg, net price 5 = £9.00; 250 mg, 5 = £12.00. Label: 3, 8, counselling, blood, hepatic or skin disorder symptoms (see above), driving (see notes above)

Dose

Epilepsy for short-term use (max. 7 days) when oral therapy temporarily not possible

Note Suppositories of 125 mg may be considered to be approximately equivalent in therapeutic effect to tablets of 100 mg but final adjustment should always depend on clinical response (plasma concentration monitoring recommended); max. dose *by rectum* 250 mg 4 times daily

Modified release

Carbagen® SR (Generics) PoM
Tablets, m/r, f/c, both scored, carbamazepine 200 mg, net price 56-tab pack = £4.81; 400 mg, 56-tab pack = £9.47. Label: 3, 8, 25, counselling, blood, hepatic or skin disorder symptoms (see above), driving (see notes above)

Dose

Child over 5 years as above; total daily dose given in 1–2 divided doses

Tegretol® Retard (Novartis) PoM
Tablets, m/r, both scored, carbamazepine 200 mg (beige-orange), net price 56-tab pack = £5.26; 400 mg (brown-orange), 56-tab pack = £10.34. Label: 3, 8, 25, counselling, blood, hepatic or skin disorder symptoms (see above), driving (see notes above)

Dose

Child over 5 years as above, total daily dose given in 2 divided doses

Administration *Tegretol® Retard* tablets can be halved but should not be chewed

OXCARBAZEPINE

Cautions hypersensitivity to carbamazepine; avoid abrupt withdrawal; hyponatraemia (monitor plasma-sodium concentration in patients at risk), heart failure (monitor body-weight), cardiac conduction disorders; avoid in porphyria (section 9.8.2); **interactions:** Appendix 1 (oxcarbazepine)

Hepatic impairment manufacturer advises caution in severe impairment—no information available

Renal impairment use half initial dose if creatinine clearance less than 30 mL/minute/1.73m^2, increase according to response at intervals of at least 1 week

Pregnancy see Antiepileptics: pregnancy and breast feeding, p. 254

Breast-feeding present in milk; amount probably too small to be harmful but manufacturer advises avoid

Blood, hepatic or skin disorders Children or their carers should be told how to recognise signs of blood, liver, or skin disorders, and advised to seek immediate medical attention if symptoms such as lethargy, confusion, muscular twitching, fever, sore throat, rash, blistering, mouth ulcers, bruising, or bleeding develop

Side-effects nausea, vomiting, constipation, diarrhoea, abdominal pain, dizziness, headache, drowsiness, agitation, amnesia, asthenia, ataxia, confusion, impaired concentration, depression, tremor, hyponatraemia, acne, alopecia, rash, nystagmus, visual disorders including diplopia; *less commonly* urticaria, leucopenia; *very rarely* hepatitis, pancreatitis, arrhythmias, hypersensitivity reactions, thrombocytopenia, systemic lupus erythematosus, Stevens-Johnson syndrome, and toxic epidermal necrolysis

Indication and dose

Monotherapy and adjunctive therapy of partial seizures with or without secondarily generalisation of a partial seizure

- **By mouth**

Child 6–12 years initially 4–5 mg/kg twice daily, increased according to response in steps of up to 5 mg/kg twice daily at weekly intervals (usual maintenance dose for adjunctive therapy 15 mg/kg twice daily); max. 23 mg/kg twice daily

Child 12–18 years initially 4–5 mg/kg (max. 300 mg) twice daily increased according to response by 300 mg twice daily at weekly intervals (usual maintenance dose range 0.3–1.2 g twice daily); max. 23 mg/kg twice daily

Note In adjunctive therapy the dose of concomitant antiepileptics may need to be reduced when using high doses of oxcarbazepine

Trileptal® (Novartis) PoM
Tablets, f/c, scored, oxcarbazepine 150 mg (green), net price 50-tab pack = £10.00; 300 mg (yellow), 50-tab pack = £20.00; 600 mg (pink), 50-tab pack = £40.00. Label: 3, 8, counselling, blood, hepatic or

OXCARBAZEPINE (*continued*)

skin disorders (see above), driving (see notes above)

Oral suspension, sugar-free, oxcarbazepine 300 mg/5 mL, net price 250 mL (with oral syringe) = £40.00. Label: 3, 8, counselling, blood, hepatic or skin disorders (see above), driving (see notes above)

Excipients: include propylene glycol

Ethosuximide

Ethosuximide is sometimes used in typical absence seizures; it may also be used in myoclonic seizures and in atypical absence, atonic, and tonic seizures.

ETHOSUXIMIDE

Cautions see notes above; avoid abrupt withdrawal; hepatic impairment; renal impairment; avoid in porphyria (section 9.8.2); **interactions:** Appendix 1 (ethosuximide)

Pregnancy may be teratogenic but see Antiepileptics: pregnancy and breast-feeding, p. 254

Breast-feeding present in milk but unlikely to be harmful; manufacturer advises avoid

Blood disorders Children or their carers should be told how to recognise signs of blood disorders, and advised to seek immediate medical attention if symptoms such as fever, sore throat, mouth ulcers, bruising or bleeding develop

Side-effects gastro-intestinal disturbances (including nausea, vomiting, abdominal pain, and anorexia); *less frequently* headache, fatigue, drowsiness, dizziness, hiccup, ataxia, mild euphoria; *rarely* tongue swelling, sleep disturbances, night terrors, depression, psychosis, photophobia, dyskinesia, increased libido, vaginal bleeding, myopia, gingival hypertrophy, and rash; also reported, hyperactivity, blood disorders such as leucopenia and aplastic anaemia (blood counts required if features of infection), systemic lupus erythematosus, and Stevens-Johnson syndrome

Pharmacokinetics ethosuximide-plasma concentration for optimum response in simple absence seizures 40–100 mg/litre (300–700 micromol/litre)

Indication and dose

Absence seizures, atypical absence, myoclonic seizures

- **By mouth**

  Child 1 month–12 years initially 5 mg/kg (max. 250 mg) twice daily, increased gradually over 2–3 weeks up to maintenance dose of 10–20 mg/kg (max. 1 g) twice daily; total daily dose may rarely be given in 3 divided doses

  Child 12–18 years initially 250 mg twice daily, increased by 250 mg at intervals of 4–7 days to usual dose of 500–750 mg twice daily; occasionally up to 1 g twice daily may be needed

Emeside® (Chemidex) PoM

Capsules, ethosuximide 250 mg, net price 56-cap pack = £38.23. Label: 8, counselling, blood disorders (see above), driving (see notes above)

Syrup, black currant, ethosuximide 250 mg/5 mL, net price 200-mL pack = £6.60. Label: 8, counselling, blood disorders (see above), driving (see notes above)

Zarontin® (Parke-Davis) PoM

Syrup, yellow, ethosuximide 250 mg/5 mL, net price 200-mL pack = £4.48. Label: 8, counselling, blood disorders (see above), driving (see notes above)

Gabapentin

Gabapentin can be given as adjunctive therapy in partial epilepsy with or without secondary generalisation.

GABAPENTIN

Cautions avoid sudden withdrawal (may cause anxiety, insomnia, nausea, pain, and sweating—taper off over at least 1 week); history of psychotic illness, diabetes mellitus, false positive readings with some urinary protein tests; **interactions:** Appendix 1 (gabapentin)

Renal impairment reduce dose if creatinine clearance less than 80 mL/minute/1.73 m^2; consult product literature

Pregnancy see Antiepileptics: pregnancy and breast-feeding, p. 254; no evidence of teratogenicity in *animal* studies, but manufacturer advises use only if potential benefit outweighs risk

Breast-feeding present in milk—manufacturer advises avoid

Side-effects diarrhoea, dry mouth, dyspepsia, nausea, vomiting; peripheral oedema; dizziness, drowsiness, anxiety, abnormal gait, amnesia, ataxia, nystagmus, tremor, asthenia, paraesthesia, emotional lability, hyperkinesia; weight gain; dysarthria, arthralgia; diplopia, amblyopia; rash, purpura; *less commonly* constipation, flatulence, dyspnoea, confusion, impotence, and leucopenia; *rarely* depression, psychosis, headache, and myalgia; hepatitis, jaundice, chest pain, palpitation, movement disorders, thrombocytopenia, tinnitus, acute renal failure, and alopecia also reported

Licensed use not licensed for use in children under 6 years

GABAPENTIN (*continued*)

Indication and dose

Adjunctive treatment of partial seizures with or without secondary generalisation not satisfactorily controlled with other antiepileptics

- By mouth

Child 2–12 years 10 mg/kg on day 1, then 10 mg/kg twice daily on day 2, then 10 mg/kg 3 times daily on day 3, increased to a usual maintenance dose of 10–20 mg/kg 3 times daily; (body-weight 26–36 kg, 900 mg daily; body-weight 37–50 kg, 1.2 g daily)

Note Some children may not tolerate daily increments; longer intervals (up to weekly) may be more appropriate

Child 12–18 years 300 mg on day 1, then 300 mg twice daily on day 2, then 300 mg 3 times daily on day 3 (approx. every 8 hours), then increased according to response in steps of 100 mg 3 times daily to a usual maintenance of 300–800 mg 3 times daily

Administration capsules can be opened but the bitter taste is difficult to mask

Gabapentin (Non-proprietary) PoM

Capsules, gabapentin 100 mg, net price 100-cap pack = £22.92; 300 mg, 100-cap pack = £50.18; 400 mg, 100-cap pack = £53.60. Label: 3, 5, 8, counselling, driving (see notes above)

Tablets, gabapentin 600 mg, net price 100-tab pack = £106.00; 800 mg, 100-tab pack= £121.48. Label: 3, 5, 8, counselling, driving (see notes above)

Neurontin® (Pfizer) PoM

Capsules, gabapentin 100 mg (white), net price 100-cap pack = £22.86; 300 mg (yellow), 100-cap pack = £53.00; 400 mg (orange), 100-cap pack = £61.33; titration pack of 40 × 300-mg (yellow) capsules with 10 × 600-mg tablets = £31.80. Label: 3, 5, 8, counselling, driving (see notes above)

Tablets, f/c, gabapentin 600 mg, net price 100-tab pack = £106.00; 800 mg, 100-tab pack = £122.66. Label: 3, 5, 8, counselling, driving (see notes above)

Lamotrigine

Lamotrigine is an antiepileptic for partial seizures and primary and secondarily generalised tonic-clonic seizures. It may be tried for atypical absence, atonic, and tonic seizures particularly in children with Lennox-Gastaut syndrome. Lamotrigine may cause serious skin rash; dose recommendations should be adhered to closely.

Lamotrigine is used either as sole treatment or as an adjunct to treatment with other antiepileptic drugs. Valproate increases plasma-lamotrigine concentration whereas the enzyme inducing antiepileptics reduce it; care is therefore required in choosing the appropriate initial dose and subsequent titration. Where the potential for interaction is not known, treatment should be initiated with lower doses such as those used with valproate.

LAMOTRIGINE

Cautions closely monitor (including hepatic, renal and clotting function) and consider withdrawal if rash, fever, or signs of hypersensitivity syndrome develop; avoid abrupt withdrawal (taper off over 2 weeks or longer) unless serious skin reaction occurs; **interactions:** see p. 253 and Appendix 1 (lamotrigine)

Hepatic impairment halve dose in moderate disease; quarter dose in severe disease

Renal impairment metabolite may accumulate in moderate or severe impairment

Pregnancy see Antiepileptics: pregnancy and breast-feeding, p. 254; no evidence of teratogenicity in animal studies, but manufacturer advises avoid unless potential benefit outweighs risk

Breast-feeding present in milk, but limited data suggest no harmful effect on neonate

Blood disorders The CSM has advised prescribers to be alert for symptoms and signs suggestive of bone-marrow failure such as anaemia, bruising, or infection. Aplastic anaemia, bone-marrow depression and pancytopenia have been associated rarely with lamotrigine.

Side-effects rash (see Skin reactions below); hypersensitivity syndrome (possibly including rash, fever, lymphadenopathy, hepatic dysfunction, blood disorders, disseminated intravascular coagulation and multi-organ dysfunction); nausea, vomiting, diarrhoea, hepatic dysfunction; headache, fatigue, dizziness, sleep disturbances, tremor, movement disorders, agitation, confusion, hallucinations; blood disorders (including leucopenia, thrombocytopenia, pancytopenia); lupus erythematosus-like effect; photosensitivity; nystagmus, diplopia, blurred vision, conjunctivitis

Skin reactions Serious skin reactions including Stevens-Johnson syndrome and toxic epidermal necrolysis (rarely with fatalities) have developed especially in children; most rashes occur in the first 8 weeks. Rash is sometimes associated with hypersensitivity syndrome (see Side-effects above). Consider withdrawal if rash or signs of hypersensitivity syndrome develop. The CSM has advised that factors associated with increased risk of serious skin reactions include concomitant use of valproate, initial lamotrigine dosing higher than recommended, and more rapid dose escalation than recommended.

Counselling Warn children and their carers to see their doctor immediately if rash or signs or symptoms of hypersensitivity syndrome develop

LAMOTRIGINE (*continued*)

Indication and dose

Monotherapy and adjunctive treatment of partial seizures and primary and secondarily generalised tonic-clonic seizures; seizures associated with Lennox-Gastaut syndrome

- By mouth

Adjunctive therapy *with valproate*

Child 2–12 years initially 150 micrograms/kg once daily for 14 days (those weighing under 13 kg may receive 2 mg on alternate days for first 14 days) then 300 micrograms/kg once daily for further 14 days, thereafter increased by max. of 300 micrograms/kg daily every 7–14 days; usual maintenance 1–5 mg/kg daily in 1–2 divided doses (max. single dose 100 mg)

Child 12–18 years initially 25 mg on alternate days for 14 days then 25 mg daily for further 14 days, thereafter increased by max. of 25–50 mg daily every 7–14 days; usual maintenance 100–200 mg daily in 1–2 divided doses

Adjunctive therapy (with enzyme inducing drugs) *without valproate*

Child 2–12 years initially 300 micrograms/kg twice daily for 14 days then 600 micrograms/kg twice daily for further 14 days, thereafter increased by max. of 1.2 mg/kg daily every 7–14 days; usual maintenance 2.5–7.5 mg/kg (max. single dose 200 mg) twice daily

Child 12–18 years initially 50 mg daily for 14 days then 50 mg twice daily for further 14 days, thereafter increased by max. of 100 mg daily every 7–14 days; usual maintenance 100–200 mg twice daily (up to 700 mg daily has been required)

Monotherapy

Child 12–18 years initially 25 mg daily for 14 days, increased to 50 mg daily for further 14 days, then increased by max. of 50–100 mg daily every 7–14 days; usual maintenance as monotherapy, 100–200 mg daily in 1–2 divided doses (up to 500 mg daily has been required)

Safe Practice Do not confuse the different combinations; see also notes above

Lamotrigine (Non-proprietary) PoM

Tablets, lamotrigine 25 mg, net price 56-tab pack = £17.35; 50 mg, 56-tab pack = £29.50; 100 mg, 56-tab pack = £50.88; 200 mg, 30-tab pack = £46.34, 56-tab pack = £86.50. Label: 8, counselling, driving (see notes above), skin reactions

Dispersible tablets, lamotrigine 5 mg, net price 28-tab pack = £8.04; 25 mg, 56-tab pack = £20.31; 100 mg, 56-tab pack = £59.76. Label: 8, 13, counselling, driving (see notes above), skin reactions

Lamictal® (GSK) PoM

Tablets, all yellow, lamotrigine 25 mg, net price 21-tab pack (*'Valproate Add-on therapy' Starter Pack*) = £7.65, 42-tab pack (*'Monotherapy' Starter Pack*) = £15.30, 56-tab pack = £20.41; 50 mg, 42-tab pack (*'Non-valproate Add-on therapy' Starter Pack*) = £26.02, 56-tab pack = £34.70; 100 mg, 56-tab pack = £59.86; 200 mg, 56-tab pack = £101.76. Label: 8, counselling, driving (see notes above), skin reactions

Dispersible tablets, chewable, lamotrigine 2 mg, net price 30-tab pack = £ 8.71; 5 mg, 28-tab pack = £8.14; 25 mg, 56-tab pack = £20.41; 100 mg, 56-tab pack = £59.86. Label: 8, 13, counselling, driving (see notes above), skin reactions

Levetiracetam

Levetiracetam is used for the adjunctive treatment of partial seizures.

LEVETIRACETAM

Cautions avoid sudden withdrawal

Hepatic impairment halve dose in severe hepatic impairment if creatinine clearance less than 70 mL/minute/1.73 m²

Renal impairment reduce dose if creatinine clearance less than 80 mL/minute/1.73 m²

Pregnancy see Antiepileptics: pregnancy and breast-feeding, p. 254; manufacturer advises use only if potential benefit outweighs risk—toxicity in *animal* studies

Breast-feeding present in milk—manufacturer advises avoid; see also notes above

Side-effects nausea, vomiting, dyspepsia, diarrhoea; cough; drowsiness, asthenia, amnesia, ataxia, convulsions, dizziness, headache, tremor, hyperkinesia, depression, emotional lability, insomnia, anxiety, anorexia; diplopia; rash; *also reported* confusion, irritability, psychosis, suicidal ideation, leucopenia, pancytopenia, thrombocytopenia, and alopecia

Indication and dose

Adjunctive treatment of partial seizures with or without secondary generalisation

- By mouth

Child 4–18 years, body-weight under 50 kg initially 10 mg/kg twice daily, adjusted in steps of not exceeding 10 mg/kg twice daily every 2 weeks; max. 30 mg/kg twice daily

Body-weight over 50 kg initially 500 mg twice daily, adjusted in steps of 500 mg twice daily every 2–4 weeks; max. 1.5 g twice daily

Keppra® (UCB Pharma) ▼ PoM

Tablets, f/c, levetiracetam 250 mg (blue), net price 60-tab pack = £29.70; 500 mg (yellow), 60-tab pack = £52.30; 750 mg (orange), 60-tab pack = £89.10; 1 g (white), 60-tab pack = £101.10. Label: 3, 8

Oral solution, sugar-free, levetiracetam 100 mg/mL, net price 300 mL = £71.80. Label: 3, 8

4 Central nervous system

Phenobarbital and other barbiturates

Phenobarbital (phenobarbitone) is effective for tonic-clonic, partial seizures and neonatal seizures but may cause behavioural disturbances and hyperkinesia. It may be tried for atypical absence, atonic, and tonic seizures. Rebound seizures may be a problem on withdrawal. Monitoring plasma concentrations is less useful than with other drugs because tolerance occurs.

Primidone is largely converted to phenobarbital and this is probably responsible for its antiepileptic action. It is used rarely in children.

PHENOBARBITAL
(Phenobarbitone)

Cautions see also notes above; debilitated, respiratory depression (avoid if severe), avoid sudden withdrawal; avoid in porphyria (see section 9.8.2); **interactions:** see p. 253 and Appendix 1 (barbiturates)

Hepatic impairment may precipitate coma

Renal impairment avoid large doses in severe impairment

Pregnancy see Antiepileptics: pregnancy and breast-feeding, p. 254

Breast-feeding avoid if possible; drowsiness may occur

Side-effects drowsiness, lethargy, mental depression, ataxia and allergic skin reactions; hyperkinesia; megaloblastic anaemia (may be treated with folic acid); **overdosage:** see Emergency Treatment of Poisoning, p. 35

Pharmacokinetics trough plasma concentration for optimum response 15–40 mg/litre (60–180 micromol/litre)

Indication and dose

All forms of epilepsy except absence seizures
- **By mouth or by intravenous injection**

Neonate initially 20 mg/kg *by slow intravenous injection* then 2.5–5 mg/kg once daily either *by slow intravenous injection* or *by mouth*; dose and frequency adjusted according to response

Child 1 month–12 years initially 1–1.5 mg/kg twice daily, increased by 2 mg/kg daily as required; usual maintenance dose 2.5–4 mg/kg once or twice daily

Child 12–18 years initially 60–180 mg twice daily; usual maintenance dose 60–180 mg once daily

Status epilepticus section 4.8.2

Note For therapeutic purposes phenobarbital and phenobarbital sodium may be considered equivalent in effect

Administration for administration *by mouth*, tablets may be crushed

For *intravenous injection*, dilute to concentration of 20 mg/mL with Water for Injections; give over 20 minutes (no faster than 1 mg/minute).

Phenobarbital (Non-proprietary) CD

Tablets, phenobarbital 15 mg, net price 28-tab pack = 63p; 30 mg, 28-tab pack = 65p; 60 mg, 28-tab pack = 71p. Label: 2, 8, counselling, driving (see notes above)

Elixir, phenobarbital 15 mg/5 mL in a suitable flavoured vehicle, containing alcohol 38%, net price 100 mL = 77p. Label: 2, 8, counselling, driving (see notes above)

Note Some hospitals supply **alcohol-free** formulations of varying phenobarbital strengths

Injection, phenobarbital sodium 200 mg/mL in propylene glycol 90% and water for injections 10%, net price 1-mL amp = £1.74

Note Must be diluted before intravenous administration (see under Administration)

PRIMIDONE

Cautions see under Phenobarbital; **interactions:** see p. 253 and Appendix 1 (primidone)

Hepatic impairment reduce dose, may precipitate coma

Renal impairment see Phenobarbital

Pregnancy see Phenobarbital

Breast-feeding see Phenobarbital

Side-effects see under Phenobarbital; also nausea and visual disturbances; *less commonly* vomiting, headache, and dizziness; *rarely* personality changes arthralgia, and osteomalacia

Pharmacokinetics monitor plasma concentrations of derived phenobarbital. Optimum range as for phenobarbital

Indication and dose

All forms of epilepsy except absence seizures (but see notes above)
- **By mouth**

Child under 2 years initially 125 mg daily at bedtime, increased by 125 mg every 3 days according to response; usual maintenance, 125–250 mg twice daily

Child 2–5 years initially 125 mg daily at bedtime, increased by 125 mg every 3 days according to response; usual maintenance, 250–375 mg twice daily

Child 5–9 years initially 125 mg daily at bedtime, increased by 125 mg every 3 days according to response; usual maintenance, 375–500 mg twice a day

PRIMIDONE (*continued*)

Child 9–18 years initially 125 mg daily at bedtime, increased by 125 mg every 3 days to 250 mg twice daily, then increased according to response by 250 mg every 3 days to max. 750 mg twice daily

Mysoline® (Acorus) PoM
Tablets, scored, primidone 250 mg, net price 100-tab pack = £12.60. Label: 2, 8, counselling, driving (see notes above)

Phenytoin

Phenytoin is effective in tonic-clonic, partial, and neonatal seizures but it may worsen myoclonus. It has a narrow therapeutic index and the relationship between dose and plasma concentration is non-linear; small dosage increases in some children may produce large rises in plasma concentrations with acute toxic side-effects. Monitoring of plasma concentration greatly assists dosage adjustment. A few missed doses or a small change in drug absorption may result in a marked change in plasma concentration.

Phenytoin may cause coarse facies, acne, hirsutism, and gingival hyperplasia and so may be particularly undesirable in adolescent patients.

When only parenteral administration is possible, **fosphenytoin** (section 4.8.2), a pro-drug of phenytoin, may be convenient to give. Whereas phenytoin can be given intravenously only, fosphenytoin may also be given by intramuscular injection.

PHENYTOIN

Cautions see notes above; avoid abrupt withdrawal; manufacturer recommends blood counts (but evidence of practical value unsatisfactory); avoid in porphyria (section 9.8.2); **interactions:** see p. 253 and Appendix 1 (phenytoin)

Hepatic impairment reduce dose

Pregnancy see Antiepileptics: pregnancy and breast-feeding, p. 254; changes in plasma protein binding may make interpretation of plasma-phenytoin concentrations difficult; increased doses may be required in the third trimester

Breast-feeding small amounts present in milk, but not known to be harmful

Blood or skin disorders Children and their carers should be told how to recognise signs of blood or skin disorders, and advised to seek immediate medical attention if symptoms such as fever, sore throat, rash, mouth ulcers, bruising, or bleeding develop. Leucopenia which is severe, progressive, or associated with clinical symptoms requires withdrawal (if necessary under cover of suitable alternative)

Side-effects nausea, vomiting, constipation; insomnia, transient nervousness, tremor, paraesthesia, dizziness, headache, anorexia; gingival hypertrophy and tenderness; rash (discontinue; if mild re-introduce cautiously but discontinue immediately if recurrence), acne, hirsutism, coarse facies; *rarely* hepatoxicity, peripheral neuropathy, dyskinesia, lymphadenopathy, osteomalacia, blood disorders (including megaloblastic anaemia (may be treated with folic acid), leucopenia, thrombocytopenia, and aplastic anaemia), polyarteritis nodosa, lupus erythematosis, Stevens-Johnson syndrome, and toxic epidermal necrolysis; also reported pneumonitis and interstitial nephritis; *with excessive dosage* nystagmus, diplopia, slurred speech, ataxia, confusion, and hyperglycaemia

Pharmacokinetics therapeutic plasma-phenytoin concentrations reduced in first 3 months of life because of reduced protein binding

Plasma concentration for optimum response:

Neonate–3 months, 6–15 mg/litre (25–60 micromol/litre)

Child 3 months–18 years, 10–20 mg/litre (40–80 micromol/litre)

Licensed use licensed for use in children (age range not specified by manufacturer)

Indication and dose

All forms of epilepsy except absence seizures
- **By intravenous injection (over 20–30 minutes) and by mouth**

Neonate initial loading dose *by slow intravenous injection* (section 4.8.2) 20 mg/kg then *by mouth* 2–4 mg/kg twice daily adjusted according to response and plasma-phenytoin concentration (usual max. 7.5 mg/kg twice daily)

- **By mouth**

Child 1 month–12 years initially 1.5–2.5 mg/kg twice daily, then adjusted according to response and plasma-phenytoin concentration to 2.5–5 mg/kg twice daily (usual max. 7.5 mg/kg twice daily *or* 300 mg daily)

Child 12–18 years initially 75–150 mg twice daily then adjusted according to response and plasma-phenytoin concentration to 150–200 mg twice daily (usual max. 300 mg twice daily)

Status epilepticus, acute symptomatic seizures associated with head trauma or neurosurgery
section 4.8.2

Administration for administration *by mouth*, interrupt enteral feeds for at least 1–2 hours before and after giving phenytoin; give with water to enhance absorption

For administration by *intravenous injection* and *intravenous infusion*, see p. 272

Phenytoin (Non-proprietary) PoM
Tablets, coated, phenytoin sodium 100 mg, net price 28-tab pack = £9.82. Label: 8, counsel-

PHENYTOIN (*continued*)

ling, administration, blood or skin disorder symptoms (see Cautions above), driving (see notes above)
Note On the basis of single dose tests there are no clinically relevant differences in bioavailability between available phenytoin sodium tablets and capsules but there may be a pharmacokinetic basis for maintaining the same brand of phenytoin in some patients

Epanutin® (Pfizer) PoM
Capsules, phenytoin sodium 25 mg (white/purple), net price 28-cap pack = 66p; 50 mg (white/pink), 28-cap pack = 67p; 100 mg (white/orange), 84-cap pack = £2.83; 300 mg (white/green), 28-cap pack = £2.83. Label: 8, counselling, administration, blood or skin disorder symptoms (see Cautions above), driving (see notes above)

Infatabs® (= chewable tablets), yellow, scored, phenytoin 50 mg, net price 112= £7.38. Label: 8, 24, counselling, blood or skin disorder symptoms (see Cautions above), driving (see notes above)
Note Contain phenytoin 50 mg (as against phenytoin sodium) therefore care is needed on changing to capsules or tablets containing phenytoin sodium

Suspension, red, phenytoin 30 mg/5 mL, net price 500 mL = £4.27. Label: 8, counselling, administration, blood or skin disorder symptoms (see Cautions above), driving (see notes above)
Note Suspension of phenytoin 90 mg in 15 mL may be considered to be approximately equivalent in therapeutic effect to capsules or tablets containing phenytoin sodium 100 mg, but nevertheless care is needed in making changes

Parenteral preparations
Section 4.8.2

Tiagabine

Tiagabine is used as adjunctive treatment for partial seizures, with or without secondary generalisation.

TIAGABINE

Cautions avoid in porphyria (section 9.8.2); avoid abrupt withdrawal; **interactions:** Appendix 1 (tiagabine)

Hepatic impairment in mild to moderate impairment, initial maintenance dose is 5–10 mg 1–2 times daily; avoid in severe impairment

Pregnancy see Antiepileptics: pregnancy and breast-feeding, p. 254; no evidence of teratogenicity in *animal* studies, but manufacturer advises use only if potential benefit outweighs risk

Breast-feeding manufacturer advises avoid unless potential benefit outweighs risk

Driving May impair performance of skilled tasks (e.g. driving)

Side-effects diarrhoea, dizziness, tiredness, nervousness, tremor, concentration difficulties, emotional lability, speech impairment; *rarely* confusion, depression, drowsiness, psychosis, non-convulsive status epilepticus; leucopenia reported

Indication and dose

Adjunctive treatment *with enzyme-inducing drugs* for partial seizures with or without secondary generalisation not satisfactorily controlled by other antiepileptics
- By mouth

Child 12–18 years initially 5 mg twice daily for 1 week then increased at weekly intervals in steps of 5–10 mg daily; usual maintenance dose 30–45 mg daily in 2–3 divided doses (doses above 30 mg daily given in 3 divided doses)

Adjunctive treatment *with non-enzyme-inducing drugs* for partial seizures with or without secondary generalisation not satisfactorily controlled by other antiepileptics
- By mouth

Child 12–18 years initially 5 mg twice daily for 1 week then increased at weekly intervals in steps of 5–10 mg daily; initial maintenance dose 15–30 mg daily in 2–3 divided doses (doses above 30 mg daily given in 3 divided doses)

Gabitril® (Cephalon) PoM
Tablets, f/c, scored, tiagabine (as hydrochloride) 5 mg, net price 100-tab pack = £43.37; 10 mg, 100-tab pack = £86.74; 15 mg, 100-tab pack = £130.11. Label: 21

Topiramate

Topiramate can be given alone or as adjunctive treatment in generalised tonic-clonic seizures or partial seizures with or without secondary generalisation. It can also be used as adjunctive treatment for seizures associated with Lennox-Gastaut syndrome. Topiramate is also licensed for prophylaxis of migraine (section 4.7.4.2).

TOPIRAMATE

Cautions avoid abrupt withdrawal; ensure adequate hydration (especially if predisposition to nephrolithiasis or in strenuous activity or warm environment); avoid in porphyria (section 9.8.2); **interactions:** see p. 253 and Appendix 1 (topiramate)

Hepatic impairment use with caution—clearance may be decreased

Renal impairment longer time to steady-state plasma concentrations in moderate to severe impairment

Pregnancy see Antiepileptics: pregnancy and breast-feeding, p. 254; manufacturer advises avoid unless potential benefit outweighs risk—toxicity in *animal* studies

Breast-feeding manufacturer advises avoid—present in milk

CSM advice Topiramate has been associated with acute myopia with secondary angle-closure glaucoma, typically occurring within 1 month of starting treatment. Choroidal effusions resulting in anterior displacement of the lens and iris have also been reported. The CSM advises that if raised intra-ocular pressure occurs:

- seek specialist ophthalmological advice;
- use appropriate measures to reduce intra-ocular pressure;
- stop topiramate as rapidly as feasible

Side-effects nausea, abdominal pain, dyspepsia, diarrhoea, dry mouth, taste disturbances, weight loss, anorexia; paraesthesia, hypoaesthesia, headache, fatigue, dizziness, speech disorder, drowsiness, insomnia, impaired memory and concentration, anxiety, depression; visual disturbances; *less commonly* suicidal ideation; *rarely* reduced sweating, metabolic acidosis; serious skin reactions

Indication and dose

Monotherapy of generalised tonic-clonic seizures or partial seizures with or without secondary generalisation

- **By mouth**

  Child 6–16 years initially 0.5–1 mg/kg at night for 1 week then increased in steps of 250–500 micrograms/kg twice daily at intervals of 1–2 weeks; usual dose 1.5–3 mg/kg twice daily; max. 8 mg/kg twice daily

  Child 16–18 years initially 25 mg at night for 1 week then increased in steps of 12.5–25 mg twice daily at intervals of 1–2 weeks; usual dose 50 mg twice daily; max. 200 mg twice daily

Adjunctive treatment of generalised tonic-clonic seizures or partial seizures with or without secondary generalisation, adjunctive treatment of seizures in Lennox-Gastaut syndrome

- **By mouth**

  Child 2–16 years initially 25 mg at night for 1 week then increased in steps of 0.5–1.5 mg/kg twice daily at intervals of 1–2 weeks; usual dose 2.5–4.5 mg/kg twice daily; max. 15 mg/kg twice daily

  Child 16–18 years initially 25 mg at night for 1 week then increased in steps of 12.5–25 mg twice daily at intervals of 1–2 weeks; usual dose 100–200 mg twice daily; max. 400 mg twice daily

Migraine prophylaxis

- **By mouth**

  Child 16–18 years initially 25 mg daily at night for 1 week then increased in steps of 25 mg daily at intervals of 1 week; usual dose 50–100mg daily in 2 divided doses

Note If child cannot tolerate titration regimens recommended above then smaller steps or longer interval between steps may be used

Topamax® (Janssen-Cilag) ▼ PoM

Tablets, f/c, topiramate 25 mg, net price 60-tab pack = £20.92; 50 mg (light yellow), 60-tab pack = £34.36; 100 mg (yellow), 60-tab pack = £61.56; 200 mg (salmon), 60-tab pack = £119.54. Label: 3, 8, counselling, driving (see notes above)

Sprinkle capsules, topiramate 15 mg, net price 60-cap pack = £16.04; 25 mg, 60-cap pack = £24.05; 50 mg, 60-cap pack = £39.52. Label: 3, 8, counselling, administration, driving (see notes above)

Counselling Swallow whole or open capsule and sprinkle contents on soft food

Valproate

Valproate (as either sodium valproate or valproic acid) is effective in controlling tonic-clonic seizures, particularly in primary generalised epilepsy. It is a drug of choice in primary generalised epilepsy, generalised absences and myoclonic seizures, and may be tried in atypical absence, atonic, and tonic seizures. Controlled trials in partial epilepsy suggest that it has similar efficacy to that of carbamazepine and phenytoin. Valproate should generally be avoided in children under 2 years especially if they are on other antiepileptics, but may be required in infants with continuing epileptic tendency. Plasma-valproate concentrations are not a useful index of efficacy, therefore routine monitoring is unhelpful. The drug has widespread metabolic effects, and may have dose-related side-effects.

Valproic acid (as semisodium valproate) (section 4.2.3) is licensed for acute mania associated with bipolar disorder.

SODIUM VALPROATE

Cautions see notes above; monitor liver function before therapy and during first 6 months especially in children most at risk (see also below); measure full blood count and ensure no undue potential for bleeding before starting and before surgery; systemic lupus erythematosus; false-positive urine tests for ketones; avoid sudden withdrawal; **interactions:** see p. 253 and Appendix 1 (valproate)

Hepatic impairment avoid if possible; see also Contra-indications and Liver Toxicity below

Renal impairment reduce dose in mild to moderate impairment; in severe disease alter dosage according to free serum valproic acid concentration

Pregnancy see Antiepileptics: pregnancy and breast-feeding, p. 254; neonatal bleeding (related to hypofibrinaemia) and neonatal hepatotoxicity also reported

Breast-feeding amount too small to be harmful

Liver toxicity Liver dysfunction (including fatal hepatic failure) has occurred in association with valproate (especially in children under 3 years and in those with metabolic or degenerative disorders, organic brain disease or severe seizure disorders associated with mental retardation) usually in first 6 months and usually involving multiple antiepileptic therapy. Raised liver enzymes during valproate treatment are usually transient but patients should be reassessed clinically and liver function (including prothrombin time) monitored until return to normal—discontinue if abnormally prolonged prothrombin time (particularly in association with other relevant abnormalities). Any concomitant use of salicylates should be stopped.

Blood or hepatic disorders Children and their carers should be told how to recognise signs of blood or liver disorders and advised to seek immediate medical attention if symptoms develop.

Pancreatitis Children and their carers should be told how to recognise signs and symptoms of pancreatitis and advised to seek immediate medical attention if symptoms such as abdominal pain, nausea and vomiting develop; discontinue if pancreatitis is diagnosed

Contra-indications active liver disease, family history of severe hepatic dysfunction, porphyria (section 9.8.2)

Side-effects nausea, gastric irritation, diarrhoea; increased appetite, weight gain; hyperammonaemia, thrombocytopenia; transient hair loss (regrowth may be curly); less frequently increased alertness, aggression, hyperactivity, behavioural disturbances, ataxia, tremor, and vasculitis; *rarely* hepatic dysfunction (see under Cautions; withdraw treatment immediately if persistent vomiting and abdominal pain, anorexia, jaundice, oedema, malaise, drowsiness, or loss of seizure control), lethargy, drowsiness, confusion, stupor, hallucinations, menstrual disturbances, anaemia, leucopenia, pancytopenia, and rash; *very rarely* pancreatitis (see under Cautions), peripheral oedema, increase in bleeding time, extrapyramidal symptoms, encephalopathy, coma, gynaecomastia, Fanconi's syndrome, hirsutism, acne, toxic epidermal necrolysis, and Stevens-Johnson syndrome

Licensed use *Epilim Chrono*® not licensed for use in children under 20 kg

Indication and dose

All forms of epilepsy, infantile spasms

- By mouth or by rectum

Neonate initially 20 mg/kg once daily; usual maintenance dose 10 mg/kg twice daily

Child 1 month–12 years initially 5–7.5 mg/kg twice daily; usual maintenance dose 12.5–15 mg/kg twice daily (up to 30 mg/kg twice daily in infantile spasms; monitor clinical chemistry and haematological parameters if dose exceeds 20 mg/kg twice daily)

Child 12–18 years initially 300 mg twice daily increased in steps of 200 mg daily at 3-day intervals; usual maintenance dose 0.5–1 g twice daily; max. 1.25 g twice daily

Note If switching from oral therapy to intravenous therapy, the intravenous dose should be the same as the established oral dose

- By intravenous injection over 3–5 minutes

Neonate 10 mg/kg twice daily

Child 1 month–18 years 10 mg/kg twice daily

- By continuous intravenous infusion

Child 1 month–12 years initially 10 mg/kg *by intravenous injection* then *by continuous intravenous infusion* 20–40 mg/kg daily

Child 12–18 years initially 10 mg/kg *by intravenous injection* then up to max. 2.5 g daily *by continuous intravenous infusion*

Administration for *rectal administration*, sodium valproate oral solution may be given rectally and retained for 15 minutes (may require dilution with water to prevent rapid expulsion).

For *intravenous injection*, may be diluted in Glucose 5% *or* Sodium Chloride 0.9%.

For *continuous intravenous infusion*, dilute injection solution with Glucose 5% *or* Sodium Chloride 0.9%

Sodium Valproate (Non-proprietary) PoM

Tablets (crushable), scored, sodium valproate 100 mg, net price 20 = 78p. Label: 8, counselling, blood or hepatic disorder symptoms (see above), driving (see notes above)

Tablets, e/c, sodium valproate 200 mg, net price 20 = £1.29; 500 mg, 20 = £3.02. Label: 5, 8, 25, counselling, blood or hepatic disorder symptoms (see above), driving (see notes above)

Brands include *Orlept*®

Oral solution, sodium valproate 200 mg/5 mL, net price 300 mL = £8.00. Label: 8, counselling, blood or hepatic disorder symptoms (see above), driving (see notes above)

Brands include *Orlept*® sugar-free

Epilim® (Sanofi-Synthelabo) PoM

Tablets (crushable), scored, sodium valproate 100 mg, net price 20 = 78p. Label: 8, counselling, blood or hepatic disorder symptoms (see above), driving (see notes above)

SODIUM VALPROATE (*continued*)

Tablets, both e/c, lilac, sodium valproate 200 mg, net price 20 = £1.28; 500 mg, 20 = £3.21. Label: 5, 8, 25, counselling, blood or hepatic disorder symptoms (see above), driving (see notes above)

Liquid, red, sugar-free, sodium valproate 200 mg/5 mL, net price 300-mL pack = £6.48. Label: 8, counselling, blood or hepatic disorder symptoms (see above), driving (see notes above)

Syrup, red, sodium valproate 200 mg/5 mL, net price 300-mL pack = £6.48. Label: 8, counselling, blood or hepatic disorder symptoms (see above), driving (see notes above)

Epilim® Intravenous (Sanofi-Synthelabo) PoM
Injection, powder for reconstitution, sodium valproate, net price 400-mg vial (with 4-mL amp water for injections) = £9.65

Modified release

Epilim Chrono® (Sanofi-Synthelabo) PoM
Tablets, m/r, all lilac, sodium valproate 200 mg (as sodium valproate and valproic acid), net price 100-tab pack = £8.09; 300 mg, 100-tab pack = £12.13; 500 mg, 100-tab pack = £20.21. Label: 8, 25, counselling, blood or hepatic disorder symptoms (see above), driving (see notes above)

Dose

Child, body-weight over 20 kg as above, total daily dose given in 1–2 divided doses

Valproic acid

Convulex® (Pharmacia) PoM
Capsules, e/c, valproic acid 150 mg, net price 100-cap pack = £3.68; 300 mg, 100-cap pack = £7.35; 500 mg, 100-cap pack = £12.25. Label: 8, 25, counselling, blood or hepatic disorder symptoms (see above), driving (see notes above)

Dose

Child , doses as for sodium valproate, total daily dose given in 2–4 divided doses

Equivalence to sodium valproate Manufacturer advises that *Convulex®* has a 1:1 dose relationship with products containing sodium valproate, but nevertheless care is needed in making changes.

4 Central nervous system

Vigabatrin

For partial epilepsy with or without secondary generalisation, **vigabatrin** is given in combination with other antiepileptic treatment; its use is restricted to children in whom all other combinations are inadequate or are not tolerated. It can be used as sole therapy in the management of infantile spasms.

About one-third of those treated with vigabatrin have suffered visual field defects; counselling and **careful monitoring** for this side-effect are required (see also Visual Field Defects under Cautions below). Vigabatrin has prominent behavioural side-effects in some children.

VIGABATRIN

Cautions closely monitor neurological function; avoid sudden withdrawal (taper off over 2–4 weeks); history of psychosis, depression or behavioural problems; absence seizures (may be exacerbated); **interactions:** see p. 253 and Appendix 1 (vigabatrin)

Renal impairment reduced maintenance dose may be required if creatinine clearance less than 60 mL/minute/1.73m^2

Pregnancy see Antiepileptics: pregnancy and breast-feeding, p. 254

Breast-feeding see notes above; present in milk—manufacturer advises avoid

Visual field defects Vigabatrin is associated with visual field defects. The CSM has advised that onset of symptoms varies from 1 month to several years after starting. In most cases, visual field defects have persisted despite discontinuation. Product literature advises visual field testing before treatment and at 6-month intervals; a procedure for testing visual fields in those with a developmental age of less than 9 years is available from the manufacturers. Children and their carers should be warned to report any new visual symptoms that develop and those with symptoms should be referred for an urgent ophthalmological opinion. Gradual withdrawal of vigabatrin should be considered.

Contra-indications visual field defects

Side-effects drowsiness (rarely encephalopathic symptoms consisting of marked sedation, stupor, and confusion with non-specific slow wave EEG—reduce dose or withdraw), fatigue, visual field defects (see also under Cautions), dizziness, nervousness, irritability, behavioural effects such as excitation and agitation; depression, abnormal thinking, headache, nystagmus, ataxia, tremor, paraesthesia, impaired concentration; *less commonly* confusion, aggression, psychosis, mania, memory disturbance, visual disturbance (e.g. diplopia); also weight gain, oedema, gastrointestinal disturbances, alopecia, rash; *less commonly*, urticaria, occasional increase in seizure frequency (especially if myoclonic), decrease in liver enzymes, slight decrease in haemoglobin; photophobia and retinal disorders (e.g. peripheral retinal atrophy); optic neuritis, optic atrophy, hallucinations also reported

Indication and dose

Adjunctive treatment of partial seizures with or without secondary generalisation not satisfactorily controlled with other antiepileptics
- By mouth

Neonate initially 15–20 mg/kg twice daily increased over 2–3 weeks to usual maintenance dose 30–40 mg/kg twice daily; max.150 mg/kg daily

Child 1 month–12 years initially 15–20 mg/kg twice daily increased over 2–3 weeks to usual maintenance dose 30–40 mg/kg twice daily; max. 150 mg/kg daily

VIGABATRIN (*continued*)

Child 12–18 years initially 1 g twice daily increased over 2–3 weeks to usual maintenance dose 1–1.5 g twice daily
Administration Tablets may be crushed and dispersed in liquid

- **By rectum**

Child 1 month–18 years dose as for oral therapy, see above
Administration dissolve contents of sachet in small amount of water and administer rectally

Infantile spasms as monotherapy
- **By mouth**

Neonate initially 15–25 mg/kg twice daily adjusted according to response over 7 days to usual maintenance dose 40–50 mg/kg twice daily; max. 75 mg/kg twice daily

Child 1 month–2 years initially 15–25 mg/kg twice daily adjusted according to response over 7 days to usual maintenance dose 40–50 mg/kg twice daily; max. 75 mg/kg twice daily

Sabril® (Aventis Pharma) PoM
Tablets, f/c, scored, vigabatrin 500 mg, net price 100-tab pack = £30.84. Label: 3, 8, counselling, driving (see notes above)

Powder, sugar-free, vigabatrin 500 mg/sachet. Net price 50-sachet pack = £17.08. Label: 3, 8, 13, counselling, driving (see notes above)
Note The contents of a sachet should be dissolved in water or a soft drink immediately before taking

Benzodiazepines

Clonazepam is occasionally used in tonic-clonic or partial seizures, but its sedative side-effects may be prominent. **Clobazam** may be used as adjunctive therapy in the treatment of epilepsy, but the effectiveness of these and other **benzodiazepines** may wane considerably after weeks or months of continuous therapy.

CLOBAZAM

Cautions see under Diazepam (section 4.1.2)
Hepatic impairment may precipitate coma
Renal impairment increased cerebral sensitivity—start with small doses in severe impairment
Pregnancy avoid regular use (risk of neonatal withdrawal symptoms); use only if clear indication such as seizure control (high doses during late pregnancy or labour may cause neonatal hypothermia, hypotonia and respiratory depression)
Breast-feeding present in milk—avoid if possible

Contra-indications see under Diazepam (section 4.1.2)

Side-effects see under Diazepam (section 4.1.2)

Licensed use not licensed for use in children under 3 years (only for use in child 6 months–3 years in exceptional cases)

Indication and dose

Adjunctive therapy for epilepsy, monotherapy under specialist supervision for catamenial (menstruation) seizures (usually for 7–10 days each month, just before and during menstruation), cluster seizures
- **By mouth**

Child 1 month–12 years initially 125 micrograms/kg twice daily increased every 5 days to usual maintenance dose of 250 micrograms/kg twice daily; max. 500 micrograms/kg twice daily, not exceeding 15 mg twice daily

Child 12–18 years initially 10 mg twice daily increased every 5 days to usual maintenance dose of 10–15 mg twice daily; max. 30 mg twice daily

[1]**Clobazam** (Non-proprietary) PoM NHS
Tablets, clobazam 10 mg. Net price 30-tab pack = £9.74. Label: 2 or 19, 8, counselling, driving (see notes above)
Brands include *Frisium®* NHS

Tablets, clobazam 5 mg available on a named patient basis

1. NHS except for epilepsy and endorsed 'SLS'

Extemporaneous formulations available see Extemporaneous Preparations, p. 8

CLONAZEPAM

Cautions see notes above; respiratory disease; spinal or cerebellar ataxia; myasthenia gravis (avoid if unstable); history of alcohol or drug abuse, depression or suicidal ideation; debilitated; avoid sudden withdrawal; porphyria (section 9.8.2); **interactions:** see p. 253 and Appendix 1 (anxiolytics and hypnotics)
Hepatic impairment can precipitate coma; reduce dose in mild to moderate impairment; avoid in severe impairment

CLONAZEPAM (*continued*)

Renal impairment start with small doses; increased cerebral sensitivity

Pregnancy avoid regular use (risk of neonatal withdrawal symptoms); use only if clear indication such as seizure control (high doses during late pregnancy or labour may cause neonatal hypothermia, hypotonia and respiratory depression)

Breast-feeding present in milk—avoid if possible

Driving Drowsiness may affect performance of skilled tasks (e.g. driving); effects of alcohol enhanced

Contra-indications respiratory depression; acute pulmonary insufficiency; sleep apnoea syndrome

Side-effects drowsiness, fatigue, dizziness, muscle hypotonia, coordination disturbances; also poor concentration, restlessness, confusion, amnesia, dependence, and withdrawal; salivary or bronchial hypersecretion in infants and small children; *rarely* gastro-intestinal symptoms, respiratory depression, headache, paradoxical effects including aggression and anxiety, sexual dysfunction, urinary incontinence, urticaria, pruritus, reversible hair loss, skin pigmentation changes; dysarthria, and visual disturbances on long-term treatment; blood disorders reported; **overdosage:** see Emergency Treatment of Poisoning, p. 40

Indication and dose

All forms of epilepsy

- By mouth

Child 1 month–1 year initially 250 micrograms at night for 4 nights increased over 2–4 weeks to usual maintenance dose of 0.5–1 mg in 3–4 divided doses; may be given as a single bedtime dose when maintenance dose established

Child 1–5 years initially 250 micrograms at night for 4 nights, increased over 2–4 weeks to usual maintenance of 1–3 mg daily in 3–4 divided doses; may be given as a single bedtime dose when maintenance dose established

Child 5–12 years initially 500 micrograms at night for 4 nights increased over 2–4 weeks to usual maintenance dose of 3–6 mg daily in 3–4 divided doses; may be given as a single bedtime dose when maintenance dose established

Child 12–18 years initially 1 mg at night for 4 nights increase over 2–4 weeks to usual maintenance dose of 4–8 mg daily in 3–4 divided doses; max. 20 mg daily; may be given as a single bedtime dose when maintenance dose established

Administration for administration *by mouth*, injection solution may be given orally

Rivotril® (Roche) PoM

Tablets, both scored, clonazepam 500 micrograms (beige), net price 100 = £3.92; 2 mg (white), 100 = £5.23. Label: 2, 8, counselling, driving (see notes above)

Injection, section 4.8.2

Liquid, clonazepam 2.5 mg/mL

Available from specialist importing companies

Extemporaneous formulations available see Extemporaneous Preparations, p. 8

NITRAZEPAM

Cautions avoid abrupt withdrawal; respiratory disease; porphyria (section 9.8.2); muscle weakness and myasthenia gravis; **interactions:** Appendix 1 (anxiolytics and hypnotics)

Hepatic impairment can precipitate coma; avoid in severe hepatic impairment

Renal impairment start with small doses; increased cerebral sensitivity

Contra-indications respiratory depression, acute pulmonary insufficiency, sleep apnoea syndrome; marked neuromuscular respiratory weakness including myasthenia gravis

Side-effects drowsiness, confusion, ataxia; see also under Diazepam (section 4.1.2); **overdosage:** see Emergency Treatment of Poisoning p. 40

Licensed use not licensed for use in children

Indication and dose

Infantile spasms

- By mouth

Child 1 month–2 years initially 125 micrograms/kg twice daily, adjusted according to response over 2–3 weeks to 250 micrograms/kg twice daily; max. 500 micrograms/kg (not exceeding 5 mg) twice daily; total daily dose may alternatively be given in 3 divided doses

Nitrazepam (Non-proprietary) PoM

Oral suspension, nitrazepam 2.5 mg/5 mg, net price 150mL = £5.30. Label: 1, 8

Brands include *Somnite®* NHS

Other drugs

Acetazolamide (section 11.6), a carbonic anhydrase inhibitor, has a specific role in treating epilepsy associated with menstruation. It can also be used in conjunction with other antiepileptics for tonic-clonic or partial seizures.

Piracetam is used as adjunctive treatment for cortical myoclonus.

4.8.2 Drugs used in status epilepticus

Initial management of status epilepticus includes positioning the child to avoid injury, supporting respiration including the provision of oxygen, maintaining blood pressure, and the correction of any hypoglycaemia. **Pyridoxine** should be administered if the status epilepticus is caused by pyridoxine deficiency.

Convulsive status epilepticus is treated initially with **midazolam** given into the buccal cavity or intranasally, or with **diazepam** administered as a rectal solution; the intranasal or buccal routes may be more acceptable in children.

In hospital, where resuscitation facilities are immediately available, status epilepticus is treated with intravenous **lorazepam**. Intravenous **diazepam** is effective but it is associated with a high risk of venous thrombophlebitis (reduced by using an emulsion formulation of diazepam injection).

Clonazepam can also be used as an alternative.

If seizures recur or fail to respond after 30 minutes, phenytoin sodium, fosphenytoin, or phenobarbital sodium should be used.

Phenytoin sodium may be given by slow intravenous injection, with ECG monitoring, followed by the maintenance dosage. Intramuscular use of phenytoin is not recommended (absorption is slow and erratic).

Alternatively, **fosphenytoin**, a pro-drug of phenytoin, can be given more rapidly and when given intravenously causes fewer injection-site reactions compared to phenytoin. Intravenous administration requires ECG monitoring. Although it can also be given intramuscularly, absorption is too slow by this route for treatment of status epilepticus. Doses of fosphenytoin should be expressed in terms of phenytoin sodium.

Alternatively, **phenobarbital sodium** can be given by intravenous injection.

Paraldehyde given rectally causes little respiratory depression and is therefore useful where facilities for resuscitation are poor.

If the above measures fail to control seizures, anaesthesia with thiopental (section15.1.1) should be instituted with full intensive care support. Lidocaine infusion has also been used but requires specialist management.

CLONAZEPAM

Cautions see section 4.8.1; facilities for reversing respiratory depression with mechanical ventilation must be at hand (but see also notes above)

Intravenous infusion Intravenous infusion of clonazepam is potentially hazardous (especially if prolonged), calling for close and constant observation and best carried out in specialist centres with intensive care facilities. Prolonged infusion may lead to accumulation and delay recovery

Contra-indications see section 4.8.1; avoid injections containing benzyl alcohol in neonates (see under preparations below)

Side-effects see section 4.8.1; hypotension and apnoea

Indication and dose

Status epilepticus

- **By intravenous injection over at least 2 minutes**

Neonate 100 micrograms/kg repeated after 24 hours if necessary

Child 1 month–12 years 50 micrograms/kg (max. 1 mg) repeated if necessary

Child 12–18 years 1 mg repeated if necessary

- **By intravenous infusion**

Child 1 month–12 years initially 50 micrograms/kg (max. 1 mg) *by intravenous injection* then *by intravenous infusion* 10 micrograms/kg/hour adjusted according to response; max. 60 micrograms/kg/hour

Child 12–18 years initially 1 mg *by intravenous injection* then *by intravenous infusion* 10 micrograms/kg/hour adjusted according to response; max. 60 micrograms/kg/hour

Administration for *intravenous injection*, dilute to a concentration of 500 micrograms/mL with Water for Injections

For *intravenous infusion*, dilute to a concentration of 12 micrograms/mL with Glucose 5% *or* Sodium Chloride 0.9%; incompatible with bicarbonate; absorbed on PVC—glass infusion apparatus preferred (if PVC apparatus used, complete infusion within 2 hours)

Rivotril® (Roche) PoM

Injection, clonazepam 1 mg/mL in solvent, for dilution with 1 mL water for injections immediately before injection or as described above. Net price 1-mL amp (with 1 mL water for injections) = 63p

Excipients: include benzyl alcohol (avoid in neonates, see Excipients, p. 3), ethanol, propylene glycol

Oral preparations

Section 4.8.1

DIAZEPAM

Cautions see section 4.1.2; when given intravenously facilities for reversing respiratory depression with mechanical ventilation must be at hand (but see also notes above)

Contra-indications see section 4.1.2

Side-effects see section 4.1.2; hypotension and apnoea

Licensed use *Diazepam Rectubes*® and *Stesolid Rectal Tubes*® not licensed for use in children under 1 year

Indication and dose

Safe Practice Parenteral preparations containing benzyl alcohol should not be used in neonates—associated with a fatal toxic syndrome in preterm neonates

Status epilepticus, febrile convulsions, convulsions caused by poisoning
- By intravenous injection over 3–5 minutes

Neonate 300–400 micrograms/kg repeated after 10 minutes if necessary

Child 1 month–12 years 300–400 micrograms/kg repeated after 10 minutes if necessary

Child 12–18 years 10–20 mg repeated after 10 minutes if necessary

- By rectum (as rectal solution)

Neonate 1.25–2.5 mg repeated after 5 minutes if necessary

Child 1 month–2 years 5 mg repeated after 5 minutes if necessary

Child 2–12 years 5–10 mg repeated after 5 minutes if necessary

Child 12–18 years 10 mg repeated after 5 minutes if necessary

Diazepam (Non-proprietary) PoM

Injection (solution), diazepam 5 mg/mL. Net price 2-mL amp = 32p

Injection (emulsion), diazepam 5 mg/mL (0.5%). Net price 2-mL amp = 84p

Excipients: include benzyl alcohol (avoid in neonates, see Excipients, p. 3), ethanol, propylene glycol

Brands include *Diazemuls*®

Rectal tubes (= rectal solution), diazepam 2 mg/mL, net price 1.25-mL (2.5-mg) tube = 90p, 2.5-mL (5-mg) tube = £1.28; 4 mg/mL, 2.5-mL (10-mg) tube = £1.34

Brands include *Diazepam Rectubes*®, *Stesolid*®

Oral preparations

Section 4.1.2

FOSPHENYTOIN SODIUM

Note Fosphenytoin is a pro-drug of phenytoin

Cautions see Phenytoin Sodium; resuscitation facilities must be available; **interactions:** see p. 253 and Appendix 1 (phenytoin)

Hepatic impairment consider 10–25% reduction in dose or infusion rate (except initial dose for status epilepticus)

Renal impairment consider 10–25% reduction in dose or infusion rate (except initial dose for status epilepticus)

Pregnancy see Phenytoin (section 4.8.1)

Breast-feeding see Phenytoin (section 4.8.1)

Contra-indications see Phenytoin Sodium

Side-effects see Phenytoin Sodium

CSM advice Intravenous infusion of fosphenytoin has been associated with severe cardiovascular reactions including asystole, ventricular fibrillation, and cardiac arrest. Hypotension, bradycardia, and heart block have also been reported. The CSM advises:

- monitor heart rate, blood pressure, and respiratory function for duration of infusion
- observe patient for at least 30 minutes after infusion
- if hypotension occurs, reduce infusion rate or discontinue
- reduce dose or infusion rate in renal or hepatic impairment

Licensed use not licensed for use in children under 5 years

Indication and dose

Expressed as **phenytoin sodium equivalent** (PE); fosphenytoin sodium 1.5 mg ≡ phenytoin sodium 1 mg

Status epilepticus
- By intravenous infusion (at a rate of 2–3 mg(PE)/kg/minute)

Child 5–18 years initially 15 mg(PE)/kg, then (at a rate of 1–2 mg(PE)/kg/minute) 4–5 mg(PE)/kg; total daily dose may be given in 1–4 divided doses; adjusted according to response and trough plasma-phenytoin concentration

Prophylaxis or treatment of seizures associated with neurosurgery or head injury
- By intravenous infusion (at a rate of 1–2 mg(PE)/kg/minute)

Child 5–18 years initially 10–15 mg(PE)/kg then 4–5 mg(PE)/kg daily; total daily dose may be given in 1–4 divided doses; adjusted according to response and trough plasma-phenytoin concentration

Temporary substitution for oral phenytoin
- By intravenous infusion (at a rate of 1–2 mg(PE)/kg/minute)

Child 5–18 years same dose and dosing frequency as oral phenytoin therapy

Note Prescriptions for fosphenytoin sodium should state the dose in terms of phenytoin sodium equivalent (PE)

Administration for *intermittent intravenous infusion*, dilute to a concentration of 1.5–25 mg (PE)/mL with Glucose 5% *or* Sodium Chloride 0.9%

FOSPHENYTOIN SODIUM (*continued*)

Pro-Epanutin® (Pfizer) PoM
Injection, fosphenytoin sodium 75 mg/mL (equivalent to phenytoin sodium 50 mg/mL), net price 10-mL vial = £40.00
Electrolytes phosphate 3.7 micromol/mg fosphenytoin sodium (phosphate 5.6 micromol/mg phenytoin sodium)

LORAZEPAM

Cautions see under Diazepam, section 4.1.2; facilities for reversing respiratory depression with mechanical ventilation must be at hand

Contra-indications see under Diazepam, section 4.1.2

Side-effects see under Diazepam, section 4.1.2; hypotension and apnoea

Indication and dose

Status epilepticus
- **By slow intravenous injection or by rectum or by sublingual administration**

Neonate 100 micrograms/kg as a single dose (repeated once if initial dose ineffective)

Child 1 month–12 years 100 micrograms/kg (max. 4 mg) as a single dose (repeated once if initial dose ineffective)

Child 12–18 years 4 mg as a single dose (repeated once if initial dose ineffective)

Administration for *intravenous injection*, dilute with an equal volume of Sodium Chloride 0.9% *or* Water for Injections (for neonates, dilute injection solution to a concentration of 100 micrograms/mL); give slowly into a large vein at a rate not exceeding 50 micrograms/kg over 3–5 minutes. For *rectal* or *sublingual administration*, injection solution may be used

Preparations
Section 15.1.4.1

MIDAZOLAM

Cautions section 15.1.4

Contra-indications section 15.1.4

Side-effects section 15.1.4

Licensed use *injection* not licensed for use in status epilepticus

Indication and dose

Status epilepticus
- **By buccal administration (preferred) or by intranasal administration (if excessive salivation)**

Neonate 300 micrograms/kg as a single dose

Child 1–6 months 300 micrograms/kg (max. 2.5 mg) as a single dose

Child 6 months–1 year 2.5 mg as a single dose

Child 1–5 years 5 mg as a single dose

Child 5–10 years 7.5 mg as a single dose

Child 10–18 years 10 mg as a single dose

- **By intravenous administration**

Neonate initially *by intravenous injection* 150–200 micrograms/kg followed *by continuous infusion* of 1 microgram/kg/minute (increased by 1 microgram/kg/minute every 15 minutes until seizure controlled; max. 5 micrograms/kg/minute)

Child 1 month–18 years initially *by intravenous injection* 150–200 micrograms/kg followed *by continuous intravenous infusion* of 1 microgram/kg/minute (increased by 1 microgram/kg/minute every 15 minutes) until seizure controlled; max. 5 micrograms/kg/minute

Administration for *intravenous injection*, dilute with Glucose 5% or Sodium Chloride 0.9%; rapid intravenous injection (less than 2 minutes) may cause seizure-like myoclonus in preterm neonate. Buccal liquid may be given intranasally; injection solution may be given bucally, intranasally or by mouth

Preparations
Section 15.1.4
Epistatus® (midazolam buccal liquid 10 mg/mL) is available from specialist manufacturers

PARALDEHYDE

Cautions bronchopulmonary disease, hepatic impairment; **interactions:** Appendix 1 (paraldehyde)

Pregnancy manufacturer advises avoid—crosses placenta

Breast-feeding present in milk—manufacturer advises avoid unless essential

Contra-indications gastric disorders; rectal administration in colitis

Side-effects rashes; rectal irritation after enema

Licensed use not licensed for use in children as an enema

PARALDEHYDE (*continued*)

Indication and dose

Status epilepticus
- By rectum

Neonate 0.4 mL/kg (max. 0.5 mL) as a single dose

Child 1–3 months 0.5 mL as a single dose

Child 3–6 months 1 mL as a single dose

Child 6 months–1 year 1.5 mL as a single dose

Child 1–2 years 2 mL as a single dose

Child 2–5 years 3–4 mL as a single dose

Child 5–18 years 5–10 mL as a single dose

Administration for *rectal administration,* dilute 1 part paraldehyde with 9 parts Sodium Chloride 0.9% (some centres mix paraldehyde with an equal volume of olive oil or sunflower oil instead)

Note Do not use paraldehyde if it has a brownish colour or an odour of acetic acid. Avoid contact with rubber and plastics.

Paraldehyde (Non-proprietary) PoM
Injection, sterile paraldehyde, net price 5-mL amp = £9.49

Enema available from a specials manufacturer

PHENOBARBITAL SODIUM

Phenobarbitone sodium

Cautions see under Phenobarbital (section 4.8.1)

Side-effects see under Phenobarbital (section 4.8.1)

Indication and dose

Status epilepticus
- By slow intravenous injection

Neonate initially 20 mg/kg then 2.5–5 mg.kg once or twice daily

Child 1 month–12 years initially 20 mg/kg then 2.5–5 mg/kg once or twice daily

Child 12–18 years initially 20 mg/kg (max. 1 g) then 300 mg twice daily

Other forms of epilepsy (section 4.8.1)

Note For therapeutic purposes phenobarbital and phenobarbital sodium may be considered equivalent in effect

Administration for *intravenous injection,* dilute to a concentration of 20 mg/mL with Water for Injections; give over 20 minutes (no faster than 1 mg/kg/minute)

Phenobarbital (Non-proprietary) CD
Injection, phenobarbital sodium 200 mg/mL, net price 1-mL amp = £1.82
Excipients: include propylene glycol 90%
Note Must be diluted before intravenous administration (see Administration)

Oral preparations
Section 4.8.1

PHENYTOIN SODIUM

Cautions hypotension and heart failure; resuscitation facilities must be available; injection solutions alkaline (irritant to tissues); see also p. 262; **interactions:** see p. 253 and Appendix 1 (phenytoin)

Contra-indications sinus bradycardia, sino-atrial block, and second- and third-degree heart block; Stokes-Adams syndrome; porphyria (section 9.8.2)

Side-effects intravenous injection may cause cardiovascular and CNS depression (particularly if injection too rapid) with arrhythmias, hypotension, and cardiovascular collapse; alterations in respiratory function (including respiratory arrest); injection-site reactions, see also p. 262

Indication and dose

Status epilepticus, acute symptomatic seizures associated with trauma or neurosurgery
- By slow intravenous injection or infusion (with blood-pressure and ECG monitoring)

Neonate initially 20 mg/kg as a loading dose then 2.5–5 mg/kg twice daily

Child 1 month–12 years initially 18 mg/kg as a loading dose then 2.5–5 mg/kg twice daily

Child 12–18 years initially 18 mg/kg as a loading dose then up to 100 mg 3–4 times daily

- By intramuscular injection

Not recommended (see notes above)

Administration before and after administration flush intravenous line with Sodium Chloride 0.9%.

For *intravenous injection,* give at rate not exceeding 1 mg/kg/minute (max. 50 mg/minute).

For *intravenous infusion,* dilute to a concentration not exceeding 10 mg/mL with Sodium Chloride 0.9% and give through an in-line filter (0.22–0.50 micron) at a rate not exceeding 1 mg/kg/minute (max. 50 mg/minute); complete administration within 1 hour of preparation

Phenytoin (Non-proprietary) PoM
Injection, phenytoin sodium 50 mg/mL with propylene glycol 40% and alcohol 10% in water for injections, net price 5-mL amp = £3.40

Epanutin® Ready-Mixed Parenteral (Parke-Davis) PoM
Injection, phenytoin sodium 50 mg/mL with propylene glycol 40% and alcohol 10% in water for injections. Net price 5-mL amp = £4.88

Oral preparations
Section 4.8.1

4.8.3 Febrile convulsions

Brief febrile convulsions need only simple treatment such as removing clothes, tepid sponging, or antipyretic medication e.g. **paracetamol** (section 4.7.1). *Prolonged febrile convulsions* (those lasting 15 minutes or longer), *recurrent convulsions*, or those occurring in a child at known risk must be treated more actively, as there is the possibility of resulting brain damage. **Diazepam** (section 4.8.2) is the drug of choice given either by slow intravenous injection or preferably rectally in solution, repeated if necessary. The rectal solution is generally preferred as satisfactory absorption is achieved within minutes and administration is much easier. Suppositories are not suitable because absorption is too slow.

Intermittent prophylaxis (i.e. the anticonvulsant administered at the onset of fever) is possible in only a small proportion of children; rectal administration of **diazepam** is the treatment of choice.

The exact role of continuous prophylaxis in children at risk from prolonged or complex febrile convulsions is controversial. It is probably indicated in only a small proportion of children, including those whose first seizure occurred at under 14 months or who have pre-existing neurological abnormalities or who have had previous prolonged or focal convulsions. Thus long-term anticonvulsant prophylaxis is rarely indicated.

4.9 Drugs used in dystonias and related disorders

Dystonias may result from conditions such as cerebral palsy or may be related to a deficiency of the neurotransmitter dopamine as in Segawa syndrome.

4.9.1 Dopaminergic drugs used in dystonias

Levodopa, the amino-acid precursor of dopamine, acts by replenishing depleted striatal dopamine. It is given with an extracerebral **dopa-decarboxylase inhibitor** that reduces the peripheral conversion of levodopa to dopamine, thereby limiting side-effects such as nausea, vomiting and cardiovascular effects; additionally, effective brain-dopamine concentrations can be achieved with lower doses of levodopa. The extracerebral dopa-decarboxylase inhibitor most commonly used in children is carbidopa (in **co-careldopa**).

Levodopa therapy should be initiated at a low dose and increased in small steps; the final dose should be as low as possible. Intervals between doses should be chosen to suit the needs of the individual child.

In severe dystonias related to cerebral palsy, improvement can be expected within 2 weeks. Children with Segawa syndrome are particularly sensitive to levodopa; they may even become symptom free on small doses. Levodopa also has a role in treating metabolic disorders such as defects in tetrahydrobiopterin synthesis and dihydrobiopterin reductase deficiency. For the use of tetrahydrobiopterin in metabolic disorders see section 9.4.1.

Children may experience nausea within 2 hours of taking a dose; nausea and vomiting with co-careldopa is rarely dose-limiting but domperidone (section 4.6) may be useful in controlling these effects.

In dystonic cerebral palsy treatment with larger doses of levodopa is associated with the development of potentially troublesome motor complications including response fluctuations and dyskinesias. Response fluctuations are characterised by large variations in motor performance, with normal function during the 'on' period, and weakness and restricted mobility during the 'off' period.

Sudden onset of sleep

Excessive daytime sleepiness and sudden onset of sleep can occur with co-careldopa.

Children starting treatment with these drugs, and their carers, should be warned of the possibility of these effects and of the need to exercise caution when performing skilled tasks e.g. driving or operating machinery.

Children who have suffered excessive sedation or sudden onset of sleep should refrain from performing skilled tasks until those effects have stopped recurring.

CO-CARELDOPA

A mixture of carbidopa and levodopa; the proportions are expressed in the form *x/y* where *x* and *y* are the strengths in milligrams of carbidopa and levodopa respectively

Cautions see also notes above; pulmonary disease, peptic ulceration, cardiovascular disease, diabetes mellitus, osteomalacia, open-angle glaucoma, history of skin melanoma (risk of activation), psychiatric illness (avoid if severe); warn children and carers about excessive drowsiness (see notes above); in prolonged therapy, psychiatric, hepatic, haematological, renal, and cardiovascular surveillance is advisable; warn patients to resume normal activities gradually; avoid abrupt withdrawal; **interactions:** Appendix 1 (levodopa)

Contra-indications closed-angle glaucoma

Pregnancy manufacturers advise toxicity in *animal* studies

Breast-feeding may suppress lactation; present in milk—manufacturers advise avoid

Side-effects see also notes above; anorexia, nausea and vomiting, insomnia, agitation, postural hypotension (rarely labile hypertension), dizziness, tachycardia, arrhythmias, reddish discoloration of urine and other body fluids, rarely hypersensitivity; abnormal involuntary movements and psychiatric symptoms which include hypomania and psychosis may be dose-limiting; depression, drowsiness, headache, flushing, sweating, gastro-intestinal bleeding, peripheral neuropathy, taste disturbance, pruritus, rash, and liver enzyme changes also reported; syndrome resembling neuroleptic malignant syndrome reported on withdrawal

Licensed use not licensed for use in children

Indication and dose

Dopamine-sensitive dystonias including Segawa syndrome and dystonias related to cerebral palsy

- **By mouth, expressed as levodopa**

Child 3 months–18 years initially 250 micrograms/kg 2–3 times daily of a preparation containing 1:4 carbidopa:levodopa; increased according to response every 2–3 days to max. 1 mg/kg three times daily

Treatment of defects in tetrahydrobiopterin synthesis and dihydrobiopterin reductase deficiency

- **By mouth, expressed as levodopa**

Neonate initially 250–500 micrograms/kg 4 times daily of a preparation containing 1:4 carbidopa:levodopa; increased according to reponse every 4–5 days to maintenance dose of 2.5–3 mg/kg 4 times daily; at higher doses consider preparation containing 1:10 carbidopa:levodopa; review regularly (every 3–6 months)

Child 1 month–18 years initially 250–500 micrograms/kg 4 times daily of a preparation containing 1:4 carbidopa:levodopa; increased according to reponse every 4–5 days to maintenance dose of 2.5–3 mg/kg 4 times daily; at higher doses consider preparation containing 1:10 carbidopa:levodopa; review regularly (every 3–6 months in early childhood)

Sinemet® (Bristol-Myers Squibb) PoM

Sinemet-62.5® tablets, yellow, scored, co-careldopa 12.5/50 (carbidopa 12.5 mg (as monohydrate), levodopa 50 mg), net price 90-tab pack = £7.03. Label: 14, counselling, driving, see notes above

Note 2 tablets *Sinemet-62.5®* ≡ 1 tablet *Sinemet Plus®*; *Sinemet-62.5®* previously known as *Sinemet LS®*

Sinemet-110® tablets, blue, scored, co-careldopa 10/100 (carbidopa 10 mg (as monohydrate), levodopa 100 mg), net price 90-tab pack = £6.84. Label: 14, counselling, driving, see notes above

Sinemet-Plus® tablets, yellow, scored, co-careldopa 25/100 (carbidopa 25 mg (as monohydrate), levodopa 100 mg), net price 90-tab pack = £10.05. Label: 14, counselling, driving, see notes above

Sinemet-275® tablets, blue, scored, co-careldopa 25/250 (carbidopa 25 mg (as monohydrate), levodopa 250 mg), net price 90-tab pack = £14.28. Label: 14, counselling, driving, see notes above

4.9.2 Antimuscarinic drugs used in dystonias

Antimuscarinic drugs help to control dystonias.

The antimuscarinic drugs, **benzatropine**, **procyclidine**, and **trihexyphenidyl** (benzhexol), reduce the symptoms of dystonias, including those induced by antipsychotic drugs; there is no justification for giving them routinely in the absence of dystonic symptoms. Tardive dyskinesia is not improved by antimuscarinic drugs and may be made worse.

No important differences exist between the antimuscarinic drugs, but some children tolerate one better than another.

Benzatropine may be given parenterally and it is effective emergency treatment for acute drug-induced dystonic reactions.

BENZATROPINE MESILATE

(Benztropine mesylate)

Cautions see Trihexyphenidyl Hydrochloride

Side-effects see Trihexyphenidyl Hydrochloride, but causes sedation rather than stimulation; also tachycardia, dizziness, depression, hyperthermia

Indication and dose

Dystonia

- **By intravenous injection or intramuscular injection**

Child 3–12 years 20–100 micrograms/kg (max. 2 mg) as a single dose

Child 12–18 years 1–2 mg as a single dose

Cogentin® (MSD) PoM
Injection, benzatropine mesilate 1 mg/mL, net price 2-mL amp = 92p

PROCYCLIDINE HYDROCHLORIDE

Cautions see Trihexyphenidyl Hydrochloride

Side-effects see Trihexyphenidyl Hydrochloride

Licensed use not licensed for use in children

Indication and dose

Dystonias

- **By mouth**

Child 7–12 years 1.25 mg 3 times daily

Child 12–18 years 2.5 mg 3 times daily

Acute dystonia

- **By intramuscular or intravenous injection**

Child under 2 years 0.5–2 mg as a single dose

Child 2–10 years 2–5 mg as a single dose

Child 10–18 years 5–10 mg (occasionally more than 10 mg)

Note Usually effective in 5–10 minutes but may need 30 minutes for relief

Procyclidine (Non-proprietary) PoM
Tablets, procyclidine hydrochloride 5 mg, net price 28-tab pack = £2.72. Counselling, driving

Arpicolin® (Rosemont) PoM
Syrup, sugar-free, procyclidine hydrochloride 2.5 mg/5 mL, net price 150 mL = £4.22; 5 mg/5 mL, 150 mL pack = £7.54. Counselling, driving

Kemadrin® (GSK) PoM
Tablets, scored, procyclidine hydrochloride 5 mg, net price 20 = 94p. Counselling, driving

Kemadrin® (Auden Mckenzie) PoM
Injection, procyclidine hydrochloride 5 mg/mL, net price 2-mL amp = £1.49

TRIHEXYPHENIDYL HYDROCHLORIDE

(Benzhexol hydrochloride)

Cautions cardiovascular disease, angle-closure glaucoma, gastro-intestinal obstruction, untreated urinary retention; avoid abrupt withdrawal; liable to abuse; hepatic impairment; renal impairment; pregnancy; breast-feeding; **interactions:** Appendix 1 (antimuscarinics)

Driving May affect performance of skilled tasks (e.g. driving)

Side-effects constipation, dry mouth; blurred vision; *less commonly* nausea, vomiting, agitation, confusion, hallucinations, euphoria, insomnia, restlessness, urinary retention; paranoid delusions and impaired memory also reported

Licensed use not licensed for use in children

Indication and dose

Dystonia

- **By mouth**

Child 1 month–18 years 1–2 mg daily in 1–2 divided doses, adjusted according to response

Trihexyphenidyl (Non-proprietary) PoM
Tablets, trihexyphenidyl hydrochloride 2 mg, net price 20 = 52p; 5 mg, 20 = 79p. Counselling, before or after food (see notes above), driving

Broflex® (Alliance) PoM
Syrup, pink, trihexyphenidyl hydrochloride 5 mg/5 mL. Net price 200 mL = £6.20. Counselling, before or after food (see notes above), driving

4.9.3 Drugs used in essential tremor, chorea, tics, and related disorders

Haloperidol may be useful in improving motor tics and symptoms of Gilles de la Tourette syndrome and related choreas (see section 4.2.1). **Pimozide** (section 4.2.1), and **sulpiride** (section 4.2.1) are also used in Gilles de la Tourette syndrome.

Propranolol or another beta-adrenoceptor blocking drug (section 2.4) may be useful in treating essential tremor or tremors associated with anxiety or thyrotoxicosis.

Torsion dystonias and other involuntary movements

BOTULINUM A TOXIN-HAEMAGGLUTININ COMPLEX

Cautions history of dysphagia

Pregnancy manufacturers advise avoid unless essential—toxicity in *animal* studies

Breast-feeding manufacturers advise avoid (or avoid unless essential)—no information available

Contra-indications generalised disorders of muscle activity (e.g. myasthenia gravis)

Side-effects increased electrophysiologic jitter in some distant muscles; misplaced injections may paralyse nearby muscle groups and excessive doses may paralyse distant muscles; influenza-like symptoms, *rarely* arrhythmias, myocardial infarction, seizures, hypersensitivity reactions including rash, pruritus and anaphylaxis, antibody formation (substantial deterioration in response), and injection-site reactions

Specific side-effects in paediatric cerebral palsy Drowsiness, paraesthesia, urinary incontinence, myalgia

Indication and dose

In children over 2 years for dynamic equinus foot deformity caused by spasticity in ambulant paediatric cerebral palsy for dose consult product literature (**important**: information specific to **each individual preparation** and **not interchangeable**)

Botox® (Allergan) PoM

Injection, powder for reconstitution, botulinum A neurotoxin complex, net price 100-unit vial = £128.93

Dysport® (Ipsen) PoM

Injection, powder for reconstitution, botulinum A toxin-haemagglutinin complex, net price 500-unit vial = £153.21

4.10 Drugs used in substance dependence

This section includes drugs used in the treatment of neonatal abstinence syndrome and cigarette smoking.

Treatment of alcohol or opioid dependence in children requires specialist management. The health departments of the UK have produced a report, *Drug Misuse and Dependence* which contains guidelines on clinical management.

Drug Misuse and Dependence, London, The Stationery Office, 1999 can be obtained from:

The Publications Centre
PO Box 276
London, SW8 5DT.
Tel: (087) 0600 5522
Fax: (087) 0600 5533

or from The Stationery Office bookshops and through all good booksellers.

Neonatal abstinence syndrome Neonatal abstinence syndrome occurs at birth as a result of intra-uterine exposure to opioids or high-dose benzodiazepines.

Treatment is usually initiated if:

- feeding becomes a problem and tube feeding is required;
- there is profuse vomiting or watery diarrhoea;
- the baby remains very unsettled after two consecutive feeds despite gentle swaddling and the use of a pacifier.

Treatment involves weaning the baby from the drug on which it is dependent. **Morphine** or **methadone** (section 4.7.2) can be used in babies of mothers who have been taking opioids. Morphine is widely used because the dose can be easily adjusted, but methadone may provide smoother control of symptoms. Weaning babies from opioids usually takes 7–10 days.

Weaning babies from benzodiazepines that have a long half-life is difficult to manage; **chlorpromazine** (section 4.2.1) may be used in these situations but excessive sedation may occur. For babies who are dependent on barbiturates, phenobarbital (section 4.8.1) may be tried, although it does not control gastro-intestinal symptoms.

Cigarette smoking

Smoking cessation interventions are a cost-effective way of reducing ill health and prolonging life. Smokers should be advised to stop and offered help if interested in doing so, with follow-up where appropriate.

Where possible, smokers should have access to a smoking cessation clinic for behavioural support. **Nicotine replacement therapy** is an effective aid to smoking cessation for those smoking more than 10 cigarettes a day. It is regarded as the pharmacological treatment of choice in the management of smoking cessation.

Cigarette smoking should stop completely before starting a smoking cessation regimen including nicotine replacement therapy. If complete smoking cessation is not possible some nicotine preparations are licensed for use as part of a programme to reduce smoking before stopping completely; the smoking cessation regimen can be followed during a quit attempt.

NICE guidance (nicotine replacement therapy for smoking cessation)
NICE has recommended (March 2002) that nicotine replacement therapy should be prescribed only for a smoker who commits to a target stop date. The smoker should be offered advice and encouragement to aid smoking cessation.

Therapy to aid smoking cessation is chosen according to the smoker's likely compliance, availability of counselling and support, previous experience of smoking-cessation aids, contra-indications and adverse effects of the products, and the smoker's preferences.

Initial supply of the prescribed smoking-cessation therapy should be sufficient to last only 2 weeks after the target stop date. A second prescription should be issued only if the smoker demonstrates a continuing attempt to stop smoking.

If an attempt to stop smoking is unsuccessful, the NHS should not normally fund a further attempt within 6 months.

NICOTINE

Cautions severe or unstable cardiovascular disease (including hospitalisation for severe arrhythmias, recent myocardial infarction, or recent cerebrovascular accident)—initiate under medical supervision; uncontrolled hyperthyroidism; diabetes mellitus (monitor blood-glucose concentration closely when initiating treatment); phaeochromocytoma; *oral preparations*, oesophagitis, gastritis, peptic ulcers; *patches*, exercise may increase absorption and side-effects, skin disorders (patches should not be placed on broken skin)

Hepatic impairment manufacturers advise caution in moderate to severe hepatic impairment

Renal impairment manufacturers advise caution in severe renal impairment

Pregnancy use only if smoking cessation without nicotine replacement therapy fails; intermittent therapy preferred but avoid liquorice-flavoured nicotine products

Breast-feeding present in milk; intermittent therapy preferred

Note Most warnings under Cautions also apply to continuation of cigarette smoking

Side-effects nausea, dizziness, headache and cold and influenza-like symptoms, palpitation, dyspepsia and other gastro-intestinal disturbances, hiccups, insomnia, vivid dreams, myalgia; other side-effects reported include chest pain, blood pressure changes, anxiety and irritability, somnolence and impaired concentration, abnormal hunger, dysmenorrhoea, rash; *with patches*, skin reactions (discontinue if severe)—vasculitis also reported; *with spray*, nasal irritation, nose bleeds, watering eyes, ear sensations; *with gum, lozenges, sublingual tablets* or *inhalator*, aphthous ulceration (sometimes with swelling of tongue); *with spray, inhalator, lozenges, sublingual tablets* or *gum*, throat irritation; *with inhalator*, cough, rhinitis, pharyngitis, stomatitis, sinusitis, dry mouth; *with lozenges* or *sublingual tablets*, unpleasant taste

Indication and dose

See under preparations, below

Nicorette® (Pharmacia)
Nicorette Microtab (sublingual), nicotine (as a cyclodextrin complex) 2 mg, net price starter

NICOTINE (*continued*)

pack of 2 × 15-tablet discs with dispenser = £3.57; refill pack of 7 × 15-tablet discs = £9.84. Label: 26

Dose

Smoking cessation
- **By sublingual administration**

Child 12–18 years individuals smoking *20 cigarettes or less daily*, 2 mg each hour; for patients who fail to stop smoking or have significant withdrawal symptoms, consider increasing to 4 mg each hour; individuals smoking *more than 20 cigarettes daily*, 4 mg each hour. Max. 80 mg daily; treatment continued for up to 8 weeks followed by gradual reduction over 4 weeks; review treatment if abstinence not achieved within 3 months

Nicorette chewing gum, sugar-free, nicotine (as resin) 2 mg, net price pack of 15 = £1.71, pack of 30 = £3.25, pack of 105 = £8.89; 4 mg, net price pack of 15 = £2.11, pack of 30 = £3.99, pack of 105 = £10.83

Note Also available in freshmint flavour

Dose

Smoking cessation
- **By mouth**

Child 12–18 years individuals *smoking 20 cigarettes or less daily*, initially chew one 2-mg piece slowly for approx. 30 minutes when urge to smoke occurs; individuals smoking *more than 20 cigarettes daily* or needing more than 15 pieces of 2-mg gum daily should use the 4-mg gum; max. 15 pieces of 4-mg gum daily; treatment continued for up to 8 weeks followed by gradual reduction over 4 weeks; review treatment if abstinence not achieved within 3 months

Smoking reduction
- **By mouth**

Child 12–18 years chew one piece when urge to smoke occurs between smoking episodes; reduce smoking within 6 weeks and attempt smoking cessation within 6 months; review treatment if abstinence not achieved within 9 months

Note Children under 18 years should consult a healthcare professional before starting smoking-reduction regimen

Nicorette patches, self-adhesive, all beige, nicotine, *'5 mg' patch* (releasing approx. 5 mg/16 hours), net price 7 = £9.07; *'10 mg' patch* (releasing approx. 10 mg/16 hours), 7 = £9.07; *'15 mg' patch* (releasing approx. 15 mg/16 hours), 2 = £2.85, 7 = £9.07

Dose

Smoking cessation
- **By transdermal route**

Child 12–18 years apply on waking to dry, non-hairy skin on hip, chest or upper arm, removing after approx. 16 hours, usually when retiring to bed; site next patch on different area (avoid using same area on consecutive days); initially '15-mg' patch for 16 hours daily for 8 weeks then if abstinence achieved '10-mg' patch for 16 hours daily for 2 weeks then '5-mg' patch for 16 hours daily for 2 weeks; review treatment if abstinence not achieved within 3 months

Nicorette nasal spray, nicotine 500 micrograms/metered spray, net price 200-spray unit = £10.99

Dose

Smoking cessation
- **Intranasally**

Child 12–18 years apply 1 spray into each nostril as required to max. twice an hour for 16 hours daily (max. 64 sprays daily) for 8 weeks, then reduce gradually over next 4 weeks (reduce by half at end of first 2 weeks, stop altogether at end of next 2 weeks); review treatment if abstinence not achieved within 3 months

Nicorette inhalator (nicotine-impregnated plug for use in inhalator mouthpiece), nicotine 10 mg/cartridge, net price 6-cartridge (starter) pack = £3.39, 42-cartridge (refill) pack = £11.37

Dose

Smoking cessation
- **By inhalation**

Child 12–18 years inhale when urge to smoke occurs; initially use between 6 and 12 cartridges daily for up to 8 weeks, then reduce gradually over 4 weeks (reduce by half over first 2 weeks, stop altogether at end of next 2 weeks); review treatment if abstinence not achieved within 3 months

Smoking reduction
- **By inhalation**

Child 12–18 years inhale when urge to smoke occurs between smoking episodes; reduce smoking within 6 weeks and atempt smoking cessation within 6 months; review treatment if abstinence not achieved within 9 months

Note Children under 18 years should consult a healthcare professional before starting smoking-reduction regimen

Nicotinell® (Novartis Consumer Health)

Chewing gum, sugar-free, nicotine 2 mg, net price pack of 12 = £1.59, pack of 24 = £3.01, pack of 96 = £8.26; 4 mg, pack of 12 = £1.70, pack of 24 = £3.30, pack of 96 = £10.26

Note Also available in fruit, liquorice, and mint flavours

Dose

Smoking cessation
- **By mouth**

Child 12–18 years initially one 2-mg or 4-mg piece chewed slowly for approx. 30 minutes when urge to smoke occurs; max. 60 mg daily; withdraw gradually; review treatment if abstinence not achieved within 3 months

Nicotinell mint lozenge, sugar-free, nicotine (as bitartrate) 1 mg, net price pack of 12 = £1.71, pack of 36 = £4.27, pack of 96 = £9.12; 2 mg, net price pack of 12 = £1.99, pack of 36 = £4.95, pack of 96 = £10.60. Label: 24

Excipients: include aspartame (section 9.4.1)

Dose

Smoking cessation
- **By mouth**

Child 12–18 years initially 1 lozenge every 1–2 hours when urge to smoke occurs; max. 30 mg daily; withdraw gradually; review treatment if abstinence not achieved within 3 months

TTS Patches, self-adhesive, all yellowish-ochre, nicotine, *'10' patch* (releasing approx. 7 mg/24 hours), net price 7 = £9.12; *'20' patch* (releasing approx. 14 mg/24 hours), net price 2 = £2.57, 7 = £9.40; *'30' patch* (releasing approx. 21 mg/24 hours), net price 2 = £2.85, 7 = £9.97, 21 = £24.51

Dose

Smoking cessation
- **By transdermal route**

Child 12–18 years apply to dry, non-hairy skin on trunk or upper arm, removing after 24 hours and siting replacement patch on a different area (avoid using the same area for several days); individuals smoking *less than 20 cigarettes daily*, initially '20' patch daily; individuals smoking *20 or more cigarettes daily*, initially '30' patch daily; withdraw gradually, reducing dose every 3–4 weeks; review treatment if abstinence not achieved within 3 months

NICOTINE (*continued*)

NiQuitin CQ® (GSK Consumer Healthcare)

Chewing gum, sugar-free, mint-flavour, nicotine 2 mg, net price pack of 12 = £1.71, pack of 24 = £3.25, pack of 96 = £9.97; 4 mg, net price pack of 12 = £1.71, pack of 24 = £3.25, pack of 96 = £9.97

Dose

Smoking cessation
- **By mouth**

Child 12–18 years initially 1 piece chewed slowly for approx. 30 minutes, when urge to smoke occurs; max. 15 pieces daily; withdraw gradually; review treatment if abstinence not achieved within 3 months

Lozenges, sugar-free, nicotine (as polacrilex) 2 mg, net price pack of 36 = £5.12, pack of 72 = £9.97; 4 mg, pack of 36 = £5.12, pack of 72 = £9.97. Contains 0.65 mmol Na^+/lozenge

Excipients: include aspartame (section 9.4.1)

Dose

Smoking cessation
- **By mouth**

Child 12–18 years initially 1 lozenge every 1–2 hours when urge to smoke occurs (max. 15 lozenges daily) for 6 weeks, then 1 lozenge every 2–4 hours for 3 weeks, then 1 lozenge every 4–8 hours for 3 weeks; withdraw gradually; review treatment if abstinence not achieved within 3 months

Patches, self-adhesive, pink/beige, nicotine *'7 mg' patch* (releasing approx. 7 mg/24 hours), net price 7 = £9.97; *'14 mg' patch* (releasing approx. 14 mg/24 hours), 7 = £9.97; *'21 mg' patch* (releasing approx. 21 mg/24 hours), 7 = £9.97, 14 = £18.79

Note Also available as a clear patch

Dose

Smoking cessation
- **By transdermal route**

Child 12–18 years apply on waking to dry, non-hairy skin, removing after 24 hours and siting replacement patch on different area (avoid using same area for 7 days); individuals smoking *10 or more cigarettes daily*, initially '21-mg' patch daily for 6 weeks then '14-mg' patch daily for 2 weeks then '7-mg' patch daily for 2 weeks. Individuals smoking *less than 10 cigarettes daily*, initially '14-mg' patch daily for 6 weeks then '7-mg' patch daily for 2 weeks; review treatment if abstinence not achieved within 3 months

Note Patients using the '21-mg' patch who experience excessive side-effects, which do not resolve within a few days, should change to '14-mg' patch for the remainder of the initial 6 weeks before switching to the '7-mg' patch for the final 2 weeks

4.11 Drugs for dementia

Classification not used in BNF for Children.

5 Infections

This chapter includes advice on the drug management of the following:

anthrax, p. 342
bacterial infections (summary of treatment and prophylaxis), p. 283–293
Lyme disease, p. 297
MRSA infections, p. 295
oral infections, p. 282 and p. 287

Notifiable diseases

Doctors must notify the Proper Officer of the local authority (usually the consultant in communicable disease control) when attending a patient suspected of suffering from any of the diseases listed below; a form is available from the Proper Officer.

Anthrax	Ophthalmia neonatorum
Cholera	Paratyphoid fever
Diphtheria	Plague
Dysentery (amoebic or bacillary)	Poliomyelitis, acute
Encephalitis, acute	Rabies
Food poisoning	Relapsing fever
Haemorrhagic fever (viral)	Rubella
Hepatitis, viral	Scarlet fever
Leprosy	Smallpox
Leptospirosis	Tetanus
Malaria	Tuberculosis
Measles	Typhoid fever
Meningitis	Typhus
Meningococcal septicaemia (without meningitis)	Whooping cough
Mumps	Yellow fever

Note It is good practice for doctors to also inform the consultant in communicable disease control of instances of other infections (e.g. psittacosis) where there could be a public health risk.

5.1 Antibacterial drugs

Choice of a suitable drug Before selecting an antibacterial the clinician must first consider two factors—the child and the known or likely causative organism. Factors related to the child which must be considered include history of allergy, renal and hepatic function, susceptibility to infection (i.e. whether immunocompromised), ability to tolerate drugs by mouth, severity of illness, ethnic origin, age and, if an adolescent female, whether pregnant, breast-feeding or taking an oral contraceptive.

The known or likely organism and its antibacterial sensitivity, in association with the above factors, will suggest one or more antibacterials, the final choice depending on the microbiological, pharmacological, and toxicological properties.

The principles involved in selection of an antibacterial must allow for a number of variables including age, changing renal and hepatic function, increasing bacterial resistance, and new information on side-effects. Duration of therapy, dosage, and route of administration depend on site, type and severity of infection and response.

Antibacterial policies Local policies often limit the antibacterials that may be used to achieve reasonable economy consistent with adequate cover, and to reduce the development of resistant organisms. A policy may indicate a range of drugs for general use, and permit other drugs only on the advice of the microbiologist or paediatric infectious diseases specialist.

Before starting therapy The following principles should be considered before starting:

- Viral infections should not be treated with antibacterials. However, antibacterials are occasionally helpful in controlling secondary bacterial infection (e.g. acute necrotising ulcerative gingivitis secondary to herpes simplex infections);
- Samples should be taken for culture and sensitivity testing whenever possible; **'blind'** antibacterial prescribing for unexplained pyrexia usually leads to further difficulty in establishing the diagnosis;
- Knowledge of **prevalent organisms** and their current **sensitivity** is of great help in choosing an antibacterial before bacteriological confirmation is available;
- The **dose** of an antibacterial varies according to a number of factors including age, weight, hepatic function, renal function, and severity of infection. The prescribing of the so-called 'standard' dose in serious infections may result in failure of treatment or even death of the patient; therefore it is important to prescribe a dose appropriate to the condition. An inadequate dose may also increase the likelihood of antibacterial resistance. On the other hand, for an antibacterial with a narrow margin between the toxic and therapeutic dose (e.g. an aminoglycoside) it is also important to avoid an excessive dose and the concentration of the drug in the plasma may need to be monitored;
- The **route** of administration of an antibacterial often depends on the severity of the infection. Life-threatening infections often require intravenous therapy. Antibacterials that are well absorbed may be given by mouth even for some serious infections. Parenteral administration is also appropriate when the oral route cannot be used (e.g. because of vomiting) or if absorption is inadequate (e.g. in neonates and young children). Whenever possible painful intramuscular injections should be avoided in children;
- **Duration** of therapy depends on the nature of the infection and the response to treatment. Courses should not be unduly prolonged because they encourage resistance, they may lead to side-effects and they are costly. However, in certain infections such as tuberculosis or chronic osteomyelitis it is necessary to treat for prolonged periods.

Oral bacterial infections Antibacterial drugs should only be prescribed for the *treatment* of oral infections on the basis of defined need. They may be used in conjunction with (but not as an alternative to) other appropriate measures, such as providing drainage or extracting a tooth.

The 'blind' prescribing of an antibacterial for unexplained pyrexia, cervical lymphadenopathy, or facial swelling can lead to difficulty in establishing the diagnosis. Bacteriological sampling should always be carried out in severe oral infections.

Oral infections which call for antibacterial treatment include acute suppurative pulpitis, acute periapical or periodontal abscess, cellulitis, oral-antral fistula (and acute sinusitis), severe pericoronitis, localised osteitis, acute necrotising ulcerative gingivitis, and destructive forms of chronic periodontal disease. Most of these infections are readily resolved by the early establishment of drainage and removal of the cause (typically an infected necrotic pulp). Antibacterials may be indicated if treatment has to be delayed and they are essential in immunocompromised patients or in those with conditions such as diabetes. Certain rarer infections including bacterial sialadenitis, osteomyelitis, actinomycosis, and infections involving fascial spaces such as Ludwig's angina, require antibiotics and specialist hospital care.

Antibacterial drugs may also be useful after dental surgery in some cases of spreading infection. Infection may spread to involve local lymph nodes, to fascial spaces (where it can cause airway obstruction), or into the bloodstream (where it can lead to cavernous sinus thrombosis and other serious complications). Extension of an infection can also lead to maxillary sinusitis; osteomyelitis is a complication, which usually arises when host resistance is reduced.

If the oral infection fails to respond to antibacterial treatment within 48 hours the antibacterial should be changed, preferably on the basis of bacteriological investigation. Failure to respond may also suggest an incorrect diagnosis, lack of essential additional measures (such as drainage), poor host resistance, or poor patient compliance.

Combination of a penicillin (or erythromycin) with metronidazole may sometimes be helpful for the treatment of severe or resistant oral infections.

See also **Penicillins** (section 5.1.1), **Cephalosporins** (section 5.1.2), **Tetracyclines** (section 5.1.3), **Macrolides** (section 5.1.5), **Clindamycin** (section 5.1.6), **Metronidazole** (section 5.1.11), **Fusidic acid** (section 13.10.1.2) .

Superinfection In general, broad-spectrum antibacterial drugs such as the cephalosporins are more likely to be associated with adverse reactions related to the selection of resistant organisms e.g. *fungal infections* or *antibiotic-associated colitis* (pseudomembranous colitis); other problems associated with superinfection include vaginitis and pruritus ani.

Therapy Suggested treatment is shown in Table 1. When the pathogen has been isolated treatment may be changed to a more appropriate antibacterial if necessary. If no bacterium is cultured the antibacterial can be continued or stopped on clinical grounds. Infections for which prophylaxis is useful are listed in table 2.

Switching from parenteral to oral treatment The ongoing parenteral administration of an antibacterial should be reviewed regularly. In older children it may be possible to switch to an oral antibacterial; in neonates and infants this should be done more cautiously because of the relatively high incidence of bacteraemia and the possibility of variable oral absorption.

Prophylaxis Infections for which antibacterial prophylaxis is useful are listed in Table 2. In most situations, only a short course of prophylactic antibacterial is needed. Longer-term antibacterial prophylaxis is appropriate in specific indications such as vesico-ureteric reflux

Table 1. Summary of antibacterial therapy

If treating a patient suspected of suffering from a notifiable disease, the consultant in communicable disease control should be informed (see p. 281)

Gastro-intestinal system

Gastro-enteritis

Antibacterial not usually indicated

Frequently self-limiting and may not be bacterial

Campylobacter enteritis

Erythromycin[1] *or* ciprofloxacin

Salmonella

Ciprofloxacin *or* cefotaxime

Treat invasive or severe infection; treat less severe infection in those at risk of developing invasive infection (e.g. immunocompromised, haemoglobinopathy, or child under 3 months)

Shigellosis

Azithromycin [unlicensed indication] *or* ciprofloxacin

Antibacterial not indicated for mild cases. Amoxicillin or trimethoprim may be used if organism sensitive

Typhoid fever

Ciprofloxacin *or* cefotaxime[2]

Chloramphenicol may be an alternative; infections from Indian subcontinent, Middle-East, and South-East Asia may be multiple-antibacterial-resistant and sensitivity should be tested—azithromycin [unlicensed indication] may be an option in disease caused by multiple-antibacterial-resistant organisms

Antibiotic-associated colitis (pseudomembranous colitis)

Oral metronidazole *or* oral vancomycin

Give metronidazole by intravenous infusion if oral treatment inappropriate

Necrotising enterocolitis in neonates

Benzylpenicillin + gentamicin + intravenous metronidazole (*or* intravenous amoxicillin + cefotaxime + metronidazole)

1. Where erythromycin is suggested another macrolide (e.g. azithromycin or clarithromycin) may be used.
2. Where cefotaxime is suggested ceftriaxone may be used

Peritonitis

A cephalosporin (*or* amoxicillin + gentamicin) + metronidazole (*or* clindamycin)

Peritoneal dialysis-associated peritonitis

Either vancomycin[1] + ceftazidime added to dialysis fluid *or* vancomycin added to dialysis fluid + ciprofloxacin by mouth

Treat for 14 days or longer

Cardiovascular system

Endocarditis: initial 'blind' therapy

Flucloxacillin (*or* benzylpenicillin if symptoms less severe) + gentamicin

Substitute flucloxacillin (or benzylpenicillin) with vancomycin + rifampicin if cardiac prostheses present, or if penicillin-allergic, or if meticillin-resistant *Staphylococcus aureus* suspected

Endocarditis caused by staphylococci

Flucloxacillin (*or* vancomycin + rifampicin if penicillin-allergic or if meticillin-resistant *Staphylococcus aureus*)

Treat for at least 4 weeks; treat prosthetic valve endocarditis for at least 6 weeks and if using flucloxacillin add rifampicin for at least 2 weeks

Endocarditis caused by streptococci (e.g. viridans streptococci)

Benzylpenicillin (*or* vancomycin[1] if penicillin- allergic or highly penicillin-resistant) + gentamicin

Treat endocarditis caused by fully sensitive streptococci with benzylpenicillin or vancomycin alone for 4 weeks *or* (if no cardiac or embolic complications) with benzylpenicillin + gentamicin for 2 weeks; treat more resistant organisms for 4–6 weeks (stopping gentamicin after 2 weeks for organisms moderately sensitive to penicillin); if aminoglycoside cannot be used and if streptococci moderately sensitive to penicillin, treat with benzylpenicillin alone for 4 weeks; treat prosthetic valve endocarditis for at least 6 weeks (stopping gentamicin after 2 weeks if organisms fully sensitive to penicillin)

Endocarditis caused by enterococci (e.g. *Enterococcus faecalis*)

Amoxicillin[2] (*or* vancomycin[1] if penicillin-allergic or penicillin-resistant) + gentamicin

Treat for at least 4 weeks (at least 6 weeks for prosthetic valve endocarditis); if gentamicin-resistant, substitute gentamicin with streptomycin

Endocarditis caused by haemophilus, actinobacillus, cardiobacterium, eikenella, and kingella species ('HACEK' organisms)

Amoxicillin[2] (*or* ceftriaxone if amoxicillin-resistant) + gentamicin

Treat for 4 weeks (6 weeks for prosthetic valve endocarditis); stop gentamicin after 2 weeks

Respiratory system

***Haemophilus influenzae* epiglottitis**

Cefotaxime[3] *or* chloramphenicol

Give intravenously

Uncomplicated community-acquired pneumonia

Neonate and child under 6 months, treat as for severe community acquired pneumonia of unknown aetiology

Child 6 months–5 years, oral amoxicillin[2] or oral erythromycin[4]

Child 5–18 years, oral erythromycin[4] (*or* oral amoxicillin[2] if *Streptococcus pneumoniae* suspected)

Add flucloxacillin if staphylococci suspected, e.g. in influenza or measles; treat for 7 days (14–21 days for infections caused by staphylococci); pneumococci with decreased penicillin sensitivity being isolated but not yet common in UK; use erythromycin[4] if atypical pathogens suspected (more common in children over 5 years) or if penicillin-allergic

Severe community-acquired pneumonia of unknown aetiology

Neonate, benzylpenicillin + gentamicin

Child 1 month–18 years, cefuroxime *or* co-amoxiclav (or benzylpenicillin if lobar or *Streptococcus pneumoniae* suspected)

Use erythromycin[4] if atypical pathogens such as mycoplasma (more common in children over 5 years) or chlamydia suspected or if penicillin allergic; in pneumococcal infection add vancomycin to beta-lactam antibacterial if organism highly penicillin- and cephalosporin-resistant; add flucloxacillin if staphylococci suspected; treat for 10 days (14–21 days if staphylococci, legionella, or Gram-negative enteric bacilli suspected)

1. Where vancomycin is suggested teicoplanin may be used.
2. Where amoxicillin is suggested ampicillin may be used.
3. Where cefotaxime is suggested ceftriaxone may be used
4. Where erythromycin is suggested another macrolide (e.g. azithromycin or clarithromycin) may be used.

Pneumonia possibly caused by atypical pathogens

Erythromycin[1]

Severe Legionella infections may require addition of rifampicin; tetracycline is an alternative for chlamydial and mycoplasma infections in children over 12 years; treat for at least 14 days (14–21 days for legionella)

Hospital-acquired pneumonia

A broad-spectrum cephalosporin (e.g. cefotaxime or ceftazidime) *or* an antipseudomonal penicillin or another antipseudomonal beta-lactam

An aminoglycoside may be added in severe illness

Cystic fibrosis

Staphylococcal lung infection in cystic fibrosis

Flucloxacillin (*or* erythromycin[1] *or* clindamycin if penicillin-allergic)

In severe exacerbation use flucloxacillin or a broad-spectrum cephalosporin (e.g. cefuroxime); substitute with vancomycin[2] if meticillin-resistant *Staphylococcus aureus* suspected, and if necessary, add either rifampicin or sodium fusidate

Haemophilus influenzae lung infection in cystic fibrosis

Amoxicillin *or* a broad-spectrum cephalosporin

In severe exacerbation use a third-generation cephalosporin (e.g. cefotaxime)

Pseudomonal lung infection in cystic fibrosis

Ciprofloxacin + *nebulised* colistin

In severe exacerbation treat with a parenteral aminoglycoside and an antipseudomonal beta-lactam antibacterial

Central nervous system

Meningitis: Initial 'blind' therapy

- Transfer patient urgently to hospital.
- If bacterial meningitis and especially if *meningococcal disease* suspected, general practitioners should give benzylpenicillin (see p. 294 for dose) before urgent transfer to hospital; cefotaxime (section 5.1.2) may be an alternative in penicillin allergy; chloramphenicol (section 5.1.7) may be used if history of anaphylaxis to penicillin or to cephalosporins
- Consider adjunctive treatment with dexamethasone starting before or with first dose of antibacterial; avoid dexamethasone in septic shock, suspected meningococcal disease, or if immunocompromised, or in meningitis following surgery
- In hospital, if aetiology unknown:
  Neonate and Child 1–3 months, cefotaxime[3] + amoxicillin[4]
  Child 3 months–18 years, cefotaxime[3]

Meningitis caused by group B streptococcus

Benzylpenicillin + gentamicin *or* cefotaxime[3] alone

Treat for 14 days

Meningitis caused by meningococci

Benzylpenicillin *or* cefotaxime[3]

Treat for at least 5 days; substitute chloramphenicol if history of anaphylaxis to penicillin or to cephalosporins; to eliminate nasopharyngeal carriage in patients treated with benzylpenicillin or chloramphenicol see Table 2, section 5.1.

Meningitis caused by pneumococci

Cefotaxime[3]

Treat for 10–14 days; substitute benzylpenicillin if organism penicillin-sensitive; if organism highly penicillin- and cephalosporin-resistant, add vancomycin and if necessary rifampicin; consider early adjunctive treatment with dexamethasone (but may reduce penetration of vancomycin into cerebrospinal fluid; section 6.3.2)

Meningitis caused by *Haemophilus influenzae*

Cefotaxime[3]

Treat for at least 10 days; substitute chloramphenicol if history of anaphylaxis to penicillin or to cephalosporins or if organism resistant to cefotaxime; consider early adjunctive treatment with dexamethasone (section 6.3.2); for *H. influenzae* type b give rifampicin for 4 days before hospital discharge

Meningitis caused by Listeria

Amoxicillin[4] + gentamicin

Treat for at least 14 days. Consider stopping gentamicin after one week

1. Where erythromycin is suggested another macrolide (e.g. azithromycin or clarithromycin) may be used.
2. Where vancomycin is suggested teicoplanin may be used.
3. Where cefotaxime is suggested ceftriaxone may be used
4. Where amoxicillin is suggested ampicillin may be used.

Urinary tract

Urinary-tract infection

Mildly unwell child over 3 months of age, trimethoprim *or* oral cephalosporin *or* nitrofurantoin *or* co-amoxiclav

Treat for 5–7 days but a short course (e.g. 3 days) of trimethoprim or amoxicillin is usually adequate for uncomplicated urinary-tract infections in adolescent females

Child under 3 months of age or seriously unwell child over 3 months of age, i/v amoxicillin[1] + gentamicin *or* i/v cephalosporin alone

Genital system

Syphilis

Neonatal congenital syphilis, benzylpenicillin *or* procaine benzylpenicillin [unlicensed]

Treat for 10 days

Other syphilis infections, procaine benzylpenicillin [unlicensed] *or* doxycycline *or* erythromycin

Doxycycline is an option in children over 12 years; treat early syphilis for 14 days (10 days with procaine benzylpenicillin); treat late latent syphilis (asymptomatic infection of more than 2 years) with procaine benzylpenicillin for 17 days (or with doxycycline for 28 days); treat asymptomatic contacts of patients with infectious syphilis with doxycycline for 14 days; contact tracing recommended

Uncomplicated gonorrhoea

Child under 12 years, ceftriaxone

Child 12–18 years, cefixime [unlicensed indication] *or* ciprofloxacin

Single dose treatment in uncomplicated infection; choice depends on locality where infection acquired; pharyngeal infection requires treatment with ceftriaxone; use ciprofloxacin only if organism sensitive; contact-tracing recommended; remember chlamydia

Uncomplicated genital chlamydial infection, non-gonococcal urethritis and non-specific genital infection

Child under 12 years, erythromycin for 14 days

Child 12–18 years, single dose of azithromycin *or* doxycycline for 7 days

Contact tracing recommended

Blood

Septicaemia: Initial 'blind' therapy

Neonate less than 48 hours old, benzylpenicillin + gentamicin *or* amoxicillin[1] + cefotaxime

Neonate more than 48 hours old, flucloxacillin + gentamicin *or* amoxicillin[1] + cefotaxime

Child 1 month–18 years, community-acquired septicaemia, aminoglycoside + amoxicillin[1] *or* cefotaxime[2] alone

Use aminoglycoside + broad spectrum antipseudomonal beta-lactam antibacterial if pseudomonas suspected; add metronidazole if anaerobic infection suspected; add flucloxacillin *or* vancomycin[3] if Gram-positive infection suspected

Child 1 month–18 years, hospital-acquired septicaemia, a broad-spectrum antipseudomonal beta-lactam antibacterial (e.g. ceftazidime, *Tazocin®*, *Timentin®*, imipenem (with cilastatin as *Primaxin®*) or meropenem)

Add aminoglycoside if pseudomonas suspected, or if multiple-resistant organisms suspected, or if severe sepsis; add vancomycin[3] if meticillin-resistant *Staphylococcus aureus* suspected; add metronidazole to broad-spectrum cephalosporin if anaerobic infection suspected

Septicaemia related to vascular catheter

Vancomycin[3]

Add an aminoglycoside + a broad-spectrum antipseudomonal beta-lactam if Gram-negative sepsis suspected, especially in the immunocompromised; consider removing vascular catheter, particularly if infection caused by *Staphylococcus aureus*, pseudomonas, or candida

Meningococcal septicaemia

Benzylpenicillin *or* cefotaxime[2]

If meningococcal disease suspected, general practitioners advised to give a single dose of benzylpenicillin before urgent transfer to hospital (see under Benzylpenicillin, section 5.1.1.1); cefotaxime (section 5.1.2) may be an alternative in penicillin allergy; chloramphenicol may be used if history of anaphylaxis to penicillin or to cephalosporins; give rifampicin or ciprofloxacin to eliminate nasopharyngeal carriage before hospital discharge

1. Where amoxicillin is suggested ampicillin may be used.
2. Where cefotaxime is suggested ceftriaxone may be used
3. Where vancomycin is suggested teicoplanin may be used.

Musculoskeletal system

Osteomyelitis

Flucloxacillin *or* clindamycin if penicillin-allergic (*or* vancomycin[1] if resistant *Staphylococcus epidermidis* or meticillin-resistant *Staph. aureus*)

Treat acute infection for 4–6 weeks and chronic infection for at least 12 weeks; if child under 5 years of age and not immunised against *Haemophilus influenzae*, add cefotaxime[2] to flucloxacillin; combine vancomycin[1] with either fusidic acid or rifampicin if prostheses present or if life-threatening condition

Septic arthritis

Flucloxacillin + fusidic acid *or* clindamycin alone if penicillin-allergic (*or* vancomycin[1] if resistant *Staphylococcus epidermidis* or meticillin-resistant *Staph. aureus*)

Treat usually for 6 weeks (longer if infection complicated or if prosthesis is present); if child under 5 years of age and not immunised against *Haemophilus influenzae*, use cefotaxime[2] + flucloxacillin; combine vancomycin[1] with either fusidic acid or rifampicin if prosthesis present or if life-threatening condition

Eye

Purulent conjunctivitis

Neonate, neomycin eye drops

Child 1 month–18 years, chloramphenicol *or* gentamicin eye-drops

Congenital chlamydial conjunctivitis

Erythromycin (by mouth)

Treat for 14 days

Congenital gonococcal conjunctivitis

Ceftriaxone

Single-dose treatment

Ear, nose, and oropharynx

Pericoronitis

Metronidazole *or* amoxicillin

Antibacterial required only in presence of systemic features of infection or of trismus or persistent swelling despite local treatment; treat for 3 days or until symptoms resolve

Acute necrotising ulcerative gingivitis

Metronidazole *or* amoxicillin

Antibacterial required only if systemic features of infection; treat for 3 days or until symptoms resolve

Periapical or periodontal abscess

Amoxicillin *or* metronidazole

Antibacterial required only in severe disease with cellulitis or if systemic features of infection; treat for 5 days

Periodontitis

Metronidazole *or* doxycycline

Antibacterial required for severe disease or disease unresponsive to local treatment; doxycycline is an option in children over 12 years

Throat infections

Phenoxymethylpenicillin (*or* erythromycin[3] if penicillin-allergic)

Most throat infections are caused by viruses and many do not require antibacterial therapy; consider prescribing antibacterial for beta-haemolytic streptococcal pharyngitis (treat for 10 days), if history of valvular heart disease, if marked systemic upset, if peritonsillar cellulitis or if at increased risk from acute infection (e.g. in immunosuppression, diabetes); **avoid** amoxicillin if possibility of glandular fever, see section 5.1.1.3; initial parenteral therapy (in severe infection) with benzylpenicillin, then oral therapy with phenoxymethylpenicillin *or* amoxicillin[4]

Sinusitis

Amoxicillin[4] *or* erythromycin[3]

Antibacterial should usually be used only for persistent symptoms and purulent discharge lasting at least 7 days or if severe symptoms; treat for 7 days. Consider oral co-amoxiclav if no improvement after 48 hours. Initial parenteral therapy with co-amoxiclav or cefuroxime may be required in severe infections

Otitis externa

Flucloxacillin (*or* erythromycin[3] if penicillin-allergic)

Use ciprofloxacin (or an aminoglycoside) if pseudomonas suspected, see section 12.1.1

---

1. Where vancomycin is suggested teicoplanin may be used.
2. Where cefotaxime is suggested ceftriaxone may be used
3. Where erythromycin is suggested another macrolide (e.g. azithromycin or clarithromycin) may be used.
4. Where amoxicillin is suggested ampicillin may be used.

Otitis media

Amoxicillin[1] (*or* erythromycin[2] if penicillin-allergic).

Many infections caused by viruses; most uncomplicated cases resolve without antibacterial treatment; in children without systemic features, antibacterial treatment may be started after 72 hours if no improvement (earlier in immunocompromised patients, children under 2 years, or if deterioration); treat for 5 days (longer if severely ill); consider co-amoxiclav if no improvement after 48 hours; initial parenteral therapy in severe infection with co-amoxiclav or cefuroxime

Skin

Impetigo

Topical fusidic acid (*or* mupirocin if meticillin-resistant *Staphylococcus aureus*); oral flucloxacillin *or* erythromycin[2] if widespread

Topical treatment for 7 days usually adequate; max. duration of topical treatment 10 days; seek local microbiology advice before using topical treatment in hospital; oral treatment for 7 days; add phenoxymethylpenicillin to flucloxacillin if streptococcal infection suspected

Erysipelas

Phenoxymethylpenicillin (or erythromycin[2] if penicillin-allergic)

Add flucloxacillin to phenoxymethylpenicillin if staphylococcus suspected; substitute benzylpenicillin for phenoxymethylpenicillin if parenteral treatment required

Cellulitis

Benzylpenicillin + flucloxacillin (or erythromycin[2] alone if penicillin-allergic)

Substitute phenoxymethylpenicillin for benzylpenicillin if oral treatment appropriate; discontinue flucloxacillin if streptococcal infection confirmed. Substitute treatment with broad-spectrum antibacterials if patients at risk from anaerobic or Gram-negative infections (e.g. use co-amoxiclav alone for facial infection, orbital infection, or infection caused by animal or human bites. Use ceftazidime + clindamycin in immunocompromised patients)

Animal and human bites

Co-amoxiclav alone (*or* clindamycin if penicillin-allergic)

Cleanse wound thoroughly; for tetanus-prone wound, give human tetanus immunoglobulin (with adsorbed diphtheria [low dose] and tetanus vaccine if necessary, according to immunisation history and risk of infection), see under Tetanus Vaccines, section 14.4; consider rabies prophylaxis (section 14.4) for bites from animals in endemic countries; assess risk of blood-borne viruses

Acne—see section 13.6

Paronychia or 'septic spots' in neonate

Flucloxacillin

Add aminoglycoside if systemically unwell

Surgical wound infection

Flucloxacillin *or* co-amoxiclav

5 Infections

Table 2. Summary of antibacterial prophylaxis

Prevention of recurrence of rheumatic fever

Phenoxymethylpenicillin by mouth

Child 1 month–6 years 125 mg twice daily

Child 6–18 years 250 mg twice daily

or

Erythromycin by mouth

Child 1 month–2 years 125 mg twice daily

Child 2–18 years 250 mg twice daily

Prevention of secondary case of group A streptococcal infection

Phenoxymethylpenicillin by mouth

Child 1 month–1 year 62.5 mg every 6 hours for 10 days

Child 1–6 years 125 mg every 6 hours for 10 days

Child 6–12 years 250 mg every 6 hours for 10 days

Child 12–18 years 250–500 mg every 6 hours for 10 days

or

Erythromycin[2] (if penicillin-allergic) by mouth

Child 1 month–2 years 125 mg every 6 hours for 10 days

Child 2–8 years 250 mg every 6 hours for 10 days

Child 8–18 years 250–500 mg every 6 hours for 10 days

1. Where amoxicillin is suggested ampicillin may be used.
2. Where erythromycin is suggested another macrolide (e.g. azithromycin or clarithromycin) may be used.

Prevention of secondary case of meningococcal meningitis[1]

Rifampicin by mouth

Neonate 5 mg/kg every 12 hours for 2 days

Child 1 month–1 year 5 mg/kg every 12 hours for 2 days

Child 1–12 years 10 mg/kg (max. 600 mg) every 12 hours for 2 days

Child 12 -18 years 600 mg every 12 hours for 2 days

or

Ciprofloxacin by mouth [not licensed for this indication]

Child 5–12 years 250 mg as a single dose

Child 12–18 years 500 mg as a single dose

or

Ceftriaxone by intramuscular injection [not licensed for this indication] (preferred if pregnant)

Child 1 month–12 years 125 mg as a single dose

Child 12–18 years 250 mg as a single dose

Prevention of secondary case of Haemophilus influenzae type b disease[1]

Rifampicin by mouth

Child 1–3 months 10 mg/kg once daily for 4 days

Child 3 months–12 years 20 mg/kg (max. 600 mg) once daily for 4 days

Child 12–18 years 600 mg once daily for 4 days

Prevention of secondary case of diphtheria in non-immune patient

Erythromycin by mouth

Child 1 month–2 years 125 mg every 6 hours for 7 days

Child 2–8 years 250 mg every 6 hours for 7 days

Child 8–18 years 500 mg every 6 hours for 7 days

Treat for further 10 days if nasopharyngeal swabs positive after first 7 days' treatment

Prevention of secondary case of pertussis in non-immune patient or partially immune patient

Erythromycin[2] by mouth

Child 1 month–2 years 125 mg every 6 hours for 7 days

Child 2–8 years 250 mg every 6 hours for 7 days

Child 8–18 years 250–500 mg every 6 hours for 7 days

Note Pertussis vaccine inappropriate for outbreak since 3 injections required for protection

Prevention of pneumococcal infection in asplenia or in patients with sickle cell disease

Phenoxymethylpenicillin by mouth

Child 1 month–6 years 125 mg every 12 hours

Child 6–12 years 250 mg every 12 hours

Child 12–18 years 500 mg every 12 hours

If cover also needed for *H. influenzae* in child give amoxicillin instead

Child 1 month–5 years 125 mg every 12 hours

Child 5–12 years 250 mg every 12 hours

Child 12–18 years 500 mg every 12 hours

Note Antibiotic prophylaxis is not fully reliable; for vaccines in asplenia see p. 676

Prevention of *Staphylococcus aureus* lung infection in cystic fibrosis

Flucloxacillin[3] by mouth

Child 1 month–1 year 500 mg twice daily

Child 1–7 years 1 g twice daily

Child 7–18 years 2 g twice daily

1. For details of those who should receive chemoprophylaxis contact a consultant in communicable disease control (or a consultant in infectious diseases or the local Health Protection Agency service). Unless there has been mouth-to-mouth contact (or direct exposure to infectious droplets from a patient with meningococcal disease), healthcare workers do not generally require chemoprophylaxis.
2. Where erythromycin is suggested another macrolide (e.g. azithromycin or clarithromycin) may be used.
3. Use cefradine if flucloxacillin cannot be used

Prevention of endocarditis[1]

Dental and oral procedures [2,3] (including cosmetic piercing[4] involving tongue and oral mucosa)
either oral **amoxicillin** 1 hour before procedure,
Child under 5 years 750 mg
Child 5–10 years 1.5 g
Child 10–18 years 3 g
or i/v **amoxicillin** at induction of anaesthesia or just before procedure,
Child under 5 years 250 mg
Child 5–10 years 500 mg
Child 10–18 years 1 g
or if child *penicillin-allergic*, oral **clindamycin** [5] 1 hour before procedure,
Child under 5 years 150 mg
Child 5–10 years 300 mg
Child 10–18 years 600 mg
or if *penicillin-allergic* child unable to swallow capsules, oral **azithromycin**[6] 1 hour before procedure,
Child under 5 years 200 mg
Child 5–10 years 300 mg
Child 10–18 years 500 mg
or if child *penicillin-allergic*, i/v **clindamycin** [5] over at least 10 minutes, at induction of anaesthesia or just before procedure,
Child under 5 years 75 mg
Child 5–10 years 150 mg
Child 10–18 years 300 mg

Upper respiratory-tract procedure (including tonsillectomy, adenoidectomy), as for dental procedures

Nasal packing or intubation i/v **flucloxacillin** at induction of anaesthesia or just before procedure,
Child under 2 years 250 mg
Child 2–10 years 500 mg
Child 10–18 years 1 g
or if child *penicillin-allergic*, i/v **clindamycin** over at least 10 minutes (give 600 mg over at least 20 minutes), at induction of anaesthesia or just before procedure,
Child under 5 years 75 mg
Child 5–10 years 150 mg
Child 10–16 years 300 mg
Child 16–18 years 600 mg

1. Advice on the prevention of endocarditis reflects the recommendations of a Working Party of the British Society for Antimicrobial Chemotherapy. The Working Party recommends antibacterial prophylaxis for dental or non-dental procedures in children with a history of infective endocarditis, or who have had cardiac valve replacement surgery (including mechanical or biological prosthetic valves), or who have a surgically constructed systemic or pulmonary shunt or conduit. Antibacterial prophylaxis also recommended for non-dental procedures in children with complex congenital heart disease (except secundum atrial septal defects), or complex left ventricular outflow abnormalities (including aortic stenosis and bicuspid aortic valves), or acquired valvulopathy or mitral valve prolapse (with substantial pathology and regurgitation)
2. Antibacterial prophylaxis should be prescribed for all dental procedures involving dento-gingival manipulation or endodontics. It may be supplemented with *chlorhexidine gluconate gel 1%* or *chlorhexidine gluconate mouthwash 0.2 %* used 5 minutes before procedure
3. Multistage dental procedures should ideally be scheduled at intervals of at least 14 days to allow mucosal healing. If further dental procedures cannot be delayed, antibacterial prophylaxis should alternate between amoxicillin and clindamycin; expert advice should be obtained if child is penicillin-allergic
4. A Working Party of the British Society for Antimicrobial Chemotherapy advises that cosmetic piercing involving tongue or oral mucosa should be discouraged in children at risk of endocarditis
5. **Clindamycin** is not licensed for use in endocarditis prophylaxis but it is recommended by the Endocarditis Working Party
6. Azithromycin is not licensed for use in endocarditis prophylaxis but it is recommended by the Endocarditis Working Party

Gastro-intestinal procedures[1] (including endoscopic retrograde cholangiopancreatography, hepatic or biliary surgery, lithotripsy, surgery involving intestinal mucosa, sclerotherapy of oesophageal varices, oesophageal stricture dilatation, oesophageal laser therapy), i/v **amoxicillin** and i/v **gentamicin** at induction of anaesthesia or just before procedure,

Child under 5 years i/v amoxicillin 250 mg + i/v gentamicin 1.5 mg/kg

Child 5–10 years i/v amoxicillin 500 mg + i/v gentamicin 1.5 mg/kg

Child 10–18 years i/v amoxicillin 1 g + i/v gentamicin 1.5 mg/kg

or if child *penicillin-allergic*, i/v **teicoplanin** and i/v **gentamicin** at induction of anaesthesia or just before procedure,

Child under 14 years i/v teicoplanin 6 mg/kg (max. 400 mg) + i/v gentamicin 1.5 mg/kg

Child 14–18 years i/v teicoplanin 400 mg + i/v gentamicin 1.5 mg/kg

Genito-urinary procedures (including cytoscopy, urethral dilatation), as for gastro-intestinal procedures

Obstetric and gynaecological procedures[2] (including vaginal hysterectomy, caesarean section), as for gastro-intestinal procedures

Joint prostheses and dental treatment

Advice of a Working Party of the British Society for Antimicrobial Chemotherapy is that patients with prosthetic joint implants (including total hip replacements) do not require antibacterial prophylaxis for dental treatment. The Working Party considers that it is unacceptable to expose patients to the adverse effects of antibacterials when there is no evidence that such prophylaxis is of any benefit, but that those who develop any intercurrent infection require prompt treatment with antibacterials to which the infecting organisms are sensitive.

The Working Party has commented that joint infections have rarely been shown to follow dental procedures and are even more rarely caused by oral streptococci.

Dermatological procedures

Advice of a Working Party of the British Society for Antimicrobial Chemotherapy is that patients who undergo dermatological procedures[3] do not require antibacterial prophylaxis against endocarditis.

Immunosuppression and indwelling intraperitoneal catheters

Advice of a Working Party of the British Society for Antimicrobial Chemotherapy is that patients who are immunosuppressed (including transplant patients) and patients with indwelling intraperitoneal catheters do not require antibacterial prophylaxis for dental treatment provided there is no other indication for prophylaxis.

The Working Party has commented that there is little evidence that dental treatment is followed by infection in immunosuppressed and immunodeficient patients nor is there evidence that dental treatment is followed by infection in patients with indwelling intraperitoneal catheters.

1. For banding of oesophageal varices, upper endoscopy, sigmoidoscopy, colonoscopy, percutaneous endoscopic gastrostomy, transoesophageal echocardiography, barium enema or percutaneous liver biopsy, antibacterial prophylaxis recommended only for children who have a history of infective endocarditis, or who have had cardiac valve replacement surgery (including mechanical or biological prosthetic valves), or who have a surgically constructed systemic or pulmonary shunt or conduit
2. For patients undergoing vaginal delivery, therapeutic abortion, insertion or removal of intrauterine device, antibacterial prophylaxis required if infection suspected (antibacterial treatment also required) or in prolonged rupture of membranes
3. The British Association of Dermatologists Therapy Guidelines and Audit Subcommittee advise that such dermatological procedures include skin biopsies and excision of moles or of malignant lesions

Prevention of gas-gangrene in high lower-limb amputations or following major trauma

i/v benzylpenicillin

Child 1 month–12 years 25 mg/kg (max. 600mg) every 6 hours for 5 days

Child 12–18 years 300–600 mg every 6 hours for 5 days

or if penicillin-allergic i/v or oral metronidazole

Child 1 month–12 years 7.5mg/kg (max. 500mg) every 8 hours for 5 days

Child 12–18 years 400–500 mg every 8 hours for 5 days

Prevention of tuberculosis in susceptible close contacts or those who have become tuberculin positive[1]

Isoniazid for 6 months

Neonate 5 mg/kg daily

Child 1 month –12 years 5 mg/kg daily (max. 300 mg daily)

Child 12–18 years 300 mg daily

or isoniazid + rifampicin for 3 months

Child 1 month–12 years isoniazid 5 mg/kg daily (max. 300 mg daily) + rifampicin 10 mg/kg daily (max. 600 mg daily)

Child 12–18 years isoniazid 300 mg daily + rifampicin 600 mg daily (rifampicin 450 mg daily if body-weight less than 50 kg)

or (if contact infected with isoniazid-resistant tuberculosis) rifampicin for 6 months

Child 1 month–12 years 10 mg/kg daily (max. 600 mg daily)

Child 12–18 years 600 mg daily (450 mg daily if body-weight under 50 kg)

Prevention of infection in gastro-intestinal procedures

Operations on stomach or oesophagus

Single dose[2] of i/v gentamicin *or* i/v cefuroxime

Open biliary surgery

Single dose[2] of i/v cefuroxime + i/v metronidazole[3] *or* i/v gentamicin + i/v metronidazole[3]

Resections of colon and rectum, and resections in inflammatory bowel disease, and appendicectomy

Single dose[2] of i/v gentamicin + i/v metronidazole[3] *or* i/v cefuroxime + i/v metronidazole[3] *or* i/v co-amoxiclav alone

Endoscopic retrograde cholangiopancreatography

Single dose of i/v gentamicin *or* oral or i/v ciprofloxacin

Prophylaxis particularly recommended if bile stasis, pancreatic pseudocyst, previous cholangitis or neutropenia

Prevention of infection in orthopaedic surgery

Management of fractures

Single dose[2] of i/v cefuroxime or i/v flucloxacillin

Substitute i/v vancomycin if history of allergy to penicillins or to cephalosporins; use cefuroxime + metronidazole for complex open fractures with extensive soft-tissue damage; prophylaxis continued for 24 hours in open fractures (longer if complex open fractures)

---

1. For details of those who should receive chemoprophylaxis contact the lead clinician for local tuberculosis services (or a consultant in communicable disease control). See also section 5.1.9, for advice on immunocompromised patients and on prevention of tuberculosis
2. Additional intra-operative or postoperative doses of antibacterial may be given for prolonged procedures or if there is major blood loss
3. Metronidazole may alternatively be given by suppository but to allow adequate absorption, it should be given 2 hours before surgery

Prevention of infection in obstetric surgery

Termination of pregnancy

Single dose[1] of oral metronidazole

If genital chlamydial infection cannot be ruled out, give doxycycline (section 5.1.3) postoperatively

Prevention of infection in vascular surgery

Reconstructive arterial surgery of abdomen, pelvis or legs

Single dose[1] of i/v cefuroxime or i/v gentamicin

Add i/v metronidazole for patients at risk from anaerobic infections including those with diabetes, gangrene or undergoing amputation; add i/v vancomycin if high risk of meticillin-resistant *Staphylococcus aureus*

5.1.1 Penicillins

The penicillins are bactericidal and act by interfering with bacterial cell wall synthesis. They diffuse well into body tissues and fluids, but penetration into the cerebrospinal fluid is poor except when the meninges are inflamed. They are excreted in the urine in therapeutic concentrations.

The most important side-effect of the penicillins is hypersensitivity which causes rashes and anaphylaxis and can be fatal. Allergic reactions to penicillins occur in 1–10% of exposed individuals; anaphylactic reactions occur in fewer than 0.05% of treated patients. Individuals with a history of anaphylaxis, urticaria, or rash immediately after penicillin administration are at risk of immediate hypersensitivity to a penicillin; these individuals should not receive a penicillin, a cephalosporin or another beta-lactam antibacterial. Children who are allergic to one penicillin will be allergic to all because the hypersensitivity is related to the basic penicillin structure. Individuals with a history of a minor rash (i.e. non-confluent rash restricted to a small area of the body) or a rash that occurs more than 72 hours after penicillin administration are probably not allergic to penicillin and in these individuals a penicillin should not be withheld unnecessarily for serious infections; the possibility of an allergic reaction should, however, be borne in mind.

A rare but serious toxic effect of the penicillins is encephalopathy due to cerebral irritation. This may result from excessively high doses or in patients with severe renal failure. The penicillins should **not** be given by intrathecal injection because they can cause encephalopathy which may be fatal.

Another problem relating to high doses of penicillin, or normal doses given to patients with renal failure, is the accumulation of electrolyte since most injectable penicillins contain either sodium or potassium.

Diarrhoea frequently occurs during oral penicillin therapy. It is most common with broad-spectrum penicillins, which can also cause antibiotic-associated colitis.

5.1.1.1 Benzylpenicillin and phenoxymethylpenicillin

Benzylpenicillin (Penicillin G) remains an important and useful antibiotic but is inactivated by bacterial beta-lactamases. It is effective for many streptococcal (including pneumococcal), gonococcal, and meningococcal infections and also for anthrax (section 5.1.12), diphtheria, gas-gangrene, leptospirosis, and treatment of Lyme disease (section 5.1.1.3) in children. It is also used in combination with gentamicin for the empirical treatment of sepsis in neonates less than 48 hours old. Pneumococci, meningococci, and gonococci which have decreased sensitiv-

1. Additional intra-operative or postoperative doses of antibacterial may be given for prolonged procedures or if there is major blood loss

ity to penicillin have been isolated; **benzylpenicillin is no longer the drug of first choice for pneumococcal meningitis**. Although benzylpenicillin is effective in the treatment of tetanus, metronidazole (section 5.1.11) is preferred. Benzylpenicillin is inactivated by gastric acid and absorption from the gastro-intestinal tract is low; therefore it must be given by injection.

Procaine benzylpenicillin (procaine penicillin) (available on a named-patient basis from specialist importing companies) is used for the treatment of early syphilis and late latent syphilis.

Phenoxymethylpenicillin (Penicillin V) has a similar antibacterial spectrum to benzylpenicillin, but is less active. It is gastric acid-stable, so is suitable for oral administration. It should not be used for serious infections because absorption can be unpredictable and plasma concentrations variable. It is indicated principally for respiratory-tract infections in children, for streptococcal tonsillitis, and for continuing treatment after one or more injections of benzylpenicillin when clinical response has begun. It should not be used for meningococcal or gonococcal infections. Phenoxymethylpenicillin is used for prophylaxis against streptococcal infections following rheumatic fever and against pneumococcal infections following splenectomy or in sickle cell disease.

Oral infections Phenoxymethylpenicillin is effective for dentoalveolar abscess.

BENZYLPENICILLIN

(Penicillin G)

Cautions history of allergy; false-positive urinary glucose (if tested for reducing substances); **interactions:** Appendix 1 (penicillins)

Renal impairment neurotoxicity—high doses may cause convulsions. Creatinine clearance 10–50 mL/min/1.73m², use normal dose every 8–12 hours; creatinine clearance less than 10 mL/min/1.73m² use normal dose every 12 hours

Pregnancy not known to be harmful

Breast-feeding trace amounts in breast milk—not known to be harmful but be alert for hypersensitivity in infant

Contra-indications penicillin hypersensitivity

Side-effects hypersensitivity reactions including urticaria, fever, joint pains, rashes, angioedema, anaphylaxis, serum sickness-like reactions; *rarely* CNS toxicity including convulsions (especially with high doses or in severe renal impairment), interstitial nephritis, haemolytic anaemia,leucopenia, thrombocytopenia and coagulation disorders; also reported diarrhoea (including antibiotic-associated colitis)

Indication and dose

Mild to moderate susceptible infections (including throat infections, otitis media, pneumonia, cellulitis, neonatal sepsis, Table 1, section 5.1)

- **By intramuscular injection or by slow intravenous injection or infusion (intravenous route recommended in neonates and infants)**

Preterm neonate and neonate under 7 days 25 mg/kg every 12 hours; dose doubled in severe infection

Neonate 7–28 days 25 mg/kg every 8 hours; dose doubled in severe infection

Child 1 month–18 years 25 mg/kg every 6 hours; increased to 50 mg/kg every 4–6 hours (max. 2.4 g every 4 hours) in severe infection

Endocarditis (combined with another antibacterial if necessary, see Table 1, section 5.1)

- **By slow intravenous injection or infusion**

Child 1 month–18 years 25 mg/kg every 4 hours, increased if necessary to 50 mg/kg (max. 2.4 g) every 4 hours

Meningitis, meningococcal disease

- **By slow intravenous injection or infusion**

Preterm neonate and neonate under 7 days 50 mg/kg every 12 hours

Neonate 7–28 days 50 mg/kg every 8 hours

Child 1 month–18 years 50 mg/kg every 4–6 hours (max. 2.4 g every 4 hours)

Important. If bacterial meningitis and especially if meningococcal disease is suspected general practitioners are advised to give a single injection of benzylpenicillin by intravenous injection (or by intramuscular injection) before transferring the patient urgently to hospital. Suitable doses are: **Infant under 1 year** 300 mg; **Child** 1–9 years 600 mg, 10 years and over 1.2 g. In penicillin allergy, cefotaxime (section 5.1.2) may be an alternative; chloramphenicol may be used if there is a history of anaphylaxis to penicillins

Treatment or prevention of neonatal group B streptococcus infection

- **By slow intravenous injection or infusion**

Preterm neonate and neonate under 7 days 50 mg/kg every 12 hours

Neonate 7–28 days 50 mg/kg every 8 hours

Prophylaxis in limb amputation Table 2, section 5.1

- **By intrathecal injection**

not recommended

Administration Intravenous route recommended in neonates and infants. Intermittent intravenous infusion in glucose 5% *or* sodium chloride 0.9%. Give over 15–30 minutes. Longer administration time is particularly important when using doses of 50 mg/kg to avoid CNS toxicity

BENZYLPENICILLIN (*continued*)

Crystapen® (Britannia) PoM
Injection, powder for reconstitution, benzylpenicillin sodium (unbuffered), net price 600-mg vial = 43p, 2-vial 'GP pack' = £1.90; 1.2-g vial = 87p
Electrolytes Na^+ 1.68 mmol/600-mg vial; 3.36 mmol/1.2-g vial

PHENOXYMETHYLPENICILLIN
(Penicillin V)

Cautions see under Benzylpenicillin; **interactions:** Appendix 1 (penicillins)

Renal impairment no dose adjustment required

Contra-indications see under Benzylpenicillin

Side-effects see under Benzylpenicillin

Indication and dose

Susceptible infections including oral infections, tonsillitis, otitis media, erysipelas, cellulitis

- **By mouth**

  Child 1 month–1 year 62.5 mg 4 times daily; increased in severe infection to ensure at least 12.5 mg/kg 4 times daily

  Child 1–6 years 125 mg 4 times daily; increased in severe infection to ensure at least 12.5 mg/kg 4 times daily

  Child 6–12 years 250 mg 4 times daily; increased in severe infection to ensure at least 12.5 mg/kg 4 times daily

  Child 12–18 years 500 mg 4 times daily; increased in severe infection up to 1 g 4 times daily

Prevention of pneumococcal infection in asplenia or sickle cell disease, see Table 2, section 5.1

Prevention of recurrence of rheumatic fever, see Table 2, section 5.1

Phenoxymethylpenicillin (Non-proprietary) PoM
Tablets, phenoxymethylpenicillin (as potassium salt) 250 mg, net price 28-tab pack = £1.67. Label: 9, 23

Oral solution, phenoxymethylpenicillin (as potassium salt) for reconstitution with water, net price 125 mg/5 mL, 100 mL = £1.59; 250 mg/5 mL, 100 mL = £2.22. Label: 9, 23

Dental prescribing on NHS Phenoxymethylpenicillin Tablets and Oral Solution may be prescribed

5.1.1.2 Penicillinase-resistant penicillins

Most staphylococci are now resistant to benzylpenicillin because they produce penicillinases. **Flucloxacillin**, however, is not inactivated by these enzymes and is thus effective in infections caused by penicillin-resistant staphylococci, which is the main indication for its use. Flucloxacillin is acid-stable and can, therefore, be given by mouth as well as by injection.

Flucloxacillin is well absorbed from the gut. For CSM warning on cholestatic jaundice see under Flucloxacillin.

MRSA *Staphylococcus aureus* strains resistant to meticillin [now discontinued] (meticillin-resistant *Staph. aureus*, MRSA) and to flucloxacillin have emerged; some of these organisms may be sensitive to vancomycin or teicoplanin (section 5.1.7). Strains may be susceptible to rifampicin, sodium fusidate, tetracyclines, aminoglycosides, macrolides and clindamycin. Rifampicin or sodium fusidate should not be used alone because resistance may develop rapidly. Trimethoprim alone may be used for less serious infections caused by some MRSA strains including urinary tract infections. Linezolid (section 5.1.7) and the combination of the streptogramin antibacterials quinupristin and dalfopristin (section 5.1.7) are active against MRSA; these antibacterial drugs should be reserved for organisms resistant to other antibacterials, for children who cannot tolerate other antibacterial drugs or who are not responding to vancomycin or teicoplanin. Treatment is guided by the sensitivity of the infecting strain. It is important that hospitals have infection control guidelines to minimise MRSA transmission, including policies on isolation and treatment of MRSA carriers, and on hand hygiene. For eradication of nasal carriage of MRSA see section 12.2.3.

FLUCLOXACILLIN

Cautions see under Benzylpenicillin (section 5.1.1.1); also hepatic impairment (see CSM advice below)

> CSM advice (hepatic disorders) CSM has advised that very rarely cholestatic jaundice and hepatitis may occur up to several weeks after treatment with flucloxacillin has been stopped. Administration for more than 2 weeks and increasing age are risk factors. CSM has reminded that:
> - flucloxacillin should not be used in patients with a history of hepatic dysfunction associated with flucloxacillin;
> - flucloxacillin should be used with caution in patients with hepatic impairment;
> - careful enquiry should be made about hypersensitivity reactions to beta-lactam antibacterials.

Renal impairment use normal dose every 8 hours if creatinine clearance less than 10 mL/minute/1.73m^2

Pregnancy not known to be harmful

Breast-feeding trace amounts in breast milk—not known to be harmful but be alert for hypersensitivity in infant

Contra-indications see under Benzylpenicillin (section 5.1.1.1)

Side-effects see under Benzylpenicillin (section 5.1.1.1); also gastro-intestinal disturbances; *very rarely* hepatitis and cholestatic jaundice reported (see also CSM advice above)

Indication and dose

Infections due to beta-lactamase-producing staphylococci including otitis externa; adjunct in pneumonia, impetigo, cellulitis
- By mouth

Neonate under 7 days 25 mg/kg twice daily

Neonate 7–21 days 25 mg/kg 3 times daily

Neonate 21–28 days 25 mg/kg 4 times daily

Child 1 month–2 years 62.5–125 mg 4 times daily

Child 2–10 years 125–250 mg 4 times daily

Child 10–18 years 250–500 mg 4 times daily

- By intramuscular injection

Child 1 month–18 years 12.5–25 mg/kg every 6 hours (max. 500 mg every 6 hours)

- By slow intravenous injection or by intravenous infusion

Neonate under 7 days 25 mg/kg every 12 hours; may be doubled in severe infection

Neonate 7–21 days 25 mg/kg every 8 hours; may be doubled in severe infection

Neonate 21–28 days 25 mg/kg every 6 hours; may be doubled in severe infection

Child 1 month–18 years 12.5–25 mg/kg every 6 hours (max. 1 g every 6 hours); may be doubled in severe infection

Osteomyelitis (Table 1, section 5.1), cerebral abscess, staphylococcal meningitis
- By slow intravenous injection or by intravenous infusion

Neonate under 7 days 50–100 mg/kg every 12 hours

Neonate 7–21 days 50–100 mg/kg every 8 hours

Neonate 21–28 days 50–100 mg/kg every 6 hours

Child 1 month–18 years 50 mg/kg (max. 2 g) every 6 hours

Endocarditis (Table 1, section 5.1)
- By slow intravenous injection or by intravenous infusion

Child 1 month–18 years 50 mg/kg (max. 2 g) every 6 hours

Prevention of Staphylococcal lung infection in cystic fibrosis

Table 2, section 5.1

Staphylococcal lung infection in cystic fibrosis
- By mouth

Child 1 month–18 years 12.5–25 mg/kg (max. 1 g) 4 times daily; total daily dose may alternatively be given in 3 divided doses

Administration for *intermittent intravenous infusion*, dilute reconstituted solution in Glucose 5% *or* Sodium Chloride 0.9% and give over 30–60 minutes; alternatively, may be given *via drip tubing* in Glucose 5% *or* Sodium Chloride 0.9% *or* Ringer's Solution *or* Compound Sodium Lactate

Flucloxacillin (Non-proprietary) PoM

Capsules, flucloxacillin (as sodium salt) 250 mg, net price 20 = £2.17; 500 mg, 20 = £3.78. Label: 9, 23
Brands include *Fluclomix®*, *Galfloxin®*, *Ladropen®*

Oral solution (= elixir or syrup), flucloxacillin (as sodium salt) for reconstitution with water, 125 mg/5 mL, net price 100 mL = £3.88; 250 mg/5 mL, 100 mL = £6.97. Label: 9, 23
Brands include *Ladropen®*

Injection, powder for reconstitution, flucloxacillin (as sodium salt). Net price 250-mg vial = 91p; 500-mg vial = £1.81; 1-g vial = £3.63

Floxapen® (GSK) PoM

Capsules, both black/caramel, flucloxacillin (as sodium salt) 250 mg, net price 28-cap pack = £6.31; 500 mg, 28-cap pack = £12.66. Label: 9, 23

Syrup, tutti-frutti- and menthol-flavoured, flucloxacillin (as magnesium salt) for reconstitution with water, 125 mg/5 mL, net price 100 mL = £3.25; 250 mg/5 mL, 100 mL = £6.48. Label: 9, 23
Excipients: include sucrose

Injection, powder for reconstitution, flucloxacillin (as sodium salt). Net price 250-mg vial = 91p; 500-mg vial = £1.81; 1-g vial = £3.63
Electrolytes Na^+ 0.57 mmol/250-mg vial, 1.13 mmol/500-mg vial, 2.26 mmol/1-g vial

5.1.1.3 Broad-spectrum penicillins

Ampicillin is active against certain Gram-positive and Gram-negative organisms but is inactivated by penicillinases including those produced by *Staphylococcus aureus* and by common Gram-negative bacilli such as *Escherichia coli*. Ampicillin is also active against *Listeria* spp. and enterococci.. Almost all staphylococci, 50% of *E. coli* strains and 15% of *Haemophilus influenzae* strains are now resistant. The likelihood of resistance should therefore be considered before using ampicillin for the 'blind' treatment of infections; in particular, it should not be used for hospital patients without checking sensitivity.

Ampicillin can be given by mouth, but less than half the dose is absorbed and absorption is further decreased by the presence of food in the gut. Ampicillin is well excreted in the bile and urine.

Amoxicillin (amoxycillin) is a derivative of ampicillin and has a similar antibacterial spectrum. It is better absorbed than ampicillin when given by mouth, producing higher plasma and tissue concentrations; unlike ampicillin, absorption is not affected by the presence of food in the stomach.

Amoxicillin or ampicillin are principally indicated for the treatment of community-acquired pneumonia and middle ear infections, both of which may be due to *Streptococcus pneumoniae* and *H. influenzae*, and for urinary-tract infections (section 5.1.13). They are also used in the treatment of endocarditis and listerial meningitis. Amoxicillin is used for endocarditis prophylaxis (Table 2, section 5.1); it may also be used for the treatment of Lyme disease [not licensed], see below.

Maculopapular rashes occur commonly with ampicillin (and amoxicillin) but are not usually related to true penicillin allergy. They often occur in children with glandular fever; broad-spectrum penicillins should not therefore be used for 'blind' treatment of a sore throat. Rashes are also common in children with acute or chronic lymphocytic leukaemia or in cytomegalovirus infection.

Co-amoxiclav consists of amoxicillin with the beta-lactamase inhibitor clavulanic acid. Clavulanic acid itself has no significant antibacterial activity but, by inactivating beta-lactamases, it makes the combination active against beta-lactamase-producing bacteria that are resistant to amoxicillin. These include resistant strains of *Staph. aureus*, *E. coli*, and *H. influenzae*, as well as many *Bacteroides* and *Klebsiella* spp. Co-amoxiclav should be reserved for infections likely, or known, to be caused by amoxicillin-resistant beta-lactamase-producing strains; for CSM warning on cholestatic jaundice see under Co-amoxiclav.

A combination of ampicillin with flucloxacillin (as co-fluampicil) is available to treat infections involving either streptococci or staphylococci (e.g. cellulitis).

Lyme disease Lyme disease should generally be treated by those experienced in its management. In children over 12 years of age **doxycycline** (p. 314) is the antibacterial of choice for *early Lyme disease*. **Amoxicillin** [unlicensed indication], **cefuroxime axetil**, or **azithromycin** [unlicensed indication] are alternatives if doxycycline is contra-indicated. Intravenous administration of **cefotaxime**, **ceftriaxone** (section 5.1.2), or **benzylpenicillin** (p. 294) is recommended for Lyme disease associated with moderate to severe *cardiac* or *neurological* abnormalities, *late Lyme disease*, and *Lyme arthritis*. The duration of treatment is generally 2–4 weeks; Lyme arthritis requires longer treatment with oral antibacterial drugs.

Oral infections Amoxicillin or ampicillin are as effective as phenoxymethylpenicillin (section 5.1.1.1) but they are better absorbed; however, they may encourage emergence of resistant organisms.

Like phenoxymethylpenicillin, amoxicillin and ampicillin are ineffective against bacteria that produce beta-lactamases. Amoxicillin is also used for prophylaxis of endocarditis (Table 2, section 5.1)

AMOXICILLIN
(Amoxycillin)

Cautions see under Ampicillin; maintain adequate hydration with high doses (particularly during parenteral therapy)

Renal impairment risk of crystalluria with high doses (particularly during parenteral therapy) in mild to moderate impairment; reduce dose in severe impairment; rashes more common and risk of crystalluria

Contra-indications see under Ampicillin

Side-effects see under Ampicillin

5 Infections

AMOXICILLIN (*continued*)

Indication and dose

Susceptible infections including urinary-tract infections, sinusitis; *Haemophilus influenzae* infections
- **By mouth**

Neonate under 7 days 30 mg/kg (max. 62.5 mg) twice daily; dose doubled in severe infection

Neonate 7–28 days 30 mg/kg (max. 62.5 mg) 3 times daily; dose doubled in severe infection

Child 1 month–1 year 62.5 mg 3 times daily; dose doubled in severe infection

Child 1–5 years 125 mg 3 times daily; dose doubled in severe infection

Child 5–12 years 250 mg 3 times daily; dose doubled in severe infection

Child 12–18 years 500 mg 3 times daily; dose doubled in severe infection

- **By intramuscular injection**

Child 1 month–18 years 30 mg/kg every 8 hours (max. 500mg every 8 hours)

- **By intravenous injection or infusion**

Neonate under 7 days 30 mg/kg every 12 hours; dose doubled in severe infection

Neonate 7–28 days 30 mg/kg every 8 hours; dose doubled in severe infection

Child 1 month–18 years 20–30 mg/kg (maximum 500 mg) every 8 hours; dose doubled in severe infection (max. 4 g daily)

Uncomplicated community-acquired pneumonia (Table 1, section 5.1), invasive salmonellosis
- **By mouth**

Child 1 month–1 year 125 mg 3 times daily

Child 1–5 years 250 mg 3 times daily

Child 5–18 years 500 mg 3 times daily

- **By slow intravenous injection or by intravenous infusion**

Neonate under 7 days 50 mg/kg every 12 hours

Neonate 7–28 days 50 mg/kg every 8 hours

Child 1 month–18 years 50 mg/kg (max.1 g) every 8 hours

Listerial meningitis (in combination with another antibacterial, Table 1, section 5.1), group B streptococcal infection, enterococcal endocarditis (in combination with another antibiotic)
- **By intravenous infusion**

Neonate under 7 days 50 mg/kg every 12 hours; dose may be doubled in meningitis

Neonate 7–28 days 50 mg/kg every 8 hours; dose may be doubled in meningitis

Child 1 month–18 years 50 mg/kg every 4–6 hours (max. 2 g every 4 hours)

Otitis media
- **By mouth**

Child 1 month–18 years 40 mg/kg daily in 3 divided doses (max. 3 g daily in 3 divided doses)

Cystic fibrosis (treatment of asymptomatic *H. influenzae* carriage or mild exacerbations)
- **By mouth**

Child 1 month–1 year 125 mg 3 times daily

Child 1–7 years 250 mg 3 times daily

Child 7–18 years 500 mg 3 times daily

Endocarditis prophylaxis Table 2, section 5.1

Helicobacter pylori eradication section 1.3

Administration Displacement value may be significant when reconstituting injection, consult local guidelines. Dilute intravenous injection to a concentration of 50 mg/mL (100 mg/mL for neonates). May be further diluted with Glucose 5% *or* Glucose 10% *or* Sodium chloride 0.9% *or* 0.45% for intravenous infusion. Give intravenous infusion over 30 minutes when using high doses.

Amoxicillin (Non-proprietary) PoM

Capsules, amoxicillin (as trihydrate) 250 mg, net price 21 = £1.29; 500 mg, 21 = £1.69. Label: 9
Brands include *Amix®*, *Amoram®*, *Amoxident®*, *Galenamox®*, *Rimoxallin®*

Oral suspension, amoxicillin (as trihydrate) for reconstitution with water, 125 mg/5 mL, net price 100 mL = £1.23; 250 mg/5 mL, 100 mL = £1.75. Label: 9
Note Sugar-free versions are available and can be ordered by specifying 'sugar-free' on the prescription
Brands include *Amix®*, *Amoram®*, *Galenamox®*, *Rimoxallin®*

Sachets, sugar-free, amoxicillin (as trihydrate) 3 g/sachet, net price 2-sachet pack = £5.12, 14-sachet pack = £31.94. Label: 9, 13

Injection, powder for reconstitution, amoxicillin (as sodium salt), net price 250-mg vial = 32p; 500-mg vial = 58p; 1-g vial = £1.16

Dental prescribing on NHS Amoxicillin Capsules and Oral Suspension may be prescribed. Amoxicillin Sachets may be prescribed as Amoxicillin Oral Powder

Amoxil® (GSK) PoM

Capsules, both maroon/gold, amoxicillin (as trihydrate), 250 mg, net price 21-cap pack = £3.59; 500 mg, 21-cap pack = £7.19. Label: 9

Syrup SF, both sugar-free, peach- strawberry- and lemon-flavoured, amoxicillin (as trihydrate) for reconstitution with water, 125 mg/5 mL, net price 100 mL = 59p; 250 mg/5 mL, 100 mL = 59p. Label: 9

Paediatric suspension, amoxicillin 125 mg (as trihydrate)/1.25 mL when reconstituted with water, net price 20 mL (peach- strawberry- and lemon-flavoured) = £3.38. Label: 9, counselling , use of pipette
Excipients: include sucrose 600 mg/1.25 mL

Sachets SF, powder, sugar-free, amoxicillin (as trihydrate) 3 g/sachet, 2-sachet pack (peach- strawberry- and lemon-flavoured) = £2.99. Label: 9, 13

AMOXICILLIN (*continued*)

Injection, powder for reconstitution, amoxicillin (as sodium salt), net price 500-mg vial = 58p; 1-g vial = £1.16
Electrolytes Na^+ 3.3 mmol/g

AMPICILLIN

Cautions history of allergy; erythematous rashes common in glandular fever, cytomegalovirus infection, and acute or chronic lymphocytic leukaemia (see notes above); **interactions:** Appendix 1 (penicillins)

Renal impairment if creatinine clearance less than 10 mL/minute/1.73m² reduce dose or frequency—rashes more common

Pregnancy not known to be harmful

Breast-feeding trace amounts in breast milk—not known to be harmful but be alert for hypersensitivity in infant

Contra-indications penicillin hypersensitivity

Side-effects nausea, vomiting, diarrhoea; rashes (discontinue treatment); rarely, antibiotic-associated colitis; see also under Benzylpenicillin (section 5.1.1.1)

Indication and dose

Susceptible infections including urinary-tract infections, otitis media, sinusitis, oral infections (Table 1, section 5.1), *Haemophilus influenzae* infections, invasive salmonellosis

- By mouth

Neonate under 7 days 30 mg/kg (max. 62.5 mg) twice daily; dose doubled in severe infection

Neonate 14–21 days 30 mg/kg (max. 62.5 mg) 3 times daily; dose doubled in severe infection

Neonate 21–28 days 30 mg/kg (max. 62.5 mg) 4 times daily; dose doubled in severe infection

Child 1 month–1 year 62.5 mg 4 times daily; dose doubled in severe infection

Child 1–5 years 125mg 4 times daily; dose doubled in severe infection

Child 5–12 years 250mg 4 times daily; dose doubled in severe infection

Child 12–18 years 500 mg 4 times daily; dose doubled in severe infection

- By intramuscular injection

Child 1 month–18 years 25 mg/kg (max. 500 mg) every 6 hours

- By intravenous injection or infusion

Neonate under 7 days 30 mg/kg every 12 hours; dose doubled in severe infection

Neonate 7–21 days 30 mg/kg every 8 hours; dose doubled in severe infection

Neonate 21–28 days 30 mg/kg every 6 hours; dose doubled in severe infection

Child 1 month–18 years 25 mg/kg (max. 1 g) every 6 hours; dose doubled in severe infection

Uncomplicated community-acquired pneumonia (Table 1, section 5.1), invasive salmonellosis

- By mouth

Child 1 month–1 year 125 mg 4 times daily

Child 1–5 years 250 mg 4 times daily

Child 5–18 years 500 mg 4 times daily

- By slow intravenous injection or by intravenous infusion

Neonate under 7 days 50 mg/kg every 12 hours

Neonate 7–21 days 50 mg/kg every 8 hours

Neonate 21–28 days 50 mg/kg every 6 hours

Child 1 month–18 years 50 mg/kg (max.1 g) every 6 hours

Listerial meningitis, group B streptococcal infection, enterococcal endocarditis (in combination with another antibacterial, see Table 1, section 5.1)

- By intravenous infusion

Neonate under 7 days 50 mg/kg every 12 hours; dose doubled in meningitis

Neonate 7–21 days 50 mg/kg every 8 hours; dose doubled in meningitis

Neonate 21–28 days 50 mg/kg every 6 hours; dose doubled in meningitis

Child 1 month–18 years 50 mg/kg every 4–6 hours (max. 2 g every 4 hours)

Administration *Oral*: administer at least 30 minutes before food

Injection: displacement value may be significant when reconstituting injection, consult local guidelines. Dilute intravenous injection to a concentration of 50–100 mg/mL. May be further diluted with glucose 5% or 10% or sodium chloride 0.9% or 0.45% for infusion. Give over 30 minutes when using doses of greater than 50 mg/kg to avoid CNS toxicity including convulsions.

Ampicillin (Non-proprietary) PoM

Capsules, ampicillin 250 mg, net price 20 = £2.30; 500 mg, 20 = £3.15. Label: 9, 23
Brands include *Rimacillin®*

Oral suspension, ampicillin 125 mg/5 mL when reconstituted with water, net price 100 mL = £2.63; 250 mg/5 mL, 100 mL = £4.56. Label: 9, 23
Brands include *Rimacillin®*

Injection, powder for reconstitution, ampicillin (as sodium salt), net price 500-mg vial = 68p

Dental prescribing on NHS Ampicillin Capsules and Oral Suspension may be prescribed

AMPICILLIN (*continued*)

Penbritin® (Chemidex) PoM
Capsules, both grey/red, ampicillin (as trihydrate) 250 mg, net price 28-cap pack = £2.10; 500 mg, 28-cap pack = £5.28. Label: 9, 23

With flucloxacillin

Co-fluampicil (Non-proprietary) PoM
Capsules, co-fluampicil 250/250 (flucloxacillin 250 mg as sodium salt, ampicillin 250 mg as trihydrate), net price 28-cap pack = £8.86. Label: 9, 22
Brands include *Flu-Amp®*

Magnapen® (CP) PoM
Capsules, black/turquoise, co-fluampicil 250/250 (flucloxacillin 250 mg as sodium salt, ampicillin 250 mg as trihydrate), net price 20-cap pack = £6.15. Label: 9, 22

Syrup, co-fluampicil 125/125 (flucloxacillin 125 mg as magnesium salt, ampicillin 125 mg as trihydrate)/5 mL when reconstituted with water, net price 100 mL = £4.99. Label: 9, 22
Excipients: include sucrose 3.14 g/5 mL

Injection 500 mg, powder for reconstitution, co-fluampicil 250/250 (flucloxacillin 250 mg as sodium salt, ampicillin 250 mg as sodium salt), net price per vial = £1.33
Electrolytes Na^+ 1.3 mmol/vial

CO-AMOXICLAV

A mixture of amoxicillin (as the trihydrate or as the sodium salt) and clavulanic acid (as potassium clavulanate); the proportions are expressed in the form *x*/*y* where *x* and *y* are the strengths in milligrams of amoxicillin and clavulanic acid respectively

Cautions see under Ampicillin and notes above; also caution in hepatic impairment (monitor hepatic function); maintain adequate hydration with high doses (particularly during parenteral therapy)

Cholestatic jaundice CSM has advised that cholestatic jaundice can occur either during or shortly after the use of co-amoxiclav. An epidemiological study has shown that the risk of acute liver toxicity was about 6 times greater with co-amoxiclav than with amoxicillin; these reactions have only rarely been reported in children. Jaundice is usually self-limiting and very rarely fatal. The duration of treatment should be appropriate to the indication and should not usually exceed 14 days

Hepatic impairment monitor liver function in liver disease. See also Cholestatic Jaundice above

Renal impairment *Oral*: use normal dose every 12 hours if creatinine clearance 10–30 mL/minute/1.73m². Use half normal dose every 12 hours if creatinine clearance less than 10 mL/minute/1.73m². *Augmentin-Duo®* not recommended if creatinine clearance less than 30 mL/minute/1.73m².

Intravenous: use normal initial dose and then use half dose every 12 hours if creatinine clearance 10–30 mL/minute/1.73m²; use normal initial dose and then use half normal dose every 24 hours if creatinine clearance less than 10mL/minute/1.73m²

Pregnancy not known to be harmful

Breast-feeding trace amounts present in breast milk—not known to be harmful but be alert for hypersensitivity in the infant

Contra-indications penicillin hypersensitivity, history of co-amoxiclav-associated or penicillin-associated jaundice or hepatic dysfunction

Side-effects see under Ampicillin; hepatitis, cholestatic jaundice (see above); Stevens-Johnson syndrome, toxic epidermal necrolysis, exfoliative dermatitis, vasculitis reported; rarely prolongation of bleeding time, dizziness, headache, convulsions (particularly with high doses or in renal impairment); superficial staining of teeth with suspension, phlebitis at injection site

Indication and dose

Infections due to beta-lactamase-producing strains (where amoxicillin alone not appropriate) including respiratory-tract infections, genito-urinary and abdominal infections, cellulitis, animal bites

- **By mouth, expressed as co-amoxiclav (see also under *Augmentin-Duo®* preparation below)**

Neonate 0.25 mL/kg of *125/31* suspension 3 times daily

Child 1 month–1 year 0.25 mL/kg of *125/31* suspension 3 times daily; dose doubled in severe infection

Child 1–6 years 5 mL of *125/31* suspension 3 times daily *or* 0.25 mL/kg of *125/31* suspension 3 times daily; dose doubled in severe infection

Child 6–12 years 5 mL of *250/62* suspension 3 times daily *or* 0.15 mL/kg of *250/62* suspension 3 times daily; dose doubled in severe infection

Child 12–18 years one *250/125* strength tablet 3 times daily; increased in severe infections to one *500/125* strength tablet, 3 times daily

- **By intravenous injection over 3–4 minutes or by intravenous infusion, expressed as co-amoxiclav**

Preterm neonate and neonate under 7 days 30 mg/kg every 12 hours

Neonate 7–28 days 30 mg/kg every 8 hours

Child 1–3 months 30 mg/kg every 8 hours

Child 3 months–12 years 30 mg/kg every 8 hours increased in more serious infections to 30 mg/kg every 6 hours

Child 12–18 years 1.2 g every 8 hours increased in more serious infections to 1.2 g every 6 hours

Severe dental infections (but not generally first-line, see notes above), expressed as co-amoxiclav

- **By mouth**

Child 12–18 years one *250/125* strength tablet every 8 hours for 5 days

Administration for *intermittent intravenous infusion* dilute reconstituted solution to a concentration of 10mg/mL with Sodium Chloride 0.9% or Water for Injections; give over 30–40 minutes and

CO-AMOXICLAV (*continued*)

complete infusion within 4 hours of reconstitution.

Co-amoxiclav (Non-proprietary) PoM

Tablets, co-amoxiclav 250/125 (amoxicillin 250 mg as trihydrate, clavulanic acid 125 mg as potassium salt), net price 21-tab pack = £4.47. Label: 9

Tablets, co-amoxiclav 500/125 (amoxicillin 500 mg as trihydrate, clavulanic acid 125 mg as potassium salt), net price 21-tab pack = £11.30. Label: 9

Oral suspension, co-amoxiclav 125/31 (amoxicillin 125 mg as trihydrate, clavulanic acid 31.25 mg as potassium salt)/5 mL when reconstituted with water, net price 100 mL = £4.18. Label: 9

Oral suspension, co-amoxiclav 250/62 (amoxicillin 250 mg as trihydrate, clavulanic acid 62.5 mg as potassium salt)/5 mL when reconstituted with water, net price 100 mL = £5.48. Label: 9

Injection 500/100, powder for reconstitution, co-amoxiclav 500/100 (amoxicillin 500 mg as sodium salt, clavulanic acid 100 mg as potassium salt), net price per vial = £1.49

Injection 1000/200, powder for reconstitution, co-amoxiclav 1000/200 (amoxicillin 1 g as sodium salt, clavulanic acid 200 mg as potassium salt), net price per vial = £2.97

Augmentin® (GSK) PoM

Tablets 375 mg, f/c, co-amoxiclav 250/125 (amoxicillin 250 mg as trihydrate, clavulanic acid 125 mg as potassium salt), net price 21-tab pack = £4.45. Label: 9

Tablets 625 mg, f/c, co-amoxiclav 500/125 (amoxicillin 500 mg as trihydrate, clavulanic acid 125 mg as potassium salt). Net price 21-tab pack = £8.49. Label: 9

Dispersible tablets, sugar-free, co-amoxiclav 250/125 (amoxicillin 250 mg as trihydrate, clavulanic acid 125 mg as potassium salt). Net price 21-tab pack = £10.22. Label: 9, 13

Suspension '125/31 SF', sugar-free, co-amoxiclav 125/31 (amoxicillin 125 mg as trihydrate, clavulanic acid 31 mg as potassium salt)/5 mL when reconstituted with water. Net price 100 mL (raspberry- and orange-flavoured) = £4.25. Label: 9
Excipients: include aspartame 12.5 mg/5 mL (section 9.4.1)

Suspension '250/62 SF', sugar-free, co-amoxiclav 250/62 (amoxicillin 250 mg as trihydrate, clavulanic acid 62 mg as potassium salt)/5 mL when reconstituted with water. Net price 100 mL (raspberry- and orange-flavoured) = £5.97. Label: 9
Excipients: include aspartame 12.5 mg/5 mL (section 9.4.1)

Injection 600 mg, powder for reconstitution, co-amoxiclav 500/100 (amoxicillin 500 mg as sodium salt, clavulanic acid 100 mg as potassium salt). Net price per vial = £1.38
Electrolytes Na^+ 1.35 mmol, K^+ 0.5 mmol/600-mg vial

Injection 1.2 g, powder for reconstitution, co-amoxiclav 1000/200 (amoxicillin 1 g as sodium salt, clavulanic acid 200 mg as potassium salt). Net price per vial = £2.76
Electrolytes Na^+ 2.7 mmol, K^+ 1 mmol/1.2-g vial

Augmentin-Duo® (GSK) PoM

Suspension '400/57', sugar-free, strawberry-flavoured, co-amoxiclav 400/57 (amoxicillin 400 mg as trihydrate, clavulanic acid 57 mg as potassium salt)/5 mL when reconstituted with water. Net price 35 mL = £4.38, 70 mL = £6.15. Label: 9
Excipients: include aspartame 12.5 mg/5 mL (section 9.4.1)

Dose

Child 2 months–2 years 0.15 mL/kg twice daily, doubled in severe infection

Child 2–6 years (13–21 kg) 2.5 mL twice daily, doubled in severe infection

Child 7–12 years (22–40 kg) 5 mL twice daily, doubled in severe infections

5.1.1.4 Antipseudomonal penicillins

The carboxypenicillin, **ticarcillin**, is principally indicated for serious infections caused by *Pseudomonas aeruginosa* although it also has activity against certain other Gram-negative bacilli including *Proteus* spp. and *Bacteroides fragilis.*

Ticarcillin is now available only in combination with clavulanic acid (section 5.1.1.3); the combination (*Timentin®*) is active against beta-lactamase-producing bacteria resistant to ticarcillin.

Tazocin® contains the ureidopenicillin **piperacillin** with the beta-lactamase inhibitor tazobactam. Piperacillin is more active than ticarcillin against *Ps. aeruginosa*. The spectrum of activity of *Tazocin®* and *Timentin®* is comparable to that of the carbapenems, imipenem and meropenem (section 5.1.2).

These antipseudomonal penicillins may be used for the empirical treatment of septicaemia in immunocompromised children but otherwise should generally be reserved for serious infections resistant to other antibacterials. For pseudomonas septicaemias (especially in neutropenia or endocarditis) these antipseudomonal penicillins should be given with an aminoglycoside (e.g. gentamicin or netilmicin, section 5.1.4) since they have a synergistic effect. Penicillins and aminoglycosides must not, however, be mixed in the same syringe or infusion.

Tazocin® is used in cystic fibrosis for the treatment of *Ps. aeruginosa* colonisation when ciprofloxacin and nebulised colistin have been ineffective, or in infective exacerbations, when it is combined with an aminoglycoside.

Owing to the sodium content of many of these antibiotics, high doses may lead to hypernatraemia.

PIPERACILLIN

Cautions see under Benzylpenicillin (section 5.1.1.1)

Contra-indications see under Benzylpenicillin (section 5.1.1.1)

Renal impairment reduce dose if creatinine clearance less than 40 mL/minute/1.73m^2 (child under 12 years) or if creatinine clearance less than 20 mL/minute/1.73m^2 (child 12–18 years); consult product literature

Pregnancy manufacturer advises use only if potential benefit outweighs risk

Breast-feeding present in milk—manufacturer advises use only if potential benefit outweighs risk

Side-effects see under Benzylpenicillin (section 5.1.1.1); also nausea, vomiting, diarrhoea; *less commonly* stomatitis, dyspepsia, constipation, jaundice, hypotension, headache, insomnia, and injection-site reactions; *rarely* abdominal pain, hepatitis, oedema, fatigue and eosinophilia; *very rarely* hypoglycaemia, hypokalaemia, pancytopenia, Stevens-Johnson syndrome, and toxic epidermal necrolysis

Licensed use *Tazocin®* not licensed for use in children under 12 years (except for children with neutropenia and complicated appendicitis)

Indication and dose

See preparations

With tazobactam

Tazocin® (Lederle) PoM

Injection 2.25 g, powder for reconstitution, piperacillin 2 g (as sodium salt), tazobactam 250 mg (as sodium salt). Net price per vial = £7.96

Electrolytes Na^+ 4.69 mmol/2.25-g vial

Injection 4.5 g, powder for reconstitution, piperacillin 4 g (as sodium salt), tazobactam 500 mg (as sodium salt). Net price per vial = £15.79

Electrolytes Na^+ 9.37 mmol/4.5-g vial

Dose

(Expressed as a combination of piperacillin and tazobactam combined)

Lower respiratory tract, urinary tract, intra-abdominal and skin infections, and bacterial septicaemia
- **By intravenous injection over 3–5 minutes or by intravenous infusion**

Neonate 90 mg/kg every 8 hours

Child 1 month–12 years 90 mg/kg every 6–8 hours; (max 4.5 g every 6 hours)

Child 12–18 years 2.25–4.5 g every 6–8 hours, usually 4.5 g every 8 hours

Infections in children with neutropenia in combination with an aminoglycoside
- **By intravenous injection over 3–5 minutes or by intravenous infusion**

Child 1 month–18 years 90 mg/kg every 6 hours; (max 4.5 g every 6 hours)

Complicated appendicitis
- **By intravenous injection over 3–5 minutes or by intravenous infusion**

Child 2–12 years 112.5 mg/kg every 8 hours (max 4.5 g every 8 hours) for 5–14 days

Administration for *intermittent infusion,* dilute reconstituted solution further to at least 90 mg/mL with Glucose 5%, Sodium Chloride 0.9% or Water for Injections; give over 20–30 minutes

TICARCILLIN

Cautions see under Benzylpenicillin (section 5.1.1.1)

Hepatic impairment cholestatic jaundice, see under Co-amoxiclav

Renal impairment reduce dose in mild renal impairment

Pregnancy not known to be harmful

Breast-feeding trace amounts present in breast milk—not known to be harmful but be alert for hypersensitivity in the infant

Contra-indications see under Benzylpenicillin (section 5.1.1.1)

Side-effects see under Benzylpenicillin (section 5.1.1.1); also nausea, vomiting, coagulation disorders, haemorrhagic cystitis (more frequent in children), injection-site reactions, Stevens-Johnson syndrome, toxic epidermal necrolysis, hypokalaemia, eosinophilia

Indication and dose

See under preparation

With clavulanic acid

Note For a CSM warning on cholestatic jaundice possibly associated with clavulanic acid, see under Co-amoxiclav

Timentin® (GSK) PoM

Injection 3.2 g, powder for reconstitution, ticarcillin 3 g (as sodium salt), clavulanic acid 200 mg (as potassium salt). Net price per vial = £5.66

Electrolytes Na^+ 16 mmol, K^+ 1 mmol /3.2-g vial

Dose

(Expressed as a combination of ticarcillin and clavulanic acid)

Infections due to *Pseudomonas* and *Proteus* spp. see notes above
- **By intravenous infusion**

Neonate under 7 days 80 mg/kg every 12 hours

Neonate 7–28 days 80 mg/kg every 8 hours

Child 1 month–18 years 80 mg/kg (max 3.2 g) every 6–8 hours increased to every 4 hours in more severe infections

Administration Displacement value may be important, consult local guidelines. For intermittent infusion, dilute reconstituted solution further to a concentration of 16–32 mg/mL with glucose 5% *or* to a concentration of 32 mg/mL with water for injections; infuse over 30–40 minutes.

5.1.1.5 Mecillinams

Pivmecillinam has significant activity against many Gram-negative bacteria including *Escherichia coli*, klebsiella, enterobacter, and salmonellae. It is not active against *Pseudomonas aeruginosa* or enterococci. Pivmecillinam is hydrolysed to mecillinam, which is the active drug.

PIVMECILLINAM HYDROCHLORIDE

Cautions see under Benzylpenicillin (section 5.1.1.1); also liver and renal function tests required in long-term use; avoid in porphyria (section 9.8.2); **interactions:** Appendix 1 (penicillins)

Renal impairment reduce dose

Pregnancy not known to be harmful

Contra-indications see under Benzylpenicillin (section 5.1.1.1); also carnitine deficiency, oesophageal strictures, gastro-intestinal obstruction, infants under 3 months

Side-effects see under Benzylpenicillin (section 5.1.1.1); nausea, vomiting, dyspepsia; also reduced serum and total body carnitine (especially with long-term or repeated use)

Licensed use not licensed for use in children under 3 months

Indication and dose

Acute uncomplicated cystitis
- By mouth

Child body-weight over 40 kg initially 400 mg then 200 mg every 8 hours for 3 days

Chronic or recurrent bacteriuria

Child body-weight over 40 kg 400 mg every 6–8 hours

Urinary-tract infections

Child body-weight under 40 kg 5–10 mg/kg every 6 hours; total daily dose may alternatively be given in 3 divided doses

Salmonellosis not recommended therefore no dose stated

Counselling Tablets should be swallowed whole with plenty of fluid during meals while sitting or standing

Selexid® (Leo) PoM
Tablets, f/c, pivmecillinam hydrochloride 200 mg, net price 10-tab pack = £4.50. Label 9, 21, 27, counselling, posture (see Dose above)

5.1.2 Cephalosporins and other beta-lactams

Antibiotics in this section include the **cephalosporins**, such as cefotaxime, ceftazidime, cefuroxime, cefalexin and cefradine, the **monobactam**, aztreonam, and the **carbapenems**, imipenem (a thienamycin derivative) and meropenem.

Cephalosporins

The cephalosporins are broad-spectrum antibacterials which are used for the treatment of septicaemia, pneumonia, meningitis, biliary-tract infections, peritonitis, and urinary-tract infections. The pharmacology of the cephalosporins is similar to that of the penicillins, excretion being principally renal. Cephalosporins penetrate the cerebrospinal fluid poorly unless the meninges are inflamed; cefotaxime and ceftriaxone are suitable cephalosporins for infections of the CNS (e.g meningitis).

The principal side-effect of the cephalosporins is hypersensitivity and about 10% of penicillin-sensitive patients will also be allergic to the cephalosporins.

Cefradine (cephradine) has generally been replaced by the newer cephalosporins.

Cefuroxime is a 'second generation' cephalosporin that is less susceptible than the earlier cephalosporins to inactivation by beta-lactamases. It is, therefore, active against certain bacteria that are resistant to the other drugs and has greater activity against *Haemophilus influenzae* and *Neisseria gonorrhoeae*.

Cefotaxime, **ceftazidime** and **ceftriaxone** are 'third generation' cephalosporins with greater activity than the 'second generation' cephalosporins against certain Gram-negative bacteria. However, they are less active than cefuroxime against Gram-positive bacteria, most notably *Staphylococcus aureus*. Their broad antibacterial spectrum may encourage superinfection with resistant bacteria or fungi.

Ceftazidime has good activity against pseudomonas. It is also active against other Gram-negative bacteria.

Ceftriaxone has a longer half-life and therefore needs to be given only once daily. Indications include serious infections such as septicaemia, pneumonia, and meningitis. The calcium salt of ceftriaxone forms a precipitate in the gall bladder which may rarely cause symptoms but these usually resolve when the antibacterial is stopped. In neonates, ceftriaxone may displace bilirubin from plasma-albumin and should be avoided in neonates with unconjugated hyperbilirubinaemia, hypoalbuminaemia, acidosis or impaired bilirubin binding.

Orally active cephalosporins The orally active 'first generation' cephalosporins, **cefalexin** (cephalexin), **cefradine**, and **cefadroxil** and the 'second generation' cephalosporins, **cefaclor** and **cefprozil**, have a similar antimicrobial spectrum. They are useful for urinary-tract infections which do not respond to other drugs or which occur in pregnancy, respiratory-tract infections, otitis media, sinusitis, and skin and soft-tissue infections. Cefaclor has good activity against *H. influenzae*, but it is associated with protracted skin reactions especially in children. Cefadroxil has a long duration of action and can be given twice daily; it has poor activity against *H. influenzae*. **Cefuroxime axetil**, an ester of the 'second generation' cephalosporin cefuroxime, has the same antibacterial spectrum as the parent compound; it is poorly absorbed and needs to be given with food to maximise absorption.

Cefixime has a longer duration of action than the other cephalosporins that are active by mouth. It is presently only licensed for acute infections.

Cefpodoxime proxetil is more active than the other oral cephalosporins against respiratory bacterial pathogens and it is licensed for upper and lower respiratory-tract infections.

For treatment of Lyme disease, see section 5.1.1.3.

Oral infections The cephalosporins offer little advantage over the penicillins in dental infections, often being less active against anaerobes. Infections due to oral streptococci (often termed viridans streptococci) which become resistant to penicillin are usually also resistant to cephalosporins. This is of importance in the case of children who have had rheumatic fever and are on long-term penicillin therapy. Cefalexin and cefradine have been used in the treatment of oral infections.

CEFACLOR

Cautions sensitivity to beta-lactam antibacterials (avoid if history of immediate hypersensitivity reaction); false positive urinary glucose (if tested for reducing substances) and false positive Coombs' test; **interactions:** Appendix 1 (cephalosporins)

Renal impairment no dosage adjustment required, manufacturer advises caution

Pregnancy not known to be harmful

Breast-feeding present in milk in low concentration, considered compatible with breast-feeding

Contra-indications cephalosporin hypersensitivity; porphyria (section 9.8.2)

Side-effects diarrhoea and rarely antibiotic-associated colitis (CSM has warned both more likely with higher doses), nausea and vomiting, abdominal discomfort, headache; allergic reactions including rashes, pruritus, urticaria, serum sickness-like reactions with rashes, fever and arthralgia, and anaphylaxis; Stevens-Johnson syndrome, toxic epidermal necrolysis reported; disturbances in liver enzymes, transient hepatitis and cholestatic jaundice; other side-effects reported include eosinophilia and blood disorders (including thrombocytopenia, leucopenia, agranulocytosis, aplastic anaemia and haemolytic anaemia); reversible interstitial nephritis, hyperactivity, nervousness, sleep disturbances, hallucinations, confusion, hypertonia, and dizziness

Indication and dose

Infections due to sensitive Gram-positive and Gram-negative bacteria but see notes above

- **By mouth**

Child 1 month–12 years 20 mg/kg daily in 3 divided doses, doubled for severe infection (usual max. 1 g daily)

or

Child 1 month–1 year 62.5 mg 3 times daily; dose doubled for severe infections

Child 1–5 years 125 mg 3 times daily; dose doubled for severe infections

Child 5–12 years 250 mg 3 times daily; dose doubled for severe infections

Child 12–18 years 250 mg 3 times daily; dose doubled for severe infections (max. 4 g daily)

Asymptomatic carriage of *Haemophilus influenzae* or mild exacerbations in cystic fibrosis

- **By mouth**

Child 1 month–1 year 125 mg every 8 hours

Child 1–7 years 250 mg 3 times daily

Child 7–18 years 500 mg 3 times daily

CEFACLOR (*continued*)

Cefaclor (Non-proprietary) PoM

Capsules, cefaclor (as monohydrate) 250 mg, net price 21-cap pack = £5.69; 500 mg 50-cap pack = £26.27. Label: 9

Brands include *Keftid®*

Suspension, cefaclor (as monohydrate) for reconstitution with water, 125 mg/5 mL, net price 100 mL = £4.23; 250 mg/5 mL, 100 mL = £7.38. Label: 9

Note Sugar-free versions are available and can be ordered by specifying 'sugar-free' on the prescription

Brands include *Keftid®*

Distaclor® (Flynn) PoM

Capsules, cefaclor (as monohydrate) 500 mg (violet/grey), net price 20 = £17.33. Label: 9

Suspension, both pink, cefaclor (as monohydrate) for reconstitution with water, 125 mg/5 mL, net price 100 mL = £4.13; 250 mg/5 mL, 100 mL = £8.26. Label: 9

Distaclor MR® (Flynn) PoM

Tablets, m/r, both blue, cefaclor (as monohydrate) 375 mg. Net price 14-tab pack = £6.93. Label: 9, 21, 25

Dose

Susceptible infections

Child 12–18 years 375 mg every 12 hours with food, dose doubled for pneumonia

Lower urinary-tract infections

Child 12–18 years 375 mg every 12 hours with food

CEFADROXIL

Cautions see under Cefaclor

Renal impairment reduce dose in moderate impairment

Pregnancy not known to be harmful

Breast-feeding present in milk in low concentrations

Contra-indications see under Cefaclor

Side-effects see under Cefaclor

Indication and dose

Infections due to sensitive Gram-positive and Gram-negative bacteria but see notes above

- By mouth

Child 1 month–1 year 12.5 mg/kg twice daily

Child 1–6 years 250 mg twice daily

Child 6–18 years

Body-weight under 40 kg 500 mg twice daily;

Body-weight over 40 kg 0.5–1 g twice daily (1 g once daily for skin, soft tissue and uncomplicated urinary-tract infections)

Cefadroxil (Non-proprietary) PoM

Capsules, cefadroxil (as monohydrate) 500 mg, net price 20-cap pack = £5.64. Label: 9

Baxan® (Bristol-Myers Squibb) PoM

Capsules, cefadroxil (as monohydrate) 500 mg, net price 20-cap pack = £5.64. Label: 9

Suspension, cefadroxil (as monohydrate) for reconstitution with water, 125 mg/5 mL, net price 60 mL = £1.75; 250 mg/5 mL, 60 mL = £3.48; 500 mg/5 mL, 60 mL = £5.21. Label: 9

CEFALEXIN
(Cephalexin)

Cautions see under Cefaclor

Renal impairment dose reduction recommended in severe renal impairment

Pregnancy not known to be harmful

Breast-feeding present in milk in low concentrations, considered compatible with breast feeding

Contra-indications see under Cefaclor

Side-effects see under Cefaclor

Indication and dose

Infections due to sensitive Gram-positive and Gram-negative bacteria but see notes above

- By mouth

Neonate under 7 days 25 mg/kg (max. 125 mg) twice daily

Neonate 7–21 days 25 mg/kg (max. 125 mg) 3 times daily

Neonate 21–28 days 25 mg/kg (max. 125 mg) 4 times daily

Child 1 month–12 years 12.5 mg/kg twice daily; dose doubled in severe infection; max. 25 mg/kg 4 times daily (max. 1 g 4 times daily) *or*

Child 1 month–1 year 125 mg twice daily

Child 1–5 years 125 mg 3 times daily

Child 5–12 years 250 mg 3 times daily

Child 12–18 years 500 mg 2–3 times daily, increased to 1–1.5 g 3–4 times daily for severe infection

Prophylaxis of recurrent urinary-tract infection

- By mouth

Child 1 month–18 years 12.5mg/kg at night (max. 125mg at night)

Cefalexin (Non-proprietary) PoM

Capsules, cefalexin 250 mg, net price 28-cap pack = £2.68; 500 mg, 21-cap pack = £3.29. Label: 9

Tablets, cefalexin 250 mg, net price 28-tab pack = £2.20; 500 mg, 21-tab pack = £3.88. Label: 9

Oral suspension, cefalexin for reconstitution with water, 125 mg/5 mL, net price 100 mL = £1.891; 250 mg/5 mL, 100 mL = £2.74. Label: 9

Dental prescribing on NHS Cefalexin Capsules, Tablets, and Oral Suspension may be prescribed

CEFALEXIN (*continued*)

Ceporex® (Galen) PoM
Capsules, both caramel/grey, cefalexin 250 mg, net price 28-cap pack = £4.02; 500 mg, 28-cap pack = £7.85. Label: 9

Tablets, all pink, f/c, cefalexin 250 mg, net price 28-tab pack = £4.02; 500 mg, 28-tab pack = £7.85. Label: 9

Syrup, all orange, cefalexin for reconstitution with water, 125 mg/5 mL, net price 100 mL = £1.43; 250 mg/5 mL, 100 mL = £2.87; 500 mg/5 mL, 100 mL = £5.57. Label: 9

Keflex® (Flynn) PoM
Capsules, cefalexin 250 mg (green/white), net price 28-cap pack = £1.76; 500 mg (pale green/dark green), 21-cap pack = £2.66. Label: 9

Tablets, both peach, cefalexin 250 mg, net price 28-tab pack = £2.09; 500 mg (scored), 21-tab pack = £2.47. Label: 9

Suspension, cefalexin for reconstitution with water, 125 mg/5 mL, net price 100 mL = 88p; 250 mg/5 mL, 100 mL = £1.51. Label: 9

CEFIXIME

Cautions see under Cefaclor

Renal impairment reduce dose in moderate to severe impairment

Pregnancy not known to be harmful

Breast-feeding manufacturer advises avoid—no information available

Contra-indications see under Cefaclor

Side-effects see under Cefaclor

Indication and dose

Acute infections due to sensitive Gram-positive and Gram-negative bacteria, but see notes above
- **By mouth**
  Child 6 months–1 year 75 mg daily
  Child 1–5 years 100 mg daily
  Child 5–10 years 200 mg daily
  Child 10–18 years 200–400 mg daily *or* 100–200 mg twice daily

Gonorrhoea [unlicensed indication, see also Table 1, section 5.1]
- **By mouth**
  Child 12–18 years 400 mg as a single dose

Suprax® (Rhône-Poulenc Rorer) PoM
Tablets, f/c, scored, cefixime 200 mg. Net price 7-tab pack = £13.23. Label: 9

Paediatric oral suspension, cefixime 100 mg/5 mL when reconstituted with water, net price 50 mL (with double-ended spoon for measuring 3.75 mL or 5 mL since dilution not recommended) = £10.53, 100 mL = £18.91. Label: 9

CEFOTAXIME

Cautions see under Cefaclor

Renal impairment usual initial dose, then use half normal dose if creatinine clearance less than 5 mL/minute/1.73m^2

Pregnancy not known to be harmful

Breast-feeding present in milk in low concentration, considered compatible with breast-feeding

Contra-indications see under Cefaclor

Side-effects see under Cefaclor; rarely arrhythmias following rapid injection reported

Indication and dose

Infections due to sensitive Gram-positive and Gram-negative bacteria, surgical prophylaxis, Haemophilus epiglottitis and meningitis (Table 1, section 5.1) see also notes above
- **By intramuscular or by intravenous injection or intravenous infusion**
  Neonate under 7 days 25 mg/kg every 12 hours; dose doubled in severe infection and meningitis
  Neonate 7–21 days 25 mg/kg every 8 hours; dose doubled in severe infection and meningitis
  Neonate 21–28 days 25 mg/kg every 6–8 hours; dose doubled in severe infection and meningitis
  Child 1 month–18 years 50 mg/kg every 8–12 hours; increase to every 6 hours in very severe infections and meningitis (max. 12 g daily)

Important. If bacterial meningitis and especially if meningococcal disease is suspected the patient should be transferred urgently to hospital. If benzylpenicillin cannot be given (e.g. because of an allergy), a single dose of cefotaxime may be given (if available) before urgent transfer to hospital. Suitable doses of cefotaxime by intravenous injection (or by intramuscular injection) are **Child under 12 years** 50 mg/kg; **Child over 12 years** 1 g; chloramphenicol (section 5.1.7) may be used if there is a history of anaphylaxis to penicillins or cephalosporins

Gonorrhoea
- **By intramuscular or by intravenous injection or intravenous infusion**
  Child 12–18 years 500 mg as a single dose

Severe exacerbations of *Heamophilus influenzae* infection in cystic fibrosis
- **By intravenous injection or intravenous infusion**
  Child 1 month–18 years 50 mg/kg every 6–8 hours (max. 12 g daily)

Administration Displacement value may be significant, consult local guidelines. For intermittent intravenous infusion dilute in glucose 5% *or* sodium chloride 0.9% *or* compound sodium

CEFOTAXIME (*continued*)

lactate *or* water for injections; administer over 20–60 minutes

Cefotaxime (Non-proprietary) PoM

Injection, powder for reconstitution, cefotaxime (as sodium salt), net price 500-mg vial = £2.14; 1-g vial = £4.31; 2-g vial = £8.57

Claforan® (Aventis Pharma) PoM

Injection, powder for reconstitution, cefotaxime (as sodium salt), net price 500-mg vial = £2.14; 1-g vial (with or without infusion connector) = £4.31; 2-g vial (with or without infusion connector) = £8.57

Electrolytes Na^+ 2.09 mmol/g

CEFPODOXIME

Cautions see under Cefaclor

Renal impairment increase dose interval to every 24 hours if creatinine clearance 10–40 mL/minute/1.73m^2. Increase dose interval to every 48 hours if creatinine clearance less than10 mL/minute/1.73m^2

Pregnancy not known to be harmful

Breast-feeding present in milk in low concentration

Contra-indications see under Cefaclor

Side-effects see under Cefaclor

Indication and dose

Upper respiratory-tract infections (but in pharyngitis and tonsillitis reserved for infections which are recurrent, chronic, or resistant to other antibacterials), lower respiratory-tract infections (including bronchitis and pneumonia), skin and soft tissue infections, uncomplicated urinary-tract infections

- By mouth

Child 15 days–6 months 4 mg/kg twice daily

Child 6 months–2 years 40 mg twice daily

Child 3–8 years 80 mg twice daily

Child 9–12 years 100 mg twice daily

Child 12–18 years 100 mg twice daily (increased to 200 mg twice daily in sinusitis, skin and soft tissue infections, uncomplicated upper urinary tract infections and if necessary in lower respiratory tract infections)

Uncomplicated gonorrhoea

- By mouth

Child 12–18 years 200 mg as a single dose

Orelox® (Hoechst Marion Roussel) PoM

Tablets, f/c, cefpodoxime 100 mg (as proxetil), net price 10-tab pack = £10.18. Label: 5, 9, 21

Oral suspension, cefpodoxime (as proxetil) for reconstitution with water, 40 mg/5 mL, net price 100 mL = £11.97. Label: 5, 9, 21

Excipients: include aspartame (section 9.4.1)

CEFPROZIL

Cautions see under Cefaclor

Renal impairment usual initial dose then use half normal dose if creatinine clearance less than 30 mL/minute/1.73m^2

Pregnancy not known to be harmful

Breast-feeding present in milk in low concentrations, considered compatible with breast feeding

Contra-indications see under Cefaclor

Side-effects see under Cefaclor

Indication and dose

Upper respiratory-tract infections and skin and soft tissue infections

- By mouth

Child 6 months–12 years 20 mg/kg (max. 500 mg) once daily usually for 10 days

Child 12–18 years 500 mg once daily usually for 10 days

Otitis media

- By mouth

Child 6 months–12 years 20 mg/kg (max. 500 mg) twice daily

Cefzil® (Bristol-Myers Squibb) PoM

Tablets, cefprozil, 250 mg (orange), net price 20-tab pack = £14.95; 500 mg, 10-tab pack = £14.95. Label: 9

Suspension, cefprozil, 250 mg/5 mL when reconstituted with water, net price 100 mL = £15.22. Label: 9

Excipients: include aspartame equivalent to phenylalanine 28 mg/5 mL (section 9.4.1)

CEFRADINE
(Cephradine)

Cautions see under Cefaclor

Renal impairment reduce dose in moderate to severe impairment

Pregnancy not known to be harmful

Breast-feeding present in milk in low concentrations

Contra-indications see under Cefaclor

Side-effects see under Cefaclor

Licensed use not licensed for use in children for prophylaxis in urinary-tract infections or for prevention of *Staphylococcus aureus* lung infection in cystic fibrosis

Indication and dose

Infections due to sensitive Gram-positive and Gram-negative bacteria but see notes above

- By mouth

Child 1 month–12 years 12.5–25 mg/kg twice daily (total daily dose may alternatively be given in 3–4 divided doses)

CEFRADINE (*continued*)

Child 12–18 years 0.5–1 g twice daily *or* 250–500 mg 4 times daily; up to 1 g 4 times daily in severe infections

- **By deep intramuscular injection or by intravenous injection over 3–5 minutes or by intravenous infusion**

  Child 1 month–12 years 12.5–25 mg/kg every 6 hours

  Child 12–18 years 0.5–1 g every 6 hours, increased to 2 g every 6 hours in severe infection

Surgical prophylaxis

- **By deep intramuscular injection or by intravenous injection over 3-5 minutes**

  Child 12–18 years 1–2 g at induction

Prevention of *Staphylococcus aureus* lung infection in cystic fibrosis

- **By mouth**

  Child 1 month–1 year 500 mg twice daily

  Child 1–7 years 1 g twice daily

  Child 7–18 years 2 g twice daily

Prophylaxis in urinary-tract infection

- **By mouth**

  Child 1 month–12 years 3 mg/kg at night.

Administration Displacement value may be significant when reconstituting injections, consult local guidelines. For continuous *or* intermittent intravenous infusion dilute reconstituted solution further in Glucose 5% *or* Glucose 10% or Sodium chloride 0.9% or Ringer's solution or Compound sodium lactate

Cefradine (Non-proprietary) PoM

Capsules, cefradine 250 mg, net price 20-cap pack = £4.26; 500 mg, 20-cap pack = £7.92. Label: 9

Brands include *Nicef*®

Dental prescribing on NHS Cefradine Capsules may be prescribed

Velosef® (Squibb) PoM

Capsules, cefradine 250 mg (orange/blue), net price 20-cap pack = £3.55; 500 mg (blue), 20-cap pack = £7.00. Label: 9

Syrup, cefradine 250 mg/5 mL when reconstituted with water. Net price 100 mL = £4.22. Label: 9

Dental prescribing on NHS *Velosef*® syrup may be prescribed as Cefradine Oral Solution

Injection, powder for reconstitution, cefradine. Net price 500-mg vial = 99p; 1-g vial = £1.95

CEFTAZIDIME

Cautions see under Cefaclor

Renal impairment reduce dose if creatinine clearance less than 50 mL/minute/1.73m^2

Pregnancy not known to be harmful

Breast-feeding present in milk in low concentration, considered compatible with breast-feeding

Contra-indications see under Cefaclor

Side-effects see under Cefaclor

Licensed use nebulised route unlicensed

Indication and dose

Infections due to sensitive Gram-positive and Gram-negative bacteria but see notes above

- **By intravenous injection or infusion**

  Neonate under 7 days 25 mg/kg every 24 hours; dose doubled in severe infection and meningitis

  Neonate 7–21 days 25 mg/kg every 12 hours; dose doubled in severe infection and meningitis

  Neonate 21–28 days 25 mg/kg every 8 hours; dose doubled in severe infection and meningitis

  Child 1 month–18 years 25 mg/kg every 8 hours; dose doubled in severe infection, febrile neutropenia and meningitis (max. 6g daily)

Pseudomonal lung infection in cystic fibrosis

- **By intravenous injection or infusion or by deep intramuscular injection**

  Child 1 month–18 years 50 mg/kg every 8 hours (max. 9 g daily)

Chronic *Burkholderia cepacia* infection in cystic fibrosis

- **By inhalation of nebulised solution**

  Child 1 month–18 years 1 g twice daily

Administration For parenteral administration, intravenous route recommended in children. Displacement value may be significant, consult local guidelines. For intermittent intravenous infusion dilute reconstituted solution further to a concentration of not more than 40 mg/mL in Glucose 5% or Glucose 10% or Sodium chloride 0.9% or Compound sodium lactate.

For nebulisation, dissolve dose in 3 mL of water for injection

Ceftazidime (Non-proprietary) PoM

Injection, powder for reconstitution, ceftazidime (as pentahydrate), with sodium carbonate, net price 1-g vial = £8.50; 2-g vial = £17.00

Fortum® (GSK) PoM

Injection, powder for reconstitution, ceftazidime (as pentahydrate), with sodium carbonate, net price 250-mg vial = £2.20, 500-mg vial = £4.40, 1-g vial = £8.79, 2-g vial (for injection and for infusion, both) = £17.59, 3-g vial (for injection or infusion) = £25.76; *Monovial*, 2 g vial (with transfer needle) = £17.59

Electrolytes Na^+ 2.3 mmol/g

Kefadim® (Flynn) PoM

Injection, powder for reconstitution, ceftazidime (as pentahydrate), with sodium carbonate, net price 1-g vial = £7.92; 2-g vial = £15.84

Electrolytes Na^+ 2.3 mmol/g

CEFTRIAXONE

Cautions see under Cefaclor; preterm neonates; may displace bilirubin from serum albumin, administer over 60 minutes in neonates (see also Contra-indications); treatment longer than 14 days, renal failure, dehydration, or concomitant parenteral nutrition—risk of ceftriaxone precipitation in gall bladder

Hepatic impairment if hepatic impairment is accompanied by severe renal impairment, reduce dose and monitor plasma concentration

Renal impairment max. 50 mg/kg daily (max.2 g daily) in severe renal impairment; also monitor plasma concentration if hepatic impairment accompanied by severe renal impairment

Pregnancy not known to be harmful

Breast-feeding present in milk in low concentration, considered compatible with breast-feeding

Contra-indications see under Cefaclor; neonates with jaundice, hypoalbuminaemia, acidosis or impaired bilirubin binding

Side-effects see under Cefaclor; calcium ceftriaxone precipitates in urine (particularly in very young, dehydrated or those who are immobilised) or in gall bladder—consider discontinuation if symptomatic; rarely prolongation of prothrombin time, pancreatitis

Indication and dose

Infections due to sensitive Gram-positive and Gram-negative bacteria

- **By intravenous infusion over 60 minutes**

Neonate 20–50 mg/kg once daily

- **By deep intramuscular injection, or by intravenous injection over 2–4 minutes, or by intravenous infusion**

Child 1 month–12 years

Body-weight under 50 kg 50 mg/kg once daily; up to 80 mg/kg daily in severe infections and meningitis; intramuscular doses over 1 g divided between more than one site; doses of 50 mg/kg and over by intravenous infusion only

Body-weight 50 kg and over dose as for child 12–18 years

Child 12–18 years 1 g daily; 2–4 g daily in severe infections and meningitis; intramuscular doses over 1 g divided between more than one site; single intravenous doses above 1 g by intravenous infusion only

Uncomplicated gonorrhoea

- **By deep intramuscular injection**

Child 12–18 years 250 mg as a single dose

Surgical prophylaxis

- **By deep intramuscular injection or by intravenous injection over at least 2–4 minutes, or (for colorectal surgery) by intravenous infusion**

Child 12–18 years 1 g at induction; colorectal surgery, 2 g at induction; intramuscular doses over 1 g divided between more than one site

Prophylaxis of meningococcal meningitis Table 2, section 5.1

Administration Displacement value may be significant, consult local guidelines. For *intravenous infusion*, dilute reconstituted solution with Glucose 5% or 10% *or* Sodium Chloride 0.9%; give over at least 30 minutes (60 minutes in neonates). Not to be given with infusion fluids containing calcium.

For *intramuscular injection* ceftriaxone may be mixed with 1% Lidocaine Hydrochloride Injection to reduce pain at intramuscular injection site; final concentration 250–350 mg/mL.

Ceftriaxone (Non-proprietary) PoM

Injection, powder for reconstitution, ceftriaxone (as sodium salt), net price 1-g vial = £10.17; 2-g vial = £20.36

Rocephin® (Roche) PoM

Injection, powder for reconstitution, ceftriaxone (as sodium salt), net price 250-mg vial = £2.55; 1-g vial = £10.17; 2-g vial = £20.36

Electrolytes Na^+ 3.6 mmol /g

CEFUROXIME

Cautions see under Cefaclor

Renal impairment reduce parenteral dose in moderate to severe renal impairment

Pregnancy not known to be harmful

Breast-feeding present in milk in low concentration

Contra-indications see under Cefaclor

Side-effects see under Cefaclor

Indication and dose

Infections due to sensitive Gram-positive and Gram-negative bacteria

- **By mouth (as cefuroxime axetil),**

Child 3 months–2 years 10 mg/kg (max. 125 mg) twice daily

Child 2–12 years 15 mg/kg (max. 250 mg) twice daily

Child 12–18 years 250 mg twice daily; dose doubled in severe lower respiratory-tract infections, or if pneumonia suspected; dose reduced to 125mg twice daily in lower urinary-tract infection

- **By intravenous injection or infusion or by intramuscular injection**

Neonate under 7 days 25 mg/kg every 12 hours; dose doubled in severe infection, intravenous route only

Neonate 7–21 days 25 mg/kg every 8 hours; dose doubled in severe infection, intravenous route only

CEFUROXIME (*continued*)

Neonate 21–28 days 25 mg/kg every 6 hours; dose doubled in severe infection, intravenous route only

Child 1 month–18 years 20 mg/kg (max. 750 mg) every 8 hours; increase to 50–60 mg/kg (max. 1.5 g) every 6–8 hours in severe infection and cystic fibrosis

Lyme disease
- By mouth

Child 12–18 years 500 mg twice daily for 20 days

Surgical prophylaxis
- By intravenous injection

Child 1 month–18 years 50 mg/kg (max. 1.5 g) at induction, up to 3 further doses of 30 mg/kg (max. 750 mg) may be given by *intramuscular or intravenous injection* every 8 hours for high-risk procedures

Administration Single doses over 750mg should be administered by the intravenous route only. Displacement value may be significant when reconstituting injection, consult local guidelines. For intermittent intravenous infusion, dilute reconstituted solution further in glucose 5% *or* sodium chloride 0.9% *or* compound sodium lactate; give over 30 minutes.

Zinacef® (GSK) PoM

Injection, powder for reconstitution, cefuroxime (as sodium salt). Net price 250-mg vial = 94p; 750-mg vial = £2.34; 1.5-g vial = £4.70

Electrolytes Na^+ 1.8 mmol/750-mg vial

Zinnat® (GSK) PoM

Tablets, both f/c, cefuroxime (as axetil) 125 mg, net price 14-tab pack = £4.84; 250 mg, 14-tab pack = £9.67. Label: 9, 21, 25

Suspension, cefuroxime (as axetil) 125 mg/5 mL when reconstituted with water, net price 70 mL (tutti-frutti-flavoured) = £5.52. Label: 9, 21

Excipients: include aspartame (section 9.4.1)

Other beta-lactam antibiotics

Aztreonam is a monocyclic beta-lactam ('monobactam') antibiotic with an antibacterial spectrum limited to Gram-negative aerobic bacteria including *Pseudomonas aeruginosa*, *Neisseria meningitidis*, and *Haemophilus influenzae*; it should not be used alone for 'blind' treatment since it is not active against Gram-positive organisms. Aztreonam is also effective against *Neisseria gonorrhoeae* (but not against concurrent chlamydial infection). Side-effects are similar to those of the other beta-lactams although aztreonam may be less likely to cause hypersensitivity in penicillin-sensitive patients.

Imipenem, a carbapenem, has a broad spectrum of activity which includes many aerobic and anaerobic Gram-positive and Gram-negative bacteria. Imipenem is partially inactivated in the kidney by enzymatic activity and is therefore administered in combination with **cilastatin**, a specific enzyme inhibitor, which blocks its renal metabolism. Side-effects are similar to those of other beta-lactam antibiotics; neurotoxicity has been observed at very high dosage or in renal failure.

Meropenem is similar to imipenem but is stable to the renal enzyme which inactivates imipenem and therefore can be given without cilastatin. Meropenem has less seizure-inducing potential and can be used to treat central nervous system infection.

Ertapenem has a broad spectrum of activity that covers Gram-positive and Gram-negative organisms and anaerobes. It is licensed for treating abdominal and gynaecological infections and for community-acquired pneumonia, but it is not active against penicillin-resistant pneumococci. Unlike imipenem and meropenem, ertapenem is not active against *Pseudomonas* or against *Acinetobacter* spp.

Carbapenems in paediatrics are generally restricted to serious hospital acquired infections unresponsive to standard therapy.

AZTREONAM

Cautions hypersensitivity to beta-lactam antibiotics; **interactions:** Appendix 1 (aztreonam)

Hepatic impairment experience limited, monitor liver function

Renal impairment usual initial dose, then half normal dose if creatinine clearance 10–30 ml/minute/1.73m^2, usual initial dose, then one-quarter normal dose if creatinine clearance less than 10 ml/minute/1.73m^2

Breast-feeding present in milk in low concentration, considered compatible with breast-feeding

Contra-indications aztreonam hypersensitivity

Pregnancy manufacturer advises avoid—crosses placenta and no further information available

AZTREONAM (*continued*)

Side-effects nausea, vomiting, diarrhoea, abdominal cramps; mouth ulcers, altered taste; jaundice and hepatitis; flushing; hypersensitivity reactions; blood disorders (including thrombocytopenia and neutropenia); rashes, injection-site reactions; *rarely* hypotension, seizures, asthenia, confusion, dizziness, headache, halitosis, and breast tenderness; *very rarely* antibiotic-associated colitis, gastro-intestinal bleeding, and toxic epidermal necrolysis

Licensed use not licensed for use in children under 7 days

Indication and dose

Gram-negative infections including *Pseudomonas aeruginosa, Haemophilus influenzae,* and *Neisseria meningitidis*
- **By intravenous injection over 3–5 minutes or by intravenous infusion**

Neonate under 7 days 30 mg/kg every 12 hours

Neonate 7–28 days 30 mg/kg every 6–8 hours

Child 1 month–2 years 30 mg/kg every 6–8 hours

Child 2–12 years 30 mg/kg every 6–8 hours increased to 50 mg/kg every 6–8 hours in severe infection and cystic fibrosis (max 2 g every 6 hours)

Child 12–18 years 1 g every 8 hours or 2 g every 12 hours; 2 g every 6–8 hours for severe infections (including systemic *Ps. aeruginosa* and lung infections in cystic fibrosis)

Administration Displacement value may be significant, consult local guidelines. For intermittent intravenous infusion, dilute reconstituted solution further in Glucose 5% *or* Sodium chloride 0.9% *or* Ringer's solution *or* Compound sodium lactate to a concentration of less than 20 mg/mL; to be given over 20–60 minutes

Azactam® (Squibb) PoM
Injection, powder for reconstitution, aztreonam. Net price 500-mg vial = £4.48; 1-g vial = £8.95; 2-g vial = £17.90

ERTAPENEM

Cautions **interactions:** Appendix 1 (ertapenem)

Renal impairment avoid if creatinine clearance less than 30 mL/minute/1.73 m^2

Pregnancy manufacturer advises avoid unless potential benefit outweighs risk

Contra-indications hypersensitivity to beta-lactam antibiotics

Breast-feeding present in milk—manufacturer advises avoid

Side-effects diarrhoea, nausea, vomiting, headache, injection-site reactions, rash, pruritus, raised platelet count; *less commonly* dry mouth, taste disturbances, dyspepsia, abdominal pain, anorexia, constipation, melaena, antibiotic-associated colitis, hypotension, chest pain, oedema, pharyngeal discomfort, dyspnoea, dizziness, sleep disturbances, confusion, asthenia, seizures, vaginitis, raised glucose, petechiae; *rarely* dysphagia, cholecystitis, liver disorder (including jaundice), arrhythmia, increase in blood pressure, syncope, nasal congestion, cough, wheezing, hypersensitivity reactions, anxiety, depression, agitation, tremor, pelvic peritonitis, renal impairment, muscle cramp, scleral disorder, blood disorders (including neutropenia, thrombocytopenia, haemorrhage), hypoglycaemia, electrolyte disturbances; *very rarely* hallucinations

Indication and dose

Abdominal infections, acute gynaecological infections, community-acquired pneumonia
- **By intravenous infusion**

Child 3 months–13 years 15 mg/kg every 12 hours (max. 1 g daily)

Child 13–18 years 1 g once daily

Administration reconstitute 1 g with 10 mL Water for Injections or Sodium Chloride 0.9%; for *intermittent intravenous infusion,* dilute requisite dose in Sodium Chloride 0.9% to a final concentration not exceeding 20 mg/mL; incompatible with glucose solutions

Invanz® (MSD) ▼ PoM
Intravenous infusion, powder for reconstitution, ertapenem (as sodium salt), net price 1-g vial = £31.65
Electrolytes Na^+ 6 mmol/1-g vial

IMIPENEM WITH CILASTATIN

Cautions CNS disorders (e.g. epilepsy); hypersensitivity to beta-lactam antibacterials (avoid if history of immediate hypersensitivity reaction); **interactions:** Appendix 1 (imipenem with cilastatin)

Renal impairment not licensed for use in children with renal impairment. Reduce dose in mild, moderate, and severe impairment

Pregnancy manufacturer advises avoid unless potential benefit outweighs risk (toxicity in *animal* studies)

Breast-feeding present in milk but unlikely to be absorbed (however, manufacturer advises avoid)

Side-effects nausea, vomiting, diarrhoea (antibiotic-associated colitis reported), taste disturbances, tooth or tongue discoloration, hearing loss; blood disorders, positive Coombs' test; allergic reactions (with rash, pruritus, urticaria, Stevens-Johnson syndrome, fever, anaphylactic reactions, rarely toxic epidermal necrolysis, exfoliative dermatitis); myoclonic activity, convulsions, confusion and mental disturbances reported; slight increases in liver enzymes and bilirubin reported, rarely hepatitis; increases in serum creatinine and blood urea; red coloration of urine in children reported; local reactions:

5 Infections

IMIPENEM WITH CILASTATIN (*continued*)

erythema, pain and induration, and thrombophlebitis

Licensed use not licensed for use in children under 3 months

Indication and dose

Aerobic and anaerobic Gram-positive and Gram-negative infections, hospital-acquired septicaemia Table 1, section 5.1; not indicated for CNS infections

- **By intravenous infusion**

expressed in terms of imipenem

Neonate under 7 days 20 mg/kg every 12 hours

Neonate 7–21 days 20 mg/kg every 8 hours

Neonate 21–28 days 20 mg/kg every 6 hours

Child 1–3 months 20 mg/kg every 6 hours

Child 3 months–18 years

Body-weight under 40 kg 15 mg/kg (max. 500 mg) every 6 hours

Body-weight over 40 kg 250–500 mg every 6 hours; less sensitive organisms up to 12.5 mg/kg (max. 1 g) every 6 hours; total daily dose may alternatively be given in 3 divided doses

Cystic fibrosis

- **By intravenous infusion**

Child 1 month–18 years

Body-weight under 40 kg 22.5 mg/kg every 6 hours

Body-weight over 40 kg 1 g every 6–8 hours

Administration for intermittent intravenous infusion dilute to a concentration of 5 mg (as imipenem)/mL in sodium chloride 0.9% *or* sodium chloride and glucose; give up to 500 mg over 20–30 minutes; give 1 g over 40–60 minutes

Primaxin® (MSD) PoM

Intravenous infusion, powder for reconstitution, imipenem (as monohydrate) 500 mg with cilastatin (as sodium salt) 500 mg, net price per vial = £12.00; *Monovial* (vial with transfer needle) = £12.00

Electrolytes Na^+ 1.72 mmol/vial

MEROPENEM

Cautions hypersensitivity to beta-lactam antibacterials (avoid if history of immediate hypersensitivity reaction); **interactions:** Appendix 1 (meropenem)

Hepatic impairment monitor transaminase and bilirubin concentrations

Renal impairment use normal dose every 12 hours if creatinine clearance 26–50 ml/minute/1.73m², use half normal dose every 12 hours if creatinine clearance 10–25 ml/minute/1.73m², use half normal dose every 24 hours if creatinine clearance less than 10 ml/minute/1.73m²

Pregnancy manufacturer advises use only if potential benefit outweighs risk—no information available

Breast-feeding unlikely to be absorbed (but manufacturer advises avoid unless potential benefit outweighs risk)

Side-effects nausea, vomiting, diarrhoea (antibiotic-associated colitis reported), abdominal pain; disturbances in liver function tests; thrombocytopenia (reduction in partial thromboplastin time reported), positive Coombs' test, eosinophilia, leucopenia, neutropenia; headache, paraesthesia; hypersensitivity reactions including rash, pruritus, urticaria, angioedema, and anaphylaxis; also reported, convulsions, Stevens-Johnson syndrome and toxic epidermal necrolysis; local reactions including pain and thrombophlebitis at injection site

Licensed use not licensed for use in children for infection in neutropenia; not licensed for use in children under 3 months

Indication and dose

Aerobic and anaerobic Gram-positive and Gram-negative infections, hospital-acquired septicaemia Table 1, section 5.1

- **By intravenous injection over 5 minutes or by intravenous infusion**

Neonate under 7 days 20 mg/kg every 12 hours, dose doubled in severe infection

Neonate 7–28 days 20 mg/kg every 8 hours; dose doubled in severe infection

Child 1 month–12 years

Body-weight under 50 kg 10 mg/kg every 8 hours dose doubled in hospital-acquired pneumonia, peritonitis, septicaemia and infections in neutropenic patients

Body-weight over 50 kg dose as for child 12–18 years

Child 12–18 years 500 mg every 8 hours; dose doubled in hospital-acquired pneumonia, peritonitis, septicaemia and infections in neutropenic patients

Meningitis

- **By intravenous injection over 5 minutes or by intravenous infusion**

Neonate under 7 days 40 mg/kg every 12 hours

Neonate 7–28 days 40 mg/kg every 8 hours

Child 1 month–12 years

Body-weight under 50 kg 40 mg/kg every 8 hours

Body-weight over 50 kg dose as for child 12–18 years

Child 12–18 years 2 g every 8 hours

MEROPENEM (*continued*)

Exacerbations of chronic lower respiratory-tract infections in cystic fibrosis
- **By intravenous injection over 5 minutes or by intravenous infusion**

 Child 1 month–18 years 40 mg/kg every 8 hours (max. 2 g every 8 hours)

Administration Displacement value may be significant, consult local guidelines. For intermittent intravenous infusion dilute reconstituted solution further in glucose 5% *or* glucose 10% *or* sodium chloride 0.9% and give over 15–30 minutes

Meronem® (AstraZeneca) PoM
Injection, powder for reconstitution, meropenem (as trihydrate), net price 500-mg vial = £14.33; 1-g vial = £28.65
Electrolytes Na^+ 3.9 mmol/g

5.1.3 Tetracyclines

The tetracyclines are broad-spectrum antibiotics whose value has decreased owing to increasing bacterial resistance. In children over 12 years of age they are useful for infections caused by chlamydia (trachoma, psittacosis, salpingitis, urethritis, and lymphogranuloma venereum), rickettsia (including Q-fever), brucella (doxycycline with either streptomycin or rifampicin), and the spirochaete, *Borrelia burgdorferi* (Lyme disease—see section 5.1.1.3). They are also used in respiratory and genital mycoplasma infections, in acne, in destructive (refractory) periodontal disease, in exacerbations of chronic respiratory diseases (because of their activity against *Haemophilus influenzae*), and for leptospirosis in penicillin hypersensitivity (as an alternative to erythromycin).

Microbiologically, there is little to choose between the various tetracyclines, the only exception being **minocycline** which has a broader spectrum; it is active against *Neisseria meningitidis* and has been used for meningococcal prophylaxis but is no longer recommended because of side-effects including dizziness and vertigo (see Table 2, section 5.1 for current recommendations). *Deteclo®* (a combination of tetracycline, chlortetracycline and demeclocycline) does not have any advantages over preparations containing a single tetracycline.

Oral infections In children over 12 years of age, tetracyclines can be effective against oral anaerobes but the development of resistance (especially by oral streptococci) has reduced their usefulness for the treatment of acute oral infections; they may still have a role in the treatment of destructive (refractory) forms of periodontal disease. Doxycycline has a longer duration of action than tetracycline or oxytetracycline and need only be given once daily; it is reported to be more active against anaerobes than some other tetracyclines.

For the use of doxycycline in the treatment of recurrent aphthous ulceration, oral herpes, or as an adjunct to gingival scaling and root planing for periodontitis, see section 12.3.1 and section 12.3.2.

Cautions Tetracyclines should be used with caution in patients receiving potentially hepatotoxic drugs. Tetracyclines may increase muscle weakness in patients with myasthenia gravis, and exacerbate systemic lupus erythematosus. Antacids, and aluminium, calcium, iron, magnesium and zinc salts decrease the absorption of tetracyclines; milk also reduces the absorption of demeclocycline, oxytetracycline, and tetracycline. Other **interactions:** Appendix 1 (tetracyclines).

Hepatic impairment: avoid (or use with caution); tetracycline, demeclocycline, and *Deteclo®* max. 1 g daily in divided doses

Renal impairment: with the exception of doxycycline and minocycline, the tetracyclines may exacerbate renal failure and should not be given to patients with mild, moderate, or severe renal impairment. Doxycyline or minocycline may be used cautiously (avoid excessive doses)

Pregnancy: avoid in pregnancy. In the first trimester, effects on skeletal development in *animal* studies. In the second and third trimester, dental discolouration.

Breast-feeding: avoid (although absorption and therefore discolouration of teeth in infant probably usually prevented by chelation with calcium in milk)

Contra-indications Deposition of tetracyclines in growing bone and teeth (by binding to calcium) causes staining and occasionally dental hypoplasia, and they should **not** be given to children under 12 years, or to pregnant or breast-feeding women. However, doxycycline may be used in children for treatment and post-exposure prophylaxis of anthrax when an alternative antibacterial cannot be given [unlicensed indication].

Side-effects Side-effects of the tetracyclines include nausea, vomiting, diarrhoea (antibiotic-associated colitis reported occasionally), dysphagia, and oesophageal irritation. Other rare side-effects include hepatotoxicity, pancreatitis, blood disorders, photosensitivity (particularly with demeclocycline), and hypersensitivity reactions (including rash, exfoliative dermatitis, Stevens-Johnson syndrome, urticaria, angioedema, anaphylaxis, pericarditis). Headache and visual disturbances may indicate benign intracranial hypertension (discontinue treatment); bulging fontanelles have been reported in infants.

TETRACYCLINE

Cautions see notes above

Contra-indications see notes above

Side-effects see notes above; also reported, pancreatitis, acute renal failure, skin discoloration

Indication and dose

Susceptible infections see notes above
- By mouth

  Child 12–18 years 250 mg 4 times daily, increased in severe infections to 500 mg 3–4 times daily

Acne section 13.6.2

Non-gonococcal urethritis
- By mouth

  Child 12–18 years 500 mg 4 times daily for 7–14 days (21 days if failure or relapse after first course)

Tetracycline (Non-proprietary) PoM

Tablets, coated, tetracycline hydrochloride 250 mg, net price 28-tab pack = £1.91. Label: 7, 9, 23, counselling, posture

Dental prescribing on NHS Tetracycline Tablets may be prescribed

Compound preparations

Deteclo® (Goldshield) PoM

Tablets, blue, f/c, tetracycline hydrochloride 115.4 mg, chlortetracycline hydrochloride 115.4 mg, demeclocycline hydrochloride 69.2 mg, net price 14-tab pack = £1.83. Label: 7, 9, 11, 23, counselling, posture

Dose
- By mouth

  Child 12–18 years 1 tablet every 12 hours; 3–4 tablets daily in more severe infections

DEMECLOCYCLINE HYDROCHLORIDE

Cautions see notes above, but photosensitivity more common (avoid exposure to sunlight or sun lamps)

Contra-indications see notes above

Side-effects see notes above; also reversible nephrogenic diabetes insipidus, acute renal failure

Indication and dose

Susceptible infections see notes above
- By mouth

  Child 12–18 years 150 mg 4 times daily *or* 300 mg twice daily

Ledermycin® (Goldshield) PoM

Capsules, red, demeclocycline hydrochloride 150 mg, net price 28-cap pack = £6.94. Label: 7, 9, 11, 23

DOXYCYCLINE

Cautions see notes above, but may be used in renal impairment; alcohol dependence; photosensitivity reported (avoid exposure to sunlight or sun lamps); avoid in porphyria (section 9.8.2)

Contra-indications see notes above

Side-effects see notes above; also anorexia, flushing, tinnitus

Licensed use not licensed for use in children under 12 years

Indication and dose

Susceptible infections see notes above
- By mouth

  Child 12–18 years 200 mg on first day, then 100 mg daily; severe infections (including refractory urinary-tract infections) 200 mg daily

Early syphilis
- By mouth

  Child 12–18 years 100 mg twice daily for 14 days

Late latent syphilis
- By mouth

  Child 12–18 years 200 mg twice daily for 14 days

Uncomplicated genital chlamydia, non-gonococcal urethritis, pelvic inflammatory disease Table 1, section 5.1
- By mouth

  Child 12–18 years 100 mg twice daily for 7 days (14 days in pelvic inflammatory disease)

DOXYCYCLINE (*continued*)

Anthrax (treatment or post-exposure prophylaxis) see also section 5.1.12
- **By mouth**

Child under 12 years (only if alternative antibacterial cannot be given) 2.5 mg/kg twice daily (max. 100 mg twice daily)

Child 12–18 years 100 mg twice daily

Acne section 13.6.2

Counselling Capsules should be swallowed whole with plenty of fluid during meals while sitting or standing

Note Doxycycline doses in BNF for Children may differ from those in product literature

Doxycycline (Non-proprietary) PoM
Capsules, doxycycline (as hyclate) 50 mg, net price 28-cap pack = £3.47; 100 mg, 8-cap pack = £1.71. Label: 6, 9, 11, 27, counselling, posture
Brands include *Doxylar®*
Dental prescribing on NHS Doxycycline Capsules 100 mg may be prescribed

Vibramycin® (Pfizer) PoM
Capsules, doxycycline (as hyclate) 50 mg (green/ivory), net price 28-cap pack = £7.74. Label: 6, 9, 11, 27, counselling, posture

Vibramycin-D® (Pfizer) PoM
Dispersible tablets, yellow, scored, doxycycline 100 mg, net price 8-tab pack = £4.91. Label: 6, 9, 11, 13

LYMECYCLINE

Cautions see notes above

Contra-indications see notes above

Side-effects see notes above

Indication and dose

Susceptible infections see notes above
- **By mouth**

Child 12–18 years 408 mg twice daily, increased to 1.224–1.632 g daily in severe infections

Acne
- **By mouth**

Child 12–18 years 408 mg daily for at least 8 weeks

Tetralysal 300® (Galderma) PoM
Capsules, red/yellow, lymecycline 408 mg (= tetracycline 300 mg). Net price 28-cap pack = £7.16, 56-cap pack = £14.26. Label: 6, 9

MINOCYCLINE

Cautions see notes above, but may be used in renal impairment; if treatment continued for longer than 6 months, monitor every 3 months for hepatotoxicity, pigmentation and for systemic lupus erythematosus—discontinue if these develop or if pre-existing systemic lupus erythematosus worsens

Contra-indications see notes above

Side-effects see notes above; also anorexia, dizziness, tinnitus and vertigo (more common in women), acute renal failure; pigmentation (sometimes irreversible), discoloration of conjunctiva, tears and sweat, systemic lupus erythematosus

Indication and dose

Susceptible infections see notes above
- **By mouth**

Child 12–18 years 100 mg twice daily

Acne section 13.6.2

Counselling Tablets or capsules should be swallowed whole with plenty of fluid while sitting or standing

Minocycline (Non-proprietary) PoM
Capsules, minocycline (as hydrochloride) 50 mg, net price 56-cap pack = £17.20; 100 mg, 28-cap pack = £14.74. Label: 6, 9, counselling, posture
Brands include *Aknemin®*

Tablets, minocycline (as hydrochloride) 50 mg, net price 28-tab pack = £7.59, 84-tab pack = £16.20; 100 mg, 28-tab pack = £11.78. Label: 6, 9, counselling, posture

Minocin MR® (Lederle) PoM
Capsules, m/r, orange/brown (enclosing yellow and white pellets), minocycline (as hydrochloride) 100 mg. Net price 56-cap pack = £21.14. Label: 6, 25

Dose

Acne
- **By mouth**

Child 12–18 years 1 capsule daily

Sebomin MR® (Alpharma) PoM
Capsules, m/r, orange, minocycline (as hydrochloride) 100 mg, net price 56-cap pack = £21.14. Label: 6, 25

Dose

Acne
- **By mouth**

Child 12–18 years 1 capsule daily

OXYTETRACYCLINE

Cautions see notes above; porphyria (section 9.8.2)

Contra-indications see notes above

Side-effects see notes above

Indication and dose

Susceptible infections see notes above

- By mouth

Child 12–18 years 250–500 mg 4 times daily

Acne section 13.6.2

Oxytetracycline (Non-proprietary) PoM

Tablets, coated, oxytetracycline dihydrate 250 mg, net price 28-tab pack = 81p. Label: 7, 9, 23

Brands include *Oxymycin®*, *Oxytetramix®*

Dental prescribing on NHS Oxtetracycline Tablets may be prescribed

5.1.4 Aminoglycosides

These include amikacin, gentamicin, neomycin, netilmicin, streptomycin, and tobramycin. All are bactericidal and active against some Gram-positive and many Gram-negative organisms. Amikacin, gentamicin, and tobramycin are also active against *Pseudomonas aeruginosa*; streptomycin is active against *Mycobacterium tuberculosis* and is now almost entirely reserved for tuberculosis (section 5.1.9).

The aminoglycosides are not absorbed from the gut (although there is a risk of absorption in inflammatory bowel disease and liver failure) and must therefore be given by injection for systemic infections.

Excretion is principally via the kidney and accumulation occurs in renal impairment.

Most side-effects of this group of antibiotics are dose-related therefore care must be taken with dosage and whenever possible treatment should not exceed 7 days. The important side-effects are ototoxicity, and nephrotoxicity; they occur most commonly in children with renal failure.

If there is impairment of renal function (or high pre-dose serum concentrations) the interval between doses must be increased; if the renal impairment is severe the dose itself should be reduced as well.

Aminoglycosides may impair neuromuscular transmission and should not be given to children with myasthenia gravis; large doses given during surgery have been responsible for a transient myasthenic syndrome in patients with normal neuromuscular function.

Aminoglycosides should preferably not be given with potentially ototoxic diuretics (e.g. furosemide (frusemide)); if concurrent use is unavoidable administration of the aminoglycoside and of the diuretic should be separated by as long a period as practicable.

Serum concentrations Serum concentration monitoring avoids both excessive and subtherapeutic concentrations thus preventing toxicity and ensuring efficacy. In children with normal renal function, aminoglycoside concentration should be measured initially after 3 or 4 doses for multiple daily dose regimens; children with renal impairment may require earlier and more frequent measurement of aminoglycoside concentration.

Blood samples should be taken approximately 1 hour after intramuscular or intravenous administration ('peak' concentration, not necessary for once daily dosing in children over 1 month) and also just before the next dose ('trough' concentration).

Serum-aminoglycoside concentration should be measured in all children and **must** be determined in infants, in neonates, in obesity, and in cystic fibrosis, *or* if high doses are being given, *or* if there is renal impairment.

Once daily dosage Although aminoglycosides may be given in 2–3 divided doses during the 24 hours, *once daily administration* is more convenient (while ensuring adequate serum concentration) but local guidelines on dosage and serum concentrations should be consulted.

Cystic fibrosis A higher dose of parenteral aminoglycoside is often required in children with cystic fibrosis because renal clearance of the aminoglycoside is increased. For the role of aminoglycosides in the treatment of pseudomonal lung infections in cystic fibrosis see Table 1, section 5.1. Nebulised tobramycin is used for chronic pseudomonal lung infection in cystic fibrosis; however, resistance may develop, and some children do not respond to treatment. Gentamicin can be used similarly [unlicensed use].

Endocarditis **Gentamicin** is used in combination with other antibiotics for the treatment of bacterial endocarditis (Table 1, section 5.1). Serum-gentamicin concentration should be determined twice each week (more often in renal impairment). **Streptomycin** may be used as an alternative in gentamicin-resistant enterococcal endocarditis.

Gentamicin is the aminoglycoside of choice in the UK and is used widely for the treatment of serious infections. It has a broad spectrum but is inactive against anaerobes and has poor activity against haemolytic streptococci and pneumococci. When used for the 'blind' therapy of undiagnosed serious infections it is usually given in conjunction with a penicillin or metronidazole (or both). Gentamicin is used together with another antibiotic for the treatment of endocarditis (see above and Table 1, section 5.1).

Loading and maintenance doses may be calculated on the basis of the patient's weight and renal function (e.g. using a nomogram); adjustments are then made according to serum-gentamicin concentrations. High doses are occasionally indicated for serious infections, especially in the neonate, children with cystic fibrosis or the immunocompromised patient; whenever possible treatment should not exceed 7 days.

Amikacin is more stable than gentamicin to enzyme inactivation. Amikacin is used in the treatment of serious infections caused by gentamicin-resistant Gram-negative bacilli.

Netilmicin has similar activity to gentamicin, but may cause less ototoxicity in those needing treatment for longer than 10 days. Netilmicin is active against a number of gentamicin-resistant Gram-negative bacilli but is less active against *Ps. aeruginosa* than gentamicin or tobramycin.

Tobramycin has similar activity to gentamicin. It is slightly more active against *Ps. aeruginosa* but shows less activity against certain other Gram-negative bacteria. Tobramycin may be administered by nebuliser for the treatment of *Ps. aeruginosa* infection in cystic fibrosis (see Cystic Fibrosis, above).

Neomycin is too toxic for parenteral administration and can only be used for infections of the skin or mucous membranes or to reduce the bacterial population of the colon prior to bowel surgery or in hepatic failure. Oral administration may lead to malabsorption. Small amounts of neomycin may be absorbed from the gut in children with hepatic failure and, as these children may also be uraemic, cumulation may occur with resultant ototoxicity.

Neonates As aminoglycosides are eliminated principally via the kidney, neonatal treatment must reflect the changes in glomerular filtration that occur with increasing gestational and postnatal age. In patients on single daily dose regimens it may become necessary to prolong the dose interval to more than 24 hours if the trough concentration is high.

GENTAMICIN

Cautions neonates, infants (adjust dose and monitor renal, auditory and vestibular function together with serum gentamicin concentrations); avoid prolonged use; conditions characterised by muscular weakness; obesity (use ideal weight for height to calculate dose and monitor serum-gentamicin concentration closely); see also notes above; **interactions:** Appendix 1 (aminoglycosides)

Renal impairment reduce dose frequency; monitor serum concentrations; see notes above

Pregnancy *second, third trimesters*: auditory or vestibular nerve damage; risk greatest with streptomycin; probably very small with gentamicin and tobramycin, but avoid unless essential (if given, serum-aminoglycoside concentration monitoring essential)

Contra-indications myasthenia gravis

Side-effects vestibular and auditory damage, nephrotoxicity; rarely, hypomagnesaemia on prolonged therapy, antibiotic-associated colitis; also reported, nausea, vomiting, rash, blood disorders; see also notes above

Licensed use not licensed for nebulisation

Pharmacokinetics *Extended interval dose regimen in neonates or multiple daily dose regimen*: one-hour ('peak') serum concentration should be 5–10 mg/litre (3–5 mg/litre for endocarditis, 8–12 mg/litre in cystic fibrosis); pre-dose ('trough') concentration should be less than 2 mg/litre (less than

GENTAMICIN (*continued*)

1 mg/litre for endocarditis)
Once daily dose regimen: pre-dose ('trough') concentration should be less than 1 mg/litre
Intrathecal/intraventricular injection: cerebrospinal fluid concentration should not exceed 10 mg/litre

Indication and dose

Neonatal sepsis
- **Extended interval dose regimen by slow intravenous injection or intravenous infusion**

Neonate less than 32 weeks postmenstrual age 4–5 mg/kg every 36 hours

Neonate 32 weeks and over postmenstrual age 4–5 mg/kg every 24 hours

- **Multiple daily dose regimen by slow intravenous injection**

Neonate less than 29 weeks postmenstrual age 2.5 mg/kg every 24 hours

Neonate 29-35 weeks postmenstrual age 2.5 mg/kg every 18 hours

Neonate over 35 weeks postmenstrual age 2.5 mg/kg every 12 hours

Septicaemia, meningitis and other CNS infections, biliary-tract infection, acute pyelonephritis, endocarditis (see notes above), pneumonia in hospital patients, adjunct in listerial meningitis (Table 1, section 5.1)
- **Multiple daily dose regimen by intramuscular or by slow intravenous injection over at least 3 minutes**

Child 1 month–12 years 2.5 mg/kg every 8 hours

Child 12–18 years 2 mg/kg every 8 hours

- **Once daily dose regimen (not for endocarditis or meningitis) by intravenous infusion**

Child 1 month–18 years initially 7 mg/kg, then adjusted according to serum-gentamicin concentration

Pseudomonal lung infection in cystic fibrosis
- **By slow intravenous injection over at least 3 minutes or by intravenous infusion**

Child 1 month–18 years 3 mg/kg every 8 hours

- **By inhalation of nebulised solution**

Child 1 month–2 years 40 mg twice daily

Child 2–8 years 80 mg twice daily

Child 8–18 years 160 mg twice daily

Bacterial ventriculitis and CNS infection (supplement to systemic therapy)
- **By intrathecal or intraventricular injection, seek specialist advice**

Neonate seek specialist advice

Child 1 month–18 years 1 mg daily (increased if necessary to 5 mg daily)
Note only preservative-free, intrathecal preparation should be used

Endocarditis prophylaxis Table 2, section 5.1

Eye section 11.3.1

Ear section 12.1.1

Note Local guidelines may vary. See Pharmacokinetics above for serum-concentration monitoring. In obese or severely oedematous children use ideal weight for height to calculate the dose

Administration for *intravenous infusion*, dilute in Glucose 5% or Sodium Chloride 0.9%; give over 30 minutes
For *nebulisation*, dilute preservative-free preparation in 3 mL sodium chloride 0.9%. Administer after physiotherapy and bronchodilators
For *intrathecal* or *intraventricular injection*, use preservative-free intrathecal preparations only

Gentamicin (Non-proprietary) PoM
Injection, gentamicin (as sulphate), net price 40 mg/mL, 1-mL amp = £1.40, 2-mL amp = £1.54, 2-mL vial = £1.48
Paediatric injection, gentamicin (as sulphate) 10 mg/mL, net price 2-mL vial = £1.80
Intrathecal injection, gentamicin (as sulphate) 5 mg/mL, net price 1-mL amp = 74p

Cidomycin® (Beacon) PoM
Injection, gentamicin (as sulphate) 40 mg/mL. Net price 2-mL amp or vial = £1.48

Genticin® (Roche) PoM
Injection, gentamicin (as sulphate) 40 mg/mL. Net price 2-mL amp = £1.40

Isotonic Gentamicin Injection (Baxter) PoM
Intravenous infusion, gentamicin (as sulphate) 800 micrograms/mL in sodium chloride intravenous infusion 0.9%. Net price 100-mL (80-mg) *Viaflex®* bag = £1.61
Electrolytes Na^+ 15.4 mmol/100-mL bag

AMIKACIN

Cautions see under Gentamicin

Contra-indications see under Gentamicin

Side-effects see under Gentamicin

Pharmacokinetics *Multiple dose regimen*: one-hour ('peak') serum concentration should not exceed 30 mg/litre; pre-dose ('trough') concentration should be less than 10 mg/litre
Once daily dose regimen: pre-dose ('trough') concentration should be less than 1 mg/litre

Licensed use dose for cystic fibrosis not licensed

Indication and dose

Neonatal sepsis
- **Extended interval dose regimen by slow intravenous injection over 3–5 minutes or by intravenous infusion**

Neonate 15 mg/kg every 24 hours

5 Infections

AMIKACIN (*continued*)

- **Multiple daily dose regimen by intramuscular or by slow intravenous injection or by infusion**

Neonate loading dose of 10 mg/kg then 7.5 mg/kg every 12 hours

Serious Gram-negative infections resistant to gentamicin
- **By slow intravenous injection over 3–5 minutes**

Child 1 month–18 years 7.5 mg/kg every 12 hours

Child 12–18 years 7.5 mg/kg every 12 hours, increased to 7.5 mg/kg every 8 hours in severe infections, max. 500 mg every 8 hours for up to 10 days (max. cumulative dose 15 g)

Once daily dose regimen (not for endocarditis or meningitis)
- **By intravenous injection or infusion**

Child 1 month–18 years initially 15 mg/kg, then adjusted according to serum-amikacin concentration

Pseudomonal lung infection in cystic fibrosis
- **Multiple daily dose regimen by slow intravenous injection or infusion**

Child 1 month–18 years 10 mg/kg every 8 hours (max. 500 mg every 8 hours)

Note Local dosage guidelines may vary. For monitoring guidelines see Pharmacokinetics above. In obese or severely oedematous children use ideal weight for height to calculate the dose

Administration for *intravenous infusion*, dilute with Glucose 5% *or* Sodium Chloride 0.9% *or* Compound Sodium Lactate; give over 30 minutes

Amikacin (Non-proprietary) PoM
Injection, amikacin (as sulphate) 250 mg/mL. Net price 2-mL vial = £10.14
Electrolytes Na^+ 0.56 mmol/500-mg vial

Amikin® (Bristol-Myers Squibb) PoM
Injection, amikacin (as sulphate) 250 mg/mL. Net price 2-mL vial = £10.14
Electrolytes $Na^+ < 0.5$ mmol/vial

Paediatric injection, amikacin (as sulphate) 50 mg/mL. Net price 2-mL vial = £2.36
Electrolytes $Na^+ < 0.5$ mmol/vial

NETILMICIN

Cautions see under Gentamicin

Contra-indications see under Gentamicin

Side-effects see under Gentamicin

Pharmacokinetics *Extended interval dose regimen in neonates or multiple daily dose regimen:* one-hour ('peak') serum concentration should not exceed 12 mg/litre; pre-dose ('trough') concentration should be less than 2 mg/litre

Once daily dose regimen: pre-dose ('trough') concentration should be less than 1 mg/litre

Indication and dose

Neonatal sepsis
- **Extended interval dose regimen by intravenous injection or intravenous infusion**

Neonate less than 32 weeks postmenstrual age 6 mg/kg every 36 hours

Neonate 32 weeks and over postmenstrual age 6 mg/kg every 24 hours

- **Multiple daily dose regimen by intramuscular injection or by intravenous injection over 3–5 minutes or by intravenous infusion**

Neonate under 7 days 3 mg/kg every 12 hours

Neonate 7–28 days 2.5–3 mg/kg every 8 hours

Serious Gram-negative infections resistant to gentamicin
- **By slow intravenous injection over 3–5 minutes**

Child 1 month–1 year 2.5–3 mg/kg every 8 hours

Child 1–18 years 2–2.5 mg/kg every 8 hours

- **Once daily dosage regimen (not for endocarditis or meningitis) by slow intravenous injection or by intravenous infusion**

Child 1 month–18 years initially 7 mg/kg, then adjusted according to serum-netilmicin concentration

Note Local dose guidelines may vary. For serum-concentration monitoring see Pharmacokinetics above. In obese or severely oedematous children use ideal weight for height to calculate the dose

Administration for *intravenous infusion*, dilute with Glucose 5% or 10% *or* Sodium Chloride 0.9%; give over 30–120 minutes

Netillin® (Schering-Plough) PoM
Injection, netilmicin (as sulphate) 10 mg/mL, net price 1.5-mL (15-mg) amp = £1.42; 50 mg/mL, 1-mL (50-mg) amp = £2.11; 100 mg/mL, 1-mL (100-mg) amp = £2.75; 1.5-mL (150-mg) amp = £3.92, 2-mL (200-mg) amp = £5.09

TOBRAMYCIN

Cautions see under Gentamicin

Specific cautions for inhaled treatment Other inhaled drugs should be administered before tobramycin; monitor for bronchospasm with initial dose, measure peak flow before and after nebulisation—if bronchospasm occurs, repeat test using bronchodilator; monitor renal function before treatment and then annually; severe haemoptysis

Contra-indications see under Gentamicin

Side-effects see under Gentamicin; *on inhalation*, mouth ulcers, voice alteration, cough, bronchospasm (see Cautions)

Pharmacokinetics *Intravenous extended interval dose regimen in neonates or multiple daily dose regimen:* one-hour ('peak') serum concentration should not exceed 10 mg/litre (8–12 mg/litre in cystic fibrosis); pre-dose ('trough') concentration

TOBRAMYCIN (*continued*)

should be less than 2 mg/litre

Once daily dose regimen: pre-dose ('trough') concentration should be less than 1 mg/litre

Indication and dose

Neonatal sepsis

- **Extended interval dose regimen by intravenous injection over 3–5 minutes or by intravenous infusion**

  Neonate less than 32 weeks postmenstrual age 4–5 mg/kg every 36 hours

  Neonate 32 weeks and over postmenstrual age 4–5 mg/kg every 24 hours

- **Multiple daily dose regimen by intramuscular injection or by slow intravenous injection or by intravenous infusion**

  Neonate under 7 days 2 mg/kg every 12 hours

  Neonate 7–28 days 2–2.5 mg/kg every 8 hours

Septicaemia, meningitis and other CNS infections, biliary-tract infection, acute pyelonephritis, pneumonia in hospital patients

- **Multiple daily dose regimen by slow intravenous injection over 3–5 minutes**

  Child 1 month–12 years 2–2.5 mg/kg every 8 hours

  Child 12–18 years 1 mg/kg every 8 hours; in severe infections up to 5 mg/kg daily in divided doses every 6–8 hours (reduced to 3 mg/kg daily as soon as clinically indicated)

- **Once daily dose regimen by intravenous infusion**

  Child 1 month–18 years initially 7 mg/kg, then adjusted according to serum-tobramycin concentration

Pseudomonal lung infection in cystic fibrosis

- **Multiple daily dose regimen by slow intravenous injection over 3–5 minutes**

  Child 1 month–18 years 8–10 mg/kg/daily in 3 divided doses

- **Once daily dose regimen by intravenous infusion over 30 minutes**

  Child 5–18 years initially 10 mg/kg (max. 660 mg), then adjusted according to serum-tobramycin concentration

- **By inhalation**

  see under preparations

Note Local dosage guidelines may vary. In obese or severely oedematous children use ideal weight for height to calculate the dose. For serum concentration monitoring guidelines see Pharmacokinetics above

Administration for *intravenous infusion*, dilute with Glucose 5% *or* Sodium Chloride 0.9%; give over 20–60 minutes

Tobramycin (Non-proprietary) PoM

Injection, tobramycin (as sulphate) 40 mg/mL, net price 1-mL (40-mg) vial = £2.73, 2-mL (80-mg) vial = £4.16, 6-mL (240-mg) vial = £12.47

Tobi® (Chiron) PoM

Nebuliser solution, tobramycin 60 mg/mL, net price 56 × 5-mL (300-mg) unit = £1484.00

Dose

Chronic pulmonary *Pseudomonas aeruginosa* infection in cystic fibrosis patients

- **By inhalation of nebulised solution**

  Child 6–18 years 300 mg every 12 hours for 28 days, courses repeated after 28-day intervals

5.1.5 Macrolides

Erythromycin has an antibacterial spectrum that is similar but not identical to that of penicillin; it is thus an alternative in penicillin-allergic patients.

Indications for erythromycin include respiratory infections, whooping cough, legionnaires' disease, and campylobacter enteritis. It is active against many penicillin-resistant staphylococci but some are now also resistant to erythromycin; it has poor activity against *Haemophilus influenzae*. Erythromycin is also active against chlamydia and mycoplasmas.

Erythromycin causes nausea, vomiting, and diarrhoea in some children; in mild to moderate infections this can be avoided by giving a lower dose or the total dose in 4 divided doses but if a more serious infection, such as Legionella pneumonia, is suspected higher doses are needed.

Clarithromycin is an erythromycin derivative with slightly greater activity than the parent compound. Tissue concentrations are higher than with erythromycin. It is given twice daily.

Azithromycin is a macrolide with slightly less activity than erythromycin against Gram-positive bacteria but enhanced activity against some Gram-negative organisms including *H. influenzae*. Plasma concentrations are very low but tissue concentrations are much higher. It has a long tissue half-life and once daily dosage is recommended. For treatment of Lyme disease, see section 5.1.1.3. Azithromycin is also used in the treatment of trachoma [unlicensed indication] (section 11.3.1).

Azithromycin and clarithromycin cause fewer gastro-intestinal side-effects than erythromycin.

Spiramycin is also a macrolide (section 5.4.7).

For prophylaxis of infective endocarditis in patients allergic to penicillin, a single-dose of oral clindamycin is used; see Table 2, section 5.1. Single-dose azithromycin is used for prophylaxis of endocarditis in those unable to take clindamycin [unlicensed indication].

Oral infections Erythromycin is an alternative for oral infections in penicillin-allergic patients or where a beta-lactamase producing organism is involved. However, many organisms are now resistant to erythromycin or rapidly develop resistance; its use should therefore be limited to short courses. Metronidazole (section 5.1.11) may be preferred as an alternative to a penicillin.

ERYTHROMYCIN

Cautions predisposition to QT interval prolongation (including electrolyte disturbances, concomitant use of drugs that prolong QT interval); porphyria (section 9.8.2); **interactions**: Appendix 1 (macrolides)

Hepatic impairment may cause idiosyncratic hepatotoxicity

Renal impairment reduce dose in severe renal impairment (ototoxicity)

Pregnancy not known to be harmful

Breast-feeding only small amounts in milk—not known to be harmful

Side-effects nausea, vomiting, abdominal discomfort, diarrhoea (antibiotic-associated colitis reported); less frequently urticaria, rashes and other allergic reactions; reversible hearing loss reported after large doses; cholestatic jaundice, pancreatitis, cardiac effects (including chest pain and arrhythmias), myasthenia-like syndrome, Stevens-Johnson syndrome, and toxic epidermal necrolysis also reported

Indication and dose

Alternative to penicillin in hypersensitive patients, oral infections (see notes above), campylobacter enteritis, respiratory-tract infections (including legionnaires' disease), chlamydial ophthalmia

- **By mouth**

Neonate 12.5 mg/kg every 6 hours

Child 1 month–2 years 125 mg 4 times daily; dose doubled in severe infections

Child 2–8 years 250 mg 4 times daily; dose doubled in severe infections

Child 8–18 years 250–500 mg 4 times daily; dose doubled in severe infections

Note Total daily dose may be given in two divided doses

- **By intravenous infusion**

Neonate 10–12.5 mg/kg every 6 hours

Child 1 month–18 years 12.5 mg/kg every 6 hours; dose doubled in severe infections (max 4 g daily)

- **By continuous intravenous infusion**

Child 1 month–18 years 25 mg/kg daily, dose doubled in severe infection (max 4 g daily)

Early syphilis

- **By mouth**

Child 12–18 years 500 mg 4 times daily for 14 days

Uncomplicated genital chlamydia, non-gonococcal urethritis

- **By mouth**

Child 12–18 years 500 mg twice daily for 14 days

Prophylaxis against pneumococcal infection

- **By mouth**

Child 1 month–2 years 125 mg twice daily

Child 2–8 years 250 mg twice daily

Child 8–18 years 500 mg twice daily

Gastric stasis section 1.2

Acne vulgaris section 13.6

Diphtheria, whooping cough prophylaxis Table 2, section 5.1

Administration Dilute reconstituted solution further in glucose 5% (neutralised with Sodium bicarbonate) or sodium chloride 0.9% to a concentration of 1 mg/mL for continuous infusion and 1–5 mg/mL for intermittent infusion; give intermittent infusion over 20–60 minutes

Concentration of up to 10 mg/mL may be used in fluid-restriction if administered via a central venous catheter

Erythromycin (Non-proprietary) PoM

Capsules, enclosing e/c microgranules, erythromycin 250 mg, net price 28-cap pack = £4.92. Label: 5, 9, 25

Brands include *Tiloryth®*

Tablets, e/c, erythromycin 250 mg, net price 20 = £1.92. Label: 5, 9, 25

Brands include *Rommix®*

Dental prescribing on NHS Erythromycin Tablets e/c may be prescribed

Erythromycin Ethyl Succinate (Non-proprietary) PoM

Oral suspension, erythromycin (as ethyl succinate) for reconstitution with water 125 mg/5 mL, net

ERYTHROMYCIN (*continued*)

price 100 mL = £2.20; 250 mg/5 mL, 100 mL = £2.72; 500 mg/5 mL, 100 mL = £4.44. Label: 9

Note Sugar-free versions are available and can be ordered by specifying 'sugar-free' on the prescription

Brands include *Primacine®*

Dental prescribing on NHS Erythromycin Ethyl Succinate Oral Suspension may be prescribed

Erythromycin Lactobionate (Non-proprietary) PoM

Intravenous infusion, powder for reconstitution, erythromycin (as lactobionate), net price 1-g vial = £9.98

Erymax® (Zeneus) PoM

Capsules, opaque orange/clear orange, enclosing orange and white e/c pellets, erythromycin 250 mg, net price 28-cap pack = £5.95, 112-cap pack = £23.80. Label: 5, 9, 25

Erythrocin® (Abbott) PoM

Tablets, both f/c, erythromycin (as stearate), 250 mg, net price 20 = £2.92; 500 mg, 20 = £6.01. Label: 9

Dental prescribing on NHS May be prescribed as Erythromycin Stearate Tablets

Erythroped® (Abbott) PoM

Suspension SF, sugar-free, banana-flavoured, erythromycin (as ethyl succinate) for reconstitution with water, 125 mg/5 mL (*Suspension PI SF*), net price 140 mL = £3.18; 250 mg/5 mL, 140 mL = £6.20; 500 mg/5 mL (*Suspension SF Forte*), 140 mL = £10.99. Label: 9

Erythroped A® (Abbott) PoM

Tablets, yellow, f/c, erythromycin 500 mg (as ethyl succinate). Net price 28-tab pack = £8.29. Label: 9

Dental prescribing on NHS May be prescribed as Erythromycin Ethyl Succinate Tablets

AZITHROMYCIN

Cautions see under Erythromycin; **interactions:** Appendix 1 (macrolides)

Pregnancy manufacturer advises use only if adequate alternatives not available

Breast-feeding present in milk; manufacturer advises use only if no suitable alternative

Contra-indications

Hepatic impairment avoid, jaundice reported

Side-effects see under Erythromycin; also anorexia, dyspepsia, flatulence, constipation, pancreatitis, hepatitis, syncope, dizziness, headache, drowsiness, agitation, anxiety, hyperactivity, asthenia, paraesthesia, convulsions, mild neutropenia, thrombocytopenia, interstitial nephritis, acute renal failure, arthralgia, photosensitivity; *rarely* taste disturbances, tongue discoloration, and hepatic failure

Licensed use not licensed for typhoid fever and prophylaxis of endocarditis

Indication and dose

Respiratory-tract infections, otitis media, skin and soft-tissue infections

• By mouth

Child over 6 months 10 mg/kg once daily (max. 500 mg once daily) for 3 days *or*

Child over 6 months Body-weight 15–25 kg 200 mg once daily for 3 days

Body-weight 26–35 kg 300 mg once daily for 3 days

Body-weight 36–45 kg 400 mg once daily for 3 days

Body-weight over 45 kg 500 mg once daily for 3 days

Infection in cystic fibrosis

• By mouth

Child 6 months–18 years 10 mg/kg once daily (max. 500 mg once daily) for 3 days; course repeated after 1 week, then repeat as necessary

Uncomplicated genital chlamydial infections and non-gonococcal urethritis

• By mouth

Child 12–18 years 1 g as a single dose

Mild to moderate typhoid due to multiple-antibacterial resistant organisms

• By mouth

Child 6 months–18 years 10 mg/kg once daily (max. 500 mg) for 7 days

Prophylaxis of endocarditis Table 2, section 5.1

Zithromax® (Pfizer) PoM

Capsules, azithromycin (as dihydrate) 250 mg, net price 4-cap pack = £8.95, 6-cap pack = £13.43. Label: 5, 9, 23

Oral suspension, cherry/banana-flavoured, azithromycin (as dihydrate) 200 mg/5 mL when reconstituted with water. Net price 15-mL pack = £5.08, 22.5-mL pack = £7.62, 30-mL pack = £13.80. Label: 5, 9

Dental prescribing on NHS May be prescribed as Azithromycin Oral Suspension 200 mg/5 mL

CLARITHROMYCIN

Cautions see under Erythromycin; **interactions:** Appendix 1 (macrolides)

Hepatic impairment hepatic dysfunction including jaundice reported

Renal impairment use half normal dose if creatinine clearance less than 30 mL/minute/1.73 m^2; avoid *Klaricid XL®* if creatinine clearance less than 30 mL/minute/1.73 m^2

Pregnancy manufacturer advises avoid unless potential benefit outweighs risk

Breast-feeding manufacturer advises avoid unless potential benefit outweighs risk—present in milk

CLARITHROMYCIN (*continued*)

Side-effects see under Erythromycin; also dyspepsia, tooth and tongue discoloration, smell and taste disturbances, stomatitis, glossitis, and headache; *less commonly* hepatitis, arthralgia, and myalgia; *rarely* tinnitus; *very rarely* pancreatitis, dizziness, insomnia, nightmares, anxiety, confusion, psychosis, paraesthesia, convulsions, hypoglycaemia, renal failure, leucopenia, and thrombocytopenia; on intravenous infusion, local tenderness, phlebitis

Licensed use intravenous route not licensed for use in children

Indication and dose

Respiratory-tract infections, mild to moderate skin and soft tissue infections, otitis media
- **By mouth**

  Neonate 7.5 mg/kg twice daily

  Child 1 month–12 years Body-weight under 8 kg 7.5 mg/kg twice daily

  Body-weight 8–11 kg 62.5 mg twice daily

  Body-weight 12–19 kg 125 mg twice daily

  Body-weight 20–29 kg 187.5 mg twice daily

  Body-weight 30–40 kg 250 mg twice daily

  Child 12–18 years 250 mg twice daily for 7 days, increased if necessary in severe infections to 500 mg every 12 hours for up to 14 days

- **By intravenous infusion into large proximal vein**

  Child 1 month–12 years 7.5 mg/kg every 12 hours

  Child 12–18 years 500 mg every 12 hours

Helicobacter pylori eradication section 1.3

Administration for intermittent intravenous infusion dilute reconstituted solution further in Glucose 5% *or* Sodium chloride 0.9% *or* Ringer's solution *or* Compound sodium lactate to a concentration of 2 mg/mL; give into large proximal vein over 60 minutes

Clarithromycin (Non-proprietary) PoM
Tablets, clarithromycin 250 mg, net price 14-tab pack = £10.94; 500 mg, 14-tab pack = £21.90. Label: 9

Clarosip® (Grünenthal) PoM
Granules, clarithromycin 125 mg/straw, net price 14-straw pack = £6.70; 187.5 mg/straw, 14-straw pack = £9.70; 250 mg/straw, 14-straw pack = £12.70. Label: 9, counselling, administration
Counselling. Place straw in cold or warm drink such as water, carbonated drink, or tea (but **not** full fat milk, milkshake, or drink with solid particles) and sip drink through straw; several sips may be required to obtain full dose

Klaricid® (Abbott) PoM
Tablets, both yellow, f/c, clarithromycin 250 mg, net price 14-tab pack = £10.94; 500 mg, 14-tab pack = £21.90, 20-tab pack = £31.29. Label: 9

Paediatric suspension, clarithromycin for reconstitution with water 125 mg/5 mL, net price 70 mL = £5.58, 100 mL = £9.60; 250 mg/5 mL, 70 mL = £11.16. Label: 9

Granules, clarithromycin 250 mg/sachet, net price 14-sachet pack = £11.68. Label: 9, 13

Intravenous infusion, powder for reconstitution, clarithromycin. Net price 500-mg vial = £11.46
Electrolytes $Na^+ < 0.5$ mmol/500-mg vial

Klaricid XL® (Abbott) PoM
Tablets, m/r, yellow, clarithromycin 500 mg, net price 7-tab pack = £9.90, 14-tab pack = £19.81. Label: 9, 21, 25

Dose
- **By mouth**
  Child 12–18 years 500 mg once daily (doubled in severe infections) for 7–14 days

5.1.6 Clindamycin

Clindamycin is active against Gram-positive cocci, including penicillin-resistant staphylococci and also against many anaerobes, especially *Bacteroides fragilis.* It is well concentrated in bone and excreted in bile and urine.

Clindamycin is recommended for staphylococcal joint and bone infections such as osteomyelitis, and intra-abdominal sepsis.

Clindamycin is used for prophylaxis of endocarditis in patients allergic to penicillin [unlicensed indication], see Table 2, section 5.1.

Clindamycin has been asssociated with antibiotic-associated colitis (section 1.5), which may be fatal. Although it can occur with most antibacterials, antibiotic-associated colitis occurs more frequently with clindamycin. Children should therefore discontinue treatment immediately if diarrhoea develops.

Oral infections Clindamycin should not be used routinely for the treatment of oral infections because it may be no more effective than penicillins against anaerobes and there may be cross-resistance with erythromycin-resistant bacteria. Clindamycin can be used for the treatment of dentoalveolar abcess that has not responded to penicillin or to metronidazole.

CLINDAMYCIN

Cautions discontinue immediately if diarrhoea or colitis develops; monitor liver and renal function on prolonged therapy and in neonates and infants; avoid rapid intravenous administration; **interactions:** Appendix 1 (clindamycin)

Hepatic impairment reduce dose

Renal impairment half-life may be prolonged, reduce dose

Pregnancy not known to be harmful

Breast-feeding amount probably too small to be harmful; bloody diarrhoea reported in 1 infant

Contra-indications diarrhoeal states; avoid injections containing benzyl alcohol in neonates (see under preparations below)

Side-effects diarrhoea (discontinue treatment), abdominal discomfort, oesophagitis, nausea, vomiting, antibiotic-associated colitis; jaundice; leucopenia, eosinophilia, and thrombocytopenia reported; rash, pruritus, urticaria, anaphylactoid reactions, Stevens-Johnson syndrome, exfoliative and vesiculobullous dermatitis reported; pain, induration, and abscess after intramuscular injection; thrombophlebitis after intravenous injection

Licensed use not licensed for prophylaxis of endocarditis

Indication and dose

Endocarditis prophylaxis section 5.1

Staphylococcal bone and joint infections, peritonitis see notes above

- **By mouth**

Neonate under 14 days 3–6 mg/kg 3 times daily

Neonate 14–28 days 3–6 mg/kg 4 times daily

Child 1 month–12 years 3–6 mg/kg 4 times daily (body-weight under 10 kg, minimum dose 37.5 mg 3 times daily)

Child 12–18 years 150–300 mg 4 times daily; in severe infections 450 mg 4 times daily

- **By deep intramuscular injection or by intravenous infusion**

Child 1 month–12 years 3.75–6.25 mg/kg 4 times daily; increased up to 10 mg/kg 4 times daily in severe infections; total daily dose may alternatively be given in 3 divided doses

Child 12–18 years 150–675 mg 4 times daily; total daily dose may alternatively be given in 2–3 divided doses; in life-threatening infection up to 1.2 g 4 times daily; single doses above 600 mg by intravenous infusion only; single doses by intravenous infusion not to exceed 1.2 g

Administration for *intravenous infusion*, dilute to a concentration of not more than 18 mg/mL with Glucose 5% *or* Sodium Chloride 0.9%; give over 10–60 minutes at a max. rate of 20 mg/kg/hour

Staphylococcal lung infection in cystic fibrosis

- **By mouth**

Child 1 month–18 years 5–7 mg/kg (max. 600 mg) 4 times daily

Treatment of falciparum malaria, p. 375

Clindamycin (Non-proprietary) PoM

Capsules, clindamycin (as hydrochloride) 150 mg, net price 24-cap pack = £13.72. Label: 9, 27, counselling, see above (diarrhoea)

Dental prescribing on NHS Clindamycin Capsules may be prescribed

Liquid, 75 mg/5 mL available from specialist importing companies

Dalacin C® (Pharmacia) PoM

Capsules, clindamycin (as hydrochloride) 75 mg (lavender), net price 24-cap pack = £7.45; 150 mg, (lavender/maroon), 24-cap pack = £13.72. Label: 9, 27, counselling, see above (diarrhoea)

Dental prescribing on NHS May be prescribed as Clindamycin Capsules

Injection, clindamycin (as phosphate) 150 mg/mL, net price 2-mL amp = £6.20; 4-mL amp = £12.35

Excipients: include benzyl alcohol (avoid in neonates, see Excipients, p. 3)

5.1.7 Some other antibacterials

Antibacterials discussed in this section include chloramphenicol, fusidic acid, glycopeptide antibiotics (vancomycin and teicoplanin), linezolid, the streptogramins (quinupristin and dalfopristin) and the polymyxin, colistin.

Chloramphenicol

Chloramphenicol is a potent broad-spectrum antibiotic; however, it is associated with serious haematological side-effects when given systemically and should therefore be reserved for the treatment of life-threatening infections, particularly those caused by *Haemophilus influenzae*, and also for typhoid fever. Chloramphenicol is also used in cystic fibrosis for the treatment of respiratory *Burkholderia cepacia* infection resistant to other antibacterials.

Grey baby syndrome may follow excessive doses in neonates with immature hepatic metabolism; monitoring of plasma concentrations is recommended.

Chloramphenicol eye drops (section 11.3.1) and chloramphenicol ear drops (section 12.1.1) are also available.

CHLORAMPHENICOL

Cautions avoid repeated courses and prolonged treatment; blood counts required before and periodically during treatment; monitor plasma-chloramphenicol concentration in neonates (see below); **interactions:** Appendix 1 (chloramphenicol)

Hepatic impairment avoid if possible—increased risk of bone-marrow depression; reduce dose and monitor plasma-chloramphenicol concentration

Renal impairment avoid in severe impairment unless no alternative; dose-related depression of haematopoiesis

Contra-indications porphyria (section 9.8.2)

Pregnancy neonatal grey-baby syndrome if used in third trimester

Breast-feeding use another antibiotic; may cause bone-marrow toxicity in infant; concentration in milk usually insufficient to cause 'grey-baby syndrome'

Side-effects blood disorders including reversible and irreversible aplastic anaemia (with reports of resulting leukaemia), peripheral neuritis, optic neuritis, headache, depression, urticaria, erythema multiforme, nausea, vomiting, diarrhoea, stomatitis, glossitis, dry mouth; nocturnal haemoglobinuria reported; grey syndrome (abdominal distension, pallid cyanosis, circulatory collapse) may follow excessive doses in neonates with immature hepatic metabolism (see Pharmacokinetics below)

Pharmacokinetics plasma concentration monitoring required in neonates and preferred in those under 4 years of age, and in hepatic impairment; recommended peak plasma concentration (approx. 1 hour after end of intravenous injection or infusion or 2 hours after oral administration) 15–25 mg/litre; pre-dose ('trough') concentration should not exceed 15 mg/litre

Indication and dose

See notes above

- **By intravenous injection**

  Neonate up to 14 days 12.5 mg/kg twice daily

  Neonate 14–28 days 12.5 mg/kg 2–4 times daily

  Note Check dosage carefully; overdosage can be fatal (see also pharmacokinetics above)

- **By mouth or by intravenous injection or infusion**

  Child 1 month–18 years 12.5 mg/kg every 6 hours; dose may be doubled in severe infections such as septicaemia, meningitis and epiglottitis providing plasma-chloramphenicol concentrations are measured and high doses reduced as soon as indicated

Administration Displacement value may be significant for injection, consult local guidelines. For intermittent intravenous infusion, dilute reconstituted solution further in glucose 5% *or* sodium chloride 0.9%

Chloramphenicol (Non-proprietary) PoM

Capsules, chloramphenicol 250 mg. Net price 60 = £377.00

Extemporaneous formulations available see Extemporaneous Preparations, p. 8

Kemicetine® (Pharmacia) PoM

Injection, powder for reconstitution, chloramphenicol (as sodium succinate). Net price 1-g vial = £1.39

Electrolytes Na^+ 3.14 mmol/g

Fusidic acid

Fusidic acid and its salts are narrow-spectrum antibiotics. The only indication for their use is in infections caused by penicillin-resistant staphylococci, especially osteomyelitis, as they are well concentrated in bone; they are also used for staphylococcal endocarditis. A second antistaphylococcal antibiotic is usually required to prevent emergence of resistance during treatment.

SODIUM FUSIDATE

Cautions monitor liver function with high doses, on prolonged therapy or in hepatic impairment; elimination may be reduced in hepatic impairment or biliary disease or biliary obstruction; **interactions:** Appendix 1 (fusidic acid)

Hepatic impairment impaired biliary excretion, avoid or reduce dose; possibly increased risk of hepatotoxicity, monitor liver function

Pregnancy not known to be harmful; manufacturer advises use only if potential benefit outweighs risk

Breast-feeding present in milk; manufacturer advises caution

Side-effects nausea, vomiting, reversible jaundice, especially after high dosage or rapid infusion (withdraw therapy if persistent); rarely hypersensitivity reactions, acute renal failure (usually with jaundice), blood disorders

Indication and dose

Penicillin-resistant staphylococcal infection including osteomyelitis, staphylococcal endocarditis in combination with other antibacterials see under Preparations, below

SODIUM FUSIDATE (*continued*)

Sodium fusidate (Leo) PoM
Intravenous infusion, powder for reconstitution, sodium fusidate 500 mg (= fusidic acid 480 mg), with buffer, net price per vial (with diluent) = £70.04
Electrolytes Na^+ 3.1 mmol/vial when reconstituted with buffer

Dose

As sodium fusidate

- **By intravenous infusion**

Neonate 10 mg/kg every 12 hours

Child 1 month–18 years 6–7 mg/kg (max. 500 mg) every 8 hours

Administration reconstitute with buffer solution provided; further dilute to 1 mg/mL with Sodium chloride 0.9% *or* Glucose 5% intravenous infusion (but see below); infuse over at least 6 hours via a superficial vein or 2 hours via a central venous line; incompatible in solution of pH less than 7.4

Fucidin® (Leo) PoM
Tablets, f/c, sodium fusidate 250 mg, net price 10-tab pack = £6.02. Label: 9

Dose

as sodium fusidate

Child 12–18 years 500 mg every 8 hours, dose doubled for severe infections

Skin infection as sodium fusidate

Child 12–18 years 250 mg every 12 hours for 5–10 days

Suspension, off-white, banana- and orange-flavoured, fusidic acid 250 mg/5 mL, net price 50 mL = £6.73. Label: 9, 21

Dose

As fusidic acid

Neonate 15 mg/kg 3 times daily

Child 1 month–1 year 15 mg/kg 3 times daily

Child 1–5 years 250 mg 3 times daily

Child 5–12 years 500 mg 3 times daily

Child 12–18 years 750 mg 3 times daily

Note Fusidic acid is incompletely absorbed and doses recommended for suspension are proportionately higher than those for sodium fusidate tablets

Vancomycin and teicoplanin

The glycopeptide antibiotics vancomycin and teicoplanin have bactericidal activity against aerobic and anaerobic Gram-positive bacteria including multi-resistant *Staphylococci*. However, there are reports of *Staphylococcus aureus* with reduced suseptibility to glycopeptides. There are increasing reports of glycopeptide-resistant *Enterococci*.

Vancomycin is used *by the intravenous route* in the prophylaxis and treatment of endocarditis and other serious infections caused by Gram-positive cocci. It has a relatively long duration of action and can therefore be given every 12 hours; less frequent administration may be necessary in premature neonates with immature renal function. Vancomycin is principally excreted via the kidney and dose reduction is necessary in renal impairment.

Penetration in to cerebrospinal fluid is poor; vancomycin may be administered by the intrathecal or intraventricular route for treatment of meningitis [unlicensed]. Vancomycin (added to dialysis fluid) is also used in the treatment of peritonitis associated with peritoneal dialysis [unlicensed route] (Table 1 section 5.1).

Vancomycin given *by mouth* for 7–10 days is effective in the treatment of antibiotic-associated colitis (pseudomembranous colitis, see also section 1.5); low doses (see below) are considered adequate (higher dose may be considered if the infection fails to respond or if it is severe). Vancomycin is also used by mouth in prophylaxis of neonatal necrotising enterocolitis. Vancomycin should **not** be given by mouth for systemic infections since it is not significantly absorbed.

Teicoplanin is very similar to vancomycin but has a significantly longer duration of action allowing once-daily administration. Plasma concentration monitoring is not usually necessary, but may help optimise therapy. Unlike vancomycin, teicoplanin can be given by intramuscular as well as by intravenous injection; it is not given by mouth.

VANCOMYCIN

Cautions avoid rapid infusion (risk of anaphylactoid reactions, see Side-effects); rotate infusion sites; avoid if history of deafness; all patients require plasma-vancomycin measurement (after 3 or 4 doses if renal function normal, earlier if renal impairment), blood counts, urinalysis, and

VANCOMYCIN (*continued*)

renal function tests; monitor auditory function in renal impairment; systemic absorption may follow oral administration especially in inflammatory bowel disorders or following multiple doses; **interactions:** Appendix 1 (vancomycin)

Renal impairment reduce dose—monitor plasma-vancomycin concentration and renal function regularly

Pregnancy manufacturer advises use only if potential benefit outweighs risk—plasma-vancomycin concentration monitoring essential to reduce risk of fetal toxicity

Breast-feeding present in milk—significant absorption following oral administration unlikely

Side-effects after parenteral administration: nephrotoxicity including renal failure and interstitial nephritis; ototoxicity (discontinue if tinnitus occurs); blood disorders including neutropenia (usually after 1 week or high cumulative dose), rarely agranulocytosis and thrombocytopenia; nausea; chills, fever; eosinophilia, anaphylaxis, rashes (including exfoliative dermatitis, Stevens-Johnson syndrome, toxic epidermal necrolysis, and vasculitis); phlebitis (irritant to tissue); on rapid infusion, severe hypotension (including shock and cardiac arrest), wheezing, dyspnoea, urticaria, pruritus, flushing of the upper body ('red man' syndrome), pain and muscle spasm of back and chest

Pharmacokinetics plasma concentration monitoring required; pre-dose ('trough') concentration should be 5–10 mg/litre (10–15 mg/litre in endocarditis)

Licensed use not licensed for intraventricular use

Indication and dose

Infections due to Gram-positive bacteria including osteomyelitis, septicaemia and soft tissue infections see notes above

- **By intravenous infusion**

Neonate less than 29 weeks postmenstrual age 15 mg/kg every 24 hours

Neonate 29-35 weeks postmenstrual age 15 mg/kg every 12 hours

Neonate over 35 weeks postmenstrual age 15 mg/kg every 8 hours

Child 1 month–18 years 15 mg/kg every 8 hours (maximum daily dose 2 g), adjusted according to plasma concentration

Antibiotic-associated colitis (see also notes above)

- **By mouth**

Child 1 month–5 years 5 mg/kg 4 times daily for 7–10 days

Child 5–12 years 62.5 mg 4 times daily for 7–10 days

Child 12–18 years 125 mg 4 times daily for 7–10 days

Prophylaxis of necrotising enterocolitis in neonates

- **By mouth**

Neonate 15 mg/kg 3 times daily

CNS infection e.g. ventriculitis

- **By intraventricular administration, seek specialist advice**

Neonate 10 mg once every 24 hours

Child 1 month–18 years 10 mg once every 24 hours

Note for all children reduce to 5 mg daily if ventricular size reduced or increase to 15–20 mg once daily if ventricular size increased. Adjust dose according to CSF concentration after 3-4 days; aim for pre-dose ('trough') concentration less than 10 mg/litre. If CSF not draining freely reduce dose frequency to once every 2–3 days

Peritonitis associated with peritoneal dialysis
Add to each bag of dialysis fluid to achieve a concentration of 20–25 mg/litre

Endocarditis prophylaxis Table 2, section 5.1

Note Vancomycin doses in BNF for Children may differ from those in product literature

Administration Displacement value may be significant, consult product literature and local guidelines. For intermittent intravenous infusion, the reconstituted preparation should be further diluted in sodium chloride 0.9% *or* glucose 5% to a concentration of up to 5 mg/mL; give over at least 60 minutes (rate not to exceed 10 mg/minute for doses over 500 mg); use continuous infusion only if intermittent not available (limited evidence); 10 mg/mL can be used if infused via a central venous line over at least 1 hour

Injection may be given orally; flavouring syrups may be added to the solution at the time of administration.

Safe Practice For intraventricular administration, seek specialist advice

Vancomycin (Non-proprietary) PoM

Capsules, vancomycin (as hydrochloride) 125 mg, net price 28-cap pack = £66.23; 250 mg, 28-cap pack = £132.47. Label: 9

Injection, powder for reconstitution, vancomycin (as hydrochloride), for use as an infusion, net price 500-mg vial = £8.05; 1-g vial = £16.11

Note Can be used to prepare solution for oral administration

Vancocin® (Flynn) PoM

Matrigel capsules, vancomycin (as hydrochloride) 125 mg, net price 20-cap pack = £63.08. Label: 9

Injection, powder for reconstitution, vancomycin (as hydrochloride), for use as an infusion, net price 500-mg vial = £8.05; 1-g vial = £16.11

Note Can be used to prepare solution for oral administration

5 Infections

TEICOPLANIN

Cautions vancomycin sensitivity; blood counts and liver and kidney function tests required—monitor renal and auditory function on prolonged administration during renal impairment or if other nephrotoxic or neurotoxic drugs given; **interactions:** Appendix 1 (teicoplanin)

Renal impairment reduce dose on day 4: use half normal dose if creatinine clearance is 40–60 mL/minute/1.73m^2 and use one-third normal dose if creatinine clearance is less than 40 mL/minute/1.73m^2

Pregnancy manufacturer advises use only if potential benefit outweighs risk

Breast-feeding no information available

Side-effects nausea, vomiting, diarrhoea; rash, pruritus, fever, bronchospasm, rigors, urticaria, angioedema, anaphylaxis; dizziness, headache; blood disorders including eosinophilia, leucopenia, neutropenia, and thrombocytopenia; disturbances in liver enzymes, transient increase of serum creatinine, renal failure; tinnitus, mild hearing loss, and vestibular disorders also reported; rarely exfoliative dermatitis, Stevens-Johnson syndrome, toxic epidermal necrolysis; local reactions include erythema, pain, thrombophlebitis, injection site abscess and rarely flushing with infusion

Indication and dose

Potentially serious Gram-positive infections including endocarditis, and serious infections due to Staphylococcus aureus

- **By intravenous injection or intravenous infusion over 30 minutes**

Neonate initially 16 mg/kg for one dose followed 24 hours later by 8 mg/kg once daily (intravenous infusion only)

Child 1 month–18 years in moderate infections initially 10 mg/kg (max. 400 mg) every 12 hours for 3 doses, then 6 mg/kg (max. 200 mg) once daily; in severe infections or in neutropenia initially 10 mg/kg (max. 400 mg) every 12 hours for 3 doses then 10 mg/kg (max. 400 mg) once daily; after first 3 doses, subsequent doses can be given by intramuscular injection if necessary although intravenous route preferable for children

Endocarditis prophylaxis Table 2, section 5.1

Administration For intermittent intravenous infusion, dilute reconstituted solution further in sodium chloride 0.9% *or* glucose 5% *or* compound sodium lactate intravenous infusion; give over 30 minutes. Intermittent intravenous infusion preferred in neonates

Targocid® (Aventis Pharma) PoM

Injection, powder for reconstitution, teicoplanin, net price 200-mg vial (with diluent) = £17.58; 400-mg vial (with diluent) = £35.62

Electrolytes Na^+ < 0.5 mmol/200- and 400-mg vial

Linezolid

Linezolid, an oxazolidinone antibacterial, is active against Gram-positive bacteria including meticillin-resistant *Staphylococcus aureus* (MRSA), and glycopeptide-resistant enterococci. Resistance to linezolid can develop with prolonged treatment or if the dose is less than that recommended. Linezolid should be reserved for infections resistant to other antibacterials or when other antibacterials are not tolerated. Linezolid is not sufficiently active against common Gram-negative organisms. There is limited information on use in children and expert advice should be sought.

LINEZOLID

Cautions monitor full blood count (including platelet count) weekly (see also CSM Advice below); unless close observation and blood-pressure monitoring possible, avoid in uncontrolled hypertension, phaeochromocytoma, carcinoid tumour, thyrotoxicosis, bipolar depression, schizophrenia, or acute confusional states; **interactions:** Appendix 1 (MAOIs)

Hepatic impairment no dose adjustment necessary but in severe hepatic impairment use only if potential benefit outweighs risk

Renal impairment no dose adjustment necessary but metabolites may accumulate if creatinine clearance less than 30 mL/minute/1.73m^2

Pregnancy manufacturer advises use only if potential benefit outweighs risk—no information available

CSM advice Haematopoietic disorders (including thrombocytopenia, anaemia, leucopenia, and pancytopenia) have been reported in patients receiving linezolid. It is recommended that full blood counts are monitored weekly. Close monitoring is recommended in patients who:

- receive treatment for more than 10–14 days;
- have pre-existing myelosuppression;
- are receiving drugs that may have adverse effects on haemoglobin, blood counts, or platelet function;
- have severe renal impairment.

If significant myelosuppression occurs, treatment should be stopped unless it is considered essential, in which case intensive monitoring of blood counts and appropriate management should be implemented.

Monoamine oxidase inhibition Linezolid is a reversible, non-selective monoamine oxidase inhibitor (MAOI). Patients should avoid consuming large amounts of tyramine-rich foods (such as mature cheese, yeast extracts,

LINEZOLID (*continued*)

undistilled alcoholic beverages, and fermented soya bean products). In addition, linezolid should not be given with another MAOI or within 2 weeks of stopping another MAOI. Unless close observation and blood-pressure monitoring is possible, avoid in those receiving SSRIs, $5HT_1$ agonists ('triptans'), tricyclic antidepressants, sympathomimetics, dopaminergics, buspirone, pethidine and possibly other opioid analgesics. For other interactions see Appendix 1 (MAOIs)

Contra-indications see also Monoamine oxidase inhibition above

Breast-feeding manufacturer advises avoid—present in milk in animal studies

Side-effects diarrhoea (antibiotic-associated colitis reported), nausea, vomiting, taste disturbances, headache; *less commonly* thirst, dry mouth, glossitis, stomatitis, tongue discoloration, abdominal pain, dyspepsia, gastritis, constipation, pancreatitis, hypertension, fever, fatigue, dizziness, insomnia, hypoaesthesia, paraesthesia, tinnitus, polyuria, anaemia, leucopenia, thrombocytopenia, eosinophilia, electrolyte disturbances, blurred vision, rash, pruritus, diaphoresis, and injection-site reactions; *very rarely* renal failure, pancytopenia and Stevens-Johnson syndrome; also reported, lactic acidosis; peripheral and optic neuropathy reported on prolonged therapy

Licensed use not licensed for use in children

Indication and dose

Pneumonia, complicated skin and soft-tissue infections caused by Gram-positive bacteria (initiated under expert supervision)

- By mouth or by intravenous infusion over 30–120 minutes

Neonate under 7 days 10 mg/kg every 12 hours, increase to every 8 hours if poor response

Neonate over 7 days 10 mg/kg every 8 hours

Child 1 month–12 years 10 mg/kg (max. 600 mg) every 8 hours

Child 12–18 years 600 mg every 12 hours

Zyvox (Pharmacia) ▼ PoM

Tablets, f/c, linezolid 600 mg, net price 10-tab pack = £445.00. Label: 9, 10, patient information leaflet

Suspension, yellow, linezolid 100 mg/5 mL when reconstituted with water, net price 150 mL (orange-flavoured) = £222.50. Label: 9, 10 patient information leaflet

Excipients: include aspartame 20 mg/5 mL (section 9.4.1)

Intravenous infusion, linezolid 2 mg/mL, net price 300-mL *Excel*® bag = £44.50

Excipients: include Na^+ 5 mmol/300-mL bag, glucose 13.71 g/300-mL bag

Quinupristin and dalfopristin

A combination of the streptogramin antibiotics, **quinupristin** and **dalfopristin** (as *Synercid*®) is licensed in adults for infections due to Gram-positive bacteria; there is limited information on use in children and expert advice should be sought. The combination should be reserved for treating infections which have failed to respond to other antibacterials (e.g. meticillin-resistant *Staphylococcus aureus*, MRSA) or for patients who cannot be treated with other antibacterials. Quinupristin and dalfopristin are not active against *Enterococcus faecalis* and they need to be given in combination with other antibacterials for mixed infections which also involve Gram-negative organisms.

QUINUPRISTIN WITH DALFOPRISTIN

A mixture of quinupristin and dalfopristin (both as mesilate salts) in the proportions 3 parts to 7 parts

Cautions predisposition to cardiac arrhythmias (including congenital QT syndrome, concomitant use of drugs that prolong QT interval, cardiac hypertrophy, dilated cardiomyopathy, hypokalaemia, hypomagnesaemia, bradycardia); **interactions**: Appendix 1 (quinupristin with dalfopristin)

Hepatic impairment consider reducing dose to 5 mg/kg every 8 hours in moderate impairment, adjusted according to clinical response; avoid in severe hepatic impairment or if plasma-bilirubin concentration greater than 3 times upper limit of reference range

Pregnancy manufacturer advises avoid unless potential benefit outweighs risk—no information available

Contra-indications plasma-bilirubin concentration greater than 3 times upper limit of reference range

Breast-feeding manufacturer advises avoid—present in milk in *animal* studies

Side-effects nausea, vomiting, diarrhoea, headache, arthralgia, myalgia, asthenia, rash, pruritus, anaemia, leucopenia, eosinophilia, raised urea and creatinine; injection-site reactions on peripheral venous administration; less frequently oral candidiasis, stomatitis, constipation, abdominal pain, antibiotic-associated colitis, anorexia, peripheral oedema, hypotension, chest pain, arrhythmias, dyspnoea, hypersensitivity reactions (including anaphylaxis and urticaria), insomnia, anxiety, confusion, dizziness, paraesthesia, hypertonia, hepatitis, jaundice, pancreatitis, gout; also reported, thrombocytopenia, pancytopenia, electrolyte disturbances

Licensed use not licensed for use in children

QUINUPRISTIN WITH DALFOPRISTIN (*continued*)

Indication and dose

Serious Gram-positive infections where no alternative antibacterial is suitable including hospital-acquired pneumonia, skin and soft-tissue infections, infections due to vancomycin-resistant *Enterococcus faecium* Dose expressed as a combination of quinupristin and dalfopristin (in a ratio of 3:7)

- **By intravenous infusion into central vein**

  Child 1 month–18 years 7.5 mg/kg every 8 hours for 7 days in skin and soft-tissue infections; for 10 days in hospital-acquired pneumonia; duration of treatment in *E. faecium* infection depends on site of infection

Administration Reconstitute 500 mg with 5 mL water for injections or glucose 5%; gently swirl vial without shaking to dissolve; allow to stand for at least 2 minutes until foam disappears; *for intravenous infusion* dilute requisite dose with glucose 5% intravenous infusion to a concentration of 5 mg/mL and give over 60 minutes via central venous catheter. In an emergency, first dose may be diluted to 2 mg/mL and given over 60 minutes via peripheral line; flush line with glucose 5% before and after infusion; incompatible with sodium chloride solutions

Synercid® (Aventis Pharma) PoM

Intravenous infusion, powder for reconstitution, quinupristin (as mesilate) 150 mg, dalfopristin (as mesilate) 350 mg, net price 500-mg vial = £37.00

Electrolytes Na^+ approx. 16 mmol/500-mg vial

Polymyxins

The polymyxin antibiotic, **colistin**, is active against Gram-negative organisms, including *Pseudomonas aeruginosa.* It is **not** absorbed by mouth and thus needs to be given by injection to obtain a systemic effect; however, it is toxic and has few indications for systemic use except in the treatment of respiratory infections with multi-resistant organisms in cystic fibrosis.

Colistin is used by mouth in bowel sterilisation regimens in neutropenic patients (usually with nystatin); it is **not** recommended for gastro-intestinal infections. It is also given by inhalation of a nebulised solution as an adjunct to standard antibacterial therapy in patients with cystic fibrosis.

Both colistin and polymyxin B are included in some preparations for topical application.

COLISTIN

Cautions porphyria (section 9.8.2); risk of bronchospasm on inhalation—may be prevented or treated with a selective $beta_2$ agonist; **interactions:** Appendix 1 (polymyxins)

Renal impairment monitor plasma-colistin concentration during parenteral treatment in all grades of impairment. Reduce parenteral dose in moderate to severe impairment

Contra-indications myasthenia gravis

Pregnancy avoid—possible risk of fetal toxicity especially in 2nd and 3rd trimesters

Breast-feeding present in milk but poorly absorbed from gut; manufacturers advise avoid (or use only if potential benefit outweighs risk)

Side-effects neurotoxicity reported especially with excessive doses (including apnoea, perioral and peripheral paraesthesia, vertigo; rarely vasomotor instability, slurred speech, confusion, psychosis, visual disturbances); nephrotoxicity; hypersensitivity reactions including rash; injection-site reactions; inhalation may cause sore throat, sore mouth, cough, bronchospasm

Pharmacokinetics see notes above; plasma concentration monitoring required for intravenous treatment in renal impairment and cystic fibrosis; recommended 'peak' plasma-colistin concentration (approx. 30 minutes after intravenous injection or infusion) 10–15 mg/litre (125–200 units/mL); colistin sulphate may be absorbed from the gastro-intestinal tract in infants under 6 months old

Indication and dose

Pseudomonas aeruginosa infection in cystic fibrosis

- **By intravenous injection into a totally implantable venous access device, or by intravenous infusion (but see notes above)**

  Child 1 month–18 years

  Body-weight under 60 kg 16 666–25 000 units/kg every 8 hours

  Body-weight over 60 kg 1–2 million units every 8 hours

- **By inhalation of nebulised solution**

  Child 1 month–2 years 500 000–1 million units twice daily

  Child 2–18 years 1–2 million units twice daily

Administration For *intravenous infusion*, dilute to a concentration of 40 000 units/mL with Sodium Chloride 0.9%; give over 30 minutes

For *slow intravenous injection* into a totally implantable venous access device, dilute to a concentration of 90 000 units/mL for child under 12 years (200 000 units/mL for child over 12 years)

For *nebulisation* administer required dose in 2–4 mL of sodium chloride 0.9% (or water for

COLISTIN (*continued*)

injections). Colistin must not be mixed with tobramycin as they are chemically unstable together; it may be mixed with gentamicin if used immediately

Colomycin® (Forest) PoM
Injection, powder for reconstitution, colistimethate sodium (colistin sulphomethate sodium). Net price 500 000-unit vial = £1.14; 1 million-unit vial = £1.68; 2 million-unit vial = £3.09
Electrolytes (before reconstitution) Na^+ < 0.5 mmol/500 000-unit, 1 million-unit, and 2 million-unit vial
Note *Colomycin®* Injection (dissolved in physiological saline) may be used for nebulisation

Promixin® (Profile) PoM
Powder for nebuliser solution, colistimethate sodium (colistin sulphomethate sodium), net price 1 million-unit vial = £4.60.

Injection, powder for reconstitution, colistimethate sodium (colistin sulphomethate sodium), net price 1 million unit-vial = £2.30
Electrolytes (before reconstitution) Na^+ < 0.5 mmol/1 million-unit vial

5.1.8 Sulphonamides and trimethoprim

The importance of the sulphonamides has decreased as a result of increasing bacterial resistance and their replacement by antibacterials which are generally more active and less toxic.

Sulfamethoxazole (sulphamethoxazole) and trimethoprim are used in combination (as **co-trimoxazole**) because of their synergistic activity. However, co-trimoxazole is associated with rare but serious side-effects e.g. Stevens-Johnson syndrome and blood dyscrasias, notably bone marrow depression and agranulocytosis (see CSM recommendations below). Co-trimoxazole should be avoided in children less than 6 weeks of age (except for treatment and prophylaxis of *pneumocystis pneumonia*) because of the risk of kernicterus. There is a risk of haemolytic anaemia if used in children with glucose-6-phosphate dehydrogenase (G6PD) deficiency (section 9.1.5).

CSM recommendations. Co-trimoxazole should be limited to the role of drug of choice in *Pneumocystis jiroveci* (*Pneumocystis carinii*) pneumonia; it is also indicated for *toxoplasmosis* and *nocardiasis.* It should now only be considered for use in *acute exacerbations of chronic bronchitis* and *infections of the urinary tract* when there is good bacteriological evidence of sensitivity to co-trimoxazole and good reason to prefer this combination to a single antibacterial; similarly it should only be used in *acute otitis media in children* when there is good reason to prefer it.

Trimethoprim can be used alone for urinary- and respiratory-tract infections and for shigellosis and invasive salmonella infections. Trimethoprim has side-effects similar to co-trimoxazole but they are less severe and occur less frequently.

For *topical preparations* of sulphonamides used in the treatment of burns see section 13.10.1.1.

CO-TRIMOXAZOLE

A mixture of trimethoprim and sulfamethoxazole in the proportions of 1 part to 5 parts

Cautions maintain adequate fluid intake; avoid in blood disorders (unless under specialist supervision); monitor blood counts on prolonged treatment; discontinue immediately if blood disorders or rash develop; predisposition to folate deficiency; asthma; G6PD deficiency (section 9.1.5); avoid in infants under 6 weeks (except for treatment or prophylaxis of pneumocystis pneumonia); **interactions:** Appendix 1 (trimethoprim, sulfamethoxazole)

Hepatic impairment manufacturer advises avoid in severe liver disease

Renal impairment use half normal dose if creatinine clearance 15–30 mL/minute/1.73m²; avoid if creatinine clearance less than 15 mL/minute/1.73m² and if plasma-sulfamethoxazole concentration cannot be monitored

Pregnancy teratogenic risk (trimethoprim a folate antagonist) in first trimester neonatal haemolysis and methaemoglobinaemia in 3rd trimester; fear of increased risk of kernicterus in neonates appears to be unfounded

Breast-feeding small risk of kernicterus in jaundiced infants and of haemolysis in G6PD-deficient infants (due to sulfamethoxazole)

Contra-indications porphyria (section 9.8.2)

Side-effects nausea, diarrhoea; headache; rash (*very rarely* including Stevens-Johnson syndrome, toxic epidermal necrolysis, photosensitivity)—discontinue immediately; *less commonly* vomiting; *very rarely* glossitis, stomatitis, anorexia, liver damage (including jaundice and hepatic necrosis), pancreatitis, antibiotic-associated colitis, myocarditis, cough and shortness of breath, pulmonary infiltrates, aseptic meningitis, depression, convulsions, peripheral neuropathy,

CO-TRIMOXAZOLE (*continued*)

ataxia, tinnitus, vertigo, hallucinations, hypoglycaemia, blood disorders (including leucopenia, thrombocytopenia, megaloblastic anaemia, eosinophilia), hyperkalaemia, hyponatraemia, renal disorders including interstitial nephritis, arthralgia, myalgia, vasculitis, and systemic lupus erythematosus

Pharmacokinetics plasma concentration monitoring may be required with high doses or during moderate to severe renal impairment; seek expert advice

Licensed use not licensed for use in children under 6 weeks

Indication and dose

Treatment of general infections (but see notes above) dose expressed as co-trimoxazole

- **By mouth**

  Child 6 weeks–12 years 24 mg/kg twice daily *or*

  Child 6 weeks–6 months 120 mg twice daily

  Child 6 months–6 years 240 mg twice daily

  Child 6–12 years 480 mg twice daily

  Child 12–18 years 960 mg twice daily

- **By intravenous infusion**

  Child 6 weeks–18 years 18 mg/kg every 12 hours; increased in severe infection to 27 mg/kg (max. 1.44 g) every 12 hours

Treatment of *Pneumocystis jiroveci* (*P. carinii*) infections (undertaken where facilities for appropriate monitoring available—consult microbiologist and product literature)

- **By mouth or by intravenous infusion**

  Child 1 month–18 years 60 mg/kg every 12 hours for 14 days; total daily dose may alternatively be given in 3–4 divided doses

  Note oral route preferred

Prophylaxis of *Pneumocystis jiroveci* (*P. carinii*) infections

- **By mouth**

  Child 1 month–18 years 450 mg/m^2 (max 960 mg) twice daily for three days of the week (either consecutively or on alternate days)

  Note dose regimens may vary, consult local guidelines

Note 480 mg of co-trimoxazole consists of sulfamethoxazole 400 mg and trimethoprim 80 mg

Administration for intermittent intravenous infusion may be further diluted in glucose 5% and 10% or sodium chloride 0.9% or Ringer's intravenous solution. Dilute contents of 1 ampoule (5 mL) to 125 mL, 2 ampoules (10 mL) to 250 mL or 3 ampoules (15 mL) to 500 mL; suggested duration of infusion 60–90 minutes (but may be adjusted according to fluid requirements); if fluid restriction necessary, 1 ampoule (5 mL) may be diluted with 75 mL glucose 5% and the required dose infused over max. 60 minutes; check container for haze or precipitant during administration. In severe fluid restriction may be given undiluted via a central venous line

Co-trimoxazole (Non-proprietary) PoM

Tablets, co-trimoxazole 480 mg, net price 28-tab pack = £5.19; 960 mg, 20 = £4.69. Label: 9
Brands include *Fectrim®*, *Fectrim® Forte*

Paediatric oral suspension, co-trimoxazole 240 mg/5 mL, net price 100 mL = £1.12. Label: 9

Oral suspension, co-trimoxazole 480 mg/5 mL. Net price 100 mL = £4.41. Label: 9

Strong sterile solution, co-trimoxazole 96 mg/mL. For dilution and use as an intravenous infusion. Net price 5-mL amp = £1.58, 10-mL amp = £3.06

Septrin® (GSK) PoM

Tablets, co-trimoxazole 480 mg. Net price 20 = £3.10. Label: 9

Forte tablets, scored, co-trimoxazole 960 mg. Net price 20 = £4.69. Label: 9

Adult suspension, co-trimoxazole 480 mg/5 mL. Net price 100 mL (vanilla-flavoured) = £4.41. Label: 9

Paediatric suspension, sugar-free, co-trimoxazole 240 mg/5 mL. Net price 100 mL (banana- and vanilla-flavoured) = £2.45. Label: 9

Intravenous infusion, co-trimoxazole 96 mg/mL. To be diluted before use. Net price 5-mL amp = £1.48

Excipients: include propylene glycol, sulphites

TRIMETHOPRIM

Cautions predisposition to folate deficiency; manufacturer recommends blood counts on long-term therapy (but evidence of practical value unsatisfactory); neonates (specialist supervision required); porphyria (section 9.8.2); **interactions:** Appendix 1 (trimethoprim)

Renal impairment use half normal dose after 3 days if creatinine clearance 15–30 mL/minute/1.73 m^2; use half normal dose immediately if creatinine clearance less than 15 mL/minute/1.73 m^2 (monitor plasma-trimethoprim concentration if creatinine clearance less than 10 mL/minute/1.73 m^2)

Breast-feeding present in milk—short-term use not known to be harmful

Blood disorders On long-term treatment, patients and their carers should be told how to recognise signs of blood disorders and advised to seek immediate medical attention if symptoms such as fever, sore throat, rash, mouth ulcers, purpura, bruising or bleeding develop

Contra-indications blood dyscrasias

Pregnancy teratogenic risk (folate antagonist) in first trimester; manufacturers advise avoid

TRIMETHOPRIM (*continued*)

Side-effects gastro-intestinal disturbances including nausea and vomiting, pruritus, rashes, hyperkalaemia, depression of haematopoiesis; rarely erythema multiforme, toxic epidermal necrolysis, photosensitivity and other allergic reactions including angioedema and anaphylaxis; aseptic meningitis reported

Licensed use not licensed for use in children under 6 weeks

Indication and dose

Urinary-tract infections; respiratory-tract infections
- By mouth

Neonate initially 3 mg/kg as a single dose then 1–2mg/kg twice daily

Child 1 month–18 years 4 mg/kg (max. 200 mg) twice daily

Chronic infections; prophylaxis of urinary tract infection
- By mouth

Neonate 2 mg/kg once daily at night

Child 1 month–12 years 2 mg/kg (max. 100 mg) once daily at night

Child 12–18 years 100 mg once daily at night

Pneumocystis pneumonia, p. 390

Trimethoprim (Non-proprietary) PoM

Tablets, trimethoprim 100 mg, net price 20 = 73p; 200 mg, 14-tab pack = 99p. Label: 9

Brands include *Trimopan®*

Suspension, trimethoprim 50 mg/5 mL, net price 100 mL = £1.77. Label: 9

5.1.9 Antituberculous drugs

Tuberculosis is treated in two phases—an *initial phase* using 4 drugs and a *continuation phase* using two drugs in fully sensitive cases. Treatment requires specialised knowledge, particularly where the disease involves resistant organisms or non-respiratory organs.

The regimens given below are recommended for the treatment of tuberculosis in the UK; variations occur in other countries. Either the unsupervised regimen or the supervised regimen described below should be used; the two regimens should **not** be used concurrently. Compliance with therapy is a major determinant of its success. Treatment needs to be carefully monitored in families in whom concordance may be problematic.

Initial phase The concurrent use of 4 drugs during the initial phase is designed to reduce the bacterial population as rapidly as possible and to prevent the emergence of drug-resistant bacteria. The drugs are best given as combination preparations, provided the respective dose of each drug is appropriate, unless the child is unable to swallow the tablets or one of the components cannot be given because of resistance or intolerance. The treatment of choice for the initial phase is the daily use of isoniazid, rifampicin, pyrazinamide and ethambutol. However, care is needed in young children receiving ethambutol because of the difficulty in testing eyesight and in obtaining reports of visual symptoms (see below). Streptomycin is rarely used in the UK although it may be used in the initial phase of treatment if resistance to isoniazid has been established before therapy is commenced and ethambutol is contra-indicated. Treatment should be started without waiting for culture results if clinical features, or histology results are consistent with tuberculosis; treatment should be continued even if culture results are negative. The initial phase drugs should be continued for 2 months. Where a positive culture for *M. tuberculosis* has been obtained, but susceptibility results are not available after 2 months, treatment with pyrazinamide and ethambutol should be continued until full susceptibility is confirmed, even if this is for longer than 2 months.

Continuation phase After the initial phase, treatment is continued for a further 4 months with isoniazid and rifampicin (preferably given as a combination preparation). Longer treatment is necessary for meningitis, direct spinal cord involvement, and for resistant organisms which may also require modification of the regimen.

Unsupervised treatment The following regimen should be used for those who are likely to take antituberculous drugs reliably **without supervision**. Children and families who are unlikely to comply with daily administration of antituberculous drugs should be treated with the regimen described under Supervised Treatment.

Recommended dosage for standard unsupervised 6-month treatment

Isoniazid (for 2-month initial and 4-month continuation phases)
Child 1 month–18 years 5–10 mg/kg (max. 300 mg) once daily

Rifampicin (for 2-month initial and 4–month continuation phase)
Child 1 month–18 years 10 mg/kg once daily (max. 450 mg if body-weight under 50 kg; if body-weight 50 kg and over max. 600 mg)

Pyrazinamide (for 2-month initial phase only)
Child 1 month–18 years 35 mg/kg once daily (max. 1.5 g if body-weight under 50 kg; if body-weight 50 kg and over max. 2 g)

Ethambutol (for 2-month initial phase only)
Child 1 month–18 years 15 mg/kg once daily

Note In general, doses should be rounded up to facilitate administration of suitable volumes of liquid or an appropriate strength of tablet. The exception is ethambutol due to the risk of toxicity. Doses may also need to be recalculated to allow for weight gain in younger children.
The fixed-dose combination preparations (*Rifater*®, *Rifinah*®, *Rimactazid*®) are unlicensed for use in children. Consideration may be given to use of these preparations in older children, provided the respective dose of each drug is appropriate for the weight of the child.

Pregnancy and breast-feeding The standard regimen (above) may be used during pregnancy and breast-feeding. Streptomycin should not be given in pregnancy.

Neonates Congenital tuberculosis is acquired from maternal extrapulmonary sites at birth, particularly the genital tract; if infection is suspected, the baby will require treatment with isoniazid 10 mg/kg once daily, rifampicin 10 mg/kg once daily, pyrazinamide 35 mg/kg once daily, and ethambutol 15 mg/kg once daily.

Supervised treatment Drug administration needs to be **fully supervised** (directly observed therapy, DOT) in children or families who cannot comply reliably with the treatment regimen. These patients are given isoniazid, rifampicin, pyrazinamide and ethambutol (or streptomycin) 3 times a week under supervision for the first 2 months followed by isoniazid and rifampicin 3 times a week for a further 4 months.

Recommended dosage for intermittent supervised 6-month treatment

Isoniazid (for 2-month initial and 4-month continuation phases)
Child 1 month–18 years, 15 mg/kg (max. 900 mg) 3 times a week

Rifampicin (for 2-month initial and 4-month continuation phases)
Child 1 month–18 years, 15 mg/kg (max. 900 mg) 3 times a week

Pyrazinamide (for 2-month initial phase only)
Child 1 month–18 years, 50 mg/kg (max. 2 g 3 times a week if body-weight under 50 kg; max. 2.5 g 3 times a week if body-weight 50 kg and over)

Ethambutol (for 2-month initial phase only)
Child 1 month–18 years, 30 mg/kg 3 times a week

Note In general, doses should be rounded up to facilitate administration of suitable volumes of liquid or an appropriate strength of tablet. The exception is ethambutol due to the risk of toxicity. Doses may also need to be recalculated to allow for weight gain in younger children.
The fixed-dose combination preparations (*Rifater*®, *Rifinah*®, *Rimactazid*®) are unlicensed for use in children. Consideration may be given to use of these preparations in older children, provided the respective dose of each drug is appropriate for the weight of the child.

Immunocompromised patients Multi-resistant *Mycobacterium tuberculosis* may be present in immunocompromised children. The organism should always be cultured to confirm its type and drug sensitivity. Confirmed *M. tuberculosis* infection sensitive to first-line drugs should be treated with a standard 6-month regimen; after completing treatment, children should be closely monitored. The regimen may need to be modified if infection is caused by resistant organisms, and specialist advice is needed.

Specialist advice should be sought about tuberculosis treatment or chemoprophylaxis in a HIV-positive individual; care is required in choosing the regimen and in avoiding potentially hazardous interactions. Starting antiretroviral treatment in the first 2 months of antituberculosis treatment increases the risk of immune reconstitution syndrome.

Infection may also be caused by other mycobacteria e.g. *M. avium* complex in which case specialist advice on management is needed.

Corticosteroids A corticosteroid should be given (in addition to antituberculosis therapy) for meningeal or pericardial tuberculosis.

Prevention of tuberculosis Chemoprophylaxis may be required in children who are close contacts of a case of smear-positive pulmonary tuberculosis and who are severely immunosuppressed (including congenital immunodeficiencies, cytotoxic or immunosuppressive therapy) and in those who have evidence of latent tuberculosis and require treatment with immunosuppressants; expert advice should be sought.

Chemoprophylaxis involves use of either isoniazid alone for 6 months or of isoniazid and rifampicin for 3 months (see Table 2, section 5.1).

For prevention of tuberculosis in susceptible close contacts or those who have become tuberculin-positive, see Table 2, section 5.1. For advice on immunisation against tuberculosis and tuberculin testing, see section 14.4.

Monitoring Since isoniazid, rifampicin and pyrazinamide are associated with liver toxicity (see Appendix 2), *hepatic function* should be checked before treatment with these drugs. Those with pre-existing liver disease should have frequent checks particularly in the first 2 months. If there is no evidence of liver disease (and pre-treatment liver function is normal), further checks are only necessary if the patient develops fever, malaise, vomiting, jaundice or unexplained deterioration during treatment. In view of the need to comply fully with antituberculous treatment on the one hand and to guard against serious liver damage on the other, children and their carers should be informed carefully how to recognise signs of liver disorders and advised to discontinue treatment and seek **immediate** medical attention should symptoms of liver disease occur.

Renal function should be checked before treatment with antituberculous drugs and appropriate dosage adjustments made. Streptomycin or ethambutol should preferably be avoided in patients with renal impairment, but if used, the dose should be reduced and the plasma-drug concentration monitored.

Visual acuity should be tested before ethambutol is used (see below).

Major causes of treatment failure are incorrect prescribing by the physician and inadequate compliance by the child or their carer. Monthly tablet counts and urine examination (rifampicin imparts an orange-red coloration) may be useful indicators of compliance with treatment. Avoid both excessive and inadequate dosage. Treatment should be supervised by a specialist paediatrician.

Isoniazid is cheap and highly effective. Like rifampicin it should always be included in any antituberculous regimen unless there is a specific contra-indication. Its only common side-effect is peripheral neuropathy which is more likely to occur where there are pre-existing risk factors such as diabetes, chronic renal failure, malnutrition and HIV infection. In these circumstances, and in breast-fed infants treated with isoniazid, pyridoxine (section 9.6.2) should be given prophylactically from the start of treatment. Other side-effects such as hepatitis (important: see Monitoring above) and psychosis are rare.

Rifampicin, a rifamycin, is a key component of any antituberculous regimen. Like isoniazid it should always be included unless there is a specific contra-indication.

During the first two months ('initial phase') of rifampicin administration transient disturbance of liver function with elevated serum transaminases is common but generally does not require interruption of treatment. Occasionally more serious liver toxicity requires a change of treatment particularly in those with pre-existing liver disease (important: see Monitoring above).

On intermittent treatment six toxicity syndromes have been recognised—influenza-like, abdominal, and respiratory symptoms, shock, renal failure, and thrombocytopenic purpura—and can occur in 20 to 30% of patients.

Rifampicin induces hepatic enzymes which accelerate the metabolism of several drugs including oestrogens, corticosteroids, phenytoin, sulphonylureas, and anticoagulants; **interactions**: Appendix 1 (rifamycins). **Important**: the effectiveness of hormonal contraceptives is reduced and alternative family planning advice should be offered.

Rifabutin is indicated in adults for *prophylaxis* against *M. avium* complex infections in patients with a low CD4 count; it is also licensed in adults for the *treatment* of non-tuberculous mycobacterial disease and pulmonary tuberculosis. There is limited experience in children. As with rifampicin it induces hepatic enzymes and the effectiveness of hormonal contraceptives is reduced requiring alternative family planning methods.

Pyrazinamide is a bactericidal drug only active against intracellular dividing forms of *Mycobacterium tuberculosis*; it exerts its main effect only in the first two or three months. It is particularly useful in tuberculous meningitis because of good meningeal penetration. It is not active against *M. bovis*. Serious liver toxicity may occasionally occur (important: see Monitoring above).

Ethambutol is included in a treatment regimen if isoniazid resistance is suspected; it can be omitted if the risk of resistance is low.

Side-effects of ethambutol are largely confined to visual disturbances in the form of loss of acuity, colour blindness, and restriction of visual fields. These toxic effects are more common where excessive dosage is used or if the child's renal function is impaired. The earliest features of ocular toxicity are subjective and children and their carers should be advised to discontinue therapy immediately if deterioration in vision develops and promptly seek further advice. Early discontinuation of the drug is almost always followed by recovery of eyesight. Those who cannot understand warnings about visual side-effects should, if possible, be given an alternative drug. In particular, ethambutol should be used with caution in children until they are at least 5 years old and capable of reporting symptomatic visual changes accurately.

Where possible visual acuity should be tested by Snellen chart before treatment with ethambutol.

Streptomycin is now rarely used in the UK except for resistant organisms. Plasma-drug concentration should be measured in patients with impaired renal function in whom streptomycin must be used with great care. Side-effects increase after a cumulative dose of 100 g, which should only be exceeded in exceptional circumstances.

Drug-resistant tuberculosis should be treated by a specialist paediatrician with experience in such cases, and where appropriate facilities for infection-control exist. Second-line drugs available for infections caused by resistant organisms, or when first-line drugs cause unacceptable side-effects, include amikacin, capreomycin, cycloserine, newer macrolides (e.g. azithromycin and clarithromycin), quinolones (e.g. moxifloxacin) and protionamide (prothionamide) (no longer on UK market). Availability of suitable formulations may limit choice in children.

CYCLOSERINE

Cautions monitor haematological, renal, and hepatic function; **interactions:** Appendix 1 (cycloserine)

Renal impairment reduce dose in mild to moderate renal impairment; avoid in severe renal impairment

Pregnancy manufacturer advises use only if potential benefit outweighs risk—crosses the placenta

Breast-feeding present in milk—amount too small to be harmful

Contra-indications epilepsy, depression, severe anxiety, psychotic states, alcohol dependence, porphyria (section 9.8.2)

Side-effects mainly neurological, including headache, dizziness, vertigo, drowsiness, tremor, convulsions, confusion, psychosis, depression (discontinue or reduce dose if symptoms of CNS toxicity); rashes, allergic dermatitis (discontinue or reduce dose); megaloblastic anaemia; changes in liver function tests; heart failure at high doses reported

Pharmacokinetics blood concentration should not exceed a peak concentration of 30 mg/litre (measured 3–4 hours after the dose); penetrates CNS

Licensed use licensed for use in children (age range not specified by manufacturer)

CYCLOSERINE (*continued*)

Indication and dose

Tuberculosis resistant to first-line drugs, used in combination with other drugs

- By mouth

  Child 2–12 years initially 5 mg/kg twice daily, adjusted according to blood concentration and response

  Child 12–18 years initially 250 mg twice daily for 2 weeks adjusted according to blood concentration and response to max. 500 mg twice daily

Cycloserine (King) PoM

Capsules, red/grey cycloserine 250 mg, net price 100-cap pack = £220.69. Label: 2, 8

ETHAMBUTOL HYDROCHLORIDE

Cautions test visual acuity before treatment and warn patients to report visual changes—see notes above; young children (see notes above)—routine ophthalmological monitoring recommended

Renal impairment reduce dose; if creatinine clearance less than 30 mL/minute/1.73m^2 monitor plasma-ethambutol concentration; risk of optic nerve damage

Pregnancy not known to be harmful; see notes above

Breast-feeding amount too small to be harmful

Contra-indications optic neuritis, poor vision

Side-effects optic neuritis, red/green colour blindness, peripheral neuritis, rarely rash, pruritus, urticaria, thrombocytopenia

Pharmacokinetics 'peak' concentration (2–2.5 hours after dose) should be 2–6 mg/litre (7–22 micromol/litre); 'trough' (pre-dose) concentration should be less than 1 mg/litre (4 micromol/litre); for advice on laboratory assay of ethambutol contact the Poisons Unit at New Cross Hospital (Tel (020) 7771 5360)

Indication and dose

Tuberculosis, used in combination with other drugs see notes above

Ethambutol (Non-proprietary) PoM

Tablets, ethambutol hydrochloride 100 mg (yellow), net price 56-tab pack = £11.50; 400 mg (grey), 56-tab pack = £42.73. Label: 8

Extemporaneous formulations available see Extemporaneous Preparations, p. 8

ISONIAZID

Cautions slow acetylator status (increased risk of side-effects); epilepsy; history of psychosis; alcohol dependence, malnutrition, diabetes mellitus, HIV infection (risk of peripheral neuritis); porphyria (section 9.8.2); **interactions:** Appendix 1 (isoniazid)

Hepatic impairment use with caution; monitor liver function regularly and particularly frequently in the first 2 months

Renal impairment reduce dose in severe renal impairment; risk of peripheral neuropathy

Pregnancy not known to be harmful; see notes above

Breast-feeding monitor infant for possible toxicity; theoretical risk of convulsions and neuropathy; prophylactic pyridoxine advisable in mother and infant

Hepatic disorders Children and their carers should be told how to recognise signs of liver disorder, and advised to discontinue treatment and seek immediate medical attention if symptoms such as persistent nausea, vomiting, malaise or jaundice develop

Contra-indications drug-induced liver disease

Side-effects nausea, vomiting, constipation, dry mouth; peripheral neuritis with high doses (pyridoxine prophylaxis, see notes above), optic neuritis, convulsions, psychotic episodes, vertigo; hypersensitivity reactions including fever, erythema multiforme, purpura; blood disorders including agranulocytosis, haemolytic anaemia, aplastic anaemia; hepatitis; systemic lupus erythematosus-like syndrome, pellagra, hyperreflexia, difficulty with micturition, hyperglycaemia, and gynaecomastia reported

Indication and dose

Tuberculosis, used in combination with other drugs see notes above

Isoniazid (Non-proprietary) PoM

Tablets, isoniazid 50 mg, net price 56-tab pack = £5.78; 100 mg, 28-tab pack = £5.77. Label: 8, 22

Injection, isoniazid 25 mg/mL, net price 2-mL amp = £7.39

Extemporaneous formulations available see Extemporaneous Preparations, p. 8

PYRAZINAMIDE

Cautions diabetes; **interactions:** Appendix 1 (pyrazinamide)

Hepatic disorders Children and their carers should be told how to recognise signs of liver disorder, and advised to discontinue treatment and seek immediate medical attention if symptoms such as persistent nausea, vomiting, malaise or jaundice develop

Hepatic impairment monitor hepatic function—idiosyncratic hepatotoxicity more common; avoid in severe hepatic impairment

Pregnancy manufacturer advises use only if potential benefit outweighs risk; see also notes above

Breast-feeding amount too small to be harmful

Contra-indications porphyria (section 9.8.2)

Side-effects hepatotoxicity including fever, anorexia, hepatomegaly, splenomegaly, jaundice, liver failure; nausea, vomiting, dysuria, arthralgia,

PYRAZINAMIDE (*continued*)

sideroblastic anaemia, rash and occasionally photosensitivity

Licensed use not licensed

Indication and dose

Tuberculosis in combination with other drugs
see notes above

Pyrazinamide (Non-proprietary) PoM
Tablets, scored, pyrazinamide 500 mg. Label: 8
Available on named-patient basis from specialist importing companies

Extemporaneous formulations available see Extemporaneous Preparations, p. 8

RIFABUTIN

Cautions see under Rifampicin; porphyria (section 9.8.2)

Hepatic impairment reduce dose in severe hepatic impairment

Renal impairment use half normal dose if creatinine clearance less than 30 mL/minute/1.73m^2

Pregnancy manufacturer advises avoid—no information available

Breast-feeding manufacturer advises avoid—no information available

Side-effects nausea, vomiting; leucopenia, thrombocytopenia, anaemia, rarely haemolysis; raised liver enzymes, jaundice, rarely hepatitis; uveitis following high doses or administration with drugs which raise plasma concentration—see also **interactions:** Appendix 1 (rifamycins); arthralgia, myalgia, influenza-like syndrome, dyspnoea; also hypersensitivity reactions including fever, rash, eosinophilia, bronchospasm, shock; skin, urine, saliva and other body secretions coloured orange-red; asymptomatic corneal opacities reported with long-term use

Licensed use not licensed for use in children

Indication and dose

Prophylaxis of *Mycobacterium avium* complex infections in immunosuppressed patients with low CD4 count (see product literature) Also see notes above
- By mouth
  Child 1–12 years 5 mg/kg (max. 300 mg) once daily
  Child 12–18 years 300 mg once daily

Treatment of non-tuberculous mycobacterial disease, in combination with other drugs
- By mouth
  Child 1month–12 years 5 mg/kg once daily for up to 6 months after cultures negative
  Child 12–18 years 450–600 mg once daily for up to 6 months after cultures negative

Treatment of pulmonary tuberculosis, in combination with other drugs
- By mouth
  Child 12–18years 150–450 mg once daily for at least 6 months

Mycobutin® (Pharmacia) PoM
Capsules, red-brown, rifabutin 150 mg. Net price 30-cap pack = £90.38. Label: 8, 14, counselling, lenses, see under Rifampicin

Extemporaneous formulations available see Extemporaneous Preparations, p. 8

RIFAMPICIN

Cautions liver function tests and blood counts in hepatic disorders, and on prolonged therapy, see also below; porphyria (section 9.8.2); **important:** advise those on oral contraceptives to use additional means; discolours soft contact lenses; see also notes above; **interactions:** Appendix 1 (rifamycins)

Note If treatment interrupted re-introduce with low dosage and increase gradually; discontinue permanently if serious side-effects develop

Hepatic disorders Children and their carers should be told how to recognise signs of liver disorder, and advised to discontinue treatment and seek immediate medical attention if symptoms such as persistent nausea, vomiting, malaise or jaundice develop

Hepatic impairment impaired elimination; monitor liver function; avoid or do not exceed 8 mg/kg daily

Pregnancy manufacturers advise very high doses teratogenic in *animal* studies in 3rd trimester; risk of neonatal bleeding may be increased; see also notes above

Breast-feeding amount too small to be harmful

Contra-indications jaundice

Side-effects gastro-intestinal symptoms including anorexia, nausea, vomiting, diarrhoea (antibiotic-associated colitis reported); headache, drowsiness; those occurring mainly on intermittent therapy include influenza-like symptoms (with chills, fever, dizziness, bone pain), respiratory symptoms (including shortness of breath), collapse and shock, haemolytic anaemia, acute renal failure, and thrombocytopenic purpura; alterations of liver function, jaundice; flushing, urticaria, and rashes; other side-effects reported include oedema, muscular weakness and myopathy, exfoliative dermatitis, toxic epidermal necrolysis, pemphigoid reactions, leucopenia, eosinophilia, menstrual disturbances; urine, saliva, and other body secretions coloured

RIFAMPICIN (*continued*)

orange-red; thrombophlebitis reported if infusion used for prolonged period

Licensed use not licensed for use in children for pruritus due to cholestasis

Indication and dose

Tuberculosis, in combination with other drugs see notes above

Prophylaxis of meningococcal meningitis and *Haemophilus influenzae* (type b) infection Table 2, section 5.1

Brucellosis, legionnaires disease, serious staphylococcal infections, in combination with other antibacterials
- By mouth or by intravenous infusion

Neonates 5–10 mg/kg twice daily

Child 1 month–1 year 5–10 mg/kg twice daily

Child 1–18 years 10 mg/kg (max. 600 mg) twice daily

Pruritus due to cholestasis
- By mouth or by intravenous infusion

Child 1 month–18 years 5–10 mg/kg (max. 600 mg) once daily

Administration Owing to risk of contact sensitisation care must be taken to avoid contact during preparation and infusion. Displacement value may be significant, consult local reconstitution guidelines; reconstitute with solvent provided. May be further diluted with glucose 5% and 10% or sodium chloride 0.9% or Ringer's solution to a final concentration of 1.2 mg/mL; in fluid restricted patients up to 6 mg/mL may be used. Infuse over 2–3 hours.

Rifampicin (Non-proprietary) PoM
Capsules, rifampicin 150 mg, net price 20 = £5.27; 300 mg, 20 = £10.16. Label: 8, 14, 22, counselling, see contact lenses above

Rifadin® (Aventis Pharma) PoM
Capsules, rifampicin 150 mg (blue/red), net price 20 = £3.81; 300 mg (red), 20 = £7.62. Label: 8, 14, 22, counselling, see contact lenses above

Syrup, red, rifampicin 100 mg/5 mL (raspberry-flavoured). Net price 120 mL = £3.70. Label: 8, 14, 22, counselling, see contact lenses above
Excipients: include sucrose

Intravenous infusion, powder for reconstitution, rifampicin. Net price 600-mg vial (with solvent) = £7.98
Electrolytes Na^{+} < 0.5 mmol/vial

Rimactane® (Sandoz) PoM
Capsules, rifampicin 150 mg (red), net price 60-cap pack = £11.35; 300 mg (red/brown), 60-cap pack = £22.69. Label: 8, 14, 22, counselling, see contact lenses above

Combined preparations
See notes above

Rifater® (Aventis Pharma) PoM
Tablets, pink, s/c, rifampicin 120 mg, isoniazid 50 mg, pyrazinamide 300 mg. Net price 20 = £4.39. Label: 8, 14, 22, counselling, see contact lenses above

Rifinah 150® (Aventis Pharma) PoM
Tablets, pink, s/c, rifampicin 150 mg, isoniazid 100 mg, net price 84-tab pack = £16.55. Label: 8, 14, 22, counselling, see contact lenses above

Rifinah 300® (Aventis Pharma) PoM
Tablets, orange, s/c, rifampicin 300 mg, isoniazid 150 mg, net price 56-tab pack = £21.87. Label: 8, 14, 22, counselling, see contact lenses above

Rimactazid 300® (Sandoz) PoM
Tablets, orange, s/c, rifampicin 300 mg, isoniazid 150 mg, net price 60-tab pack = £38.77. Label: 8, 14, 22, counselling, see contact lenses above

STREPTOMYCIN

Cautions see under Aminoglycosides, section 5.1.4; measure plasma-concentration in renal impairment; **interactions:** Appendix 1 (aminoglycosides)

Contra-indications see under Aminoglycosides, section 5.1.4

Side-effects see under Aminoglycosides, section 5.1.4; also hypersensitivity reactions, paraesthesia of mouth

Pharmacokinetics one-hour ('peak') concentration should be 15–40 mg/litre; pre-dose ('trough') concentration should be less than 5 mg/litre (less than 1 mg/litre in renal impairment)

Licensed use not licensed for use in children

Indication and dose

Tuberculosis, resistant to other treatment, in combination with other drugs
- By deep intramuscular injection

Child 1 month–18 years 20–30 mg/kg (max. 1 g) once daily

Adjunct to doxycycline in brucellosis, expert advice essential
- By deep intramuscular injection

Child 1 month–18 years 5–10 mg/kg every 6 hours; total daily dose may alternatively be given in 2–3 divided doses

Streptomycin Sulphate (Non-proprietary) PoM
Injection, powder for reconstitution, streptomycin (as sulphate), net price 1-g vial = £8.25
Available on named-patient basis from Celltech

5.1.10 Antileprotic drugs

Classification not used in BNF for children.

5.1.11 Metronidazole

Metronidazole is an antimicrobial drug with high activity against anaerobic bacteria and protozoa. It is also used for surgical and gynaecological sepsis in which its activity against colonic anaerobes, especially *Bacteroides fragilis*, is important. Metronidazole is also effective in the treatment of antibiotic-associated colitis (pseudomembranous colitis, see also section 1.5). Metronidazole is well absorbed orally and the intravenous route is normally reserved for severe infections. Metronidazole by the rectal route is an effective alternative to the intravenous route when oral administration is not possible. Intravenous metronidazole is used for the treatment of established cases of tetanus; diazepam (section 10.2.2) and tetanus immunoglobulin (section 14.5) are also used.

Topical metronidazole (section 13.10.1.2) reduces the odour produced by anaerobic bacteria in fungating tumours; it is also used in the management of rosacea (section 13.6).

Oral infections Metronidazole is an alternative to a penicillin for the treatment of many oral infections where the patient is allergic to penicillin or the infection is due to beta-lactamase-producing anaerobes (Table 1, section 5.1). It is the drug of first choice for the treatment of acute necrotising ulcerative gingivitis (Vincent's infection) and pericoronitis; suitable alternatives are amoxicillin (section 5.1.1.3) and erythromycin (section 5.1.5). For these purposes treatment with metronidazole for 3 days is sufficient, but the duration of treatment may need to be longer in pericoronitis. Tinidazole is licensed for the treatment of acute ulcerative gingivitis.

METRONIDAZOLE

Cautions disulfiram-like reaction with alcohol, clinical and laboratory monitoring advised if treatment exceeds 10 days; **interactions:** Appendix 1 (metronidazole)

Hepatic impairment in severe liver disease reduce total daily dose to one-third, and give once daily; use with caution in hepatic encephalopathy

Pregnancy manufacturer advises avoidance of high-dose regimens; use only if potential benefit outweighs risk

Breast-feeding significant amount in milk; manufacturer advises avoid large single doses though otherwise compatible; may give milk a bitter taste

Side-effects gastro-intestinal disturbances (including nausea and vomiting), taste disturbances, furred tongue, oral mucositis, anorexia; *very rarely* hepatitis, jaundice, pancreatitis, drowsiness, dizziness, headache, ataxia, psychotic disorders, darkening of urine, thrombocytopenia, pancytopenia, myalgia, arthralgia, visual disturbances, rash, pruritus, and erythema multiforme; on prolonged or intensive therapy peripheral neuropathy, transient epileptiform seizures, and leucopenia

Licensed use not licensed for use in neonates or children under 1 year

Indication and dose

Protozoal infections section 5.4.2

Anaerobic infections (usually treated for 7 days and for 10 days in antibiotic-associated colitis)

- **By mouth**

Neonate initially 15 mg/kg then 7.5 mg/kg twice daily

Child 1 month–12 years 7.5 mg/kg (max. 400 mg) every 8 hours

Child 12–18 years 400 mg every 8 hours

- **By rectum**

Child 1 month–1 year 125 mg 3 times daily for 3 days, then twice daily thereafter

Child 1–-5 years 250 mg 3 times daily for 3 days, then twice daily thereafter

Child 5–12 years 500 mg 3 times daily, for 3 days, then twice daily thereafter

Child 12–18 years 1 g 3 times daily for 3 days, then twice daily thereafter

- **By intravenous infusion over 20-30 minutes**

Neonate 15 mg/kg as a single loading dose, followed after 24 hours by 7.5 mg/kg every 12 hours thereafter

Child 1 month–18 years 7.5 mg/kg (max. 500 mg) every 8 hours

Pelvic inflammatory disease (see also Table 1, section 5.1)

- **By mouth**

Child 12–18 years 400 mg twice daily for 14 days

METRONIDAZOLE (*continued*)

Acute ulcerative gingivitis and other acute dental infections
- **By mouth**
  Child 1–3 years 50 mg every 8 hours
  Child 3–7 years 100 mg every 12 hours
  Child 7–10 years 100 mg every 8 hours
  Child 10–18 years 200 mg every 8 hours

Helicobacter pylori eradication section 1.3

Surgical prophylaxis
- **By mouth or by intravenous infusion**
  Child 1 month–12 years 7.5 mg/kg 2 hours before surgery; up to 3 further doses of 7.5 mg/kg may be given every 8 hours for high-risk procedures
  Child 12–18 years 400–500 mg 2 hours before surgery; up to 3 further doses of 400–500 mg may be given every 8 hours for high-risk procedures
- **By rectum**
  Child 5–10 years 500 mg 2 hours before surgery; up to 3 further doses of 500 mg may be given every 8 hours for high-risk procedures
  Child 10–18 years 1 g 2 hours before surgery; up to 3 further doses of 1 g may be given every 8 hours for high-risk procedures

Note Metronidazole doses in BNF for Children may differ from those in product literature

Metronidazole (Non-proprietary) PoM
Tablets, metronidazole 200 mg, net price 21-tab pack = £1.17; 400 mg, 21-tab pack = £1.41. Label: 4, 9, 21, 25, 27
Brands include *Vaginyl®*

Tablets, metronidazole 500 mg, net price 21-tab pack = £5.36. Label: 4, 9, 21, 25, 27

Suspension, metronidazole (as benzoate) 200 mg/5 mL. Net price 100 mL = £7.70. Label: 4, 9, 23
Brands include *Norzol®*

Intravenous infusion, metronidazole 5 mg/mL. Net price 20-mL amp = £1.53, 100-mL container = £3.41

Dental prescribing on NHS Metronidazole Tablets and Oral Suspension may be prescribed

Flagyl® (Winthrop) PoM
Tablets, both f/c, ivory, metronidazole 200 mg, net price 21-tab pack = £3.62; 400 mg, 14-tab pack = £5.12. Label: 4, 9, 21, 25, 27

Suppositories, metronidazole 500 mg, net price 10 = £12.25; 1 g, 10 = £18.60. Label: 4, 9

Flagyl® (Aventis Pharma) PoM
Intravenous infusion, metronidazole 5 mg/mL, net price 100-mL *Viaflex®* bag = £3.41
Electrolytes Na^+ 13.6 mmol/100-mL bag

Flagyl S® (Winthrop) PoM
Suspension, orange- and lemon-flavoured, metronidazole (as benzoate) 200 mg/5 mL. Net price 100 mL = £9.01. Label: 4, 9, 23

Metrolyl® (Sandoz) PoM
Intravenous infusion, metronidazole 5 mg/mL, net price 100-mL Steriflex® bag = £1.22
Electrolytes Na^+ 14.53 mmol/100-mL bag

Suppositories, metronidazole 500 mg, net price 10 = £12.34; 1 g, 10 = £18.34. Label: 4, 9

5.1.12 Quinolones

Nalidixic acid and **norfloxacin** are effective in uncomplicated urinary-tract infections.

Ciprofloxacin is active against both Gram-positive and Gram-negative bacteria. It is particularly active against Gram-negative bacteria, including salmonella, shigella, campylobacter, neisseria, and pseudomonas. Ciprofloxacin has only moderate activity against Gram-positive bacteria such as *Streptococcus pneumoniae* and *Enterococcus faecalis*; it should not be used for pneumococcal pneumonia. It is active against chlamydia and some mycobacteria. Most anaerobic organisms are not susceptible. Ciprofloxacin is licensed for pseudomonal infections in cystic fibrosis (in children above 5 years), and for treatment and prophylaxis of inhalation anthrax. When the benefits of treatment outweigh the risks, ciprofloxacin is licensed for infections of the respiratory tract, the urinary tract, and of the gastro-intestinal system (including typhoid fever). It is also used in the treatment of septicaemia caused by multi-resistant organisms (usually hospital acquired) and gonorrhoea (although resistance is increasing). Ciprofloxacin is also used in the prophylaxis of meningococcal disease.

Ofloxacin eye drops are used in ophthalmic infections (section 11.3.1).

There is much less experience of the other quinolones in children; expert advice should be sought.

Anthrax *Inhalation* or *gastro-intestinal anthrax* should be treated initially with either **ciprofloxacin** or, in children over 12 years, **doxycycline** [unlicensed indication] (section 5.1.3) combined with one or two other antibacterials (such as amoxicillin, benzylpenicillin, chloramphenicol, clarithromycin, clindamycin, imipenem with cilastatin, rifampicin [unlicensed indication], and vancomycin). When the condition improves and the sensitivity of the *Bacillus anthracis* strain is known, treatment may be switched to a single antibacterial. Treatment should continue for 60 days because germination may be delayed.

Cutaneous anthrax should be treated with either ciprofloxacin [unlicensed indication] or doxycycline [unlicensed indication] (section 5.1.3) for 7 days. Treatment may be switched to amoxicillin (section 5.1.1.3) if the infecting strain is susceptible. Treatment may need to be extended to 60 days if exposure is due to aerosol. A combination of antibacterials for 14 days is recommended for cutaneous anthrax with systemic features, extensive oedema, or lesions of the head or neck.

Ciprofloxacin or doxycycline may be given for *post-exposure prophylaxis.* If exposure is confirmed, antibacterial prophylaxis should continue for 60 days. Antibacterial prophylaxis may be switched to amoxicillin after 10–14 days if the strain of *B. anthracis* is susceptible. Vaccination against anthrax (section 14.4) may allow the duration of antibacterial prophylaxis to be shortened.

Cautions Quinolones should be used with caution in children with a history of epilepsy or conditions that predispose to seizures, in G6PD deficiency (section 9.1.5), myasthenia gravis (risk of exacerbation). Exposure to excessive sunlight should be avoided (discontinue if photosensitivity occurs). The CSM has warned that quinolones may induce **convulsions** in patients with or without a history of convulsions; taking NSAIDs at the same time may also induce them. Other **interactions:** Appendix 1 (quinolones).

Quinolones cause arthropathy in the weight-bearing joints of immature *animals* and are therefore generally not recommended in children and growing adolescents. However, the significance of this effect in humans is uncertain and in some specific circumstances short-term use of a quinolone in children is justified. **Nalidixic acid** is used for resistant urinary-tract infections in children over 3 months of age.

CSM advice (tendon damage)

Tendon damage (including rupture) has been reported rarely in patients receiving quinolones. Tendon rupture may occur within 48 hours of starting treatment. The CSM has reminded that:

- quinolones are contra-indicated in patients with a history of tendon disorders related to quinolone use;
- elderly patients are more prone to tendinitis;
- the risk of tendon rupture is increased by the concomitant use of corticosteroids;
- if tendinitis is suspected, the quinolone should be discontinued immediately.

Side-effects Side-effects of the quinolones include nausea, vomiting, dyspepsia, abdominal pain, diarrhoea (rarely antibiotic-associated colitis), headache, dizziness, sleep disorders, rash (rarely Stevens-Johnson syndrome and toxic epidermal necrolysis), and pruritus. Less frequent side-effects include anorexia, increase in blood urea and creatinine; drowsiness, restlessness, asthenia, depression, confusion, hallucinations, convulsions, paraesthesia; photosensitivity, hypersensitivity reactions including fever, urticaria, angioedema, arthralgia, myalgia, and anaphylaxis; blood disorders (including eosinophilia, leucopenia, thrombocytopenia); disturbances in vision, taste, hearing and smell. Also isolated reports of tendon inflammation and damage (especially in those taking corticosteroids, see also CSM advice above). Other side-effects that have been reported include haemolytic anaemia, renal failure, interstitial nephritis, and hepatic dysfunction (including hepatitis and cholestatic jaundice). The drug should be **discontinued** if psychiatric, neurological or hypersensitivity reactions (including severe rash) occur.

CIPROFLOXACIN

Cautions see notes above; avoid excessive alkalinity of urine and ensure adequate fluid intake (risk of crystalluria); **interactions:** Appendix 1 (quinolones)

Skilled tasks May impair performance of skilled tasks (e.g. driving)

Renal impairment if creatinine clearance less than 20 mL/minute/1.73m^2 use half normal dose

Breast-feeding avoid unless necessary—high concentrations in breast milk

Contra-indications

Pregnancy avoid—arthropathy in *animal* studies; safer alternatives available

Side-effects see notes above; also reported flatulence, dysphagia, tremor, hyperglycaemia, vasculitis, erythema nodosum, petechiae, haemorrhagic bullae, tinnitus, tenosynovitis, tachycardia, oedema, syncope, hot flushes and sweating; pain and phlebitis at injection site

Licensed use licensed for use in children over 5 years for pseudomonal lower respiratory-tract infections in cystic fibrosis; licensed for use in children for prophylaxis and treatment of inhalational anthrax; licensed for use in children for other infections where the benefit is considered to outweigh the potential risks; suspension not licensed for use in children under 2 years; not licensed for use in children for gastro-intestinal anthrax; not licensed for use in children for prophylaxis of meningococcal meningitis; not licensed for use in neonates

Indication and dose

Respiratory-tract infections, urinary-tract infections, gastro-intestinal infections; see notes above

- **By mouth**

Neonate 7.5 mg/kg twice daily

Child 1 month–18 years 5–7.5 mg/kg twice daily; dose doubled in severe infection (max. 750 mg twice daily)

- **By intravenous infusion (over 30–60 minutes; 400 mg over 60 minutes)**

Neonate 5 mg/kg every 12 hours

Child 1 month–18 years 4 mg/kg every 12 hours; dose doubled in severe infection (max. 400 mg every 12 hours)

Pseudomonal lower respiratory-tract infection in cystic fibrosis

- **By mouth**

Child 1 month–5 years 5–15 mg/kg twice daily

Child 5–18 years 20 mg/kg (max. 750 mg) twice daily

- **By intravenous infusion over 30–60 minutes (400 mg over 60 minutes)**

Child 1 month–5 years 4–8 mg/kg every 12 hours

Child 5–18 years 10 mg/kg (max. 400 mg) every 8 hours

Gonorrhoea

- **By mouth**

Child 12–18 years 500 mg as a single dose

Anthrax (treatment and post-exposure prophylaxis, see notes above)

- **By mouth**

Child 1 month–18 years 15 mg/kg (max. 500 mg) twice daily

- **By intravenous infusion (over 30–60 minutes; 400 mg over 60 minutes)**

Child 1 month–18 years 10 mg/kg (max. 400 mg) every 12 hours

Eye infections section 11.3.1

Prophylaxis of meningococcal meningitis Table 2, section 5.1

Ciprofloxacin (Non-proprietary) PoM

Tablets, ciprofloxacin (as hydrochloride) 100 mg, net price 6-tab pack = £1.50; 250 mg, 10-tab pack = £1.75, 20-tab pack = £2.32; 500 mg, 10-tab pack = £2.05, 20-tab pack = £2.47; 750 mg, 10-tab pack = £3.00. Label: 7, 9, 25, counselling, driving

Ciproxin® (Bayer) PoM

Tablets, all f/c, ciprofloxacin (as hydrochloride) 100 mg, net price 6-tab pack = £2.80; 250 mg (scored), 10-tab pack = £7.50, 20-tab pack = £15.00; 500 mg (scored), 10-tab pack = £14.20, 20-tab pack = £28.40; 750 mg, 10-tab pack = £20.00. Label: 7, 9, 25, counselling, driving

Suspension, strawberry-flavoured, ciprofloxacin for reconstitution with diluent provided, 250 mg/ 5 mL, net price 100 mL = £15.00. Label: 7, 9, 25, counselling, driving

Intravenous infusion, ciprofloxacin (as lactate) 2 mg/mL, in sodium chloride 0.9%, net price 50-mL bottle = £8.65, 100-mL bottle = £16.89, 200-mL bottle = £25.70

Electrolytes Na^+ 15.4 mmol/100-mL bottle

5 Infections

NALIDIXIC ACID

Cautions see notes above; avoid in porphyria (section 9.8.2); false positive urinary glucose (if tested for reducing substances); monitor blood counts, renal and liver function if treatment exceeds 2 weeks; **interactions:** Appendix 1 (quinolones)

Hepatic impairment manufacturer advises caution in liver disease

Renal impairment use half normal dose if creatinine clearance 20 mL/minute/1.73^2 or less; ineffective in renal failure because concentration in urine is inadequate

Breast-feeding risk to infant very small but one case of haemolytic anaemia reported

NALIDIXIC ACID (*continued*)

Contra-indications

Pregnancy avoid—arthropathy in *animal* studies; safer alternatives available

Side-effects see notes above; also reported toxic psychosis, increased intracranial pressure, cranial nerve palsy, metabolic acidosis

Licensed use not licensed for use in children under 3 months of age

Indication and dose

Urinary tract infection resistant to other antibiotics

- **By mouth**

Child 3 months–12 years 12.5 mg/kg 4 times daily for 7 days, reduced to 7.5 mg/kg 4 times daily in prolonged therapy or 15 mg/kg twice daily for prophylaxis

Child 12–18 years 900 mg 4 times daily for 7 days, reduced in chronic infections to 600 mg 4 times daily

Uriben® (Rosemont) PoM

Suspension, pink, nalidixic acid 300 mg/5 mL, net price 150 mL (raspberry- and strawberry-flavoured) = £11.42. Label: 9, 11

Excipients: include sucrose 450 mg/5mL

5.1.13 Urinary-tract infections

Urinary-tract infection is more common in adolescent girls than in boys; when it occurs in adolescent boys there is frequently an underlying abnormality of the renal tract. Recurrent episodes of infection are an indication for radiological investigation especially in children in whom untreated pyelonephritis may lead to permanent kidney damage.

Escherichia coli is the most common cause of urinary-tract infection; *Staphylococcus saprophyticus* is also common in sexually active young women. Less common causes include Proteus and Klebsiella spp. *Pseudomonas aeruginosa* infections usually occur in the hospital setting and may be associated with functional or anatomical abnormalities of the renal tract. *Staphylococcus epidermidis* and *Enterococcus faecalis* infection may complicate catheterisation or instrumentation.

Whenever possible a specimen of urine should be collected for culture and sensitivity testing before starting antibacterial therapy. The antibacterial chosen should reflect current local bacterial sensitivity to antibacterials.

Urinary-tract infections in children require prompt antibacterial treatment to minimise the risk of renal scarring. For the first infection, treatment may be initiated with trimethoprim, a first generation cephalosporin, or co-amoxiclav and the choice of antibacterial is reviewed when sensitivity results are available; full doses of the antibacterial drug should be given for 5–7 days. Antibacterial prophylaxis with low doses of trimethoprim or nitrofurantoin should then be given if further investigations are considered necessary. Antibacterial prophylaxis should be continued until investigations are complete; long-term prophylaxis may be necessary in some cases (e.g. vesicoureteric reflux or renal scarring). Nitrofurantoin is contra-indicated in children under 3 months of age because of the theoretical possibility of haemolytic anaemia.

Children under 3 months of age or seriously unwell children over 3 months of age should be transferred to hospital and treated initially with intravenous antibacterial drugs such as ampicillin with gentamicin, or cefotaxime alone, until the infection responds; full doses of oral antibacterials are then given for a further period. Antibacterial prophylaxis should then be given as above.

Short-course antibacterial therapy A short course (e.g. 3 days) of trimethoprim or amoxicillin may be adequate for uncomplicated infections in adolescent females.

Resistant infections Widespread bacterial resistance, especially to amoxicillin, ampicillin, and trimethoprim has increased the importance of urine culture before therapy. Alternatives for resistant organisms include co-amoxiclav (amoxicillin with clavulanic acid), an oral cephalosporin, pivmecillinam, or a quinolone.

Acute pyelonephritis can lead to septicaemia and is best treated initially by injection of a broad-spectrum antibacterial such as cefotaxime, ceftriaxone, or a quinolone especially if the patient is severely ill; gentamicin can also be used.

Patients with *heart-valve lesions* undergoing instrumentation of the urinary tract should be given a parenteral antibacterial to prevent bacteraemia and endocarditis (Table 2, section 5.1).

Pregnancy Urinary-tract infection in *pregnancy* may be asymptomatic and requires prompt treatment to prevent progression to acute pyelonephritis. Penicillins and cephalosporins are suitable for treating urinary-tract infection during pregnancy. Nitrofurantoin may also be used but it should be avoided at term. Sulphonamides, quinolones, and tetracyclines should be avoided during pregnancy; trimethoprim should also preferably be avoided particularly in the first trimester.

Renal impairment In *renal failure* antibacterials normally excreted by the kidney accumulate with resultant toxicity unless the dose is reduced. This applies especially to the aminoglycosides which should be used with great caution; tetracyclines, methamine, and nitrofurantoin should be avoided altogether.

NITROFURANTOIN

Cautions anaemia; diabetes mellitus; electrolyte imbalance; vitamin B and folate deficiency; pulmonary disease; monitor lung and liver function on long-term therapy (discontinue if deterioration in lung function); susceptibility to peripheral neuropathy; false positive urinary glucose (if tested for reducing substances); urine may be coloured yellow or brown; **interactions**: Appendix 1 (nitrofurantoin)

Hepatic impairment cholestatic jaundice and chronic active hepatitis reported

Pregnancy may produce neonatal haemolysis if used at term

Contra-indications infants less than 3 months old, G6PD deficiency, porphyria (section 9.8.2)

Renal impairment avoid; risk of peripheral neuropathy; ineffective because of inadequate urine concentrations

Breast-feeding avoid; only small amounts in milk but enough to produce haemolysis in G6PD-deficient infants (section 9.1.5)

Side-effects anorexia, nausea, vomiting, and diarrhoea; acute and chronic pulmonary reactions (pulmonary fibrosis reported; possible association with lupus erythematosus-like syndrome); peripheral neuropathy; also reported, hypersensitivity reactions (including angioedema, anaphylaxis, sialadenitis, urticaria, rash and pruritus); rarely, cholestatic jaundice, hepatitis, exfoliative dermatitis, erythema multiforme, pancreatitis, arthralgia, blood disorders (including agranulocytosis, thrombocytopenia, and aplastic anaemia), benign intracranial hypertension, and transient alopecia

Indication and dose

Acute uncomplicated urinary tract infection
- By mouth

Child 3 months–12 years 750 micrograms/kg 4 times daily for 7 days

Child 12–18 years 50 mg 4 times daily for 7 days; increased to 100 mg 4 times daily in severe chronic recurrent infections

Prophylaxis of urinary tract infection (but see Cautions)
- By mouth

Child 3 months–12 years 1 mg/kg at night

Child 12–18 years 50–100 mg at night

Nitrofurantoin (Non-proprietary) PoM

Tablets, nitrofurantoin 50 mg, net price 20 = £1.65; 100 mg, 20 = £3.04. Label: 9, 14, 21

Oral suspension, nitrofurantoin 25 mg/5 mL, net price 300 mL = £65.00. Label: 9, 14, 21

Furadantin® (Goldshield) PoM

Tablets, all yellow, scored, nitrofurantoin 50 mg, net price 20 = £1.96; 100 mg, 20 = £3.62. Label: 9, 14, 21

Macrobid® (Goldshield) PoM

Capsules, m/r, blue/yellow, nitrofurantoin 100 mg (as nitrofurantoin macrocrystals and nitrofurantoin monohydrate). Net price 14-cap pack = £4.89. Label: 9, 14, 21, 25

Dose

Uncomplicated urinary-tract infection

Child 12–18 years 1 capsule twice daily with food

Genito-urinary surgical prophylaxis

Child 12–18 years 1 capsule twice daily on day of procedure and for 3 days after

Macrodantin® (Goldshield) PoM

Capsules, nitrofurantoin 50 mg (yellow/white), net price 30-cap pack = £3.05; 100 mg (yellow/white), 20 = £3.84. Label: 9, 14, 21

5 Infections

5.2 Antifungal drugs

Treatment of fungal infections

The systemic treatment of common fungal infections is outlined below; specialist treatment is required in most forms of systemic or disseminated fungal infections. For local treatment of fungal infections, see section 7.2.2 (genital), section 7.4.4 (bladder), section 11.3.2 (eye), section 12.1.1 (ear), section 12.3.2 (oropharynx), and section 13.10.2 (skin).

Aspergillosis Aspergillosis most commonly affects the respiratory tract but in severely immunocompromised patients, invasive forms can affect the sinuses, heart, brain, and skin. **Amphotericin** by intravenous infusion is the drug of choice but response varies; liposomal amphotericin, **itraconazole**, or **voriconazole** are alternatives in children in whom initial treatment has failed. Itraconazole is used as an adjunct in the treatment of allergic bronchopulmonary aspergillosis. **Caspofungin** is licensed in adults for invasive aspergillosis unresponsive to amphotericin or to itraconazole, or in patients who cannot tolerate amphotericin or itraconazole; information on use in children is limited.

Candidiasis Many superficial candidal infections are treated locally including infections of the skin (section 13.10.2). Vaginal candidiasis (section 7.2.2) can be treated with locally acting antifungals; alternatively, fluconazole can be given by mouth. Systemic antifungal treatment is required in widespread or intractable infection.

Oropharyngeal candidiasis generally responds to topical therapy (section 12.3.2); fluconazole is given by mouth for unresponsive infections; it is reliably absorbed and is effective. Itraconazole may be used for fluconazole-resistant infections.

For *deep and disseminated candidiasis*, **amphotericin** by intravenous infusion is used alone or (especially when good CNS penetration is required) with **flucytosine** by intravenous infusion. Alternatively **fluconazole** is given alone for *Candida albicans* infection, particularly in HIV-infected children and in neonates. **Voriconazole** is licensed in children over 2 years of age for infections caused by fluconazole-resistant *Candida* spp. (including *C. krusei*). The use of **caspofungin** should be restricted to treating fluconazole-resistant *Candida* infections that have not responded to amphotericin or in children intolerant of amphotericin.

Cryptococcosis Cryptococcosis is uncommon but infection in the immunocompromised, especially HIV-infected children, can be life-threatening; cryptococcal meningitis is the most common form of fungal meningitis. The treatment of choice in cryptococcal meningitis is **amphotericin** by intravenous infusion with **flucytosine** by intravenous infusion for 2 weeks, followed by **fluconazole** by mouth for 8 weeks. In cryptococcosis, **fluconazole** given alone is an alternative in AIDS patients with no disturbances of consciousness.

Histoplasmosis Histoplasmosis is rare in temperate climates; it can be life-threatening, particularly in HIV-infected children. **Itraconazole** can be used for the treatment of immunocompetent children with indolent non-meningeal infection including chronic pulmonary histoplasmosis; **ketoconazole** is an alternative in immunocompetent children. **Amphotericin** by intravenous infusion is preferred in children with fulminant or severe infections. Following successful treatment, itraconazole can be used for prophylaxis against relapse.

Skin and nail infections Mild localised fungal infections of the skin (including tinea corporis, tinea cruris, and tinea pedis) respond to topical therapy (section 13.10.2). Systemic therapy (itraconazole, fluconazole, or terbinafine) is appropriate if topical therapy fails, if many areas are affected, or if the site of infection is difficult to treat such as in infections of the nails (onychomycosis) and of the scalp (tinea capitis).

Griseofulvin is used for tinea capitis in children but not neonates; it was used extensively in tinea of various other sites but has largely been replaced by newer antifungals. **Terbinafine** may be preferred because it has a broader spectrum of activity and requires a shorter duration of treatment. The role of terbinafine in the management of *Microsporum* spp. (cat or dog ringworm) is uncertain.

Pityriasis versicolor (section 13.10.2) may be treated with **itraconazole** by mouth if topical therapy is ineffective; **fluconazole** by mouth is an alternative. Oral **terbinafine** is **not** effective for pityriasis versicolor.

Terbinafine and **itraconazole** have largely replaced griseofulvin for the systemic treatment of onychomycosis, particularly of the toenail. Terbinafine is not licensed for use in children but may be used under specialist advice. Itraconazole can be administered as intermittent 'pulse' therapy.

Immunocompromised children Immunocompromised children are at particular risk of fungal infections and may receive antifungal drugs prophylactically; oral imidazole or triazole antifungals are the drugs of choice for prophylaxis. **Fluconazole** is more reliably absorbed than itraconazole and ketoconazole and is considered less toxic than ketoconazole on long-term use.

Amphotericin by intravenous infusion is used for the empirical *treatment* of serious fungal infections. Fluconazole is used for treatment of *Candida albicans* infection.

Caspofungin is licensed for the empirical treatment of systemic fungal infections (such as those involving *Candida* spp. or *Aspergillus* spp.) in adults with neutropenia.

Drugs used in fungal infections

Polyene antifungals The polyene antifungals include amphotericin and nystatin; neither drug is absorbed when given by mouth. They are used for oral, oropharyngeal, and perioral infections by local application in the mouth (section 12.3.2).

Amphotericin by intravenous infusion is used for the treatment of systemic fungal infections and is active against most fungi and yeasts. It is highly protein bound and penetrates poorly into body fluids and tissues. When given parenterally amphotericin is toxic and side-effects are common. Lipid formulations of amphotericin (*Abelcet®*, *AmBisome®*, and *Amphocil®*) are significantly less toxic and are recommended when the conventional formulation of amphotericin is contra-indicated because of toxicity, especially nephrotoxicity, or when response to conventional amphotericin is inadequate; lipid formulations are more expensive.

Nystatin is used principally for *Candida albicans* infections of the skin (section 13.10.2) and mucous membranes, including oesophageal and intestinal candidiasis.

Imidazole antifungals The imidazole antifungals include clotrimazole, econazole, sulconazole, and tioconazole. They are used for the local treatment of vaginal candidiasis (section 7.2.2) and for dermatophyte infections (section 13.10.2).

Ketoconazole is better absorbed by mouth than other imidazoles. It has been associated with fatal hepatotoxicity; the CSM has advised that prescribers should weigh the potential benefits of ketoconazole treatment against the risk of liver damage and should carefully monitor patients both clinically and biochemically. It should not be used by mouth for superficial fungal infections.

Miconazole can be used locally for oral infections; it is also effective in intestinal infections. Systemic absorption may follow use of miconazole oral gel and may result in significant drug interactions.

Triazole antifungals **Fluconazole** is very well absorbed after oral administration. It also achieves good penetration into the cerebrospinal fluid to treat fungal meningitis.

Itraconazole is active against a wide range of dermatophytes. There is limited information available on use in children. Itraconazole capsules require an acid environment in the stomach for optimal absorption.

Itraconazole has been associated with liver damage and should be avoided or used with caution in children with liver disease; fluconazole is less frequently associated with hepatotoxicity.

Voriconazole is a broad-spectrum antifungal drug which is licensed in adults for the treatment of life-threatening infections.

Other antifungals **Caspofungin** is active against *Aspergillus* spp. and *Candida* spp. It is given by intravenous infusion for invasive infection resistant to other antifungals.

Flucytosine is often used with amphotericin in a synergistic combination. Bone marrow depression can occur which limits its use, particularly in children with AIDS; weekly blood counts are necessary during prolonged therapy. Resistance to flucytosine can develop during therapy and sensitivity testing is essential before and during treatment.

Griseofulvin is effective for widespread or intractable dermatophyte infections but has been superseded by newer antifungals, particularly for nail infections. Griseofulvin is used in the treatment of tinea capitis. It is the drug of choice for trichophyton infections in children. Duration of therapy is dependent on the site of the infection and may extend to a number of months.

Terbinafine is the drug of choice for fungal nail infections and is also used for ringworm infections where oral treatment is considered appropriate.

AMPHOTERICIN
(Amphotericin B)

Cautions when given parenterally, toxicity common (close supervision necessary and close observation required for at least 30 minutes after test dose; see Anaphylaxis below); hepatic and renal-function tests, blood counts and plasma electrolyte (including plasma-potassium and magnesium concentration) monitoring required; corticosteroids (avoid except to control reactions); avoid rapid infusion (risk of arrhythmias); **interactions:** Appendix 1 (amphotericin)

Renal impairment use only if no alternative; nephrotoxicity may be reduced with use of lipid formulation

Pregnancy not known to be harmful, but manufacturers advise avoid unless potential benefit outweighs risk

Anaphylaxis The CSM has advised that anaphylaxis occurs rarely with any intravenous amphotericin product and a test dose is advisable before the first infusion; the patient should be carefully observed for at least 30 minutes after the test dose. Prophylactic antipyretics or hydrocortisone should only be used in patients who have previously experienced acute adverse reactions (in whom continued treatment with amphotericin is essential)

Side-effects when given parenterally, anorexia, nausea and vomiting, diarrhoea, epigastric pain; febrile reactions, headache, muscle and joint pain; anaemia; disturbances in renal function (including hypokalaemia and hypomagnesaemia) and renal toxicity; also cardiovascular toxicity (including arrhythmias), blood disorders, neurological disorders (including hearing loss, diplopia, convulsions, peripheral neuropathy), abnormal liver function (discontinue treatment), rash, anaphylactoid reactions (see Anaphylaxis, above); pain and thrombophlebitis at injection site

Licensed use *suspension* licensed for treatment of intestinal candidiasis in children over 1 month and for prophylaxis in neonate; intravenous conventional formulation amphotericin (*Fungizone®*) is licensed for use in children (age range not specified by manufacturer); lipid formulations (*Abelcet®*, *Ambisome®*, *Amphocil®*) are licensed for use in children (age range not specified by manufacturers)

Indication and dose

Intestinal candidiasis
- By mouth

Child 1 month–12 years 100 mg 4 times daily

Child 12–18 years 100–200 mg 4 times daily

Prophylaxis of neonatal intestinal candidiasis
- By mouth

Neonate 100 mg once daily

Oral and perioral infections section 12.3.2

Systemic fungal infections
- By intravenous infusion

see preparations

Fungilin® (Squibb) PoM
Suspension, yellow, sugar-free, amphotericin 100 mg/mL, net price 12 mL = £2.15. Label: 9, counselling, use of pipette

Fungizone® (Squibb) PoM
Intravenous infusion, powder for reconstitution, amphotericin (as sodium deoxycholate complex). Net price 50-mg vial = £3.16
Electrolytes Na^+ < 0.5 mmol/vial

Dose

Systemic fungal infection
- By intravenous infusion

Neonate initial test dose of 100 micrograms/kg included as part of first dose of 250 micrograms/kg daily, increased over 2–4 days if tolerated to max. 1 mg/kg once daily

Child 1 month–18 years initial test dose of 100 micrograms/kg (max. 1 mg) included as part of first dose of 250 micrograms/kg daily; increased over 2–4 days if tolerated to 1 mg/kg daily; in severe infection max. 1.5 mg/kg daily or on alternate days

Note prolonged treatment usually necessary; if interrupted for longer than 7 days recommence at 250 micrograms/kg daily and increase gradually

Administration For *intravenous infusion*, reconstitute each vial with 10 mL Water for Injections and shake immediately to produce a 5 mg/mL colloidal solution; dilute further in Glucose 5% to a concentration of 100 micrograms/mL (in fluid-restricted children, up to 400 micrograms/mL given via a central line); pH of glucose solution must not be below 4.2 (check each container—

AMPHOTERICIN (*continued*)

consult product literature for details of buffer); infuse over 4–6 hours, or if tolerated over a minimum of 2 hours (initial test dose given over 20–30 minutes); begin infusion immediately after dilution and protect from light; incompatible with Sodium Chloride solutions—flush existing intravenous line with Glucose 5% or use separate line; an in-line filter (pore size no less than 1 micron) may be used

Lipid formulations

Abelcet® (Zeneus) PoM

Intravenous infusion, amphotericin 5 mg/mL as lipid complex with L-α-dimyristoylphosphatidylcholine and L-α-dimyristoylphosphatidylglycerol. Net price 20-mL vial = £82.13 (hosp. only)

Dose

Severe invasive candidiasis; severe systemic fungal infections in children not responding to conventional amphotericin or to other antifungal drugs or where toxicity or renal impairment precludes conventional amphotericin, including invasive aspergillosis, cryptococcal meningitis and disseminated cryptococcosis in children with HIV

- **By intravenous infusion**

  Child 1 month–18 years initial test dose of 100 micrograms/kg (max. 1 mg) then 5 mg/kg daily as a single dose

Administration for *intravenous infusion*, allow suspension to reach room temperature, shake gently to ensure no yellow settlement, withdraw requisite dose (using 17–19 gauge needle) into one or more 20-mL syringes; replace needle on syringe with a 5-micron filter needle provided (fresh needle for each syringe) and dilute in Glucose 5% to a concentration of 1 mg/mL (2 mg/mL in fluid restriction); preferably give *via* an infusion pump at a rate of 2.5 mg/kg/hour (initial test dose given over 15 minutes); an in-line filter (pore size no less than 15 micron) may be used; do not use sodium chloride or other electrolyte solutions—flush existing intravenous line with Glucose 5% or use separate line

AmBisome® (Gilead) PoM

Intravenous infusion, powder for reconstitution, amphotericin 50 mg encapsulated in liposomes. Net price 50-mg vial = £96.69

Electrolytes Na^+ < 0.5 mmol/vial

Excipients: include sucrose 900 mg/vial

Dose

Severe systemic or deep mycoses where toxicity (particularly nephrotoxicity) precludes use of conventional amphotericin

- **By intravenous infusion**

  Neonate initial test dose 100 micrograms/kg then 1 mg/kg daily as a single dose, increased if necessary in steps of 1 mg/kg daily; max. 3 mg/kg daily as a single dose (empirical) or 5 mg/kg daily as a single dose (proven infection)

  Child 1 month–18 years initial test dose 100 micrograms/kg (max. 1 mg) then 1 mg/kg daily as a single dose; increased if necessary in steps of 1 mg/kg daily; max. 3 mg/kg daily as a single dose (empirical) or 5 mg/kg daily as a single dose (proven infection)

Fever in neutropenic patients unresponsive to broad-spectrum antibacterials

- **By intravenous infusion**

  Child 1 month–18 years initial test dose 100 micrograms/kg (max. 1 mg) then 3 mg/kg daily as a single dose until afebrile for 3 consecutive days; max. period of treatment 42 days

Visceral leishmaniasis see section 5.4.5 and product literature

Administration for *intravenous infusion*, reconstitute each vial with 12 mL Water for Injections and shake vigorously to produce a preparation containing 4 mg/mL; withdraw requisite dose from vial and introduce into Glucose 5% through the 5-micron filter provided to produce a final concentration of 0.2–2 mg/mL; infuse over 30–60 minutes (initial test dose given over 10 minutes); incompatible with sodium chloride solutions—flush existing intravenous line with Glucose 5% or use separate line

Amphocil® (Cambridge) PoM

Intravenous infusion, powder for reconstitution, amphotericin as a complex with sodium cholesteryl sulphate. Net price 50-mg vial = £96.81, 100-mg vial = £190.05

Electrolytes Na^+ < 0.5 mmol/vial

Dose

Severe systemic or deep mycoses where toxicity or renal failure precludes use of conventional amphotericin

- **By intravenous infusion**

  Child 1 month–18 years initial test dose 100 micrograms/kg (max. 2 mg) over 10 minutes then 30 minutes later 1 mg/kg daily, increased gradually if necessary to 3–4 mg/kg daily as a single dose; max. 6 mg/kg daily

Administration for *intravenous infusion*, initially reconstitute with Water for Injections (50 mg in 10 mL, 100 mg in 20 mL) shaking gently to dissolve (fluid may be opalescent) then dilute to a concentration of 625 micrograms/mL with Glucose 5% (1 volume of reconstituted solution with 7 volumes of infusion fluid); give at a rate of 1–2 mg/kg/hour or slower if not tolerated (for initial test dose use a 100 microgram/mL solution and give over 10 minutes); incompatible with sodium chloride or other electrolyte solutions, flush existing intravenous line with Glucose 5% or use separate line

CASPOFUNGIN

Cautions interactions: Appendix 1 (caspofungin)

Hepatic impairment 70 mg on first day then 35 mg once daily in moderate hepatic impairment; no information available for severe hepatic impairment

Pregnancy manufacturer advises avoid unless essential—toxicity in *animal* studies

Contra-indications

Breast-feeding present in milk in *animal* studies—manufacturer advises avoid

Side-effects nausea, vomiting, abdominal pain, diarrhoea; tachycardia, flushing; dyspnoea; fever, headache; anaemia, decrease in serum potassium, hypomagnesaemia; rash, pruritus, sweating; injection-site reactions; *less commonly* hypercalcaemia; also reported, hepatic dysfunc-

CASPOFUNGIN (*continued*)

tion, oedema, acute respiratory distress syndrome, hypersensitivity reactions (including anaphylaxis)

Licensed use not licensed for use in children

Indication and dose

Invasive aspergillosis either unresponsive to amphotericin or itraconazole or in patients intolerant of amphotericin or itraconazole; invasive candidiasis (see notes above); empirical treatment of systemic fungal infections in patients with neutropenia

- By intravenous infusion

Child 2–18 years 50 mg/m² (max. 70 mg) once daily

Administration for *intravenous infusion*, allow vial to reach room temperature; initially reconstitute each vial with 10.5 mL Water for Injections, mixing gently to dissolve then dilute requisite dose in 250 mL Sodium Chloride 0.9% *or* Compound Sodium Lactate (Hartmann's solution) (35 mg or 50 mg doses may be diluted in 100 mL infusion fluid if necessary); give over 60 minutes; incompatible with glucose solutions

Cancidas® (MSD) PoM

Intravenous infusion, powder for reconstitution, caspofungin (as acetate), net price 50-mg vial = £327.67; 70-mg vial = £416.78

FLUCONAZOLE

Cautions monitor liver function—discontinue if signs or symptoms of hepatic disease (risk of hepatic necrosis); susceptibility to QT interval prolongation; **interactions:** Appendix 1 (antifungals, triazole)

Hepatic impairment toxicity with related drugs

Renal impairment usual initial dose then halve subsequent doses if creatinine clearance less than 50 mL/min/1.73m²

Pregnancy manufacturer advises avoid—multiple congenital abnormalities reported with long-term high doses

Breast-feeding present in milk—risk to infant probably small but manufacturer advises avoid

Side-effects nausea, abdominal discomfort, diarrhoea, flatulence, headache, rash (discontinue treatment or monitor closely if infection invasive or systemic); less frequently dyspepsia, vomiting, taste disturbance, hepatic disorders, angioedema, anaphylaxis, dizziness, seizures, alopecia, pruritus, toxic epidermal necrolysis, Stevens-Johnson syndrome (severe cutaneous reactions more likely in AIDS patients), hyperlipidaemia, leucopenia, thrombocytopenia, and hypokalaemia reported

Licensed use not licensed for tinea infections in children

Indication and dose

Mucosal candidiasis (except genital)

- By mouth or by intravenous infusion

Neonate under 2 weeks 3–6 mg/kg on first day then 3 mg/kg every 72 hours

Neonate 2–4 weeks 3–6 mg/kg on first day then 3 mg/kg every 48 hours

Child 1 month–12 years 3–6 mg/kg on first day then 3 mg/kg (max. 100 mg) daily for 7–14 days in oropharyngeal candidiasis (max. 14 days except in severely immunocompromised patients); for 14–30 days in other mucosal infections (e.g. oesophagitis, candiduria, non-invasive bronchopulmonary infections)

Child 12–18 years 50 mg daily (100 mg daily in unusually difficult infections) given for 7–14 days in oropharyngeal candidiasis (max. 14 days except in severely immunocompromised patients); for 14–30 days in other mucosal infections (e.g. oesophagitis, candiduria, non-invasive bronchopulmonary infections)

Vaginal candidiasis (see also Recurrent Vulvovaginal Candidiasis, section 7.2.2) and candidal balanitis

- By mouth

Child 16–18 years a single dose of 150 mg

Tinea pedis, corporis, cruris, pityriasis versicolor, and dermal candidiasis

- By mouth

Child 1 month–18 years 3 mg/kg (max. 50 mg) daily for 2–4 weeks (for up to 6 weeks in tinea pedis); max. duration of treatment 6 weeks

Invasive candidal infections (including candidaemia and disseminated candidiasis) and cryptococcal infections (including meningitis)

- By mouth or by intravenous infusion

Neonate under 2 weeks 6–12 mg/kg every 72 hours, treatment continued according to response (at least 8 weeks for cryptococcal meningitis)

Neonate 2–4 weeks 6–12 mg/kg every 48 hours, treatment continued according to response (at least 8 weeks for cryptococcal meningitis)

Child 1 month–18 years 6–12 mg/kg (max. 400 mg) daily, treatment continued according to response (at least 8 weeks for cryptococcal meningitis)

Prevention of fungal infections in immunocompromised patients

- By mouth or by intravenous infusion

Neonate under 2 weeks according to extent and duration of neutropenia, 3–12 mg/kg every 72 hours

Neonate 2–4 weeks according to extent and duration of neutropenia, 3–12 mg/kg every 48 hours

Child 1 month–18 years according to extent and duration of neutropenia, 3–12 mg/kg (max. 400 mg) daily; 12 mg/kg (max. 400 mg) daily if high risk of systemic infections e.g. following

FLUCONAZOLE (*continued*)

bone-marrow transplantation; commence treatment before anticipated onset of neutropenia and continue for 7 days after neutrophil count in desirable range

Administration for *intravenous infusion*, give over 10–30 minutes; do not exceed an infusion rate of 5–10 mL/minute

Fluconazole (Non-proprietary) PoM

[1]Capsules, fluconazole 50 mg, net price 7-cap pack = £2.89; 150 mg, single-capsule pack = £1.65; 200 mg, 7-cap pack = £5.39. Label: 9, (50 and 200 mg)

Dental prescribing on NHS Fluconazole Capsules 50 mg may be prescribed

Intravenous infusion, fluconazole 2 mg/mL, net price 25-mL bottle = £7.32; 100-mL bottle = £29.28

Diflucan® (Pfizer) PoM

[1]Capsules, fluconazole 50 mg (blue/white), net price 7-cap pack = £16.61; 150 mg (blue), single-capsule pack = £7.12; 200 mg (purple/white), 7-cap pack = £66.42. Label: 9, (50 and 200 mg)

Oral suspension, orange-flavoured, fluconazole for reconstitution with water, 50 mg/5 mL, net price 35 mL = £16.61; 200 mg/5 mL, 35 mL = £66.42. Label: 9

Dental prescribing on NHS May be prescribed as Fluconazole Oral Suspension 50 mg/5 mL

Intravenous infusion, fluconazole 2 mg/mL in sodium chloride intravenous infusion 0.9%, net price 25-mL bottle = £7.32; 100-mL bottle = £29.28

Electrolytes Na^+ 15 mmol/100-mL bottle

FLUCYTOSINE

Cautions blood disorders; liver- and kidney-function tests and blood counts required (weekly in renal impairment or blood disorders); **interactions**: Appendix 1 (flucytosine)

Renal impairment use normal dose every 12 hours if creatinine clearance 20–40 mL/minute/1.73m²; use normal dose every 24 hours if creatinine clearance 10–20 mL/minute/1.73m²; use initial normal dose if creatinine clearance less than 10 mL/minute/1.73m² and then adjust dose according to plasma-flucytosine concentration

Pregnancy teratogenic in *animal* studies; manufacturer advises use only if potential benefit outweighs risk

Breast-feeding manufacturer advises avoid—although risk to infant probably small

Side-effects nausea, vomiting, diarrhoea, rashes; less frequently cardiotoxicity, confusion, hallucinations, convulsions, headache, sedation, vertigo, alterations in liver function tests (hepatitis and hepatic necrosis reported), and toxic epidermal necrolysis; blood disorders including thrombocytopenia, leucopenia, and aplastic anaemia reported

Pharmacokinetics for plasma-concentration monitoring blood should be taken shortly before starting the next infusion. Plasma concentration for optimum response 25–50 mg/litre (200–400 micromol/litre)—should not be allowed to exceed 80 mg/litre (620 micromol/litre)

Licensed use *tablets* unlicensed in UK

Indication and dose

Systemic yeast and fungal infections; adjunct to amphotericin (or fluconazole) in cryptococcal meningitis (see Cryptococcosis, p. 346), adjunct to amphotericin in severe systemic candidiasis and in other severe or long-standing infections

- **By intravenous infusion or by mouth**

Neonate 50 mg/kg every 12 hours

Child 1 month–18 years 50 mg/kg every 6 hours; extremely sensitive organisms, 25–37.5 mg/kg every 6 hours may be sufficient; treatment continued usually for not more than 7 days; treat for 2 weeks in cryptococcal meningitis (see Cryptococcosis, p. 346)

Administration for *intravenous infusion*, give over 20–40 minutes through a giving set with a 15-micron filter

Ancotil® (Valeant) PoM

Intravenous infusion, flucytosine 10 mg/mL. Net price 250-mL infusion bottle = £30.33 (hosp. only)

Electrolytes Na^+ 34.5 mmol/250-mL bottle

Note Flucytosine tablets may be available on a named-patient basis from Bell and Croyden

Extemporaneous formulations available see Extemporaneous Preparations, p. 8

GRISEOFULVIN

Cautions **interactions**: Appendix 1 (griseofulvin)

Skilled tasks May impair performance of skilled tasks; effects of alcohol enhanced

Contra-indications systemic lupus erythematosus (risk of exacerbation); porphyria (section 9.8.2)

Hepatic impairment avoid in severe liver disease

Pregnancy avoid pregnancy *during* and for *1 month* after treatment (fetotoxicity and teratogenicity in *animals*); effective contraception required during and for at least 1 month after administration (**important**: effectiveness of oral contraceptives reduced); also males should avoid fathering a child during and for at least 6 months after treatment

Breast-feeding avoid—no information available

Side-effects nausea, vomiting, diarrhoea; headache; less frequently hepatotoxicity, dizziness, confusion, fatigue, sleep disturbances, impaired

1. Capsules can be sold to the public for vaginal candidiasis and associated candidal balanitis in those aged 16–18 years, in a container or packaging containing not more than 150 mg and labelled to show a max. dose of 150 mg

GRISEOFULVIN (*continued*)

co-ordination, peripheral neuropathy, leucopenia, systemic lupus erythematosus, rash (including rarely erythema multiforme, toxic epidermal necrolysis), and photosensitivity

Licensed use *tablets* licensed for use in children (age range not specified by manufacturer); *suspension* not licensed in UK

Indication and dose

Dermatophyte infections where topical therapy has failed or is inappropriate
- By mouth

Child 1 month–12 years 10 mg/kg (max. 500 mg) once daily or in divided doses; in severe infection dose may be doubled, reducing when response occurs

Child 12–18 years 500 mg once daily or in divided doses; in severe infection dose may be doubled, reducing when response occurs

Tinea capitis caused by *Trichophyton tonsurans*
- By mouth

Child 1 month–12 years 15–20 mg/kg (max. 1 g) once daily or in divided doses

Child 12–18 years 1 g once daily or in divided doses

Griseofulvin (Non-proprietary) PoM

Tablets, griseofulvin 125 mg, net price 20 = £6.76; 500 mg, 20 = £1.79. Label: 9, 21, counselling, skilled tasks

Suspension, griseofulvin 125 mg/5 mL. Label: 9, 21, counselling, skilled tasks

Available via specialist importing companies

Grisovin® (Chemidex) PoM

Tablets, both f/c, griseofulvin 125 mg, net price 20 = 48p; 500 mg, 20 = £1.79. Label: 9, 21, counselling, skilled tasks

ITRACONAZOLE

Cautions absorption reduced in AIDS and neutropenia (monitor plasma-itraconazole concentration and increase dose if necessary); susceptibility to congestive heart failure (see also CSM advice, below); **interactions:** Appendix 1 (antifungals, triazole)

Hepatotoxicity Potentially life-threatening hepatotoxicity reported very rarely. Monitor liver function—discontinue if signs of hepatitis develop; avoid or use with caution if history of hepatotoxicity with other drugs or in active liver disease; use with caution in patients receiving other hepatotoxic drugs

Counselling Children or their carers should be told how to recognise signs of liver disorder and advised to seek immediate medical attention if symptoms such as anorexia, nausea, vomiting, fatigue, abdominal pain or dark urine develop

Hepatic impairment use only if potential benefit outweighs risk of hepatotoxicity (see hepatotoxicity above); dose reduction may be necessary

Renal impairment risk of congestive heart failure; bioavailability of oral formulations possibly reduced; use intravenous infusion with caution if creatinine clearance 30–50 mL/minute/1.73m^2 (monitor renal function); avoid intravenous infusion if creatinine clearance less than 30 mL/minute/1.73m^2

Pregnancy manufacturer advises use only in life-threatening situations (toxicity at high doses in *animal* studies); ensure effective contraception during treatment and until the next menstrual period following end of treatment

Breast-feeding small amounts present in milk—may accumulate; manufacturer advises avoid unless potential benefit outweighs risk

CSM advice (heart failure) Following rare reports of heart failure, the CSM has advised caution when prescribing itraconazole to patients at high risk of heart failure. Those at risk include:
- patients receiving high doses and longer treatment courses;
- those with cardiac disease;
- patients receiving treatment with negative inotropic drugs, e.g. calcium channel blockers.

Side-effects *very rarely* nausea, vomiting, dyspepsia, abdominal pain, diarrhoea, constipation, jaundice, hepatitis (see also Hepatotoxicity above), heart failure (see CSM advice above), pulmonary oedema, headache, dizziness, peripheral neuropathy (discontinue treatment), menstrual disorder, hypokalaemia, rash, pruritus, Stevens-Johnson syndrome, and alopecia; *with intravenous injection, very rarely* hypertension and hyperglycaemia

Licensed use *Sporanox®* capsules and *Sporanox® Pulse* are not licensed for use in children under 12 years; *Sporanox®* liquid and *Sporanox®* infusion are not licensed for use in children (age range not specified by manufacturer)

Indication and dose

Oropharyngeal candidiasis
- By mouth

Child 1 month–12 years 3–5 mg/kg once daily; max 100 mg daily (200 mg daily in AIDS or neutropenia) for 15 days

Child 12–18 years 100 mg once daily (200 mg once daily in AIDS or neutropenia) for 15 days

Pityriasis versicolor
- By mouth

Child 1 month–12 years 3–5 mg/kg (max. 200 mg) once daily for 7 days

Child 12–18 years 200 mg once daily for 7 days

Tinea corporis and tinea cruris
- By mouth

Child 1 month–12 years 3–5 mg/kg (max. 100 mg) once daily for 15 days

Child 12–18 years *either* 100 mg once daily for 15 days *or* 200 mg once daily for 7 days

ITRACONAZOLE (*continued*)

Tinea pedis and tinea manuum
- **By mouth**

Child 1 month–12 years 3–5 mg/kg (max. 100 mg) once daily for 30 days

Child 12–18 years *either* 100 mg once daily for 30 days *or* 200 mg twice daily for 7 days

Onychomycosis
- **By mouth**

Child 12–18 years *either* 200 mg once daily for 3 months *or* course ('pulse') of 200 mg twice daily for 7 days, subsequent courses repeated after 21-day interval; fingernails 2 courses, toenails 3 courses

Systemic aspergillosis, candidiasis and cryptococcosis including cryptococcal meningitis where other antifungal drugs inappropriate or ineffective (limited information available)
- **By mouth**

Child 1 month–18 years 5 mg/kg (max. 200 mg) once daily; increased in invasive or disseminated disease and in cryptococcal meningitis to 5 mg/kg (max. 200 mg) twice daily

- **By intravenous infusion**

Child 1 month–18 years 2.5 mg/kg (max. 200 mg) every 12 hours for 2 days, then 2.5 mg/kg (max. 200 mg) once daily for max. 12 days

Histoplasmosis
- **By mouth**

Child 1 month–18 years 5 mg/kg (max. 200 mg) 1–2 times daily

Maintenance in AIDS patients to prevent relapse of underlying fungal infection and prophylaxis in neutropenia when standard therapy inappropriate
- **By mouth**

Child 1 month–18 years 5 mg/kg (max. 200 mg) once daily, increased to 5 mg/kg (max. 200 mg) twice daily if low plasma-itraconazole concentration (see Cautions)

Prophylaxis of deep fungal infections (when standard therapy inappropriate) in patients with haematological malignancy or undergoing bone-marrow transplantation who are expected to become neutropenic
- **By mouth (liquid preparation only)**

Child 1 month–18 years 2.5 mg/kg twice daily starting before transplantation or before chemotherapy (taking care to avoid interaction with cytotoxic drugs) and continued until neutrophil count recovers

Administration For *intravenous infusion*, dilute 250 mg with 50 mL Sodium Chloride 0.9% and give requisite dose through an in-line filter (0.2 micron) over 60 minutes

Sporanox® (Janssen-Cilag) PoM

Capsules, blue/pink, enclosing coated beads, itraconazole 100 mg, net price 4-cap pack = £3.98; 15-cap pack = £14.93; 28-cap pack (*Sporanox®-Pulse*) = £27.88; 60-cap pack = £59.75. Label: 5, 9, 21, 25

Oral liquid, sugar-free, itraconazole 10 mg/mL, net price 150 mL (with 10-mL measuring cup) = £49.67. Label: 9, 23, counselling, administration

Counselling Do not take with food; swish around mouth and swallow, do not rinse afterwards

Concentrate for intravenous infusion, itraconazole 10 mg/mL. For dilution before use. Net price 25-mL amp (with infusion bag and filter) = £67.86

Excipients: include propylene glycol

KETOCONAZOLE

Cautions monitor liver function clinically and biochemically—for treatment lasting longer than 14 days perform liver function tests before starting, 14 days after starting, then at monthly intervals (for details consult product literature)—for CSM advice see p. 347; avoid in porphyria (section 9.8.2); **interactions:** Appendix 1 (antifungals, imidazole)

Contra-indications

Hepatic impairment avoid

Pregnancy avoid—manufacturer advises teratogenicity in *animal* studies

Breast-feeding manufacturer advises avoid

Side-effects nausea, vomiting, abdominal pain; headache; rashes, urticaria, pruritus; rarely angioedema, thrombocytopenia, paraesthesia, photophobia, dizziness, alopecia, gynaecomastia and oligospermia; fatal liver damage—see also under Cautions, risk of developing hepatitis greater if given for longer than 14 days

Licensed use not licensed for children under 1 year

Indication and dose

Systemic mycoses, serious chronic resistant mucocutaneous candidiasis, serious resistant gastro-intestinal mycoses, resistant dermatophyte infections of skin or finger nails (not toe nails)
- **By mouth**

Child 1–12 years 3 mg/kg once daily with food

Child 12–18 years 200 mg once daily with food, increased if necessary to 400 mg daily

Note treatment usually for 14 days; if response inadequate after 14 days continue until at least 1 week after symptoms have cleared and cultures negative

Chronic resistant vaginal candidiasis
- **By mouth**

Child 12–18 years 400 mg once daily with food for 5 days

KETOCONAZOLE (*continued*)

Prophylaxis and maintenance treatment in immunosuppressed patients
- By mouth

Child 1–12 years 3 mg/kg once daily with food

Child 12–18 years 200 mg once daily with food

Nizoral® (Janssen-Cilag) PoM
Tablets, scored, ketoconazole 200 mg. Net price 30-tab pack = £14.91. Label: 5, 9, 21

Extemporaneous formulations available see Extemporaneous Preparations, p. 8

MICONAZOLE

Cautions avoid in porphyria (section 9.8.2); **interactions:** Appendix 1 (antifungals, imidazole)

Pregnancy manufacturer advises avoid unless potential benefit outweighs risk—toxicity in *animal* studies at high doses

Breast-feeding manufacturer advises caution—no information available, but unlikely to be harmful to infant

Contra-indications

Hepatic impairment avoid

Side-effects nausea and vomiting, diarrhoea (usually on long-term treatment); rarely allergic reactions; isolated reports of hepatitis

Licensed use not licensed for use in neonates

Indication and dose

Prevention and treatment of oral and intestinal fungal infections
- By mouth

Neonate (oral fungal infections only) 1 mL 2–4 times daily smeared around the mouth after feeds

Child 1 month–2 years 2.5 mL twice daily in the mouth after food; retain near lesions before swallowing

Child 2–6 years 5 mL twice daily in the mouth after food; retain near lesions before swallowing

Child 6–12 years 5 mL 4 times daily in the mouth after food; retain near lesions before swallowing

Child 12–18 years 5–10 mL 4 times daily in the mouth after food; retain near lesions before swallowing

Localised lesions smear a small amount of gel on affected area with clean finger up to four times a day; continue treatment for 48 hours after lesions have resolved

[1]**Daktarin®** (Janssen-Cilag) PoM
Oral gel, sugar-free, orange-flavoured, miconazole 24 mg/mL (20 mg/g). Net price 15-g tube = £2.45, 80-g tube = £4.75. Label: 9, counselling, hold in mouth, after food
Excipients: include alcohol

1. 15-g tube can be sold to public for prevention and treatment of oral fungal infections in children

NYSTATIN

Side-effects nausea, vomiting, diarrhoea at high doses; oral irritation and sensitisation; rash (including urticaria) and rarely Stevens-Johnson syndrome reported

Licensed use *suspension* not licensed for treatment of intestinal candidiasis in neonates; *suspension* licensed for prophylaxis in neonates as once daily dose; *tablets* not licensed for use in children (age range not specified by manufacturer)

Indication and dose

Treatment of intestinal candidiasis
- By mouth

Neonate 100 000 units 4 times daily after feeds

Child 1 month–12 years 100 000 units 4 times daily; immunocompromised children may require higher doses (e.g. 500 000 units 4 times daily)

Child 12–18 years 500 000 units 4 times daily; doubled in severe infections

Vaginal infection section 7.2.2

Oral infection section 12.3.2

Skin infection section 13.10.2

Nystan® (Squibb) PoM
Tablets, brown, s/c, nystatin 500 000 units, net price 56-tab pack = £4.70. Label: 9

Suspension, yellow, nystatin 100 000 units/mL, net price 30 mL with pipette = £2.05. Label: 9, counselling, use of pipette
Excipients: include alcohol

TERBINAFINE

Cautions psoriasis (risk of exacerbation); autoimmmune disease (risk of lupus-erythematosus-like effect) **interactions:** Appendix 1 (terbinafine)

Hepatic impairment manufacturer advises avoid—elimination reduced

Renal impairment use half normal dose if creatinine clearance less than 50 mL/minute/1.73m^2

Pregnancy manufacturer advises use only if benefit outweighs risk—no information available

Breast-feeding present in milk—manufacturer advises avoid

TERBINAFINE (*continued*)

Side-effects abdominal discomfort, anorexia, nausea, diarrhoea; headache; rash and urticaria occasionally with arthralgia or myalgia; *less commonly* taste disturbance; *rarely* liver toxicity (including jaundice, cholestasis and hepatitis)—discontinue treatment, angioedema, dizziness, malaise, paraesthesia, hypoaesthesia, photosensitivity, serious skin reactions (including Stevens-Johnson syndrome and toxic epidermal necrolysis) —discontinue treatment if progressive skin rash; *very rarely* psychiatric disturbances, blood disorders (including leucopenia and thrombocytopenia), lupus erythematosus-like effect, and exacerbation of psoriasis

Licensed use not licensed for use in children

Indication and dose

Dermatophyte infections of the nails, ringworm infections (including tinea pedis, cruris, corporis, and capitas) where oral therapy appropriate (due to site, severity or extent)

- By mouth

Child over 1 year; body-weight 10–20 kg 62.5 mg once daily

Child body-weight 20–40 kg 125 mg once daily

Child body-weight over 40 kg 250 mg once daily

Note treatment usually for 2 weeks in tinea capitis, 2–6 weeks in tinea pedis, 2–4 weeks in tinea cruris, 4 weeks in tinea corporis, 6 weeks–3 months in nail infections (occasionally longer in toenail infections)

Fungal skin infections section 13.10.2

Terbinafine (Non-proprietary) PoM

Tablets, terbinafine (as hydrochloride) 250 mg, net price 14-tab pack = £23.15, 28-tab pack = £44.65. Label: 9

Lamisil® (Novartis) PoM

Tablets, off-white, scored, terbinafine (as hydrochloride) 250 mg, net price 14-tab pack = £23.16, 28-tab pack = £44.66. Label: 9

VORICONAZOLE

Cautions monitor liver function before treatment and during treatment; haematological malignancy (increased risk of hepatic reactions); monitor renal function; electrolyte disturbances, cardiomyopathy, bradycardia, symptomatic arrhythmias, history of QT interval prolongation, concomitant use with other drugs that prolong QT interval; avoid exposure to sunlight; **interactions:** Appendix 1 (antifungals, triazole)

Hepatic impairment in mild to moderate hepatic cirrhosis use usual initial dose then halve subsequent doses; no information available for severe hepatic cirrhosis—manufacturer advises use only if potential benefit outweighs risk

Renal impairment excipient in intravenous infusion solution may accumulate if creatinine clearance less than 50 mL/minute/1.73m^2—manufacturer advises use intravenous infusion only if potential benefit outweighs risk and monitor renal function; alternatively, use tablets or oral suspension (no dose adjustment required)

Pregnancy toxicity in *animal* studies—manufacturer advises avoid unless potential benefit outweighs risk; effective contraception required during treatment

Contra-indications

Breast-feeding manufacturer advises avoid—no information available

Side-effects gastro-intestinal disturbances (including nausea, vomiting, abdominal pain, diarrhoea), jaundice; oedema, hypotension, chest pain; respiratory distress syndrome, sinusitis; headache, dizziness, asthenia, anxiety, depression, confusion, agitation, hallucinations, paraesthesia, tremor; influenza-like symptoms; hypoglycaemia; haematuria; blood disorders (including anaemia, thrombocytopenia, leucopenia, pancytopenia), acute renal failure, hypokalaemia; visual disturbances including altered perception, blurred vision, and photophobia; rash, pruritus, photosensitivity, alopecia, cheilitis; injection-site reactions; *less commonly* taste disturbances, cholecystitis, pancreatitis, hepatitis, constipation, arrhythmias (including QT interval prolongation), syncope, raised serum cholesterol, hypersensitivity reactions (including flushing), ataxia, nystagmus, hypoaesthesia, adrenocortical insufficiency, arthritis, blepharitis, optic neuritis, scleritis, glossitis, gingivitis, psoriasis, and Stevens-Johnson syndrome; *rarely* pseudomembranous colitis, convulsions, sleep disturbances, tinnitis, hearing disturbances, extrapyramidal effects, hypertonia, hypothyroidism, hyperthyroidism, discoid lupus erythematosus, toxic epidermal necrolysis, retinal haemorrhage, and optic atrophy

Indication and dose

Invasive aspergillosis; serious infections caused by *Scedosporium* spp., *Fusarium* spp., or invasive fluconazole-resistant *Candida* spp. (including *C. krusei*)

- By mouth

Child 2–12 years (oral suspension recommended) 200 mg every 12 hours

Child 12–18 years, body-weight under 40 kg 200 mg every 12 hours for 2 doses then 100 mg every 12 hours, increased if necessary to 150 mg every 12 hours

Child 12–18 years, body-weight over 40 kg 400 mg every 12 hours for 2 doses then 200 mg every 12 hours, increased if necessary to 300 mg every 12 hours

VORICONAZOLE (*continued*)

- **By intravenous infusion**
  Child 2–12 years 7 mg/kg every 12 hours (reduced to 4 mg/kg every 12 hours if not tolerated)
  Child 12–18 years 6 mg/kg every 12 hours for 2 doses, then 4 mg/kg every 12 hours (reduced to 3 mg/kg every 12 hours if not tolerated) for max. 6 months

Administration For *intravenous infusion,* reconstitute each 200 mg with 19 mL Water for Injections to produce a 10 mg/mL solution; dilute dose to concentration of 0.5–5 mg/mL with Glucose 5% *or* Sodium Chloride 0.9% *or* Compound Sodium Lactate and give at a rate not exceeding 3 mg/kg/hour

Vfend® (Pfizer) PoM
Tablets, f/c, voriconazole 50 mg, net price 28-tablet pack = £227.84; 200 mg, 28-tab pack = £911.36. Label: 11, 23

Oral suspension, voriconazole 200 mg/5 mL when reconstituted with water, net price 75 mL (orange-flavoured) = £501.25. Label: 11, 23

Intravenous infusion, powder for reconstitution, voriconazole, net price 200-mg vial = £77.14
Excipients: include sulphobutylether beta cyclodextrin sodium (risk of accumulation in renal impairment)
Electrolytes Na^+ 9.62 mmol/vial

5.3 Antiviral drugs

The majority of virus infections resolve spontaneously in immunocompetent subjects. A number of specific treatments for viral infections are available, particularly for the immunocompromised. This section includes notes on herpes simplex and varicella-zoster, human immunodeficiency virus, cytomegalovirus, respiratory syncytial virus, viral hepatitis and influenza.

5.3.1 HIV infection

There is no cure for infection caused by the human immunodeficiency virus (HIV) but a number of drugs slow or halt disease progression. Drugs for HIV infection (antiretrovirals) increase life expectancy considerably but they are toxic.

The natural progression of HIV disease is different in children compared to adults; drug treatment should only be undertaken by specialists within a formal paediatric HIV clinical network. Guidelines and dose regimens are under constant review and for this reason specific dose recommendations have not been included in *BNF for Children*.

Further information on the management of children with HIV can be obtained from the Children's HIV Association (CHIVA) http://www.bhiva.org/chiva; and further information on antiretroviral use and toxicity can be obtained from the Paediatric European Network for Treatment of AIDS (PENTA) website http://www.ctu.mrc.ac.uk/penta.

Principles of treatment Treatment is aimed at suppressing viral replication for as long as possible; it should be started before the immune system is irreversibly damaged. The need for early drug treatment should, however, be balanced against the development of toxicity. Commitment to treatment and strict adherence over many years are required; the regimen chosen should take into account convenience and the child's tolerance of treatment. The development of drug resistance is reduced by using a combination of drugs; such combinations should have synergistic or additive activity while ensuring that their toxicity is not additive. It is recommended that viral sensitivity to antiretroviral drugs is established before starting treatment or before switching drugs if the infection is not responding.

Initiation of treatment Treatment is based on child's age, CD4 cell count, viral load, and symptoms. The choice of antiviral treatment for children should take into account the method and frequency of administration, risk of side-effects, compatibility of drugs with food, palatability, and the appropriateness of the formulation. Initiating treatment with a combination of drugs ('highly active antiretroviral therapy' which includes 2 nucleoside reverse transcriptase inhibitors with *either* a non-nucleoside reverse transcriptase inhibitor *or* a boosted protease inhibitor) is recommended. The metabolism of many antiretrovirals can vary in young children; it may therefore be necessary to adjust the dose according to the plasma-drug concentration.

Switching therapy Deterioration of the condition (including clinical, virological changes, and CD4 cell changes) may require a complete change of therapy. The choice of an alternative regimen depends on factors such as the response to previous treatment, tolerance, and the possibility of cross-resistance.

Pregnancy Treatment of HIV infection in pregnancy aims to minimise the viral load and disease progression in the mother and reduce the risk of toxicity to the fetus (but the teratogenic potential of most antiretroviral drugs is unknown). Combination antiretroviral therapy represents optimal treatment but all options require **careful assessment** by a specialist. Consideration also needs to be given to preventing transmission of the infection to the newborn (see below).

Prevention of transmission to neonate Zidovudine given in the perinatal period to the mother and the neonate reduces transmission to the baby. However, optimal treatment of the mother's HIV infection with combination treatment maximises the chance of preventing transmission. Local protocols and national guidelines (www.bhiva.org) should be consulted for recommendations on treatment during pregnancy and the perinatal period.

Breast-feeding Breast-feeding by HIV-positive mothers may cause HIV infection in the infant and should be avoided.

Post-exposure prophylaxis Children exposed to HIV-infection through needlestick injury or by another route should be sent to an accident and emergency department for post-exposure prophylaxis [unlicensed indication]. Antiretrovirals for prophylaxis are chosen on the basis of efficacy and potential for toxicity.

Drugs used for HIV infection **Zidovudine**, a nucleoside reverse transcriptase inhibitor (or 'nucleoside analogue'), was the first anti-HIV drug to be introduced. Other nucleoside reverse transcriptase inhibitors include **abacavir**, **didanosine**, **emtricitabine**, **lamivudine**, **stavudine**, and **tenofovir**. Stavudine, especially with didanosine, is associated with a higher risk of lipodystrophy and lactic acidosis and should be used only if alternative regimens are not suitable.

The protease inhibitors include **amprenavir**, **atazanavir**, **fosamprenavir** (a prodrug of amprenavir), **indinavir**, **lopinavir**, **nelfinavir**, **ritonavir**, and **saquinavir**. Ritonavir in low doses boosts the activity of amprenavir, atazanavir, indinavir, lopinavir, and saquinavir increasing the persistence of plasma concentrations of these drugs; at such a low dose, ritonavir has no intrinsic antiviral activity. A combination of lopinavir with low-dose ritonavir is available for use in children over 2 years. The protease inhibitors are metabolised by cytochrome P450 enzyme systems and therefore have a significant potential for drug interactions. Protease inhibitors are associated with lipodystrophy and metabolic effects (see below).

The non-nucleoside reverse transcriptase inhibitors **efavirenz** and **nevirapine** are active against the subtype HIV-1 but not HIV-2, a subtype prevalent mainly in Africa. These drugs may interact with a number of drugs metabolised in the liver. Nevirapine can occasionally cause rash (including, very rarely, Stevens-Johnson syndrome) and fatal hepatitis. Rash is also associated with efavirenz but it is usually milder.

Enfuvirtide, which inhibits HIV from fusing to the host cell, is licensed for managing infection that has failed to respond to a regimen of other antiretroviral drugs. Enfuvirtide should be combined with other potentially active antiretroviral drugs; it is given by subcutaneous injection.

Improvement in immune function as a result of antiretroviral treatment may provoke an inflammatory reaction against residual opportunistic organisms.

Lipodystrophy syndrome Metabolic effects associated with antiretroviral treatment include *fat redistribution*, *insulin resistance* and *dyslipidaemia*; collectively these have been termed *lipodystrophy syndrome*. Insulin resistance and hyperglycaemia occur only rarely in children.

Fat redistribution (with loss of subcutaneous fat, increased abdominal fat, 'buffalo hump' and breast enlargement) is associated with regimens containing protease inhibitors and nucleoside reverse transcriptase inhibitors.

Dyslipidaemia (with adverse effects on body lipids) is associated with antiretroviral treatment, particularly with protease inhibitors; in children, hypercholesterolaemia appears to be more common than hypertriglyceridaemia. Protease inhibitors are associated with insulin resistance and hyperglycaemia but they occur rarely in children. Plasma lipids and blood glucose should be taken into account before prescribing regimens containing a protease inhibitor; children receiving protease inhibitors should be monitored for changes in plasma lipids and blood glucose.

Nucleoside reverse transcriptase inhibitors

Cautions Nucleoside reverse transcriptase inhibitors should be used with caution in children with hepatic impairment (greater risk of hepatic side-effects, see also Lactic Acidosis below). However, some nucleoside reverse transcriptase inhibitors are used in children who also have chronic hepatitis B. They should also be used with caution in renal impairment and in pregnancy (see also p. 357).

Lactic acidosis Life-threatening lactic acidosis associated with hepatomegaly and hepatic steatosis has been reported with nucleoside reverse transcriptase inhibitors. They should be used with caution in children with hepatomegaly, hepatitis (especially hepatitis C treated with interferon alfa and ribavirin), liver-enzyme abnormalities and with other risk factors for liver disease and hepatic steatosis. Treatment with the nucleoside reverse transcriptase inhibitor should be **discontinued** in case of symptomatic hyperlactataemia, lactic acidosis, progressive hepatomegaly or rapid deterioration of liver function.

Side-effects Side-effects of the nucleoside reverse transcriptase inhibitors include gastro-intestinal disturbances (such as nausea, vomiting, abdominal pain, flatulence and diarrhoea), anorexia, pancreatitis, liver damage (see also Lactic Acidosis, above), dyspnoea, cough, headache, insomnia, dizziness, fatigue, blood disorders (including anaemia, neutropenia, and thrombocytopenia), myalgia, arthralgia, rash, urticaria, and fever. See notes above for metabolic effects and lipodystrophy (Lipodystrophy Syndrome).

5 Infections

ABACAVIR

Cautions see notes above; **interactions**: Appendix 1 (abacavir)

Hepatic impairment avoid in moderate to severe impairment

Renal impairment manufacturer advises avoid in severe impairment

Hypersensitivity reactions Life-threatening hypersensitivity reactions reported (more common in Caucasians)—characterised by fever or rash and possibly nausea, vomiting, diarrhoea, abdominal pain, dyspnoea, cough, lethargy, malaise, headache, and myalgia; less frequently mouth ulceration, oedema, hypotension, sore throat, acute respiratory distress syndrome, anaphylaxis, paraesthesia, arthralgia, conjunctivitis, lymphadenopathy, lymphocytopenia and renal failure (CSM has identified hypersensitivity reactions presenting as sore throat, influenza-like illness, cough and breathlessness); rarely myolysis; laboratory abnormalities may include raised liver function tests (see below) and creatine phosphokinase; symptoms usually appear in the first 6 weeks, but may occur at any time; monitor for symptoms every 2 weeks for 2 months; discontinue immediately if any symptom of hypersensitivity develops and do not rechallenge (risk of more severe hypersensitivity reaction); discontinue if hypersensitivity cannot be ruled out, even when other diagnoses possible—if rechallenge necessary it must be carried out in hospital setting; if abacavir is stopped for any reason other than hypersensitivity, exclude hypersensitivity reaction as the cause and rechallenge only if medical assistance is readily available; care needed with concomitant use of drugs which cause skin toxicity

Counselling Children and carers should be told the importance of regular dosing (intermittent therapy may increase the risk of sensitisation), how to recognise signs of hypersensitivity, and advised to seek immediate medical attention if symptoms develop or before re-starting treatment; children or their carers should be advised to keep Alert Card with them at all times

Contra-indications

Pregnancy manufacturer advises avoid (toxicity in *animal* studies); see also Pregnancy , p. 357

Breast-feeding avoid (see notes above)

Side-effects see notes above; also hypersensitivity reactions (see above); *very rarely* Stevens-

ABACAVIR (*continued*)

Johnson syndrome and toxic epidermal necrolysis; rash and gastro-intestinal disturbances more common in children

Licensed use *Ziagen*® not licensed for use in children under 3 months; *Kivexa*® not licensed for use in children under 12 years; *Trizivir*® not licensed for use in children

Indication and dose

HIV infection in combination with other antiretroviral drugs ; for dose consult Guidelines

Ziagen® (GSK) PoM

Tablets, yellow, f/c, abacavir (as sulphate) 300 mg, net price 60-tab pack = £221.81. Counselling, hypersensitivity reactions

Oral solution, sugar-free, banana and strawberry flavoured, abacavir (as sulphate) 20 mg/mL, net price 240-mL = £59.15. Counselling, hypersensitivity reactions

Excipients: include propylene glycol

With lamivudine

For cautions, contra-indications and side-effects see under individual drugs

Kivexa® (GSK) ▼ PoM

Tablets, orange, f/c, abacavir (as sulphate) 600 mg, lamivudine 300 mg, net price 30-tab pack = £373.94. Counselling, hypersensitivity reactions

With lamivudine and zidovudine

Note use only if child is stabilised (for 6–8 weeks) on the individual components in the same proportions. For cautions, contra-indications and side-effects see under individual drugs

Trizivir® (GSK) PoM

Tablets, blue-green, f/c, abacavir (as sulphate) 300 mg, lamivudine 150 mg, zidovudine 300 mg, net price 60-tab pack = £540.40. Counselling, hypersensitivity reactions

DIDANOSINE

(ddI, DDI)

Cautions see notes above; also history of pancreatitis (preferably avoid, otherwise extreme caution, see also below); peripheral neuropathy or hyperuricaemia (see under Side-effects); dilated retinal examinations recommended (especially in children) every 6 months, or if visual changes occur; **interactions:** Appendix 1 (didanosine)

Renal impairment reduce dose in mild impairment

Hepatic impairment insufficient information but monitor for toxicity

Pregnancy manufacturer advises avoid—no information available

Pancreatitis If symptoms of pancreatitis develop or if serum lipase is raised and pancreatitis is confirmed, discontinue treatment. Whenever possible avoid concomitant treatment with other drugs known to cause pancreatic toxicity (e.g. intravenous pentamidine isetionate); monitor closely if concomitant therapy unavoidable. Since significant elevations of triglycerides cause pancreatitis monitor closely if triglycerides elevated

Contra-indications

Breast-feeding avoid (see notes above)

Side-effects see notes above; also pancreatitis (less common in children, see also under cautions), liver failure, anaphylactic reactions, peripheral neuropathy—suspend (reduced dose may be tolerated when symptoms resolve), diabetes mellitus, hypoglycaemia, acute renal failure, rhabdomyolysis, dry eyes, retinal and optic nerve changes, dry mouth, parotid gland enlargement, sialadenitis, alopecia, hyperuricaemia (suspend if raised significantly)

Licensed use *tablets* not licensed for use in children under 3 months; *EC* capsules not licensed for use in children under 6 years

Indication and dose

HIV infection in combination with other antiretroviral drugs ; for dose consult Guidelines (see notes above)

Videx® (Bristol-Myers Squibb) PoM

Tablets, both with calcium and magnesium antacids, didanosine 25 mg, net price 60-tab pack = £26.60; 200 mg, 60-tab pack = £163.68. Label: 23, counselling, administration, see below

Excipients: include aspartame equivalent to phenylalanine 36.5 mg per tablet (section 9.4.1)

Note Antacids in formulation may affect absorption of other drugs—see **interactions:** Appendix 1 (antacids)

Administration to ensure sufficient antacid, each dose to be taken as 2 tablets (**CHILD** under 1 year 1 tablet) chewed thoroughly, crushed or dispersed in water; clear apple juice may be added for flavouring; tablets to be taken 2 hours after atazanavir with ritonavir

Videx® EC capsules, enclosing e/c granules, didanosine 125 mg, net price 30-cap pack = £51.15; 200 mg, 30-cap pack = £81.84; 250 mg, 30-cap pack = £102.30; 400 mg, 30-cap pack = £163.68. Label: 25, counselling, administration, see below

Administration capsules should be swallowed whole and taken at least 2 hours before or 2 hours after food

EMTRICITABINE

Cautions see notes above; also on discontinuation, monitor patients with hepatitis B (risk of exacerbation of hepatitis); **interactions:** Appendix 1 (emtricitabine)

Renal impairment reduce dose or increase dosage interval in mild impairment

Pregnancy manufacturer advises avoid—no information available

Contra-indications

Breast-feeding avoid (see notes above)

Side-effects see notes above; also abnormal dreams, pruritus, and hyperpigmentation

Licensed use not licensed for use in children under 4 months

EMTRICITABINE (*continued*)

Indication and dose

HIV infection in combination with other antiretroviral drugs ; for dose, consult Guidelines (see notes above)

Emtriva® (Gilead) ▼ PoM
Capsules, white/blue, emtricitabine 200 mg, net price 30-cap pack = £163.50

Oral solution, orange, emtricitabine 10 mg/mL, net price 170-mL pack = £46.50
Excipients: include propylene glycol
Note 240 mg oral solution ≡ 200 mg capsule; where appropriate the capsule may be used instead of the oral solution

With tenofovir
See under Tenofovir

LAMIVUDINE
(3TC)

Cautions see notes above; **interactions:** Appendix 1 (lamivudine)

Renal impairment reduce dose in mild impairment

Pregnancy manufacturer advises avoid during first trimester; see also p. 357

Chronic hepatitis B Recurrent hepatitis in patients with chronic hepatitis B may occur on discontinuation of lamivudine. When treating chronic hepatitis B with lamivudine, monitor liver function tests at least every 3 months and serological markers of hepatitis B every 6 months, more frequently in patients with advanced liver disease or following transplantation (monitoring to continue after discontinuation)—consult product literature

Contra-indications

Breast-feeding avoid (see notes above)

Side-effects see notes above; also peripheral neuropathy, muscle disorders including rhabdomyolysis, nasal symptoms, alopecia

Licensed use *Epivir®* not licensed for use in children under 3 months; *Zeffix®* not licensed for use in children (age range not specified by manufacturer)

Indication and dose

See preparations, below

Epivir® (GSK) PoM
Tablets, f/c, lamivudine 150 mg (white), net price 60-tab pack = £152.14; 300 mg (grey), 30-tab pack = £167.21

Oral solution, banana- and strawberry-flavoured, lamivudine 50 mg/5 mL, net price 240-mL pack = £41.41
Excipients: include propylene glycol, sucrose 1 g/5 mL

Dose

Epivir® **for HIV infection in combination with other antiretroviral drugs** for dose, consult Guidelines (see notes above)

Zeffix® (GSK) PoM
Tablets, brown, f/c, lamivudine 100 mg, net price 28-tab pack = £78.09

Oral solution, banana and strawberry flavoured, lamivudine 25 mg/5 mL, net price 240-mL pack = £22.79
Excipients: include propylene glycol, sucrose 1 g/5 mL

Dose

Zeffix® **for chronic hepatitis B infection with** ***either*** **compensated liver disease (with evidence of viral replication and histology of active liver inflammation or fibrosis),** ***or*** **decompensated liver disease** for dose, seek specialist advice; children receiving lamivudine for concomitant HIV infection should continue to receive lamivudine in a dose appropriate for HIV infection

With abacavir
See under Abacavir

With zidovudine
See under Zidovudine

With abacavir and zidovudine
See under Abacavir

STAVUDINE
(d4T)

Cautions see notes above; also history of peripheral neuropathy (see below); history of pancreatitis or concomitant use with other drugs associated with pancreatitis; **interactions:** Appendix 1 (stavudine)

Renal impairment reduce dose to 50% if creatinine clearance 25–50 mL/minute/1.73m²; reduce dose to 25% if creatinine clearance less than 25 mL/minute/1.73m²

Pregnancy manufacturer advises avoid—risk of hepatic steatosis and lactic acidosis

Peripheral neuropathy Switch to another antiretroviral if peripheral neuropathy develops—characterised by persistent numbness, tingling or pain in feet or hands; if stavudine needs to be continued, resume treatment at half previous dose

Contra-indications

Breast-feeding avoid (see notes above)

Side-effects see notes above; also peripheral neuropathy, abnormal dreams, cognitive dysfunction, drowsiness, depression, pruritus; *less commonly* anxiety, gynaecomastia

Licensed use *capsules* not licensed for use in children under 3 months

Indication and dose

HIV infection in combination with other antiretroviral drugs ; for dose, consult Guidelines (see notes above)

Zerit® (Bristol-Myers Squibb) PoM
Capsules, stavudine 15 mg (yellow/red), net price 56-cap pack = £143.10; 20 mg (brown), 56-cap pack = £148.05; 30 mg (light orange/dark orange), 56-cap pack = £155.25; 40 mg (dark orange), 56-cap pack = £159.94 (all hosp. only)

Oral solution, cherry-flavoured, stavudine for reconstitution with water, 1 mg/mL, net price 200 mL = £24.35

5 Infections

TENOFOVIR DISOPROXIL

Cautions see notes above; also test renal function and serum phosphate before treatment, then every 4 weeks (more frequently if at increased risk of renal impairment) for 1 year and then every 3 months, interrupt treatment if renal function deteriorates or serum phosphate decreases; **interactions:** Appendix 1 (tenofovir)

Renal impairment increase dose interval in mild impairment

Pregnancy manufacturer advises avoid—no information available

Contra-indications

Breast-feeding avoid (see notes above)

Side-effects see notes above; also hypophosphataemia, reduced bone density, polyuria, and renal failure

Licensed use not licensed for use in children

Indication and dose

HIV infection in combination with other antiretroviral drugs ; for dose, consult Guidelines (see notes above)

Viread® (Gilead) ▼ PoM

Tablets, f/c, blue, tenofovir disoproxil (as fumarate) 245 mg, net price 30-tab pack = £255.00. Label: 21, counselling, administration

Counselling Patients with swallowing difficulties may disperse tablet in half a glass of water, grape juice, or orange juice (but very bitter taste)

With emtricitabine

For **cautions, contra-indications**, and **side-effects** see under individual drugs

Truvada® (Gilead) ▼ PoM

Tablets, blue, f/c, tenofovir disoproxil (as fumarate) 245 mg, emtricitabine 200 mg, net price 30-tab pack = £418.50. Label: 21, Counselling, administration

Patients with swallowing difficulties may disperse tablet in half a glass of water, orange juice, or grape juice (but very bitter taste)

ZIDOVUDINE

(Azidothymidine, AZT)

Note The abbreviation AZT which is sometimes used for zidovudine has also been used for another drug

Cautions see notes above; also haematological toxicity particularly with high dose and advanced disease (blood tests at least every 2 weeks for first 3 months then at least once a month, early disease with good bone marrow reserves may require less frequent tests e.g. every 1–3 months); vitamin B_{12} deficiency (increased risk of neutropenia); reduce dose or interrupt treatment according to product literature if anaemia or myelosuppression; **interactions:** Appendix 1 (zidovudine)

Renal impairment reduce dose in severe impairment—consult product information

Pregnancy limited information available; manufacturer advises use only if clearly indicated; see also p. 357

Contra-indications abnormally low neutrophil counts or haemoglobin values (consult product literature); neonates with hyperbilirubinaemia requiring treatment other than phototherapy, or with raised transaminase (consult product literature)

Breast-feeding avoid (see notes above)

Side-effects see notes above; also anaemia (may require transfusion), taste disturbance, chest pain, influenza-like symptoms, paraesthesia, neuropathy, convulsions, dizziness, drowsiness, insomnia, anxiety, depression, loss of mental acuity, myopathy, gynaecomastia, urinary frequency, sweating, pruritus, pigmentation of nails, skin and oral mucosa

Licensed use *Combivir®* is not licensed for use in children under 12 years

Indication and dose

HIV infection in combination with other antiretroviral drugs; prevention of maternal-fetal HIV transmission (see notes above under Prevention of Transmission to Neonate)

Administration for *intermittent intravenous infusion*, dilute to a concentration of 2 mg/mL or 4 mg/mL with Glucose 5% and give over 1 hour

Retrovir® (GSK) PoM

Capsules, zidovudine 100 mg (white/blue band), net price 100-cap pack = £110.98; 250 mg (blue/white/dark blue band), 40-cap pack = £110.98

Oral solution, sugar-free, strawberry-flavoured, zidovudine 50 mg/5 mL, net price 200-mL pack with 10-mL oral syringe = £22.20

Injection, zidovudine 10 mg/mL. For dilution and use as an intravenous infusion. Net price 20-mL vial = £11.14

With lamivudine

For cautions, contra-indications, and side-effects of lamivudine, see Lamivudine

Combivir® (GSK) PoM

Tablets, f/c, zidovudine 300 mg, lamivudine 150 mg, net price 60-tab pack = £318.60

With abacavir and lamivudine

See under Abacavir

5 Infections

Protease inhibitors

Cautions Protease inhibitors should be used with caution in diabetes (see also Lipodystrophy Syndrome, p. 357). Caution is also needed in children with haemophilia who may be at increased risk of bleeding and in hepatic impairment; the risk of hepatic side-effects is increased in children with chronic hepatitis B or C. Atazanavir and fosamprenavir may be used at usual doses in children with renal impairment, but other protease inhibitors should be used with caution in renal impairment. Indinavir is rarely used in children because of the risk of nephrolithiasis. Protease inhibitors should also be used with caution during pregnancy.

Side-effects Side-effects of the protease inhibitors include gastro-intestinal disturbances (including diarrhoea, nausea, vomiting, abdominal pain, flatulence), anorexia, hepatic dysfunction, pancreatitis; blood disorders including anaemia, neutropenia, and thrombocytopenia; sleep disturbances, fatigue, headache, dizziness, paraesthesia, myalgia, myositis, rhabdomyolysis; taste disturbances; rash, pruritus, Stevens-Johnson syndrome, hypersensitivity reactions including anaphylaxis; see also notes on p. 357 for lipodystrophy and metabolic effects.

AMPRENAVIR

Cautions see notes above; **interactions:** Appendix 1 (amprenavir)

Hepatic impairment avoid oral solution due to high propylene glycol content; reduce dose of capsules in moderate to severe impairment

Renal impairment use oral solution with caution in mild to moderate impairment due to high propylene glycol content; avoid oral solution in severe impairment

Pregnancy avoid oral solution due to high propylene glycol content; manufacturer advises use capsules only if potential benefit outweighs risk

Rash Rash may occur, usually in the second week of therapy; discontinue permanently if severe rash with systemic or allergic symptoms or, mucosal involvement; if rash mild or moderate, may continue without interruption—rash usually resolves within 2 weeks and may respond to antihistamines

Contra-indications

Breast-feeding avoid (see p. 357)

Side-effects see notes above; also reported, rash including rarely Stevens-Johnson syndrome (see also Rash above); tremors, oral or perioral paraesthesia, mood disorders including depression

Licensed use not licensed for use in children under 4 years

Indication and dose

HIV infection in combination with other antiretroviral drugs in children previously treated with other protease inhibitors for dose, consult Guidelines (see notes above)

Agenerase® (GSK) PoM

Capsules, ivory, amprenavir 50 mg, net price 480-cap pack = £139.50. Label: 5

Excipients: include vitamin E 36 units/50 mg amprenavir (avoid vitamin E supplements)

Oral solution, grape-bubblegum- and peppermint-flavoured, amprenavir 15 mg/mL, net price 240-mL pack = £33.48. Label: 4, 5

Excipients: include vitamin E 46 units/mL (avoid vitamin E supplements), propylene glycol 550 mg/mL (see Excipients, p. 3)

Electrolytes potassium 30 micromol/mL, sodium 200 micromol/mL

Note The bioavailability of *Agenerase®* oral solution is lower than that of capsules; the two formulations are **not** interchangeable on a milligram-for-milligram basis

ATAZANAVIR

Cautions see notes above; concomitant use with drugs that prolong PR interval; cardiac conduction disorders; **interactions:** Appendix 1 (atazanavir)

Hepatic impairment use with caution in mild impairment; avoid in moderate to severe impairment

Pregnancy manufacturer advises avoid—theoretical risk of hyperbilirubinaemia in neonate if used at term

Contra-indications

Breast-feeding avoid (see p. 357)

Side-effects see notes above; also mouth ulcers, jaundice, hepatosplenomegaly, hypertension, oedema, palpitation, syncope, chest pain, dyspnoea, peripheral neurological symptoms, abnormal dreams, amnesia, depression, anxiety, gynaecomastia, weight changes, increased appetite, nephrolithiasis, urinary frequency, haematuria, proteinuria, arthralgia, alopecia

Licensed use not licensed for use in children under 18 years

Indication and dose

HIV infection in combination with other antiretroviral drugs in children previously treated with antiretrovirals for dose, consult Guidelines (see notes above)

Reyataz® (Bristol-Myers Squibb) ▼ PoM

Capsules, atazanavir (as sulphate) 100 mg (dark blue/white), net price 60-cap pack = £315.69; 150 mg (dark blue/light blue), 60-cap pack = £315.69; 200 mg (dark blue), 60-cap pack = £315.69. Label: 5, 21

5 Infections

FOSAMPRENAVIR

Note Fosamprenavir is a pro-drug of amprenavir

Cautions see notes above and under Amprenavir

Hepatic impairment Manufacturer advises caution in mild to moderate hepatic impairment; avoid in severe hepatic impairment

Pregnancy Toxicity in *animal* studies; manufacturer advises use only if potential benefit outweighs risk

Contra-indications

Breast-feeding avoid (see p. 357)

Side-effects see notes above and under Amprenavir

Licensed use not licensed for use in children under 18 years

Indication and dose

HIV infection in combination with other antiretroviral drugs for dose, consult Guidelines (see notes above)

Note 700 mg fosamprenavir is equivalent to approx. 600 mg amprenavir

Telzir® (GSK) ▼ PoM

Tablets, f/c, pink, fosamprenavir (as calcium) 700 mg, net price 60-tab pack = £274.92

Oral suspension, fosamprenavir (as calcium) 50 mg/mL, net price 225-mL pack (grape-bubble-gum-and peppermint-flavoured) (with 10-mL oral syringe) = £73.31. Label: 23

Excipients: include propylene glycol

INDINAVIR

Cautions see notes above; ensure adequate hydration (risk of nephrolithiasis); children at risk of nephrolithiasis (monitor for nephrolithiasis); avoid in porphyria (section 9.8.2); **interactions:** Appendix 1 (indinavir)

Hepatic impairment increased risk of nephrolithiasis; reduce dose in mild to moderate impairment; not studied in severe impairment

Pregnancy toxicity in *animal* studies, manufacturer advises avoid; theoretical risk of hyperbilirubinaemia and renal stones in neonate if used at term

Contra-indications

Breast-feeding avoid (see p. 357); contra-indicated in neonates (risk of hyperbilirubinaemia)

Side-effects see notes above; also reported, dry mouth, hypoaesthesia, dry skin, hyperpigmentation, alopecia, paronychia, interstitial nephritis (with medullary calcification and cortical atrophy in asymptomatic severe leucocyturia), nephrolithiasis (may require interruption or discontinuation), dysuria, haematuria, crystalluria, proteinuria, pyuria; haemolytic anaemia

Licensed use not licensed for use in children under 4 years

Indication and dose

HIV infection in combination with nucleoside reverse transcriptase inhibitors for dose, consult Guidelines (see notes above)

Crixivan® (MSD) PoM

Capsules, indinavir (as sulphate), 200 mg, net price 360-cap pack = £226.28; 400 mg, 90-cap pack = £113.15, 180-cap pack = £226.28. Label: 27, counselling, administration

Counselling Administer 1 hour before or 2 hours after a meal; may be administered with a low-fat light meal (may be mixed with apple sauce); in combination with didanosine tablets, allow 1 hour between each drug (antacids in didanosine tablets reduce absorption of indinavir); in combination with low-dose ritonavir, give with food

Note Dispense in original container (contains desiccant)

LOPINAVIR WITH RITONAVIR

Cautions see notes above; concomitant use with drugs that prolong QT interval; pancreatitis (see below); **interactions:** Appendix 1 (lopinavir, ritonavir)

Hepatic impairment avoid oral solution—high propylene glycol content; manufacturer advises avoid capsules in severe impairment

Renal impairment use with caution in severe impairment; avoid oral solution due to high propylene glycol content

Pregnancy manufacturer advises avoid (toxicity in *animal* studies); oral solution has high propylene glycol content

Pancreatitis Signs and symptoms suggestive of pancreatitis (including raised serum amylase and lipase) should be evaluated—discontinue if pancreatitis diagnosed

Contra-indications

Breast-feeding avoid (see p. 357)

Side-effects see notes and Cautions above; also electrolyte disturbances; *less commonly* dysphagia, appetite changes, weight changes, cholecystitis, hypertension, myocardial infarction, palpitation, thrombophlebitis, vasculitis, chest pain, oedema, dyspnoea, cough, agitation, anxiety, amnesia, ataxia, hypertonia, confusion, depression, abnormal dreams, extrapyramidal effects, neuropathy, influenza-like syndrome, Cushing's syndrome, hypothyroidism, menorrhagia, sexual dysfunction, breast enlargement, dehydration, hypercalciuria, lactic acidosis, arthralgia, hyperuricaemia, abnormal vision, otitis media, tinnitus, dry mouth, sialadenitis, mouth ulceration, peridontitis, acne, alopecia, dry

LOPINAVIR WITH RITONAVIR (*continued*)

skin, sweating, skin discoloration, nail disorders; *rarely* prolonged PR interval

Licensed use not licensed for use in children under 2 years

Indication and dose

HIV infection in combination with other antiretroviral drugs for dose, consult Guidelines (see notes above)

Kaletra® (Abbott) PoM

Capsules, orange, lopinavir 133.3 mg, ritonavir 33.3 mg, net price 180-cap pack = £307.39. Label: 21

Oral solution, lopinavir 400 mg, ritonavir 100 mg/5 mL, net price 5×60-mL packs = £307.39. Label: 21

Excipients: include propylene glycol 153 mg/mL (see Excipients, p. 3), alcohol 42%

Counselling oral solution tastes bitter

Note 5 mL oral solution ≡ 3 capsules; where appropriate, capsules may be used instead of oral solution

NELFINAVIR

Cautions see notes above; **interactions:** Appendix 1 (nelfinavir)

Hepatic impairment manufacturer advises caution—no information available

Renal impairment manufacturer advises caution—no information available

Pregnancy manufacturer advises avoid—no information available

Contra-indications

Breast-feeding avoid (see p. 357)

Side-effects see notes above; also reported, fever

Licensed use not licensed for use in children under 3 years

Indication and dose

HIV infection in combination with other antiretroviral drugs for dose, consult Guidelines (see notes above)

Viracept® (Roche) PoM

Tablets blue, f/c, nelfinavir (as mesilate) 250 mg, net price 300-tab pack = £273.16. Label: 21

Oral powder, nelfinavir (as mesilate) 50 mg/g. Net price 144 g (with 1-g and 5-g scoop) = £28.72. Label: 21, counselling, administration

Excipients: include aspartame (section 9.4.1)

Counselling Powder may be mixed with water, milk, formula feeds or pudding; it should **not** be mixed with acidic foods or juices owing to its taste

If given with didanosine, nelfinavir should be given 1 hour before or 2 hours after didanosine

RITONAVIR

Cautions see notes above; avoid in porphyria (section 9.8.2); pancreatitis (see below); **interactions:** Appendix 1 (ritonavir)

Hepatic impairment avoid in severe hepatic impairment

Pregnancy manufacturer advises avoid—toxicity in *animal* studies

Pancreatitis Signs and symptoms suggestive of pancreatitis (including raised serum amylase and lipase) should be evaluated—discontinue if pancreatitis diagnosed

Contra-indications

Breast-feeding avoid (see p. 357)

Side-effects see notes and Cautions above; also reported, diarrhoea (may impair absorption—close monitoring required), throat irritation, vasodilatation, syncope, hypotension; drowsiness, circumoral and peripheral paraesthesia, hyperaesthesia, seizures, raised uric acid, dry mouth and ulceration, cough, anxiety, fever, decreased blood thyroxine concentration, menorrhagia, sweating, electrolyte disturbances, increased prothrombin time

Licensed use licensed for use in children 2–18 years

Indication and dose

Progressive or advanced HIV infection in combination with nucleoside reverse transcriptase inhibitors; low doses used to increase effect of some protease inhibitors for dose, consult Guidelines (see notes above)

Norvir® (Abbott) PoM

Capsules, ritonavir 100 mg, net price 336-cap pack = £377.39. Label 21

Excipients: include alcohol 12%

Oral solution, sugar-free, ritonavir 400 mg/5 mL, net price 5 × 90-mL packs (with measuring cup) = £403.20. Label: 21, counselling, administration

Excipients: include alcohol, propylene glycol

Counselling Oral solution contains 43% alcohol; bitter taste can be masked by mixing with chocolate milk; do not mix with water, measuring cup must be dry

Administration of ritonavir and didanosine should be separated by at least 2 hours

With lopinavir

See under Lopinavir with ritonavir

5 Infections

SAQUINAVIR

Cautions see notes above; concomitant use of garlic (avoid garlic capsules—reduces plasma-saquinavir concentration); **interactions**: Appendix 1 (saquinavir)

Hepatic impairment manufacturer advises caution in moderate impairment; avoid in severe impairment

Renal impairment manufacturer advises caution in severe impairment—dose adjustment possibly required

Pregnancy manufacturer advises avoid

Contra-indications

Breast-feeding avoid (see p. 357)

Side-effects see notes above; also buccal and mucosal ulceration, taste disturbance, chest pain, peripheral neuropathy, hypoaesthesia, paraesthesia, mood changes, fever, changes in libido, verrucae, nephrolithiasis, pruritus, Stevens-Johnson syndrome; *rarely* sleep disturbances, convulsions

Licensed use not licensed for use in children under 16 years

Indication and dose

HIV infection in combination with other antiretroviral drugs for dose, consult Guidelines (see notes above)

Note To avoid confusion between the different formulations of saquinavir, prescribers should specify the brand to be dispensed; absorption from *Fortovase®* [now discontinued] is much greater than from *Invirase®*.

Counselling in combination with low-dose ritonavir, take within 2 hours of a meal

Invirase® (Roche) PoM

Capsules, brown/green, saquinavir (as mesilate) 200 mg, net price 270-cap pack = £240.06. Label: 21

Tablets, orange, f/c, saquinavir (as mesilate) 500 mg, net price 120-tab pack = £266.73. Label: 21

Non-nucleoside reverse transcriptase inhibitors

EFAVIRENZ

Cautions chronic hepatitis B or C (greater risk of hepatic side-effects); history of mental illness or seizures; **interactions**: Appendix 1 (efavirenz)

Hepatic impairment in mild to moderate liver disease, monitor for dose-related side-effects (e.g. CNS effects) and liver function; avoid in severe hepatic impairment

Renal impairment in severe impairment manufacturer advises caution—no information available

Pregnancy manufacturer advises avoid unless no alternative available

Rash Rash, usually in the first 2 weeks, is the most common side-effect; discontinue if severe rash with blistering, desquamation, mucosal involvement or fever; if rash mild or moderate, may continue without interruption—rash usually resolves within 1 month

Psychiatric disorders Children or their carers should be advised to seek immediate medical attention if symptoms such as severe depression, psychosis or suicidal ideation occur

Contra-indications

Breast-feeding avoid (see p. 357)

Side-effects rash including Stevens-Johnson syndrome (see Rash above); abdominal pain, diarrhoea, nausea, vomiting; anxiety, depression, sleep disturbances, abnormal dreams, dizziness, headache, fatigue, impaired concentration (administration at bedtime especially in first 2–4 weeks reduces CNS effects); pruritus; *less commonly* pancreatitis, hepatitis, psychosis, mania, suicidal ideation, amnesia, ataxia, convulsions, and blurred vision; also reported hepatic failure, raised serum cholesterol, gynaecomastia, photosensitivity

Licensed use *Capsules* and *oral solution* not licensed for use in children under 3 years and body-weight under 13 kg; *tablets* not licensed for use in children with body-weight under 40 kg

Indication and dose

HIV infection in combination with other antiretroviral drugs for dose, consult Guidelines (see notes above)

Sustiva (Bristol-Myers Squibb) PoM

Capsules, efavirenz 50 mg (yellow/white), net price 30-cap pack = £17.41; 100 mg (white), 30-cap pack = £34.77; 200 mg (yellow), 90-cap pack = £208.40. Label: 23

Administration Capsules may be opened and contents added to food (contents have a peppery taste) [unlicensed use]

Tablets, f/c, yellow, efavirenz 600 mg, net price 30-tab pack = £208.40. Label: 23

Oral solution, sugar-free, strawberry and mint flavour, efavirenz 30 mg/mL, net price 180-mL pack = £56.02

Note The bioavailability of *Sustiva®* oral solution is lower than that of the capsules and tablets; the oral solution is **not** interchangeable with either capsules or tablets on a milligram-for-milligram basis

NEVIRAPINE

Cautions chronic hepatitis B or C, high CD4 cell count, and females (all at greater risk of hepatic side-effects); **interactions**: Appendix 1 (nevirapine)

Hepatic impairment manufacturer advises caution in moderate hepatic impairment; avoid in severe hepatic impairment; see also Hepatic Disease, below

Pregnancy manufacturer advises avoid

Hepatic disease Potentially life-threatening hepatotoxicity including fatal fulminant hepatitis reported usually in first 6 weeks; close monitoring required during first 18 weeks; monitor liver function before treatment then every

NEVIRAPINE (*continued*)

2 weeks for 2 months then after 1 month and then regularly; discontinue permanently if abnormalities in liver function tests accompanied by hypersensitivity reaction (rash, fever, arthralgia, myalgia, lymphadenopathy, hepatitis, renal impairment, eosinophilia, granulocytopenia); suspend if severe abnormalities in liver function tests but no hypersensitivity reaction—discontinue permanently if significant liver function abnormalities recur; monitor patient closely if mild to moderate abnormalities in liver function tests with no hypersensitivity reaction

Rash Rash, usually in first 6 weeks, is most common side-effect; incidence reduced if introduced at low dose and dose increased gradually; monitor closely for skin reactions during first 18 weeks; discontinue permanently if severe rash or if rash accompanied by blistering, oral lesions, conjunctivitis, facial oedema, general malaise or hypersensitivity reactions; if rash mild or moderate may continue without interruption but dose should not be increased until rash resolves

Counselling Children and carers should be told how to recognise hypersensitivity reactions and advised to discontinue treatment and seek immediate medical attention if severe skin reaction, hypersensitivity reactions or symptoms of hepatitis develop

Contra-indications severe hepatic impairment; post-exposure prophylaxis

Breast-feeding avoid (see p. 357)

Side-effects rash including Stevens-Johnson syndrome and rarely, toxic epidermal necrolysis (see also Cautions above); nausea, hepatitis (see also Hepatic Disease above), headache; *less commonly* vomiting, abdominal pain, fatigue, fever, and myalgia; *rarely* diarrhoea, angioedema, anaphylaxis, hypersensitivity reactions (may involve hepatic reactions and rash, see Hepatic Disease above), arthralgia, anaemia, and granulocytopenia; *very rarely* neuropsychiatric reactions

Licensed use *oral solution*, not licensed for use in children under 2 months; *tablets*, not licensed for use in children weighing less than 50 kg

Indication and dose

Progressive or advanced HIV infection, in combination with at least two other antiretroviral drugs for dose, consult Guidelines (see notes above)

Note If treatment interrupted for more than 7 days re-introduce using low dose and increase dose cautiously

Viramune® (Boehringer Ingelheim) PoM

Tablets, nevirapine 200 mg, net price 60-tab pack = £160.00. Counselling, hypersensitivity reactions

Suspension, nevirapine 50 mg/5 mL, net price 240-mL pack = £50.40. Counselling, hypersensitivity reactions

Other antiretrovirals

ENFUVIRTIDE

Cautions chronic hepatitis B or C (possibly greater risk of hepatic side-effects)

Hepatic impairment manufacturer advises caution—no information available

Renal impairment manufacturer advises caution if creatinine clearance less than 35 mL/minute/1.73m^2—no information available

Pregnancy manufacturer advises avoid

Hypersensitivity reactions Hypersensitivity reactions including rash, fever, nausea, vomiting, chills, rigors, low blood pressure, respiratory distress, glomerulonephritis, and raised liver enzymes reported; discontinue immediately if any signs or symptoms of systemic hypersensitivity develop and do not rechallenge

Counselling Children and carers should be told how to recognise signs of hypersensitivity, and advised to discontinue treatment and seek immediate medical attention if symptoms develop

Contra-indications

Breast-feeding avoid (see p. 357)

Side-effects injection-site reactions; pancreatitis, gastro-oesophageal reflux disease, anorexia, weight loss; hypertriglyceridaemia; peripheral neuropathy, asthenia, tremor, anxiety, nightmares, irritability, impaired concentration, vertigo; pneumonia, sinusitis, influenza-like illness; diabetes mellitus; haematuria; renal calculi, lymphadenopathy; myalgia; conjunctivitis; dry skin, acne, erythema, skin papilloma; *less commonly* hypersensitivity reactions (see Cautions)

Licensed use not licensed for use in children under 6 years

Indication and dose

HIV infection in combination with other antiretroviral drugs for resistant infection or for children intolerant to other antiretroviral regimens for dose, consult Guidelines (see notes above)

Administration for *subcutaneous injection*, reconstitute with 1.1 mL Water for Injections and allow to stand (for up to 45 minutes) to dissolve; do **not** shake or invert vial

Fuzeon® (Roche) ▼ PoM

Injection, powder for reconstitution, enfuvirtide 108 mg (= enfuvirtide 90 mg/mL when reconstituted), net price 108-mg vial = £19.13 (with Water for Injections, syringe, and alcohol swabs). Counselling, hypersensitivity reactions

5 Infections

5.3.2 Herpesvirus infections

5.3.2.1 Herpes simplex and varicella–zoster infection

The two most important herpesvirus pathogens are herpes simplex virus (herpesvirus hominis) and varicella–zoster virus.

Herpes simplex infections Herpes infection of the mouth and lips and in the eye is generally associated with herpes simplex virus serotype 1 (HSV-1); other areas of the skin may also be infected, especially in immunodeficiency. Genital infection is most often associated with HSV-2 and also HSV-1. Treatment of herpes simplex infection should start as early as possible and usually within 5 days of the appearance of the infection.

In individuals with good immune function, mild infection of the eye (ocular herpes, section 11.3.3) and of the lips (herpes labialis or cold sores, section 13.10.3) is treated with a topical antiviral drug. Primary herpetic gingivostomatitis is managed by changes to diet and with analgesics (section 12.3.2). Severe infection, neonatal herpes infection or infection in immunocompromised individuals requires treatment with a systemic antiviral drug. Primary or recurrent genital herpes simplex infection is treated with an antiviral drug given by mouth. Persistance of a lesion or recurrence in an immunocompromised child may signal the development of resistance.

Specialist advice should be sought for systemic treatment of herpes simplex infection in pregnancy.

Varicella–zoster infections Regardless of immune function and the use of any immunoglobulins, neonates with *chickenpox* should be treated with a parenteral antiviral to reduce the risk of severe disease. Oral therapy is not recommended as absorption is variable.

Chickenpox in otherwise healthy children between 1 month and 12 years is usually mild and antiviral treatment is not usually required. Chickenpox is more severe in adolescents than in children; antiviral treatment started within 24 hours of the onset of rash may reduce the duration and severity of symptoms in otherwise healthy adolescents. Antiviral treatment is generally recommended in immunocompromised patients and those at special risk (e.g. because of severe cardiovascular or respiratory disease or chronic skin disorder); an antiviral is given for 10 days with at least 7 days of parenteral treatment.

In pregnancy severe chickenpox may cause complications, especially varicella pneumonia. Specialist advice should be sought for the treatment of chickenpox during pregnancy.

In *herpes zoster* (shingles) systemic antiviral treatment can reduce the severity and duration of pain, reduce complications, and reduce viral shedding. Treatment with the antiviral should be started within 72 hours of the onset of rash and is usually continued for 7–10 days.

Immunocompromised patients at high risk of disseminated or severe infection should be treated with a parenteral antiviral drug. Chronic pain which persists after the rash has healed (postherpetic neuralgia) requires specific management (section 4.7.3).

Neonates and children who have been exposed to chickenpox and are at special risk of complications may require prophylaxis with varicella-zoster immunoglobulin (see under Specific Immunoglobulins, section 14.5).

Choice **Aciclovir** is active against herpesviruses but does not eradicate them. Uses of aciclovir include systemic treatment of varicella–zoster and the systemic and topical treatment of herpes simplex infections of the skin (section 13.10.3) and mucous membranes (section 7.2.2). It is used by mouth for severe herpetic stomatitis (see also p. 604). Aciclovir eye ointment (section 11.3.3) is used for herpes simplex infections of the eye; it is combined with systemic treatment for ophthalmic zoster.

Famciclovir, a prodrug of penciclovir, is similar to aciclovir and is licensed in adults for use in herpes zoster and genital herpes; there is limited information available on use in children. Penciclovir itself is used as a cream for herpes simplex labialis (section 13.10.3).

Valaciclovir is an ester of aciclovir, licensed in adults for herpes zoster and herpes simplex infections of the skin and mucous membranes (including genital herpes); it is also licensed in children over 12 years for preventing cytomegalovirus disease following renal transplantation. Valaciclovir may be used for the treatment of mild herpes zoster in immunocompromised children over 12 years; treatment should be initiated under specialist supervision. Valaciclovir once daily may reduce the risk of transmitting genital herpes to heterosexual partners—specialist advice should be sought.

ACICLOVIR

(Acyclovir)

Cautions maintain adequate hydration (especially with infusion or high doses); **interactions:** Appendix 1 (aciclovir)

Renal impairment use normal intravenous dose every 12 hours if creatinine clearance 25–50 mL/minute/1.73 m^2 (every 24 hours if creatinine clearance 10–25 mL/minute/1.73 m^2); consult product literature for intravenous dose if creatinine clearance less than 10 mL/minute/1.73 m^2; for herpes zoster, use normal oral dose every 8 hours if creatinine clearance 10–25 mL/minute/1.73 m^2 (every 12 hours if creatinine clearance less than 10 mL/minute/1.73 m^2); for herpes simplex, use normal oral dose every 12 hours if creatinine clearance less than 10 mL/minute/1.73 m^2

Pregnancy not known to be harmful but manufacturers advise avoid unless potential benefit outweighs risk; limited absorption from topical preparations

Breast-feeding significant amount in milk after systemic administration; not known to be harmful but manufacturers advise caution

Side-effects nausea, vomiting, abdominal pain, diarrhoea, headache, fatigue, rash, urticaria, pruritus, photosensitivity; *very rarely* hepatitis, jaundice, dyspnoea, neurological reactions (including dizziness, confusion, hallucinations convulsions, and drowsiness), acute renal failure, anaemia, thrombocytopenia, and leucopenia; on *intravenous infusion*, severe local inflammation (sometimes leading to ulceration), and *very rarely* agitation, tremors, psychosis and fever

Licensed use *Tablets* and *suspension* not licensed for treatment of herpes zoster in children (age range not specified by manufacturer); *intravenous infusion* not licensed for herpes zoster in children under 18 years; *tablets* and *suspension* not licensed for attenuation of chickenpox (if varicella-zoster immunoglobulin not indicated) in children under 18 years

Indication and dose

Herpes simplex treatment

- **By mouth**

Child 1 month–2 years 100 mg 5 times daily, usually for 5 days (longer if new lesions appear during treatment or if healing incomplete); dose doubled if immunocompromised or if absorption impaired

Child 2–18 years 200 mg 5 times daily, usually for 5 days (longer if new lesions appear during treatment or if healing incomplete); dose doubled if immunocompromised or if absorption impaired

- **By intravenous infusion**

Neonate with disseminated herpes simplex 20 mg/kg every 8 hours for 14 days (21 days if CNS involvement)

Child 1–3 months with disseminated herpes simplex 20 mg/kg every 8 hours for 14 days (21 days if CNS involvement)

Child 3 months–12 years 250 mg/m^2 every 8 hours usually for 5 days, dose doubled if CNS involvement (given for up to 21 days) or if immunosuppressed

Child 12–18 years 5 mg/kg every 8 hours usually for 5 days, dose doubled if CNS involvement (given for up to 21 days) or if immunosuppressed

Note To avoid excessive dose in obese patients parenteral dose should be calculated on the basis of ideal weight for height

Herpes simplex prophylaxis in the immunocompromised

- **By mouth**

Child 1 month–2 years 100–200 mg 4 times daily

Child 2–18 years 200–400 mg 4 times daily

Chickenpox and herpes zoster infection

- **By mouth**

Child 1 month–12 years 20 mg/kg (max. 800 mg) 4 times daily for 5 days

Child 12–18 years 800 mg 5 times daily for 7 days

- **By intravenous infusion**

Neonate 10–20 mg/kg every 8 hours for at least 7 days

Child 1–3 months 10–20 mg/kg every 8 hours for at least 7 days

Child 3 months–12 years 250 mg/m^2 every 8 hours usually for 5 days, dose doubled if immunocompromised

Child 12–18 years 5 mg/kg every 8 hours usually for 5 days, dose doubled if immunocompromised

Note To avoid excessive dose in obese patients parenteral dose should be calculated on the basis of ideal weight for height

ACICLOVIR (*continued*)

Attenuation of chickenpox if varicella–zoster immunoglobulin not indicated
- **By mouth**

  Child 1 month–18 years 10 mg/kg 4 times daily for 7 days starting 1 week after exposure

Herpesvirus skin infections section 13.10.3

Herpesvirus eye infections section 11.3.3

Administration for *intravenous infusion*, reconstitute to 25 mg/mL with Water for Injections or Sodium Chloride 0.9% then dilute to concentration of 5 mg/mL with Sodium Chloride 0.9% *or* Sodium Chloride and Glucose *or* Compound Sodium Lactate and give over 1 hour; alternatively, may be administered in a concentration of 25 mg/mL using a suitable infusion pump and central venous access and given over 1 hour

Aciclovir (Non-proprietary) PoM
Tablets, aciclovir 200 mg, net price 25-tab pack = £4.01; 400 mg, 56-tab pack = £7.31; 800 mg, 35-tab pack = £9.53. Label: 9
Brands include *Virovir®*
Dental prescribing on NHS Aciclovir Tablets 200 mg may be prescribed

Dispersible tablets, aciclovir 200 mg, net price 25-tab pack = £2.82; 400 mg, 56-tab pack = £8.30; 800 mg, 35-tab pack = £9.53. Label: 9

Intravenous infusion, powder for reconstitution, aciclovir (as sodium salt). Net price 250-mg vial = £10.91; 500-mg vial = £20.22
Electrolytes Na^+ 1.1 mmol/250-mg vial

Intravenous infusion, aciclovir (as sodium salt), 25 mg/mL, net price 10-mL (250-mg) vial = £10.37; 20-mL (500-mg) vial = £19.21; 40-mL (1-g) vial = £40.44
Electrolytes Na^+ 1.16 mmol/250-mg vial

Zovirax® (GSK) PoM
Tablets, all dispersible, f/c, aciclovir 200 mg (blue), net price 25-tab pack = £18.80; 400 mg (pink), 56-tab pack = £68.98; 800 mg (scored, *Shingles Treatment Pack*), 35-tab pack = £69.85. Label: 9
Suspension, both off-white, sugar-free, aciclovir 200 mg/5 mL (banana-flavoured), net price 125 mL = £29.56; 400 mg/5 mL (*Double Strength Suspension*, orange-flavoured) 100 mL = £33.02. Label: 9
Dental prescribing on NHS May be prescribed as Aciclovir 200 mg/5 mL Oral Suspension
Intravenous infusion, powder for reconstitution, aciclovir (as sodium salt). Net price 250-mg vial = £10.15; 500-mg vial = £18.81
Electrolytes Na^+ 1.1 mmol/250-mg vial

VALACICLOVIR

Note Valaciclovir is a pro-drug of aciclovir

Cautions see under Aciclovir

Hepatic impairment manufacturer advises caution with high doses used for preventing cytomegalovirus disease—no information available in children

Renal impairment for herpes zoster, 1 g every 12 hours if creatinine clearance 15–30 mL/minute/1.73 m² (every 24 hours if creatinine clearance less than 15 mL/minute/1.73 m²); reduce dose according to creatinine clearance for cytomegalovirus prophylaxis following renal transplantation

Side-effects see under Aciclovir but neurological reactions more frequent with high doses

Licensed use not licensed for use in children except for CMV prophylaxis in children over 12 years

Indication and dose

Herpes zoster in immunocompromised
- **By mouth**

  Child 12–18 years 1 g 3 times daily for 7 days

Prevention of cytomegalovirus disease following renal transplantation (preferably starting within 72 hours of transplantation)
- **By mouth**

  Child 12–18 years 2 g 4 times daily usually for 90 days

Valtrex® (GSK) PoM
Tablets, f/c, valaciclovir (as hydrochloride) 500 mg, net price 10-tab pack = £21.86, 42-tab pack = £91.61. Label: 9

5 Infections

5.3.2.2 Cytomegalovirus infection

Recommendations for the optimum maintenance therapy of cytomegalovirus (CMV) infections and the duration of treatment are subject to rapid change.

Ganciclovir is related to aciclovir but it is more active against cytomegalovirus; it is also much more toxic than aciclovir and should therefore be prescribed under specialist supervision and only when the potential benefit outweighs the risks. Ganciclovir is administered by intravenous infusion for the *initial treatment* of CMV retinitis. The use of ganciclovir may also be considered for symptomatic congenital CMV infection. Ganciclovir causes profound myelosuppression when given with zidovudine; the two should not normally be given together particularly during initial ganciclovir therapy. The likelihood of ganciclovir resistance increases in patients with a high viral load or in those who receive the drug over a long duration; cross-resistance to cidofovir is common.

Valaciclovir (section 5.3.2.1) is licensed for use in children over 12 years for prevention of cytomegalovirus disease following renal transplantation.

Foscarnet is also active against cytomegalovirus; it is toxic and can cause renal impairment.

Cidofovir is given in combination with probenecid for CMV retinitis in AIDS patients when ganciclovir and foscarnet are contra-indicated. Cidofovir is nephrotoxic. There is limited information on its use in children.

For local treatment of CMV retinitis, see section 11.3.3.

GANCICLOVIR

Cautions close monitoring of full blood count (severe deterioration may require correction and possibly treatment interruption); history of cytopenia; low platelet count; potential carcinogen and teratogen; radiotherapy; ensure adequate hydration during intravenous administration; vesicant—infuse into vein with adequate flow preferably using plastic cannula; possible risk of long-term carcinogenic or reproductive toxicity; **interactions:** Appendix 1 (ganciclovir)

Renal impairment reduce dose—consult product literature

Contra-indications hypersensitivity to ganciclovir or aciclovir; abnormally low haemoglobin, neutrophil, or platelet counts (consult product literature)

Pregnancy avoid—teratogenic risk (ensure effective contraception during treatment and barrier contraception for males during and for at least 90 days after treatment)

Breast-feeding avoid—no information available

Side-effects diarrhoea, nausea, vomiting, dyspepsia, abdominal pain, constipation, flatulence, dysphagia, hepatic dysfunction; dyspnoea, chest pain, cough; headache, insomnia, convulsions, dizziness, neuropathy, depression, anxiety, confusion, abnormal thinking, fatigue, weight loss, anorexia; infection, fever, night sweats; anaemia, leucopenia, thrombocytopenia, pancytopenia, renal impairment; myalgia, arthralgia; macular oedema, retinal detachment, vitreous floaters, eye pain; ear pain, taste disturbance; dermatitis, pruritus; injection-site reactions; *less commonly* mouth ulcers, pancreatitis, arrhythmias, hypotension, anaphylactic reactions, psychosis, tremor, male infertility, haematuria, disturbances in hearing and vision, and alopecia

Indication and dose

Life-threatening or sight-threatening cytomegalovirus infections in immunocompromised patients only; prevention of cytomegalovirus disease during immunosuppressive therapy following organ transplantation

- **By intravenous infusion**

Child 1 month–18 years initially (induction) 5 mg/kg every 12 hours for 14–21 days for treatment or for 7–14 days for prevention; for maintenance dose, see below

Maintenance (for patients at risk of relapse of retinitis)

- **By intravenous infusion**

Child 1 month–18 years 6 mg/kg daily on 5 days per week *or* 5 mg/kg daily until adequate recovery of immunity; if retinitis progresses initial induction treatment may be repeated

Local treatment of CMV retinitis section 11.3.3

Administration for *intravenous infusion*, reconstitute with Water for Injections (500 mg/10 mL) then dilute to a concentration of not more than 10 mg/mL with Glucose 5% *or* Sodium Chloride 0.9% *or* Compound Sodium Lactate and give over 1 hour

Cymevene® (Roche) PoM

Intravenous infusion, powder for reconstitution, ganciclovir (as sodium salt). Net price 500-mg vial = £31.60

Electrolytes Na^+ 2 mmol/500-mg vial

Caution in handling Ganciclovir is toxic and personnel should be adequately protected during handling and administration; if solution comes into contact with skin or mucosa, wash off immediately with soap and water

FOSCARNET SODIUM

Cautions monitor electrolytes, particularly calcium and magnesium; monitor serum creatinine every second day during induction and every week during maintenance; ensure adequate hydration; avoid rapid infusion; **interactions**: Appendix 1 (foscarnet)

Renal impairment reduce dose—consult product literature

Contra-indications

Pregnancy avoid

Breast-feeding avoid—present in milk in *animal* studies

Side-effects nausea, vomiting, diarrhoea (occasionally constipation and dyspepsia), abdominal pain, anorexia; changes in blood pressure and ECG; headache, fatigue, mood disturbances (including psychosis), asthenia, paraesthesia, convulsions, tremor, dizziness, and other neurological disorders; rash; impairment of renal function including acute renal failure; hypocalcaemia (sometimes symptomatic) and other electrolyte disturbances; abnormal liver function tests; decreased haemoglobin concentration, leucopenia, granulocytopenia, thrombocytopenia; thrombophlebitis if given undiluted by per-

FOSCARNET SODIUM (*continued*)

ipheral vein; genital irritation and ulceration (due to high concentrations excreted in urine); isolated reports of pancreatitis

Licensed use not licensed for use in children (age range not specified by manufacturer)

Indication and dose

CMV retinitis
- **By intravenous infusion**
  Child 1 month–18 years induction 60 mg/kg every 8 hours for 2–3 weeks then maintenance 60 mg/kg daily, increased to 90–120 mg/kg if tolerated; if retinitis progresses on maintenance dose, repeat induction regimen

Mucocutaneous herpes simplex infection
- **By intravenous infusion**
  Child 1 month–18 years 40 mg/kg every 8 hours for 2–3 weeks or until lesions heal

Administration for *intravenous infusion*, give undiluted solution via a central venous catheter; alternatively dilute with Glucose 5% to a concentration of 12 mg/mL for administration via a peripheral vein; infuse over at least 1 hour

Foscavir® (AstraZeneca) PoM
Intravenous infusion, foscarnet sodium hexahydrate 24 mg/mL, net price 250-mL bottle = £34.49

5.3.3 Viral hepatitis

Treatment for viral hepatitis should be initiated by a specialist in hepatology or infectious diseases. The management of uncomplicated acute viral hepatitis is largely symptomatic. Hepatitis B and hepatitis C viruses are major causes of chronic hepatitis. For details on immunisation against hepatitis A and B infections, see section 14.4 (active immunisation) and section 14.5 (passive immunisation).

Chronic hepatitis B **Interferon alfa** (section 8.2.4), **peginterferon alfa-2a**, **lamivudine** (section 5.3.1), and **adefovir dipivoxil** have a role in the treatment of chronic hepatitis B in adults but their role in children has not been established. Specialist supervision is required for the management of chronic hepatitis B.

Chronic hepatitis C A combination of **ribavirin** (section 5.3.5) and **interferon alfa** (section 8.2.4) is licensed for use in children over 3 years with chronic hepatitis C. Specialist supervision is required and the regimen is chosen according to the genotype of the infecting virus and the viral load. A combination of **peginterferon alfa** (BNF Section 8.2.4) and ribavirin may be preferred.

5.3.4 Influenza

For advice on immunisation against influenza, see section 14.4.

Oseltamivir and **zanamivir** reduce replication of influenza A and B viruses by inhibiting viral neuraminidase. They are most effective for the treatment of influenza if started within a few hours of the onset of symptoms; they are licensed for use within 48 hours of the first symptoms. In otherwise healthy individuals they reduce the duration of symptoms by about 1–1.5 days. The effect of oseltamivir or zanamivir on hospitalisation or on mortality is not clear in those at risk of serious complications from influenza. Oseltamivir is not licensed for use in a child under 1 year because of concerns about neurotoxicity but it may be used under specialist supervision if the child under 1 year is seriously ill. In children over 1 year, oseltamivir is also licensed for prophylaxis when used within 48 hours of exposure to influenza and when influenza is circulating in the community and in exceptional circumstances (e.g. when vaccination does not cover the infecting strain) to prevent influenza in an epidemic. Where prophylaxis against influenza A or B is required and oseltamivir cannot be used, zanamivir is an alternative [unlicensed indication].

Amantadine is licensed for prophylaxis and treatment of influenza A but it is no longer recommended (see NICE guidance).

NICE guidance (oseltamivir, zanamivir, and amantadine for prophylaxis and treatment of influenza)
NICE has recommended (February and September 2003) that the drugs described here are not a substitute for vaccination, which remains the most effective way of preventing illness from influenza. When influenza A or influenza B is circulating in the community:

- amantadine is **not** recommended for post-exposure prophylaxis, seasonal prophylaxis, or treatment of influenza;
- oseltamivir and zanamivir are **not** recommended for seasonal prophylaxis against influenza;
- oseltamivir or zanamivir are **not** recommended for post-exposure prophylaxis, or treatment of otherwise healthy individuals with influenza;
- oseltamivir is recommended for post-exposure prophylaxis in at-risk adolescents over 13 years [oseltamivir is now licensed for children over 1 year[1]] who are not effectively protected by influenza vaccine and who can commence oseltamivir within 48 hours of close contact with someone suffering from influenza-like illness; prophylaxis is also recommended for residents in care establishments (regardless of influenza vaccination) who can commence oseltamivir within 48 hours if influenza-like illness is present in the establishment;
- oseltamivir and zanamivir are recommended (in accordance with UK licensing) to treat at-risk adults who can start treatment within 48 hours of the onset of symptoms; oseltamivir is recommended for at-risk children who can start treatment within 48 hours of the onset of symptoms;

At-risk patients are those who have one or more of the following conditions:

- chronic respiratory disease (including asthma) [but see cautions under Zanamivir below];
- significant cardiovascular disease (excluding hypertension);
- chronic renal disease;
- immunosuppression;
- diabetes mellitus.

Community-based virological surveillance schemes including those run by the Health Protection Agency and the Royal College of General Practitioners should be used to indicate when influenza is circulating in the community.

1. The Department of Health in England has advised (February 2006) that it is appropriate to apply these recommendations to children over 1 year

OSELTAMIVIR

Cautions

Renal impairment reduce dose if creatinine clearance 10–30 mL/minute/1.73m²; avoid if creatinine clearance less than 10 mL/minute/1.73m²

Pregnancy avoid unless potential benefit outweighs risk

Breast-feeding avoid unless potential benefit outweighs risk; present in milk in *animal* studies

Side-effects nausea, vomiting, abdominal pain, dyspepsia, diarrhoea; headache, fatigue, insomnia, dizziness; conjunctivitis, epistaxis; rash; *very rarely* hepatitis, Stevens-Johnson syndrome, and toxic epidermal necrolysis

Indication and dose

Prevention of influenza
- **By mouth**

Child 1–13 years

Body-weight under 15 kg 30 mg once daily for 10 days for post-exposure prophylaxis; for up to 6 weeks during an epidemic

Body-weight 15–23 kg 45 mg once daily for 10 days for post-exposure prophylaxis; for up to 6 weeks during an epidemic

Body-weight 23–40 kg 60 mg once daily for 10 days for post-exposure prophylaxis; for up to 6 weeks during an epidemic

Body-weight over 40 kg 75 mg once daily for 10 days for post-exposure prophylaxis; for up to 6 weeks during an epidemic

Child 13–18 years 75 mg once daily for 10 days for post-exposure prophylaxis; for up to 6 weeks during an epidemic

Treatment of influenza
- **By mouth**

Child 1–13 years

Body-weight under 15 kg 30 mg twice daily for 5 days

Body-weight 15–23 kg 45 mg twice daily for 5 days

Body-weight 23–40 kg 60 mg twice daily for 5 days

Body-weight over 40 kg 75 mg twice daily for 5 days

Child 13–18 years 75 mg twice daily for 5 days

OSELTAMIVIR (*continued*)

[1]**Tamiflu®** (Roche) ▼ PoM
Capsules, grey/yellow, oseltamivir (as phosphate) 75 mg, net price 10-cap pack = £16.36. Label: 9

Suspension, sugar-free, tutti-frutti-flavoured, oseltamivir (as phosphate) for reconstitution with water, 60 mg/5 mL, net price 75 mL = £16.36. Label: 9
Excipients: include sorbitol 1.7 g/5 mL

1. NHS except for the treatment and prophylaxis of influenza as indicated in the notes above and NICE guidance; endorse prescription 'SLS'

ZANAMIVIR

Cautions asthma and chronic pulmonary disease (risk of bronchospasm—short-acting bronchodilator should be available; avoid in severe asthma unless close monitoring possible and appropriate facilities available to treat bronchospasm); uncontrolled chronic illness; other inhaled drugs should be administered before zanamivir

Pregnancy only use if potential benefit outweighs risk—no information available

Contra-indications

Breast-feeding avoid—present in milk in *animal* studies

Side-effects *very rarely* bronchospasm, respiratory impairment, angioedema, urticaria, and rash

Licensed use not licensed for use in children under 12 years

Indication and dose

Treatment of influenza
- **By inhalation of powder**
  Child 12–18 years 10 mg twice daily for 5 days

[1]**Relenza®** (GSK) PoM
Dry powder for inhalation disks containing 4 blisters of zanamivir 5 mg/blister, net price 5 disks with *Diskhaler®* device = £24.55

1. NHS except for the treatment and prophylaxis of influenza as indicated in the notes above and NICE guidance; endorse prescription 'SLS'

5.3.5 Respiratory syncytial virus

Ribavirin (tribavirin) inhibits a wide range of DNA and RNA viruses. It is licensed for administration by inhalation for the treatment of severe bronchiolitis caused by the respiratory syncytial virus (RSV) in infants, especially when they have other serious diseases. However, there is no evidence that ribavirin produces clinically relevant benefit in RSV bronchiolitis. Ribavirin is given by mouth with peginterferon alfa or interferon alfa for the treatment of chronic hepatitis C infection (see Viral Hepatitis, section 5.3.3). Ribavirin is also effective in Lassa fever and has also been used parenterally in the treatment of life-threatening RSV, parainfluenza virus, and adenovirus infections in immunocompromised children [unlicensed indications].

Palivizumab is a monoclonal antibody licensed for preventing serious lower respiratory-tract disease caused by respiratory syncytial virus in children at high risk of the disease; it should be prescribed under specialist supervision and on the basis of the likelihood of hospitalisation. Palivizumab should be considered for children under 6 months with haemodynamically significant left-to-right shunt congenital heart disease or who have pulmonary hypertension. It should also be considered for children under 2 years *either* with chronic lung disease who are using oxygen at home (or have been on prolonged oxygen treatment) *or* with severe congenital immunodeficiency. Palivizumab may also be used for the first 6–12 months of life in a child born at under 35 weeks gestation, if the child is considered by the specialist to be at special risk of hospitalisation. It is licensed for monthly use during the RSV season; the first dose should be administered before the start of the RSV season.

PALIVIZUMAB

Cautions moderate to severe acute infection or febrile illness; thrombocytopenia; serum-palivizumab concentration may be reduced after cardiac surgery

Contra-indications hypersensitivity to humanised monoclonal antibodies

Side-effects fever, injection-site reactions, nervousness; *less commonly* diarrhoea, vomiting, constipation, haemorrhage, rhinitis, cough, wheeze, pain, drowsiness, asthenia, hyperkinesia, leucopenia, and rash; *rarely* apnoea, hypersensitivity reactions (including anaphylaxis)

Licensed use Not licensed in children with congenital immunodeficiency or in children born at 35 weeks gestation or less and older than 6 months (licensed in children under 6 months)

PALIVIZUMAB (continued)

Indication and dose

Prevention of serious disease following respiratory syncytial virus infection (see notes above)

- **By intramuscular injection (preferably in anterolateral thigh)**

  Child 1 month–2 years 15 mg/kg once a month during season of RSV risk (child undergoing cardiac bypass surgery, 15 mg/kg as soon as stable after surgery, then once a month during season of risk); injection volume over 1 mL should be divided between 2 or more sites

Synagis® (Abbott) ▼ PoM

Injection, powder for reconstitution, palivizumab, net price 50-mg vial = £360.40; 100-mg vial = £600.10

RIBAVIRIN

(Tribavirin)

Cautions

Specific cautions for inhaled treatment Maintain standard supportive respiratory and fluid management therapy; monitor electrolytes closely; monitor equipment for precipitation; pregnant women (and those planning pregnancy) should avoid exposure to aerosol

Specific cautions for systemic treatment Exclude pregnancy before treatment in females of childbearing age; effective contraception essential during treatment and for 6 months after treatment (7 months after intravenous treatment) in females and in males of childbearing age; routine monthly pregnancy tests recommended; condoms must be used if partner of male patient is pregnant (ribavirin excreted in semen); cardiac disease (assessment including ECG recommended before and during treatment—discontinue if deterioration); determine full blood count, platelets, electrolytes, serum creatinine, liver function tests and uric acid before starting treatment and then on weeks 2 and 4 of treatment, then as indicated clinically—adjust dose if adverse reactions or laboratory abnormalities develop (consult product literature); test thyroid function before treatment and then every 3 months

Interactions: Appendix 1 (Ribavirin)

Hepatic impairment no dosage adjustment required; avoid oral administration in severe hepatic dysfunction or decompensated cirrhosis

Renal impairment Plasma-ribavirin concentration increased; manufacturer advises avoid oral ribavirin if creatinine clearance less than 50 mL/minute/1.73 m^2; manufacturer advises use intravenous preparation with caution if creatinine clearance less than 30 mL/minute/1.73 m^2

Contra-indications

Pregnancy avoid (**important teratogenic risk**: see Cautions)

Breast-feeding avoid

Specific contra-indications for systemic treatment Haemoglobinopathies; severe debilitating medical conditions; severe hepatic dysfunction or decompensated cirrhosis; autoimmune disease (including autoimmune hepatitis); history of severe psychiatric condition

Side-effects

Specific side-effects for inhaled treatment Worsening respiration, bacterial pneumonia, and pneumothorax reported; rarely non-specific anaemia and haemolysis

Specific side-effects for systemic treatment Haemolytic anaemia (anaemia may be improved by epoetin); also (in combination with interferon alfa-2b) nausea, vomiting, dry mouth, stomatitis, glossitis, tooth disorders, dyspepsia, abdominal pain, diarrhoea, constipation, pancreatitis, anorexia, chest pain, tachycardia, palpitation, syncope, peripheral oedema, flushing, Raynaud's disease, hypertriglyceridaemia; dyspnoea, cough, rhinitis, pharyngitis, interstitial pneumonitis; growth retardation (including decrease in height and weight), increased appetite, sleep disturbances, headache, dizziness, irritability, depression, suicidal ideation, agitation, anxiety, confusion, impaired concentration, abnormal dreams, dysphonia, hyperkinesia, tremor, peripheral neuropathy; influenza-like symptoms; thyroid disorders, menstrual disturbances, virilism, reduced libido, impotence, testicular pain; micturition disorders; neutropenia, thrombocytopenia, lymphadenopathy; myalgia, arthralgia, hyperuricaemia; eye changes including blurred vision; rash, pruritus, urticaria, photosensitivity, acne, psoriasis, alopecia, dry skin, skin discoloration, increased sweating; additional side-effects reported with intravenous therapy include bradyarrythmia, rigors, and injection-site reactions

Licensed use inhalation licensed for use in children (age range not specified by manufacturer); intravenous preparation unlicensed

Indication and dose

Bronchiolitis

- **By aerosol inhalation or nebulisation (via small particle aerosol generator)**

  Child 1 month–2 years inhale solution containing 20 mg/mL for 12–18 hours for at least 3 days; max. 7 days

Life-threatening RSV, parainfluenza virus, and adenovirus infection in immunocompromised children (seek expert advice)

- **By intravenous infusion over 15 minutes**

  Child 1 month–18 years 33 mg/kg as a single dose, then 16 mg/kg every 6 hours for 4 days, then 8 mg/kg every 8 hours for 3 days

Chronic hepatitis C (in combination with interferon alfa-2b) in previously untreated children without liver decompensation

- **By mouth**

  Child over 3 years; body-weight under 47 kg 15 mg/kg daily in 2 divided doses

  Child body-weight 47–49 kg 200 mg in the morning and 400 mg in the evening

  Child body-weight 50–65 kg 400 mg twice daily

  Child body-weight 65–85 kg 400 mg in the morning and 600 mg in the evening

  Child body-weight over 85 kg 600 mg twice daily

Rebetol® (Schering-Plough) PoM

Capsules, ribavirin 200 mg, net price 84-cap pack = £275.65, 140-cap pack = £459.42, 168-cap pack = £551.30. Label: 21

Virazole® (Valeant) PoM

Inhalation, ribavirin 6 g for reconstitution with 300 mL water for injections. Net price 3 × 6-g vials = £349.00

Intravenous infusion, available on a named-patient basis from Valeant

5.4 Antiprotozoal drugs

Advice on specific problems available from:

HPA (Health Protection Agency) Malaria Reference Laboratory (for healthcare professionals **only**)	(020) 7636 3924 (prophylaxis only)
National Travel Health Network and Centre (for healthcare professionals **only**)	0845 602 6712
Scottish Centre for Infection and Environmental Health (registered users of Travax only) www.travax.scot.nhs.uk (for registered users of the NHS Travax website only)	(0141) 300 1130 (weekdays 2–4 p.m. only)
Birmingham	(0121) 424 0357
Liverpool	(0151) 708 9393
London	0845 155 5000 (treatment)
Oxford	(01865) 225 430

Advice for travellers

HPA Malaria Reference Laboratory Recorded advice for Travellers (£1.00/minute standard rate)	09065 508 908
Hospital for Tropical Diseases, Travel Healthline (50p/minute)	09061 337 733
NHS advice for travellers www.fitfortravel.scot.nhs.uk	
WHO advice on international travel and health www.who.int/ith	

5.4.1 Antimalarials

Recommendations on the prophylaxis and treatment of malaria reflect guidelines agreed by UK malaria specialists. Choice will depend on the age of the child (see below).

The centres listed above should be consulted for advice on special problems.

Treatment of malaria

If the infective species is **not known**, or if the infection is **mixed**, initial treatment should be as for *falciparum malaria* with quinine, *Malarone®* (proguanil with atovaquone), or *Riamet®* (artemether with lumefantrine). Falciparum malaria can progress rapidly in unprotected children and antimalarial treatment should be considered in those with features of severe malaria and possible exposure, even if the initial blood tests for the organism are negative.

Falciparum malaria (treatment)

Falciparum malaria (malignant malaria) is caused by *Plasmodium falciparum*. In most parts of the world *P. falciparum* is now resistant to chloroquine which should not therefore be given for treatment.

Quinine, ***Malarone®*** (proguanil with atovaquone), or ***Riamet®*** (artemether with lumefantrine) can be given *by mouth* if the child can swallow and retain tablets and there are no serious manifestations (e.g. impaired consciousness); quinine should be given *by intravenous infusion* (see below) if the child is seriously ill or unable to take tablets. **Mefloquine** is now rarely used for treatment because of concerns about resistance. Specialist advice should be sought in difficult cases since other drugs such as **artesunate** (given intravenously) and intramuscular **artemether** may be available for 'named-patient use'.

Oral. **Quinine** is well tolerated by children although the salts are bitter.

The dosage regimen for quinine *by mouth* is:

10 mg/kg (of quinine salt[1]) every 8 hours for 7 days

followed by

either clindamycin 7–13 mg/kg every 8 hours (max. 1.35 g daily) for 5 days [unlicensed indication]

or, in children over 12 years, doxycycline 200 mg once daily *or* 100 mg twice daily for at least 7 days

If the parasite is likely to be sensitive, *Fansidar®* as a single dose may be given instead of either clindamycin or doxycyline after a course of quinine. The dose regimen for *Fansidar®* by mouth is:

Child up to 4 years ½ tablet as a single dose

Child 5–6 years 1 tablet as a single dose

Child 7–9 years 1½ tablets as a single dose

Child 10–14 years 2 tablets as a single dose

Child 14–18 years 3 tablets as a single dose

Alternatively, ***Malarone®***, or ***Riamet®*** may be given instead of quinine. It is not necessary to give doxycycline, clindamycin, or *Fansidar®* after *Malarone®* or *Riamet®* treatment.

The dose regimen for *Malarone® by mouth* is:

Child body-weight 5–8 kg, 2 'paediatric' tablets once daily for 3 days

Child body-weight 9–10 kg, 3 'paediatric' tablets once daily for 3 days

Child body-weight 11–20 kg, 1 'standard' tablet once daily for 3 days

Child body-weight 21–30 kg, 2 'standard' tablets once daily for 3 days

Child body-weight 31–40 kg, 3 'standard' tablets once daily for 3 days

Child body-weight over 40 kg, 4 'standard' tablets once daily for 3 days

The dose regimen for *Riamet® by mouth* is:

Child 12–18 years and body-weight over 35 kg, 4 tablets initially followed by 5 further doses of 4 tablets each given at 8, 24, 36, 48, and 60 hours (total 24 tablets over 60 hours)

Parenteral. If the child is seriously ill, **quinine** should be given *by intravenous infusion.* The dose regimen for quinine *by intravenous infusion* is calculated on a mg/kg basis:

Neonates and children, loading dose[2] of 20 mg/kg[3] (up to maximum 1.4 g) of quinine salt[1] infused over 4 hours *then after 8 hours* maintenance dose of 10 mg/kg[4] (up to maximum 700 mg) of quinine salt[1] infused over 4 hours every 8 hours (until child can swallow tablets to complete the 7-day course) *followed by either Fansidar® or* doxycycline as above.

Pregnancy Falciparum malaria is particularly dangerous in pregnancy, especially in the last trimester. The treatment doses of oral and intravenous quinine given above (including the loading dose) can safely be given in pregnancy. Clindamycin, 450 mg every 8 hours for 5 days [unlicensed indication] should be given after quinine. Doxycycline should be avoided in pregnancy (affects teeth and skeletal development in fetus); *Fansidar®*, *Malarone®*, and *Riamet®* are also best avoided until more information is available.

1. Valid for quinine hydrochloride, dihydrochloride, and sulphate; not valid for quinine bisulphate which contains a correspondingly smaller amount of quinine.
2. In intensive care units the loading dose can alternatively be given as quinine salt[1] 7 mg/kg infused over 30 minutes followed immediately by 10 mg/kg over 4 hours then (after 8 hours) maintenance dose as described.
3. **Important:** the loading dose of 20 mg/kg should **not** be used if the patient has received quinine (or quinidine) or mefloquine during the previous 24 hours
4. Maintenance dose should be reduced to 5–7 mg/kg of quinine salt in children with renal impairment or if parenteral treatment is required for more than 48 hours.

Benign malarias (treatment)

Benign malaria is usually caused by *Plasmodium vivax* and less commonly by *P. ovale* and *P. malariae*. **Chloroquine**[1] is the drug of choice for the treatment of benign malarias (but chloroquine-resistant *P. vivax* infection has been reported from New Guinea and some adjacent islands).

Chloroquine alone is adequate for *P. malariae* infections but in the case of *P. vivax* and *P. ovale*, a *radical cure* (to destroy parasites in the liver and thus prevent relapses) is required. This is achieved with **primaquine**[2] given after the chloroquine.

The dosage regimen of chloroquine *by mouth* for benign malaria in children is:

initial dose of 10 mg/kg of base (max. 600 mg) *then*

a single dose of 5 mg/kg of base (max. 300 mg) after 6–8 hours *then*

a single dose of 5 mg/kg of base (max. 300 mg) daily for 2 days

For a *radical cure* children are then given **primaquine**[2] in a dose of 250 micrograms/kg daily for 14 days.

Pregnancy Treatment doses of chloroquine can be given for benign malaria. In the case of *P. vivax* or *P. ovale*, however, the radical cure with primaquine should be **postponed** until the pregnancy is over; instead chloroquine should be continued at a dose of 10 mg/kg (max. 600 mg) each week during the pregnancy.

Prophylaxis against malaria

The recommendations on prophylaxis reflect guidelines agreed by UK malaria specialists; the advice is aimed at residents of the UK who travel to endemic areas. The choice of drug for a particular child should take into account:

- risk of exposure to malaria;
- extent of drug resistance;
- efficacy of the recommended drugs;
- side-effects of the drugs;
- patient-related factors (e.g. age, pregnancy, renal or hepatic impairment).

Prophylactic doses are based on guidelines agreed by UK malaria experts and may differ from advice in product literature. **Weight is a better guide than age**. If in doubt obtain advice from specialist centre, see p. 375.

Protection against bites **Prophylaxis is not absolute**, and breakthrough infection can occur with any of the drugs recommended. Personal protection against being bitten is very important. Mosquito nets impregnated with permethrin provide the most effective barrier protection against insects (infants should sleep with a mosquito net stretched over the cot or baby carrier); coils, mats and vaporised insecticides are also useful. Diethyltoluamide (DEET) in lotions, sprays or roll-on formulations is safe and effective in children over 2 months of age when applied to the skin but the protective effect only lasts for a few hours. Long sleeves and trousers worn after dusk also provide protection.

Length of prophylaxis In order to determine tolerance and to establish habit, prophylaxis should generally be started one week (preferably 2½ weeks in the case of mefloquine) before travel into an endemic area (or if not possible at earliest opportunity up to 1 or 2 days before travel); *Malarone*® prophylaxis should be started 1–2 days before travel. Prophylaxis should be continued for **4 weeks after leaving** (except for *Malarone*® prophylaxis which should be stopped 1 week after leaving).

In those requiring long-term prophylaxis, chloroquine and proguanil may be used for periods of over 5 years. Mefloquine is licensed for use up to 1 year (although it has been used for up to 3 years without undue problems). Doxycycline can be used for up to 2 years while *Malarone*® is licensed for up to 28 days but can

1. Alternatives to chloroquine for the treatment of benign malaria are *Malarone*® [unlicensed indication], quinine, mefloquine, or *Riamet*® [unlicensed indication]; as with chloroquine, primaquine should be given for radical cure.
2. Before starting primaquine blood should be tested for glucose-6-phosphate dehydrogenase (G6PD) activity since the drug can cause haemolysis in G6PD-deficient patients. In G6PD deficiency primaquine, in a dose 500–750 micrograms/kg (max. 30 mg) once a week for 8 weeks, has been found useful and without undue harmful effects.

probably be used for up to 3 months (and possibly 6 months or longer). Specialist advice should be sought for long-term prophylaxis.

Return from malarial region It is important to be aware that **any illness** that occurs within 1 year and **especially within 3 months of return might be malaria** even if all recommended precautions against malaria were taken. Travellers and carers of children should be **warned** of this and told that if they develop any illness **particularly within 3 months** of their return they should go **immediately** to a doctor and specifically mention their exposure to malaria.

Epilepsy Both chloroquine and mefloquine are unsuitable for malaria prophylaxis in children with a history of epilepsy. In areas *without chloroquine resistance*, proguanil alone is recommended; in areas *with chloroquine resistance*, doxycycline or *Malarone®* may be considered. The metabolism of doxycycline may be influenced by antiepileptics (see **interactions:** Appendix 1 (tetracyclines)).

Asplenia Asplenic children (or those with severe splenic dysfunction) are at particular risk of severe malaria. If travel to malarious areas is unavoidable, rigorous precautions are required against contracting the disease.

Renal impairment Avoidance (or dosage reduction) of proguanil is recommended since it is excreted by the kidneys. *Malarone®* should not be used for prophylaxis in children with creatinine clearance less than 30 mL/minute/1.73 m^2. Chloroquine is only partially excreted by the kidneys and reduction of the dose for prophylaxis is not required except in severe impairment. Mefloquine is considered to be appropriate to use in renal impairment and does not require dosage reduction. Doxycycline is also considered to be appropriate.

Pregnancy Travel to malarious areas should be avoided during pregnancy; if travel is unavoidable, effective prophylaxis must be used. Chloroquine and proguanil may be given in usual doses in areas where *P. falciparum* strains are sensitive; in the case of proguanil, folic acid 5 mg daily should be given. The manufacturer advises that prophylaxis with mefloquine should be avoided as a matter of principle but studies of mefloquine in pregnancy (including use in the first trimester) indicate that it can be considered for travel to chloroquine-resistant areas. Doxycycline is contra-indicated during pregnancy. *Malarone®* should be avoided during pregnancy unless there is no suitable alternative. The centres listed on p. 375 should be consulted for advice on prophylaxis in resistant areas.

Breast-feeding Prophylaxis is required in **breast-fed infants**; although antimalarials are present in milk, the amounts are too variable to give reliable protection.

Specific recommendations

Where a journey requires two regimens, the regimen for the higher risk area should be used for the whole journey. Those travelling to remote or little-visited areas may require expert advice.

Risk may vary in different parts of a country—check under all risk levels

Warning Settled immigrants and their carers (or long-term visitors) to the UK may be unaware that they will have **lost some of their immunity** and also that the areas where they previously lived **may now be malarious**

North Africa, the Middle East, and Central Asia

Very low risk Risk *very low* in Algeria, Egypt (tourist areas malaria-free), Georgia (south-east, July–October), Kyrgystan (but *Low Risk* in south-west, see below), Libya, rural Morocco, most tourist areas of Turkey, Uzbekistan (extreme south-east only):

chemoprophylaxis not recommended but avoid mosquito bites and consider malaria if fever presents

Low risk Risk *low* in Armenia (June–October), Azerbaijan (southern border areas, June–September), Egypt (El Fayoum only, June–October), rural north Iraq and Basrah Province (May–November), Kyrgystan (south-west, May–October), north border of Syria (May–October), Turkey (plain around Adana, Side, south-east Anatolia, March–November), Turkmenistan (south-east only, June–October):

preferably

chloroquine *or* (if chloroquine not appropriate) proguanil hydrochloride

---

Risk Risk *present* and *chloroquine resistance present* in Afghanistan (below 2000 m, May–November), Iran, Oman (remote rural areas only), Saudi Arabia (except northern, eastern and central provinces, Asir plateau, and western border cities where very little risk, no risk in Mecca), Tajikistan (June–October), Yemen (no risk in Sana'a):

chloroquine + proguanil hydrochloride *or* (if chloroquine + proguanil not appropriate and child over 12 years) doxycyline

Sub-Saharan Africa

No chemoprophylaxis recommended for Cape Verde and non-rural areas of Mauritius (but avoid mosquito bites and consider malaria if fever presents); *chloroquine prophylaxis* appropriate for rural areas of **Mauritius**

Very high risk Risk *very high* (or *locally very high*) and *chloroquine resistance very widespread* in Angola, Benin, Botswana (northern half November–June), Burkina Faso, Burundi, Cameroon, Central African Republic, Chad, Comoros, Congo, Democratic Republic of the Congo (formerly Zaïre), Djibouti, Equatorial Guinea, Eritrea, Ethiopia (below 2200 m; no risk in Addis Ababa), Gabon, Gambia, Ghana, Guinea, Guinea-Bissau, Ivory Coast, Kenya, Liberia, Madagascar, Malawi, Mali, Mauritania (all year in south; July–November in north), Mozambique, Namibia (all year along Kavango and Kunene rivers; November–June in northern third), Niger, Nigeria, Principe, Rwanda, São Tomé, Senegal, Sierra Leone, Somalia, South Africa (Kruger Park, north-east, low-altitude areas of Northern Province and Mpumalanga, and north-east KwaZulu-Natal as far south as Tugela river), Sudan, Swaziland, Tanzania, Togo, Uganda, Zambia, Zimbabwe (all year in Zambezi valley; November–June in other areas below 1200 m; risk negligible in Harare and Bulawayo):

mefloquine *or* doxycycline (if child over 12) *or Malarone*®

Note In Zimbabwe and neighbouring countries, pyrimethamine with dapsone (also known as *Deltaprim*®) prophylaxis is used by local residents (sometimes with chloroquine).

South Asia

Variable risk Risk *variable* and *chloroquine resistance usually moderate* in Bangladesh (except in Chittagong Hill Tracts, see below; no risk in Dhaka city), southern districts of Bhutan, India (no risk in parts of mountain states of north; *High Risk* in Assam), Nepal (below 1500 m, especially Terai districts; no risk in Kathmandu), Pakistan (below 2000 m), Sri Lanka (no risk in and just south of Colombo):

chloroquine + proguanil hydrochloride *or* (if chloroquine + proguanil not appropriate) mefloquine *or* doxycycline *or Malarone*®

High risk Risk *high* and *chloroquine resistance high* in Bangladesh (only in Chittagong Hill Tracts), India (Assam only):

mefloquine *or* doxycycline (if child over 12) *or Malarone*®

South-East Asia

Very low risk Risk *very low* in Bali, main tourist areas of China (but *substantial risk* in Yunnan and Hainan, see below; *chloroquine prophylaxis* appropriate for other remote areas), Hong Kong, Korea (both Democratic People's Republic and Republic), Malaysia (but *substantial risk* in Sabah, and *variable risk* in deep forests, see below), Sarawak (but *variable risk* in deep forests, see below), Thailand (Bangkok, main tourist centres—**important:** regional risk exists, see under *Great risk*, below):

> chemoprophylaxis not recommended but avoid mosquito bites and consider malaria if fever presents

Variable risk Risk *variable* and *some chloroquine resistance* in Indonesia (very low risk in Bali, and cities but *substantial risk* in Irian Jaya [West Papua] and Lombok, see below), rural Philippines below 600 m (no risk in cities, Cebu, Bohol, and Catanduanes), deep forests of peninsular Malaysia and Sarawak (but *substantial risk* in Sabah, see below):

> chloroquine + proguanil hydrochloride *or* (if chloroquine + proguanil not appropriate) mefloquine *or Malarone®*

Substantial risk Risk *substantial* and *drug resistance common* in Cambodia (no risk in Phnom Penh; for western provinces, see below), China (Yunnan and Hainan; *chloroquine prophylaxis* appropriate for other remote areas), East Timor, Irian Jaya [West Papua], Laos (no risk in Vientiane), Lombok, Malaysia (Sabah; see also *Very low risk* and *Variable risk* above), Myanmar (formerly Burma; see also *Great risk* below), Vietnam (no risk in cities, Red River delta area, coastal plain north of Nha Trang):

> mefloquine *or* doxycycline (if child over 12) *or Malarone®*

Great risk and drug resistance present Risk *great and mefloquine resistance present* in western provinces of Cambodia, borders of Thailand with Cambodia and Myanmar, and Ko Chang, Myanmar (eastern Shan State):

> doxycycline (if child over 12) *or Malarone®*

Oceania

Risk Risk *high* and *chloroquine resistance high* in Papua New Guinea (below 1800 m), Solomon Islands, Vanuatu:

> doxycycline (if child over 12) *or* mefloquine *or Malarone®*

Central and South America and the Caribbean

Variable to low risk Risk *variable to low* in Argentina (rural areas along northern borders only), rural Belize (except Belize district), rural Costa Rica (below 500 m), Dominican Republic, El Salvador (Santa Ana province in west), Guatemala (below 1500 m), Haiti, Honduras, some rural areas of Mexico (not regularly visited by tourists), Nicaragua, Panama (west of Panama Canal but *variable to high risk* east of Panama Canal, see below), rural Paraguay:

> chloroquine *or* (if chloroquine not appropriate) proguanil hydrochloride

Variable to high risk Risk *variable to high* and *chloroquine resistance present* in rural areas of Bolivia (below 2500 m), Ecuador (below 1500 m; no malaria in

Galapagos Islands and Guayaquil; see below for Esmeraldas Province), Panama (east of Panama Canal), rural areas of Peru (below 1500 m; see below for Amazon basin area), rural areas of Venezuela (except on coast, Caracas free of malaria):

> chloroquine + proguanil hydrochloride *or* (if chloroquine + proguanil not appropriate) mefloquine *or* doxycycline (if child over 12) *or Malarone*®

High risk Risk *high* and *marked chloroquine resistance* in Bolivia (Amazon basin area), Brazil (throughout 'Legal Amazon' area which includes the Amazon basin area, Mato Grosso and Maranhao only; elsewhere *very low risk*—no chemoprophylaxis), Colombia (most areas below 800 m), Ecuador (Esmeraldas Province), French Guiana, all interior regions of Guyana, Peru (Amazon basin area), Surinam (except Paramaribo and coast), Venezuela (Amazon basin area):

> mefloquine *or* doxycycline (if child over 12) *or Malarone*®

Standby treatment [unlicensed]

> Children and their carers travelling for prolonged periods to areas of chloroquine-resistance who are unlikely to have easy access to medical care should carry a standby treatment course. Self-medication should be **avoided** if medical help is accessible; prophylaxis should be continued during and after the attack.
>
> In order to avoid excessive self-medication, the traveller should be provided with **written instructions** that urgent medical attention should be sought if fever (38°C or more) develops 7 days (or more) after arriving in a malarious area and that self-treatment is indicated if medical help is not immediately available or the condition is worsening.
>
> In view of the continuing emergence of resistant strains and of the different regimens required for different areas expert advice should be sought on the best treatment course for an individual traveller. A drug used for chemoprophylaxis should not be considered for standby treatment for the same traveller.

Artemether with lumefantrine

Artemether with lumefantrine is licensed for the *treatment of acute uncomplicated falciparum malaria.*

ARTEMETHER WITH LUMEFANTRINE

Cautions electrolyte disturbances, concomitant use with other drugs known to cause QT-interval prolongation; monitor patients unable to take food (greater risk of recrudescence); **interactions:** Appendix 1 (artemether with lumefantrine)

Hepatic impairment manufacturer advises caution in severe impairment—monitor ECG and plasma potassium concentration

Renal impairment manufacturer advises caution in severe impairment—monitor ECG and plasma potassium concentration

Pregnancy toxicity in *animal* studies with artemether; manufacturer advises use only if potential benefit outweighs risk

Skilled tasks Dizziness may affect performance of skilled tasks

Contra-indications history of arrhythmias, of clinically relevant bradycardia, and of congestive heart failure accompanied by reduced left ventricular ejection fraction; family history of sudden death or of congenital QT interval prolongation

Breast-feeding Manufacturer advises avoid breast-feeding for at least 1 week after last dose; present in milk in *animal* studies

Side-effects abdominal pain, anorexia, diarrhoea, vomiting, nausea, palpitation, cough, headache, dizziness, sleep disturbances, asthenia, arthralgia, myalgia, pruritus and rash

Licensed use unlicensed for use in children under 12 years and body-weight under 35 kg

ARTEMETHER WITH LUMEFANTRINE *(continued)*

Indication and dose

Treatment of acute uncomplicated falciparum malaria for dose, see p. 375

Treatment of benign malaria see p. 377

Riamet® (Novartis) ▼ PoM
Tablets, yellow, artemether 20 mg, lumefantrine 120 mg, net price 24-tab pack = £22.50. Label: 21, counselling, skilled tasks

Chloroquine

Chloroquine is used for the *prophylaxis of malaria* in areas of the world where the *risk of chloroquine-resistant falciparum malaria is still low*. It is also used with proguanil when chloroquine-resistant falciparum malaria is present but this regimen may not give optimal protection (see specific recommendations by country, p. 378).

Chloroquine is **no longer recommended** for the *treatment of falciparum malaria* owing to widespread resistance, nor is it recommended if the infective species is *not known* or if the infection is *mixed*; in these cases treatment should be with quinine, *Malarone®*, or *Riamet®* (for details, see p. 375). It is still recommended for the *treatment of benign malarias* (for details, see p. 377).

CHLOROQUINE

Cautions may exacerbate psoriasis, neurological disorders (avoid for prophylaxis if history of epilepsy, see notes above), may aggravate myasthenia gravis, severe gastro-intestinal disorders, G6PD deficiency (see section 9.1.5); ophthalmic examination with long-term therapy; avoid concurrent therapy with hepatotoxic drugs—other **interactions:** Appendix 1 (chloroquine and hydroxychloroquine)

Renal impairment mild to moderate, reduce dose (but for malaria prophylaxis see p. 378); severe, avoid (but for malaria prophylaxis see p. 378)

Pregnancy *first, third trimesters:* benefit of prophylaxis and treatment in malaria outweighs risk; **important:** *see also* Falciparum Malaria (Treatment), Benign Malarias (Treatment), and Prophylaxis Against Malaria

Breast-feeding amount probably too small to be harmful when used for malaria prophylaxis; inadequate for reliable protection against malaria in breast-fed infant, *see* p. 378; avoid breast-feeding when used for rheumatic diseases

Side-effects gastro-intestinal disturbances, headache; also hypotension, convulsions, visual disturbances, depigmentation or loss of hair, skin reactions (rashes, pruritus); rarely, bone-marrow suppression, hypersensitivity reactions such as urticaria and angioedema; other side-effects (not usually associated with malaria prophylaxis or treatment), see under Antimalarials, section 10.1.3; very toxic in **overdosage**—immediate advice from poisons centres essential (see also p. 39)

Indication and dose

Prophylaxis of malaria
- **By mouth**

Dose (expressed as chloroquine base) preferably started 1 week before entering endemic area and continued for 4 weeks after leaving (see notes above)

Child up to 12 weeks, body-weight under 6 kg 37.5 mg once weekly
Child 12 weeks–1 year, body-weight 6–10 kg 75 mg once weekly
Child 1–4 years, body-weight 10–16 kg 112.5 mg once weekly
Child 4–8 years, body-weight 16–25 kg 150 mg once weekly
Child 8–13 years, body-weight 25–45 kg 225 mg once weekly
Child over 13 years, body-weight over 45 kg 300 mg once weekly

Counselling Warn travellers about **importance** of avoiding mosquito bites, **importance** of taking prophylaxis regularly, and **importance** of immediate visit to doctor if ill within 1 year and **especially** within 3 months of return. For details, see notes above

Treatment of benign malaria see p. 377

Note Chloroquine doses in BNFC may differ from those in product literature

Chloroquine sulphate (Beacon) PoM
Injection, chloroquine sulphate 54.5 mg/mL (≡ chloroquine base 40 mg/mL), net price 5-mL amp = 79p
Administration for *intravenous infusion*, dilute in Sodium Chloride 0.9% and give over 8 hours

[1]**Avloclor®** (AstraZeneca) PoM
Tablets, scored, chloroquine phosphate 250 mg (≡ chloroquine base 155 mg). Net price 20-tab pack = £1.22. Label: 5, counselling, prophylaxis, see above

Malarivon® (Wallace Mfg) PoM
Syrup, chloroquine phosphate 80 mg/5 mL (≡ chloroquine base 50 mg/5 mL), net price 75 mL = £3.35. Label: 5, counselling, prophylaxis, see above

1. Can be sold to the public provided it is licensed and labelled for the prophylaxis of malaria. Drugs for malaria prophylaxis not prescribable on the NHS; health authorities may investigate circumstances under which antimalarials are prescribed

CHLOROQUINE (*continued*)

[1]**Nivaquine®** (Beacon)
Syrup, golden, chloroquine sulphate 68 mg/5 mL (≡ chloroquine base 50 mg/5 mL), net price 100 mL = £5.15. Label: 5, counselling, prophylaxis, see above

With proguanil
For cautions and side-effects of proguanil see Proguanil; for dose see above

Paludrine/Avloclor® (AstraZeneca)
Tablets, travel pack of 14 tablets of chloroquine phosphate 250 mg (≡ chloroquine base 155 mg) and 98 tablets of proguanil hydrochloride 100 mg, net price 112-tab pack = £8.79. Label: 5, 21, counselling, prophylaxis, see above

Mefloquine

Mefloquine is used for the *prophylaxis of malaria* in areas of the world where there is a *high risk of chloroquine-resistant falciparum malaria* (for details, see specific recommendations by country, p. 378).

Mefloquine is now rarely used for the *treatment of falciparum malaria* because of increased resistance. It is effective for the *treatment of benign malarias*, but is not required as chloroquine is usually effective. Mefloquine should not be used for treatment if it has been used for prophylaxis.

The CSM has advised that travellers should be informed about adverse reactions of mefloquine and, if they occur, medical advice should be sought on alternative antimalarials before the next dose is due; the patient information leaflet, which describes adverse reactions should always be provided when dispensing mefloquine.

MEFLOQUINE

Cautions cardiac conduction disorders; epilepsy (avoid for prophylaxis); not recommended in infants under 3 months (5 kg); **interactions:** Appendix 1 (mefloquine)

Hepatic impairment avoid for chemoprophylaxis in severe liver disease

Pregnancy (see Prophylaxis against Malaria, p. 378)—manufacturer advises **avoid** pregnancy during and for 3 months after (teratogenicity in *animal* studies)

Breast-feeding present in milk but risk to infant minimal

Skilled tasks Dizziness or a disturbed sense of balance may affect performance of skilled tasks; effects may persist for up to 3 weeks

Contra-indications history of neuropsychiatric disorders, including depression, or convulsions; hypersensitivity to quinine

Side-effects nausea, vomiting, diarrhoea, abdominal pain; dizziness, loss of balance, headache, sleep disorders (insomnia, drowsiness, abnormal dreams); also neuropsychiatric reactions (including sensory and motor neuropathies, tremor, ataxia, anxiety, depression, suicidal ideation, panic attacks, agitation, hallucinations, psychosis, convulsions), tinnitus and vestibular disorders, visual disturbances, circulatory disorders (hypotension and hypertension), chest pain, tachycardia, bradycardia, cardiac conduction disorders, dyspnoea, muscle weakness, myalgia, arthralgia, rash, urticaria, pruritus, alopecia, asthenia, malaise, fatigue, fever, loss of appetite, leucopenia or leucocytosis, thrombocytopenia; rarely Stevens-Johnson syndrome, AV block, encephalopathy and anaphylaxis

Licensed use not licensed for use in children under 5 kg body-weight and under 3 months

Indication and dose

Prophylaxis of malaria preferably started 2½ weeks before entering endemic area and continued for 4 weeks after leaving (see notes above)

- **By mouth**

Child body-weight 6–16 kg 62.5 mg once weekly

Child body-weight 16–25 kg 125 mg once weekly

Child body-weight 25–45 kg 187.5 mg once weekly

Child body-weight over 45 kg 250 mg once weekly

Long-term chemoprophylaxis Mefloquine prophylaxis can be taken for up to 1 year

Counselling See CSM advice in notes above. Also warn travellers and carers of children travelling about **importance** of avoiding mosquito bites, **importance** of taking prophylaxis regularly, and **importance** of immediate visit to doctor if ill within 1 year and **especially** within 3 months of return. For details, see notes above

Treatment of chloroquine-resistant vivax malaria see Benign Malaria, p. 377

[2]**Lariam®** (Roche) PoM
Tablets, scored, mefloquine (as hydrochloride) 250 mg. Net price 8-tab pack = £14.53. Label: 21, 25, 27, counselling, skilled tasks, prophylaxis, see above

1. Can be sold to the public provided it is licensed and labelled for the prophylaxis of malaria. Drugs for malaria prophylaxis not prescribable on the NHS; health authorities may investigate circumstances under which antimalarials are prescribed
2. Drugs for malaria prophylaxis not prescribable on the NHS; health authorities may investigate circumstances under which antimalarials prescribed

5 Infections

Primaquine

Primaquine is used to eliminate the liver stages of *P. vivax or P. ovale following chloroquine treatment* (for details, see p. 377).

PRIMAQUINE

Cautions G6PD deficiency (test blood, see under Benign Malarias (treatment) above); systemic diseases associated with granulocytopenia (e.g. juvenile idiopathic arthritis, lupus erythematosus); **interactions:** Appendix 1 (primaquine)

Pregnancy risk of neonatal haemolysis and methaemoglobinaemia in third trimester; see also Benign Malaria (treatment)

Side-effects nausea, vomiting, anorexia, abdominal pain; *less commonly* methaemoglobinaemia, haemolytic anaemia especially in G6PD deficiency, leucopenia

Licensed use not licensed

Indication and dose

Adjunct in the treatment of *Plasmodium vivax* and *P. ovale* malaria (eradication of liver stages) for dose see Benign Malaria, p. 377

Primaquine (Non-proprietary)
Tablets, primaquine (as phosphate) 7.5 mg or 15 mg
Available from specialist importing companies, see p. 848

Proguanil

Proguanil is used (usually *with chloroquine*, but occasionally *alone*) for the *prophylaxis of malaria*, (for details, see specific recommendations by country, p. 378).

Proguanil used alone is not suitable for the *treatment of malaria*; *Malarone®* (a combination of atovaquone with proguanil) is, however, licensed for the treatment of acute uncomplicated falciparum malaria.

Malarone® is also used for the *prophylaxis of falciparum malaria* in areas of *widespread mefloquine or chloroquine resistance*. *Malarone®* is also used as an alternative to mefloquine or doxycycline. *Malarone®* is particularly suitable for short trips to highly chloroquine-resistant areas because it needs to be taken only for 7 days after leaving an endemic area.

PROGUANIL HYDROCHLORIDE

Cautions **interactions:** Appendix 1 (proguanil)

Renal impairment (see notes under Prophylaxis against malaria) reduce dose as follows:

mild: use half normal dose

moderate: use one-quarter normal dose on alternate days

severe: use one-quarter normal dose once weekly; increased risk of haematological toxicity

Pregnancy benefit of prophylaxis in malaria outweighs risk. Adequate folate supplements should be given to mother; see also Prophylaxis Against Malaria

Breast-feeding amount probably too small to be harmful and inadequate for reliable protection against malaria in breast-fed infant

Side-effects mild gastric intolerance, diarrhoea and constipation; occasionally mouth ulcers and stomatitis; *very rarely* cholestasis, vasculitis, skin reactions and hair loss

Indication and dose

Prophylaxis of malaria preferably started 1 week before entering endemic area and continued for 4 weeks after leaving (see notes above)

- **By mouth**

Child up to 12 weeks, body-weight under 6 kg 25 mg once daily

Child 12 weeks–1 year, body-weight 6–10 kg 50 mg once daily

Child 1–4 years, body-weight 10–16 kg 75 mg once daily

Child 4–8 years, body-weight 16–25 kg 100 mg once daily

Child 8–13 years, body-weight 25–45 kg 150 mg once daily

Child over 13 years, body-weight over 45 kg 200 mg once daily

Counselling Warn travellers and carers of children travelling about **importance** of avoiding mosquito bites, **importance** of taking prophylaxis regularly, and **importance** of immediate visit to doctor if ill within 1 year and **especially** within 3 months of return. For details, see notes above

Note Proguanil doses in BNFC may differ from those in product literature

[1]**Paludrine®** (AstraZeneca)
Tablets, scored, proguanil hydrochloride 100 mg. Net price 98-tab pack = £7.43. Label: 21, counselling, prophylaxis, see above

With chloroquine
See under Chloroquine

1. Drugs for malaria prophylaxis not prescribable on the NHS; health authorities may investigate circumstances under which antimalarials prescribed

PROGUANIL HYDROCHLORIDE WITH ATOVAQUONE

Cautions diarrhoea or vomiting (reduced absorption of atovaquone); efficacy not evaluated in cerebral or complicated malaria (including hyperparasitaemia, pulmonary oedema or renal failure); **interactions**: see Appendix 1 (proguanil, atovaquone)

Renal impairment avoid for malaria prophylaxis and, if possible for treatment, if creatinine clearance less than 30 mL/minute/1.73m^2

Pregnancy manufacturer advises avoid unless essential

Breast-feeding avoid—no information available

Side-effects abdominal pain, nausea, vomiting, diarrhoea; cough; headache, dizziness, insomnia, anorexia, fever; rash, pruritus; *less commonly* mouth ulcers, stomatitis, blood disorders, hyponatraemia, and hair loss

Indication and dose

See under preparations

Counselling Warn travellers about **importance** of avoiding mosquito bites, **importance** of taking prophylaxis regularly, and **importance** of immediate visit to doctor if ill within 1 year and **especially** within 3 months of return. For details, see notes above

[1]**Malarone®** (GSK) PoM
Tablets ('standard'), pink, f/c, proguanil hydrochloride 100 mg, atovaquone 250 mg. Net price 12-tab pack = £22.92. Label: 21, counselling, prophylaxis, see above

Dose

Prophylaxis of malaria started 1–2 days before entering endemic area and continued for 1 week after leaving
- By mouth
  - **Child body-weight over 40 kg** 1 tablet daily

Treatment of falciparum malaria
- By mouth
  - **Child body-weight 11–20 kg** 1 tablet daily for 3 days
  - **Child body-weight 21–30 kg** 2 tablets once daily for 3 days
  - **Child body-weight 31–40 kg** 3 tablets once daily for 3 days
  - **Child body-weight over 40 kg** 4 tablets once daily for 3 days

[1]**Malarone® Paediatric** (GSK) ▼ PoM
Paediatric tablets, pink, f/c proguanil hydrochloride 25 mg, atovaquone 62.5 mg, net price 12-tab pack = £7.64. Label: 21, counselling, prophylaxis, see above

Dose

Prophylaxis of malaria started 1–2 days before entering endemic area and continued for 1 week after leaving
- By mouth
  - **Child body-weight 11–20 kg** 1 tablet once daily
  - **Child body-weight 21–30 kg** 2 tablets once daily
  - **Child body-weight 31–40 kg** 3 tablets once daily
  - **Child body-weight over 40 kg** use *Malarone®* ('standard') tablets, see above

Treatment of falciparum malaria
- By mouth
  - **Child body-weight 5–8 kg** 2 tablets once daily for 3 days
  - **Child body-weight 9–10 kg** 3 tablets once daily for 3 days
  - **Child body-weight over 11 kg** use *Malarone®* ('standard') tablets, see above

Administration tablets may be crushed and mixed with food or milky drink just before administration

Pyrimethamine

Pyrimethamine should not be used alone, but is used with sulfadoxine (in *Fansidar®*).

Fansidar® is not recommended for the *prophylaxis of malaria*, but it is used in the treatment of *falciparum malaria* and can be used *after treatment with quinine*.

PYRIMETHAMINE WITH SULFADOXINE

Cautions see under Pyrimethamine (section 5.4.7) and under Co-trimoxazole (section 5.1.8); not recommended for prophylaxis (severe side-effects on long-term use); **interactions**: Appendix 1 (pyrimethamine, sulphonamides)

Pregnancy possible teratogenic risk in *first trimester* as pyrimethamine is a folate antagonist; in *third trimester*—risk of neonatal haemolysis and methaemoglobinaemia; fears of increased risk of neonatal kernicterus appear unfounded

Breast-feeding small risk of neonatal kernicterus in jaundiced infants; risk of haemolysis in G6PD-deficient child due to sulfadoxine

Contra-indications see under Pyrimethamine (section 5.4.7) and under Co-trimoxazole (section 5.1.8); sulphonamide allergy

Side-effects see under Pyrimethamine (section 5.4.7) and under Co-trimoxazole (section 5.1.8); pulmonary infiltrates (e.g. eosinophilic or allergic alveolitis) reported—discontinue if cough or shortness of breath

Licensed use not licensed for use in children of body-weight under 5 kg

Indication and dose

Adjunct to quinine in treatment of *Plasmodium falciparum* malaria see notes above

Prophylaxis not recommended by UK malaria experts

Fansidar® (Roche) PoM
Tablets, scored, pyrimethamine 25 mg, sulfadoxine 500 mg, net price 3-tab pack = 74p

1. Drugs for malaria prophylaxis not prescribable on the NHS; health authorities may investigate circumstances under which antimalarials prescribed

Quinine

Quinine is not suitable for the *prophylaxis of malaria*.

Quinine is used for the *treatment of falciparum malaria* or if the infective species is *not known* or if the infection is *mixed* (for details see p. 375).

QUININE

Cautions atrial fibrillation, conduction defects, heart block, monitor blood glucose and electrolyte concentration during parenteral treatment; G6PD deficiency (see section 9.1.5); **interactions:** Appendix 1 (quinine)

Renal impairment reduce parenteral maintenance dose for malaria treatment, see p. 376

Pregnancy risk of teratogenesis with high doses in *first trimester*, but in malaria benefit of treatment outweighs risk

Contra-indications haemoglobinuria, myasthenia gravis, optic neuritis

Side-effects cinchonism, including tinnitus, headache, hot and flushed skin, nausea, abdominal pain, rashes, visual disturbances (including temporary blindness), confusion; hypersensitivity reactions including angioedema, blood disorders (including thrombocytopenia and intravascular coagulation), and acute renal failure; hypoglycaemia (especially after parenteral administration); cardiovascular effects (see Cautions); very toxic in **overdosage**—immediate advice from poisons centres essential (see also p. 39)

Indication and dose

Treatment of falciparum malaria see p. 375

Note Quinine (anhydrous base) 100 mg ≡ quinine bisulphate 169 mg ≡ quinine dihydrochloride 122 mg ≡ quinine hydrochloride 122 mg ≡ quinine sulphate 121 mg. Quinine bisulphate 300-mg tablets are available but provide less quinine than 300 mg of the dihydrochloride, hydrochloride, or sulphate

Administration for *intravenous infusion*, dilute to a concentration of 2 mg/mL (max. 30 mg/mL in fluid restriction) with Glucose 5% *or* Sodium Chloride 0.9% and give over 4 hours

Quinine Sulphate (Non-proprietary) PoM

Tablets, coated, quinine sulphate 200 mg, net price 28-tab pack = £2.13; 300 mg, 28-tab pack = £2.20

Quinine Dihydrochloride (Non-proprietary) PoM

Injection, quinine dihydrochloride 300 mg/mL. For dilution and use as an infusion. 1- and 2-mL amps

Available as a manufactured special, see p. 861

Note Intravenous injection of quinine is so hazardous that it has been superseded by infusion

Administration *intravenous infusion* dilute to 2 mg/mL with sodium chloride 0.9% *or* glucose 5% intravenous infusion (in fluid restriction max. concentration 30 mg/mL); give over 4 hours

Tetracyclines

Doxycycline (section 5.1.3) is used in children over 12 years for the *prophylaxis of malaria* in areas of *widespread mefloquine or chloroquine resistance*. Doxycycline is also used as an alternative to mefloquine or *Malarone®* (for details, see specific recommendations by country, p. 378).

Doxycycline is also used as an *adjunct to quinine in the treatment of falciparum malaria* (for details see p. 375).

DOXYCYCLINE

Cautions section 5.1.3

Contra-indications section 5.1.3

Side-effects section 5.1.3

Licensed use not licensed for use in children under 12 years

Indication and dose

Prophylaxis of malaria preferably started 1 week before entering endemic area and continued for 4 weeks after leaving (see notes above)

- By mouth

  Child over 12 years 100 mg once daily

Treatment of falciparum malaria see p. 375

Preparations

Section 5.1.3

5.4.2 Amoebicides

Metronidazole is the drug of choice for *acute invasive amoebic dysentery* since it is very effective against vegetative forms of *Entamoeba histolytica* which can cause ulceration of the large intestine. **Tinidazole** is also effective. Metronidazole and tinidazole are also active against amoebae which may have migrated to the liver. Treatment with metronidazole (or tinidazole) is followed by a 10-day course of diloxanide furoate.

5 Infections

Diloxanide furoate is the drug of choice for asymptomatic patients with *E. histolytica* cysts in the faeces; metronidazole and tinidazole are relatively ineffective. Diloxanide furoate is relatively free from toxic effects and the usual course is of 10 days, given alone for chronic infections or following metronidazole or tinidazole treatment.

For *amoebic abscesses* of the liver **metronidazole** is effective; tinidazole is an alternative. The course may be repeated after 2 weeks if necessary. Aspiration of the abscess is indicated where it is suspected that it may rupture or where there is no improvement after 72 hours of metronidazole; the aspiration may need to be repeated. Aspiration aids penetration of metronidazole and, for abscesses with large volume of pus, if carried out in conjunction with drug therapy, may reduce the period of disability.

Diloxanide furoate is not effective against hepatic amoebiasis, but a 10-day course should be given at the completion of metronidazole or tinidazole treatment to destroy any amoebae in the gut.

DILOXANIDE FUROATE

Contra-indications

Pregnancy manufacturer advises avoid—no information available

Breast-feeding manufacturer advises avoid—no information available

Side-effects flatulence, vomiting, urticaria, pruritus

Licensed use not licensed for use in children under 25 kg body-weight

Indication and dose

Chronic amoebiasis and as adjunct to metronidazole or tinidazole in acute amoebiasis
- **By mouth**

Child 1 month–12 years 6.6 mg/kg 3 times daily for 10 days

Child 12–18 years 500 mg 3 times daily for 10 days

Diloxanide (Sovereign) PoM
Tablets, diloxanide furoate 500 mg, net price 30-tab pack = £32.95. Label: 9

Extemporaneous formulations available see Extemporaneous Preparations, p. 8

METRONIDAZOLE

Cautions section 5.1.11
Side-effects section 5.1.11
Indication and dose

Anaerobic infections section 5.1.11

Invasive intestinal amoebiasis
- **By mouth**

Child 1–3 years 200 mg every 8 hours for 5 days

Child 3–7 years 200 mg every 6 hours for 5 days

Child 7–10 years 400 mg every 8 hours for 5 days

Child 10–18 years 800 mg every 8 hours for 5 days

Extra-intestinal amoebiasis (including liver abscess) and asymptomatic amoebic cyst passers
- **By mouth**

Child 1–3 years 100–200 mg 3 times daily for 5–10 days

Child 3–7 years 100–200 mg 4 times daily for 5–10 days

Child 7–10 years 200–400 mg 3 times daily for 5–10 days

Child 10–18 years 400–800 mg 3 times daily for 5–10 days

Urogenital trichomoniasis
- **By mouth**

Child 1–3 years 50 mg 3 times daily for 7 days

Child 3–7 years 100 mg twice daily for 7 days

Child 7–10 years 100 mg 3 times daily for 7 days

Child 10–18 years 200 mg 3 times daily for 7 days *or* 400–500 mg twice daily for 5–7 days, *or* 2 g as a single dose

Giardiasis
- **By mouth**

Child 1–3 years 500 mg once daily for 3 days

Child 3–7 years 600–800 mg once daily for 3 days

Child 7–10 years 1 g once daily for 3 days

Child 10–18 years 2 g once daily for 3 days *or* 400 mg 3 times daily for 5 days *or* 500 mg twice daily for 7–10 days

Preparations
Section 5.1.11

TINIDAZOLE

Cautions see under Metronidazole (section 5.1.11); avoid in porphyria (section 9.8.2); **interactions:** Appendix 1 (tinidazole)

Pregnancy manufacturer advises avoid in first trimester

Breast-feeding present in milk—manufacturer advises avoid breast-feeding during and for 3 days after stopping treatment

Side-effects see under Metronidazole (section 5.1.11)

Licensed use licensed for use in children (age range not specified by manufacturer)

Indication and dose

Intestinal amoebiasis
- **By mouth**

  Child 1 month–12 years 50–60 mg/kg (max. 2 g) once daily for 3 days

  Child 12–18 years 2 g once daily for 2–3 days

Amoebic involvement of liver
- **By mouth**

  Child 1 month–12 years 50–60 mg/kg (max. 2 g) once daily for 5 days

  Child 12–18 years 1.5–2 g once daily for 3–6 days

Urogenital trichomoniasis and giardiasis
- **By mouth**

  Child 1 month–12 years single dose of 50–75 mg/kg (max. 2 g) (repeated once if necessary)

  Child 12–18 years single dose of 2 g (repeated once if necessary)

Fasigyn® (Pfizer) PoM

Tablets, f/c. tinidazole 500 mg. Net price 20-tab pack = £13.80. Label: 4, 9, 21, 25

5.4.3 Trichomonacides

Metronidazole (section 5.4.2) is the treatment of choice for *Trichomonas vaginalis* infection. Contact tracing is recommended and sexual contacts should be treated simultaneously. If metronidazole is ineffective, **tinidazole** (section 5.4.2) may be tried.

5.4.4 Antigiardial drugs

Metronidazole (section 5.4.2) is the treatment of choice for *Giardia lamblia* infections. **Tinidazole** (section 5.4.2) may be used as an alternative to metronidazole.

5.4.5 Leishmaniacides

Cutaneous leishmaniasis frequently heals spontaneously but if skin lesions are extensive or unsightly, treatment is indicated, as it is in visceral leishmaniasis (kala-azar).

Sodium stibogluconate, an organic pentavalent antimony compound, is the treatment of choice for visceral leishmaniasis. The dose is 20 mg/kg daily (max. 850 mg) for at least 20 days by intramuscular or intravenous injection; the dosage varies with different geographical regions and expert advice should be obtained. Skin lesions are treated for 10 days.

Amphotericin is used with or after an antimony compound for visceral leishmaniasis unresponsive to the antimonial alone; side-effects may be reduced by using liposomal amphotericin (*AmBisome®*—section 5.2) at a dose of 1–3 mg/kg daily for 10–21 days to a cumulative dose of 21–30 mg/kg. An alternative regimen in immunocompetent patients is 3 mg/kg daily for 5 days then 3 mg/kg on days 14 and 21; the course may be repeated if parasitic clearance is not achieved. Other lipid formulations of amphotericin (*Abelcet®* and *Amphocil®*) are also likely to be effective but less information is available.

Pentamidine isetionate (pentamidine isethionate) (section 5.4.8) has been used in antimony-resistant visceral leishmaniasis, but although the initial response is often good, the relapse rate is high; it is associated with serious side-effects. Other treatments include paromomycin (available from specialist importing companies).

SODIUM STIBOGLUCONATE

Cautions intravenous injections must be given slowly over 5 minutes (to reduce risk of local thrombosis) and stopped if coughing or substernal pain; mucocutaneous disease (see below); monitor ECG before and during treatment; heart disease (withdraw if conduction disturbances occur); treat intercurrent infection (e.g. pneumonia)

Hepatic impairment use with caution in hepatic disease

Pregnancy avoid unless potential benefit outweighs risk

Mucocutaneous disease Successful treatment of mucocutaneous leishmaniasis may induce severe inflammation around the lesions (may be life-threatening if pharyngeal or tracheal involvement)—may require corticosteroid

SODIUM STIBOGLUCONATE (*continued*)

Contra-indications

Renal impairment avoid in severe impairment

Breast-feeding avoid

Side-effects anorexia, nausea, vomiting, abdominal pain; ECG changes; coughing (see Cautions); headache, lethargy, arthralgia, myalgia; *rarely* jaundice, flushing, bleeding from nose or gum, substernal pain (see Cautions), vertigo, fever, sweating, and rash; also reported pancreatitis and anaphylaxis; pain and thrombosis on intravenous administration, intramuscular injection also painful

Licensed use licensed for use in children (age range not specified by manufacturer)

Indication and dose

Leishmaniasis for dose, see notes above

Pentostam® (GSK) PoM

Injection, sodium stibogluconate equivalent to pentavalent antimony 100 mg/mL. Net price 100-mL bottle = £66.43

5.4.6 Trypanocides

The prophylaxis and treatment of trypanosomiasis is difficult and differs according to the strain of organism. Expert advice should therefore be obtained.

5.4.7 Drugs for toxoplasmosis

Most infections caused by *Toxoplasma gondii* are self-limiting, and treatment is not necessary. Exceptions are children with eye involvement (toxoplasma choroidoretinitis), and those who are immunosuppressed. Toxoplasmic encephalitis is a common complication of AIDS. The treatment of choice is a combination of **pyrimethamine** and **sulfadiazine** (sulphadiazine), given for several weeks (expert advice **essential**). Pyrimethamine is a folate antagonist, and adverse reactions to this combination are relatively common (folinic acid supplements and weekly blood counts needed). Alternative regimens use combinations of pyrimethamine with clindamycin or clarithromycin or azithromycin. Long-term secondary prophylaxis is required after treatment of toxoplasmosis in AIDS.

If toxoplasmosis is acquired in pregnancy, transplacental infection may lead to severe disease in the fetus; specialist advice should be sought on management. Spiramycin may reduce the risk of transmission of maternal infection to the fetus. When there is evidence of placental or fetal infection, pyrimethamine may be given with sulfadiazine and folinic acid after the first trimester.

In neonates without signs of toxoplasmosis, but born to mothers known to have become infected, spiramycin is given while awaiting laboratory results. If toxoplasmosis is confirmed in the infant, pyrimethamine and sulfadiazine are given for 12 months, together with folinic acid.

PYRIMETHAMINE

Cautions blood counts required with prolonged treatment; history of seizures—avoid large loading doses; **interactions:** Appendix 1 (pyrimethamine)

Hepatic impairment manufacturer advises caution

Renal impairment manufacturer advises caution

Pregnancy theoretical teratogenic risk in first trimester (folate antagonist); adequate folate supplement should be given to mother

Breast-feeding present in milk—avoid breast-feeding during toxoplasmosis treatment; avoid other folate antagonists

Side-effects depression of haematopoiesis with high doses, rashes, insomnia

Licensed use not licensed for use in children under 5 years

Indication and dose

Toxoplasmosis in pregnancy (in combination with sulfadiazine and folinic acid (section 8.1)), see notes above

- **By mouth**

Adolescent 12–18 years 50 mg once daily until delivery

Congenital toxoplasmosis (in combination with sulfadiazine and folinic acid (section 8.1)),

- **By mouth**

Neonate 1 mg/kg twice daily for 2 days, *then* 1 mg/kg once daily for 6 months, *then* 1 mg/kg 3 times a week for 6 months

Malaria no dose stated because not recommended alone

Daraprim® (GSK) PoM

Tablets, scored, pyrimethamine 25 mg. Net price 30-tab pack = £2.17

Extemporaneous formulations available see Extemporaneous Preparations, p. 8

SPIRAMYCIN

Cautions cardiac disease, arrhythmias (including predisposition to QT interval prolongation)

Hepatic impairment use with caution

Breast-feeding present in breast milk

Contra-indications sensitivity to other macrolides

Side-effects gastro-intestinal disturbances including nausea, vomiting, diarrhoea; dizziness, headache; rash; hepatotoxicity; *rarely*, prolongation of QT interval, thrombocytopenia and vasculitis

Licensed use not licensed

Indication and dose

Toxoplasmosis in pregnancy see notes above
- By mouth

Adolescent 12–18 years 1.5 g twice daily until delivery

Chemoprophylaxis of congenital toxoplasmosis
- By mouth

Neonate 50 mg/kg twice daily

Spiramycin (Non-proprietary)

Tablets, spiramycin 750 000 units (250 mg); 1.5 million units (500 mg); 3 million units (1 g)

Syrup, spiramycin 75 000 units/mL (25 mg/mL)

Note 3000 units ≡ 1 mg spiramycin

Available from specialist importing companies, see p. 848

SULFADIAZINE

Cautions see under Co-trimoxazole, section 5.1.8

Pregnancy risk of neonatal haemolysis and methaemoglobinaemia in third trimester; fear of increased risk of kernicterus in neonates appears to be unfounded

Breast-feeding small risk of kernicterus in jaundiced infants and of haemolysis in G6PD-deficient infants

Contra-indications see under Co-trimoxazole, section 5.1.8

Renal impairment avoid in severe impairment—high risk of crystalluria

Side-effects see under Co-trimoxazole, section 5.1.8

Licensed use not licensed for use in toxoplasmosis

Indication and dose

Toxoplasmosis in pregnancy (in combination with pyrimethamine and folinic acid (section 8.1)) , see notes above
- By mouth

Adolescent 12–18 years 1 g 3 times daily until delivery

Congenital toxoplasmosis (in combination with pyrimethamine and folinic acid (section 8.1))
- By mouth

Neonate 50 mg/kg twice daily for 12 months

Sulfadiazine (Non-proprietary) PoM

Tablets, sulfadiazine 500 mg, net price 56-tab pack = £17.60. Label: 9, 27

Injection, sulfadiazine (as sodium salt) 250 mg/mL, net price 4-mL amp = £4.97

Extemporaneous formulations available see Extemporaneous Preparations, p. 8

5.4.8 Drugs for pneumocystis pneumonia

Pneumonia caused by *Pneumocystis jiroveci* (*Pneumocystis carinii*) occurs in immunosuppressed children; it is a common cause of pneumonia in AIDS. Pneumocystis pneumonia should generally be treated by those experienced in its management. Blood gas measurement is used to assess disease severity.

Treatment

Mild to moderate disease **Co-trimoxazole** (section 5.1.8) in high dosage is the drug of choice for the treatment of mild to moderate pneumocystis pneumonia.

A combination of **dapsone** with **trimethoprim** 5 mg/kg every 6–8 hours (section 5.1.8) is given by mouth for the treatment of mild to moderate disease [unlicensed indication] in children who cannot tolerate co-trimoxazole.

A combination of **clindamycin** (section 5.1.6) and **primaquine** (section 5.4.1) may be used in the treatment of mild to moderate disease [unlicensed indication]; this combination is associated with considerable toxicity.

Inhaled **pentamidine isetionate** is sometimes used for mild disease. It is better tolerated than parenteral pentamidine but systemic absorption may still occur.

Severe disease **Co-trimoxazole** (section 5.1.8) in high dosage, given by mouth or by intravenous infusion, is the drug of choice for the treatment of severe pneumocystis pneumonia. **Pentamidine isetionate** given by intravenous infusion is an alternative for children who cannot tolerate co-trimoxazole, or who have not responded to it. Pentamidine isetionate is a potentially toxic drug that can cause severe hypotension during or immediately after infusion.

Corticosteroid treatment can be lifesaving in those with severe pneumocystis pneumonia (see Adjunctive Therapy below).

Adjunctive therapy In moderate to severe pneumocystis infections associated with HIV infection, prednisolone (section 6.3.2) is given by mouth in a dose of 2 mg/kg (max. 80 mg daily) for 5 days (alternatively, hydrocortisone may be given parenterally); the dose is then reduced over the next 16 days and then stopped. Corticosteroid treatment should ideally be started at the same time as the anti-pneumocystis therapy and certainly no later than 24–72 hours afterwards. The corticosteroid should be withdrawn before anti-pneumocystis treatment is complete.

Prophylaxis

Prophylaxis against pneumocystis pneumonia should be given to all children with a history of the infection. Prophylaxis against pneumocystis pneumonia should also be considered for severely immunocompromised children. Prophylaxis should continue until immunity recovers sufficiently. It should not be discontinued if the child has oral candidiasis, continues to lose weight, or is receiving cytotoxic therapy or long-term immunosuppressant therapy.

Co-trimoxazole (section 5.1.8) by mouth is the drug of choice for prophylaxis against pneumocystis pneumonia. Co-trimoxazole may be used in infants born to mothers with a high risk of transmission of infection.

Intermittent inhalation of **pentamidine isetionate** is used for prophylaxis against pneumocystis pneumonia in children unable to tolerate co-trimoxazole. It is effective but children may be prone to extrapulmonary infection. Alternatively, **dapsone** can be used.

DAPSONE

Cautions cardiac or pulmonary disease; anaemia (treat severe anaemia before starting); susceptibility to haemolysis including G6PD deficiency (section 9.1.5); avoid in porphyria (section 9.8.2); **interactions:** Appendix 1 (dapsone)

Pregnancy risk of neonatal haemolysis and methaemoglobinaemia in third trimester; folic acid 5 mg daily should be given to mother

Breast-feeding haemolytic anaemia; although significant amount in milk, risk to infant very small unless infant is G6PD deficient

Blood disorders On long-term treatment, children and their carers should be told how to recognise signs of blood disorders and advised to seek immediate medical attention if symptoms such as fever, sore throat, rash, mouth ulcers, purpura, bruising or bleeding develop

Side-effects haemolysis, methaemoglobinaemia, neuropathy, allergic dermatitis (rarely including toxic epidermal necrolysis and Stevens-Johnson syndrome), anorexia, nausea, vomiting, tachycardia, headache, insomnia, psychosis, hepatitis, agranulocytosis; dapsone syndrome (rash with fever and eosinophilia)—discontinue immediately (may progress to exfoliative dermatitis, hepatitis, hypoalbuminaemia, psychosis and death)

Licensed use not licensed for treatment of *P. jiroveci* pneumonia; monotherapy not licensed for children for prophylaxis of *P. jiroveci* pneumonia

Indication and dose

Treatment of *Pneumocystis jiroveci (P. carinii)* pneumonia (in combination with trimethoprim)
- **By mouth**

Child 1 month–12 years 2 mg/kg (max. 100 mg) once daily

Child 13–18 years 100 mg once daily

Prophylaxis of *Pneumocystis jiroveci (P. carinii)* pneumonia
- **By mouth**

Child 1 month–18 years 2 mg/kg (max. 100 mg) once daily

Dapsone (Non-proprietary) PoM

Tablets, dapsone 50 mg, net price 28-tab pack = £3.12; 100 mg 28-tab pack = £4.23. Label: 8

PENTAMIDINE ISETIONATE

Cautions risk of severe hypotension following administration (establish baseline blood pressure and administer with child lying down; monitor blood pressure closely during administration, and at regular intervals, until treatment concluded); hypokalaemia, hypomagnesaemia, coronary heart disease, bradycardia, history of ventricular arrhythmias, concomitant use with other drugs known to prolong Q-T interval; hypertension or hypotension; hyperglycaemia or hypoglycaemia;

PENTAMIDINE ISETIONATE (*continued*)

leucopenia, thrombocytopenia, or anaemia; carry out laboratory monitoring according to product literature; care required to protect personnel during handling and administration; **interactions:** Appendix 1 (pentamidine isetionate)

Hepatic impairment use with caution

Renal impairment reduce dose in mild renal impairment; consult product literature

Pregnancy manufacturer advises avoid unless essential

Breast-feeding manufacturer advises avoid unless essential

Side-effects severe reactions, sometimes fatal, due to hypotension, hypoglycaemia, pancreatitis, and arrhythmias; also leucopenia, thrombocytopenia, acute renal failure, hypocalcaemia; also reported: azotaemia, abnormal liver-function tests, anaemia, hyperkalaemia, nausea and vomiting, dizziness, syncope, flushing, hyperglycaemia, rash, and taste disturbances; Stevens-Johnson syndrome reported; on inhalation, bronchoconstriction (may be prevented by prior use of bronchodilators), cough and shortness of breath; discomfort, pain, induration, abscess formation, and muscle necrosis at injection site

Licensed use *nebuliser solution* not licensed for use in children

Indication and dose

Pneumocystis jiroveci (Pneumocystis carinii) pneumonia

- **By intravenous infusion**

Child 1 month–18 years 4 mg/kg once daily for at least 14 days

- **By inhalation of nebulised solution (using suitable equipment—consult product literature)**

Child 1 month–18 years 600 mg pentamidine isetionate once daily for 3 weeks; secondary prevention, 300 mg every 4 weeks *or* 150 mg every 2 weeks

Visceral leishmaniasis (kala-azar, section 5.4.5)

- **By deep intramuscular injection**

Child 1–18 years 3–4 mg/kg on alternate days to max. total of 10 injections; course may be repeated if necessary

Cutaneous leishmaniasis

- **By deep intramuscular injection**

Child 1–18 years 3–4 mg/kg once or twice weekly until condition resolves (but see also section 5.4.5)

Trypanosomiasis

- **By deep intramuscular injection or intravenous infusion**

Child 1–18 years 4 mg/kg daily or on alternate days to total of 7–10 injections

Administration Direct intravenous injection should be avoided whenever possible and **never** given rapidly; intramuscular injections should be deep and preferably given into the buttock.

For *intravenous infusion*, reconstitute 300 mg with 3–5 mL Water for Injections (displacement value may be significant), then dilute required dose with 50–250 mL Glucose 5% *or* Sodium Chloride 0.9% intravenous infusion; give over at least 60 minutes

Pentacarinat® (JHC) PoM

Injection, powder for reconstitution, pentamidine isetionate, net price 300-mg vial = £31.04

Nebuliser solution, pentamidine isetionate, net price 300-mg bottle = £32.84

Caution in handling Pentamidine isetionate is toxic and personnel should be adequately protected during handling and administration—consult product literature

5.5 Anthelmintics

Advice on prophylaxis and treatment of helminth infections is available from the following specialist centres:

Birmingham	(0121) 424 0357
Scottish Centre for Infection and Environmental Health (registered users of Travax only)	(0141) 300 1130 (weekdays 2–4 p.m. only)
Liverpool	(0151) 708 9393
London	(020) 7387 9300 (treatment advice only)

5.5.1 Drugs for threadworms (pinworms, *Enterobius vermicularis*)

Anthelmintics are effective in threadworm infections, but their use needs to be combined with hygienic measures to break the cycle of auto-infection. All members of the family require treatment.

Adult threadworms do not live for longer than 6 weeks and for development of fresh worms, ova must be swallowed and exposed to the action of digestive juices in the upper intestinal tract. Direct multiplication of worms does not take place in the large bowel. Adult female worms lay ova on the perianal skin which causes pruritus; scratching the area then leads to ova being transmitted on fingers to the mouth, often via food eaten with unwashed hands. Washing hands and scrubbing nails before each meal and after each visit to the toilet is essential. A bath taken immediately after rising will remove ova laid during the night.

Mebendazole is the drug of choice for treating threadworm infection in children over 6 months. It is given as a single dose; as reinfection is very common, a second dose may be given after 2 weeks.

Piperazine is available in combination with sennosides as a single-dose preparation.

MEBENDAZOLE

Cautions interactions: Appendix 1 (mebendazole)

Pregnancy manufacturer advises avoid—toxicity in *animal* studies

Breast-feeding amount present in milk too small to be harmful but manufacturer advises avoid

Note The patient information leaflet in the *Vermox*® pack includes the statement that it is not suitable for women known to be pregnant or for children under 2 years

Side-effects *very rarely* abdominal pain, diarrhoea; convulsions (in infants) and rash (including Stevens-Johnson syndrome and toxic epidermal necrolysis) reported

Licensed use not licensed for use in children under 2 years

Indication and dose

Threadworms
- By mouth

Child 6 months–18 years 100 mg as a single dose; if reinfection occurs second dose may be needed after 2 weeks

Whipworms
- By mouth

Child 1–18 years 100 mg twice daily for 3 days

Roundworms section 5.5.2

Hookworms section 5.5.4

[1]Mebendazole (Non-proprietary) PoM

Tablets, chewable, mebendazole 100 mg

1. Can be sold to the public if supplied for oral use in the treatment of enterobiasis in children over 2 years provided its container or package is labelled to show a max. single dose of 100 mg and it is supplied in a container or package containing not more than 800 mg

Vermox® (Janssen-Cilag) PoM

Tablets, orange, scored, chewable, mebendazole 100 mg. Net price 6-tab pack = £1.45

Suspension, mebendazole 100 mg/5 mL. Net price 30 mL = £1.68

PIPERAZINE

Cautions epilepsy

Hepatic impairment manufacturer advises avoid

Renal impairment avoid in severe renal impairment—risk of neurotoxicity

Pregnancy not known to be harmful but manufacturer advises avoid in first trimester

Breast-feeding present in milk—manufacturer advises avoid breast-feeding for 8 hours after dose (express and discard milk during this time)

Note Packs on sale to the general public carry a warning to avoid in epilepsy, liver or kidney disease, and to seek medical advice in pregnancy

Side-effects nausea, vomiting, colic, diarrhoea, allergic reactions including urticaria, bronchospasm, and rare reports of arthralgia, fever, Stevens-Johnson syndrome and angioedema; rarely dizziness, muscular inco-ordination ('worm wobble'); drowsiness, nystagmus, vertigo, blurred vision, confusion and clonic contractions in children with neurological or renal abnormalities

Indication and dose

See under preparation, below

Piperazine Citrate (Non-proprietary)

Syrup, piperazine hydrate 750 mg/5 mL (as citrate)
Brands include *Ascalix*®

Dose

Consult product literature

Syrup, piperazine hydrate 4 g/30 mL (as citrate)
Brands include *Ascalix*®

Dose

Consult product literature

5 Infections

PIPERAZINE (*continued*)

With sennosides

For cautions, contra-indications, side-effects of senna see section 1.6.2

Pripsen® (Thornton & Ross)
Oral powder, piperazine phosphate 4 g, total sennosides (calculated as sennoside B) 15.3 mg/sachet. Net price two-dose sachet pack = £1.36. Label: 13

Dose

(Stirred into milk or water)

Threadworms
• By mouth
Child 3 months–1 year 1 level 2.5-mL spoonful as a single dose in the morning, repeated after 14 days
Child 1–6 years 1 level 5-mL spoonful as a single dose in the morning, repeated after 14 days
Child 6–18 years content of 1 sachet as a single dose (in the morning), repeated after 14 days

Roundworms first dose as for threadworms; repeat at monthly intervals for up to 3 months if reinfection risk

5.5.2 Ascaricides (common roundworm infections)

Levamisole (available from specialist importing companies) is very effective against *Ascaris lumbricoides* and is generally considered to be the drug of choice, although supplies may be difficult to obtain. It is very well tolerated; mild nausea or vomiting has been reported in about 1% of treated patients.

Mebendazole (section 5.5.1) is also active against ascaris; the usual dose in children over 1 year is 100 mg twice daily for 3 days.

Piperazine may be given in a single dose, see Piperazine, above.

LEVAMISOLE

Cautions epilepsy; juvenile idiopathic arthritis; Sjögren's syndrome

Hepatic impairment use with caution—dose adjustment may be necessary

Pregnancy embryotoxic in *animal* studies, avoid if possible

Breast-feeding no information available

Contra-indications blood disorders

Side-effects nausea, vomiting, diarrhoea; dizziness, headache; on *prolonged treatment* taste disturbances, insomnia, convulsions, influenza-like syndrome, blood disorders, vasculitis, arthralgia, myalgia, rash

Licensed use not licensed

Indication and dose

Roundworm (*Ascaris lumbricoides*)
• By mouth
Child 1 month–18 years 2.5–3 mg/kg (max. 150 mg) as a single dose

Hookworm
• By mouth
Child 1 month–18 years 2.5 mg/kg (max. 150 mg) as a single dose repeated after 7 days if severe

Nephrotic syndrome (specialist supervision section 6.3.2)
• By mouth
Child 1month–18 years 2.5 mg/kg (max. 150 mg) on alternate days

Levamisole (Non-proprietary) PoM
Tablets, levamisole (as hydrochloride) 50 mg
Label: 4
Available from specialist importing companies, see p. 848

5.5.3 Drugs for tapeworm infections

Taenicides

Niclosamide (available from specialist importing companies) is the most widely used drug for tapeworm infections and side-effects are limited to occasional gastro-intestinal upset, lightheadedness, and pruritus; it is not effective against larval worms. Fears of developing cysticercosis in *Taenia solium* infections have proved unfounded. All the same, a laxative may be given 2 hours after the dose; an antiemetic may be given before treatment.

Praziquantel (available on named-patient basis from Merck (*Cysticide®*)) is as effective as niclosamide and is given to children over 4 years of age as a single dose of 10–20 mg/kg after a light breakfast (*or* as a single dose of 25 mg/kg for *Hymenolepis nana*).

Hydatid disease

Cysts caused by *Echinococcus granulosus* grow slowly and asymptomatic children do not always require treatment. Surgical treatment remains the method of choice in many situations. **Albendazole** (available from specialist importing companies) is used in conjunction with surgery to reduce the risk of recurrence or as primary treatment in inoperable cases. Albendazole is given to children over 2 years of age in a dose of 7.5 mg/kg (max. 400 mg twice daily) twice daily for 28 days followed by 14-day break and then repeated for up to 2–3 cycles. Alveolar echinococcosis due to *E. multilocularis* is usually fatal if untreated. Surgical removal with albendazole cover is the treatment of choice, but where effective surgery is impossible, repeated cycles of albendazole (for a year or more) may help. Careful monitoring of liver function is particularly important during drug treatment.

5.5.4 Drugs for hookworms (ancylostomiasis, necatoriasis)

Hookworms live in the upper small intestine and draw blood from the point of their attachment to their host. An iron-deficiency anaemia may thereby be produced and, if present, effective treatment of the infection requires not only expulsion of the worms but treatment of the anaemia.

Mebendazole (section 5.5.1) has a useful broad-spectrum activity, and is effective against hookworms; the usual dose for children over 1 year of age is 100 mg twice daily for 3 days. **Levamisole** is also effective (section 5.5.2), but supplies may be difficult to obtain.

5.5.5 Schistosomicides (bilharziasis)

Adult *Schistosoma haematobium* worms live in the genito-urinary veins and adult *S. mansoni* in those of the colon and mesentery. *S. japonicum* is more widely distributed in veins of the alimentary tract and portal system.

Praziquantel (available on named-patient basis from Merck (*Cysticide®*)) is effective against all human schistosomes. In children over 4 years the dose is 20 mg/kg followed after 4–6 hours by a further dose of 20 mg/kg (20 mg/kg 3 times daily for one day for *S. japonicum* infections). No serious toxic effects have been reported. Of all the available schistosomicides, it has the most attractive combination of effectiveness, broad-spectrum activity, and low toxicity.

5.5.6 Filaricides

Diethylcarbamazine (available from specialist importing companies) is effective against microfilariae and adult worms of *Loa loa*, *Wuchereria bancrofti*, and *Brugia malayi*. To minimise reactions, treatment in children over 1 month is commenced with a dose of diethylcarbamazine citrate 1 mg/kg in divided doses on the first day and increased gradually over 3 days to 6 mg/kg daily (3 mg/kg daily if child under 10 years) in divided doses; length of treatment varies according to infection type, and usually gives a radical cure for these infections. Close medical supervision is necessary particularly in the early phase of treatment. In heavy infections there may be a febrile reaction, and in heavy *Loa loa* infection there is a small risk of encephalopathy. In such cases treatment must be given under careful in-patient supervision and stopped at the first sign of cerebral involvement (and specialist advice sought).

Ivermectin (available from specialist importing companies) is very effective in *onchocerciasis* and it is now the drug of choice. In children over 5 years, a single dose of 150 micrograms/kg by mouth produces a prolonged reduction in microfilarial levels. Retreatment at intervals of 6 to 12 months depending on symptoms must be given until the adult worms die out. Reactions are usually slight and most commonly take the form of temporary aggravation of itching and rash. Diethylcarbamazine or suramin should no longer be used for onchocerciasis because of their toxicity.

5.5.7 Drugs for cutaneous larva migrans (creeping eruption)

Dog and cat hookworm larvae may enter human skin where they produce slowly extending itching tracks usually on the foot. Single tracks can be treated with topical tiabendazole (no commercial preparation available). Multiple infections respond to **ivermectin**, **albendazole** (*Zentel*®) or **tiabendazole** (thiabendazole) (*Mintezol*®, *Triasox*®) by mouth—all available from specialist importing companies.

5.5.8 Drugs for strongyloidiasis

Adult forms of *Strongyloides stercoralis* live in the gut and produce larvae which penetrate the gut wall and invade the tissues, setting up a cycle of auto-infection. **Tiabendazole** (thiabendazole) (*Mintezol*®, *Triasox*®) is the drug of choice; it is given to children over 1 month at a dosage of 25 mg/kg (max. 1.5 g) every 12 hours for 2–3 days, or 5–7 days in disseminated infection. **Albendazole** (*Zentel*®) is an alternative with fewer side-effects; it is given to children over 2 years of age in a dose of 400 mg once or twice daily for 3 days, repeated after 3 weeks if necessary. **Ivermectin** given to children over 5 years in a dose of 200 micrograms/kg daily for 2 days, may be the most effective drug for chronic *Strongyloides* infection.

All of these drugs are available from specialist importing companies.

6 Endocrine system

This chapter includes advice on the drug management of the following:

Adrenal suppression during illness, trauma or surgery, p. 423
Serious infections in patients taking corticosteroids, p. 423
Nephrotic syndrome, p. 425
Delayed puberty, p. 430
Prococious puberty, p. 434
Diabetes insipidus, p. 441

6.1 Drugs used in diabetes

Diabetes mellitus occurs because of a lack of insulin or resistance to its action. It is diagnosed by measuring fasting or random blood-glucose concentration (and occasionally by glucose tolerance test). Although there are many subtypes, the two principle classes of diabetes are type 1 diabetes and type 2 diabetes.

Type 1 diabetes Type 1 diabetes, also referred to as insulin-dependent diabetes mellitus (IDDM), is due to a deficiency of insulin following autoimmune destruction of pancreatic beta cells and is the most common form of diabetes in children. Children with type 1 diabetes require administration of insulin.

Type 2 diabetes Type 2 diabetes, also referred to as non-insulin-dependent diabetes mellitus (NIDDM), is rare in children but the incidence is increasing, particularly in adolescents, as obesity increases. It results from reduced secretion of insulin or from peripheral resistance to the action of insulin. Although children may be controlled on diet alone, many require oral antidiabetic drugs or insulin to maintain satisfactory control. There is limited information available on the use of oral anti-diabetics in children (see section 6.1.2). In overweight individuals, type 2 diabetes may be prevented by losing weight and increasing physical activity.

Maturity-onset diabetes of the young (MODY) describes a number of rare disease states, distinct from type 2 diabetes, that are also characterised by impaired glucose tolerance. A sulphonylurea such as glicazide (p. 410) may be effective in certain forms of MODY.

Treatment of diabetes should be aimed at alleviating symptoms and minimising the risk of long-term complications by appropriate control of diabetes.

Diabetes is a strong risk factor for cardiovascular disease later in life. Other risk factors for cardiovascular disease (smoking, hypertension, obesity and hyperlipidaemia) should be addressed. The use of an ACE inhibitor (section 2.5.5.1) and of a lipid-regulating drug (section 2.12) can be beneficial in children with diabetes and a high cardiovascular risk. For reference to the use of an ACE inhibitor in the management of diabetic nephropathy, see section 6.1.5.

Prevention of diabetic complications Although rare, retinopathy, neuropathy and nephropathy can occur in children with diabetes. Screening for complications should begin 5 years after diagnosis of diabetes or from 12 years of age. Optimal glycaemic control in both type 1 diabetes and type 2 diabetes reduces, in the long term, the risk of microvascular complications including retinopathy, development of proteinuria and to some extent neuropathy.

A measure of the total glycated (or glycosylated) haemoglobin (HbA_1) or a specific fraction (HbA_{1c}) provides a good indication of long-term glycaemic control. The ideal HbA_{1c} concentration is between 6.5 and 7.5% but this cannot always be achieved, and for those on insulin there are significantly increased risks of severe hypoglycaemia. Tight control of blood pressure in hypertensive children with diabetes may reduce mortality significantly and protects visual acuity (by reducing considerably the risks of maculopathy and retinal photocoagulation) (see also section 2.5).

6.1.1 Insulins

Insulin plays a key role in the regulation of carbohydrate, fat, and protein metabolism. It is a polypeptide hormone of complex structure. There are differences in the amino-acid sequence of animal insulins, human insulins and the human insulin analogues. Human sequence insulin may be produced semisynthetically by enzymatic modification of porcine insulin (emp) or biosynthetically by recombinant DNA technology using bacteria (crb, prb) or yeast (pyr).

Immunological resistance to insulin action is uncommon. Preparations of human sequence insulin should theoretically be less immunogenic than other insulin preparations, but no real advantage has been shown in trials.

Insulin is inactivated by gastro-intestinal enzymes, and must therefore be given by injection; the subcutaneous route is ideal in most circumstances. Insulin is usually injected into the thighs, buttocks, or abdomen; absorption from a limb site may be increased if the limb is used in strenuous exercise after the injection. Generally subcutaneous insulin injections cause few problems; fat hypertrophy does however occur and is a factor in poor glycaemic control. Fat hypertrophy can be minimised by using different injection sites in rotation. Local allergic reactions are rare.

Insulin should be given to all children with type 1 diabetes; it may also be needed to treat type 2 diabetes either when other methods cannot control the condition or during periods of acute illness or peri-operatively. Insulin is required in all instances of ketoacidosis (section 6.1.3), which can develop rapidly in children.

Management of diabetes with insulin The aim of treatment is to achieve the best possible control of blood-glucose concentration without making the child or carer obsessional and to avoid disabling hypoglycaemia; close co-operation is needed between the child or carer and the medical team to achieve good control and thereby reduce the risk of complications. Mixtures of insulin preparations may be required and appropriate combinations have to be determined for the individual child. For severely ill children with diabetes of recent onset, treatment should be started with several doses of soluble insulin given throughout the day with medium-acting insulin generally given at bedtime. For those less severely ill, treatment may be started with a mixture of premixed short- and medium-acting insulins given twice daily. The dose of insulin is increased gradually taking care to avoid troublesome hypoglycaemia. The proportion of the short-acting soluble component can be increased in those with excessive postprandial hyperglycaemia.

Initiation of insulin may be followed by a partial remission phase or 'honeymoon period' when lower doses of insulin may be required than are subsequently necessary to maintain glycaemic control.

There are 3 main types of insulin preparations:

- those of **short** duration which have a relatively rapid onset of action, namely soluble insulin, insulin lispro, and insulin aspart (section 6.1.1.1);
- those with an **intermediate** action, e.g. isophane insulin and insulin zinc suspension (section 6.1.1.2); and
- those whose action is slower in onset and lasts for **long** periods, e.g. insulin zinc suspension, insulin detemir, and insulin glargine (section 6.1.1.2)

The duration of action of a particular type of insulin varies considerably from one child to another, and needs to be assessed individually.

Examples of insulin regimens

- Twice-daily isophane insulin: often the initial regimen; soluble insulin is added if necessary;
- Twice-daily mixture of soluble insulin and isophane insulin: either mixed before administration or given as a pre-mixed combination e.g. 20:80 or 30:70 of soluble insulin:isophane insulin;
- Three-times-daily combination of soluble insulin and isophane insulin in the morning, soluble insulin only before evening meal, and isophane insulin only at bedtime; suitable for children who have at least 2 hours between the last 2 injections of the day;
- Multiple injection regimen: either soluble insulin or a rapid-acting insulin before meals and long—acting insulin at bedtime; suitable for those who need flexibility. New long-acting insulins (insulin detemir or insulin glargine) may be useful for this regimen.

Insulin requirements Most prepubertal children require around 0.6–0.8 units/kg/day of insulin after the initial temporary remission phase. Unless the child leads a very sedentary life-style, a requirement for higher doses may indicate poor compliance, poor absorption of insulin from the injection site (e.g. because of lipohypertrophic sites) or the beginning of puberty. During puberty up to 1.5–2 units/kg/day of insulin may be required, especially during growth spurts. Around 1 year after menarche or after the growth spurt in boys, the dose may need to be adjusted to avoid excessive weight gain. Insulin requirements may be *increased* by infection, stress, accidental or surgical trauma, and during the second and third trimester of pregnancy. Insulin requirements may be *decreased* in very active individuals and in those with renal or hepatic impairment, some endocrine disorders (e.g. Addison's disease, hypopituitarism) or coeliac disease. Insulin requirements should be assessed frequently in all these circumstances. In pregnancy insulin requirement should be assessed frequently by an experienced diabetes physician.

Insulin administration Insulin is generally given by *subcutaneous injection* half-an-hour before a meal except for rapid-acting insulins, which should be given immediately before, with or even immediately after a meal (section 6.1.1.1). Injection devices ('pens') (section 6.1.1.3) which hold the insulin in a cartridge and meter the required dose are convenient to use. The conventional syringe and needle is less popular with children and carers, but may be required for insulins not available in cartridge form.

For intensive insulin regimens multiple subcutaneous injections (3 to 4 times daily) are usually recommended.

Short-acting insulins (soluble insulin, insulin aspart and insulin lispro) can also be given by *continuous subcutaneous infusion* using a portable infusion pump. This device delivers a continuous basal insulin infusion and patient-activated bolus doses at meal times. This technique is appropriate only for children who suffer recurrent hypoglycaemia or marked morning rise in blood-glucose concentration despite optimised multiple-injection regimens. NICE (February 2003) has also recommended continuous subcutaneous infusion as an option in those who suffer repeated or unpredictable hypoglycaemia despite optimal multiple-injection regimens (including the use of insulin glargine where appropriate). Children on subcutaneous insulin infusion must be highly motivated, able to monitor their blood-glucose concentration or have it monitored by a carer, and have expert training, advice and supervision from an experienced healthcare team.

Soluble insulin by the *intravenous route* is reserved for urgent treatment, and for fine control in serious illness and in the perioperative period (see under Diabetes and Surgery, below).

Monitoring Many carers and children are trained to monitor blood-glucose concentrations (section 6.1.6). Since blood-glucose concentrations vary substantially throughout the day, 'normoglycaemia' cannot always be achieved throughout a 24-hour period without causing damaging hypoglycaemia. It is therefore best to recommend that children should maintain a blood-glucose concentration of between 4 and 9 mmol/litre for most of the time (4–7 mmol/litre before meals and less than 9 mmol/litre after meals), while accepting that on occasions, for brief periods, it will be above these values; efforts should be made to prevent the blood-glucose concentration from falling below 4 mmol/litre. Carers and children should be advised to look for 'peaks' and 'troughs' of blood glucose, and to adjust the insulin dosage only once or twice weekly. Overall it is ideal to aim for an HbA_{1c} (glycosylated haemoglobin) concentration of 6.5–7.5% or less (reference range 4–6%) but this is not always possible without causing disabling hypoglycaemia. Measurement of serum-fructosamine concentration can also be used for assessment of control; this is simpler and cheaper but the measurement of HbA_{1c} is generally more reliable.

The intake of energy and of simple and complex carbohydrates should be adequate to allow normal growth and development but obesity must be avoided. The carbohydrate intake needs to be regulated and should be distributed throughout the day. Fine control of plasma glucose can be achieved by moving portions of carbohydrate from one meal to another without altering the total intake.

Hypoglycaemia Hypoglycaemia is a potential problem for all children receiving insulin and they and their carers, should be given careful instruction on how to avoid it.

Loss of warning of hypoglycaemia is common among insulin-treated children and can be a serious hazard, especially for cyclists and drivers. Very tight control of diabetes lowers the blood-glucose concentration needed to trigger hypoglycaemic symptoms; increase in the frequency of hypoglycaemic episodes reduces the warning symptoms experienced by the child.

To restore the warning signs, episodes of hypoglycaemia must be minimised; this involves appropriate adjustment of insulin type, dose and frequency together with suitable timing and quantity of meals and snacks.

Driving Information on the requirements for driving vehicles by individuals receiving treatment for diabetes is available in the BNF (section 6.1.1) or from the DVLA at www.dvla.gov.uk/at-a-glance/content.htm.

Diabetes and surgery Children with type 1 diabetes should undergo surgery in centres with facilities for the care of children with diabetes.

Children with type 1 diabetes who require surgery:

- should be admitted to hospital for general anaesthesia
- should receive insulin, even if they are fasting, to avoid ketoacidosis
- should receive glucose infusion when fasting before an anaesthetic to prevent hypoglycaemia.

Elective surgery. Surgery in children with diabetes is best scheduled early on the list, preferably in the morning. If glycaemic control is poor it is advisable to admit the child well in advance of surgery. On the *evening before surgery*, blood-glucose should be measured frequently, especially before meals and snacks and at bedtime; urine should be tested for ketones. The usual evening or bedtime insulin and bedtime snack should be given. Ketosis or severe hypoglycaemia require correction, preferably by overnight intravenous infusion (section 6.1.3 and section 6.1.4), and the surgery may need to be postponed.

For *surgery scheduled for the morning*, the usual morning dose of insulin should be omitted. Early on the day of the operation, intravenous infusion of fluids and insulin should be started (see Intravenous Fluids and Continuous Insulin Infusion below).

For *surgery scheduled for the afternoon*, one-third of the usual morning dose of insulin should be given in the morning as short-acting (or soluble) insulin. Intravenous fluids and insulin infusion should be started by midday.

For *emergency surgery*, intravenous fluids and an insulin infusion should be started immediately (see Intravenous Fluids and Continuous Insulin Infusion below). If ketoacidosis is present the recommendations for diabetic ketoacidosis should be followed (section 6.1.3).

For *minor procedures that require fasting*, a slight modification of the usual regimen may be all that is necessary e.g. for early morning procedures delay insulin and food until immediately after the procedure. In all cases the advice of a doctor or anaesthetist experienced in the management of children with diabetes should be sought.

Intravenous fluids and continuous insulin infusion. Blood-glucose and plasma-electrolyte concentrations must be measured frequently in a child receiving intravenous support. Intravenous infusion should be continued until after the child starts to eat and drink. The following infusions should be used and adjusted according to the child's fluid and electrolyte requirements:

- Constant infusion of sodium chloride 0.45% and glucose 5% intravenous infusion together with potassium chloride 20 mmol/litre (provided that plasma-potassium concentration is not raised) at a rate determined by factors such as volume depletion and age; the amount of potassium chloride infused is adjusted according to plasma electrolyte measurements
- Constant infusion of soluble insulin 1 unit/mL in sodium chloride 0.9% intravenous infusion initially at a rate of 0.025 units/kg/hour (up to 0.05 units/kg/hour if the child is unwell), then adjusted to blood-glucose concentration
- Blood-glucose concentration should be maintained between 5 and 12 mmol/litre. If the glucose concentration falls below 5 mmol/litre, glucose 10% intravenous infusion may be required; conversely, if the glucose concentration persistently exceeds 15 mmol/litre, sodium chloride 0.9% intravenous infusion should be substituted

- If the child develops overt hypoglycaemia (blood-glucose less than 3 mmol/litre) then the insulin infusion should be suspended for up to 30 minutes

The usual subcutaneous insulin regimen should be started before the first meal (but the dose may need to be 10–20% higher than usual if the child is still bedbound or unwell) and the intravenous insulin infusion stopped 1 hour later. If glycaemic control is not adequately achieved, additional insulin may be given in the following ways:

- additional doses of soluble insulin at any of the 4 injection times (before meals or bedtime) *or*
- temporary addition of intravenous insulin infusion to subcutaneous regimen *or*
- complete reversion to intravenous insulin infusion (particularly if the child is unwell).

Neonatal diabetes Neonatal diabetes is a rare condition that presents with acidosis, dehydration, hyperglycaemia and rarely ketosis; it responds to continuous insulin infusion (0.02 to 0.125 units/kg/hour); the dose should be adjusted according to blood glucose concentrations. When the neonate is stable, treatment may be switched to subcutaneous injection of insulin given once or twice a day. Treatment is normally required for 4-6 weeks in transient forms but may be required permanently in some cases.

Neonatal hyperglycaemia Newborn babies are relatively intolerant of glucose, especially in the first week of life and if premature. If intravenous glucose is necessary e.g. for total parenteral nutrition, infuse at a lower rate for 6–12 hours and the glucose intolerance should resolve. Insulin is not needed for such transient glucose intolerance, but may be needed if blood-glucose concentration is persistently high.

6.1.1.1 Short-acting insulins

Soluble insulin is a short-acting form of insulin. For maintenance regimens it is usual to inject it 15 to 30 minutes before meals.

Soluble insulin is the most appropriate form of insulin for use in diabetic emergencies and at the time of surgery. It can be given intravenously and intramuscularly, as well as subcutaneously.

When injected subcutaneously, soluble insulin has a rapid onset of action (30 to 60 minutes), a peak action between 2 and 4 hours, and a duration of action of up to 8 hours.

When injected intravenously, soluble insulin has a very short half-life of only about 5 minutes and its effect disappears within 30 minutes.

The human insulin analogues, **insulin aspart** and **insulin lispro**, have a faster onset (10–20 minutes) and shorter duration of action (2–5 hours) than soluble insulin; as a result, compared to soluble insulin, fasting and preprandial blood-glucose concentration is a little higher, postprandial blood-glucose concentration is a little lower, and hypoglycaemia occurs slightly less frequently. There is no evidence to justify switching from conventional insulin to a human insulin analogue if glycaemic control is adequate; they should only be used in children in preference to soluble insulin when a fast onset of action is required e.g. in very young children who refuse food and when timing of injections in relation to meals is difficult. They may also be useful in children prone to pre-lunch hypoglycaemia and those who eat late in the evening and are prone to nocturnal hypoglycaemia. Insulin aspart and insulin lispro may also be administered by subcutaneous infusion.

SOLUBLE INSULIN

Cautions see notes above; **interactions:** Appendix 1 (antidiabetics)

Renal impairment reduce dose in severe impairment as insulin requirements fall; compensatory response to hypoglycaemia is impaired

Pregnancy insulin requirements should be assessed frequently by an experienced diabetes physician

Side-effects see notes above; transient oedema; local reactions and fat hypertrophy at injection

SOLUBLE INSULIN (*continued*)

site; rarely hypersensitivity reactions including urticaria, rash; overdose causes hypoglycaemia

Indication and dose

Hyperglycaemia, surgery in children with diabetes

- **By intravenous infusion**

Neonate 0.01–0.1 units/kg/hour, adjusted according to blood-glucose concentration, see also notes above

Child 1 month–18 years 0.025–0.1 units/kg/hour, adjusted according to blood-glucose concentration, see also notes above

Administration For *intravenous infusion*, dilute to a concentration of 1 unit/mL with Sodium Chloride 0.9% and mix thoroughly; insulin may be adsorbed by plastics, flush giving set with at least 20 mL of infusion fluid containing insulin

Diabetes mellitus

- **By subcutaneous injection**

According to requirements (see notes above)

Note Rotate injection site to reduce local reactions and fat hypertrophy

Counselling Show container to child or carer and confirm the expected version is dispensed

Highly purified animal

Hypurin® Bovine Neutral (CP) PoM
Injection, soluble insulin (bovine, highly purified) 100 units/mL. Net price 10-mL vial = £18.48; cartridges (for *Autopen®* devices) 5 × 1.5 mL = £13.86, 5 × 3 mL = £27.72

Hypurin® Porcine Neutral (CP) PoM
Injection, soluble insulin (porcine, highly purified) 100 units/mL. Net price 10-mL vial = £16.80; cartridges (for *Autopen®* devices) 5 × 1.5 mL = £12.60, 5 × 3 mL = £25.20

Pork Actrapid® (Novo Nordisk) PoM
Injection, soluble insulin (porcine, highly purified) 100 units/mL. Net price 10-mL vial = £4.00
Note Not recommended for use in subcutaneous insulin infusion pumps—may precipitate in catheter or needle

Human sequence

Actrapid® (Novo Nordisk) PoM
Injection, soluble insulin (human, pyr) 100 units/mL. Net price 10-mL vial = £7.48
Note Not recommended for use in subcutaneous insulin infusion pumps—may precipitate in catheter or needle

Velosulin® (Novo Nordisk) PoM
Injection, soluble insulin (human, pyr) 100 units/mL. Net price 10-mL vial = £10.40

Humulin S® (Lilly) PoM
Injection, soluble insulin (human, prb) 100 units/mL. Net price 10-mL vial = £15.00; 5 × 3-mL cartridge (for most *Autopen®* devices or *HumaPen®*) = £25.56

Insuman® Rapid (Aventis Pharma) ▼ PoM
Injection, soluble insulin (human, crb) 100 units/mL, net price 5 × 3-mL cartridge (for *OptiPen® Pro 1* NHS) = £23.43; 5 × 3-mL *Insuman® Rapid OptiSet®* prefilled disposable injection devices (range 2–40 units, allowing 2-unit dosage adjustment) = £27.90
Note Not recommended for use in subcutaneous insulin infusion pumps

Mixed preparations

See Biphasic Isophane Insulin (section 6.1.1.2)

INSULIN ASPART

(Recombinant human insulin analogue)

Cautions see under Soluble Insulin; children under 6 years (use only if benefit likely compared to soluble insulin)

Pregnancy see under Soluble Insulin; limited evidence of safety

Side-effects see under Soluble Insulin

Licensed use not licensed for use in children under 6 years

Indication and dose

Diabetes mellitus

- **By subcutaneous injection**

Immediately before meals or when necessary shortly after meals, according to requirements

- **By subcutaneous infusion, intravenous injection or intravenous infusion**

According to requirements

Counselling Show container to child or carer and confirm the expected version is dispensed

Administration for *intravenous infusion*, dilute to a concentration of 0.05–1 unit/mL with Glucose 5% *or* Sodium Chloride 0.9% and mix thoroughly; adsorbed to some extent by plastics of infusion set

NovoRapid® (Novo Nordisk) PoM
Injection, insulin aspart (recombinant human insulin analogue) 100 units/mL, net price 10-mL vial = £17.27; *Penfill®* cartridge (for *Innovo®* and *NovoPen®* devices) 5 × 3-mL = £29.43; 5 × 3-mL *FlexPen®* prefilled disposable injection devices (range 1–60 units, allowing 1-unit dosage adjustment) = £32.00

INSULIN LISPRO

(Recombinant human insulin analogue)

Cautions see under Soluble Insulin; children under 12 years (use only if benefit likely compared to soluble insulin)

Pregnancy see under Soluble Insulin; limited evidence of safety

Side-effects see under Soluble Insulin

INSULIN LISPRO (*continued*)

Licensed use not licensed for use in children under 12 years

Indication and dose

Diabetes mellitus
- By subcutaneous injection
shortly before meals or when necessary shortly after meals, according to requirements
- By subcutaneous infusion, or intravenous injection, or intravenous infusion
According to requirements

Counselling Show container to child or carer and confirm the expected version is dispensed

Administration For *intravenous infusion*, dilute to a concentration of 0.1–1 unit/mL with Glucose 5% *or* Sodium Chloride 0.9% and mix thoroughly; adsorbed to some extent by plastics of infusion set—prime giving set before starting infusion

Humalog® (Lilly) PoM
Injection, insulin lispro (recombinant human insulin analogue) 100 units/mL. Net price 10-mL vial = £17.28; 5 × 3-mL cartridge (for most *Autopen®* devices or *HumaPen®*) = £29.46; 5 × 3-mL *Humalog®-Pen* prefilled disposable injection devices (range 1–60 units, allowing 1-unit dosage adjustment) = £29.46

6.1.1.2 Intermediate- and long-acting insulins

When given by subcutaneous injection, intermediate- and long-acting insulins have an onset of action of approximately 1–2 hours, a maximal effect at 4–12 hours, and a duration of 16–35 hours. Some are given twice daily in conjunction with short-acting (soluble) insulin, and others are given once daily. Soluble insulin can be mixed with intermediate and long-acting insulins (except insulin detemir and insulin glargine), essentially retaining the properties of the two components, although there may be some blunting of the initial effect of the soluble insulin component (especially on mixing with protamine zinc insulin, see below).

Close monitoring of blood glucose is essential when introducing a change to the insulin regimen; the total daily dose as well as any concomitant treatment may need to be adjusted.

Isophane insulin is a suspension of insulin with protamine which is of particular value for initiation of twice-daily insulin regimens. Isophane may be mixed with soluble insulin before injection but ready-mixed preparations may be more appropriate (**biphasic isophane insulin**, **biphasic insulin aspart**, or **biphasic insulin lispro**).

Insulin zinc suspension (crystalline) has a more prolonged duration of action; it may be used independently or in **insulin zinc suspension** (30% amorphous, 70% crystalline).

Protamine zinc insulin is usually given once daily with short-acting (soluble) insulin. It has the drawback of binding with the soluble insulin when mixed in the same syringe, and is now rarely used.

Insulin detemir and **insulin glargine** are human insulin analogues with prolonged duration of action; insulin detemir is given once or twice daily and insulin glargine is given once daily. They may help to reduce nocturnal hypoglycaemia in those using multiple daily injection regimens. There is little evidence to justify switching from conventional intermediate- or long-acting insulin to a human insulin analogue if glycaemic control is adequate.

INSULIN DETEMIR

(Recombinant human insulin analogue—long-acting)

Cautions see under Soluble Insulin (section 6.1.1.1)

Pregnancy see under Soluble Insulin; limited evidence of safety

Side-effects see under Soluble Insulin (section 6.1.1.1)

Licensed use not licensed for use in children under 6 years

Indication and dose

Diabetes mellitus
- By subcutaneous injection
Child over 6 years According to requirements
Counselling Show container to child or carer and confirm the expected version is dispensed

Levemir® (Novo Nordisk) ▼ PoM
Injection, insulin detemir (recombinant human insulin analogue) 100 units/mL, net price 5 × 3-mL cartridge (for *NovoPen®* devices) = £39.00; 5 × 3-mL *FlexPen®* prefilled disposable injection device (range 1–60 units, allowing 1-unit dosage adjustment) = £39.00.

INSULIN GLARGINE

(Recombinant human insulin analogue—long acting)

Cautions see under Soluble Insulin (section 6.1.1.1)

Pregnancy see under Soluble Insulin; limited evidence of safety

Side-effects see under Soluble Insulin (section 6.1.1.1)

Licensed use not licensed for use in children under 6 years

Indication and dose

Diabetes mellitus
- **By subcutaneous injection**

According to requirements
Counselling Show container to patient and confirm that patient is expecting the version dispensed

Lantus® (Aventis Pharma) ▼ PoM
Injection, insulin glargine (recombinant human insulin analogue) 100 units/mL, net price 10-mL vial = £26.00; 5 × 3-mL cartridge (for *OptiPen® Pro 1*) = £39.00; 5 × 3-mL *Lantus® OptiSet®* prefilled disposable injection devices (range 2–40 units, allowing 2-unit dosage adjustment) = £39.00

INSULIN ZINC SUSPENSION

(Insulin Zinc Suspension (Mixed); I. Z. S.—long acting)

A sterile neutral suspension of bovine insulin or of human insulin in the form of a complex obtained by the addition of a suitable zinc salt; consists of rhombohedral crystals (10–40 microns) and of particles of no uniform shape (not exceeding 2 microns)

Cautions see under Soluble Insulin (section 6.1.1.1)

Side-effects see under Soluble Insulin (section 6.1.1.1)

Indication and dose

Diabetes mellitus
- **By subcutaneous injection**

According to requirements
Counselling Show container to child or carer and confirm the expected version is dispensed

Highly purified animal

Hypurin® Bovine Lente (CP) PoM
Injection, insulin zinc suspension (bovine, highly purified) 100 units/mL. Net price 10-mL vial = £18.48

ISOPHANE INSULIN

(Isophane Insulin Injection; Isophane Protamine Insulin Injection; Isophane Insulin (NPH)—intermediate acting)

A sterile suspension of bovine or porcine insulin or of human insulin in the form of a complex obtained by the addition of protamine sulphate or another suitable protamine

Cautions see under Soluble Insulin (section 6.1.1.1)

Side-effects see under Soluble Insulin (section 6.1.1.1); protamine may cause allergic reactions

Indication and dose

Diabetes mellitus
- **By subcutaneous injection**

According to requirements
Counselling Show container to child or carer and confirm the expected version is dispensed

Highly purified animal

Hypurin® Bovine Isophane (CP) PoM
Injection, *isophane insulin* (bovine, highly purified) 100 units/mL. Net price 10-mL vial = £18.48; cartridges (for *Autopen®* devices) 5 × 1.5 mL = £13.86, 5 × 3 mL = £27.72

Hypurin® Porcine Isophane (CP) PoM
Injection, isophane insulin (porcine, highly purified) 100 units/mL. Net price 10-mL vial = £16.80; cartridges (for *Autopen®* devices) 5 × 1.5 mL = £12.60, 5 × 3 mL = £25.20

Pork Insulatard® (Novo Nordisk) PoM
Injection, isophane insulin (porcine, highly purified) 100 units/mL. Net price 10-mL vial = £4.00

Human sequence

Insulatard® (Novo Nordisk) PoM
Injection, isophane insulin (human, pyr) 100 units/mL. Net price 10-mL vial = £7.48; *Insulatard Penfill®* cartridge (for *Innovo®*, or *Novopen®* devices) 5 × 3 mL = £20.08; 5 × 3-mL *Insulatard InnoLet®* prefilled disposable injection devices (range 1–50 units, allowing 1-unit dosage adjustment) = £20.04

Humulin I® (Lilly) PoM
Injection, isophane insulin (human, prb) 100 units/mL. Net price 10-mL vial = £15.00; 5 × 3-mL cartridge (for most *Autopen®* devices or *HumaPen®*) = £27.22; 5 × 3-mL *Humulin I-Pen®* prefilled disposable injection devices (range 1–60 units, allowing 1-unit dosage adjustment) = £27.22

Insuman® Basal (Aventis Pharma) ▼ PoM
Injection, isophane insulin (human, crb) 100 units/mL, net price 5-mL vial = £5.84; 5 × 3-mL cartridge (for *OptiPen® Pro 1* NHS) = £23.43; 5 × 3-mL *Insuman® Basal OptiSet®* prefilled disposable injection devices (range 2–40 units, allowing 2-unit dosage adjustment) = £27.90

Mixed preparations

See Biphasic Isophane Insulin (p. 406)

PROTAMINE ZINC INSULIN

(Protamine Zinc Insulin Injection—long acting)

A sterile suspension of insulin in the form of a complex obtained by the addition of a suitable protamine and zinc chloride; this preparation was included in BP 1980 but is not included in BP 1988

Cautions see under Soluble Insulin (section 6.1.1.1); see also notes above

Side-effects see under Soluble Insulin (section 6.1.1.1); protamine may cause allergic reactions

Indication and dose

Diabetes mellitus
- **By subcutaneous injection**

  According to requirements

  Counselling Show container to child or carer and confirm the expected version is dispensed

Hypurin® Bovine Protamine Zinc (CP) PoM

Injection, protamine zinc insulin (bovine, highly purified) 100 units/mL. Net price 10-mL vial = £18.48

Biphasic insulins

Biphasic insulins are pre-mixed insulin preparations containing various combinations of short-acting (soluble) or rapid-acting (analogue) insulin and an intermediate-acting insulin.

The percentage of short-acting insulin varies from 10% to 50%. These preparations should be administered by subcutaneous injection up to 15 minutes before or soon after a meal.

BIPHASIC INSULIN ASPART

(Intermediate-acting insulin)

Cautions see under Soluble Insulin and Insulin Aspart (section 6.1.1.1)

Side-effects see under Soluble Insulin (section 6.1.1.1); protamine may cause allergic reactions

Indication and dose

Diabetes mellitus
- **By subcutaneous injection**

  Up to 10 minutes before or soon after a meal, according to requirements

  Counselling Show container to child or carer and confirm the expected version is dispensed; the proportions of the two components should be checked **carefully** (the order in which the proportions are stated may not be the same in other countries)

NovoMix® 30 (Novo Nordisk) PoM

Injection, biphasic insulin aspart (recombinant human insulin analogue), 30% insulin aspart, 70% insulin aspart protamine, 100 units/mL, net price 5 × 3-mL *Penfill®* cartridges (for *Innovo®* and *NovoPen®* devices) = £29.43; 5 × 3-mL *FlexPen®* prefilled disposable injection devices (range 1–60 units, allowing 1-unit dosage adjustment) = £32.00

BIPHASIC INSULIN LISPRO

(Intermediate-acting insulin)

Cautions see under Soluble Insulin and Insulin Lispro (section 6.1.1.1)

Side-effects see under Soluble Insulin (section 6.1.1.1); protamine may cause allergic reactions

Indication and dose

Diabetes mellitus
- **By subcutaneous injection**

  Up to 15 minutes before or soon after a meal, according to requirements

  Counselling Show container to child or carer and confirm the expected version is dispensed; the proportions of the two components should be checked **carefully** (the order in which the proportions are stated may not be the same in other countries)

Humalog® Mix25 (Lilly) PoM

Injection, biphasic insulin lispro (recombinant human insulin analogue), 25% insulin lispro, 75% insulin lispro protamine, 100 units/mL, net price 5 × 3-mL cartridge (for most *Autopen®* devices or *HumaPen®*) = £29.46; 5 × 3-mL prefilled disposable injection devices (range 1–60 units, allowing 1-unit dosage adjustment) = £30.98

Humalog® Mix50 (Lilly) PoM

Injection, biphasic insulin lispro (recombinant human insulin analogue), 50% insulin lispro, 50% insulin lispro protamine, 100 units/mL, net price 5 × 3-mL prefilled disposable injection devices (range 1–60 units, allowing 1-unit dosage adjustment) = £30.98

BIPHASIC ISOPHANE INSULIN

(Biphasic Isophane Insulin Injection—intermediate acting)

A sterile buffered suspension of either porcine or human insulin complexed with protamine sulphate (or another suitable protamine) in a solution of insulin of the same species

Cautions see under Soluble Insulin (section 6.1.1.1)

Side-effects see under Soluble Insulin (section 6.1.1.1); protamine may cause allergic reactions

BIPHASIC ISOPHANE INSULIN (*continued*)

Indication and dose

Diabetes mellitus
- **By subcutaneous injection**
  According to requirements
  Counselling Show container to child or carer and confirm the expected version is dispensed; the proportions of the two components should be checked **carefully** (the order in which the proportions are stated may not be the same in other countries)

Highly purified animal

Hypurin® Porcine 30/70 Mix (CP) PoM
Injection, *biphasic isophane insulin* (porcine, highly purified), 30% soluble, 70% isophane, 100 units/mL. Net price 10-mL vial = £16.80; cartridges (for *Autopen®* devices) 5 × 1.5 ml = £12.60, 5 × 3 mL = £25.20

Pork Mixtard 30® (Novo Nordisk) PoM
Injection, biphasic isophane insulin (porcine, highly purified), 30% soluble, 70% isophane, 100 units/mL. Net price 10-mL vial = £4.00

Human sequence

Mixtard® 10 (Novo Nordisk) PoM
Injection, biphasic isophane insulin (human, pyr), 10% soluble, 90% isophane, 100 units/mL. Net price *Mixtard 10 Penfill®* cartridge (for *Innovo®* or *Novopen®* devices) 5 × 3 mL = £20.08

Mixtard® 20 (Novo Nordisk) PoM
Injection, biphasic isophane insulin (human, pyr), 20% soluble, 80% isophane, 100 units/mL. Net price *Mixtard 20 Penfill®* cartridge (for *Innovo®* or *Novopen®* devices) 5 × 3 mL = £20.08

Mixtard® 30 (Novo Nordisk) PoM
Injection, biphasic isophane insulin (human, pyr), 30% soluble, 70% isophane, 100 units/mL. Net price 10-mL vial = £7.48; *Mixtard 30 Penfill®* cartridge (for *Innovo®* or *Novopen®* devices) 5 × 3 mL = £20.08; 5 × 3-mL *Mixtard 30 InnoLet®* prefilled disposable injection devices (range 1–50 units allowing 1-unit dosage adjustment) = £19.87

Mixtard® 40 (Novo Nordisk) PoM
Injection, biphasic isophane insulin (human, pyr), 40% soluble, 60% isophane, 100 units/mL. Net price *Mixtard 40 Penfill®* cartridge (for *Innovo®* or *Novopen®* devices) 5 × 3 mL = £20.08

Mixtard® 50 (Novo Nordisk) PoM
Injection, biphasic isophane insulin (human, pyr), 50% soluble, 50% isophane, 100 units/mL. Net price *Mixtard 50 Penfill®* cartridge (for *Innovo®* or *Novopen®* devices) 5 × 3 mL = £20.08

Humulin M3® (Lilly) PoM
Injection, biphasic isophane insulin (human, prb), 30% soluble, 70% isophane, 100 units/mL. Net price 10-mL vial = £15.00; 5 × 3-mL cartridge (for most *Autopen®* devices or *HumaPen®*) = £25.56

Insuman® Comb 15 (Aventis Pharma) ▼ PoM
Injection, biphasic isophane insulin (human, crb), 15% soluble, 85% isophane, 100 units/mL, net price 5 × 3-mL *Insuman® Comb 15 OptiSet®* prefilled disposable injection devices (range 2–40 units, allowing 2-unit dosage adjustment) = £27.90

Insuman® Comb 25 (Aventis Pharma) ▼ PoM
Injection, biphasic isophane insulin (human, crb), 25% soluble, 75% isophane, 100 units/mL, net price 5-mL vial = £5.84; 5 × 3-mL cartridge (for *OptiPen® Pro 1* NHS) = £23.43; 5 × 3-mL *Insuman® Comb 25 OptiSet®* prefilled disposable injection devices (range 2–40 units, allowing 2-unit dosage adjustment) = £27.90

Insuman® Comb 50 (Aventis Pharma) ▼ PoM
Injection, biphasic isophane insulin (human, crb), 50% soluble, 50% isophane, 100 units/mL, net price; 5 × 3-mL cartridge (for *OptiPen® Pro 1* NHS) = £23.43; 5 × 3-mL *Insuman® Comb 50 OptiSet®* prefilled disposable injection devices (range 2–40 units, allowing 2-unit dosage adjustment) = £27.90

6.1.1.3 Hypodermic equipment

Carers and children should be advised on the safe disposal of lancets, single-use syringes, and needles. Suitable arrangements for the safe disposal of contaminated waste must be made before these products are prescribed for patients who are carriers of infectious diseases.

Injection devices

Autopen® (Owen Mumford)
Injection device; *Autopen® 24* (for use with Aventis 3-mL insulin cartridges), allows adjustments of dosage in multiples of 1 unit, max. 21 units (single-unit version) *or* 2 units, max. 42 units (2 unit version), net price (both) = £14.70; *Autopen® Classic, Autopen® Special Edition*, and *Autopen® Junior* (for use with Lilly 3-mL insulin cartridges), all allow adjustment of dosage in multiples of 1 unit, max. 21 units (single-unit version) *or* 2 units, max. 42 units (2-unit version), net price = £14.92

HumaPen® Ergo (Lilly)
Injection device, for use with *Humulin®* and *Humalog®* 3-mL cartridges; allows adjustment of dosage in multiples of 1 unit, max. 60 units, net price = £22.39 (available in burgundy and teal)

HumaPen® Luxura (Lilly)
Injection device, for use with *Humulin®* and *Humalog®* 3-mL cartridges; allows adjustment of dosage in multiples of 1 unit, max. 60 units, net price = £26.36

Innovo® (Novo Nordisk)
Injection device, for use with 3-mL *Penfill®* insulin cartridges; allows adjustment of dosage in multiples of 1 unit, max. 70 units, net price = £26.88 (available in green or orange)

mhi-500® (Medical House)
Needle-free insulin delivery device NHS for use with any 10-mL vial *or* any 3-mL cartridge of insulin (except the Novo Nordisk 3 mL penfills), allows adjustment of dosage in multiples of 0.5 units, max. 50 units, net price *starter pack* NHS for 10-mL adaptor (*mhi-500®* device, 5 nozzles, 2 insulin vial adaptors) = £122.12, for 3-mL adaptor = (*mhi-*

500® device, 5 nozzles, 2 insulin cartridge adaptors) = £120.00; *3-month consumables pack* for 10-mL adaptor (13 nozzles, 5 insulin vial adaptors) = £22.54, for 3-mL adaptor (13 nozzles, 5 insulin cartridge adaptors) = £34.45; *vial adaptor pack* (6 insulin vial adaptors) = £7.51, *cartridge adaptor pack* (6 insulin cartridge adaptors) = £7.38; *nozzle pack* (6 nozzles) = £7.51

NovoPen® (Novo Nordisk)
Injection device; for use with *Penfill®* insulin cartridges; *NovoPen® Junior* (for 3-mL cartridges), allows adjustment of dosage in multiples of 0.5 units, max. 35 units, net price = £23.66; *NovoPen® 3 Demi* (for 3-mL cartridges), allows adjustment of dosage in multiples of 0.5 units, max. 35 units, net price = £24.07; *NovoPen® 3 Classic* or *Fun* (for 3-mL cartridges), allows adjustment of dosage in multiples of 1 unit, max. 70 units, net price = £24.07

OptiPen® Pro 1 (Aventis Pharma)
Injection device, for use with *Insuman®* insulin cartridges; allows adjustment of dosage in multiples of 1 unit, max. 60 units, net price = £22.00

Lancets

Lancets—sterile, single use (Drug Tariff)
Ascensia Microlet® 100 = £3.55, 200 = £6.76; *BD Micro-Fine®+* 100 = £3.16, 200 = £6.13; *Cleanlet Fine®* 100 = £3.19, 200 = £6.13; *Finepoint®* 100 = £3.48; *FreeStyle®* 200 = £6.50; *GlucoMen®* Fine 100 = £3.42, 200 = £6.61; *Hypoguard Supreme®* 100 = £2.75; *MediSense Thin®* 200 = £6.63; *Milward Steri-Let®*, 23 gauge, 100 = £3.00, 200 = £5.70, 28 gauge, 100 = £3.00, 200 = £5.70; *Monolet®* 100 = £3.28, 200 = £6.24; *Monolet Extra* 100 = £3.28; *One Touch UltraSoft®* 100 = £3.49; [1]*Softclix®* 200 = £6.93; [1]*Softclix XL®* 50 = £1.73; [2]*Unilet ComforTouch®* 100 = £3.40, 200 = £6.44; [2]*Unilet General Purpose®* 100 = £3.47, 200 = £6.59; [2]*Unilet General Purpose Superlite®* 100 = £3.46, 200 = £6.56; [3]*Unilet Superlite®* 100 = £3.46, 200 = £6.56; *Vitrex Soft®*, 23-gauge, 100 = £3.00, 200 = £5.70; *Vitrex Gentle®* 28-gauge, 100 = £3.19, 200 = £6.13
Compatible finger-pricking devices (unless indicated otherwise, see footnotes), all NHS: *B-D Lancer®*, *Glucolet®*, *Monojector®*, *Penlet II®*, *Soft Touch®*

1. Use NHS *Softclix®* finger-pricking device
2. NHS *Autolet®* and NHS *Autolet Impression®* are also compatible finger-pricking devices
3. Use NHS *Autolet®*, or NHS *Glucolet®* finger-pricking devices

Needles

Hypodermic Needle, Sterile single use (Drug Tariff)
For use with reusable glass syringe, sizes 0.5 mm (25G), 0.45 mm (26G), 0.4 mm (27G). Net price 100-needle pack = £2.53
Brands include *Microlance®*, *Monoject®*

Needles for Prefilled and Reusable Pen Injectors (Drug Tariff)
Screw on, needle length 6.1 mm or less, net price 100-needle pack = £12.08; 6.2–9.9 mm, 100-needle pack = £8.57; 10 mm or more, 100-needle pack = £8.57
Brands include *BD Micro-Fine®+*, *NovoFine®*, *Unifine® Pentips*

Snap on, needle length 6.1 mm or less, net price 100-needle pack = £11.82; 6.2–9.9 mm, 100-needle pack = £8.38; 10 mm or more, 100-needle pack = £8.38
Brands include *Penfine®*

Syringes

Hypodermic Syringe (Drug Tariff)
Calibrated glass with Luer taper conical fitting, for use with U100 insulin. Net price 0.5 mL and 1 mL = £15.18
Brands include *Abcare®*

Pre-Set U100 Insulin Syringe (Drug Tariff)
Calibrated glass with Luer taper conical fitting, supplied with dosage chart and strong box, for blind patients. Net price 1 mL = £21.99

U100 Insulin Syringe with Needle (Drug Tariff)
Disposable with fixed or separate needle for single use or single patient-use, colour coded orange. Needle length 8 mm, diameters 0.33 mm (29G), 0.3 mm (30G), net price 10 (with needle), 0.3 mL = £1.27, 0.5 mL = £1.23; needle length 12 mm, diameters 0.45 mm (26G), 0.4 mm (27G), 0.36 mm (28G), 0.33 mm (29G), net price 10 (with needle), 0.3 mL = £1.37; 0.5 mL = £1.32; 1 mL = £1.33
Brands include *BD Micro-Fine®+*, *Clinipak®*, *Insupak®*, *Monoject® Ultra*, *Omnikan®*, *Plastipak®*, *Unifine®*

Accessories

Needle Clipping (Chopping) Device (Drug Tariff)
Consisting of a clipper to remove needle from its hub and container from which cut-off needles cannot be retrieved; designed to hold 1200 needles, not suitable for use with lancets. Net price = £1.24
Brands include *BD Safe-Clip®*

Sharpsbin (Drug Tariff)
Net price 1-litre sharpsbin = 85p

6.1.2 Oral antidiabetic drugs

Oral antidiabetic drugs are used for the treatment of type 2 (non-insulin-dependent) diabetes mellitus. They should be prescribed only if the child fails to respond adequately to restriction of energy and carbohydrate intake and an increase in physical activity. They should be used to augment the effect of diet and exercise, and not to replace them.

Type 2 diabetes does not usually occur until adolescence and information on the use of oral antidiabetic drugs in children is limited. Treatment with oral antidiabetic drugs should be initiated under specialist supervision **only**; the initial dose should be at the lower end of the adult dose range and then adjusted according to response.

Metformin (section 6.1.2.2) is the oral antidiabetic drug of choice because there is most experience with this drug in children. If dietary changes and metformin do not control the diabetes adequately, either a sulphonylurea (section 6.1.2.1) or insulin (section 6.1.1) may be added.

Alternatively, oral therapy may be substituted with insulin.

When insulin is added to oral therapy, it is generally given at bedtime as isophane insulin, and when insulin replaces an oral regimen it is generally given as twice-daily injections of a biphasic insulin (or isophane insulin mixed with soluble insulin). Weight gain and hypoglycaemia may be complications of insulin therapy but weight gain may be reduced if the insulin is given in combination with metformin.

6.1.2.1 Sulphonylureas

The sulphonylureas are not the first choice oral antidiabetics in children. They act mainly by augmenting insulin secretion and consequently are effective only when some residual pancreatic beta-cell activity is present; during long-term administration they also have an extrapancreatic action. All may cause hypoglycaemia but this is uncommon and usually indicates excessive dosage. Sulphonylurea-induced hypoglycaemia may persist for many hours and must always be treated in hospital.

Sulphonylureas are considered for children in whom metformin is contra-indicated or not tolerated. Several sulphonylureas are available but experience in children is limited; choice is determined by side-effects and the duration of action as well as the child's age and renal function. The long-acting sulphonylureas chlorpropamide and glibenclamide are associated with a greater risk of hypoglycaemia and for this reason are generally avoided in children. Shorter-acting alternatives, such as **tolbutamide**, may be preferred.

Insulin therapy should be instituted temporarily during intercurrent illness (such as coma, infection, and trauma). Sulphonylureas should be omitted on the morning of surgery; insulin is often required because of the ensuing hyperglycaemia in these circumstances.

Sulphonylureas may be useful in the management of certain forms of maturity-onset diabetes of the young; there is most experience with gliclazide.

Cautions Sulphonylureas can encourage weight gain and should be prescribed only if poor control and symptoms persist despite adequate attempts at dieting; metformin (section 6.1.2.2) is considered the drug of choice in children. Caution is needed in those with mild to moderate hepatic and renal impairment because of the hazard of hypoglycaemia. The short-acting tolbutamide may be used in renal impairment but careful monitoring of blood-glucose concentration is essential; care is required to choose the smallest possible dose that produces adequate control of blood glucose.

Contra-indications Sulphonylureas should be avoided where possible in severe hepatic and renal impairment and in porphyria (section 9.8.2). They should not be used while breast-feeding and insulin therapy should be substituted during pregnancy. Sulphonylureas are contra-indicated in the presence of ketoacidosis.

Side-effects Side-effects of sulphonylureas are generally mild and infrequent and include gastro-intestinal disturbances such as nausea, vomiting, diarrhoea and constipation.

Sulphonylureas can occasionally cause a disturbance in liver function, which may rarely lead to cholestatic jaundice, hepatitis and hepatic failure. Hypersensitivity reactions can occur, usually in the first 6–8 weeks of therapy, they consist mainly of allergic skin reactions which progress rarely to erythema multiforme and exfoliative dermatitis, fever and jaundice; photosensitivity has rarely been reported with chlorpropamide and glipizide. Blood disorders are also rare but may include leucopenia, thrombocytopenia, agranulocytosis, pancytopenia, haemolytic anaemia, and aplastic anaemia.

GLIBENCLAMIDE

Cautions see notes above; **interactions**: Appendix 1 (antidiabetics)

Contra-indications see notes above

Side-effects see notes above

Licensed use not licensed for use in children

Indication and dose

Type 2 diabetes mellitus, maturity-onset diabetes of the young (specialist management only, see notes above)
- By mouth

Child 12–18 years initially 2.5 mg daily with or immediately after breakfast, adjusted according to response, max. 15 mg daily

Glibenclamide (Non-proprietary) PoM
Tablets, glibenclamide 2.5 mg, net price 28-tab pack = 78p; 5 mg, 28-tab pack = 95p

Daonil® (Hoechst Marion Roussel) PoM
Tablets, scored, glibenclamide 5 mg, net price 28-tab pack = £2.69

Semi-Daonil® (Hoechst Marion Roussel) PoM
Tablets, scored, glibenclamide 2.5 mg, net price 28-tab pack = £1.73

Euglucon® (Aventis Pharma) PoM
Tablets, glibenclamide 2.5 mg, net price 28-tab pack = £1.72

GLICLAZIDE

Cautions see notes above; **interactions**: Appendix 1 (antidiabetics)

Contra-indications see notes above

Side-effects see notes above

Licensed use not licensed for use in children

Indication and dose

Type 2 diabetes mellitus, maturity-onset diabetes of the young (specialist management only, see notes above)
- By mouth

Child 12–18 years initially 20 mg once daily with breakfast, adjusted according to response; up to 160 mg as a single dose; max. 160 mg twice daily

Gliclazide (Non-proprietary) PoM
Tablets, scored, gliclazide 80 mg, net price 28-tab pack = £1.62, 60-tab pack = £1.87
Brands include *DIAGLYK®*

Diamicron® (Servier) PoM
Tablets, scored, gliclazide 80 mg, net price 60-tab pack = £6.51

TOLBUTAMIDE

Cautions see notes above; **interactions**: Appendix 1 (antidiabetics)

Contra-indications see notes above

Side-effects see notes above; also headache, tinnitus

Licensed use not licensed in children

Indication and dose

Type 2 diabetes mellitus (see notes above), specialist management only
- By mouth

Child 12–18 years 0.5–1.5 g (max. 2 g) daily in divided doses; with or immediately after food

Tolbutamide (Non-proprietary) PoM
Tablets, tolbutamide 500 mg. Net price 28-tab pack = £1.70

Extemporaneous formulations available see Extemporaneous Preparations, p. 8

6.1.2.2 Biguanides

Metformin, the only available biguanide, has a different mode of action from the sulphonylureas, and is not interchangeable with them. It exerts its effect mainly by decreasing gluconeogenesis and by increasing peripheral utilisation of glucose; since it acts only in the presence of endogenous insulin it is effective only if there are some residual functioning pancreatic islet cells.

Metformin is the drug of first choice in children with type 2 diabetes, in whom strict dieting has failed to control diabetes. When the combination of strict diet and metformin treatment fails, other options, that may be considered under specialist management only, include:

- combining with insulin (section 6.1.1) but weight gain and hypoglycaemia can be problems (weight gain minimised if insulin given at night);
- combining with a sulphonylurea (section 6.1.2.1) (reports of increased hazard with this combination remain unconfirmed);

Insulin treatment is almost always required in medical and surgical emergencies; insulin should also be substituted before elective surgery (omit metformin on the morning of surgery and give insulin if required).

Hypoglycaemia does not usually occur with metformin; other advantages are the lower incidence of weight gain and lower plasma-insulin concentration. It does not exert a hypoglycaemic action in non-diabetic subjects unless given in overdose.

Gastro-intestinal side-effects are initially common with metformin, and may persist in some children, particularly when high doses are given. A slow increase in dose may improve tolerability.

Metformin may provoke lactic acidosis which is most likely to occur in children with renal impairment; it should not be used in children with even mild renal impairment.

METFORMIN HYDROCHLORIDE

Cautions see notes above; determine renal function before treatment and once or twice annually during treatment; **interactions:** Appendix 1 (antidiabetics)

Contra-indications ketoacidosis, withdraw if tissue hypoxia likely (e.g. sepsis, respiratory failure, hepatic impairment), use of iodine-containing X-ray contrast media (do not restart metformin until renal function returns to normal) and use of general anaesthesia (suspend metformin on the morning of surgery and restart when renal function returns to normal)

Hepatic impairment contra-indicated

Renal impairment contra-indicated

Pregnancy contra-indicated, insulin preferred

Breast-feeding manufacturer advises avoid—present in milk

Side-effects anorexia, nausea, vomiting, diarrhoea (usually transient), abdominal pain, metallic taste; *rarely* lactic acidosis (withdraw treatment), decreased vitamin-B_{12} absorption, erythema, pruritus and urticaria; hepatitis also reported

Licensed use not licensed in children under 10 years

Indication and dose

Diabetes mellitus (see notes above) specialist supervision **only**

- **By mouth**

Child 10–18 years initially 500 mg once daily adjusted according to response at intervals of not less than 1 week; max. 2 g daily in 2–3 divided doses

Metformin (Non-proprietary) PoM

Tablets, coated, metformin hydrochloride 500 mg, net price 28-tab pack = £1.31, 84-tab pack= £1.78; 850 mg, 56-tab pack = £1.88. Label: 21

Oral solution, metformin hydrochloride 500 mg/5 mL, net price 150 mL. Label: 21 (available as a manufactured special)

Glucophage® (Merck) PoM

Tablets, f/c, metformin hydrochloride 500 mg, net price 84-tab pack = £2.40; 850 mg, 56-tab pack = £2.67. Label: 21

6.1.2.3 Other antidiabetics

There is little experience of the use of **acarbose** in children. It has been used in older children; therapy should be initiated by an appropriate expert.

The use of nateglinide in combination with a sulphonylurea is generally reserved for the management of some subtypes of *maturity-onset diabetes of the young* or other syndromic diabetes and requires specialist management.

6.1.3 Diabetic ketoacidosis

The management of diabetic ketoacidosis involves the replacement of fluid and electrolytes and the administration of insulin. **Soluble insulin** is given intravenously for the management of diabetic ketoacidotic and hyperosmolar non-ketotic coma; insulin is continued until the metabolic disturbance is brought under control.

Clinically well children who are dehydrated up to 5% usually respond to oral rehydration and subcutaneous insulin. For those who do not respond, or are clinically unwell, or are dehydrated by more than 5%, insulin and replacement fluids are best given by intravenous infusion. Soluble insulin should be diluted (and **mixed thoroughly**) with sodium chloride 0.9% intravenous infusion to a concentration of 1 unit/mL and infused at a rate of 0.1 units/kg/hour. **Sodium**

chloride 0.9% intravenous infusion should also be given; **potassium chloride** is included in the infusion as appropriate to prevent the hypokalaemia induced by the insulin unless anuria is suspected. **Sodium chloride 0.45% and glucose 5%** intravenous infusion may be used as replacement fluid after 6 hours if response is adequate and plasma sodium concentrate is stable. **Sodium bicarbonate** infusion (1.26% or 2.74%) is rarely necessary and is used only in cases of extreme acidosis (blood pH less than 6.9) and shock since the acid-base disturbance is normally corrected by the insulin.

Blood glucose is expected to decrease by about 5 mmol/litre/hour; if the response is inadequate the insulin infusion rate can be increased. If the rate of decrease exceeds 5 mmol/litre/hour or blood glucose falls to 14–17 mmol/litre, **glucose intravenous infusion 5% or 10%** should be added to the replacement fluids.

The insulin infusion rate can be reduced to no less than 0.05 units/kg/hour when blood-glucose concentration has fallen below 15 mmol/litre *and* blood pH is greater than 7.3 *and* a glucose infusion has been started (see above); it is continued until the child is ready to take food by mouth. Subcutaneous insulin can then be started. The insulin infusion should not be stopped until 1 hour after starting subcutaneous soluble or long-acting insulin or 10 minutes after starting subcutaneous insulin aspart or insulin lispro.

6.1.4 Treatment of hypoglycaemia

Prompt treatment of hypoglycaemia in children from any cause is essential to prevent subsequent neurological damage. Hyperinsulinism, fatty acid oxidation disorders and glycogen storage disease are less common causes of acute hypoglycaemia in children.

Initially glucose 10–20 g is given by mouth either in liquid form or as granulated sugar or sugar lumps. Approximately 10 g of glucose is available from 2 teaspoons of sugar, 3 sugar lumps, *Glucogel®* (formerly known as *Hypostop® Gel*; glucose 9.2 g/23-g oral ampoule), and non-diet versions of *Lucozade® Sparkling Glucose Drink* 50–55 mL, *Coca-Cola®* 90 mL, *Ribena® Original* 15 mL (to be diluted). If necessary this may be repeated in 10–15 minutes. Further food is required to prevent recurrence of hypoglycaemia.

Hypoglycaemia which causes unconsciousness or fitting is an emergency. **Glucagon**, a polypeptide hormone produced by the alpha cells of the islets of Langerhans, increases plasma-glucose concentration by mobilising glycogen stored in the liver. In hypoglycaemia, if sugar cannot be given by mouth, glucagon can be given by injection. Carbohydrates should be given as soon as possible to restore liver glycogen; glucagon is not appropriate for chronic hypoglycaemia. It may be issued to parents or carers of insulin-treated children for emergency use in hypoglycaemic attacks. It is often advisable to prescribe on an 'if necessary' basis to hospitalised insulin-treated children, so that it may be given rapidly by the nurses during a hypoglycaemic emergency. If not effective in 10 minutes intravenous glucose should be given.

Alternatively, 2–5 mL/kg of glucose intravenous infusion 10% (200–500mg/kg of glucose) (section 9.2.2) may be given intravenously into a large vein through a large-gauge needle; care is required since this concentration is irritant especially if extravasation occurs. Glucose intravenous infusion 50% is **not** recommended, as it is very viscous and hypertonic. Close monitoring is necessary, particularly in the case of an overdose with a long-acting insulin because further administration of glucose may be required. Children whose hypoglycaemia is caused by an oral antidiabetic drug should be transferred to hospital because the hypoglycaemic effects of these drugs may persist for many hours.

Glucagon is not effective in the treatment of hypoglycaemia due to fatty acid oxidation or glycogen storage disorders.

Neonatal hypoglycaemia Neonatal hypoglycaemia at birth is treated with **glucose intravenous infusion 10%** given at a rate of 5 mL/kg/hour. An initial dose of 2.5 mL/kg over 5 minutes may be required if hypoglycaemia is severe enough to cause loss of consciousness or fitting. Mild asymptomatic persistent hypoglycaemia may respond to a single dose of **glucagon**. Glucagon has also been used in the short-term management of endogenous hyperinsulinism.

GLUCAGON

Cautions see notes above, insulinoma, glucagonoma; ineffective in chronic hypoglycaemia, starvation, and adrenal insufficiency; delayed hypoglycaemia when used as a diagnostic test—deaths reported (ensure a meal is eaten before discharge)

Contra-indications phaeochromocytoma

Side-effects nausea, vomiting, diarrhoea, hypokalaemia, rarely hypersensitivity reactions

Licensed use unlicensed for growth hormone test and hyperinsulinism

Indication and dose

Hypoglycaemia associated with diabetes
- **By subcutaneous, intramuscular, or intravenous injection**

Neonate 20 micrograms/kg

Child 1 month–2 years 500 micrograms

Child 2–18 years, body-weight less than 25 kg 500 micrograms; **body-weight over 25 kg** 1 mg

Endogenous hyperinsulinism
- **By intramuscular or intravenous injection**

Neonate 200 micrograms/kg (max. 1 mg) as a single dose

Child 1 month–2 years 1 mg as a single dose

- **By continuous intravenous infusion**

Neonate 1–18 micrograms/kg/hour, adjusted according to response (max. 50 micrograms/kg/hour)

Child 1 month–2 years 1–10 micrograms/kg/hour, increased if necessary

Administration Do not add to infusion fluids containing calcium—precipitation may occur

Diagnosis of growth hormone secretion specialist centre only (section 6.5.1)
- **By intramuscular injection**

Child 1month–18 years 100 micrograms/kg (max. 1 mg) as a single dose; dose may vary, consult local guidelines

Beta-blocker poisoning see p. 40

Note 1 unit of glucagon = 1 mg of glucagon

[1]**GlucaGen® HypoKit** (Novo Nordisk) PoM

Injection, powder for reconstitution, glucagon (rys) as hydrochloride with lactose, net price 1-mg vial with prefilled syringe containing water for injection = £11.52

1. PoM restriction does not apply where administration is for saving life in emergency

Chronic hypoglycaemia

Diazoxide is useful in the management of chronic hypoglycaemia due to excessive insulin secretion, either from a tumour involving the islets of Langerhans or from persisting hyperinsulinaemic hypoglycaemia of infancy (nesidioblastosis, see also glucagon above). Diazoxide has no place in the management of acute hypoglycaemia. **Chlorothiazide** 3–5mg/kg twice daily (section 2.2.1) reduces diazoxide-induced sodium and water retention and has the added benefit of potentiating the glycaemic effect of diazoxide.

If diazoxide and chlorothiazide fail to suppress excessive glucose requirements in chronic hypoglycaemia then **octreotide** or **nifedipine** (section 2.6.2) may be added. Octreotide can suppress secretion of growth hormone, but growth is unlikely to be affected in the long term.

DIAZOXIDE

Cautions ischaemic heart disease; haematological examinations and blood pressure monitoring required during prolonged treatment; growth, bone, and developmental checks; avoid the intravenous route if possible; extravasation can cause tissue necrosis and single doses of 300 mg have been associated with angina and cerebral and myocardial infarction; **interactions:** Appendix 1 (diazoxide)

Renal impairment reduce dose in severe impairment—increased sensitivity to hypotensive effect

Pregnancy prolonged use in second or third trimesters may produce alopecia and impaired glucose tolerance in neonate; inhibits uterine activity

Contra-indications see section 2.5.1

Side-effects anorexia, nausea, vomiting, hyperuricaemia, sodium and water retention, hyperglycaemia, hypotension, oedema, tachycardia, arrhythmias, extrapyramidal effects; hypertrichosis on prolonged treatment

Licensed use chronic intractable hypoglycaemia (for use in hypertensive crisis see section 2.5.1)

Indication and dose

Chronic intractable hypoglycaemia
- **By mouth or by intravenous injection**

Neonate initially 5 mg/kg twice daily to establish response, adjust dose according to response; usual maintenance dose 1.5–3 mg/kg 2–3 times daily; up to 7 mg/kg 3 times daily may be required in some cases, higher doses unlikely to be beneficial

DIAZOXIDE (*continued*)

Child 1 month–18 years initially 1.7 mg/kg 3 times daily then adjusted according to response; usual maintenance dose 1.5–3mg/kg 2–3 times daily; up to 5 mg/kg 3 times daily may be required in some cases, higher doses unlikely to be beneficial

Eudemine® (Celltech) PoM
Tablets, diazoxide 50 mg. Net price 20 = £9.29

Eudemine® (Non-proprietary)
Injection, diazoxide 15 mg/mL. Net price 20-mL amp = £30.00

Extemporaneous formulations available see Extemporaneous Preparations, p. 8

OCTREOTIDE

Cautions avoid abrupt withdrawal of short-acting octreotide—see Side-effects below; in insulinoma (risk of increased depth and duration of hypoglycaemia—monitor closely when initiating treatment and changing doses); diabetes mellitus (antidiabetic requirements may be reduced); monitor thyroid function on long-term therapy; **interactions:** Appendix 1 (octreotide)

Pregnancy possible effect on fetal growth, avoid unless benefit outweighs risk

Breast-feeding no information, avoid unless essential

Side-effects anorexia, nausea, vomiting, abdominal pain, bloating, flatulence, diarrhoea, and steatorrhoea; postprandial glucose tolerance may be impaired, rarely persistent hyperglycaemia with chronic administration; hypoglycaemia has also been reported; reduced gall bladder motility and bile flow; gallstones reported after long-term treatment; abrupt withdrawal of subcutaneous octreotide is associated with biliary colic and pancreatitis; pain and irritation at injection site—sites should be rotated; rarely, pancreatitis shortly after administration, altered liver function tests, hepatitis and transient alopecia

Licensed use not licensed in children

Indication and dose

Persistent hyperinsulinaemic hypoglycaemia unresponsive to diazoxide and glucose
- **By subcutaneous injection**

Neonate initially 2–5 micrograms/kg every 6–8 hours, adjusted according to response; up to 7 micrograms/kg every 4 hours may rarely be required

Child 1 month–18 years initially 1–2 micrograms/kg every 4–6 hours, dose adjusted according to response; up to 7 micrograms/kg every 4 hours may rarely be required

Bleeding from oesophageal or gastric varices
- **By continuous intravenous infusion**

Child 1 month–18 years 1 microgram/kg/hour, higher doses may be required initially; when no active bleeding reduce dose over 24 hours; usual max. 50 micrograms/hour

Administration *Intravenous infusion*, dilute with sodium chloride 0.9% to a concentration of 10-50%

Sandostatin® (Novartis) PoM
Injection, octreotide (as acetate) 50 micrograms/mL, net price 1-mL amp = £3.47; 100 micrograms/mL, 1-mL amp = £6.53; 200 micrograms/mL 5-mL vial = £65.10; 500 micrograms/mL, 1-mL amp = £31.65

6.1.5 Treatment of diabetic nephropathy and neuropathy

Diabetic nephropathy

Regular review of diabetic children over 12 years of age should include an annual test for microalbuminuria (the earliest sign of nephropathy). If reagent strip tests (*Micral-Test II®* NHS or *Microbumintest®* NHS) are used and prove positive, the result should be confirmed by laboratory analysis of a urine sample. Microalbuminuria may occur transiently during puberty; if it persists (at least 3 positive tests) children should be considered for treatment with an ACE inhibitor (section 2.5.5.1) or an angiotensin-II receptor antagonist (section 2.5.5.2) under specialist guidance; to minimise the risk of renal deterioration, blood pressure should be carefully controlled (section 2.5).

ACE inhibitors may potentiate the hypoglycaemic effect of insulin and oral antidiabetic drugs; this effect is more likely during the first weeks of combined treatment and in children with renal impairment.

For the treatment of hypertension in diabetes, see section 2.5.

Diabetic neuropathy

Clinical neuropathy is rare in children whose diabetes is well controlled.

6.1.6 Diagnostic and monitoring agents for diabetes mellitus

Blood glucose monitoring

Blood glucose monitoring gives a direct measure of the glucose concentration at the time of the test and can detect hypoglycaemia as well as hyperglycaemia. Carers and children should be properly trained in the use of blood glucose monitoring systems and the appropriate action to take on the results obtained. Inadequate understanding of the normal fluctuations in blood glucose may lead to confusion and inappropriate action.

Blood glucose monitoring is best carried out by means of a meter. Visual colour comparison is sometimes used but is much less satisfactory. Meters give a more precise reading and are useful for patients with poor eyesight or who are colour blind.

Note In the UK blood-glucose concentration is expressed in mmol/litre and Diabetes UK advises that these units should be used for self-monitoring of blood glucose. In other European countries units of mg/100 mL (or mg/dL) are commonly used.
It is advisable to check that the meter is pre-set in the correct units.

Test strips

Active® (Roche Diagnostics)
Reagent strips, for blood glucose monitoring, range 0.6–33.3 mmol/litre, for use with *Glucotrend®* and *Accu-Chek® Active* NHS meters only. Net price 50-strip pack = £16.13

Advantage Plus® (Roche Diagnostics)
Reagent strips, for blood glucose monitoring, range 0.6–33.3 mmol/litre, for use with *Accu-Chek® Advantage* NHS meter only. Net price 50-strip pack = £16.13

Ascensia® Autodisc (Bayer Diagnostics)
Sensor discs, for blood glucose monitoring, range 0.6–33.3 mmol/litre, for use with *Ascensia Breeze®* NHS and *Ascensia Esprit® 2* NHS meters only. Net price 5 × 10-disc pack = £15.67

Ascensia® Glucodisc (Bayer Diagnostics)
Sensor discs, for blood glucose monitoring, range 0.6–33.3 mmol/L, for use with *Ascensia Esprit®* 2 NHS meter only. Net price 5 × 10-disc pack = £15.53

Ascenia® Microfill (Bayer Diagnostics)
Sensor strips, for blood glucose monitoring, range 0.6–33.3 mmol/litre, for use with *Ascensia® Contour* NHS meter only. Net price 50-strip pack = £15.55

BM-Accutest® (Roche Diagnostics)
Reagent strips, for blood glucose monitoring, range 1.1–33.3 mmol/litre, for use with *Accutrend®* NHS meters only. Net price 50-strip pack = £15.64

Compact® (Roche Diagnostics)
Reagent strips, for blood glucose monitoring, range 0.6–33.3 mmol/litre, for use with *Accu-Chek® Compact* and *Accu-Chek® Compact Plus* NHS meters only. Net price 3 × 17-strip pack = £16.26

FreeStyle® (TheraSense)
Reagent strips, for blood glucose monitoring, range 1.1–27.8 mmol/litre, for use with *FreeStyle®* NHS meter only. Net price 50-strip pack = £15.67

GlucoMen® (Menarini Diagnostics)
Sensor strips, for blood glucose monitoring, range 1.1–33.3 mmol/litre, for use with *GlucoMen® Glycó* NHS meter only. Net price 50-strip pack = £14.94

Glucotide® (Bayer Diagnostics)
Reagent strips, for blood glucose monitoring, range 0.6–33.3 mmol/litre, for use with *Glucometer® 4* NHS meter only. Net price 50-strip pack = £15.33

Hypoguard® Supreme (Hypoguard)
Reagent strips, for blood glucose monitoring, range 2.2–27.7 mmol/litre, for use with *Hypoguard® Supreme* NHS meters. Net price 50-strip pack = £13.64

Hypoguard® Supreme Spectrum (Hypoguard)
Reagent strips, for blood glucose monitoring, visual range 2.2–27.8 mmol/litre. Net price 50-strip pack = £10.34

MediSense G2® (MediSense)
Sensor strips, for blood glucose monitoring, range 1.1–33.3 mmol/litre. for use with *MediSense Card®* NHS or *MediSense Pen®* NHS meters only. Net price 50-strip pack = £14.40

MediSense® Optium Plus (MediSense)
Sensor strips, for blood glucose monitoring, range 1.1–27.7 mmol/litre, for use with *MediSense® Optium* NHS meter only. Net price 50-strip pack = £15.30

MediSense® Soft-Sense (MediSense)
Sensor strips, for blood glucose monitoring, range 1.7–25 mmol/litre, for use with *MediSense® Soft-Sense* meter only. Net price 50-strip pack = £15.55

One Touch® (LifeScan)
Reagent strips, for blood glucose monitoring, range 0–33.3 mmol/litre, for use with *One Touch® II, Profile* and *Basic* NHS meters only. Net price 50-strip pack = £15.41

One Touch® Ultra (LifeScan)
Reagent strips, for blood glucose monitoring, range 1.1–33.3 mmol/litre, for use with *One Touch® Ultra* meter only. Net price 50-strip pack = £15.57

PocketScan® (LifeScan)
Reagent strips, for blood glucose monitoring, range 1.1–33.3 mmol/litre, for use with *PocketScan®* NHS meter only. Net price 50-strip pack = £15.21

Prestige® Smart System (DiagnoSys)
Reagent strips, for blood glucose monitoring, range 1.4–33.3 mmol/litre, for use with *Prestige® Smart System* NHS meter only. Net price 50-strip pack = £15.29

Meters

Accu-Chek® Active (Roche Diagnostics) NHS
Meter, for blood glucose monitoring (for use with *Active®* test strips). *Accu-Chek® Active* system = £7.79

Accu-Chek® Advantage (Roche Diagnostics) NHS
Meter, for blood glucose monitoring (for use with *Advantage Plus®* test strips). *Accu-Chek® Advantage* system = £7.00

Accu-Chek® Compact Plus (Roche Diagnostics) NHS
Meter, for blood glucose monitoring (for use with *Compact Plus®* test strips). *Accu-Chek® Compact Plus* system = £7.79

Ascensia Breeze® (Bayer Diagnostics) NHS
Meter, for blood glucose monitoring (for use with *Ascensia® Autodisc* test sensor discs)

Ascensia Contour (Bayer Diagnostics) NHS
Meter, for blood glucose monitoring (for use with *Ascensia® Microfill* sensor strips) = £19.97

Ascensia Esprit® 2 (Bayer Diagnostics) NHS
Meter, for blood glucose monitoring (for use with *Ascensia® Glucodisc* test sensor discs) = £17.49

FreeStyle® (TheraSense) NHS
Meter for blood glucose monitoring (for use with *FreeStyle®* test strips) = £25.00

GlucoMen® Glycó (Menarini Diagnostics) NHS
Meter, for blood glucose monitoring (for use with *GlucoMen®* sensor strips)

GlucoMen® PC (Menarini Diagnostics) NHS
Meter, for blood glucose monitoring (for use with *GlucoMen®* sensor strips)

Hypoguard® Supreme (Hypoguard) NHS
Meters, for blood glucose monitoring (for use with *Hypoguard® Supreme* test strips). *Hypoguard® Supreme Plus* meter = £35.00; *Hypoguard® Supreme Extra* meter = £45.00

MediSense® (MediSense) NHS
Meters (Sensor), for blood glucose monitoring. *MediSense Card* = £15.31, *MediSense®* card starter pack = £17.50, *MediSense®* Pen = £30.63, *MediSense®* pen starter pack = £39.38, *MediSense® Precision QID* starter pack = £12.00 (all for use with *MediSense G2®* test strips); *MediSense® Optium* starter pack (for use with *MediSense® Optium* test strips) = £17.50; *MediSense® Soft-Sense* meter (for use with *MediSense® Soft-Sense* test strips)

One Touch® (LifeScan) NHS
Meters, for blood glucose monitoring (for use with *One Touch®* test strips). *One Touch® Basic* system pack = £9.38, *One Touch® Profile* system pack = £18.38

One Touch® Ultra (LifeScan) NHS
Meter, for blood glucose monitoring (for use with *One Touch® Ultra* test strips) = £10.00

PocketScan® (LifeScan) NHS
Meter, for blood glucose monitoring (for use with *PocketScan®* test strips). *Complete PocketScan® System* = £17.50

Prestige® Smart System (DiagnoSys) NHS
Meter, for blood glucose monitoring (for use with *Prestige® Smart System* test strips) = £5.63

Urinalysis

Urine testing for glucose is useful in children who find blood glucose monitoring difficult. Tests for glucose range from reagent strips specific to glucose to reagent tablets which detect all reducing sugars. *Clinitest®* is rarely used now; *Clinistix®* is suitable for screening purposes only. It is rarely necessary for children to test themselves for ketones unless they become unwell.

Microalbuminuria can be detected with *Micral-Test II®* NHS or *Microbumintest®* NHS but this should be followed by confirmation in the laboratory, since false positive results are common.

6 Endocrine system

Glucose

Clinistix® (Bayer Diagnostics)
Meter, for blood glucose monitoring (for use with *Prestige® Smart System* test strips) = £5.63

Clinitest® (Bayer Diagnostics)
Reagent tablets, for detection of glucose and other reducing substances in urine. Pocket set (test tube, dropper and 36 tablets), net price = £4.02, 36-tab pack = £2.00, 6-test tube pack = £3.70, 6-dropper pack = £3.80

Diabur-Test 5000® (Roche Diagnostics)
Reagent strips, for detection of glucose in urine. Net price 50-strip pack = £2.69

Diastix® (Bayer Diagnostics)
Reagent strips, for detection of glucose in urine. Net price 50-strip pack = £2.71

Medi-Test® Glucose (BHR)
Reagent strips, for detection of glucose in urine. Net price 50-strip pack = £2.17

Ketones

Ketostix® (Bayer Diagnostics)
Reagent strips, for detection of ketones in urine. Net price 50-strip pack = £2.87

Ketur Test® (Roche Diagnostics)
Reagent strips, for detection of ketones in urine. Net price 50-strip pack = £2.58

Protein

Albustix® (Bayer Diagnostics)
Reagent strips, for detection of protein in urine. Net price 50-strip pack = £3.94

Medi-Test® Protein 2 (BHR)
Reagent strips, for detection of protein in urine. Net price 50-strip pack = £3.03

Other reagent strips available for urinalysis include:

Combur-3 Test® NHS (glucose and protein—Roche Diagnostics), *Clinitek Microalbumin®* NHS (albumin and creatinine—Bayer Diagnostics), *Ketodiastix®* NHS (glucose and ketones—Bayer Diagnostics), *Medi-Test Combi 2®* NHS (glucose and protein—BHR), *Micral-Test II®* NHS (albumin—Roche Diagnostics), *Microalbustix®* NHS (albumin and creatinine—Bayer Diagnostics), *Microbumintest®* NHS (albumin—Bayer Diagnostics), *Uristix®* NHS (glucose and protein—Bayer Diagnostics)

Glucose tolerance test

The **glucose** tolerance test is now rarely needed for the diagnosis of diabetes when symptoms of hyperglycaemia are present. However, it is used for the investigation of insulin resistance, glycogen storage disease, and excessive growth hormone secretion. A dose of 1.75 g/kg (max. 75 g) of anhydrous glucose is used. It is also used to establish the presence of gestational diabetes; this generally involves giving anhydrous glucose 75 g (equivalent to Glucose BP 82.5 g) by mouth to the fasting patient, and measuring blood-glucose concentrations at intervals. The appropriate amount of glucose should be given with 200–300 mL fluid. Anhydrous glucose 75 g may alternatively be given as 113 mL *Polycal*® (Nutricia Clinical) with extra fluid to administer a total volume of 200–300 mL.

6.2 Thyroid and antithyroid drugs

6.2.1 Thyroid hormones

Thyroid hormones are used in hypothyroidism (juvenile myxoedema), and also in diffuse non-toxic goitre, congenital or neonatal hypothyroidism, and Hashimoto's thyroiditis (lymphadenoid goitre). Neonatal hypothyroidism requires prompt treatment for normal development.

Levothyroxine sodium (thyroxine sodium) is the treatment of choice for *maintenance* therapy.

Doses for congenital hypothyroidism and juvenile myxoedema should be titrated according to clinical response, growth assessment, and measurement of plasma thyroxine and thyroid-stimulating hormone concentrations. In congenital hypothyroidism higher initial doses (up to 15 micrograms/kg daily) may benefit mental development.

Liothyronine sodium has a similar action to levothyroxine but is more rapidly metabolised and has a more rapid effect; 20–25 micrograms is equivalent to approximately 100 micrograms of levothyroxine. Its effects develop after a few hours and disappear within 24 to 48 hours of discontinuing treatment. It may be used in *severe hypothyroid states* when a rapid response is desired.

Liothyronine by intravenous injection is the treatment of choice in *hypothyroid coma*. Adjunctive therapy includes intravenous fluids, hydrocortisone, and treatment of infection; assisted ventilation is often required.

LEVOTHYROXINE SODIUM
(Thyroxine sodium)

Cautions panhypopituitarism or predisposition to adrenal insufficiency (initiate corticosteroid therapy before starting levothyroxine), cardiovascular disorders (pre-therapy ECG may be valuable), long-standing hypothyroidism, diabetes insipidus, diabetes mellitus (dose of antidiabetic drugs including insulin may need to be increased); **interactions:** Appendix 1 (thyroid hormones)

Pregnancy dose adjustment may be necessary, monitor maternal serum thyrotrophin

Breast-feeding minimal amount present in breast milk; unlikely to affect tests for neonatal hypothyroidism

Contra-indications thyrotoxicosis

Side-effects usually at excessive dosage (see Initial Dosage above) include anginal pain, arrhythmias, palpitation, skeletal muscle cramps, tachycardia, diarrhoea, vomiting, tremors, restlessness, excitability, insomnia, headache, flushing, sweating, fever, heat intolerance, excessive loss of weight and muscular weakness

Indication and dose

Hypothyroidism (in cardiac disease reduce dose by 50% and increase more slowly)
- By mouth

Neonate initially 15 micrograms/kg once daily, adjusted in steps of 5 micrograms/kg every 2 weeks or as necessary; usual dose 25–37.5 micrograms daily

Child 1 month–2 years initially 15 micrograms/kg once daily adjusted in steps of 25 micrograms daily every 2–4 weeks until metabolism normalised

Child 2–12 years initially 5–10 micrograms/kg once daily adjusted in steps of 25 micrograms daily every 2–4 weeks until metabolism normalised

Child 12–18 years initially 50–100 micrograms once daily adjusted in steps of 50 micrograms daily every 3–4 weeks until metabolism normalised; usual dose 100–200 micrograms daily

Levothyroxine (Non-proprietary) PoM
Tablets, levothyroxine sodium 25 micrograms, net price 28-tab pack = 93p; 50 micrograms, 28-tab pack = £1.17; 100 micrograms, 28-tab pack = £1.04
Brands include *Eltroxin*®
Liquid preparations available from specialist importing companies

Extemporaneous formulations available see Extemporaneous Preparations, p. 8
Note Bioavailability may vary in extemporaneous preparations

LIOTHYRONINE SODIUM

(L-Tri-iodothyronine sodium)

Cautions see under Levothyroxine Sodium; **interactions**: Appendix 1 (thyroid hormones)

Pregnancy does not cross the placenta in significant amounts; dose adjustments may be necessary, monitor maternal serum thyrotropin

Contra-indications see under Levothyroxine Sodium

Side-effects see under Levothyroxine Sodium

Licensed use unlicensed for use in children

Indication and dose

See Levothyroxine and notes above

Hypothyroidism
- **By mouth**

Child 12–18 years initially 10–20 micrograms daily gradually increased to 60 micrograms daily in 2–3 divided doses

- **By slow intravenous injection**

(replacement for oral levothyroxine)

Convert **daily** levothyroxine dose to liothyronine (see below) and give in 2–3 divided doses, adjusted according to response

Note 2 micrograms liothyronine equivalent to approx. 8 micrograms levothyroxine

Hypothyroid coma
- **By slow intravenous injection**

Child 1 month–12 years 2–10 micrograms every 12 hours or up to every 4 hours if necessary; reduce to 1 to 5 micrograms in patients with cardiovascular disease

Child 12–18 years 5–20 micrograms repeated every 12 hours or up to every 4 hours if necessary; reduce to 10-20 micrograms in patients with cardiovascular disease *alternatively* initially 50 micrograms then 25 micrograms every 8 hours reducing to 25 micrograms twice daily

Tertroxin® (Goldshield) PoM
Tablets, scored, liothyronine sodium 20 micrograms, net price 100-tab pack = £15.92

Triiodothyronine (Goldshield) PoM
Injection, powder for reconstitution, liothyronine sodium (with dextran). Net price 20-microgram amp = £37.92

6.2.2 Antithyroid drugs

Antithyroid drugs are used for hyperthyroidism either to prepare children for thyroidectomy or for long-term management. In the UK carbimazole is the most commonly used drug. Propylthiouracil may be used in those who suffer sensitivity reactions to carbimazole as sensitivity is not necessarily displayed to both drugs. Both drugs act primarily by interfering with the synthesis of thyroid hormones.

Treatment in children should be undertaken by a specialist.

CSM warning (neutropenia and agranulocytosis)
Doctors are reminded of the importance of recognising bone marrow suppression induced by carbimazole and the need to stop treatment promptly.

1. Children and their carers should be asked to report symptoms and signs suggestive of infection, especially sore throat.
2. A white blood cell count should be performed if there is any clinical evidence of infection.
3. Carbimazole should be stopped promptly if there is clinical or laboratory evidence of neutropenia.

Carbimazole or **propylthiouracil** are initially given in large doses to block thyroid function. This dose is continued until the child becomes euthyroid, usually after 4 to 8 weeks, and is then gradually reduced to a maintenance dose of 30–60% of the initial dose. Alternatively high-dose treatment is continued in combination with levothyroxine replacement (*blocking-replacement regimen*); this is particularly useful when dose adjustment proves difficult or relapse is a problem. Treatment is usually continued for 12 to 24 months. The blocking-replacement regimen is **not** suitable during pregnancy. Hypothyroidism should be avoided particularly during pregnancy as it can cause fetal goitre.

When substituting, carbimazole 1 mg is considered equivalent to propylthiouracil 10 mg but the dose may need adjusting according to response.

Rashes and pruritus are common with carbimazole but they can be treated with antihistamines without discontinuing therapy; alternatively propylthiouracil may be substituted. If a child on carbimazole develops a sore throat it should be reported immediately because of the rare complication of agranulocytosis (see CSM warning, above).

Iodine has been used as an adjunct to antithyroid drugs for 10 to 14 days before partial thyroidectomy; however, there is little evidence of a beneficial effect. Iodine should not be used for long-term treatment because its antithyroid action tends to diminish.

Radioactive sodium iodide (^{131}I) solution is used increasingly for the treatment of thyrotoxicosis at all ages, particularly where medical therapy or compliance is a problem, in patients with cardiac disease, and in patients who relapse after thyroidectomy.

Propranolol (section 2.4) is useful for rapid relief of thyrotoxic symptoms and may be used in conjunction with antithyroid drugs or as an adjunct to radioactive iodine. Beta-blockers are also useful in neonatal thyrotoxicosis and in supraventricular arrhythmias due to hyperthyroidism. Propranolol has been used in conjunction with iodine to prepare mildly thyrotoxic patients for surgery but it is preferable to make the patient euthyroid with carbimazole. Laboratory tests of thyroid function are not altered by beta-blockers. Most experience in treating thyrotoxicosis has been gained with propranolol but **atenolol** (section 2.4) is also used.

Thyrotoxic crisis ('thyroid storm') requires emergency treatment with intravenous administration of fluids, propranolol and hydrocortisone as sodium succinate, as well as oral iodine solution and carbimazole or propylthiouracil which may need to be administered by nasogastric tube.

Pregnancy and breast-feeding Radioactive iodine therapy is contra-indicated during pregnancy. Propylthiouracil and carbimazole can be given but the blocking-replacement regimen (see above) is **not** suitable. Both propylthiouracil and carbimazole cross the placenta and in high doses may cause fetal goitre and hypothyroidism—the lowest dose that will control the hyperthyroid state should be used (requirements in Graves' disease tend to fall during pregnancy). Rarely, carbimazole has been associated with aplasia cutis of the neonate.

Carbimazole and propylthiouracil are present in breast milk but this does not preclude breast-feeding as long as neonatal development is closely monitored and the lowest effective dose is used.

Neonatal hyperthyroidism is treated with carbimazole or propylthiouracil, usually for 8 to 12 weeks. In severe symptomatic disease iodine may be needed to block the thyroid and propranolol required to treat peripheral symptoms.

CARBIMAZOLE

Cautions

Hepatic impairment increased risk of jaundice

Pregnancy see notes above

Breast-feeding see notes above

Side-effects nausea, mild gastro-intestinal disturbances, headache, rashes and pruritus, arthralgia; rarely myopathy, alopecia, bone marrow suppression (including pancytopenia and agranulocytosis, see **CSM warning** above), jaundice

Indication and dose

Hyperthyroidism (including Graves' disease), thyrotoxic crisis, thyrotoxicosis

- By mouth

Neonate initially 250 micrograms/kg 3 times daily until euthyroid then adjust as necessary (see notes above); higher initial doses (up to 1 mg/kg daily) are occasionally required, particularly in thyrotoxic crisis

Child 1 month–12 years initially 250 micrograms/kg (max. 10 mg) 3 times daily until euthyroid then adjusted as necessary (see notes above); higher initial doses occasionally required, particularly in thyrotoxic crisis

Child 12–18 years initially 10 mg 3 times daily until euthyroid then adjusted as necessary (see notes above); higher initial doses occasionally required, particularly in thyrotoxic crisis

Counselling Warn child and carers to tell doctor **immediately** if sore throat, mouth ulcers, bruising, fever, malaise, or non-specific illness develops

Neo-Mercazole® (Roche) PoM

Tablets, both pink, carbimazole 5 mg, net price 100-tab pack = £5.05; 20 mg, 100-tab pack = £18.75. Counselling, blood disorder symptoms

Administration tablets may be crushed in water and used immediately

Extemporaneous formulations available see Extemporaneous Preparations, p. 8

IODINE AND IODIDE

Cautions not for long-term treatment

Pregnancy avoid if possible, neonatal goitre and hypothyroidism may occur

Contra-indications

Breast-feeding possibly concentrated in milk—avoid; risk of neonatal goitre and hypothyroidism

Side-effects hypersensitivity reactions including coryza-like symptoms, headache, lacrimation, conjunctivitis, pain in salivary glands, laryngitis, bronchitis, rashes; on prolonged treatment depression, insomnia, impotence; goitre in infants of mothers taking iodides

Indication and dose

See under preparation

Aqueous Iodine Oral Solution

(Lugol's Solution), iodine 5%, potassium iodide 10% in purified water, freshly boiled and cooled, total iodine 130 mg/mL. Net price 100 mL = £1.19. Label: 27

Dose

Neonatal thyrotoxicosis
- By mouth

Neonate 0.05–0.1 mL 3 times daily

Thyrotoxicosis (pre-operative)
- By mouth

Neonate 0.1–0.3 mL 3 times daily

Child 1 month–18 years 0.1–0.3 mL 3 times daily

Thyrotoxic crisis
- By mouth

Child 1 month—1 year 0.2–0.3 mL 3 times daily

Administration Dilute well with milk or water

PROPYLTHIOURACIL

Cautions see under Carbimazole

Hepatic impairment consider dose reduction

Renal impairment creatinine clearance 10–50 mL/minute/1.73 m², use 75% of normal dose; creatinine clearance less than 10 mL/minute/1.73 m², use 50% of normal dose

Pregnancy see notes above

Breast-feeding see notes above

Side-effects see under Carbimazole; leucopenia; rarely cutaneous vasculitis, thrombocytopenia, aplastic anaemia, hypoprothrombinaemia, hepatitis, encephalopathy, hepatic necrosis, nephritis, lupus erythematous-like syndromes

Licensed use not licensed for use in children under 6 years of age

Indication and dose

Hyperthyroidism (including Graves' disease), thyrotoxic crisis, thyrotoxicosis
- By mouth

Neonate initially 2.5–5 mg/kg twice daily until euthyroid then adjusted as necessary (see notes above); higher doses occasionally required, particularly in thyrotoxic crisis

Child 1 month–1 year initially 2.5 mg/kg 3 times daily until euthyroid then adjusted as necessary (see notes above); higher doses occasionally required, particularly in thyrotoxic crisis

Child 1–5 years initially 25 mg 3 times daily until euthyroid then adjusted as necessary (see notes above); higher doses occasionally required, particularly in thyrotoxic crisis

Child 5–12 years initially 50 mg 3 times daily until euthyroid then adjusted as necessary (see notes above); higher doses occasionally required, particularly in thyrotoxic crisis

Child 12–18 years initially 100 mg 3 times daily administered until euthyroid then adjusted as necessary (see notes above); higher doses occasionally required, particularly in thyrotoxic crisis

Propylthiouracil (Non-proprietary) PoM

Tablets, propylthiouracil 50 mg. Net price 56-tab pack = £24.92

Extemporaneous formulations available see Extemporaneous Preparations, p. 8

PROPRANOLOL

Cautions see section 2.4

Contra-indications see section 2.4

Side-effects see section 2.4

Licensed use see section 2.4

Indication and dose

Hyperthyroidism with autonomic symptoms, thyrotoxicosis, thyrotoxic crisis
- By mouth

Neonate initially 250–500 micrograms/kg every 6–8 hours, adjusted according to response

Child 1 month–18 years initially 250–500 micrograms/kg every 8 hours, then adjusted according to response; doses up to 1 mg/kg every 8 hours occasionally required, max. 40 mg every 8 hours

- By intravenous injection over 10 minutes

Neonate initially 20–50 micrograms/kg every 6–8 hours, adjusted according to response

Child 1 month–18 years initially 25–50 micrograms/kg (max. 5 mg) every 6–8 hours, adjusted according to response

Preparations

See section 2.4

6.3 Corticosteroids

6.3.1 Replacement therapy

The adrenal cortex normally secretes hydrocortisone (cortisol) which has glucocorticoid activity and weak mineralocorticoid activity. It also secretes the mineralocorticoid aldosterone.

In deficiency states, physiological replacement is best achieved with a combination of **hydrocortisone** (section 6.3.2) and the mineralocorticoid **fludrocortisone**; hydrocortisone alone does not usually provide sufficient mineralocorticoid activity for complete replacement.

In *Addison's disease* or following adrenalectomy, **hydrocortisone** by mouth is usually required. This is given in 2–3 divided doses, the larger in the morning and the smaller in the evening, mimicking the normal diurnal rhythm of cortisol secretion. The optimum daily dose is determined on the basis of clinical response. Glucocorticoid therapy is supplemented by fludrocortisone.

In *acute adrenocortical insufficiency*, **hydrocortisone** is given intravenously (preferably as sodium succinate) every 6 to 8 hours in sodium chloride intravenous infusion 0.9%.

In *hypopituitarism*, glucocorticoids should be given as in adrenocortical insufficiency, but since the production of aldosterone is also regulated by the renin-angiotensin system a mineralocorticoid is not usually required. Additional replacement therapy with levothyroxine (section 6.2.1) and sex hormones (section 6.4) should be given as indicated by the pattern of hormone deficiency.

In *congenital adrenal hyperplasia*, the pituitary gland increases production of corticotropin to compensate for reduced formation of cortisol; this results in excessive adrenal androgen production. Treatment is aimed at suppressing corticotropin using hydrocortisone (section 6.3.2). Careful and continual dose titration is required to avoid growth retardation and toxicity; for this reason potent, synthetic glucocorticoids such as dexamethasone are usually reserved for use in adolescents. The dose is adjusted according to clinical response and measurement of adrenal androgens and 17-hydroxyprogesterone. Salt-losing forms of congenital adrenal hyperplasia (where there is a lack of aldosterone production) require mineralocorticoid replacement. Mineralocorticoid replacement may also be beneficial even when salt-losing symptoms are not evident.

FLUDROCORTISONE ACETATE

Cautions section 6.3.2; **interactions:** Appendix 1 (corticosteroids)

Contra-indications section 6.3.2

Side-effects section 6.3.2

Indication and dose

Mineralocorticoid replacement in adrenocortical insufficiency

- **By mouth**

Neonate initially 100 micrograms once daily, adjusted according to response; usual range 50–300 micrograms daily

Child 1 month–18 years initially 50–100 micrograms once daily; maintenance 50–300 micrograms once daily, adjusted according to response

Florinef® (Squibb) PoM
Tablets, pink, scored, fludrocortisone acetate 100 micrograms. Net price 56-tab pack = £2.50. Label: 10, steroid card

Extemporaneous formulations available see Extemporaneous Preparations, p. 8
Note Bioavailability uncertain, tablets may result in more reliable absorption and may be dispersed in water

6.3.2 Glucocorticoid therapy

In comparing the relative potencies of corticosteroids in terms of their anti-inflammatory (glucocorticoid) effects it should be borne in mind that high glucocorticoid activity in itself is of no advantage unless it is accompanied by relatively low mineralocorticoid activity (see Disadvantages of Corticosteroids below). The mineralocorticoid activity of **fludrocortisone** (section 6.3.1) is so high that its anti-inflammatory activity is of no clinical relevance. The table below shows equivalent anti-inflammatory doses.

Equivalent anti-inflammatory doses of corticosteroids

This table takes no account of mineralocorticoid effects, nor does it take account of variations in duration of action

Prednisolone 1 mg	≡	Betamethasone 150 micrograms
	≡	Cortisone acetate 5 mg
	≡	Deflazacort 1.2 mg
	≡	Dexamethasone 150 micrograms
	≡	Hydrocortisone 4 mg
	≡	Methylprednisolone 800 micrograms
	≡	Triamcinolone 800 micrograms

The relatively high mineralocorticoid activity of **cortisone** and **hydrocortisone**, and the resulting fluid retention, make them unsuitable for disease suppression on a long-term basis. However, they can be used for adrenal replacement therapy (section 6.3.1); hydrocortisone is preferred because cortisone requires conversion in the liver to hydrocortisone. Hydrocortisone is used on a short-term basis by intravenous injection for the emergency management of some conditions. The relatively moderate anti-inflammatory potency of hydrocortisone also makes it a useful topical corticosteroid for the management of inflammatory skin conditions because side-effects (both topical and systemic) are less marked (section 13.4); cortisone is not active topically.

Prednisolone has predominantly glucocorticoid activity and is the corticosteroid most commonly used by mouth for long-term disease suppression.

Betamethasone and **dexamethasone** have very high glucocorticoid activity in conjunction with insignificant mineralocorticoid activity. This makes them particularly suitable for high-dose therapy in conditions where fluid retention would be a disadvantage.

Betamethasone and dexamethasone also have a long duration of action and this, coupled with their lack of mineralocorticoid action makes them particularly suitable for conditions which require suppression of corticotropin (corticotrophin) secretion. Some esters of betamethasone and of **beclometasone** (beclomethasone) exert a considerably more marked topical effect (e.g. on the skin or the lungs) than when given by mouth; use is made of this to obtain topical effects whilst minimising systemic side-effects (e.g. for skin applications and asthma inhalations).

Deflazacort has a high glucocorticoid activity; it is derived from prednisolone.

Disadvantages of corticosteroids

Overdosage or prolonged use may exaggerate some of the normal physiological actions of corticosteroids leading to mineralocorticoid and glucocorticoid side-effects.

Administration of corticosteroids may result in suppression of growth and may affect the development of puberty. It is important to use the lowest effective dose; alternate day regimens may be appropriate and limit growth reduction. For the effect of corticosteroids given in pregnancy, see Pregnancy and Breast-feeding, below.

Mineralocorticoid side-effects include hypertension, sodium and water retention and potassium loss. They are most marked with fludrocortisone, but are significant with cortisone, hydrocortisone, corticotropin, and tetracosactide (tetracosactrin). Mineralocorticoid actions are negligible with the high potency glucocorticoids, betamethasone and dexamethasone, and occur only slightly with methylprednisolone, prednisolone, and triamcinolone.

Glucocorticoid side-effects include diabetes and osteoporosis (section 6.6); in addition high doses are associated with avascular necrosis of the femoral head. Mental disturbances, such as nightmares, insomnia, irritability, and aggressive behaviour may occur; a serious paranoid state or depression with risk of suicide may be induced, particularly in children with a history of mental disorder.

Euphoria is frequently observed. Muscle wasting (proximal myopathy) may also occur. Corticosteroid therapy is also weakly linked with peptic ulceration (the potential advantage of soluble or enteric-coated preparations to reduce the risk is speculative only).

High doses of corticosteroids may cause Cushing's syndrome, with moon face, striae, and acne; it is usually reversible on withdrawal of treatment, but this must always be gradually tapered to avoid symptoms of acute adrenal insufficiency (**important:** see also Adrenal Suppression below).

Adrenal suppression

During prolonged therapy with corticosteroids, adrenal atrophy develops and may persist for years after stopping. Abrupt withdrawal after a prolonged period may lead to acute adrenal insufficiency, hypotension or death (see Withdrawal of Corticosteroids, below). Withdrawal may also be associated with fever, myalgia, arthralgia, rhinitis, conjunctivitis, painful itchy skin nodules and weight loss.

To compensate for a diminished adrenocortical response caused by prolonged corticosteroid treatment, any significant intercurrent illness, trauma, or surgical procedure requires a temporary increase in corticosteroid dose, or if already stopped, a temporary re-introduction of corticosteroid treatment. Anaesthetists **must** therefore know whether a patient is taking or has been taking a corticosteroid, to avoid a precipitous fall in blood pressure during anaesthesia or in the immediate postoperative period; a regimen for corticosteroid replacement may be necessary before and after surgery.

Children on long-term corticosteroid treatment should carry a Steroid Treatment Card (see p. 424) which gives guidance on minimising risk and provides details of prescriber, drug, dosage and duration of treatment.

Infections

Prolonged courses of corticosteroids increase susceptibility to infections and severity of infections; clinical presentation of infections may also be atypical. Serious infections e.g. *septicaemia* and *tuberculosis* may reach an advanced stage before being recognised, and *amoebiasis* or *strongyloidiasis* may be activated or exacerbated (exclude before initiating a corticosteroid in those at risk or with suggestive symptoms). Fungal or viral *ocular infections* may also be exacerbated (see also section 11.4.1).

Chickenpox Unless they have had chickenpox, children receiving oral or parenteral corticosteroids for purposes other than replacement should be regarded as being *at risk of severe chickenpox* (see Steroid Treatment Card). Manifestations of fulminant illness include pneumonia, hepatitis and disseminated intravascular coagulation; rash is not necessarily a prominent feature.

Passive immunisation with varicella–zoster immunoglobulin is needed for exposed non-immune children receiving systemic corticosteroids or for those who have used them within the previous 3 months (section 14.5); varicella–zoster immunoglobulin should preferably be given within 3 days of exposure and no later than 10 days. Confirmed chickenpox warrants specialist care and urgent treatment (section 5.3.2.1). Corticosteroids should not be stopped and dosage may need to be increased.

Topical, inhaled or rectal corticosteroids are less likely to be associated with an increased risk of severe chickenpox.

Measles Children taking corticosteroids, and their carers, should be advised to take particular care to avoid exposure to measles and to seek immediate medical advice if exposure occurs. Prophylaxis with intramuscular normal immunoglobulin (section 14.5) may be needed.

> Following concern about severe chickenpox associated with systemic corticosteroids, the CSM has issued a notice that **every** patient prescribed a *systemic* corticosteroid should receive the patient information leaflet supplied by the manufacturer.

Steroid treatment cards (see below) should also be issued where appropriate. Doctors and pharmacists can obtain supplies of the card from:

England and Wales

NHS Customer Services, Astron

Causeway Distribution Centre, Oldham Broadway Business Park, Chadderton

Oldham, OL6 9XD.

Tel: (0161) 683 2376/2382

Fax: (0161) 683 2396

Scotland

Banner Business Supplies

20 South Gyle Crescent

Edinburgh, EH12 9EB.

Tel: (01506) 448 440

Fax: (01256) 448 400

For other references to the adverse effects of corticosteroids see section 11.4 (eye) and section 13.4 (skin).

STEROID TREATMENT CARD

I am a patient on STEROID treatment which must not be stopped suddenly

- If you have been taking this medicine for more than three weeks, the dose should be reduced gradually when you stop taking steroids unless your doctor says otherwise.
- Read the patient information leaflet given with the medicine.
- Always carry this card with you and show it to anyone who treats you (for example a doctor, nurse, pharmacist or dentist). For one year after you stop the treatment, you must mention that you have taken steroids.
- If you become ill, or if you come into contact with anyone who has an infectious disease, consult your doctor promptly. If you have never had chickenpox, you should avoid close contact with people who have chickenpox or shingles. If you do come into contact with chickenpox, see your doctor urgently.
- Make sure that the information on the card is kept up to date.

Use of corticosteroids

Dosage of corticosteroids varies widely in different diseases and in different children. If the use of a corticosteroid can save or prolong life, as in exfoliative dermatitis, pemphigus, acute leukaemia or acute transplant rejection, high doses may need to be given, because the complications of therapy are likely to be less serious than the effects of the disease itself.

When long-term corticosteroid therapy is used in some chronic diseases, the adverse effects of treatment may become greater than the disabilities caused by the disease. To minimise side-effects the maintenance dose should be kept as low as possible.

When potentially less harmful measures are ineffective corticosteroids are used topically for the treatment of inflammatory conditions of the skin (section 13.4). Corticosteroids should be avoided or used only under specialist supervision in psoriasis (section 13.5).

Corticosteroids are used both topically (by rectum) and systemically (by mouth or intravenously) in the management of ulcerative colitis and Crohn's disease (section 1.5 and section 1.7.2).

Use can be made of the mineralocorticoid activity of fludrocortisone to treat postural hypotension in autonomic neuropathy.

Although very high doses of corticosteroids have been given by intravenous injection in septic shock, a study in adults of high-dose methylprednisolone sodium succinate did not demonstrate efficacy and, moreover, suggested a higher mortality in some subsets of patients given the high-dose corticosteroid therapy. However, there is evidence that administration of lower doses of hydrocortisone and fludrocortisone is of benefit in adults who have adrenocortical insufficiency as a consequence of septic shock.

The suppressive action of glucocorticoids on the hypothalamic-pituitary-adrenal axis is greatest and most prolonged when they are given at night. In most normal adults a single dose of 1 mg of dexamethasone at night, depending on weight, is sufficient to inhibit corticotropin secretion for 24 hours. This is the basis of the 'overnight dexamethasone suppression test' for diagnosing Cushing's syndrome.

Betamethasone and dexamethasone are also appropriate for conditions where water retention would be a disadvantage.

A corticosteroid may be used in the management of raised intracranial pressure or cerebral oedema that occurs as a result of malignancy (see also p. 26); high doses of betamethasone or dexamethasone are generally used. However, a corticosteroid should **not** be used for the management of head injury or stroke because it is unlikely to be of benefit and may even be harmful

In acute hypersensitivity reactions such as angioedema of the upper respiratory tract and anaphylactic shock, corticosteroids are indicated as an adjunct to emergency treatment with adrenaline (epinephrine) (section 3.4.3). In such cases hydrocortisone (as sodium succinate) by intravenous injection may be required.

Corticosteroids are preferably used by inhalation in the management of asthma (section 3.2) but systemic therapy in association with bronchodilators is required for the emergency treatment of severe acute asthma (section 3.1.1).

Dexamethasone should not be used routinely for the prophylaxis and treatment of chronic lung disease in neonates because of an association with adverse neurological effects.

Corticosteroids may be useful in conditions such as auto-immune hepatitis, rheumatoid arthritis, and sarcoidosis; they may also lead to remissions of acquired haemolytic anaemia (section 9.1.3) and thrombocytopenic purpura (section 9.1.4).

High doses of a corticosteroid (usually prednisolone) are used in the treatment of *glomerular kidney disease*, including *nephrotic syndrome*. The condition frequently recurs; a corticosteroid given in high doses and for prolonged periods may delay relapse but the higher incidence of adverse effects limits the overall benefit. Those who suffer frequent relapses may be treated with prednisolone given in a low dose (daily or on alternate days) for 3–6 months; the dose should be adjusted to minimise effects on growth and development. Other drugs used in the treatment of glomerular kidney disease include levamisole (section 5.5.2), cyclophosphamide (section 8.1.1), and ciclosporin (section 8.2.2). *Congenital nephrotic syndrome* may be resistant to corticosteroids and immunosuppressants; indometacin (section 10.1.1) and an ACE inhibitor such as captopril (section 2.5.5.1) have been used.

Corticosteroids can improve the prognosis of serious conditions such as systemic lupus erythematosus and polyarteritis nodosa; the effects of the disease process may be suppressed and symptoms relieved, but the underlying condition is not cured, although it may ultimately remit. It is usual to begin therapy in these conditions at fairly high dose and then to reduce the dose to the lowest commensurate with disease control.

For other references to the use of corticosteroids see Prescribing in Palliative Care, section 8.2.2 (immunosuppression), section 10.1.2 (rheumatic diseases), section 11.4 (eye), section 12.1.1 (otitis externa), section 12.2.1 (allergic rhinitis), and section 12.3.1 (aphthous ulcers).

Pregnancy and breast-feeding

Following a review of the data on the safety of systemic corticosteroids used in pregnancy and breast-feeding the CSM has concluded:

- corticosteroids vary in their ability to cross the placenta; betamethasone and dexamethasone cross the placenta readily while 88% of prednisolone is inactivated as it crosses the placenta;
- there is no convincing evidence that systemic corticosteroids increase the incidence of congenital abnormalities such as cleft palate or lip;
- when administration is prolonged or repeated during pregnancy, systemic corticosteroids increase the risk of intra-uterine growth restriction; there is no evidence of intra-uterine growth restriction following short-term treatment (e.g. prophylactic treatment for neonatal respiratory distress syndrome);
- any adrenal suppression in the neonate following prenatal exposure usually resolves spontaneously after birth and is rarely clinically important;
- prednisolone appears in small amounts in breast milk but maternal doses of up to 40 mg daily are unlikely to cause systemic effects in the infant; infants should be monitored for adrenal suppression if the mothers are taking a higher dose.

Administration

Whenever possible *local treatment* with creams, intra-articular injections, inhalations, eye-drops, or enemas should be used in preference to *systemic treatment*. The suppressive action of a corticosteroid on cortisol secretion is least when it is given as a single dose in the morning. In an attempt to reduce pituitary-adrenal suppression further, the total dose for two days can sometimes be taken as a single dose on alternate days; alternate-day administration has not been very successful in the management of asthma (section 3.2). Pituitary-adrenal suppression can also be reduced by means of intermittent therapy with short courses. In some conditions it may be possible to reduce the dose of corticosteroid by adding a small dose of an immunosuppressive drug (section 8.2.1).

Withdrawal of corticosteroids

The CSM has recommended that *gradual* withdrawal of systemic corticosteroids should be considered in those whose disease is unlikely to relapse and have

- recently received repeated courses (particularly if taken for longer than 3 weeks)
- taken a short course within 1 year of stopping long-term therapy
- other possible causes of adrenal suppression
- received more than 40 mg daily prednisolone (or equivalent) [in adults]
- been given repeat doses in the evening
- received more than 3 weeks' treatment

Systemic corticosteroids may be stopped abruptly in those whose disease is unlikely to relapse *and* who have received treatment for 3 weeks or less *and* who are not included in the patient groups described above.

During corticosteroid withdrawal the dose may be reduced rapidly down to physiological doses (equivalent to prednisolone 5 mg/m^2 daily) and then reduced more slowly. Assessment of the disease may be needed during withdrawal to ensure that relapse does not occur.

PREDNISOLONE

Cautions adrenal suppression and infection (see notes above), growth retardation—possibly irreversible, frequent monitoring required if history of tuberculosis (or X-ray changes), hypertension, congestive heart failure, renal impairment, diabetes mellitus including family history, osteoporosis, glaucoma (including family history), corneal perforation, severe affective disorders (particularly if history of steroid-induced psychosis), epilepsy, peptic ulcer, hypothyroidism, history of steroid myopathy; **interactions:** Appendix 1 (corticosteroids)

Hepatic impairment side-effects more common

Pregnancy benefit of treatment, e.g. in asthma, outweighs risk (see also CSM advice above); risk of intra-uterine growth restriction on prolonged or repeated systemic treatment; corticosteroid cover required by mother during labour; monitor closely if fluid retention; see also notes above

Breast-feeding see notes above

Contra-indications systemic infection (unless specific antimicrobial therapy given); avoid live virus vaccines in those receiving immunosuppressive doses (serum antibody response diminished)

Side-effects minimised by using lowest effective dose for minimum period possible; *gastro-intestinal effects* include dyspepsia, peptic ulceration (with perforation), abdominal distension, acute pancreatitis, oesophageal ulceration and candidiasis; *musculoskeletal effects* include proximal myopathy, osteoporosis, vertebral and long bone fractures, avascular osteonecrosis, tendon rupture; *endocrine effects* include adrenal suppression, menstrual irregularities and amenorrhoea, Cushing's syndrome (with high doses, usually reversible on withdrawal), hirsutism, weight gain, negative nitrogen and calcium balance, increased appetite; increased susceptibility to and severity of infection; *neuropsychiatric effects* include euphoria, psychological dependence, depression, insomnia, increased intracranial pressure with papilloedema (usually after withdrawal), psychosis and aggravation of schizophrenia, aggravation of epilepsy; *ophthalmic effects* include glaucoma, papilloedema, posterior subcapsular cataracts, corneal or scleral thinning and exacerbation of ophthalmic viral or fungal disease; *other side-effects* include impaired healing, skin atrophy, bruising, striae, telangiectasia, acne, fluid and electrolyte disturbance, leucocytosis, hypersensitivity reactions (including anaphylaxis), thromboembolism, nausea, malaise, hiccups

Indication and dose

See also notes above

Asthma see p. 176

Autoimmune inflammatory disorders (including juvenile idiopathic arthritis, connective tissue disorders and systemic lupus erythematosus)
- **By mouth**

  Child 1 month–18 years initially 1–2 mg/kg once daily (usual max. 60 mg daily), then reduced after a few days if appropriate

Autoimmune hepatitis
- **By mouth**

  Child 1 month–18 years initially 2 mg/kg once daily (max. 40 mg daily) then reduced to minimum effective dose

Corticosteroid replacement therapy
- **By mouth**

  Child 12–18 years 5 mg/m^2 daily in 1–2 divided doses adjusted according to response

Ear section 12.1.1

Epilepsy see p. 255

Eye section 11.4.1

Idiopathic thrombocytopenic purpura
- **By mouth**

  Child 1–10 years 1–2 mg/kg daily for max. 14 days *or* 4 mg/kg daily for max. 4 days

Immunosuppression see p. 477

Inflammatory bowel disease see p. 73

Nephrotic syndrome
- **By mouth**

  Child 1 month–18 years initially 60 mg/m^2 once daily (max. 80 mg daily) for 4–6 weeks until proteinuria ceases then 40 mg/m^2 on alternate days for 4–6 weeks, then withdraw by reducing dose gradually; prevention of relapse 0.5–1 mg/kg once daily or on alternate days for 3–6 months

Rheumatic disease see p. 555

Prednisolone (Non-proprietary) PoM

Tablets, prednisolone 1 mg, net price 28-tab pack = 53p; 5 mg, 28-tab pack = 68p; 25 mg, 56-tab pack = £9.67. Label: 10, steroid card, 21

Tablets, both e/c, prednisolone 2.5 mg (brown), net price 30-tab pack = 31p; 5 mg (red), 30-tab pack = 51p. Label: 5, 10, steroid card, 25
Brands include *Deltacortril Enteric*®

Soluble tablets, prednisolone 5 mg (as sodium phosphate), net price 30-tab pack = £2.20. Label: 10, steroid card, 13, 21

BETAMETHASONE

Cautions see notes above and under Prednisolone

Pregnancy transient effect on fetal movements and heart rate

Contra-indications see notes above and under Prednisolone

Side-effects see notes above and under Prednisolone

Licensed use *Betnesol*® tablets not licensed for use as mouthwash

Indication and dose

Ear (section 12.1.1); eye (section 11.4.1); nose (section 12.2.1)

Suppression of inflammatory and allergic disorders; congenital adrenal hyperplasia; see also notes above

- **By slow intravenous injection or by intravenous infusion**

  Child 1 month–1 year initially 1 mg repeated up to 4 times in 24 hours according to response

  Child 1–6 years initially 2 mg repeated up to 4 times in 24 hours according to response

  Child 6–12 years initially 4 mg repeated up to 4 times in 24 hours according to response

  Child 12–18 years initially 4–20 mg repeated up to 4 times in 24 hours according to response

Administration For *intravenous infusion*, dilute with Glucose 5% or Sodium Chloride 0.9%

Betnesol® (Celltech) PoM

Soluble tablets, pink, scored, betamethasone 500 micrograms (as sodium phosphate), net price 100-tab pack = £5.17. Label: 10, steroid card, 13, 21, (when used as mouthwash, counselling, rinse for about 1 minute, **not** to be swallowed)

Dose

Oral ulceration

Child 12–18 years 500 micrograms dissolved in 20 mL water and rinsed around the mouth 4 times daily; not to be swallowed

Injection, betamethasone 4 mg (as sodium phosphate) /mL. Net price 1-mL amp = £1.22. Label: 10, steroid card

DEFLAZACORT

Cautions see notes above and under Prednisolone

Contra-indications see notes above and under Prednisolone

Side-effects see notes above and under Prednisolone

Indication and dose

Inflammatory and allergic disorders

- **By mouth**

  Child 1 month–12 years 0.25–1.5 mg/kg once daily or on alternate days; up to 2.4 mg/kg (max. 120 mg) daily has been used in emergency situations

  Child 12–18 years 3–18 mg once daily or on alternate days; up to 2.4 mg/kg (max. 120 mg) daily has been used in emergency situations

Nephrotic syndrome

- **By mouth**

  Child 1 month–18 years initially 1.5 mg/kg once daily (max. 120 mg) reduced to lowest effective dose for maintenance

Calcort® (Shire) PoM

Tablets, deflazacort 1 mg, net price 100-tab pack = £8.00; 6 mg, 60-tab pack = £16.46; 30 mg, 30-tab pack = £22.80. Label: 5, 10, steroid card

DEXAMETHASONE

Cautions see notes above and under Prednisolone

Contra-indications see notes above and under Prednisolone

Side-effects see notes above and under Prednisolone; perineal irritation may follow intravenous administration of the phosphate ester

Licensed use not licensed for use in bacterial meningitis

Indication and dose

Croup (see p. 164); nausea and vomiting with chemotherapy (section 8.1); rheumatic disease (section 10.1.2); eye (see p. 572); see also notes above

Note Dexamethasone 1 mg ≡ dexamethasone phosphate 1.2 mg ≡ dexamethasone sodium phosphate 1.3 mg

Inflammatory and allergic disorders

- **By mouth (as dexamethasone)**

  Child 1 month–18 years 10–100 micrograms/kg daily in 1–2 divided doses, adjusted according to response; up to 300 micrograms/kg daily may be required in emergency situations

- **By intramuscular injection or slow intravenous injection or infusion (as dexamethasone phosphate)**

  Child 1 month–12 years 100–400 micrograms/kg daily in 1–2 divided doses; max. 24 mg daily

  Child 12–18 years initially 0.5–24 mg daily

Cerebral oedema associated with malignancy

- **By intravenous injection (as dexamethasone phosphate)**

  Child under 35 kg body-weight initially 20 mg, then 4 mg every 3 hours for 3 days, then 4 mg every 6 hours for 1 day, then 2 mg every 6 hours for 4 days, then decrease by 1 mg daily

  Child over 35 kg body-weight initially 25 mg, then 4 mg every 2 hours for 3 days, then 4 mg every 4 hours for 1 day, then 4 mg every 6 hours for 4 days, then decrease by 2 mg daily

DEXAMETHASONE (*continued*)

Bacterial meningitis (see section 5.1)

- **By slow intravenous injection (as dexamethasone phosphate)**

Child 2 months–18 years 150 micrograms/kg every 6 hours for 4 days starting before or with first dose of antibacterial

Physiological replacement

- **By mouth or by slow intravenous injection (as dexamethasone)**

Child 1 month–18 years 250–500 micrograms/m^2 every 12 hours, adjusted according to response

Administration for administration *by mouth* tablets may be dispersed in water or injection solution given by mouth

For *intravenous infusion* dilute with Glucose 5% or Sodium Chloride 0.9%; give over 15–20 minutes

Dexamethasone (Non-proprietary) PoM

Tablets, dexamethasone 500 micrograms, net price 20 = 67p; 2 mg, 20 = £2.42. Label: 10, steroid card, 21

Available from Organon

Oral solution, sugar-free, dexamethasone (as dexamethasone sodium phosphate) 2 mg/5 mL, net price 150-mL = £42.30. Label: 10, steroid card, 21

Brands include *Dexsol*®

Injection, dexamethasone phosphate (as dexamethasone sodium phosphate) 4 mg/mL, net price 1-mL amp = £1.00, 2-mL vial = £1.98; 24 mg/mL, 5-mL vial = £16.66. Label: 10, steroid card

Available from Mayne

Injection, dexamethasone (as dexamethasone sodium phosphate) 4 mg/mL, net price 1-mL amp = 83p, 2-mL vial = £1.27. Label: 10, steroid card

Available from Organon

HYDROCORTISONE

Cautions see notes above and under Prednisolone

Contra-indications see notes above and under Prednisolone

Side-effects see notes above and under Prednisolone; phosphate ester associated with paraesthesia and pain (particularly in the perineal region)

Indication and dose

Adrenocortical insufficiency (section 6.3.1); shock, see also notes above; hypersensitivity reactions e.g. anaphylactic shock, angioedema (section 3.4.3); inflammatory bowel disease (section 1.5); haemorrhoids (section 1.7.2); rheumatic disease (section 10.1.2); eye (section 11.4.1); skin (section 13.4)

Congenital adrenal hyperplasia (see also section 6.3.1)

- **By mouth**

Neonate 6–7 mg/m^2 every 8 hours, adjusted according to response

Child 1 month–18 years 5–6.5 mg/m^2 every 8 hours, adjusted according to response; usual maintenance 4–5 mg/m^2 every 8 hours but higher doses may be needed

Acute adrenocortical insufficiency (*Addisonian crisis*) see also notes above and section 6.3.1

- **By slow intravenous administration**

Neonate initially 10 mg as a slow intravenous injection then 100 mg/m^2 daily as a continuous infusion or in divided doses every 6–8 hours; adjusted according to response; when stable reduce over 4–5 days to oral maintenance dose

Child 1 month–12 years initially 2–4 mg/kg as a slow intravenous injection or infusion then 2–4 mg/kg every 6 hours; adjusted according to response; when stable reduce over 4–5 days to oral maintenance dose

Child 12–18 years 100 mg every 6 to 8 hours by slow intravenous injection or infusion

Adrenal hypoplasia, Addison's disease, chronic maintenance or replacement therapy

- **By mouth**

Neonate usual dose 4–5mg/m^2 every 8 hours; higher doses may be needed

Child 1 month–18 years usual dose 4–5mg/m^2 every 8 hours; higher doses may be needed

Note larger doses given in the morning and smaller doses in the evening

Severe acute asthma (see also section 3.1), acute hypersensitivity reactions, angioedema

- **By intramuscular or intravenous injection**

Child 1 month–1 year initially 25 mg 3 times daily, adjusted according to response

Child 1–6 years initially 50 mg 3 times daily, adjusted according to response

Child 6–12 years initially 100 mg 3 times daily, adjusted according to response

Child 12–18 years initially 100–500 mg 3 times daily, adjusted according to response

Hypotension resistant to inotropic treatment and volume replacement (limited evidence)

- **By intravenous injection**

Neonate initially 2.5 mg/kg repeated if necessary after 4 hours, then 2.5 mg/kg every 6 hours for 48 hours or until blood pressure recovers, then dose reduced gradually over at least 48 hours

Administration for *intravenous administration*, dilute with Glucose 5% or Sodium Chloride 0.9%; give over 20–30 minutes.

For administration *by mouth*, injection solution may be swallowed [unlicensed use] but consider phosphate content; alternatively *Corlan*® pellets (section 12.3.1) may be swallowed [unlicensed use]—pellets should not be cut as may not provide appropriate dose

HYDROCORTISONE (*continued*)

[1]**Efcortesol®** (Sovereign) PoM
Injection, hydrocortisone 100 mg (as sodium phosphate)/mL, net price 1-mL amp = 75p, 5-mL amp = £3.40. Label: 10, steroid card
Note Paraesthesia and pain (particularly in the perineal region) may follow intravenous injection of the phosphate ester
1. PoM restriction does not apply where administration is for saving life in emergency

Hydrocortone® (MSD) PoM
Tablets, scored, hydrocortisone 10 mg, net price 30-tab pack = 70p; 20 mg, 30-tab pack = £1.07. Label: 10, steroid card, 21

[1]**Solu-Cortef®** (Pharmacia) PoM
Injection, powder for reconstitution, hydrocortisone (as sodium succinate). Net price 100-mg vial = 92p, 100-mg vial with 2-mL amp water for injections = £1.16. Label: 10, steroid card
1. PoM restriction does not apply where administration is for saving life in emergency

Extemporaneous formulations available see Extemporaneous Preparations, p. 8

METHYLPREDNISOLONE

Cautions see notes above and under Prednisolone; rapid intravenous administration of large doses associated with cardiovascular collapse

Contra-indications see notes above and under Prednisolone

Side-effects see notes above and under Prednisolone

Indication and dose

See also notes above; immunosuppression (section 8.2.2); rheumatic disease (section 10.1.2); skin (section 13.4)

Inflammatory and allergic disorders
- **By mouth, slow intravenous injection or by intravenous infusion**

Child 1 month–18 years 0.5–1.7 mg/kg daily in 2–4 divided doses depending on condition and response

Treatment of graft rejection reactions
- **By intravenous injection**

Child 1 month–18 years 10–20 mg/kg or 400–600 mg/m² (max. 1 g) once daily for 3 days

Severe erythema multiforme (Stevens-Johnson syndrome), lupus nephritis, systemic onset juvenile idiopathic arthritis (section 10.1.2.1)
- **By intravenous injection**

Child 1 month–18 years 10–30 mg/kg (max. 1 g) once daily or on alternate days for up to 3 days

Administration intravenous injection given over 30 minutes; for intravenous infusion may be diluted with sodium chloride intravenous infusion 0.9% or 0.45%, or glucose intravenous infusion 5% or 10%

Medrone® (Pharmacia) PoM
Tablets, scored, methylprednisolone 2 mg (pink), net price 30-tab pack = £3.23; 4 mg, 30-tab pack = £6.19; 16 mg, 30-tab pack = £17.17; 100 mg (blue), 20-tab pack = £48.32. Label: 10, steroid card, 21

Solu-Medrone® (Pharmacia) PoM
Injection, powder for reconstitution, methylprednisolone (as sodium succinate) (all with solvent). Net price 40-mg vial = £1.58; 125-mg vial = £4.75; 500-mg vial = £9.60; 1-g vial = £17.30; 2-g vial = £32.86. Label: 10, steroid card

Intramuscular depot

Depo-Medrone® (Pharmacia) PoM
Injection (aqueous suspension), methylprednisolone acetate 40 mg/mL. Net price 1-mL vial = £2.87; 2-mL vial = £5.15; 3-mL vial = £7.47. Label: 10, steroid card

Dose
- **By deep intramuscular injection into gluteal muscle** seek specialist advice

6.4 Sex hormones

Sex hormone replacement therapy is indicated in children for the treatment of gonadotrophin deficiency, gonadal disorders or delayed puberty that interferes with quality of life. Indications include constitutional delay in puberty, congenital or acquired hypogonadotrophic hypogonadism, hypergonadotrophic hypogonadism (Turner's syndrome, Klinefelter's syndrome), endocrine disorders (Cushing's syndrome or hyperprolactinaemia), and chronic illness such as cystic fibrosis or sickle-cell disease that may affect the onset of puberty.

Replacement therapy is generally started at the appropriate age for the development of puberty and should be managed by a paediatric endocrinologist. Patients with constitutional delay, chronic illness or eating disorders may need only small doses of hormone supplements for 4 to 6 months to induce puberty and endogenous sex hormone production, which is then sustained. Patients with organic causes of hormone deficiency will require life-long replacement, adjusted to allow normal development.

Inadequate treatment may lead to poor bone mineralisation, resulting in fractures and osteoporosis.

6.4.1 Female sex hormones

6.4.1.1 Oestrogens

Oestrogens are necessary for the development of female secondary sexual characteristics. If onset of puberty is delayed because of organic pathology, puberty may be induced with ethinylestradiol in increasing doses, guided by breast staging and uterine scans. Cyclical progestogen replacement is added after 12–18 months of oestrogen treatment (see section 6.4.1.2). Once the adult dosage of oestrogen has been reached (20 micrograms ethinylestradiol daily), it may be more convenient to provide replacement either as a low-dose oestrogen containing oral contraceptive formulation [unlicensed indication] (see BNF section 7.3.1) or as a combined oestrogen and progestogen hormone replacement therapy preparation [unlicensed indication] (see BNF section 6.4.1.2). There is limited experience in the use of transdermal patches or gels in children; compliance and skin irritation are sometimes a problem.

Ethinylestradiol is occasionally used, under **specialist supervision**, for the management of hereditary haemorrhagic telangiectasia (but evidence of benefit is limited), for the prevention of tall stature, and in tests of growth hormone secretion (see below). Side-effects include nausea and fluid retention.

Topical oestrogen creams are used in the treatment of labial adhesions (for preparations, see BNF section 7.2.1)

ETHINYLESTRADIOL
(Ethinyloestradiol)

Cautions see Combined Hormonal Contraceptives (BNF section 7.3.1); **interactions**: Appendix 1 (Oestrogens)

Contra-indications cardiovascular disease (sodium retention with oedema), personal or family history of thromboembolism, porphyria; see also Combined Hormonal Contraceptives (BNF section 7.3.1)

Hepatic impairment contra-indicated in liver disease including disorders of hepatic excretion (e.g. Dubin-Johnson or Rotor syndromes), infective hepatitis (until liver function returns to normal), and jaundice

Pregnancy contra-indicated

Breast-feeding contra-indicated

Side-effects nausea, vomiting, headache, breast tenderness, changes in body weight, fluid retention, depression, chorea, skin reactions, chloasma, hypertension, may irritate contact lenses, impairment of liver function, hepatic tumours, rarely photosensitivity; see also Combined Hormonal Contraceptives (BNF section 7.3.1)

Licensed use unlicensed for use in children

Indication and dose

See notes above

Induction of sexual maturation in girls
- **By mouth**

initially 2 micrograms daily, increasing every 6 months to 5 micrograms, then to 10 micrograms, and then to 20 micrograms daily
Note after 12–18 months of treatment give progestogen for 7 days of each 28-day cycle

Maintenance of sexual maturation in girls
- **By mouth**

20 micrograms daily with cyclical progestogen for 7 days of each 28-day cycle

6 Endocrine system

ETHINYLESTRADIOL (*continued*)

Prevention of tall stature in girls
- **By mouth**
  Girls 2–12 years 20–50 micrograms daily

Pituitary priming before growth hormone secretion test in girls
- **By mouth**
  Girls with bone age above 10 years 100 micrograms daily for 3 days before test

Ethinylestradiol (Non-proprietary) PoM
Tablets, ethinylestradiol 2 micrograms (unlicensed, available on a named patient basis); 10 micrograms, net price 21-tab pack = £12.86; 50 micrograms, 21-tab pack = £15.16; 1 mg, 28-tab pack = £28.85

6.4.1.2 Progestogens

There are two main groups of progestogen, *progesterone and its analogues* (dydrogesterone and medroxyprogesterone) and *testosterone analogues* (norethisterone and norgestrel). The newer progestogens (desogestrel, norgestimate, and gestodene) are all derivatives of norgestrel; levonorgestrel is the active isomer of norgestrel and has twice its potency. Progesterone and its analogues are less androgenic than the testosterone derivatives and neither progesterone nor dydrogesterone causes virilisation.

In delayed puberty cyclical progestogen is added after 12–18 months of oestrogen therapy (section 6.4.1.1) to establish a menstrual cycle; usually levonorgestrel 30 micrograms or norethisterone 5 mg daily are used for the last 7 days of each 28 day cycle.

Norethisterone is also used to postpone menstruation during a cycle; treatment is started 3 days before the expected onset of menstruation.

NORETHISTERONE

Cautions conditions that may worsen with fluid retention e.g. epilepsy, hypertension, migraine, asthma, cardiac or renal dysfunction; susceptibility to thromboembolism (particular caution with high dose); history of depression; diabetes (monitor closely); **interactions:** Appendix 1 (progestogens)

Hepatic impairment caution; avoid if severe

Breast-feeding higher doses may suppress lactation and alter milk composition; use lowest effective dose

Contra-indications history of liver tumours, severe liver impairment; severe arterial disease, undiagnosed vaginal bleeding; porphyria (section 9.8.2); history during pregnancy of idiopathic jaundice, severe pruritus, or pemphigoid gestationis

Pregnancy contra-indicated

Side-effects menstrual disturbances, premenstrual-like syndrome (including bloating, fluid retention, breast tenderness), weight gain, nausea, headache, dizziness, insomnia, drowsiness, depression; skin reactions (including urticaria, pruritus, rash, and acne), hirsutism and alopecia; jaundice and anaphylactoid reactions also reported

Licensed use not licensed for use in children

Indication and dose

See notes above

Induction and maintenance of sexual maturation in females (combined with an oestrogen after 12–24 months oestrogen therapy)
- **By mouth**
  5 mg once daily for the last 7 days of a 28-day cycle

Postponement of menstruation
- **By mouth**
  5 mg 3 times daily, starting 3 days before expected onset of menstruation

Tablets of 5 mg

Norethisterone (Non-proprietary) PoM
Tablets, norethisterone 5 mg, net price 30-tab pack = £2.69

Primolut N® (Schering Health) PoM
Tablets, norethisterone 5 mg. Net price 30-tab pack = £2.01

Utovlan® (Pharmacia) PoM
Tablets, norethisterone 5 mg, net price 30-tab pack = £1.40, 90-tab pack = £4.21

6.4.2 Male sex hormones and antagonists

Androgens cause masculinisation; they may be used as replacement therapy in androgen deficiency, delayed puberty and in those who are hypogonadal due to either pituitary or testicular disease.

When given to patients with hypopituitarism androgens can lead to normal sexual development and potency but not to fertility. If fertility is desired, the usual treatment is with gonadotrophins or pulsatile gonadotrophin-releasing hormone (section 6.5.1) which stimulates spermatogenesis as well as androgen production.

Intramuscular depot preparations of **testosterone esters** are preferred for replacement therapy. Testosterone enantate or propionate or alternatively *Sustanon*®, which consists of a mixture of testosterone esters and has a longer duration of action, may be used. For induction of puberty, depot testosterone injections are given monthly and the doses increased every 6 to 12 months according to response. Single ester testosterone injections may need to be given more frequently. Testosterone enantate is unlicensed in children. Implants of testosterone can be used for hypogonadism; the implants are replaced every 4 to 5 months.

Oral **testosterone undecanoate** is used for induction of puberty. An alternative approach that promotes growth rather than sexual maturation uses oral oxandrolone (section 6.4.3).

Chorionic gonadotrophin (section 6.5.1) has also been used in delayed puberty in the male to stimulate endogenous testosterone production, but has little advantage over testosterone.

Caution should be used when androgens or chorionic gonadotrophin are used in treating boys with delayed puberty since the fusion of epiphyses is hastened and may result in short stature.

Testosterone patches and topical gel are also available but experience of their use in children under 15 years is limited. Topical testosterone is applied to the penis in the treatment of microphallus; an extemporaneously prepared cream should be used because the alcohol in proprietary gel formulations causes irritation.

TESTOSTERONE AND ESTERS

Cautions cardiac impairment, hypertension, epilepsy, migraine, diabetes mellitus, skeletal metastases (risk of hypercalcaemia); **interactions:** Appendix 1 (testosterone)

Hepatic impairment avoid if possible—fluid retention and dose-related toxicity

Renal impairment caution—potential for fluid retention

Contra-indications history of primary liver tumours, hypercalcaemia, nephrosis

Pregnancy avoid; causes masculinisation of female fetus

Breast-feeding avoid; may cause masculinisation in the female infant or precocious development in the male infant; high doses suppress lactation

Side-effects headache, depression, gastro-intestinal bleeding, nausea, cholestatic jaundice, changes in libido, gynaecomastia, polycythaemia, anxiety, asthenia, paraesthesia, hypertension, electrolyte disturbances including sodium retention with oedema and hypercalcaemia, weight gain; increased bone growth; androgenic effects such as hirsutism, male-pattern baldness, seborrhoea, acne, pruritus; excessive frequency and duration of penile erection, precocious sexual development and premature closure of epiphyses in pre-pubertal males, suppression of spermatogenesis in males and virilism in females; *rarely* liver tumours; sleep apnoea also reported; *with patches and gel,* local irritation and allergic reactions

Licensed use *Sustanon*® and *Virormone*® licensed for use in children; *Andropatch*® licensed for use in children over 15 years

Indication and dose

See also under preparations; specialist use only

Induction and maintenance of sexual maturation in males

- **By mouth (as testosterone undecanoate)**

Child over 12 years 40 mg on alternate days increasing according to response up to 120 mg daily

- **By deep intramuscular injection of testosterone enantate or propionate**

Child over 12 years 25–50 mg/m² every month increasing dose every 6–12 months according to response

- **Patch**

Child over 15 years apply to clean, dry, unbroken skin on back, abdomen, upper arms or thighs, removing after 24 hours and siting replacement patch on a different area (with an interval of 7 days before using the same site); initially apply patches equivalent to testosterone 5 mg/24 hours (2.5 mg/24 hours in non-virilised patients) at night (approx. 10 p.m.), then adjust to 2.5–7.5 mg every 24 hours according to plasma-testosterone concentration

Treatment of microphallus

- **Topically**

Apply 3 times daily for 3 weeks

Note Use only specially manufactured preparation (see notes above)

TESTOSTERONE AND ESTERS (*continued*)

Oral

Restandol® (Organon) PoM
Capsules, red-brown, testosterone undecanoate 40 mg in oily solution. Net price 28-cap pack = £8.30; 56-cap pack = £16.60. Label: 21, 25

Intramuscular

Testosterone Enantate (Cambridge) PoM
Injection (oily), testosterone enantate 250 mg/mL. Net price 1-mL amp = £8.33

Sustanon 100® (Organon) PoM
Injection (oily), testosterone propionate 20 mg, testosterone phenylpropionate 40 mg, and testosterone isocaproate 40 mg/mL. Net price 1-mL amp = £1.09
Excipients: include arachis (peanut) oil, benzyl alcohol (see Excipients p. 3)

Dose

Delayed puberty in males
- **By intramuscular injection**
  1 mL every month for 3 doses

Pituitary priming prior to growth hormone secretion test
- **By deep intramuscular injection**
  1 mL 3–5 days before test

Sustanon 250® (Organon) PoM
Injection (oily), testosterone propionate 30 mg, testosterone phenylpropionate 60 mg, testosterone isocaproate 60 mg, and testosterone decanoate 100 mg/mL. Net price 1-mL amp = £2.55
Excipients: include arachis (peanut) oil, benzyl alcohol (see Excipients p. 3)

Virormone® (Nordic) PoM
Injection, testosterone propionate 50 mg/mL. Net price 2-mL amp = 59p

Implant

Testosterone (Organon) PoM
Implant, testosterone 100 mg, net price = £7.40; 200 mg = £13.79

Dose

Maintenance of sexual maturation in males
Child over 16 years 100–600 mg; 600 mg usually maintains plasma-testosterone concentration within the normal range for 4–5 months

Cream

Testosterone
Cream, testosterone 5% (other strengths available)
Available as manufactured special, see guidance on unlicensed medicines for details

Transdermal preparations

Andropatch® (GSK) PoM
Patches, self-adhesive, releasing testosterone approx. 2.5 mg/24 hours, net price 60-patch pack = £49.10; releasing testosterone approx. 5 mg/24 hours, net price 30-patch pack = £49.10. Counselling, administration

Anti-androgens and precocious puberty

The gonadorelin stimulation test (section 6.5.1) is used to distinguish between *gonadotrophin-dependent (central) precocious puberty* and *gonadotrophin-independent precocious puberty*. Treatment requires specialist management.

Gonadorelin analogues, used in the management of gonadotrophin-dependent precocious puberty, delay development of secondary sexual characteristics and growth velocity.

Testolactone and **cyproterone** are used in the management of gonadotrophin-independent precocious puberty, resulting from McCune-Albright syndrome, familial male precocious puberty (testotoxicosis), hormone-secreting tumours, and ovarian and testicular disorders. Testolactone inhibits the aromatisation of testosterone, the rate limiting step in oestrogen synthesis. Cyproterone is a progestogen with anti-androgen properties.

Spironolactone (section 2.2.3) is sometimes used in combination with testolactone because it has a some androgen receptor blocking properties.

High blood concentration of sex hormones may activate release of gonadotrophin releasing hormone, leading to development of secondary, central gonadotrophin-dependent precocious puberty. This may require the addition of gonadorelin analogues to prevent progression of pubertal development and skeletal maturation.

CYPROTERONE ACETATE

Cautions blood counts initially and throughout treatment; monitor adrenocortical function regularly; diabetes mellitus (see also Contra-indications)
Skilled tasks Fatigue and lassitude may impair performance of skilled tasks (e.g. driving)

Hepatic impairment monitor hepatic function regularly—dose-related toxicity, see side-effects below

Contra-indications hepatic disease, severe diabetes (with vascular changes); sickle-cell anae-

CYPROTERONE ACETATE (*continued*)

mia, malignant or wasting disease, severe depression, history of thrombo-embolic disorders

Side-effects fatigue and lassitude, breathlessness, weight changes, reduced sebum production (may clear acne), changes in hair pattern, gynaecomastia (rarely leading to galactorrhoea and benign breast nodules); rarely hypersensitivity reactions, rash and osteoporosis; inhibition of spermatogenesis (see notes above); hepatotoxicity reported (including jaundice, hepatitis and hepatic failure)

Hepatotoxicity Direct hepatic toxicity including jaundice, hepatitis and hepatic failure have been reported (usually after several months) with cyproterone acetate 200–300 mg daily. Liver function tests should be performed before treatment and whenever symptoms suggestive of hepatotoxicity occur—if confirmed cyproterone should normally be withdrawn unless the hepatotoxicity can be explained by another cause such as metastatic disease (in which case cyproterone should be continued only if the perceived benefit exceeds the risk)

Licensed use unlicensed for use in children

Indication and dose

Specialist management only

Gonadotrophin-independent precocious puberty (see notes above)
- By mouth
  Initially 25 mg twice daily, adjusted according to response

Cyproterone Acetate (Non-proprietary) PoM
Tablets, cyproterone acetate 4 mg, 10 mg (available via specialist importing company); 50 mg, net price 56-tab pack = £31.54. Label 21, counselling, driving

Androcur® (Schering Health) PoM
Tablets, scored, cyproterone acetate 50 mg. Net price 56-tab pack = £25.89. Label: 21, counselling, driving

TESTOLACTONE

Cautions interactions: Appendix 1 (testolactone)

Contra-indications

Pregnancy avoid

Breast-feeding no information available

Side-effects nausea, vomiting, anorexia, diarrhoea; hypertension; peripheral neuropathy; weight changes; changes in hair pattern; rarely hypersensitivity reactions, rash

Indication and dose

Specialist management only, see notes above

Gonadotrophin-independent precocious puberty
- By mouth
  5 mg/kg 3–4 times daily; up to 10 mg/kg 4 times daily may be required

Testolactone PoM
Tablets, testolactone 50 mg
Available from specialist importing company

GOSERELIN

Cautions monitor bone mineral density

Contra-indications undiagnosed vaginal bleeding

Pregnancy manufacturer advises avoid

Breast-feeding manufacturer advises avoid

Side-effects changes in blood pressure, headache, mood changes including depression, hypersensitivity reactions including urticaria, pruritus, rash, asthma and anaphylaxis; changes in scalp and body hair, weight changes, withdrawal bleeding, ovarian cysts (may require withdrawal), breast swelling and tenderness (males and females), visual disturbances, paraesthesia, local reactions at injection site

Licensed use not licensed for use in children

Indication and dose

Gonadotrophin-dependent precocious puberty
see notes above; for doses, see under preparations below
Note Injections may be required more frequently in some cases

Administration Rotate injection site to prevent atrophy and nodule formation

Zoladex® (AstraZeneca) PoM
Implant, goserelin 3.6 mg (as acetate) in *Safe-System®* syringe applicator. Net price each = £84.14

Dose
- **Implant, by subcutaneous injection into anterior abdominal wall**
  3.6 mg every 4 weeks

Zoladex® LA (AstraZeneca) PoM
Implant, goserelin 10.8 mg (as acetate) in *Safe-System®* syringe applicator. Net price each = £267.48

Dose
- **Implant, by subcutaneous injection into anterior abdominal wall**
  10.8 mg every 12 weeks

LEUPRORELIN ACETATE

Cautions see Goserelin

Contra-indications see Goserelin

Pregnancy avoid—teratogenic in *animal* studies

Breast-feeding manufacturer advises avoid

Side-effects see Goserelin

Licensed use not licensed for use in children

Indication and dose

Gonadotrophin-dependent precocious puberty
see notes above; for doses, see under preparations below
Note Injections may be required more frequently in some cases

Administration Rotate injection site to prevent atrophy and nodule formation

Prostap® SR (Wyeth) PoM
Injection (microsphere powder for reconstitution), leuprorelin acetate, net price 3.75-mg vial with 1-mL vehicle-filled syringe = £125.40

Dose
- **By subcutaneous or by intramuscular injection**
  3.75 mg every four weeks (half this dose is sometimes used in children with body-weight under 20 kg)

Prostap® 3 (Wyeth) PoM
Injection (microsphere powder for reconstitution), leuprorelin acetate, net price 11.25-mg vial with 2-mL vehicle-filled syringe = £376.20

Dose
- **By subcutaneous or by intramuscular injection**
  11.25 mg every 12 weeks

TRIPTORELIN

Cautions see Goserelin

Contra-indications see Goserelin

Pregnancy manufacturer advises avoid

Breast-feeding manufacturer advises avoid

Side-effects see Goserelin

Licensed use *Decapeptyl® SR* not licensed for use in children; *Gonapeptyl® Depot* licensed for use in girls under 9 years and boys under 10 years

Indication and dose

Gonadotrophin-dependent precocious puberty
see notes above; for doses see under preparations below

Administration rotate injection site to prevent atrophy and nodule formation

Decapeptyl® SR (Ipsen) PoM
Injection, (powder for suspension), m/r, triptorelin (as acetate), net price 15-mg vial (with diluent) = £207.00

Dose
- **By intramuscular injection**
  Body-weight over 30 kg 11.25 mg every 3 months
  Note Each 15-mg vial includes an overage to allow administration of an 11.25-mg dose

Gonapeptyl® Depot (Ferring) PoM
Injection (powder for suspension), triptorelin (as acetate), net price 3.75-mg prefilled syringe (with prefilled syringe of vehicle) = £85.00

Dose
- **By subcutaneous or by intramuscular injection**
  Body-weight under 20 kg initially 1.875 mg on days 0, 14, and 28, then 1.875 mg every 4 weeks
  Body-weight 20–30 kg initially 2.5 mg on days 0, 14, and 28, then 2.5 mg every 4 weeks
  Body-weight over 30 kg initially 3.75 mg on days 0, 14, and 28, then 3.75 mg every 4 weeks; discontinue when bone maturation consistent with age over 12 years in girls and over 13 years in boys
  Note may be given every 3 weeks if necessary

6.4.3 Anabolic steroids

Anabolic steroids have some androgenic activity but they cause less virilisation than androgens in girls. They are used in the treatment of some *aplastic anaemias* (section 9.1.3). Oxandrolone may be used to stimulate late pre-pubertal growth prior to induction of sexual maturation in boys with short stature and in girls with Turner's syndrome; specialist management is required.

OXANDROLONE

Cautions see Testosterone (section 6.4.2); **interactions**: Appendix 1 (oxandrolone)

Contra-indications see Testosterone (section 6.4.2)

Side-effects see Testosterone (section 6.4.2)

Indication and dose

Stimulation of late pre-pubertal growth in boys with short stature
- **By mouth**
  Boys 10–18 years (or appropriate age) 1.25–2.5 mg daily for 3–6 months

6 Endocrine system

OXANDROLONE (*continued*)

Stimulation of late pre-pubertal growth in girls with Turner's syndrome
- **By mouth**

Girls in combination with growth hormone 0.625–2.5 mg daily

Oxandrolone
Tablets, oxandrolone 2.5 mg
Available via specialist importing company on a named-patient basis

6.5 Hypothalamic and pituitary hormones

Use of preparations in these sections requires detailed prior investigation of the patient and *should be reserved for specialist centres.*

6.5.1 Hypothalamic and anterior pituitary hormones including growth hormone

Anterior pituitary hormones

Corticotrophins

Tetracosactide (tetracosactrin), an analogue of corticotropin (adrenocorticotrophic hormone, ACTH), is used to test adrenocortical function; failure of plasma-cortisol concentration to rise after administration of tetracosactide indicates adrenocortical insufficiency. A low-dose test is considered by some clinicians to be more sensitive when used to confirm established, partial adrenal suppression.

Tetracosactide should be used with caution in patients with allergic disorders e.g. asthma and should be given only if no other ACTH preparations have been given previously. Tetracosactide depot injection (*Synacthen Depot*®) is also used in the treatment of infantile spasms (see Infantile spasms, section 4.8.1) but it is contra-indicated in neonates because of the presence of benzyl alcohol in the injection. Corticotropin-releasing factor, corticorelin, (also known as corticotropin-releasing hormone, CRH) is used to test anterior pituitary function and secretion of corticotropin.

6 Endocrine system

TETRACOSACTIDE
(Tetracosactrin)

Cautions as for corticosteroids, section 6.3.2; **important:** risk of anaphylaxis (medical supervision; consult product literature); **interactions:** Appendix 1 (corticosteroids)

Contra-indications as for corticosteroids, section 6.3.2; avoid injections containing benzyl alcohol in neonates (see under preparations)

Pregnancy avoid

Breast-feeding avoid

Side-effects as for corticosteroids, section 6.3.2

Licensed use not licensed for low-dose test for adrenocortical insufficiency or treatment of infantile spasms

Indication and dose

See notes above and under preparations below

Synacthen® (Alliance) PoM
Injection, tetracosactide 250 micrograms (as acetate)/mL. Net price 1-mL amp = £2.93

Dose

Diagnosis of adrenocortical insuffiency (30-minute test)
- **By intramuscular or intravenous injection**

Standard-dose test 145 micrograms/m^2 (max. 250 micrograms) as a single dose

Low-dose test 300 nanograms/m^2 as a single dose

Administration may be diluted in sodium chloride 0.9% to 250 nanograms/mL

Synacthen Depot® (Alliance) PoM
Injection (aqueous suspension), tetracosactide acetate 1 mg/mL, with zinc phosphate complex. Net price 1-mL amp = £4.18
Excipients: include benzyl alcohol (avoid in neonates, see Excipients p. 3)

Dose

Infantile spasms
- **By intramuscular injection**

Child over 1 month initially 500 micrograms on alternate days, adjusted according to response

CORTICORELIN

(Corticotrophin-releasing hormone, CRH)

Contra-indications
Pregnancy contra-indicated
Breast-feeding contra-indicated

Side-effects flushing of face, neck and upper body, hypotension, mild sensation of taste or smell

Licensed use not licensed

Indication and dose

Test of anterior pituitary function
- **By intravenous injection over 30 seconds**
  Child 1 month–18 years 1 microgram/kg (max. 100 micrograms) as a single dose

CRH Ferring® (Shire) PoM
Injection, corticorelin 100 micrograms

Gonadotrophins

Gonadotrophins are occasionally used in the treatment of hypogonadotrophic hypogonadism and associated oligospermia. There is no justification for their use in primary gonadal failure.

Chorionic gonadotrophin is used in the investigation of testicular function in suspected primary hypogonadism and incomplete masculinisation. It has also been used in delayed puberty in boys to stimulate endogenous testosterone production, but it has little advantage over testosterone (section 6.4.2).

CHORIONIC GONADOTROPHIN

(Human Chorionic Gonadotrophin; HCG)

A preparation of a glycoprotein fraction secreted by the placenta and obtained from the urine of pregnant women having the action of the pituitary luteinising hormone

Cautions cardiac or renal impairment, asthma, epilepsy, migraine; prepubertal boys (risk of premature epiphyseal closure or precocious puberty)

Contra-indications androgen-dependent tumours

Side-effects oedema (reduce dose), headache, tiredness, mood changes, gynaecomastia, local reactions

Licensed use unlicensed in children for test of testicular function

Indication and dose

Test of testicular function
- **By intramuscular injection**
  Short stimulation test:
  Child 1 month–18 years 1500–2000 units once daily for 3 days
  Prolonged stimulation test:
  Child 1 month–18 years 1500–2000 units twice weekly for 3 weeks

Hypogonadotrophic hypogonadism
- **By intramuscular injection**
  Child 1 month–18 years 1000–2000 units twice weekly, adjusted to response

Undescended testes
- **By intramuscular injection**
  Child 7–18 years initially 500 units 3 times weekly (1000 units twice weekly if over 17 years); adjusted to response; up to 4000 units 3 times weekly may be required; continue for 1–2 months after testicular descent

Choragon® (Ferring) PoM
Injection, powder for reconstitution, chorionic gonadotrophin. Net price 5000-unit amp (with solvent) = £3.26. For intramuscular injection

Pregnyl® (Organon) PoM
Injection, powder for reconstitution, chorionic gonadotrophin. Net price 1500-unit amp = £2.20; 5000-unit amp = £3.27 (both with solvent). For subcutaneous or intramuscular injection

Growth hormone

Growth hormone is used to treat proven deficiency of the hormone, Prader-Willi syndrome, Turner's syndrome, growth disturbance in children born small for gestational age, and chronic renal insufficiency (see NICE guidance below). Growth hormone is also used in Noonan syndrome and idiopathic short stature [unlicensed indications] under specialist management. Treatment should be initiated and monitored by a paediatrician with expertise in managing growth-hormone disorders; treatment can be continued under a shared-care protocol by a general practitioner.

Growth hormone of human origin (HGH; somatotrophin) has been replaced by a growth hormone of human sequence, **somatropin**, produced using recombinant DNA technology.

NICE guidance (somatropin in children with growth failure)
NICE has recommended (May 2002) treatment with somatropin for children with:

- proven growth-hormone deficiency;
- Turner's syndrome;
- Prader-Willi syndrome;
- chronic renal insufficiency before puberty.

Treatment should be discontinued if the response is poor (i.e. an increase in growth velocity of less than 50% from baseline) in the first year of therapy.

In children with chronic renal insufficiency, treatment should be stopped after renal transplantation and not restarted for at least a year

SOMATROPIN

(Synthetic Human Growth Hormone)

Cautions diabetes mellitus (adjustment of antidiabetic therapy may be necessary), papilloedema (see under Side-effects), relative deficiencies of other pituitary hormones (notably hypothyroidism—manufacturers recommend periodic thyroid function tests but limited evidence of clinical value), history of malignant disease, disorders of the epiphysis of the hip (monitor for limping), resolved intracranial hypertension (monitor closely), initiation of treatment close to puberty not recommended in child born small for gestational age; Silver-Russell syndrome; rotate subcutaneous injection sites to prevent lipoatrophy; **interactions:** Appendix 1 (somatropin)

Breast-feeding no information available but absorption from milk unlikely

Contra-indications evidence of tumour activity (complete antitumour therapy and ensure intracranial lesions inactive before starting); not to be used after renal transplantation or for growth promotion in children with closed epiphyses (or near closure in Prader-Willi syndrome); severe obesity or severe respiratory syndrome in Prader-Willi syndrome

Pregnancy interrupt treatment if pregnancy occurs

Side-effects headache, funduscopy for papilloedema recommended if severe or recurrent headache, visual problems, nausea and vomiting occur—if papilloedema confirmed consider benign intracranial hypertension (rare cases reported); fluid retention (peripheral oedema), arthralgia, myalgia, carpal tunnel syndrome, paraesthesia, antibody formation, hypothyroidism, insulin resistance, hyperglycaemia, hypoglycaemia, reactions at injection site; leukaemia in children with growth hormone deficiency also reported

Licensed use Genotropin® not licensed for use in Noonan syndrome; *Humatrope®*, *Nutropin Aq®*, and *Saizen®* not licensed for use in Prader–Willi syndrome, Noonan syndrome, or growth disturbance in children born small for gestational age; *Norditropin®* not licensed for use in Prader–Willi syndrome or Noonan syndrome; *Zomacton®* not licensed for use in chronic renal insufficiency, Prader–Willi syndrome, Noonan syndrome or growth disturbance in children born small for gestational age

Indication and dose

Gonadal dysgenesis (Turner's syndrome)
- **By subcutaneous injection**
  45–50 micrograms/kg daily *or* 1.4 mg/m² daily

Deficiency of growth hormone
- **By subcutaneous or intramuscular injection**
  23–39 micrograms/kg daily *or* 0.7–1 mg/m² daily

Prader-Willi syndrome
- **By subcutaneous injection**
  Children with growth velocity greater than 1 cm/year in combination with energy-restricted diet, 35 micrograms/kg daily *or* 1 mg/m² daily; max. 2.7 mg daily

Chronic renal insufficiency (renal function decreased to less than 50%)
- **By subcutaneous injection**
  45–50 micrograms/kg daily *or* 1.4 mg/m² daily (higher doses may be needed) adjusted if necessary after 6 months

Growth disturbance in children born small for gestational age who have not shown catch-up growth by 4 years of age or later; Noonan syndrome
- **By subcutaneous injection**
  35 micrograms/kg daily *or* 1 mg/m² daily

Genotropin® (Pharmacia) PoM
Injection, two-compartment cartridge containing powder for reconstitution, somatropin (rbe) and diluent, net price 5.3-mg (16-unit) cartridge = £122.87, 12-mg (36-unit) cartridge = £278.20. For use with *Genotropin® Pen* NHS device (available free of charge from clinics). For subcutaneous injection

MiniQuick injection, two-compartment single-dose syringe containing powder for reconstitution, somatropin (rbe) and diluent, net price 0.2-mg (0.6-unit) syringe = £4.64; 0.4-mg (1.2-unit) syringe = £9.27; 0.6-mg (1.8-unit) syringe = £13.91; 0.8-mg (2.4-unit) syringe = £18.55; 1-mg (3-unit) syringe = £23.18; 1.2-mg (3.6-unit) syringe = £27.82; 1.4-mg (4.2-unit) syringe = £32.46; 1.6-mg (4.8-unit) syringe = £37.09; 1.8-mg (5.4-unit) syringe = £41.73; 2-mg (6-unit) syringe = £46.37. For subcutaneous injection

SOMATROPIN (*continued*)

Humatrope® (Lilly) PoM
Injection, powder for reconstitution, somatropin (rbe), net price 6-mg (18-unit) cartridge = £137.25; 12-mg (36-unit) cartridge = £274.50; 24-mg (72-unit) cartridge = £549.00; all supplied with diluent. For subcutaneous or intramuscular injection; cartridges for subcutaneous injection

Norditropin® (Novo Nordisk) PoM
SimpleXx injection, somatropin (epr) 3.3 mg (10 units)/mL, net price 1.5-mL (5-mg, 15-unit) cartridge = £115.90; 6.7 mg (20 units)/mL, 1.5-mL (10-mg, 30-unit) cartridge = £231.80; 10 mg (30 units)/mL, 1.5-mL (15-mg, 45-unit) cartridge = £347.70. For use with appropriate *NordiPen®* NHS device (available free of charge from clinics). For subcutaneous injection

NutropinAq (Ipsen) PoM
Injection, Somatropin (rbe), net price 10 mg (30 units) 2-mL cartridge = £215.57. For use with *NutropinAq®* Pen NHS device (available free of charge from clinics). For subcutaneous injection

Saizen® (Serono) PoM
Injection, powder for reconstitution, somatropin (rmc), net price 1.33-mg (4-unit) vial (with diluent) = £29.28; 3.33-mg (10-unit) vial (with diluent) = £73.20. For subcutaneous or intramuscular injection
Excipients: include benzyl alcohol (avoid in neonates, see Excipients, p. 3)

Click.easy®, powder for reconstitution, somatropin (rmc), net price 8-mg (24-unit) vial (in *Click.easy®* device with diluent) = £175.68. For use with *One.click®* NHS autoinjector device *or Cool.Click®* NHS needle-free device (both available free of charge from clinics). For subcutaneous injection

Zomacton® (Ferring) PoM
Injection, powder for reconstitution, somatropin (rbe), net price 4-mg (12-unit) vial (with diluent) = £81.32. For use with *ZomaJet® 2* NHS needle-free device or with *Auto-Jector®* NHS (both available free of charge from clinics) or with needles and syringes. For subcutaneous injection
Excipients: include benzyl alcohol (avoid in neonates, see Excipients, p. 3)

Hypothalamic hormones

Gonadorelin when injected intravenously in post-pubertal girls leads to a rapid rise in plasma concentrations of both luteinising hormone (LH) and follicle-stimulating hormone (FSH). It has not proved to be very helpful, however, in distinguishing hypothalamic from pituitary lesions. It is used in the assessment of delayed or precocious puberty.

Protirelin is a hypothalamic releasing hormone which stimulates the release of thyrotrophin from the pituitary. It is indicated for the diagnosis of mild hyperthyroidism or hypothyroidism, but its use has been superseded by immunoassays for thyroid-stimulating hormone. Together with other tests protirelin may also be used to confirm hypopituitarism and hypothalamic disease in children with marginally lowered thyrotrophin.

Sermorelin, an analogue of growth hormone releasing hormone (somatorelin, GHRH), is licensed as a diagnostic test for secretion of growth hormone but it is not used routinely because growth hormone deficiency may be due to hypothalmic deficiency.

Other growth hormone stimulation tests involve the use of insulin, glucagon, arginine and clonidine [all unlicensed uses]. The tests should be carried out in specialist centres.

GONADORELIN

(Gonadotrophin-releasing hormone; GnRH; LH–RH)

Cautions pituitary adenoma

Contra-indications

Pregnancy avoid

Breast-feeding avoid

Side-effects rarely nausea, headache, abdominal pain, increased menstrual bleeding; rarely, hypersensitivity reaction on repeated administration of large doses; irritation at injection site

Licensed use not licensed for use in children under 1 year

Indication and dose

Assessment of anterior pituitary function; assessment of delayed puberty
- **By subcutaneous or intravenous injection**
  Child 1–18 years 2.5 micrograms/kg (max. 100 micrograms) as a single dose

HRF® (Intrapharm) PoM
Injection, powder for reconstitution, gonadorelin. Net price 100-microgram vial (with diluent) = £13.72 (hosp. only)
Excipients: include benzyl alcohol (avoid in neonates, see Excipients p. 3)

PROTIRELIN

(Thyrotrophin-releasing hormone; TRH)

Cautions severe hypopituitarism, myocardial ischaemia, bronchial asthma and obstructive airways disease

Pregnancy use with caution as limited information available

Breast-feeding breast enlargement and leakage of milk reported

Side-effects after rapid intravenous administration desire to micturate, flushing, dizziness, nausea, abnormal taste; transient increase in pulse rate and blood pressure; rarely bronchospasm

Indication and dose

Assessment of thyroid function and thyroid stimulating hormone reserve

- By intravenous injection

Neonate 1 microgram/kg as a single dose; dose may vary—consult local protocol

Child 1 month–18 years 1 microgram/kg (max. 200 micrograms) as a single dose; dose may vary—consult local protocol

Diagnosis of hypopituitarism and hypothalamic disease

- By intravenous injection

Neonate 7 micrograms/kg as a single dose (unlicensed dose); dose may vary—consult local protocol

Child 1 month–18 years 7 micrograms/kg (max. 200 micrograms) as a single dose (unlicensed dose); dose may vary—consult local protocol

Protirelin (Cambridge) PoM

Injection, protirelin 100 micrograms/mL. Net price 2-mL amp = £9.03

SERMORELIN

Cautions epilepsy; discontinue growth hormone therapy 1–2 weeks before test; untreated hypothyroidism, antithyroid drugs; obesity, hyperglycaemia, elevated plasma fatty acids; avoid preparations which affect release of growth hormone (includes those affecting release of somatostatin, insulin or glucocorticoids and cyclo-oxygenase inhibitors such as aspirin and indometacin)

Contra-indications

Pregnancy avoid

Breast-feeding avoid

Side-effects occasional facial flushing and pain at injection site

Indication and dose

Diagnostic test for secretion of growth hormone

- By intravenous injection

Child 2–18 years 1 microgram/kg in the morning after an overnight fast

Geref 50® (Serono) PoM

Injection, powder for reconstitution, sermorelin 50 micrograms (as acetate). Net price per amp (with solvent) = £48.85

6.5.2 Posterior pituitary hormones and antagonists

Posterior pituitary hormones

Diabetes insipidus Diabetes insipidus is caused by either a deficiency of antidiuretic hormone (ADH, vasopressin) secretion (cranial, neurogenic or pituitary diabetes insipidus) or by failure of the renal tubules to react to secreted antidiuretic hormone (nephrogenic diabetes insipidus).

Vasopressin (antidiuretic hormone, ADH) is used in the treatment of *pituitary diabetes insipidus* as is its analogue **desmopressin**. Dosage is tailored to produce a regular diuresis every 24 hours to avoid water intoxication. Treatment may be required permanently or for a limited period only in diabetes insipidus following trauma or pituitary surgery.

Desmopressin is more potent and has a longer duration of action than vasopressin; unlike vasopressin it has no vasoconstrictor effect. It is given by mouth or intranasally for maintenance therapy, and by injection in the postoperative period or in unconscious patients. Desmopressin is also used in the differential diagnosis of diabetes insipidus; following an intramuscular or intranasal dose, restoration of the ability to concentrate urine after water deprivation confirms a diagnosis of pituitary diabetes insipidus. Failure to respond suggests nephrogenic diabetes insipidus. Fluid input must be managed carefully to avoid hyponatraemia; this test is not usually recommended in young children.

In *nephrogenic* and *partial pituitary diabetes insipidus* benefit may be gained from the paradoxical antidiuretic effect of thiazides (section 2.2.1) e.g. chlorothiazide 10–20 mg/kg (max. 500 mg) twice daily.

Other uses Desmopressin is also used to boost factor VIII concentration in mild to moderate haemophilia and in von Willebrand's disease; it is also used to test fibrinolyte response. For a comment on use of desmopressin in nocturnal enuresis see section 7.4.2.

Vasopressin infusion is used to control variceal bleeding in portal hypertension, before introducing more definitive treatment. Terlipressin, a derivative of vasopressin, and octreotide are used similarly but experience in children is limited.

VASOPRESSIN

Cautions heart failure, hypertension, asthma, epilepsy, migraine or other conditions which might be aggravated by water retention; renal impairment (see also Contra-indications); avoid fluid overload

Pregnancy oxytocic effect in third trimester

Breast-feeding not known to be harmful

Contra-indications vascular disease (especially disease of coronary arteries) unless extreme caution, chronic nephritis (until reasonable blood nitrogen concentrations attained)

Side-effects fluid retention, pallor, tremor, sweating, vertigo, headache, nausea, vomiting, belching, abdominal cramps, desire to defaecate, hypersensitivity reactions (including anaphylaxis), constriction of coronary arteries (may cause anginal attacks and myocardial ischaemia), peripheral ischaemia and rarely gangrene

Licensed use not licensed for use in children

Indication and dose

Specialist management only

Adjunct in acute massive haemorrhage of gastro-intestinal tract or oesophageal varices

- **By continuous intravenous infusion (may also be infused directly into the superior mesenteric artery)**

  Child 1 month–18 years initially 0.3 units/kg (max. 20 units) over 20–30 minutes *then* 0.3 units/kg/hour, adjusted according to response (max. 1 unit/kg/hour); if bleeding stops, continue at same dose for 12 hours, then withdraw gradually over 24–48 hours; max. duration of treatment 72 hours

Administration for *intravenous infusion* dilute with Glucose 5% or Sodium Chloride 0.9% to a concentration of 0.2–1 unit/mL

Synthetic vasopressin

Pitressin® (Goldshield) PoM

Injection, argipressin (synthetic vasopressin) 20 units/mL. Net price 1-mL amp = £17.14 (hosp. only)

DESMOPRESSIN

Cautions see under Vasopressin; less pressor activity, but still considerable caution in cardiovascular disease and in hypertension (not indicated for nocturnal enuresis or nocturia in these circumstances); also considerable caution in cystic fibrosis; in nocturia and nocturnal enuresis limit fluid intake from 1 hour before dose until 8 hours afterwards; in nocturia periodic blood pressure and weight checks needed to monitor for fluid overload; **interactions:** Appendix 1 (desmopressin)

Renal impairment use with caution, antidiuretic effect reduced

Pregnancy small oxytocic effect in third trimester; increased risk of pre-eclampsia

Breast-feeding concentration too low to be harmful

For cautions specifically relating to the use of desmopressin in nocturnal enuresis see section 7.4.2

Hyponatraemic convulsions The CSM has advised that patients being treated for primary nocturnal enuresis should be warned to avoid fluid overload (including during swimming) and to stop taking desmopressin during an episode of vomiting or diarrhoea (until fluid balance normal). The risk of hyponatraemic convulsions can also be minimised by keeping to the recommended starting doses and by avoiding concomitant use of drugs which increase secretion of vasopressin (e.g. tricyclic antidepressants)

Contra-indications cardiac insufficiency and other conditions treated with diuretics; psychogenic polydipsia and polydipsia in alcohol dependence

Side-effects fluid retention, and hyponatraemia (in more serious cases with convulsions) on administration without restricting fluid intake; stomach pain, headache, nausea, vomiting, allergic reactions, and emotional disturbance in children also reported; epistaxis, nasal congestion, rhinitis with nasal spray

Licensed use *intranasal* preparations not licensed for use in children for assessment of antidiuretic hormone secretion, for fibrinolytic response testing, or for haemophilia and von Willebrand's disease; *DDAVP®* intranasal solution not licensed for use in children for nocturnal enuresis; *Desmomelt®* and *Desmotab®* not licensed for use in children for treatment of diabetes insipidus; *Nocutil®* not licensed for use in children for diagnosis of diabetes insipidus; *Octim®* preparations not licensed for use in children for nocturnal enuresis, renal function testing or for treatment or diagnosis of diabetes insipidus

Indication and dose

Specialist management only

Assessment of antidiuretic hormone secretion (congenital deficiency suspected)

- **Intranasally**

  Child 1 month–2 years initially 100–500 nanograms as a single dose

DESMOPRESSIN (*continued*)

Assessment of antidiuretic hormone secretion (congenital deficiency not suspected)

- **Intranasally**

  Child 1 month–2 years 1–5 micrograms as a single dose

Test for suspected diabetes insipidus (water deprivation test)

- **Intranasally**

  Neonate not recommended, use trial of treatment

  Child 1 month–2 years 5–10 micrograms as a single dose; not usually recommended, see notes above

  Child 2–12 years 10–20 micrograms as a single dose, see notes above

  Child 12–18 years 20 micrograms as a single dose, see notes above

- **By subcutaneous or intramuscular injection**

  Neonate not recommended, use trial of treatment

  Child 1 month–2 years 400 nanograms as a single dose; not usually recommended, see notes above

  Child 2–12 years 0.5–1 microgram as a single dose, see notes above

  Child 12–18 years 1–2 micrograms as a single dose, see notes above

Diabetes insipidus, treatment

- **By mouth**

  (as desmopressin acetate)

  Neonate initially 1–4 micrograms 2–3 times daily, adjusted according to response

  Child 1 month–2 years initially 10 micrograms 2–3 times daily, adjusted according to response (range 30-150 micrograms daily)

  Child 2–12 years initially 50 micrograms 2–3 times daily, adjusted according to response (range 100-800 micrograms daily)

  Child 12–18 years initially 100 micrograms 2–3 times daily, adjusted according to response (range 0.2–1.2 mg daily)

- **Sublingually**

  (as desmopressin base)

  Child 2–18 years initially 60 micrograms 3 times daily, adjusted according to response (range 40–240 micrograms 3 times daily)

- **Intranasally**

  (as desmopressin acetate)

  Neonate initially 100–500 nanograms, adjusted according to response (range 1.25–10 micrograms daily in 1–2 divided doses)

  Child 1 month–2 years initially 2.5–5 micrograms 1–2 times daily, adjusted according to response

  Child 2–12 years initially 5–20 micrograms 1–2 times daily, adjusted according to response

  Child 12–18 years initially 10–20 micrograms 1–2 times daily, adjusted according to response

- **By subcutaneous or intramuscular injection**

  Neonate initially 100 nanograms once daily, adjusted according to response (intramuscular route only)

  Child 1 month–12 years initially 400 nanograms once daily, adjusted according to response

  Child 12–18 years initially 1–4 micrograms once daily, adjusted according to response

Primary nocturnal enuresis (if urine concentrating ability normal)

- **By mouth**

  (as desmopressin acetate)

  Child 5–18 years (preferably over 7 years) 200 micrograms at bedtime, increased to 400 micrograms at bedtime only if lower dose not effective (**important**: see also Cautions), reassess after 3 months by withdrawing treatment for at least 1 week

- **Sublingually**

  (as desmopressin base)

  Child 5–18 years (preferably over 7 years) 120 micrograms at bedtime, increased to 240 micrograms at bedtime only if lower dose not effective (**important**: see also Cautions); reassess after 3 months by withdrawing treatment for at least 1 week

- **Intranasally**

  (as desmopressin acetate)

  Child 5–18 years (preferably over 7 years) initially 20 micrograms at bedtime, increased to 40 micrograms at bedtime only if lower dose not effective (**important:** see Cautions); reassess after 3 months by withdrawing treatment for at least 1 week

Fibrinolytic response testing

- **By intravenous injection over 20 minutes or by subcutaneous injection**

  Child 2–18 years 300 nanograms/kg as a single dose; blood sampled after 20 minutes for fibrinolytic activity

Mild to moderate haemophilia and von Willebrand's disease

- **By intravenous infusion over 20 minutes or by subcutaneous injection**

  Child 1 month–18 years 300 nanograms/kg as a single dose immediately before surgery or after trauma; may be repeated at intervals of 12 hours if no tachycardia

- **Intranasally**

  Child 1–18 years 4 micrograms/kg as a single dose, for pre-operative use give 2 hours before procedure

DESMOPRESSIN (*continued*)

Renal function testing

- **Intranasally**

  Child 1 month–1 year 10 micrograms (empty bladder at time of administration and restrict fluid intake to 50% at next 2 feeds to avoid fluid overload)

  Child 1–15 years 20 micrograms (empty bladder at time of administration and restrict fluid intake to 500 mL from 1 hour before until 8 hours after administration to avoid fluid overload)

  Child 15–18 years 40 micrograms (empty bladder at time of administration and restrict fluid intake to 500 mL from 1 hour before until 8 hours after administration to avoid fluid overload)

- **By subcutaneous or intramuscular injection**

  Child 1 month–1 year 400 nanograms (empty bladder at time of administration and restrict fluid intake to 50% at next 2 feeds to avoid fluid overload)

  Child 1–18 years 2 micrograms (empty bladder at time of administration and restrict fluid intake to 500 mL from 1 hour before until 8 hours after administration to avoid fluid overload)

Desmopressin acetate (Non-proprietary) PoM

Nasal spray, desmopressin acetate 10 micrograms/metered spray, net price 6-mL unit (60 metered sprays) = £26.04. Counselling, fluid intake, see above

Brands include *Presinex®*

Note Children requiring dose of less than 10 micrograms should be given *DDAVP® intranasal solution*

DDAVP® (Ferring) PoM

Tablets, both scored, desmopressin acetate 100 micrograms, net price 90-tab pack = £45.48; 200 micrograms, 90-tab pack = £90.96. Counselling, fluid intake, see above

Note Tablets may be crushed

Sublingual tablets, (*DDAVP® Melt*), desmopressin (as acetate) 60 micrograms, net price 100-tab pack = £50.53; 120 micrograms, 100-tab pack = £101.07. Label: 26, counselling, fluid intake, see notes above

Intranasal solution, desmopressin acetate 100 micrograms/mL. Net price 2.5-mL dropper bottle and catheter = £9.72. Counselling, fluid intake, see above

Administration May be diluted with sodium chloride 0.9% to a concentration of 10 micrograms/mL

Injection, desmopressin acetate 4 micrograms/mL. Net price 1-mL amp = £1.10

Administration May be administered orally [unlicensed]; for intravenous infusion, to be diluted to a concentration not less than 1 microgram/mL as adheres to surfaces if very dilute; for higher doses used in mild to moderate haemophilia and von Willebrand's disease may be diluted with 30–50 mL sodium chloride 0.9% intravenous infusion

Desmotabs® (Ferring) PoM

Tablets, scored, desmopressin acetate 200 micrograms, net price 30-tab pack = £30.34. Counselling, fluid intake, see above

Note tablets may be crushed

Desmomelt® (Ferring) PoM

Sublingual tablets desmopressin (as acetate) 120 micrograms, net price 30-tab pack = £30.34. Label: 26, counselling, fluid intake, see above

Desmospray® (Ferring) PoM

Nasal spray, desmopressin acetate 10 micrograms/metered spray. Net price 6-mL unit (60 metered sprays) = £26.04. Counselling, fluid intake, see above

Note Children requiring dose of less than 10 micrograms should be given *DDAVP® intranasal solution*

Low dose Desmospray® PoM

Nasal spray, desmopressin acetate 2.5 micrograms/metered spray

Available from Ferring on a named-patient basis

Nocutil® (Norgine) PoM

Nasal spray, desmopressin acetate 10 micrograms/metered spray, net price 5-mL unit (50 metered sprays) = £19.69. Counselling, fluid intake, see above

Octim® (Ferring) PoM

Nasal spray, desmopressin acetate 150 micrograms/metered spray, net price 2.5-mL unit (25 metered sprays) = £600.00. Counselling, fluid intake, see above

Injection, desmopressin acetate 15 micrograms/mL, net price 1-mL amp = £20.00

Administration for *intravenous infusion* dilute with 50 mL of Sodium Chloride 0.9% and give over 20 minutes

TERLIPRESSIN

Cautions see under Vasopressin

Contra-indications see under Vasopressin

Side-effects see under Vasopressin, but effects milder

Licensed use unlicensed for use in children

Indication and dose

Specialist management only

Adjunct in acute massive haemorrhage of gastro-intestinal tract or oesophageal varices specialist use only

- **By intravenous injection**

  Child 12–18 years initially 2 mg then 1–2 mg every 4–6 hours until bleeding is controlled; max. duration of treatment 72 hours

Glypressin® (Ferring) PoM

Injection, terlipressin, powder for reconstitution. Net price 1-mg vial with 5 mL diluent = £19.44 (hosp. only)

6.6 Drugs affecting bone metabolism

The two disorders of bone metabolism that occur in children are rickets and osteoporosis. The two most common forms of rickets are Vitamin D deficiency rickets (section 9.6.4) and hypophosphataemic rickets (section 9.5.2). See also calcium (section 9.5.1.1).

Osteoporosis

Osteoporosis in children may be primary (e.g. *osteogenesis imperfecta* and *idiopathic juvenile osteoporosis*), or secondary (e.g. due to inflammatory disorders, immobilisation, or corticosteroids); specialist management is required

Corticosteroid-induced osteoporosis To reduce the risk of osteoporosis doses of oral corticosteroids should be as low as possible and courses of treatment as short as possible.

6.6.1 Calcitonin

Calcitonin is involved with parathyroid hormone in the regulation of bone turnover and hence in the maintenance of calcium balance and homeostasis. **Calcitonin (salmon) (salcatonin**, synthetic or recombinant salmon calcitonin) is used to lower the plasma-calcium concentration in some patients with hypercalcaemia (notably when associated with malignant disease).

CALCITONIN (SALMON)/SALCATONIN

Cautions history of allergy (skin test advised); renal impairment; heart failure; children—use for short periods only and monitor bone growth

Pregnancy avoid unless essential, toxicity in *animal* studies

Breast-feeding avoid unless essential, may inhibit lactation

Contra-indications hypocalaemia

Side-effects nausea, vomiting, diarrhoea, abdominal pain, flushing, dizziness, headache, taste disturbances; musculoskeletal pain; with nasal spray nose and throat irritation, rhinitis, sinusitis and epistaxis; *less commonly* diuresis, oedema, cough, visual disturbances, injection-site reactions, rash, hypersensitivity reactions including pruritus

Licensed use not licensed in children

Indication and dose

Specialist management only

Hypercalcaemia (experience limited in children)
- **By subcutaneous or intramuscular injection**
  Child 1 month–18 years 2.5–5 units/kg every 12 hours, max. 400 units every 6–8 hours, adjusted according to response (no additional benefit with over 8 units/kg every 6 hours)
- **By slow intravenous infusion**
  Child 1 month–18 years 5–10 units/kg over at least 6 hours

Osteoporosis
Refer for specialist advice, experience very limited

Administration for *intravenous infusion*, dilute injection solution (e.g. 400 units in 500 mL) with Sodium Chloride 0.9% and give over at least 6 hours; glass or hard plastic containers should not be used; some loss of potency on dilution and administration—use diluted solution without delay

Miacalcic® (Novartis) PoM
Nasal spray ▼, calcitonin (salmon) 200 units/metered spray, net price 2-mL unit (approx. 14 metered sprays) = £20.99

Injection, calcitonin (salmon) 50 units/mL, net price 1-mL amp = £4.27; 100 units/mL, 1-mL amp = £8.55; 200 units/mL, 2-mL vial = £30.75

6.6.2 Bisphosphonates

Bisphosphonates are adsorbed onto hydroxyapatite crystals in bone, slowing both their rate of growth and dissolution, and therefore reducing the rate of bone turnover.

A bisphosphonate such as **disodium pamidronate** is used in the management of severe forms of *osteogenesis imperfecta* and other causes of osteoporosis in children to reduce the number of fractures; the long-term effects of bisphosphonates in children have not been established. Single doses of biphosphonates are also used to manage hypercalaemia (section 9.5.1.2). Treatment should be initiated under specialist advice **only**.

ALENDRONIC ACID

Cautions upper gastro-intestinal disorders (dysphagia, symptomatic oesophageal disease, gastritis, duodenitis, or ulcers—see also under Contra-indications and Side-effects); history (within 1 year) of ulcers, active gastro-intestinal bleeding, or surgery of the upper gastro-intestinal tract; correct disturbances of calcium and mineral metabolism (e.g. vitamin-D deficiency, hypocalcaemia) before starting and monitor serum calcium during treatment; exclude other causes of osteoporosis; **interactions:** Appendix 1 (bisphosphonates)

Renal impairment manufacturer advises avoid if creatinine clearance is less than 35 mL/minute/ 1.73 m^2

Contra-indications abnormalities of oesophagus and other factors which delay emptying (e.g. stricture or achalasia), hypocalcaemia,

Pregnancy manufacturer advises avoid

Breast-feeding no information available

Side-effects oesophageal reactions (see below), abdominal pain and distension, dyspepsia, regurgitation, melaena, diarrhoea or constipation, flatulence, musculoskeletal pain, headache; *rarely* rash, pruritus, erythema, photosensitivity, uveitis, scleritis, transient decrease in serum phosphate; nausea, vomiting, gastritis, peptic ulceration and hypersensitivity reactions (including urticaria and angioedema) also reported; myalgia, malaise and fever at initiation of treatment; *very rarely* severe skin reactions (including Stevens-Johnson syndrome)

Oesophageal reactions Severe oesophageal reactions (oesophagitis, oesophageal ulcers, oesophageal stricture and oesophageal erosions) have been reported; patients should be advised to stop taking the tablets and to seek medical attention if they develop symptoms of oesophageal irritation such as dysphagia, new or worsening heartburn, pain on swallowing or retrosternal pain

Licensed use not licensed for use in children

Indication and dose

See notes above, specialist use only

Counselling Swallow the tablets whole with a full glass of water on an empty stomach at least 30 minutes before breakfast (and any other oral medication); stand or sit upright for at least 30 minutes and do not lie down until after eating breakfast. Do not take the tablets at bedtime or before rising.

Fosamax® (MSD) PoM
Tablets, alendronic acid (as sodium alendronate) 5 mg, net price 28-tab pack = £25.43; 10 mg, 28-tab pack = £23.12. Counselling, administration

Fosamax® Once Weekly (MSD) PoM
Tablets, alendronic acid (as sodium alendronate) 70 mg, net price 4-tab pack = £22.80. Counselling, administration

DISODIUM PAMIDRONATE

Disodium pamidronate was formerly called aminohydroxypropylidenediphosphonate disodium (APD)

Cautions cardiac disease; previous thyroid surgery (risk of hypocalcaemia); monitor serum electrolytes, calcium and phosphate—possibility of convulsions due to electrolyte changes; avoid concurrent use with other bisphosphonates; **interactions:** Appendix 1 (bisphosphonates)

Hepatic impairment manufacturer advises caution in severe impairment—no information available

Renal impairment monitor renal function in renal disease or predisposition to renal impairment (e.g. in tumour-induced hypercalcaemia)

Osteonecrosis of the jaw Osteonecrosis of the jaw reported in adult cancer patients being treated with bisphosphonate; consider dental examination and preventative treatment before initiating bisphosphonate; avoid invasive dental procedures during treatment

Skilled tasks Patients should be warned against driving, cycling or performing skilled tasks immediately after treatment (somnolence or dizziness may occur)

Contra-indications

Pregnancy manufacturer advises avoid

Breast-feeding manufacturer advises avoid

Side-effects hypophosphataemia, transient rise in body temperature, fever and influenza-like symptoms (sometimes accompanied by malaise, rigors, fatigue and flushes); arthralgia, myalgia, nausea, vomiting, headache, lymphocytopenia, hypomagnesaemia; rarely muscle cramps, anorexia, abdominal pain, diarrhoea, constipation, dyspepsia, agitation, confusion, dizziness, insomnia, somnolence, lethargy, anaemia, leucopenia, hypotension or hypertension, rash, pruritus, symptomatic hypocalcaemia (paraesthesia, tetany), hyperkalaemia or hypokalaemia, hypernatraemia; osteonecrosis (see also Cautions above), isolated cases of seizures, hallucinations, thrombocytopenia, haematuria, acute renal failure, deterioration of renal disease, conjunctivitis and other ocular symptoms, reactivation of herpes simplex and zoster also reported; also local reactions at injection site

Licensed use not licensed for use in children

Indication and dose

See notes above, specialist use only

Disodium pamidronate (Non-proprietary) PoM
Concentrate for intravenous infusion, disodium pamidronate 3 mg/mL, net price 5-mL vial = £27.50, 10-mL vial = £55.00; 6 mg/mL, 10-mL vial = £110.00; 9 mg/mL, 10-mL vial = £165.00

Aredia Dry Powder® (Novartis) PoM
Injection, powder for reconstitution, disodium pamidronate, for use as an infusion. Net price 15-mg vial = £29.83; 30-mg vial = £59.66; 90-mg vial = £170.45 (all with diluent)

RISEDRONATE SODIUM

Cautions oesophageal abnormalities and other factors which delay transit or emptying (e.g. stricture or achalasia—see also under Side-effects); correct hypocalcaemia before starting, correct other disturbances of bone and mineral metabolism (e.g. Vitamin-D deficiency) at onset of treatment; interactions: Appendix 1 (bisphosphonates)

Renal impairment manufacturer advises avoid if creatinine clearance is less than 30 mL/minute/ 1.73 m^2

Contra-indications hypocalcaemia (see Cautions above)

Pregnancy manufacturer advises avoid

Breast-feeding manufacturer advises avoid

Side-effects gastro-intestinal effects (including abdominal pain, dyspepsia, nausea, diarrhoea, constipation); dizziness, headache; influenza-like symptoms, musculoskeletal pain; *rarely* oesophageal stricture, oesophagitis, oesophageal ulcer, dysphagia, gastritis, duodenitis, glossitis, peripheral oedema, weight loss, myasthenia, arthralgia, apnoea, bronchitis, sinusitis, rash, nocturia, ambylopia, corneal lesion, dry eye, tinnitus, iritis; *very rarely* hypersensitivity reactions including angioedema

Licensed use not licensed for use in children

Indication and dose

See notes above, specialist use only

Counselling Swallow tablets whole with full glass of water; on rising, take on an empty stomach at least 30 minutes before first food or drink of the day or, if taking at any other time of the day, avoid food and drink for at least 2 hours before or after risedronate (particularly avoid calcium containing products e.g. milk, also avoid iron and mineral supplements and antacids); stand or sit upright for at least 30 minutes; do not take tablets at bedtime or before rising

Actonel® (Procter & Gamble Pharm.) PoM
Tablets, f/c, risedronate sodium 5 mg (yellow), net price 28-tab pack = £19.10; 30 mg (white), 28-tab pack = £152.81. Counselling, administration, food, and calcium (see above)

Actonel Once a Week® (Procter & Gamble Pharm.) PoM
Tablets, f/c, risedronate sodium 35 mg (orange), net price 4-tab pack = £20.30. Counselling, administration, food and calcium (see above)

SODIUM CLODRONATE

Cautions monitor renal and hepatic function and white cell count; also monitor serum calcium and phosphate periodically; renal dysfunction reported in patients receiving concomitant NSAIDs; maintain adequate fluid intake during treatment; **interactions:** Appendix 1 (bisphosphonates)

Contra-indications

Renal impairment contra-indicated in moderate to severe renal impairment

Pregnancy manufacturer advises avoid

Breast-feeding no information available

Side-effects nausea, diarrhoea; skin reactions

Licensed use not licensed for use in children

Indication and dose

See notes above, specialist use only

Bonefos® (Schering Health) PoM
Capsules, yellow, sodium clodronate 400 mg. Net price 30-cap pack = £40.49, 120-cap pack = £161.97. Counselling, food and calcium (see risedronate)

Tablets, f/c, scored, sodium clodronate 800 mg. Net price 10-tab pack = £28.27; 60-tab pack = £169.62. Counselling, food and calcium (see risedronate)

Concentrate (= intravenous solution), sodium clodronate 60 mg/mL, for dilution and use as infusion. Net price 5-mL amp = £12.82

Loron® (Roche) PoM
Loron 520® tablets, f/c, scored, sodium clodronate 520 mg. Net price 60-tab pack = £161.99. Label: 10, patient information leaflet., Counselling, food and calcium

6.7 Other endocrine drugs

6.7.1 Bromocriptine and other dopaminergic drugs

Classification not used in BNF for Children

6.7.2 Drugs affecting gonadotrophins

Classification not used in BNF for Children. See section 6.4.3 for use in precocious puberty.

6.7.3 Metyrapone

Metyrapone is a competitive inhibitor of 11β-hydroxylation in the adrenal cortex; the resulting inhibition of cortisol (and to a lesser extent aldosterone) production leads to an increase in ACTH production which, in turn, leads to increased synthesis and release of cortisol precursors. It may be used as a test of anterior pituitary function.

Most types of *Cushing's syndrome* are treated surgically. Metyrapone may be useful to control the symptoms of the disease or to prepare the child for surgery. The dosages used are either low, and tailored to cortisol production, or high, in which case corticosteroid replacement therapy is also needed.

Ketoconazole (section 5.2) is also used by specialists for the management of *Cushing's syndrome* [unlicensed indication].

METYRAPONE

Cautions gross hypopituitarism (risk of precipitating acute adrenal failure); hypertension on long-term administration; hypothyroidism or hepatic impairment (delayed response); many drugs interfere with diagnostic estimation of steroids; avoid in porphyria (section 9.8.2)

Skilled tasks Drowsiness may affect the performance of skilled tasks (e.g. driving)

Contra-indications adrenocortical insufficiency (see Cautions)

Pregnancy contra-indicated

Breast-feeding contra-indicated

Side-effects occasional nausea, vomiting, dizziness, headache, hypotension, sedation; rarely abdominal pain, allergic skin reactions, hypoadrenalism, hirsutism

Licensed use licensed for use in children

Indication and dose

Differential diagnosis of ACTH-dependent Cushing's syndrome
- By mouth

Child 1 month–18 years 15 mg/kg (or 300 mg/m^2) every 4 hours for 6 doses; minimum dose 250 mg every 4 hours, max. 750 mg every 4 hours

Management of Cushing's syndrome
- By mouth

range 250 mg–6 g daily, adjusted according to cortisol production; see notes above

Metopirone® (Alliance) PoM

Capsules, ivory, metyrapone 250 mg. Net price 100-tab pack = £41.44. Label: 21, counselling, driving

6 Endocrine system

7 Obstetrics, gynaecology, and urinary-tract disorders

7.1 Drugs used in obstetrics

This section is not included in BNF-C. See BNF for management of obstetrics.

For the management of ductus arteriosus see section 2.14

7.2 Treatment of vaginal and vulval conditions

7.2.1 Preparations for vaginal atrophy
7.2.2 Vaginal and vulval infections

Pre-pubertal girls may be particularly susceptible to vulvovaginitis. Barrier preparations (section 13.2.2) applied after cleansing may be useful when the symptoms are due to non-specific irritation, but systemic drugs are required in the treatment of bacterial infection (section 5.1) or threadworm infestation (section 5.5.1). Intravaginal preparations, particularly those that require the use of an applicator, are not generally suitable for young girls, topical preparations may be useful in some adolescent girls.

In older girls symptoms are often restricted to the vulva, but infections almost invariably involve the vagina, which should also be treated; treatment should be as for adults (see BNF section 7.2).

7.2.1 Preparations for vaginal atrophy

Topical oestrogen creams are used in the treatment of labial adhesions (for preparations, see BNF section 7.2.1)

7.2.2 Vaginal and vulval infections

Effective specific treatments are available for the common vaginal infections.

Fungal infections

Vaginal fungal infections are not normally a problem in younger girls but may occur in adolescents. *Candidal vulvitis* can be treated locally with cream but is almost invariably associated with vaginal infection which should also be treated. *Vaginal candidiasis* may be treated with antifungal pessaries or cream inserted high into the vagina (including during menstruation), however, these are not recommended for younger girls and oral treatment (section 5.2) may be more appropriate. Single-dose intravaginal preparations offer an advantage when compliance is a problem. Local irritation may occur on application of vaginal antifungal products.

Imidazole drugs (clotrimazole, econazole, and miconazole) are effective against candida in short courses of 1 to 14 days according to the preparation used. Vaginal applications may be supplemented with antifungal cream for vulvitis and to treat other superficial sites of infection.

Nystatin is a well established antifungal drug. A cream is used in cases of vulvitis and infection of other superficial sites. Nystatin stains clothing yellow.

Oral treatment of vaginal infection with fluconazole or itraconazole (section 5.2) may be considered; oral ketoconazole has been associated with fatal hepatotoxicity (see section 5.2 for CSM warning).

Recurrent vulvovaginal candidiasis Recurrence of vulvovaginal candidiasis is particularly likely if there are predisposing factors such as antibacterial therapy, pregnancy, diabetes mellitus, and possibly oral contraceptive use. Reservoirs of infection may also lead to recontamination and should be treated; these include other skin sites such as the digits, nail beds, and umbilicus as well as the gastro-intestinal tract and the bladder. The sexual partner may also be the source of re-infection and, if symptomatic, should be treated with cream at the same time.

Treatment against candida may need to be extended for 6 months in recurrent vulvovaginal candidiasis. Some recommended regimens suitable for older children [all unlicensed] include:

- fluconazole (section 5.2) by mouth 100 mg (as a single dose) every week for 6 months
- clotrimazole vaginally 500-mg pessary (as a single dose) every week for 6 months.

PREPARATIONS FOR VAGINAL AND VULVAL CANDIDIASIS

Note Intravaginal preparations, particularly those that require use of an applicator, should be avoided in young girls unless there is no other alternative

Side-effects occasional local irritation

Licensed use consult product literature for the licensing status of individual preparations

Indication and dose

See notes above.

Clotrimazole (Non-proprietary)

Cream (topical), clotrimazole 1%, net price 20 g = £2.29, 50 g = £3.80
Condoms: effect on latex condoms and diaphragms not yet known

Dose

Apply to anogenital area 2–3 times daily

Pessary, clotrimazole 500 mg, net price 1 pessary with applicator = £3.26

Dose

Insert 1 at night as a single dose

Canesten® (Bayer Consumer Care)

Cream (topical), clotrimazole 1%. Net price 20 g = £2.14; 50 g = £3.80
Excipients: include benzyl alcohol, cetostearyl alcohol, polysorbates
Condoms: damages latex condoms and diaphragms

Dose

Apply to anogenital area 2–3 times daily

Thrush Cream (topical), clotrimazole 2%, net price 20 g = £3.42
Excipients: include benzyl alcohol, cetostearyl alcohol, polysorbates
Condoms: damages latex condoms and diaphragms

Dose

Apply to anogenital area 2–3 times daily

Vaginal cream (*10% VC®*) PoM, clotrimazole 10%. Net price 5-g applicator pack = £4.50
Excipients: include benzyl alcohol, cetostearyl alcohol, polysorbates
Condoms: damages latex condoms and diaphragms

Dose

Insert 5 g at night as a single dose; may be repeated once if necessary

Note Brands for sale to the public include *Canesten® Internal Cream*

Pessaries, clotrimazole 100 mg, net price 6 pessaries with applicator = £3.30; 200 mg, 3 pessaries with applicator = £3.30
Condoms: damages latex condoms and diaphragms

Dose

Insert 200 mg for 3 nights *or* 100 mg for 6 nights

Pessary, clotrimazole 500 mg. Net price 1 with applicator = £3.48
Excipients: none as listed in section 13.1.3
Condoms: damages latex condoms and diaphragms

Dose

Insert 1 at night as a single dose

Combi, clotrimazole 500-mg pessary and cream (topical) 2%. Net price 1 pessary and 10 g cream = £4.74
Condoms: damages latex condoms and diaphragms

PREPARATIONS FOR VAGINAL AND VULVAL CANDIDIASIS (*continued*)

Ecostatin® (Squibb)
Cream (topical), econazole nitrate 1%. Net price 15 g = £1.49; 30 g = £2.75
Excipients: include butylated hydroxyanisole, fragrance
Condoms: damages latex condoms and diaphragms

Dose

Apply to anogenital area twice daily

Pessaries PoM, econazole nitrate 150 mg. Net price 3 with applicator = £3.35
Excipients: none as listed in section 13.1.3
Condoms: damages latex condoms and diaphragms

Dose

Insert 1 pessary for 3 nights

Pessary (*Ecostatin 1®*) PoM, econazole nitrate 150 mg, formulated for single-dose therapy. Net price 1 pessary with applicator = £3.35
Excipients: none as listed in section 13.1.3
Condoms: damages latex condoms and diaphragms

Dose

Insert 1 pessary at night as a single dose

Twinpack PoM, econazole nitrate 150-mg pessaries and cream 1%. Net price 3 pessaries and 15 g cream = £4.35
Condoms: damages latex condoms and diaphragms

Gyno-Daktarin® (Janssen-Cilag) PoM
Intravaginal cream, miconazole nitrate 2%. Net price 78 g with applicators = £4.70
Excipients: include butylated hydroxyanisole
Condoms: damages latex condoms and diaphragms

Dose

Insert 5-g applicatorful once daily for 10–14 days *or* twice daily for 7 days; *topical*, apply to anogenital area twice daily

Pessaries, miconazole nitrate 100 mg. Net price 14 = £3.18
Excipients: none as listed in section 13.1.3
Condoms: damages latex condoms and diaphragms

Dose

Insert 1 pessary daily for 14 days or 1 pessary twice daily for 7 days

Combipack, miconazole nitrate 100-mg pessaries and cream (topical) 2%. Net price 14 pessaries and 15 g cream = £4.13
Condoms: damages latex condoms and diaphragms

Ovule (= vaginal capsule) (*Gyno-Daktarin 1®*), miconazole nitrate 1.2 g in a fatty basis. Net price 1 ovule (with finger stall) = £3.18
Excipients: include hydroxybenzoates (parabens)
Condoms: damages latex condoms and diaphragms

Dose

Insert 1 ovule at night as a single dose

Gyno-Pevaryl® (Janssen-Cilag) PoM
Cream, econazole nitrate 1%. Net price 15 g = £1.43; 30 g = £3.28
Excipients: none as listed in section 13.1.3
Condoms: damages latex condoms and diaphragms

Dose

Insert 5-g applicatorful intravaginally and apply to vulva at night for at least 14 nights

Pessaries, econazole nitrate 150 mg. Net price 3 pessaries = £3.01
Excipients: none as listed in section 13.1.3
Condoms: damages latex condoms and diaphragms

Dose

Insert 1 pessary for 3 nights

Pessary (*Gyno-Pevaryl 1®*), econazole nitrate 150 mg, formulated for single-dose therapy. Net price 1 pessary with applicator = £3.20
Excipients: none as listed in section 13.1.3
Condoms: damages latex condoms and diaphragms

Dose

Insert 1 pessary at night as a single dose

Combipack, econazole nitrate 150-mg pessaries, econazole nitrate 1% cream. Net price 3 pessaries and 15 g cream = £4.13
Condoms: damages latex condoms and diaphragms

CP pack (*Gyno-Pevaryl 1®*), econazole nitrate 150-mg pessary, econazole nitrate 1% cream. Net price 1 pessary and 15 g cream = £4.13
Condoms: damages latex condoms and diaphragms

Nizoral® (Janssen-Cilag) PoM
Cream (topical), ketoconazole 2%. Net price 30 g = £3.62
Excipients: include polysorbates, propylene glycol, stearyl alcohol

Dose

Apply to anogenital area once or twice daily

Nystan® (Squibb) PoM
Cream and Ointment, see section 13.10.2

Vaginal cream, nystatin 100 000 units/4-g application. Net price 60 g with applicator = £2.77
Excipients: include benzyl alcohol, propylene glycol
Condoms: damages latex condoms and diaphragms

Dose

Insert 1–2 applicatorfuls at night for at least 14 nights

Pessaries, yellow, nystatin 100 000 units. Net price 28-pessary pack = £1.96
Excipients: none as listed in section 13.1.3
Condoms: no evidence of damage to latex condoms and diaphragms

Dose

Insert 1–2 pessaries at night for at least 14 nights

Pevaryl® (Janssen-Cilag)
Cream, econazole nitrate 1%. Net price 30 g = £2.65
Excipients: include butylated hydroxyanisole, fragrance
Condoms: effect on latex condoms and diaphragms not yet known

Dose

Apply to anogenital area twice daily

Other infections

Trichomonal infections commonly involve the lower urinary tract as well as the genital system and need systemic treatment with metronidazole (section 5.1.11) or tinidazole (section 5.4.2).

Bacterial infections with Gram-negative organisms are particularly common in association with gynaecological operations and trauma. Metronidazole is effective against certain Gram-negative organisms, especially *Bacteroides* spp. and may be used prophylactically in gynaecological surgery.

Topical vaginal products containing povidone–iodine can be used to treat vaginitis due to candidal, trichomonal, non-specific or mixed infections; they are also used for the pre-operative preparation of the vagina. Clindamycin cream and metronidazole gel are also indicated for bacterial vaginosis.

The antiviral drugs aciclovir, famciclovir, and valaciclovir may be used in the treatment of genital infection due to *herpes simplex virus*, the HSV type 2 being a major cause of genital ulceration. They have a beneficial effect on virus shedding and healing, generally giving relief from pain and other symptoms. See section 5.3 for systemic preparations, and section 13.10.3 for topical preparations.

PREPARATIONS FOR OTHER VAGINAL INFECTIONS

Betadine® (Medlock)

Cautions avoid regular use in thyroid disorders

Renal impairment in severe impairment avoid regular application to inflamed or broken mucosa

Pregnancy avoid; sufficient iodine may be absorbed to affect the fetal thyroid

Breast-feeding avoid; iodine absorbed from vaginal preparations is concentrated in milk

Side-effects rarely sensitivity; may interfere with thyroid function

Licensed use Not licensed for use in pre-pubertal children

Vaginal Cleansing Kit, solution, povidone-iodine 10%. Net price 250 mL with measuring bottle and applicator = £2.79

Excipients: include fragrance

Condoms: effect on latex condoms and diaphragms not yet known

Dose

To be diluted and used once daily, preferably in the morning; may be used with Betadine® pessaries or vaginal gel (consult product literature)

Pessaries, brown, povidone-iodine 200 mg. Net price 28 pessaries with applicator = £6.06

Condoms: effect on latex condoms and diaphragms not yet known

Dalacin® (Pharmacia) PoM

Cream, clindamycin 2% (as phosphate). Net price 40-g pack with 7 applicators = £10.86

Excipients: include benzyl alcohol, cetostearyl alcohol, polysorbates, propylene glycol

Condoms: damages latex condoms and diaphragms

Side-effects irritation, cervicitis and vaginitis; poorly absorbed into the blood—very low likelihood of systemic effects (section 5.1.6)

Licensed use Not licensed for use in children under 12 years

Dose

Bacterial vaginosis, insert 5-g applicatorful at night for 3–7 nights

Zidoval® (3M) PoM

Vaginal gel, metronidazole 0.75%. Net price 40-g pack with 5 applicators = £4.31

Excipients: include disodium edetate, hydroxybenzoates (parabens), propylene glycol

Cautions not recommended during menstruation; some absorption may occur, see section 5.1.11 for systemic effects

Side-effects local effects including irritation, candidiasis, abnormal discharge, pelvic discomfort

Licensed use Not licensed for use in children under 18 years

Dose

Bacterial vaginosis, insert 5-g applicatorful at night for 5 nights

7.3 Contraceptives

This section is not included in BNF for Children. See BNF for full information.

7.4 Drugs for genito-urinary disorders

For drugs used in the treatment of urinary-tract infections see section 5.1.13.

7.4.1 Drugs for urinary retention

Acute retention is painful and is treated by catheterisation.

Chronic retention is painless and often long-standing. Clean intermittent catheterisation may be considered. After the cause has been established and treated, drugs may be required to increase detrusor muscle tone.

7.4.2 Drugs for urinary frequency, enuresis, and incontinence

Urinary incontinence

Involuntary detrusor contractions cause urgency and urge incontinence, usually with frequency and nocturia. Antimuscarinic drugs reduce these contractions and increase bladder capacity; **oxybutynin** also has a direct relaxant effect on urinary smooth muscle. Oxybutynin may be considered first for children under 12 years. Side-effects limit the use of oxybutynin but they may be reduced by starting at a lower dose and then slowly titrating upwards; alternatively oxybutynin can be given by intravesicular instillation. **Tolterodine** is also effective for urinary incontinence; it may be considered for children over 12 years, or for younger children who have failed to respond to oxybutynin. Modified-release preparations of oxybutynin and tolterodine are available; they may have fewer side-effects. Antimuscarinic treatment should be reviewed soon after it is commenced, and then at regular intervals; a response generally occurs within 6 months but occasionally may take longer.

Cautions Antimuscarinic drugs should be used with caution in autonomic neuropathy and in hepatic or renal impairment. Antimuscarinics may worsen hyperthyroidism, congestive heart failure, arrhythmias, and tachycardia. For **interactions** see Appendix 1 (antimuscarinics).

Contra-indications Antimuscarinic drugs should be avoided in myasthenia gravis, significant bladder outflow obstruction or urinary retention, severe ulcerative colitis, toxic megacolon, and in gastro-intestinal obstruction or intestinal atony.

Side-effects Side-effects of antimuscarinic drugs include dry mouth, gastro-intestinal disturbances including constipation, blurred vision, dry eyes, drowsiness, difficulty in micturition (less commonly urinary retention), palpitation, and skin reactions (including dry skin, rash, and photosensitivity); also headache, diarrhoea, angioedema, arrhythmias, and tachycardia. Central nervous system stimulation, such as restlessness, disorientation, hallucination, and convulsion may occur. Antimuscarinic drugs may reduce sweating leading to heat sensations and fainting in hot environments or in patients with fever.

OXYBUTYNIN HYDROCHLORIDE

Cautions see also notes above; porphyria (section 9.8.2); **interactions:** see Appendix 1 (antimuscarinics)

Hepatic impairment manufacturer advises caution

Renal impairment manufacturer advises caution

Pregnancy manufacturer advises avoid unless potential benefit outweighs risk

Breast-feeding present in milk—manufacturer advises avoid

Contra-indications see notes above

Side-effects see notes above; also anorexia, facial flushing (more marked in children) and dizziness

Licensed use not licensed for use in children under 5 years; modified-release preparation not licensed for use in children; intravesical instillation not licensed

Indication and dose

Urinary frequency, urgency and incontinence, neurogenic bladder instability

- **By mouth**

  Child 2–5 years 1.25–2.5 mg 2–3 times daily;

  Child 5–18 years 2.5–3 mg twice daily increased to 5 mg 2–3 times daily

- **By intravesical instillation**

  Child 2–18 years 5 mg 2–3 times daily

Nocturnal enuresis associated with over-active bladder

- **By mouth**

  Child 7–18 years 2.5–3 mg twice daily increased to 5 mg 2–3 times daily (last dose before bedtime)

OXYBUTYNIN HYDROCHLORIDE (*continued*)

Oxybutynin Hydrochloride (Non-proprietary) PoM
Tablets, oxybutynin hydrochloride 2.5 mg, net price 56-tab pack = £5.04; 3 mg, 56-tab pack = £9.15; 5 mg, 56-tab pack = £10.26, 84-tab pack = £3.21. Label: 3

Intravesical instillation, oxybutynin (as hydrochloride) 5 mg/30 mL, net price 30-mL vial = £3.30
Available on a named-patient basis from Sanofi-Aventis

Cystrin® (Sanofi-Synthelabo) PoM
Tablets, oxybutynin hydrochloride 3 mg, net price 56-tab pack = £9.15; 5 mg (scored), 84-tab pack = £22.88. Label: 3

Ditropan® (Sanofi-Synthelabo) PoM
Tablets, both blue, scored, oxybutynin hydrochloride 2.5 mg, net price 84-tab pack = £6.86; 5 mg, 84-tab pack = £13.34. Label: 3

Elixir, oxybutynin hydrochloride 2.5 mg/5 mL. Net price 150-mL pack= £4.78. Label: 3

Modified release

Lyrinel® XL (Janssen-Cilag) PoM
Tablets, m/r, oxybutynin hydrochloride 5 mg (yellow), net price 30-tab pack = £12.34; 10 mg (pink), 30-tab pack = £24.68. Label: 3, 25

Note Children taking immediate-release oxybutynin may be transferred to the nearest equivalent daily dose of *Lyrinel® XL*

TOLTERODINE TARTRATE

Cautions see notes above; **interactions:** see Appendix 1 (antimuscarinics)

Contra-indications see notes above

Hepatic impairment reduce dose

Renal impairment reduce dose if creatinine clearance less than 30 mL/minute/1.73 m²

Pregnancy manufacturer advises avoid—toxicity in *animal* studies

Breast-feeding manufacturer advises avoid—no information available

Side-effects see notes above; also dyspepsia, fatigue, flatulence, chest pain, dry eyes, peripheral oedema, paraesthesia

Licensed use not licensed for use in children

Indication and dose

Urinary frequency, urgency, incontinence
- **By mouth**

Child 2–18 years 1 mg once daily, increase according to response to max. 2 mg twice daily

Detrusitol® (Pharmacia) PoM
Tablets, f/c, tolterodine tartrate 1 mg, net price 56-tab pack = £29.03; 2 mg, 56-tab pack = £30.56

Modified release

Detrusitol® XL (Pharmacia) PoM
Capsules, blue, m/r, tolterodine tartrate 4 mg, net price 28-cap pack = £29.03. Label: 25

Nocturnal enuresis

Nocturnal enuresis is a common occurrence in young children but persists in as many as 5% by 10 years of age. Treatment is not appropriate in children under 5 years and it is usually not needed in those aged under 7 years and in cases where the child and parents are not anxious about the bedwetting; however, children over 10 years usually require prompt treatment. An **enuresis alarm** should be first-line treatment for well-motivated children aged over 7 years because it may achieve a more sustained reduction of enuresis than use of drugs. Use of an alarm may be combined with drug therapy if either method alone is unsuccessful.

Drug therapy is not usually appropriate for children under 7 years of age; it can be used when alternative measures have failed, preferably on a short-term basis, for example to cover periods away from home. The possible side-effects of the various drugs should be borne in mind when they are prescribed.

Desmopressin (section 6.5.2), an analogue of vasopressin, is used for nocturnal enuresis; it is given intranasally or it may be given by mouth as tablets. Particular care is needed to avoid fluid overload and treatment should not be continued for longer than 3 months without stopping for a week for full reassessment. When stopping treatment with desmopressin gradual withdrawal may be considered. An antimuscarinic drug is used for managing symptoms of detrusor overactivity (section 7.4.2); specific additional measures may be required if night-time symptoms also need to be controlled.

Tricyclics (section 4.3.1) such as **amitriptyline**, **imipramine**, and less often **nortriptyline** are also used but behaviour disturbances may occur and relapse is common after withdrawal. Treatment should not normally exceed 3 months unless a full physical examination is given and the child is fully reassessed; toxicity following overdosage with tricyclics is of particular concern.

7.4.3 Drugs used in urological pain

Lidocaine (lignocaine) gel is a useful topical application in *urethral pain* or to relieve the discomfort of catheterisation (section 15.2).

Alkalinisation of urine

Alkalinisation of urine may be undertaken with **potassium citrate**. The alkalinising action may relieve the discomfort of *cystitis* caused by lower urinary tract infections.

POTASSIUM CITRATE

Cautions renal impairment, cardiac disease; **interactions:** Appendix 1 (potassium salts)

Side-effects hyperkalaemia on prolonged high dosage, mild diuresis

Indication and dose

Relief of discomfort in mild urinary-tract infections, alkalinisation of urine
for dose see preparations below

Potassium Citrate Mixture BP (Potassium Citrate Oral Solution)
Oral solution, potassium citrate 30%, citric acid monohydrate 5% in a suitable vehicle with a lemon flavour. Extemporaneous preparations should be recently prepared according to the following formula: potassium citrate 3 g, citric acid monohydrate 500 mg, syrup 2.5 mL, quillaia tincture 0.1 mL, lemon spirit 0.05 mL, double-strength chloroform water 3 mL, water to 10 mL. Contains about 28 mmol K^+/10 mL. Label: 27

Dose

Child 1–6 years 5 mL 3 times daily well diluted with water

Child 6–18 years 10 mL 3 times daily well diluted with water

Note Concentrates for preparation of Potassium Citrate Mixture BP are available from Hillcross
Proprietary brands of potassium citrate on sale to the public for the relief of discomfort in mild urinary-tract infections include *Cystopurin*® and *Effercitrate*®

7.4.4 Bladder instillations and urological surgery

Bladder infection Various solutions are available as irrigations or washouts.

Aqueous **chlorhexidine** (section 13.11.2) may be used in the management of common infections of the bladder but it is ineffective against most *Pseudomonas* spp. Solutions containing chlorhexidine 1 in 5000 (0.02%) are used but they may irritate the mucosa and cause burning and haematuria (in which case they should be discontinued); sterile **sodium chloride solution 0.9%** (physiological saline) is usually adequate and is preferred as a mechanical irrigant.

Dissolution of blood clots Clot retention is usually treated by irrigation with sterile **sodium chloride solution 0.9%** but sterile **sodium citrate solution for bladder irrigation 3%** may also be helpful.

Maintenance of indwelling urinary catheters

The deposition which occurs in catheterised patients is usually chiefly composed of phosphate and to minimise this the catheter (if latex) should be changed at least as often as every 6 weeks. If the catheter is to be left for longer periods a silicone catheter should be used together with the appropriate use of catheter maintenance solutions. Repeated blockage usually indicates that the catheter needs to be changed.

CATHETER PATENCY SOLUTIONS

Chlorhexidine 0.02%
Brands include *Uriflex C*®, 100-mL sachet = £2.40; *Uro-Tainer Chlorhexidine*®, 100-mL sachet = £2.60

Sodium chloride 0.9%
Brands include *OptiFlo S*®, 50- and 100-mL sachets = £3.10; *Uriflex S*®, 100-mL sachet = £2.40; *Uriflex SP*®, with integral drug additive port, 100-mL sachet = £2.40; *Uro-Tainer Sodium Chloride*®, 50- and 100-mL sachets = £2.99; *Uro-Tainer M*®, with integral drug additive port, 50- and 100-mL sachets = £2.90

Solution G
Citric acid 3.23%, magnesium oxide 0.38%, sodium bicarbonate 0.7%, disodium edetate 0.01%. Brands include *OptiFlo G*®, 50- and 100-mL sachets = £3.29; *Uriflex G*®, 100-mL sachet = £2.40; *Uro-Tainer*® *Twin Suby G*, 2 × 30-mL = £4.10

Solution R
Citric acid 6%, gluconolactone 0.6%, magnesium carbonate 2.8%, disodium edetate 0.01%. Brands include *OptiFlo R*®, 50- and 100-mL sachets = £3.29; *Uriflex R*®, 100-mL sachet = £2.40; *Uro-Tainer*® *Twin Solutio R*, 2 × 30-mL = £4.10

8 Malignant disease and immunosuppression

8.1 Cytotoxic drugs

The management of childhood cancer is complex and is generally confined to specialist regional centres, and some associated shared-care units, affiliated to the United Kingdom Children's Cancer Study Group. The Group, together with other national and international organisations, develops and co-ordinates treatment protocols. In children, cytotoxic drugs are almost always administered in the context of a formal protocol.

Cytotoxic drugs have both anti-cancer activity and the potential for damage to normal tissue. In children, chemotherapy is almost always started with curative intent, but may be continued as palliation if the disease is refractory.

Chemotherapy with a combination of two or more cytotoxic drugs aims to reduce the development of resistance and to improve cytotoxic effect. Treatment protocols generally incorporate a series of treatment courses at defined intervals, with clear criteria for starting each course e.g. adequate bone-marrow recovery and renal or cardiac function. The principal component of treatment for leukaemias in children is cytotoxic therapy, whereas solid tumours may be managed with surgery or radiotherapy in addition to chemotherapy.

Handling cytotoxic drugs:

1. Trained personnel should reconstitute cytotoxics;
2. Reconstitution should be carried out in designated areas;
3. Protective clothing (including gloves) should be worn;
4. The eyes should be protected and means of first aid should be specified;
5. Pregnant staff should not handle cytotoxics;
6. Adequate care should be taken in the disposal of waste material, including syringes, containers, and absorbent material.

Only medical or nursing staff who have received appropriate training should administer parenteral cytotoxics. In most instances central venous access will be required for the intravenous administration of cytotoxics to children; care is required to avoid the risk of extravasation (see Side-effects of Cytotoxic Drugs and their Management).

> Intrathecal chemotherapy
> A Health Service Circular (HSC 2003/010) provides guidance on the introduction of safe practice in NHS Trusts where intrathecal chemotherapy is administered; written local guidance covering all aspects of national guidance must be available.
>
> Copies, and further information may be obtained from:
>
> Department of Health
> PO Box 777
> London SE1 6XH
> Fax: 01623 724524
> www.dh.gov.uk

> Because of the complexity of dosage regimens in the treatment of malignant disease, dose statements have been omitted from many of the drug entries in this chapter.

Side-effects of cytotoxic drugs and their management

Side-effects common to most cytotoxic drugs are discussed below whilst side-effects characteristic of a particular drug or class of drugs (e.g. neurotoxicity with vinca alkaloids) are mentioned in the appropriate sections. Manufacturers' product literature should be consulted for full details of side-effects of individual drugs.

Extravasation of intravenous drugs A number of cytotoxic drugs will cause severe local tissue irritation and necrosis if leakage into the extravascular compartment occurs. For information on the prevention and management of extravasation injury see section 10.3.

Gastro-intestinal effects Management of gastro-intestinal effects of cytotoxic drugs includes the use of antacids, H_2-receptor antagonists, and proton pump inhibitors to protect the gastric mucosa; laxatives to treat constipation; and enteral and parenteral nutritional support.

Oral mucositis Good mouth care keeps the mouth clean and moist, helping prevent mucositis; prevention is more effective than treatment of the complication. Preventative measures include brushing teeth with a soft small head brush 2-3 times daily and rinsing the mouth frequently. Mucositis related to chemotherapy can be extremely painful and may, in some circumstances, require opioid analgesia. Secondary infection with candida is frequent; treatment with systemically absorbed antifungals (e.g. fluconazole) has been shown to be effective.

Nausea and vomiting Nausea and vomiting cause considerable distress to many children who receive chemotherapy, and to a lesser extent abdominal radiotherapy, and may lead to refusal of further treatment. Symptoms may be acute (occurring within 24 hours of treatment), delayed (first occurring more than 24 hours after treatment) or anticipatory (occurring prior to subsequent doses). Delayed and anticipatory symptoms are more difficult to control than acute symptoms and require different management.

Susceptibility to nausea and vomiting may increase with repeated exposure to the cytotoxic drug.

Drugs may be divided according to their emetogenic potential and some examples are given below, but the symptoms vary according to the dose, to other drugs administered, and to the individual's susceptibility to emetogenic stimuli.

Mildly emetogenic treatment—fluorouracil, etoposide, low doses of methotrexate, the vinca alkaloids, and abdominal radiotherapy.

Moderately emetogenic treatment—carboplatin, doxorubicin, intermediate and low doses of cyclophosphamide, mitoxantrone (mitozantrone), and high doses of methotrexate.

Highly emetogenic treatment—cisplatin, dacarbazine, and high doses of alkylating drugs.

Anti-emetic drugs, when given regularly, help prevent or ameliorate emesis associated with chemotherapy in children.

Prevention of acute symptoms. For patients at *low risk of emesis*, pretreatment with metoclopramide (or less commonly domperidone) continued for up to 24 hours after chemotherapy, is often effective (section 4.6); a $5HT_3$ antagonist (section 4.6) may also be of benefit.

For patients at *high risk of emesis* or when other treatment is inadequate, a $5HT_3$ antagonist (section 4.6) is often highly effective. The addition of dexamethasone and other anti-emetics may also be required.

Prevention of delayed symptoms. Dexamethasone, given by mouth, is the drug of choice for preventing delayed symptoms; it is used alone or with metoclopramide. The $5HT_3$ antagonists may have a role in preventing uncontrolled symptoms.

Prevention of anticipatory symptoms. Good symptom control is the best way to prevent anticipatory symptoms. The addition of lorazepam to antiemetic therapy is helpful because of its amnesic, sedative and anxiolytic effects.

Bone-marrow suppression All cytotoxic drugs except vincristine and bleomycin cause bone-marrow depression. This commonly occurs 7 to 10 days after administration, but is delayed for certain drugs, such as melphalan. Peripheral blood counts must be checked before each treatment. The duration and severity of neutropenia can be reduced by the use of granulocyte-colony stimulating factors (section 9.1.6); their use should be reserved for children who have previously experienced severe neutropenia.

Infection in a child with neutropenia requires immediate broad-spectrum antibacterial treatment that covers all likely pathogens. Antifungal treatment may be required in a child with prolonged neutropenia or fever that has lasted longer than 4–5 days. Chickenpox can be particularly hazardous in immunocompromised children; antiviral treatment (section 5.3.2.1) or varicella–zoster immunoglobulin (section 14.5) may be indicated if the child is at risk of varicella-zoster infection.

Alopecia Reversible hair loss is a common complication, although it varies in degree between drugs and individual patients.

Pregnancy and reproductive function Before using cytotoxic drugs during pregnancy consideration should be given to both the prognosis of the patient and the fetal risk. The rapidly dividing cells of the fetus are potentially susceptible to the effects of cytotoxic drugs. Although antimetabolites are thought to be the strongest teratogens, specific risk assessment of individual cytotoxics is not possible with the available data. All of the long-term effects of cytotoxic exposure are not fully known.

The use of cytotoxic drugs during the first trimester is associated with the greatest risk of harm to the fetus; spontaneous abortion and teratogenicity are possible. If at all possible cytotoxic drugs should be avoided before week 10 of pregnancy.

In the second and third trimesters the risk of teratogenicity is negligible, but growth and developmental effects are possible. In the third trimester early induction of delivery may be considered. If cytotoxic drugs are unavoidable in older girls with reproductive potential, contraceptive advice should be offered where appropriate. Regimens containing an alkylating drug carry the risk of causing permanent male sterility (but may not affect sexual potency).

Long-term and delayed toxicity Cytotoxic drugs may produce specific organ-related toxicity in children (e.g. cardiotoxicity with doxorubicin or nephrotoxicity with cisplatin and ifosfamide). Manifestations of such toxicity may not appear for several months or even years after cancer treatment. Careful follow-up of survivors of childhood cancer is therefore vital; national and local guidelines have been developed to facilitate this.

Thromboembolism Venous thromboembolism can be a complication of cancer itself, but chemotherapy can also increase the risk.

Drugs for cytotoxic-induced side-effects

Hyperuricaemia

Hyperuricaemia, which may be present in high-grade lymphoma and leukaemia, can be markedly worsened by chemotherapy and is associated with acute renal failure.

Allopurinol is used routinely in children at low to moderate risk of hyperuricaemia. It should be started 24 hours before treatment; patients should be adequately hydrated (consideration should be given to omitting phosphate and potassium from hydration fluids). The dose of mercaptopurine or azathioprine should be reduced if allopurinol is given concomitantly (see Appendix 1).

Rasburicase is a recombinant urate oxidase used in children who are at high-risk of developing hyperuricaemia. It rapidly reduces plasma uric acid and may be of particular value in reducing complications following treatment of leukaemias or bulky lymphomas.

ALLOPURINOL

Cautions ensure adequate fluid intake; for hyperuricaemia associated with cancer therapy, allopurinol treatment should be started before cancer therapy; **interactions:** Appendix 1 (allopurinol)

Hepatic impairment reduce dose, monitor liver function

Renal impairment moderate to severe, reduce dose; increased toxicity, rashes

Pregnancy toxicity not reported; manufacturer advises use only if no safer alternative and disease carries risk for mother or child

Breast-feeding present in milk—not known to be harmful

Side-effects rashes (**withdraw** therapy; if rash mild re-introduce cautiously but **discontinue** immediately if recurrence—hypersensitivity reactions occur rarely and include exfoliation, fever, lymphadenopathy, arthralgia, and eosinophilia resembling Stevens-Johnson or Lyell's syndrome, vasculitis, hepatitis, renal impairment, and very rarely seizures); gastro-intestinal disorders; rarely malaise, headache, vertigo, drowsiness, visual and taste disturbances, hypertension, alopecia, hepatotoxicity, paraesthesia and neuropathy, blood disorders (including leucopenia, thrombocytopenia, haemolytic anaemia and aplastic anaemia)

Licensed use prophylaxis of hyperuricaemia associated with cancer chemotherapy; enzyme disorders such as Lesch-Nyhan syndrome

Indication and dose

Prophylaxis of hyperuricaemia associated with cancer chemotherapy, prophylaxis of hyperuricaemic nephropathy, enzyme disorders causing increased serum urate e.g. Lesch-Nyhan syndrome

- **By mouth**

Child 1 month–15 years 10–20 mg/kg daily (max. 400 mg daily), preferably after food

Child 15–18 years initially 100 mg daily; usual maintenance dose 100 mg 3 times daily (total daily dose may be given as a single dose if tolerated); max. 900 mg daily (doses over 300 mg daily given in divided doses); preferably after food

Allopurinol (Non-proprietary) PoM
Tablets, allopurinol 100 mg, net price 28-tab pack = 91p; 300 mg, 28-tab pack = £2.17. Label: 8, 21, 27
Brands include *Caplenal®*, *Cosuric®*, *Rimapurinol®*

Zyloric (GlaxoSmithKline) PoM
Tablets, allopurinol 100 mg, net price 100-tab pack = £10.19; 300 mg, 28-tab pack = £7.31. Label: 8, 21, 27

Extemporaneous formulations available see Extemporaneous Preparations, p. 8

RASBURICASE

Cautions monitor closely for hypersensitivity; atopic allergies; may interfere with test for uric acid—consult product literature

Contra-indications susceptibility to haemolytic anaemia including G6PD deficiency;

Pregnancy manufacturer advises avoid—no information available

Breast-feeding manufacturer advises avoid—no information available

Side-effects fever; nausea, vomiting; less frequently diarrhoea, headache, hypersensitivity reactions (including rash, bronchospasm and anaphylaxis); haemolytic anaemia, methaemoglobinaemia

Licensed use not licensed for use in children

Indication and dose

Prophylaxis and treatment of acute hyperuricaemia with initial chemotherapy for haematological malignancy

- **By intravenous infusion**

Consult local treatment protocol for details

Administration Consult local treatment protocol for details
By intravenous infusion, dilute required volume with sodium chloride 0.9%

Fasturtec (Sanofi-Synthelabo) ▼ PoM
Intravenous infusion, powder for reconstitution, rasburicase, net price 1.5-mg vial (with solvent) = £48.24; 7.5-mg vial (with solvent) = £201.00

Methotrexate-induced mucositis and myelosuppression

Folinic acid (given as calcium folinate) is used to counteract the folate-antagonist action of methotrexate and thus speed recovery from methotrexate-induced mucositis or myelosuppression.

The calcium salt of **levofolinic acid**, a single isomer of folinic acid, is also used following methotrexate administration. The dose of calcium levofolinate is generally half that of calcium folinate.

The efficacy of high dose methotrexate is enhanced by delaying initiation of folinic acid for at least 24 hours, local protocols define the correct time. Folinic acid is normally continued until the plasma-methotrexate concentration falls to 100–200 nanomol/litre (45–90 micrograms/mL).

In the treatment of methotrexate overdose, folinate should be administered immediately; other measures to enhance the elimination of methotrexate are also necessary.

CALCIUM FOLINATE

(Calcium leucovorin)

Cautions avoid simultaneous administration of methotrexate; **not** indicated for pernicious anaemia or other megaloblastic anaemias due to vitamin B_{12} deficiency; **interactions:** Appendix 1 (folates)

Pregnancy manufacturer advises use only if potential benefit outweighs risk

Breast-feeding manufacturer advises caution—no information available

Contra-indications

> Safe Practice Intrathecal injection **contra-indicated**

Side-effects hypersensitivity reactions; rarely pyrexia after parenteral use

Licensed use reduction of methotrexate-induced toxicity, treatment of methotrexate overdose; megaloblastic anaemia due to folate deficiency

Indication and dose

Reduction of methotrexate-induced toxicity
- **By mouth, by intravenous injection over 2 minutes, or by intravenous infusion**

  See notes above. Consult local treatment protocol for details.

Methotrexate overdose
- **By intravenous infusion**

  See notes above. Consult local treatment protocol for details.

Megaloblastic anaemia due to folate deficiency
- **By mouth**

  Child up to 12 years 250 microgram/kg once daily

  Child 12–18 years 15 mg once daily

Metabolic disorders leading to folate deficiency
- **By mouth or by intravenous infusion**

  Child up to 18 years 15 mg once daily; larger doses may be required in older children

Administration Consult local treatment protocol for details.

By intravenous infusion, diluted in sodium chloride 0.9% or glucose 5%, given over at least 30 minutes

By mouth, the injection may be given orally

Calcium Folinate (Non-proprietary) PoM

Tablets, scored, folinic acid (as calcium salt) 15 mg, net price 10-tab pack = £40.50, 30-tab pack = £85.74

Brands include *Refolinon®*

Note Not all strengths and pack sizes are available from all manufacturers

Injection, folinic acid (as calcium salt) 3 mg/mL, net price 1-mL amp = £2.28, 10-mL amp = £4.62; 7.5 mg/mL, net price 2-mL amp = £7.80; 10 mg/mL, net price 5-mL vial = £19.41, 10-mL vial = £35.09, 30-mL vial = £94.69, 35-mL vial = £90.98

Brands include *Lederfolin®*

Note Not all strengths and pack sizes are available from all manufacturers

Injection, powder for reconstitution, folinic acid (as calcium salt), net price 15-mg vial = £4.46; 30-mg vial = £8.36

CALCIUM LEVOFOLINATE

(Calcium levoleucovorin)

Cautions see Calcium Folinate

Side-effects see Calcium Folinate

Licensed use reduction of methotrexate induced-toxicity, treatment of methotrexate overdose

Indication and dose

Reduction of methotrexate-induced toxicity
- **By intramuscular injection, by intravenous injection over at least 3 minutes, or by intravenous infusion**

  See notes above. Consult local treatment protocol for details.

CALCIUM LEVOFOLINATE (*continued*)

Methotrexate overdose
- **By intramuscular injection, by intravenous injection over at least 3 minutes, or by intravenous infusion**

See notes above. Consult local treatment protocol for details.

Administration Consult local treatment protocol for details.

By intravenous infusion, diluted in sodium chloride 0.9% or glucose 5%

Isovorin® (Wyeth) ▼ PoM

Injection, levofolinic acid (as calcium salt) 10 mg/mL, net price 2.5-mL vial = £12.09, 5-mL vial = £26.00, 17.5-mL vial = £84.63

Urothelial toxicity

Haemorrhagic cystitis is a common manifestation of urothelial toxicity which occurs with the oxazaphosphorines, cyclophosphamide and ifosfamide; it is caused by the metabolite acrolein. Adequate hydration is essential to reduce the risk of urothelial toxicity. **Mesna** reacts specifically with acrolein in the urinary tract, preventing toxicity. Mesna is given for the same duration as cyclophosphamide or ifosfamide. It is generally given intravenously; the dose of mesna is equal to or greater than that of the oxazaphosphorine. For the role of nebulised mesna as a mucolytic in cystic fibrosis see section 3.7.

MESNA

Cautions

Pregnancy not known to be harmful

Contra-indications hypersensitivity to thiol-containing compounds

Side-effects nausea, vomiting, colic, diarrhoea, fatigue, headache, limb and joint pains, depression, irritability, rash, hypotension and tachycardia; rarely hypersensitivity reactions (more common in patients with auto-immune disorders)

Licensed use not licensed for use in children

Indication and dose

Urothelial toxicity following oxazaphosphorine therapy
- **By intravenous injection or by continuous intravenous infusion**

See notes above. Consult local treatment protocol for details.

Mucolytic in cystic fibrosis Section 3.7

Administration Consult local treatment protocol for details

For *intravenous infusion,* dilute with Glucose 5% *or* Sodium Chloride 0.9%

Uromitexan® (Baxter) PoM

Tablets, f/c, mesna 400 mg, net price 10-tab pack = £21.10; 600 mg, 10-tab pack = £27.40

Injection, mesna 100 mg/mL. Net price 4-mL amp = £1.95; 10-mL amp = £4.38

Note For oral administration contents of ampoule are taken in a flavoured drink such as orange juice or cola which may be stored in a refrigerator for up to 24 hours in a sealed container

8.1.1 Alkylating drugs

Extensive experience is available with these drugs, which are among the most widely used in cancer chemotherapy. They act by damaging DNA, thus interfering with cell replication. In addition to the side-effects common to many cytotoxic drugs (section 8.1), problems associated specifically with alkylating drugs include:

- an adverse effect on gametogenesis which may be reversible, particularly in females; amenorrhoea may also occur, which also may be reversible;
- a marked increase in the incidence of secondary tumours and leukaemia, particularly when alkylating drugs are combined with extensive irradiation;
- fluid retention with oedema and dilutional hyponatraemia in younger children; the risk of this complication is higher in the first 2 days and also when given with concomitant vinca alkaloids;
- urothelial toxicity with intravenous use; adequate hydration may reduce this risk; mesna (section 8.1) provides further protection against urotoxic effects of cyclophosphamide and ifosfamide.

BUSULFAN

(Busulphan)

Cautions see section 8.1 and notes above; monitor full blood count regularly throughout treatment; monitor liver function tests; previous mediastinal or pulmonary radiation therapy; avoid in porphyria (section 9.8.2); **interactions**: Appendix 1 (busulfan)

Pregnancy avoid (teratogenic in *animals*); manufacturers advise effective contraception during and for 6 months after administration to men or women; *see also* section 8.1

Breast-feeding discontinue breast-feeding

Side-effects see section 8.1 and notes above; skin hyperpigmentation; convulsions at higher doses (use prophylactic benzodiazepine); with prolonged treatment progressive interstitial pulmonary fibrosis (potentially irreversible); hepatic veno-occlusive disease

Licensed use *Myleran*® not licensed for conditioning before stem cell transplantation; *Busilvex*® not licensed for chronic granulocytic leukaemia

Indication and dose

Chronic granulocytic leukaemia
- By mouth
  Consult local treatment protocol for details.

Conditioning before stem cell transplantation
- By mouth or by intravenous infusion
  Consult local treatment protocol for details.

Administration Consult local treatment protocol for details

For *intravenous infusion*, dilute to a concentration of 500 micrograms/mL with Glucose 5% *or* Sodium Chloride 0.9%; give through a central venous catheter over 2 hours

Busilvex® (Fabre) ▼ PoM

Concentrate for intravenous infusion, busulfan 6 mg/mL, net price 10-mL vial = £201.25

Myleran® (GSK) PoM

Tablets, f/c, busulfan 2 mg, net price 25-tab pack = £5.20

Busulfan

Capsules, busulfan 25 mg, available as a manufactured special from Nova Laboratories

Extemporaneous formulations available see Extemporaneous Preparations, p. 8

CHLORAMBUCIL

Cautions see section 8.1 and notes above; monitor full blood count regularly throughout treatment; increased seizure risk if nephrotic syndrome or history of epilepsy; avoid in porphyria (section 9.8.2)

Hepatic impairment manufacturer advises consider dose reduction in severe hepatic impairment—limited information available

Pregnancy avoid; manufacturer advises effective contraception during administration to men or women; *see also* section 8.1

Breast-feeding discontinue breast-feeding

Side-effects see section 8.1 and notes above; irreversible bone marrow suppression possible at higher doses; hepatotoxicity and jaundice; seizures (see cautions); sterility in prepubertal and pubertal males; pulmonary fibrosis, skin rashes (possible progression to Stevens-Johnson syndrome and toxic epidermal necrolysis)

Licensed use Hodgkin's disease

Indication and dose

Hodgkin's disease
- By mouth
  Consult local treatment protocol for details.

Leukeran® (GSK) PoM

Tablets, f/c, brown, chlorambucil 2 mg, net price 25-tab pack = £8.36

Extemporaneous formulations available see Extemporaneous Preparations, p. 8

CYCLOPHOSPHAMIDE

Cautions see section 8.1 and notes above; ensure satisfactory renal and hepatic function, and full blood count prior to each course; risk of urothelial toxicity (see notes above); avoid in porphyria (section 9.8.2); **interactions**: Appendix 1 (cyclophosphamide)

Hepatic impairment reduce dose—consult local treatment protocol for details

Renal impairment reduce dose—consult local treatment protocol for details

Pregnancy avoid; manufacturer advises effective contraception during and for at least 3 months after administration to men or women; see also section 8.1

Breast-feeding discontinue breast-feeding during and for 36 hours after stopping treatment

Contra-indications concurrent acute infection particularly acute urinary-tract infection, urothelial damage

Side-effects see section 8.1 and notes above; urothelial toxicity causing haemorrhagic cystitis

Licensed use not licensed for use in children

Indication and dose

Acute lymphoblastic leukaemia, non-Hodgkin's lymphoma, retinoblastoma, stage 4 neuroblastoma, rhabdomyosarcoma, soft-tissue sarcomas, Ewing tumour, neuroectodermal tumours (including medulloblastoma), infant brain tumours, ependymona, germ cell tumour, Wilms' tumour, high-dose conditioning for bone marrow transplantation
- By mouth or by intravenous infusion
  Consult local treatment protocol for details

CYCLOPHOSPHAMIDE (*continued*)

Nephrotic syndrome (Section 6.3.2)

Administration Consult local treatment protocol for details

By intravenous infusion in glucose 5%, sodium chloride 0.9% or 0.18% with glucose 4%, over at least one hour

Cyclophosphamide (Non-proprietary) PoM

Tablets, s/c, cyclophosphamide (anhydrous) 50 mg, net price 20 = £2.12. Label: 27

Injection, powder for reconstitution, cyclophosphamide, net price 500-mg vial = £2.88; 1-g vial = £5.04

Endoxana® (Baxter) PoM

Tablets, s/c, cyclophosphamide 50 mg, net price 100-tab pack = £12.00. Label: 27

Injection, powder for reconstitution, cyclophosphamide. Net price 200-mg vial = £1.86; 500-mg vial = £3.25; 1-g vial = £5.67

Extemporaneous formulations available see Extemporaneous Preparations, p. 8

IFOSFAMIDE

Cautions see section 8.1 and notes above; ensure satisfactory full blood count and renal function before each course; risk of urothelial toxicity (see notes above); **interactions:** Appendix 1 (ifosfamide)

Renal impairment avoid in mild impairment

Pregnancy avoid (teratogenic and carcinogenic in *animals*), manufacturer advises adequate contraception during and for at least 6 months after administration to men or women; see also section 8.1

Breast-feeding discontinue breast-feeding

Contra-indications see under cyclophosphamide

Hepatic impairment avoid

Side-effects see section 8.1 and notes above; see under cyclophosphamide, urinary tract effects potentially more severe; renal toxicity (tubular dysfunction, Fanconi's syndrome or diabetes insipidus, progressive chronic renal failure following long-term high-dose treatment); drowsiness, confusion, psychosis, hallucinations; rarely convulsions, encephalopathy

Licensed use licensed for use in children (age range not specified by manufacturer)

Indication and dose

Rhabdomyosarcoma, soft-tissue sarcomas, Ewing tumour, germ cell tumour, osteogenic sarcoma

- **By intravenous infusion**

  Consult local treatment protocol for details

Administration Consult local treatment protocol for details

Intravenous infusion of solution containing not greater than 40 mg/mL (reconstituted solution of 80 mg/mL further diluted in sodium chloride 0.9%, glucose and sodium chloride, or glucose 5% solution), administered over 30–180 minutes. Ensure adequate hydration and concurrent administration of mesna (see notes above and section 8.1).

Mitoxana® (Baxter) PoM

Injection, powder for reconstitution, ifosfamide. Net price 1-g vial = £24.57; 2-g vial = £45.49 (hosp. only)

MELPHALAN

Cautions see section 8.1 and notes above; monitor full blood count before and throughout treatment; for high-dose intravenous administration establish adequate hydration (see notes above), consider use of prophylactic anti-infective agents; haematopoietic stem cell transplantation essential for high dose treatment (consult local treatment protocol for details); **interactions:** Appendix 1 (melphalan)

Renal impairment reduce dose initially, avoid high doses in moderate to severe impairment

Pregnancy avoid; manufacturer advises adequate contraception during administration to men or women; see also section 8.1

Breast-feeding discontinue breast-feeding

Side-effects see section 8.1 and notes above

Licensed use childhood neuroblastoma; oral use not licensed in children

Indication and dose

High intravenous dose with haematopoietic stem cell transplantation in the treatment of childhood neuroblastoma

- **Intravenous injection**

  Consult local treatment protocol for details

Administration Consult local treatment protocol for details

By fast intravenous injection into established large-bore line (such as central venous catheter). Administer immediately following reconstitution. May be diluted in sodium chloride 0.9% to 400 micrograms/mL. Incompatible with glucose. Max. 90 minutes between reconstitution and completion of administration.

Alkeran® (GSK) PoM

Injection, powder for reconstitution, melphalan 50 mg (as hydrochloride). Net price 50-mg vial (with solvent-diluent) = £27.61

8.1.2 Cytotoxic antibiotics

Cytotoxic antibiotics are widely used. Many act as radiomimetics and simultaneous use of radiotherapy should be **avoided** as it may enhance toxicity markedly.

Daunorubicin, doxorubicin, and epirubicin are anthracycline antibiotics. Mitoxantrone (mitozantrone) is an anthracycline derivative.

All anthracycline antibiotics have been associated with varying degrees of cardiac toxicity—this may be idiosyncratic and reversible, but is commonly related to total cumulative dose and is irreversible. Cardiac function should be monitored before and at regular intervals throughout treatment and afterwards. Anthracycline antibiotics should not normally be used in children with left ventricular dysfunction. Epirubicin and mitoxantrone are considered less toxic, and may be suitable for children who have received high cumulative doses of other anthracyclines.

BLEOMYCIN

Cautions see section 8.1; ensure monitoring of pulmonary function—investigate any shortness of breath before initiation; caution in handling—irritant to tissues

Renal impairment reduce dose in moderate impairment—consult local treatment protocol for details

Pregnancy avoid (teratogenic and carcinogenic in *animal* studies); see also section 8.1

Breast-feeding discontinue breast-feeding

Contra-indications acute pulmonary infection or significantly reduced lung function

Side-effects see section 8.1, less bone marrow suppression; anorexia; pulmonary toxicity e.g. pulmonary fibrosis (usually dose-related and delayed); fever (directly following administration), fatigue; dermatological and mucous membrane toxicity, localised skin hyperpigmentation; rarely cardiorespiratory collapse and hyperpyrexia

Licensed use not licensed for use in children

Indication and dose

Some germ cell tumours, Hodgkin's lymphoma
- By intravenous infusion

Consult local treatment protocol for details

Administration Consult local treatment protocol for details

Intravenous infusion in a suitable volume of sodium chloride 0.9% (e.g. up to 100 mL) into established intravenous line

Bleomycin (Non-proprietary) PoM

Injection, powder for reconstitution, bleomycin (as sulphate). Net price 15 000-unit vial = £15.56

Note To conform to the European Pharmacopoeia vials previously labelled as containing '15 units' of bleomycin are now labelled as containing 15 000 units. The amount of bleomycin in the vial has not changed.

Brands include *Bleo-Kyowa*®

DACTINOMYCIN
(Actinomycin D)

Cautions see section 8.1 and notes above; caution in handling—irritant to tissues

Hepatic impairment consider dose reduction if raised serum bilirubin or biliary obstruction (consult local treatment protocol for details)

Pregnancy avoid (teratogenic in *animal* studies); see also section 8.1

Breast-feeding discontinue breast-feeding

Side-effects see section 8.1 and notes above; less commonly cheilitis, dysphagia; fever, malaise, lethargy; anaemia, hypoglycaemia; myalgia; acne; rarely hepatotoxicity (possibly dose-related)

Licensed use not licensed for use in children under 12 years (use only if benefit outweighs risk)

Indication and dose

Wilms' tumour, childhood rhabdomyosarcoma and other soft tissue sarcomas, Ewing's sarcoma
- By intravenous injection

Consult local treatment protocol for details

Administration Consult local treatment protocol for details

Slow intravenous injection of 500 micrograms/mL solution over 2–3 minutes

Cosmegen Lyovac® (MSD) PoM

Injection, powder for reconstitution, dactinomycin, net price 500-microgram vial = £1.50

DAUNORUBICIN

Cautions see section 8.1 and notes above; caution in handling—irritant to tissues

Hepatic impairment reduce dose according to serum bilirubin concentration (consult local treatment protocol for details)

Renal impairment reduce dose in mild to moderate impairment

Pregnancy avoid (teratogenic and carcinogenic in *animal* studies), see also section 8.1

Breast-feeding discontinue breast-feeding

DAUNORUBICIN (*continued*)

Side-effects see section 8.1 and notes above, leucopenia, less commonly mucositis; cardiac toxicity (usually 1–6 months after initiation of therapy); fever; red urine discolouration

Licensed use liposomal preparation not licensed for use in children

Indication and dose

Acute myelogenous leukaemia, acute lymphocytic leukaemia
- By intravenous infusion
  Consult local treatment protocol for details

Daunorubicin (Non-proprietary) PoM
Injection, powder for reconstitution, daunorubicin (as hydrochloride), net price 20-mg vial = £39.26

Administration Dilute with sodium chloride 0.9% and give into the tubing or side-arm of a fast flowing infusion—consult local treatment protocol for details

Lipid formulation

DaunoXome® (Gilead) PoM
Concentrate for intravenous infusion, daunorubicin encapsulated in liposomes. For dilution before use. Net price 50-mg vial = £137.67

Administration Consult local treatment protocol for details

DOXORUBICIN HYDROCHLORIDE

Cautions see section 8.1 and notes above; caution in handling—irritant to tissues; **interactions:** Appendix 1 (doxorubicin)

Hepatic impairment reduce dose according to bilirubin concentration, consult local treatment protocol for details

Pregnancy avoid (teratogenic and toxic in *animal* studies); manufacturer of liposomal product advises effective contraception during and for at least 6 months after administration to men or women; see also section 8.1

Breast-feeding discontinue breast-feeding

Side-effects see section 8.1 and notes above; red urine discoloration; thrombophlebitis over injection site; less commonly bronchospasm, fever, amenorrhoea, and skin rash

Licensed use not licensed for use in children

Indication and dose

Paediatric malignancies including Ewing's sarcoma, osteogenic sarcoma, Wilms' tumour, neuroblastoma, retinoblastoma, some liver tumours, acute lymphoblastic leukaemia, Hodgkin's lymphoma, non-Hodgkin's lymphoma
- By intravenous infusion
  Consult local treatment protocol for details

Administration Intravenous infusion in sodium chloride 0.9%, preferably via central line—consult local treatment protocol for details

Doxorubicin (Non-proprietary) PoM
Injection, powder for reconstitution, doxorubicin hydrochloride, net price 10-mg vial = £18.28; 50-mg vial = £91.40

Note The brand name *Adriamycin®* was formerly used

Injection, doxorubicin hydrochloride 2 mg/mL, net price 5-mL vial = £18.54, 25-mL vial = £92.70, 100-mL vial = £370.80

EPIRUBICIN HYDROCHLORIDE

Cautions see section 8.1 and notes above; caution in handling—irritant to tissues

Hepatic impairment reduce dose according to bilirubin concentration (consult local treatment protocol for details)

Pregnancy avoid (carcinogenic in animal studies); see also section 8.1, Pregnancy and Reproductive function

Breast-feeding discontinue breast-feeding

Side-effects see section 8.1 and notes above; red urine discolouration; anaphylaxis

Licensed use not licensed for use in children

Indication and dose

Acute lymphoblastic leukaemia, rhabdomyosarcoma, other soft tissue tumours of childhood
- Intravenous infusion
  Consult local treatment protocol for details

Administration Intravenous infusion in sodium chloride 0.9%, preferably via central line—consult local treatment protocol for details

Pharmorubicin® Rapid Dissolution (Pharmacia) PoM
Injection, powder for reconstitution, epirubicin hydrochloride. Net price 10-mg vial = £19.31; 20-mg vial = £38.62; 50-mg vial = £96.54

Pharmorubicin® Solution for Injection (Pharmacia) PoM
Injection, epirubicin hydrochloride 2 mg/mL, net price 5-mL vial = £19.31, 25-mL vial = £96.54, 100-mL vial = £386.16

MITOXANTRONE

(Mitozantrone)

Cautions see section 8.1 and notes above

Hepatic impairment manufacturer advises caution in severe hepatic impairment

Pregnancy avoid; manufacturer advises effective contraception during and for at least 6 months after administration to men or women; see also section 8.1

Breast-feeding discontinue breast feeding

Side-effects see section 8.1 and notes above; transient blue-green discoloration of urine; less commonly gastro-intestinal bleeding, anorexia, allergic reactions, dyspnoea, fatigue, fever, amenorrhoea, and transient blue discoloration of skin and nails

Licensed use not licensed for use in children

Indication and dose

Acute myeloid leukaemia, recurrent acute lymphoblastic leukaemia
- By intravenous infusion
  Consult local treatment protocol for details

Administration Consult local treatment protocol for details

Intravenous infusion diluted with at least 50 mL sodium chloride 0.9%, glucose 5%, or sodium chloride 0.18% and glucose 4% over 6 hours into a central venous line

Mitoxantrone (Non-proprietary) PoM
Concentrate for intravenous infusion, mitoxantrone (as hydrochloride) 2 mg/mL, net price 10-mL vial = £100.00

Novantrone® (Lederle) PoM
Concentrate for intravenous infusion, mitoxantrone (as hydrochloride) 2 mg/mL, net price 10-mL vial = £139.90, 12.5-mL vial = £174.89, 15-mL vial = £209.81

Onkotrone® (Baxter) PoM
Concentrate for intravenous infusion, mitoxantrone (as hydrochloride) 2 mg/mL, net price 10-mL vial = £135.39, 12.5-mL vial = £169.25, 15-mL vial = £203.04

8.1.3 Antimetabolites

Antimetabolites are incorporated into new nuclear material or they combine irreversibly with vital cellular enzymes and prevent normal cellular division. **Cytarabine**, **fludarabine**, **mercaptopurine**, **methotrexate**, and **tioguanine** are commonly used in paediatric chemotherapy.

Methotrexate inhibits the enzyme dihydrofolate reductase, essential for the synthesis of purines and pyrimidines. It is given by mouth, intravenously, intramuscularly, or intrathecally. Methotrexate causes myelosuppression, mucositis, and rarely pneumonitis. It is **contra-indicated** in significant renal impairment because it is excreted primarily by the kidney. It is also contra-indicated in patients with severe hepatic impairment. It should also be **avoided** in the presence of significant pleural effusion or ascites because it can accumulate in these fluids, and its subsequent return to the circulation may cause myelosuppression. Systemic toxicity may follow intrathecal administration and blood counts should be carefully monitored. Folinic acid (section 8.1) following methotrexate administration helps to prevent methotrexate-induced mucositis and myelosuppression.

Cytarabine acts by interfering with pyrimidine synthesis. It is given subcutaneously, intravenously, or intrathecally. It is a potent myelosuppressant and requires careful haematological monitoring. A liposomal formulation of cytarabine for intrathecal use is available for lymphomatous meningitis.

Fludarabine is generally well tolerated but does cause myelosuppression, which may be cumulative.

> **Fludarabine** has a potent and prolonged immunosuppressive effect and only irradiated blood products should be administered to prevent potentially fatal graft-versus-host reaction. Prescribers should consult specialist literature when using highly immunosuppressive drugs.

Mercaptopurine is used as maintenance therapy for acute lymphoblastic leukaemia and in the management of ulcerative colitis and Crohn's disease (section 1.5). Azathioprine, which is metabolised to mercaptopurine, is generally used as an immunosuppressant (section 8.2.1 and section 10.1.3). The dose of both drugs should be reduced if the child is receiving allopurinol since it interferes with their metabolism. For the role of thiopurine methyltransferase (TPMT) in the metabolism of azathioprine see section 8.2.1.

Tioguanine can be given by mouth for acute lymphoblastic leukaemia and acute myeloid leukaemia. Tioguanine may cause liver dysfunction, veno-occlusive disease, and late persistent splenomegaly.

CYTARABINE

Cautions see section 8.1 and notes above; **interactions:** Appendix 1 (cytarabine)

Hepatic impairment reduce dose

Renal impairment reduce dose for high dose regimens or avoid, consult local treatment protocol for details

Pregnancy avoid (teratogenic in *animal* studies); see also section 8.1

Breast-feeding discontinue breast-feeding

Side-effects see section 8.1 and notes above; 'cytarabine syndrome'—6–12 hours after intravenous administration—characterised by fever and malaise, myalgia, bone pain, maculopapular rash, and occasionally chest pain; less commonly conjunctivitis (consider prophylactic corticosteroid eye drops), neurotoxicity, renal and hepatic dysfunction, jaundice; rarely severe spinal cord toxicity following intrathecal administration

Licensed use Licensed for use in children (age range not specified by manufacturer); *Depocyte®* suspension for injection not licensed for use in children

Indication and dose

Acute lymphoblastic leukaemia, acute myeloid leukaemia, non-Hodgkin's lymphoma
- **By intravenous injection, by intravenous infusion, or by subcutaneous injection**

Consult local treatment protocol for details

Meningeal leukaemia, meningeal neoplasms
- **By intrathecal injection**

Consult local treatment protocol for details

Note Based on weight or body-surface area, children may tolerate higher doses of cytarabine than adults

Administration Consult local treatment protocol for details

By intravenous bolus injection or intravenous infusion diluted in water for injections, sodium chloride 0.9%, or glucose 5%; check container for haze or precipitate during administration. Do not give high strength (100 mg/mL) intrathecally.

Cytarabine (Non-proprietary) PoM

Injection (for intravenous, subcutaneous or intrathecal use), cytarabine 20 mg/mL, net price 5-mL vial = £4.00

Injection (for intravenous or subcutaneous use), cytarabine 20 mg/mL, net price 5-mL vial = £3.90, 25-mL vial = £19.50

Injection (for intravenous or subcutaneous use), cytarabine 100 mg/mL, net price 1-mL vial = £4.00; 5-mL vial = £20.00; 10-mL vial = £39.00; 20-mL vial = £77.50

Note Prices from different suppliers can vary

Lipid formulation for intrathecal use

DepoCyte® (Napp) ▼ PoM

Intrathecal injection, cytarabine encapsulated in liposomes, net price 50-mg vial = £1250.00

FLUDARABINE PHOSPHATE

Cautions see section 8.1 and notes above; use irradiated blood only; monitor for neurological toxicity; **interactions:** Appendix 1 (fludarabine)

Renal impairment use 50–75% of normal dose if creatinine clearance 30–70 mL/minute/1.73 m^2; avoid if creatinine clearance less than 30 mL/minute/1.73 m^2

Contra-indications haemolytic anaemia

Pregnancy avoid (teratogenic in *animal* studies); manufacturer advises effective contraception during and for at least 6 months after administration to men or women; see also section 8.1

Breast-feeding discontinue breast-feeding

Side-effects see section 8.1 and notes above; diarrhoea, anorexia; oedema; pneumonia; peripheral neuropathy, visual disturbances; chills, fever, malaise, weakness; skin rashes; *less commonly* pulmonary toxicity (including pulmonary infiltrates, pneumonitis and fibrosis), confusion; *rarely* heart failure, arrhythmia, coma, seizures, agitation, optic neuropathy, blindness, Stevens-Johnson syndrome, toxic epidermal necrolysis, and haemorrhagic cystitis

Licensed use not licensed for use in children

Indication and dose

Poor prognosis or relapsed acute myeloid leukaemia, relapsed acute lymphoblastic leukaemia, conditioning before bone marrow transplantation
- **By mouth, by intravenous injection, or by intravenous infusion**

Consult local treatment protocol for details

Administration Consult local treatment protocol for details

Reconstitute each 50 mg powder with 2 mL Water for Injections

For *intravenous injection,* dilute requisite dose with 10 mL Sodium Chloride 0.9%

For *intravenous infusion,* dilute requisite dose with 100–125 mL Sodium Chloride 0.9%; give over 30 minutes

Fludara® (Schering Health) PoM

Tablets, f/c, pink, fludarabine phosphate 10 mg, net price 15-tab pack = £279.00, 20-tab pack = £372.00

Injection, powder for reconstitution, fludarabine phosphate. Net price 50-mg vial = £156.00

MERCAPTOPURINE

Cautions see section 8.1 and notes above; monitor liver function; **interactions**: Appendix 1 (mercaptopurine)

Hepatic impairment may need dose reduction; avoid if jaundice or hepatomegaly; consult local treatment protocol for details

Renal impairment reduce dose if creatinine clearance less than 20 mL/minute/1.73 m^2

Pregnancy avoid (teratogenic); see also section 8.1

Breast-feeding discontinue breast-feeding

Side-effects see section 8.1 and notes above; gastro-intestinal effects less common; hepatotoxicity (more frequent at higher doses); rarely intestinal ulceration, pancreatitis, fever, crystalluria with haematuria, skin rash, and hyperpigmentation

Licensed use not licensed for use in children for acute lymphoblastic lymphoma or T-cell non-Hodgkins lymphoma

Indication and dose

Acute lymphoblastic leukaemia, lymphoblastic lymphomas
- By mouth

Consult local treatment protocol for details

Ulcerative colitis and Crohn's disease Section 1.5

Puri-Nethol® (GSK) PoM

Tablets, yellow, scored, mercaptopurine 50 mg. Net price 25-tab pack = £18.78

Mercaptopurine

Capsules, mercaptopurine 10 mg

Available as a manufactured special from Nova Laboratories

Extemporaneous formulations available see Extemporaneous Preparations, p. 8

METHOTREXATE

Cautions see section 8.1 and section 10.1.3; monitor renal and hepatic function; peptic ulceration, ulcerative colitis, diarrhoea, and ulcerative stomatitis; porphyria (section 9.8.2); **interactions**: Appendix 1 (methotrexate)

Hepatic impairment consult local treatment protocol for details; avoid for all indications in severe hepatic impairment

Renal impairment accumulates; nephrotoxic; reduce dose or avoid if creatinine clearance less than 60 mL/minute/1.73 m^2

Pregnancy avoid (teratogenic; fertility may be reduced during therapy but this may be reversible); manufacturer advises effective contraception during and for at least 3 months after administration to men or women; see also section 8.1

Breast-feeding discontinue breast-feeding

Side-effects see section 8.1; also anorexia, abdominal discomfort, intestinal ulceration and bleeding, diarrhoea, toxic megacolon, hepatotoxicity (see Cautions above); pulmonary oedema, pleuritic pain, pulmonary fibrosis, interstitial pneumonitis (see also Pulmonary Toxicity, p. 559); anaphylactic reactions, urticaria; dizziness, fatigue, chills, fever, drowsiness, malaise, headache, mood changes, abnormal cranial sensations, neurotoxicity; precipitation of diabetes; menstrual disturbances, vaginitis; cystitis, azotaemia, haematuria, dysuria, renal failure; osteoporosis, arthralgia, myalgia, vasculitis; conjunctivitis, blurred vision; rash, pruritus, Stevens-Johnson syndrome, toxic epidermal necrolysis, photosensitivity, changes of skin pigmentation, telangiectasia, acne, furunculosis, ecchymosis

Indication and dose

Maintenance and remission of acute lymphoblastic leukaemia, lymphoblastic lymphoma
- By mouth

Consult local treatment protocol for details

> Important The CSM has received reports of prescription and dispensing errors including fatalities. Attention should be paid to the **strength** of methotrexate tablets prescribed and the **frequency** of dosing

Treatment of early stage Burkitt's lymphoma, non-Hodgkin's lymphoma, osteogenic sarcoma, solid tumours, intracranial germ-cell tumours, some CNS tumours including infant brain tumours, acute lymphoblastic leukaemia
- By intravenous injection or infusion

Consult local treatment protocol for details

Meningeal leukaemia, treatment and prevention of CNS involvement of leukaemia
- By intrathecal injection

Consult local treatment protocol for details

Rheumatic disease section 10.1.3

Psoriasis section 13.5.3

Administration Consult local treatment protocol for details

Intravenous bolus injection or intravenous infusion over 3 to 24 hours.

Intrathecal injection using low volume preservative-free preparation.

Methotrexate (Non-proprietary) PoM

Injection, methotrexate (as sodium salt) 2.5 mg/mL. Net price 2-mL vial = £1.68

Injection, methotrexate (as sodium salt) 25 mg/mL, net price 2-mL vial =£2.62, 20-mL vial = £25.07

Injection, methotrexate 100 mg/mL (not for intrathecal use). Net price 10-mL vial = £78.33; 50-mL vial = £380.07

Oral preparations

Section 10.1.3

TIOGUANINE
(Thioguanine)

Cautions see section 8.1 and notes above; **interactions**: Appendix 1 (tioguanine)

Hepatic impairment reduce dose; consult local treatment protocol for details

Renal impairment creatinine clearance less than 20 mL/minute/1.73 m^2, reduce dose; consult local treatment protocol for details

Pregnancy avoid (teratogenicity reported when men receiving tioguanine have fathered children); ensure effective contraception during administration to men or women; see also section 8.1

Breast-feeding discontinue breast-feeding

Side-effects see section 8.1, notes above, and under mercaptopurine, gastro-intestinal effects less common; unsteady gait

Licensed use licensed for use in children (age range not specified by manufacturer)

Indication and dose

Acute myelogenous leukaemia, acute lymphoblastic leukaemia and lymphoma, chronic granulocytic leukaemia
- **By mouth**
  Consult local treatment protocol for details

Lanvis® (GSK) PoM
Tablets, yellow, scored, tioguanine 40 mg. Net price 25-tab pack = £45.41

Extemporaneous formulations available see Extemporaneous Preparations, p. 8

8.1.4 Vinca alkaloids and etoposide

The vinca alkaloids, **vinblastine** and **vincristine** are used to treat a variety of cancers including leukaemias, lymphomas, and some solid tumours.

Neurotoxicity, usually as peripheral or autonomic neuropathy, occurs with all vinca alkaloids and is a limiting side-effect of vincristine; it occurs less often with vinblastine. Children with neurotoxicity commonly have peripheral paraesthesia, loss of deep tendon reflexes, abdominal pain, and constipation; ototoxicity has been reported. If symptoms of neurotoxicity are severe, doses should be reduced, but children generally tolerate vincristine better than adults. Motor weakness can also occur and dose reduction or discontinuation of therapy may be appropriate if motor weakness increases. Recovery from neurotoxic effects is usually slow but complete.

Myelosuppression is the dose-limiting side-effect of vinblastine; vincristine causes negligible myelosuppression. The vinca alkaloids may cause reversible alopecia. They cause severe local irritation and care must be taken to avoid extravasation. Constipation is common with vinblastine and vincristine; prophylactic use of laxatives may be considered.

> Safe Practice
> Vinblastine and vincristine are for **intravenous administration only**. Inadvertent intrathecal administration can cause severe neurotoxicity, which is usually fatal.

Etoposide, usually given by slow intravenous infusion, is used to treat acute leukaemias, lymphomas, and some solid tumours. Etoposide may also be given by mouth but it is unpredictably absorbed.

ETOPOSIDE

Cautions see section 8.1 and notes above; **interactions**: Appendix 1 (etoposide)

Renal impairment consult specialist literature and local treatment protocol for details

Pregnancy avoid (teratogenic in *animal* studies); see also section 8.1

Breast-feeding discontinue breast-feeding

Contra-indications see section 8.1; severe hepatic impairment

Side-effects see section 8.1, dose limiting myelosuppression, mucositis more common if given with doxorubicin; anaphylaxis associated with concentrated infusions; hypotension associated with rapid infusion; irritant to tissues if extravasated

Licensed use not licensed for use in children

Indication and dose

Stage 4 neuroblastoma, germ-cell tumours, intracranial germ cell tumours, rhabdomyosarcoma, soft-tissue sarcomas, neuroectodermal tumours (including medulloblastoma), relapsed Hodgkin's disease, non-Hodgkin's lymphoma, Ewing tumour
- **By mouth or by intravenous infusion**
  Consult local treatment protocol for details

Administration Intravenous infusion over 1–4 hours diluted in sodium chloride 0.9% to a concentration not exceeding 400 microgram/mL. Solubility is concentration dependent: 400 micr-

ETOPOSIDE (*continued*)

ogram/mL solution stable for 96 hours at room temperature. Do not refrigerate. Use nylon filters and PVC bags or glass bottles. Inspect solution regularly for precipitate

Etoposide (Non-proprietary) PoM
Concentrate for intravenous infusion, etoposide 20 mg/mL, net price 5-mL vial = £12.15, 10-mL vial = £29.00, 25-mL vial = £60.75
Brands include *Eposin*®
Note Prices from different suppliers can vary

Etopophos® (Bristol-Myers Squibb) PoM
Injection, powder for reconstitution, etoposide (as phosphate), net price 100-mg vial = £29.87 (hosp. only)

Vepesid® (Bristol-Myers Squibb) PoM
Capsules, both pink, etoposide 50 mg, net price 20 = £105.97; 100 mg, 10-cap pack = £92.60 (hosp. only). Label: 23

Concentrate for intravenous infusion, etoposide 20 mg/mL, net price 5-mL vial = £13.56 (hosp. only)
Excipients: include benzyl alcohol (avoid in neonates, see Excipients, p. 3)

VINBLASTINE SULPHATE

Cautions see section 8.1 and notes above; caution in handling; **interactions:** Appendix 1 (vinblastine)

Hepatic impairment dose reduction may be necessary, consult local treatment protocol for details

Pregnancy avoid (limited experience suggests fetal harm; teratogenic in *animal* studies); see also section 8.1

Breast-feeding discontinue breast-feeding

Contra-indications see section 8.1 and notes above

Safe Practice Intrathecal injection **contra-indicated**

Side-effects see section 8.1 and notes above; abdominal pain, constipation, leucopenia, muscle pain; less commonly peripheral neuropathy; rarely paralytic ileus; irritant to tissues if extravasated

Licensed use licensed for use in children (age range not specified by manufacturer)

Indication and dose

Hodgkin's disease and other lymphomas
- By intravenous injection
  Consult local treatment protocol for details

Administration Consult local treatment protocol for details

For *intravenous injection*, dilute solution containing 1 mg/mL with Sodium Chloride 0.9%; give into the tubing of a fast-running Sodium Chloride 0.9% infusion

For child over 10 years, dilute to at least 20 mL to avoid inadvertent intrathecal use.

Vinblastine (Non-proprietary) PoM
Injection, vinblastine sulphate 1 mg/mL. Net price 10-mL vial = £13.09

Velbe® (Genus) PoM
Injection, powder for reconstitution, vinblastine sulphate. Net price 10-mg amp = £14.15

VINCRISTINE SULPHATE

Cautions see section 8.1 and notes above; neuromuscular disease; ileus; caution in handling; **interactions:** Appendix 1 (vincristine)

Hepatic impairment dose reduction may be necessary, consult local treatment protocol for details

Pregnancy avoid (teratogenicity and fetal loss in *animal* studies); see also section 8.1

Breast-feeding discontinue breast-feeding

Contra-indications see section 8.1 and notes above

Safe Practice Intrathecal injection **contra-indicated**

Side-effects see section 8.1 and notes above; constipation (see notes above), paralytic ileus may occur in young children; dose-limiting neuromuscular effects (see notes above); rarely convulsions followed by coma; irritant to tissues if extravasated

Licensed use licensed for use in children (age range not specified by manufacturer)

Indication and dose

Acute leukaemias, lymphomas, paediatric solid tumours
- By intravenous injection
  Consult local treatment protocol for details

Administration Consult local treatment protocol for details

For *intravenous injection*, dilute solution containing 1 mg/mL with Sodium Chloride 0.9%; give into the tubing of a fast-running Sodium Chloride 0.9% infusion

For child over 10 years dilute to at least 20 mL to avoid inadvertent intrathecal use

Vincristine (Non-proprietary) PoM
Injection, vincristine sulphate 1 mg/mL. Net price 1-mL vial = £10.92; 2-mL vial = £21.17; 5-mL vial = £44.16

Oncovin® (Genus) PoM
Injection, vincristine sulphate 1 mg/mL, net price 1-mL vial = £14.18; 2-mL vial = £28.05

8.1.5 Other antineoplastic drugs

Amsacrine

Amsacrine has an action and toxic effects similar to those of doxorubicin (section 8.1.2) and is given *intravenously*. It is occasionally used in acute myeloid leukaemia.

AMSACRINE

Cautions see section 8.1 and notes above; consider monitoring cardiac function; monitor electrolytes (fatal arrhythmias possible if hypokalaemia); previous treatment with anthracyclines; also caution in handling—irritant to skin and tissues

Hepatic impairment reduce dose—25% initially, up to 50% in severe impairment

Renal impairment reduce dose—up to 50% in severe impairment

Pregnancy avoid (teratogenic and toxic in *animal* studies); may reduce fertility; see also section 8.1

Breast-feeding discontinue breast-feeding

Side-effects see section 8.1 mucositis, phlebitis; less commonly diarrhoea, cardiotoxicity, haematuria, renal impairment, hepatotoxicity, skin rash; rarely acute renal failure, grand mal seizures

Licensed use not licensed for use in children

Indication and dose

Acute myeloid leukaemia
- **By intravenous infusion**

Consult local treatment protocol for details

Administration Consult local treatment protocol for details

Intravenous infusion via central venous catheter over 60–90 minutes diluted in Glucose 5%. Incompatible with Sodium Chloride 0.9% (precipitation if diluent contains chloride ions). Flush line with Glucose 5% prior to and after administration.

Amsidine® (Goldshield) PoM

Concentrate for intravenous infusion, amsacrine 5 mg (as lactate)/mL, when reconstituted by mixing two solutions. Net price 1.5-mL (75-mg) amp with 13.5-mL diluent vial = £49.17 (hosp. only)

Note Use glass apparatus for reconstitution

Asparaginase

Asparaginase is used almost exclusively in the treatment of acute lymphoblastic leukaemia. Hypersensitivity reactions may occur and facilities for the management of anaphylaxis should be available. A number of different preparations of asparaginase exist and only the product specified in the treatment protocol should be used. Crisantaspase is the enzyme asparaginase produced by *Erwinia chrysanthemi*. Preparations of asparaginase derived from *Escherichia coli* are also available. Children who are hypersensitive to asparaginase derived from one organism may be hypersensitive to all preparations; however, in some circumstances cautious re-introduction of a different preparation (e.g. a pegylated product) may prove successful.

CRISANTASPASE

Cautions see section 8.1 and notes above

Pregnancy avoid; see also section 8.1

Breast-feeding discontinue breast-feeding

Side-effects seesection 8.1 and notes above; fever, CNS depression, neurotoxicity; hyperglycaemia, liver dysfunction, coagulation disorders, altered plasma lipid concentration, pancreatitis

Indication and dose

Acute lymphoblastic leukaemia, other neoplastic conditions where depletion of asparagine likely to be useful
- **By intravenous, intramuscular or subcutaneous injection**

Consult local treatment protocol for details

Erwinase® (OPi) PoM

Injection, powder for reconstitution, crisantaspase. Net price 10 000-unit vial = £194.77

Preparations

Preparations of asparaginase derived from *Escherichia coli* are available but they are not licensed, they include: *Medac®* asparaginase, *Elspar®* asparaginase, and *Oncaspar®* pegaspargase.

Dacarbazine and temozolomide

Dacarbazine is a component of a commonly used combination for Hodgkin's disease (ABVD—doxorubicin [previously *Adriamycin*®], bleomycin, vinblastine, and dacarbazine). It is given *intravenously*.

Temozolomide is structurally related to dacarbazine and is used in children for second-line treatment of malignant glioma.

DACARBAZINE

Cautions see section 8.1; caution in handling

Hepatic impairment consider dose reduction in mild to moderate impairment; avoid in severe impairment

Renal impairment consider dose reduction in mild to moderate impairment; avoid in severe impairment

Pregnancy avoid (carcinogenic and teratogenic in *animal* studies); ensure effective contraception during and for at least 6 months after administration to men or women; see also section 8.1

Breast-feeding discontinue breast-feeding

Side-effects see section 8.1; less commonly flu-like syndrome; rarely liver necrosis due to hepatic vein thrombosis; irritant to skin and tissues

Licensed use licensed for use in children (age range not specified by manufacturer)

Indication and dose

Hodgkin's disease, paediatric solid tumours
- **By intravenous injection or by intravenous infusion**

  Consult local treatment protocol for details

Administration Consult local treatment protocol for details

By slow intravenous injection, reconstitute vial with water for injections to produce solution containing 10 mg/mL, administer over 2-3 minutes.

By intravenous infusion, further dilute reconstituted solution in 125-250 mL glucose 5% or sodium chloride 0.9%, administer over 15-30 minutes. Protecting infusion set from light throughout administration reduces pain.

Dacarbazine (Non-proprietary) PoM

Injection, powder for reconstitution, dacarbazine (as citrate), net price 100-mg vial = £5.05; 200-mg vial = £7.16; 500-mg vial = £16.50; 600-mg vial = £22.50; 1-g vial = £31.80

Note Prices from different suppliers can vary

DTIC-Dome® (Bayer) PoM

Injection, powder for reconstitution, dacarbazine. Net price 200-mg vial = £7.40

TEMOZOLOMIDE

Cautions see section 8.1; **interactions:** Appendix 1 (temozolomide)

Hepatic impairment caution if severe

Renal impairment caution if severe

Pregnancy avoid (teratogenic and embryotoxic in *animal* studies); manufacturer advises adequate contraception during administration; see also section 8.1; also men should avoid fathering a child during and for at least 6 months after treatment

Breast-feeding discontinue breast-feeding

Side-effects see section 8.1

Licensed use not licensed for treatment of malignant gliomas in children under 3 years

Indication and dose

Treatment of malignant gliomas
- **By mouth**

  Consult local treatment protocol for details

Temodal® (Schering-Plough) PoM

Capsules, temozolomide 5 mg, net price 5-cap pack = £17.30; 20 mg, 5-cap pack = £69.20; 100 mg, 5-cap pack = £346.00; 250 mg, 5-cap pack = £865.00. Label: 23, 25

Mitotane

Mitotane selectively inhibits the activity of the adrenal cortex. It is used in children for the symptomatic treatment of advanced or inoperable adrenocortical carcinoma. Neuro-psychological impairment can occur, possibly secondary to hypothyroidism, and gastro-intestinal side-effects such as anorexia, nausea, and vomiting are very common. Growth retardation has also been reported in children treated with mitotane.

MITOTANE

Cautions see section 8.1; suspend treatment and administer corticosteroid in case of shock, severe trauma or infection; **interactions**: Appendix 1 (mitotane)

Skilled tasks Central nervous system toxicity may affect performance of skilled tasks

Counselling Children and their carers should be warned to contact doctor immediately if injury, infection, or illness occurs

Hepatic impairment manufacturer advises caution in mild to moderate impairment—monitoring of plasma-mitotane concentration recommended; avoid in severe impairment

Renal impairment manufacturer advises caution if creatinine clearance 30–80 mL/minute/1.73 m^2—monitoring of plasma-mitotane concentration recommended; avoid if creatinine clearance less than 30 mL/minute/1.73 m^2

Pregnancy manufacturer advises avoid—effective contraception should be used if appropriate during and after treatment; see also section 8.1

Contra-indications

Breast-feeding discontinue breast-feeding

Side-effects seesection 8.1 and notes above; *also* autoimmune hepatitis, hypercholesterolaemia, hypertriglyceridaemia, gynaecomastia, increased bleeding time, rash; *rarely* hypertension, orthostatic hypotension, flushing, haematuria, proteinuria, haemorrhagic cystitis, hypouricaemia, visual disturbances and ocular disorders; cognitive impairment reported with prolonged high doses

Licensed use not licensed for use in children

Indication and dose

Symptomatic treatment of advanced or inoperable adrenocortical carcinoma
- **By mouth**
  Consult local treatment protocol for details

Lysodren® (HRA Pharma) PoM
Tablets, scored, mitotane 500 mg, net price 100-tab pack = £460.40. Label: 2, 21, counselling, skilled tasks, adrenal suppression

Platinum compounds

Carboplatin is used in the treatment of a variety of paediatric malignancies; it is given by intravenous infusion. Carboplatin can be given in an outpatient setting and is better tolerated than cisplatin; nausea and vomiting are less severe and nephrotoxicity, neurotoxicity, and ototoxicity are much less of a problem. Carboplatin is, however, more myelosuppressive than cisplatin.

Cisplatin is of value in children with a variety of malignancies; it is given by intravenous infusion. Cisplatin requires intensive intravenous hydration; routine use of intravenous fluids containing potassium or magnesium may also be required to help control hypokalaemia and hypomagnesaemia. Treatment may be complicated by severe nausea and vomiting; delayed vomiting may occur and is difficult to control. Cisplatin has dose-related and potentially cumulative side-effects including nephrotoxicity, neurotoxicity, and ototoxicity. Baseline testing of renal function and hearing is required; for children with pre-existing renal or hearing impairment or marked bone-marrow suppression, consideration should be given to withholding treatment or using another drug.

CARBOPLATIN

Cautions see section 8.1 and notes above; consider therapeutic drug monitoring; **interactions**: Appendix 1 (platinum compounds)

Renal impairment avoid if creatinine clearance less than 20 mL/minute/1.73 m^2

Pregnancy avoid (teratogenic and embryotoxic in *animal* studies); see also section 8.1

Breast-feeding discontinue breast-feeding

Side-effects see section 8.1 and notes above; less commonly nephrotoxicity and ototoxicity

Licensed use not licensed for use in children

Indication and dose

Stage 4 neuroblastoma, germ cell tumours, low-grade gliomas (including astrocytomas), neuroectodermal tumours (including medulloblastoma), rhabdomyosarcoma (metastatic and non-metastatic disease), soft-tissue sarcomas, retinoblastoma, high risk Wilms' tumour, some liver tumours
- **By intravenous infusion**
  Consult local treatment protocol for details

Administration Consult local treatment protocol for details

By intravenous infusion, dilute with glucose 5% or sodium chloride 0.9% to a concentration no lower than 500 microgram/mL, administer over at least one hour as dictated by fluid volume.

CARBOPLATIN (*continued*)

Carboplatin (Non-proprietary) PoM
Injection, carboplatin 10 mg/mL, net price 5-mL vial = £22.86, 15-mL vial = £56.29, 45-mL vial = £168.85, 60-mL vial = £260.00
Note Prices from different suppliers can vary

Paraplatin® (Bristol-Myers Squibb) PoM
Concentrate for intravenous infusion, carboplatin 10 mg/mL, net price 5-mL vial = £21.26, 15-mL vial = £61.22, 45-mL vial = £183.66, 60-mL vial = £244.88

CISPLATIN

Cautions see section 8.1 and notes above; monitor full blood count, renal function, audiology, and plasma electrolytes; **interactions:** Appendix 1 (platinum compounds)

Renal impairment avoid if possible—nephrotoxic and neurotoxic

Pregnancy avoid (teratogenic and toxic in *animal* studies); see also section 8.1

Breast-feeding discontinue breast-feeding

Side-effects see section 8.1 and notes above; ototoxicity (may be particularly severe in children); nephrotoxicity; hypomagnesaemia, hypokalaemia, hypophosphataemia, hypocalcaemia, hyperuricaemia; less commonly peripheral neuropathy

Licensed use not licensed for use in children

Indication and dose

Osteogenic sarcoma, stage 4 neuroblastoma, some liver tumours, infant brain tumours, intracranial germ cell tumours
- By intravenous infusion
  Consult local treatment protocol for details

Administration Consult local treatment protocol for details

By intravenous infusion, dilute in sodium chloride 0.9% or sodium chloride 0.45% and glucose 2.5%, administer over at least 24 hours (48 hours for infant brain tumours). Do not refrigerate (risk of precipitation).

Ensure adequate intravenous hydration and urinary output, at least 3 hours before, during, and for at least 24 hours after administration. Mannitol routinely used to aid diuresis.

Cisplatin (Non-proprietary) PoM
Injection, cisplatin 1 mg/mL, net price 10-mL vial = £5.85, 50-mL vial = £25.37, 100-mL vial = £50.22
Note Prices from different suppliers may vary
Brands include *Platinex®*

Injection, powder for reconstitution, cisplatin, net price 50-mg vial = £17.00

Procarbazine

Procarbazine is most often used in Hodgkin's disease. It is given *by mouth*. It is a weak monoamine-oxidase inhibitor and dietary restriction is rarely considered necessary. Alcohol ingestion may cause a disulfiram-like reaction.

PROCARBAZINE

Cautions see section 8.1 and notes above; **interactions:** Appendix 1 (procarbazine)

Hepatic impairment consider dose reduction; avoid in severe impairment

Renal impairment consider dose reduction; avoid in severe impairment

Pregnancy avoid (teratogenic in *animal* studies and isolated reports in humans); see also section 8.1

Breast-feeding discontinue breast-feeding

Side-effects see section 8.1 and notes above; hypersensitivity rash (discontinue treatment)

Licensed use licensed for use in children (age range not specified by manufacturer)

Indication and dose

Hodgkin's lymphoma, gliomas
- By mouth
  Consult local treatment protocol for details

Procarbazine (Cambridge) PoM
Capsules, ivory, procarbazine (as hydrochloride) 50 mg, net price 50-cap pack = £37.44. Label: 4

Extemporaneous formulations available see Extemporaneous Preparations, p. 8

Tretinoin

Tretinoin is licensed for the induction of remission in acute promyelocytic leukaemia. It is used in previously untreated children as well as in those who have relapsed after standard chemotherapy or who are refractory to it.

TRETINOIN

Note Tretinoin is the acid form of vitamin A

Cautions monitor full blood count and coagulation profile, liver function, serum calcium and plasma lipids before and during treatment; increased risk of thrombo-embolism during first month of treatment; **interactions:** Appendix 1 (retinoids)

Hepatic impairment reduce dose; consult local treatment protocol for details

Renal impairment mild impairment—reduce dose; consult local treatment protocol for details

Pregnancy teratogenic; exclude pregnancy before starting treatment; effective contraception must be used for at least 1 month before oral treatment, during treatment and for at least 1 month after stopping; see also section 8.1

Breast-feeding discontinue treatment

Contra-indications pregnancy (**important** teratogenic risk: see Cautions)

Side-effects retinoic acid syndrome (fever, dyspnoea, acute respiratory distress, pulmonary infiltrates, pleural effusion, hyperleukocytosis, hypotension, oedema, weight gain, hepatic, renal and multi-organ failure) requires immediate treatment—consult product literature; gastrointestinal disturbances, pancreatitis; arrhythmias, flushing, oedema; headache, benign intracranial hypertension (children particularly susceptible—consider dose reduction if intractable headache), shivering, dizziness, confusion, anxiety, depression, insomnia, paraesthesia, visual and hearing disturbances (children particularly susceptible to nervous system effects); raised liver enzymes, serum creatinine and lipids; bone and chest pain, alopecia, erythema, rash, pruritus, sweating, dry skin and mucous membranes, cheilitis; thromboembolism, hypercalcaemia, and genital ulceration reported

Licensed use licensed for use in children (age range not specified by manufacturer)

Indication and dose

Acute promyelocytic leukaemia

- **By mouth**

Consult treatment protocol for details

Vesanoid® (Roche) PoM

Capsules, yellow/brown, tretinoin 10 mg. Net price 100-cap pack = £170.52. Label: 21

8.2 Drugs affecting the immune response

Immunosuppressant therapy

Immunosuppressants are used to suppress rejection in organ transplant recipients and to treat a variety of chronic inflammatory and autoimmune diseases. Solid organ transplant patients are usually maintained on a calcineurin inhibitor (ciclosporin or tacrolimus), combined with an antiproliferative drug (azathioprine or mycophenolate mofetil) and a corticosteroid. Specialist management is required and other immunomodulators may be used to initiate treatment or to treat rejection.

Impaired immune responsiveness Infections in the immunocompromised child can be severe and show atypical features. Specific local protocols should be followed for the management of infection. Corticosteroids may suppress clinical signs of infection and allow diseases such as septicaemia or tuberculosis to reach an advanced stage before being recognised. Children should be up-to-date with their childhood vaccinations before initiation of immunosuppressant therapy (e.g. before transplantation); vaccination with varicella-zoster vaccine (section 14.4) is also necessary during this period—**important:** for advice on measles and chickenpox (varicella) exposure, see Immunoglobulins (section 14.5). For advice on the use of live vaccines in individuals with impaired immune response, see section 14.1. For general comments and warnings relating to corticosteroids and immunosuppressants see section 6.3.2 (under Prednisolone).

Pregnancy Transplant patients immunosuppressed with azathioprine should not discontinue it on becoming pregnant; there is no evidence that azathioprine is teratogenic. However, there have been reports of premature birth and low birth-weight following exposure to azathioprine, particularly in combination with corticosteroids. Spontaneous abortion has been reported following maternal or paternal exposure.

There is less experience of ciclosporin in pregnancy but it does not appear to be any more harmful than azathioprine. The use of these drugs during pregnancy needs to be supervised in specialist units.

Manufacturers contra-indicate the use of tacrolimus and mycophenolate in pregnancy.

8.2.1 Antiproliferative immunosuppressants

Azathioprine is widely used for transplant recipients and it is also used to treat a number of auto-immune conditions (see section 10.1.3), usually when corticosteroid therapy alone provides inadequate control. It is metabolised to mercaptopurine, and doses should be reduced to one quarter of the original dose when allopurinol is given concurrently.

Blood tests and monitoring for signs of myelosuppression are essential in long-term treatment with azathioprine. The enzyme thiopurine methyltransferase (TPMT) metabolises azathioprine; the risk of myelosuppression is increased in those with a low activity of the enzyme, particularly in the very few individuals who are homozygous for low TPMT activity.

Mycophenolate mofetil is metabolised to mycophenolic acid which has a more selective mode of action than azathioprine. It is used in combination with a corticosteroid and either ciclosporin or tacrolimus for the prophylaxis of acute rejection in transplant recipients. Compared with similar regimens incorporating azathioprine, mycophenolate mofetil may reduce the risk of acute rejection episodes; the risk of opportunistic infections (particularly due to tissue-invasive cytomegalovirus) and the occurrence of blood disorders such as leucopenia may be higher. Children may suffer a high incidence of side-effects, particularly gastro-intestinal effects, calling for temporary reduction in dose or interruption of treatment.

Cyclophosphamide (section 8.1.1) is less commonly prescribed as an immunosuppressant.

AZATHIOPRINE

Cautions monitor for toxicity throughout treatment; monitor full blood count weekly (more frequently with higher doses or if hepatic or renal impairment) for first 4 weeks (manufacturer advises weekly monitoring for 8 weeks but evidence of practical value unsatisfactory), thereafter reduce frequency of monitoring to at least every 3 months; **interactions:** Appendix 1 (azathioprine)

Bone marrow suppression Children and their carers should be warned to report immediately any signs or symptoms of bone marrow suppression e.g. inexplicable bruising or bleeding, infection

Hepatic impairment may need dose reduction

Renal impairment reduce dose in severe renal impairment

Pregnancy see section 8.2; treatment should not normally be initiated during pregnancy

Contra-indications hypersensitivity to azathioprine or mercaptopurine

Breast-feeding contra-indicated

Side-effects hypersensitivity reactions (including malaise, dizziness, vomiting, diarrhoea, fever, rigors, myalgia, arthralgia, rash, hypotension and interstitial nephritis—calling for immediate withdrawal); dose-related bone marrow suppression (see also Cautions); liver impairment, cholestatic jaundice, hair loss and increased susceptibility to infections and colitis in patients also receiving corticosteroids; nausea; rarely pancreatitis, pneumonitis, hepatic veno-occlusive disease

Licensed use licensed for use in suppression of transplant rejection; treatment of auto-immune conditions when corticosteroid therapy alone has proved inadequate, section 10.1.3

Indication and dose

Suppression of transplant rejection

- **By mouth, or (if oral route not possible) by intravenous infusion (see also note below)**

Consult local treatment protocol for details

Child 1 month–18 years maintenance, 1–3 mg/kg once daily, adjusted according to response; total daily dose may alternatively be given in 2 divided doses

Severe inflammatory bowel disease section 1.5

Administration Consult local treatment protocol for details

By intravenous injection over at least 1 minute

By intravenous infusion dilute required dose to a concentration of 0.25–2.5 mg/mL in glucose 5% *or* sodium chloride 0.9% *or* sodium chloride and

AZATHIOPRINE (*continued*)

glucose intravenous infusion and give over 30–60 minutes

Note Intravenous injection is alkaline and very irritant. Intravenous route should therefore be used **only** if oral route not feasible and discontinued as soon as oral route can be tolerated. To reduce irritation flush line with sodium chloride 0.9% *or* glucose 4%/sodium chloride 0.18%.

Azathioprine (Non-proprietary) PoM

Tablets, azathioprine 25 mg, net price 28-tab pack = £7.88; 50 mg, 56-tab pack = £7.90. Label: 21

Brands include *Azamune®*, *Immunoprin®*

Imuran® (GSK) PoM

Tablets, both f/c, azathioprine 25 mg (orange), net price 100-tab pack = £10.99; 50 mg (yellow), 100-tab pack = £7.99. Label: 21

Injection, powder for reconstitution, azathioprine (as sodium salt). Net price 50-mg vial = £15.38

Extemporaneous formulations available see Extemporaneous Preparations, p. 8

MYCOPHENOLATE MOFETIL

Cautions full blood counts every week for 4 weeks then twice a month for 2 months then every month in the first year (possibly interrupt treatment if neutropenia develops); active gastro-intestinal disease (risk of haemorrhage, ulceration and perforation); delayed graft function; increased susceptibility to skin cancer (avoid exposure to strong sunlight); possible decreased effectiveness of vaccination—avoid live vaccines; **interactions:** Appendix 1 (mycophenolate mofetil)

Bone marrow suppression Children and their carers should be warned to report immediately any signs or symptoms of bone marrow suppression e.g. infection and inexplicable bruising or bleeding

Renal impairment consider dose reduction if creatinine clearance less than 25 mL/minute/ $1.73m^2$

Contra-indications

Pregnancy manufacturer advises avoid—toxicity in *animal* studies; effective contraception required during and for 6 weeks after discontinuation of treatment

Breast-feeding manufacturer advises avoid—present in milk in *animal* studies

Side-effects diarrhoea, abdominal discomfort, gastritis, nausea, vomiting, constipation; cough, influenza-like syndrome; headache; infections (viral, bacterial, and fungal); increased blood creatinine; leucopenia, anaemia, thrombocytopenia; *less commonly* gastro-oesophageal reflux, gastro-intestinal ulceration and bleeding, pancreatitis, abnormal liver function tests, hepatitis, tachycardia, blood pressure changes, oedema, dyspnoea, tremor, insomnia, dizziness, hyperglycaemia, increased risk of malignancies, disturbances of electrolytes and blood lipids, renal tubular necrosis, arthralgia, alopecia, acne

Licensed use by mouth, in combination with a corticosteroid and ciclosporin, for children 2 years and older for the prophylaxis of acute transplant rejection in renal transplantation

Indication and dose

Prophylaxis of acute rejection in renal transplantation in combination with a corticosteroid and ciclosporin
- **By mouth or by intravenous infusion**

Consult local treatment protocol for details

Child 1 month–18 years 600 mg/m² twice daily (max. 2 g daily)

Prophylaxis of acute rejection in renal transplantation in combination with a corticosteroid and tacrolimus
- **By mouth or by intravenous infusion**

Consult local treatment protocol for details

Child 1 month–18 years 300 mg/m² twice daily (max. 2 g daily)

Prophylaxis of acute rejection in hepatic transplantation in combination with a corticosteroid and ciclosporin or tacrolimus
- **By mouth or by intravenous infusion**

Consult local treatment protocol for details

Child 1 month–18 years 10 mg/kg twice daily, increased to 20 mg/kg twice daily (max. 2 g daily)

Note Tablets and capsules not appropriate for dose titration in young children

Administration Intravenous infusion, dilute reconstituted solution with glucose 5% to produce infusion solution containing 6 mg/mL; infuse over 2 hours

CellCept® (Roche) PoM

Capsules, blue/brown, mycophenolate mofetil 250 mg, net price 100-cap pack = £87.33

Tablets, lavender, mycophenolate mofetil 500 mg, net price 50-tab pack = £87.33

Oral suspension, mycophenolate mofetil 1 g/5 mL when reconstituted with water, net price 175 mL = £122.25

Intravenous infusion, powder for reconstitution, mycophenolate mofetil (as hydrochloride), net price 500-mg vial = £9.69

8.2.2 Corticosteroids and other immunosuppressants

The corticosteroids, prednisolone and dexamethasone, are widely used in paediatric oncology; they have a marked antitumour effect. Dexamethasone is preferred for acute lymphoblastic leukaemia whilst prednisolone may be used for

Hodgkin's disease, non-Hodgkin's lymphoma, and B-cell lymphoma and leukaemia.

Dexamethasone is the corticosteroid of choice in paediatric supportive and palliative care. For children who are not receiving a corticosteroid as a component of their chemotherapy, dexamethasone may be used to reduce raised intracranial pressure (see p. 26), or to help control emesis when combined with an appropriate anti-emetic (see p. 26). For more information on glucocorticoid therapy, including the disadvantages of treatment, see section 6.3.2.

The corticosteroids are also powerful immunosuppressants. They are used to prevent organ transplant rejection, and in high dose to treat rejection episodes.

Ciclosporin (cyclosporin), a calcineurin inhibitor, is a potent immunosuppressant which is virtually non-myelotoxic but markedly nephrotoxic. It may be used in organ and tissue transplantation, for prevention of graft rejection following bone marrow, kidney, liver, pancreas, heart, lung, and heart-lung transplantation, and for prophylaxis and treatment of graft-versus-host disease. Ciclosporin also has a role in steroid-sensitive and steroid-resistant nephrotic syndrome; in corticosteroid-sensitive nephrotic syndrome it may be given with prednisolone (section 6.3).

Tacrolimus is also a calcineurin inhibitor. Although not chemically related to ciclosporin it has a similar mode of action and side-effects.

Both ciclosporin and tacrolimus may affect glucose metabolism in children. Hypertrichosis may be a concern with ciclosporin.

Basiliximab and **daclizumab** are monoclonal antibodies that prevent T-lymphocyte proliferation; they are used for prophylaxis of acute rejection in allogeneic renal transplantation. They are given with ciclosporin and corticosteroid immunosuppression regimens; their use should be confined to specialist centres.

BASILIXIMAB

Contra-indications

Pregnancy avoid; adequate contraception must be used during treatment and for 8 weeks after last dose

Breast-feeding avoid

Side-effects *rarely* severe hypersensitivity reactions; cytokine release syndrome also reported; for side-effects of regimen see under Ciclosporin (below) and Prednisolone (section 6.3.2)

Licensed use in children over 1 year of age for prophylaxis of acute rejection in allogeneic renal transplantation when used in combination with ciclosporin and corticosteroid-containing immunosuppression regimens

Indication and dose

Prophylaxis of acute rejection in allogeneic renal transplantation used in combination with ciclosporin and corticosteroid-containing immunosuppression regimens

- **By intravenous injection or by intravenous infusion**

  Consult local treatment protocol for details

  Child over 1 year, body-weight under 35 kg 10 mg within 2 hours before transplant surgery and 10 mg 4 days after surgery

  Child body-weight over 35 kg 20 mg within 2 hours before transplant surgery and 20 mg 4 days after surgery

  Note withhold second dose if severe hypersensitivity or graft loss occurs

Administration For intravenous infusion, dilute reconstituted solution with sodium chloride 0.9% or glucose 5% to concentration not exceeding 400 micrograms/mL; give over 20–30 minutes

Simulect® (Novartis) PoM
Injection, powder for reconstitution, basiliximab, net price 10-mg vial = £758.69, 20-mg vial = £842.38 (both with water for injections) . For intravenous infusion

CICLOSPORIN
(Cyclosporin)

Cautions monitor kidney function (see also below); monitor liver function (see also below); monitor blood pressure—discontinue if hypertension develops that cannot be controlled by antihypertensives; hyperuricaemia; monitor serum potassium especially in renal dysfunction (risk of hyperkalaemia); monitor serum magnesium; measure blood lipids before treatment and thereafter as appropriate; porphyria (section 9.8.2); monitor whole blood ciclosporin concentration (trough level dependent on indication—consult local treatment protocol for details); use with tacrolimus specifically contra-indicated and apart from specialist use in transplant patients preferably avoid other immunosuppressants with the exception of corticosteroids (increased risk of

CICLOSPORIN (*continued*)

infection and lymphoma); **interactions:** Appendix 1 (ciclosporin)

Additional cautions in nephrotic syndrome *Contra-indicated* in uncontrolled hypertension, uncontrolled infections, and malignancy; in long-term management, perform renal biopsies every 1–2 years

Additional cautions Atopic Dermatitis and Psoriasis, section 13.5.3; Rheumatoid Arthritis, section 10.1.3

Hepatic impairment dosage adjustment based on bilirubin and liver enzymes may be needed

Renal impairment dose as in normal renal function but dose dependent increase in serum creatinine and urea during first few weeks may necessitate discontinuation (exclude rejection if kidney transplant); in nephrotic syndrome reduce dose by 25–50% if serum creatinine more than 30% above baseline on more than one measurement

Pregnancy see section 8.2; crosses placenta

Breast-feeding present in milk—manufacturer advises avoid

Side-effects dose-dependent increase in serum creatinine and urea during first few weeks (see also under Cautions); less commonly renal structural changes on long-term administration; also hypertrichosis, headache, tremor, hypertension (especially in heart transplant patients), hepatic dysfunction, fatigue, gingival hypertrophy, gastro-intestinal disturbances, burning sensation in hands and feet (usually during first week); *occasionally* rash (possibly allergic), coarsening of facial features, mild anaemia, hyperkalaemia, hyperuricaemia, gout, hypomagnesaemia, hypercholesterolaemia, hyperglycaemia, weight increase, oedema, pancreatitis, neuropathy, confusion, paraesthesia, convulsions, benign intracranial hypertension (discontinue), dysmenorrhoea or amenorrhoea; myalgia, muscle weakness, cramps, myopathy, gynaecomastia (in patients receiving concomitant spironolactone), colitis and cortical blindness also reported; thrombocytopenia (sometimes with haemolytic uraemic syndrome) also reported; incidence of malignancies and lymphoproliferative disorders similar to that with other immunosuppressive therapy

Pharmacokinetics monitor whole blood ciclosporin concentrations (see under Cautions)

Licensed use prevention of graft rejection following bone-marrow, kidney, liver, pancreas, heart, lung, and heart-lung transplantation; prophylaxis and treatment of graft-versus-host disease; nephrotic syndrome; atopic eczema (child over 16 years—see section 13.5.3)

Indication and dose

Prevention of graft rejection following bone-marrow, kidney, liver, pancreas, heart, lung, and heart-lung transplantation, prophylaxis and treatment of graft-versus-host disease
- **By mouth or by intravenous infusion**

  Consult local treatment protocols for details

Nephrotic syndrome see also section 6.3.2, p. 425
- **By mouth**

  Child 1 month–18 years 3 mg/kg twice daily, increase if necessary in corticosteroid-resistant disease; for maintenance reduce to lowest effective dose according to whole blood-ciclosporin concentrations, proteinuria, and renal function

Ulcerative colitis section 1.5

Severe psoriasis, severe eczema section 13.5.3

Conversion Any conversion between brands should be undertaken very carefully and the manufacturer contacted for further information. Currently only *Neoral*® remains available for oral use; *Sandimmun*® capsules and oral solution and *SangCya*® oral solution are available on named-patient basis only for children who cannot be transferred to another brand of oral ciclosporin

Because of differences in bioavailability, the brand of ciclosporin to be dispensed should be specified by the prescriber

Neoral® (Novartis) PoM

Capsules, ciclosporin 10 mg (yellow/white), net price 60-cap pack = £16.44; 25 mg (blue/grey), 30-cap pack = £12.00; 50 mg (yellow/white), 30-cap pack = £26.50; 100 mg (blue/grey), 30-cap pack = £50.00. Counselling, administration

Oral solution, yellow, sugar-free, ciclosporin 100 mg/mL, net price 50 mL = £82.00. Counselling, administration

Counselling Total daily dose should be taken in 2 divided doses. Avoid grapefruit or grapefruit juice for 1 hour before dose

Mix solution with orange juice (or squash) or apple juice (to improve taste) or with water immediately before taking (and rinse with more to ensure total dose). Do not mix with grapefruit juice. Keep medicine measure away from other liquids (including water)

Sandimmun® (Novartis) PoM

Concentrate for intravenous infusion (oily), ciclosporin 50 mg/mL. To be diluted before use. Net price 1-mL amp = £1.94; 5-mL amp = £9.17

Excipients: include polyoxyl castor oil (risk of anaphylaxis, see Excipients, p. 3)

Administration By intravenous infusion, diluted to 0.5–2.5 mg/mL in sodium chloride 0.9% or glucose 5%, over 2–6 hours; not to be used with PVC equipment; observe for at least 30 minutes after starting infusion and at frequent intervals thereafter

DACLIZUMAB

Contra-indications

Pregnancy avoid

Breast-feeding avoid

Side-effects severe hypersensitivity reactions reported rarely; for side-effects of regimen see under Ciclosporin (above) and Prednisolone (section 6.3.2)

DACLIZUMAB (*continued*)

Licensed use licensed for use in children (age range not specified by manufacturer) for prophylaxis of acute rejection in allogeneic renal transplantation when used in combination with ciclosporin and corticosteroid containing immunosuppression regimens

Indication and dose

Prophylaxis of acute rejection in allogeneic renal transplantation when used in combination with ciclosporin and corticosteroid containing immunosuppression regimens

- **By intravenous infusion**

  Consult local treatment protocol for details

  Child 1–18 years 1 mg/kg within the 24-hour period before transplantation, then 1 mg/kg every 14 days for a total of 5 doses

Zenapax® (Roche) ▼ PoM

Concentrate for intravenous infusion, daclizumab 5 mg/mL, net price 5-mL = £223.68

TACROLIMUS

Cautions see under Ciclosporin; also monitor ECG (**important:** also echocardiography, see CSM warning below), visual status, blood glucose, haematological and neurological parameters; monitor whole blood tacrolimus concentration (consult local treatment protocol for details); **interactions:** Appendix 1 (tacrolimus)

Driving May affect performance of skilled tasks (e.g. driving)

Hepatic impairment reduce dose in severe impairment

Contra-indications hypersensitivity to macrolides; avoid concurrent administration with ciclosporin (care if patient has previously received ciclosporin)

Pregnancy crosses placenta; association with pre-term delivery and intra-uterine growth retardation; contra-indicated by manufacturer; exclude pregnancy before starting—if contraception needed non-hormonal methods should be used

Breast-feeding avoid—present in milk following systemic administration

Side-effects include gastro-intestinal disturbances including dyspepsia, and inflammatory and ulcerative disorders; hepatic dysfunction, jaundice, bile-duct and gall-bladder abnormalities; hypertension (less frequently hypotension), tachycardia, angina, arrhythmias, thromboembolic and ischaemic events, rarely myocardial hypertrophy, cardiomyopathy (**important**: see CSM warning below); dyspnoea, pleural effusion, tremor, headache, insomnia, paraesthesia, confusion, depression, dizziness, anxiety, convulsions, incoordination, encephalopathy, psychosis; visual and hearing abnormalities; haematological effects including anaemia, leucocytosis, leucopenia, thrombocytopenia, coagulation disorders; altered acid-base balance and glucose metabolism, electrolyte disturbances including hyperkalaemia (less frequently hypokalaemia); altered renal function including increased serum creatinine; hypophosphataemia, hypercalcaemia, hyperuricaemia; muscle cramps, arthralgia; pruritus, alopecia, rash, sweating, acne, photosensitivity; susceptibility to lymphoma and other malignancies particularly of the skin; less commonly ascites, pancreatitis, atelectasis, kidney damage and renal failure, myasthenia, hirsutism, rarely Stevens-Johnson syndrome

CSM warning Cardiomyopathy has been reported in children given tacrolimus after transplantation. Children should be monitored carefully by echocardiography for hypertrophic changes; dose reduction or discontinuation should be considered if these occur

Indication and dose

Primary immunosuppression for prevention of graft rejection following liver transplantation, commencing 12 hours after completion of surgery

- **By mouth**

  Consult local treatment protocol for details

  Child 1 month–18 years initially 150 micrograms/kg twice daily then 75–150 micrograms/kg twice daily adjusted according to whole blood concentrations

- **By continuous intravenous infusion (only if oral route inappropriate)**

  Consult local treatment protocol for details

  Child 1 month–18 years 30–60 micrograms/kg over 24 hours

Primary immunosuppression for prevention of graft rejection following kidney transplantation, commencing within 24 hours of completion of surgery

- **By mouth**

  Consult local treatment protocol for details

  Child 1 month–18 years initially 150 micrograms/kg twice daily adjusted according to whole blood concentration

- **By continuous intravenous infusion (use only if oral route inappropriate)**

  Consult local treatment protocol for details

  Child 1 month–18 years up to 60 micrograms/kg over 24 hours adjusted according to whole blood concentration

Topical use in atopic eczema section 13.5.3

Administration By continuous intravenous infusion over 24 hours, diluted to 4–100 micrograms/mL with glucose 5% or sodium chloride 0.9%, to a

TACROLIMUS (*continued*)

total volume between 20–500 mL; incompatible with PVC

Prograf® (Astellas) PoM
Capsules, tacrolimus 500 micrograms (yellow), net price 50-cap pack = £65.69; 1 mg (white), 50-cap pack = £85.22, 100-cap pack = £170.43; 5 mg (greyish-red), 50-cap pack = £314.84. Label: 23, counselling, driving

Concentrate for intravenous infusion, tacrolimus 5 mg/mL. To be diluted before use. Net price 1-mL amp = £62.05
Excipients: include polyoxyl castor oil (risk of anaphylaxis, see Excipients, p. 3)

Extemporaneous formulations available see Extemporaneous Preparations, p. 8

8.2.3 Rituximab and alemtuzumab

Rituximab, a monoclonal antibody which causes lysis of B lymphocytes, has been used as a component of the treatment of post-transplantation lymphoproliferative disease, non-Hodgkin's lymphoma, Hodgkin's lymphoma, and severe cases of resistant immune modulated disease including idiopathic thrombocytopenia purpura, haemolytic anaemia, and systemic lupus erythematosus. Full resuscitation facilities should be at hand and as with other cytotoxics, treatment should be undertaken under the close supervision of a specialist.

Rituximab should be used with caution in children receiving cardiotoxic chemotherapy or with a history of cardiovascular disease; in adults exacerbation of angina, arrhythmia, and heart failure have been reported. Transient hypotension occurs frequently during infusion and antihypertensives may need to be withheld for 12 hours before infusion.

Infusion-related side-effects (including cytokine release syndrome) are reported commonly with rituximab and occur predominantly during the first infusion; they include fever and chills, nausea and vomiting, allergic reactions (such as rash, pruritus, angioedema, bronchospasm and dyspnoea), flushing and tumour pain. Children should be given an analgesic and an antihistamine before each dose of rituximab to reduce these effects. Premedication with a corticosteroid should also be considered. The infusion may have to be stopped temporarily and the infusion-related effects treated—consult product literature or local treatment protocol for appropriate management. Evidence of pulmonary infiltration and features of tumour lysis syndrome should be sought if infusion-related effects occur.

Fatalities following **severe** cytokine release syndrome (characterised by severe dyspnoea) and associated with features of tumour lysis syndrome have occurred 1–2 hours after infusion of rituximab. Children with a high tumour burden as well as those with pulmonary insufficiency or infiltration are at increased risk and should be monitored **very closely** (and a slower rate of infusion considered).

Alemtuzumab, another monoclonal antibody that causes lysis of B lymphocytes, has been used in children for conditioning therapy before allogeneic bone marrow transplantation. In common with rituximab, it causes infusion-related side-effects including cytokine release syndrome (see above) and premedication with an analgesic, an antihistamine, and a corticosteroid is recommended.

ALEMTUZUMAB

Cautions see notes above—for full details (including monitoring) consult product literature or local treatment protocol

Contra-indications for full details consult product literature or local treatment protocol

Pregnancy avoid; manufacturer advises effective contraception for 6 months after administration in both sexes

Breast-feeding avoid; manufacturer advises avoid breast-feeding during treatment and for at least 4 weeks after administration

Side-effects see notes above—for full details (including monitoring and management of side-effects) consult product literature

Licensed use licensed for use in children 17 years of age and older

Indication and dose

See notes above

- **By intravenous infusion**
  Consult local treatment protocol for details

Administration By intravenous infusion in glucose 5% *or* sodium chloride 0.9%. Add requisite dose through a low protein binding 5-micron filter to 100-mL infusion fluid; infuse over 2 hours

MabCampath® (Schering Health) ▼ PoM
Concentrate for intravenous infusion, alemtuzumab 30 mg/mL, net price 1-mL amp = £274.83

RITUXIMAB

Cautions see notes above—but for full details (including monitoring) consult product literature or local treatment protocol

Pregnancy avoid unless potential benefit to mother outweighs risk of B-lymphocyte depletion in fetus—effective contraception (in both sexes) required during treatment and for 12 months afterwards

Contra-indications breast-feeding

Side-effects see notes above—but for full details (including monitoring and management of side-effects) consult product literature

Licensed use not licensed for use in children

Indication and dose

See notes above

- **By intravenous infusion**
  Consult local treatment protocol for details

Administration By intravenous infusion in glucose 5% *or* sodium chloride 0.9%; dilute to 1–4 mg/mL and gently invert bag to avoid foaming

MabThera® (Roche) PoM
Concentrate for intravenous infusion, rituximab 10 mg/mL, net price 10-mL vial = £174.63, 50-mL vial = £873.15

8.2.4 Other immunomodulating drugs

Interferon alfa

Interferon alfa has shown some antitumour effect and may have a role in inducing early regression of life-threatening corticosteroid-resistant haemangiomas of infancy. Interferon alfa preparations are also used in the treatment of chronic hepatitis B, and chronic hepatitis C ideally in combination with ribavirin (section 5.3.3). Interferon alfa should always be used under the close supervision of a specialist. Side-effects are dose-related, but commonly include anorexia, nausea, influenza-like symptoms, and lethargy. Ocular side-effects and depression (including suicidal behaviour) have also been reported. Myelosuppression may occur, particularly affecting granulocyte counts. Cardiovascular problems (hypotension, hypertension, and arrhythmias), nephrotoxicity and hepatotoxicity have been reported and monitoring of hepatic function is recommended. Hypertriglyceridaemia, sometimes severe, has been observed; monitoring of lipid concentration is recommended. Other side-effects include hypersensitivity reactions, thyroid abnormalities, hyperglycaemia, alopecia, psoriasiform rash, confusion, coma and seizures, and reversible motor problems in young children. Rarely pulmonary infiltrates, pneumonitis, and pneumonia have occurred; respiratory symptoms should be investigated and if pulmonary infiltrates are suspected or lung function is impaired the discontinuation of interferon alfa should be considered.

INTERFERON ALFA

Cautions consult product literature and local treatment protocol for details; **interactions:** Appendix 1 (interferons)

Hepatic impairment close monitoring in mild to moderate hepatic impairment; avoid if severe

Renal impairment mild to moderate, monitor closely; severe, avoid

Pregnancy manufacturers recommend avoid unless compelling reasons; effective contraception required in both sexes if receiving treatment

Breast-feeding manufacturers advise avoid

Contra-indications consult product literature and local treatment protocol for details; avoid injections containing benzyl alcohol in neonates (see under preparations below)

Side-effects see notes above, consult product literature and local treatment protocols for details

Licensed use Not licensed for use in children for chronic active hepatitis B; *Roferon-A®* not licensed for use in children

Indication and dose

Induction of early regression of life-threatening corticosteroid resistant haemangiomata of infancy

- **By subcutaneous injection**
  Consult local treatment protocol for details

Chronic active hepatitis B infection see under preparations below

Chronic active hepatitis C infection see under preparations below

IntronA® (Schering-Plough) PoM
Injection, interferon alfa-2b (rbe) 10 million units/mL, net price 2.5-mL vial = £108.00. For subcutaneous or intravenous injection

Injection, powder for reconstitution, interferon alfa-2b (rbe), net price 10-million unit vial (with injection equipment and water for injections) = £53.96. For subcutaneous or intravenous injection

Injection pen, interferon alfa-2b (rbe), net price 15 million units/mL, 1.5-mL cartridge = £77.76;

INTERFERON ALFA (*continued*)

25 million units/mL, 1.5-mL cartridge = £129.60; 50 million units/mL, 1.5-mL cartridge = £259.20. For subcutaneous injection

Note Each 1.5-mL multidose cartridge delivers 6 doses of 0.2 mL i.e. a total of 1.2 mL

Dose

Chronic active hepatitis B
- **By subcutaneous injection**
  Child 2–18 years 5–10 million units/m² 3 times weekly

Chronic active hepatitis C (in combination with oral ribavirin, see p. 374)
- **By subcutaneous injection**
  Child 3–18 years 3 million units/m² 3 times weekly

Roferon-A® (Roche) PoM

Injection, interferon alfa-2a (rbe). Net price 6 million units/mL, 0.5-mL (3 million-unit) prefilled syringe = £15.07; 9 million units/mL, 0.5-mL (4.5 million-unit) prefilled syringe = £22.60; 12 million units/mL, 0.5-mL (6 million-unit) prefilled syringe = £30.12; 18 million units/mL, 0.5-mL (9 million-unit) prefilled syringe = £45.19; 36 million units/mL, 0.5-mL (18 million-unit) prefilled syringe = £90.39; 30 million units/mL, 0.6-mL (18 million-unit) cartridge = £90.39, for use with *Roferon* pen device. For subcutaneous injection (cartridges, vials, and prefilled syringes) and intramuscular injection (cartridges and vials)

Excipients: include benzyl alcohol (avoid in neonates, see Excipients, p. 3)

Dose

Chronic active hepatitis B
- **By subcutaneous injection**
  Child 2–18 years 2.5–5 million units/m² 3 times weekly; up to 10 million units/m² has been used 3 times weekly

Viraferon® (Schering-Plough) PoM

Injection, interferon alfa-2b (rbe) 6 million units/mL, net price 3-mL vial = £90.40. For subcutaneous injection

Injection pen, interferon alfa-2b (rbe), net price 15 million units/mL, 1.5-mL cartridge = £90.40. For subcutaneous injection

Note 1.5-mL multidose cartridge delivers 6 doses of 0.2 mL each

Dose

Chronic active hepatitis B
- **By subcutaneous injection**
  Child 2–18 years 5–10 million units/m² 3 times weekly

Chronic active hepatitis C (in combination with oral ribavirin, see p. 374)
- **By subcutaneous injection**
  Child 3–18 years 3 million units/m² 3 times weekly

8.3 Sex hormones and hormone antagonists in malignant disease

Classification not used in BNF for Children

9 Nutrition and blood

9.1 Anaemias and some other blood disorders

9.1.1 Iron-deficiency anaemias
9.1.2 Drugs used in megaloblastic anaemias
9.1.3 Drugs used in hypoplastic, haemolytic, and renal anaemias
9.1.4 Drugs used in platelet disorders
9.1.5 G6PD deficiency
9.1.6 Drugs used in neutropenia

Before initiating treatment for anaemia it is essential to determine which type is present. Iron salts may be harmful and result in iron overload if given alone to patients with anaemias other than those due to iron deficiency.

9.1.1 Iron-deficiency anaemias

Treatment with an iron preparation is justified only in the presence of a demonstrable iron-deficiency state. Before starting treatment, it is important to exclude any serious underlying cause of the anaemia (e.g. gastro-intestinal bleeding). The possibility of thalassaemia should be considered in children of Mediterranean or Indian subcontinent descent.

Prophylaxis with an iron preparation is justifiable in individuals who have additional risk factors for iron deficiency (e.g. poor diet). Prophylaxis may also be appropriate in malabsorption, menorrhagia, pregnancy, in haemodialysis patients, and in the management of low birth-weight infants such as preterm neonates.

9.1.1.1 Oral iron

Iron salts should be given by mouth unless there are good reasons for using another route.

Ferrous salts show only marginal differences between one another in efficiency of absorption of iron, but ferric salts are much less well absorbed. Haemoglobin regeneration rate is little affected by the type of salt used provided sufficient iron is given, and in most patients the speed of response is not critical. Choice of preparation is thus usually decided by formulation, palatability, incidence of side-effects and cost.

Dose The oral dose of elemental iron to treat deficiency is 3–6 mg/kg (max. 200 mg) daily given in 2–3 divided doses. Iron supplementation may also be required to produce an optimum response to epoetin in iron-deficient children with chronic renal failure or in preterm neonates.

Prescribing Express the dose in terms of elemental iron and iron salt and select the most appropriate preparation; specify both the iron salt and formulation on the prescription.

Iron content of different iron salts

Iron salt	Amount	Content of ferrous iron
Ferrous fumarate	200 mg	65 mg
Ferrous gluconate	300 mg	35 mg
Ferrous sulphate	300 mg	60 mg
Ferrous sulphate, dried	200 mg	65 mg
Sodium feredetate	190 mg	27.5 mg

Therapeutic response The haemoglobin concentration should rise by about 100–200 mg/100 mL (1–2 g/litre) per day *or* 2 g/100 mL (20 g/litre) over 3–4 weeks. When the haemoglobin is in the normal range, treatment should be continued for a further 3 months to replenish the iron stores. Epithelial tissue changes such as atrophic glossitis and koilonychia are usually improved, but the response is often slow. The most common reason for lack of response in children is poor compliance; poor absorption is rare in children.

Prophylaxis of iron deficiency in neonates In neonates, haemoglobin and haematocrit concentrations change rapidly. These changes are not due to iron deficiency and cannot be corrected by iron supplementation. Similarly, neonatal anaemia resulting from repeated blood sampling does not respond to iron therapy.

All babies, including preterm neonates, are born with substantial iron stores but these stores can become depleted unless dietary intake is adequate. All babies require an iron intake of 400–700 nanograms daily to maintain body stores. Iron in breast milk is well absorbed but that in artificial feeds or in cow's milk is less so. Most artificial formula feeds are sufficiently fortified with iron to prevent deficiency.

Dose Prophylactic iron supplementation (elemental iron 5 mg daily) may be required in babies of low birth-weight who are solely breast-fed; supplementation is started 4–6 weeks after birth and continued until mixed feeding is established.

Infants with a poor diet may become anaemic in the second year of life, particularly if cow's milk, rather than fortified formula feed, is a major part of the diet.

Compound preparations Some oral preparations contain ascorbic acid to aid absorption of the iron but the therapeutic advantage of such preparations is minimal and cost may be increased.

There is no justification for the inclusion of other ingredients, such as the B group of vitamins, except folic acid for pregnant women.

Side-effects Gastro-intestinal irritation may occur with iron salts. Nausea and epigastric pain are dose-related but the relationship between dose and altered bowel habit (constipation or diarrhoea) is less clear. Oral iron may exacerbate diarrhoea in patients with inflammatory bowel disease.

Iron preparations taken orally may be constipating, occasionally leading to faecal impaction.

If side-effects occur, the dose may be reduced; alternatively, another iron salt may be used but an improvement in tolerance may simply be a result of a lower content of elemental iron. The incidence of side-effects due to ferrous sulphate is no greater than with other iron salts when compared on the basis of equivalent amounts of elemental iron.

Iron preparations are an important cause of accidental overdose in children and as little as 20–30 mg/kg of elemental iron can be fatal. For the treatment of **iron overdose**, see Emergency Treatment of Poisoning, p. 40.

FERROUS SULPHATE

Cautions pregnancy (see section 9.1.1); **interactions:** Appendix 1 (iron)

Side-effects see notes above

Indication and dose

Iron-deficiency anaemia, prophylaxis of iron deficiency in neonates see notes above and preparations

Counselling Although iron preparations are best absorbed on an empty stomach they may be taken after food to reduce gastro-intestinal side-effects; they may discolour stools

Ferrous Sulphate (Non-proprietary)

Tablets, coated, dried ferrous sulphate 200 mg (65 mg iron), net price 28-tab pack = £1.59

Dose

Child 6–18 years prophylactic, 1 tablet daily; therapeutic, 1 tablet 2–3 times daily

Ironorm® Drops (Wallace Mfg)

Oral drops, ferrous sulphate 625 mg (125 mg iron)/5 mL. Net price 15 mL = £3.35

Dose

Child 1 month–6 years prophylactic 0.3 mL daily

Child 6–18 years prophylactic 0.6 mL daily

FERROUS FUMARATE

Cautions pregnancy (see section 9.1.1); **interactions:** Appendix 1 (iron)

Side-effects see notes above

Indication and dose

Iron-deficiency anaemia, prophylaxis of iron deficiency in neonates see notes above and preparations

Syrup, brown, ferrous fumarate approx. 140 mg (45 mg iron)/5 mL. Net price 200 mL = £3.00

Dose

Preterm neonate 0.6–2.4 mL/kg daily

Neonate 2.5–5 mL daily

Child 1 month–6 years 2.5–5 mL twice daily

Child 6–18 years 10 mL twice daily

Fersaday® (Goldshield)

Tablets, brown, f/c, ferrous fumarate 322 mg (100 mg iron). Net price 28-tab pack = 66p

Dose

Child 12–18 years prophylactic, 1 tablet daily; therapeutic, 1 tablet twice daily

Fersamal® (Goldshield)

Tablets, brown, ferrous fumarate 210 mg (68 mg iron). Net price 20 = 29p

Dose

Child 12–18 years 1–2 tablets 3 times daily

Galfer® (Thornton & Ross)

Capsules, red/green, ferrous fumarate 305 mg (100 mg iron). Net price 20 = 36p

Dose

Child 12–18 years 1 capsule 1–2 times daily before food

Syrup, brown, sugar-free ferrous fumarate 140 mg (45 mg iron)/5 mL. Net price 300 mL = £4.86

Dose

Child 1 month–6 years 2.5–5 mL 1–2 times daily before food

Child 6–18 years 10 mL 1–2 times daily before food

FERROUS GLUCONATE

Cautions pregnancy (see section 9.1.1); **interactions**: Appendix 1 (iron)

Side-effects see notes above

Indication and dose

Iron-deficiency anaemia see notes above and preparations

Ferrous Gluconate (Non-proprietary)

Tablets, red, coated, ferrous gluconate 300 mg (35 mg iron). Net price 20 = 73p

Dose

Child 6–12 years prophylactic and therapeutic, 1–3 tablets daily

Child 12–18 years prophylactic, 2 tablets daily before food; therapeutic, 4–6 tablets daily in divided doses before food

POLYSACCHARIDE-IRON COMPLEX

Cautions pregnancy (see section 9.1.1); **interactions**: Appendix 1 (iron)

Side-effects see notes above

Indication and dose

Iron-deficiency anaemia, prophylaxis of iron deficiency in neonates see notes above and preparations

Niferex® (Tillomed)

Elixir, brown, sugar-free, polysaccharide-iron complex equivalent to 100 mg of iron/5 mL. Net price 240-mL pack = £6.06; NHS[1] 30-mL dropper bottle for paediatric use = £2.16. Counselling, use of dropper

Dose

Neonate (from dropper bottle) 1 drop (approx. 500 micrograms iron) per 450 g body-weight 3 times daily

Child 1 month–1 year (from dropper bottle) 1 drop (approx. 500 micrograms iron) per 450 g body-weight 3 times daily

Child 1–6 years 2.5 mL daily

Child 6–12 years 5 mL daily

Child 12–18 years prophylactic, 2.5 mL daily; therapeutic, 5 mL 1–2 times daily

1. except 30 mL paediatric dropper bottle for prophylaxis and treatment of iron deficiency in infants born prematurely; endorse prescription 'SLS'

SODIUM FEREDETATE
(Sodium ironedetate)

Cautions pregnancy (see section 9.1.1); **interactions**: Appendix 1 (iron)

Side-effects see notes above

Indication and dose

Iron-deficiency anaemia, prophylaxis of iron deficiency in neonates see notes above and preparations

Sytron® (Link)

Elixir, sugar-free, sodium feredetate 190 mg equivalent to 27.5 mg of iron/5 mL. Net price 100 mL = 89p

Dose

Neonate 2.5 mL twice daily (smaller doses should be used initially)

Child 1 month–1 year 2.5 mL twice daily (smaller doses should be used initially)

Child 1–5 years 2.5 mL 3 times daily

Child 5–12 years 5 mL 3 times daily

Child 12–18 years 5–10 mL 3 times daily

9.1.1.2 Parenteral iron

Iron may be administered parenterally as iron dextran, or iron sucrose. Parenteral iron is generally reserved for use when oral therapy is unsuccessful because the child cannot tolerate oral iron, or does not take it reliably, or if there is continuing blood loss, or in malabsorption.

Also, many children with chronic renal failure who are receiving haemodialysis (and some who are receiving peritoneal dialysis) require iron by the intravenous route on a regular basis (see also Erythropoietin, section 9.1.3).

With the exception of children with severe renal failure receiving haemodialysis, parenteral iron does not produce a faster haemoglobin response than oral iron provided that the oral iron preparation is taken reliably and is absorbed adequately.

Iron dextran, a complex of ferric hydroxide with dextrans, and **iron sucrose**, a complex of ferric hydroxide with sucrose, are used for the parenteral administration of iron. Anaphylactoid reactions can occur with parenteral iron complexes and a small test dose should be given initially; facilities for cardiopulmonary resuscitation must be at hand. If children complain of acute symptoms particularly nausea, back pain, breathlessness or develop hypotension the infusion should be stopped.

IRON DEXTRAN

A complex of ferric hydroxide with sucrose containing 5% (50 mg/mL) of iron

Cautions facilities for cardiopulmonary resuscitation must be at hand; increased risk of allergic reaction in immune or inflammatory conditions; renal impairment; oral iron not to be given until 5 days after last injection

Hepatic impairment avoid in severe impairment

Pregnancy avoid in first trimester

Contra-indications history of allergic disorders including asthma and eczema; infection; active rheumatoid arthritis

Renal impairment avoid in acute renal failure

Side-effects nausea, dyspepsia, diarrhoea, chest pains, hypotension, dyspnoea, arthralgia, myalgia, pruritus, urticaria, rash, fever, shivering, flushing, headache; rarely anaphylactoid reactions; injection site reactions including phlebitis reported

Licensed use not licensed for use in children under 14 years

Indication and dose

Iron-deficiency anaemia see notes above

- **By slow intravenous injection or by intravenous infusion**

  Calculated according to body-weight and iron deficit, see notes above and consult product literature

Administration For *intravenous injection*, give test dose over 1–2 minutes followed after 15 minutes by the remaining dose. For *intravenous infusion*, dilute to a concentration of 1–2 mg/mL with Glucose 5% *or* Sodium Chloride 0.9%; give test dose over 15 minutes, then give at a rate not exceeding 3.33 mL/minute—consult product literature

CosmoFer® (Vitaline) ▼ PoM
Injection, iron (as iron dextran) 50 mg/mL, net price 2-mL amp = £7.97

IRON SUCROSE

A complex of ferric hydroxide with sucrose containing 2% (20 mg/mL) of iron

Cautions facilities for cardiopulmonary resuscitation must be at hand; oral iron therapy should not be given until 5 days after last injection

Pregnancy avoid in first trimester

Contra-indications history of allergic disorders including asthma, eczema and anaphylaxis; infection

Hepatic impairment avoid

Side-effects nausea, vomiting, taste disturbances, headache, hypotension; less frequently paraesthesia, abdominal disorders, myalgia, fever, flushing, urticaria, peripheral oedema; rarely anaphylactoid reactions; injection site reactions including phlebitis reported

Licensed use not licensed for use in children

Indication and dose

Iron-deficiency anaemia see notes above

- **By slow intravenous injection or by intravenous infusion**

  Calculated according to body-weight and iron deficit, see notes above and consult product literature

Administration For *intravenous injection*, give test dose over 1–2 minutes followed after 15 minutes by the remaining dose. For *intravenous infusion*, dilute to a concentration of 1 mg/mL with Sodium Chloride 0.9%; give test dose over 15 minutes, then give at a rate not exceeding 3.33 mg/minute—consult product literature

Venofer® (Syner-Med) PoM
Injection, iron (as iron sucrose) 20 mg/mL, net price 5-mL amp = £8.50

9.1.2 Drugs used in megaloblastic anaemias

Megaloblastic anaemia is rare in children; it may result from a lack of either vitamin B_{12} or folate, and it is essential to establish in every case which deficiency is present and the underlying cause. In emergencies, where delay might be dangerous, it is sometimes necessary to administer both substances after the bone marrow test while plasma assay results are awaited. Normally, however, appropriate treatment should be instituted only when the results of tests are available.

Vitamin B_{12} is used in the treatment of megaloblastosis caused by *prolonged nitrous oxide anaesthesia*, which inactivates the vitamin, and in the rare disorders of *congenital transcobalamin II deficiency, methylmalonic acidaemia* and *homocystinuria* (see section 9.8.1).

Vitamin B_{12} should be given prophylactically after *total ileal resection.*

Apart from dietary deficiency, all other causes of vitamin-B_{12} deficiency are attributable to malabsorption. There is little place for the use of low-dose vitamin B_{12} orally and none for vitamin B_{12} intrinsic factor complexes given by mouth. Vitamin B_{12} in large oral doses [unlicensed] may be effective.

Hydroxocobalamin has completely replaced cyanocobalamin as the form of vitamin B_{12} of choice for therapy; it is retained in the body longer than cyanocobalamin and thus for maintenance therapy can be given at intervals of up to 3 months. Treatment is generally initiated with frequent administration of intramuscular injections to replenish the depleted body stores. Thereafter, maintenance treatment, which is usually for life, can be instituted. There is no evidence that doses larger than those recommended provide any additional benefit in vitamin-B_{12} neuropathy.

Folic acid has few indications for long-term therapy since most causes of folate deficiency are self-limiting or will yield to a short course of treatment. It should not be used in undiagnosed megaloblastic anaemia unless vitamin B_{12} is administered concurrently otherwise neuropathy may be precipitated (see above).

In *folate-deficient megaloblastic anaemia* (e.g. because of poor nutrition, pregnancy, or treatment with antiepileptics), daily folic acid supplementation for 4 months brings about haematological remission and replenishes body stores; higher doses may be necessary in malabsorption states. In pregnancy, folic acid 5 mg daily is continued to term.

For *prophylaxis in chronic haemolytic states or in renal dialysis*, it is sufficient to give folic acid daily or even weekly, depending on the diet and the rate of haemolysis.

For *prophylaxis in pregnancy* the dose of folic acid is 200–500 micrograms daily. See also Prevention of Neural Tube Defects below.

Folic acid is actively excreted in breast milk and is well absorbed by the infant. It is also present in cow's milk and artificial formula feeds but is heat labile. Serum and red cell folate concentrations fall after delivery and urinary losses are high, particularly in low birth-weight neonates. Although symptomatic deficiency is rare in the absence of malabsorption or prolonged diarrhoea, it is common for neonatal units to give supplements of folic acid to all preterm neonates from 2 weeks of age until full-term corrected age is reached, particularly if heated breast milk is used without an artificial formula fortifier.

Folinic acid is also effective in the treatment of folate-deficient megaloblastic anaemia but it is normally only used in association with cytotoxic drugs (see section 8.1); it is given as calcium folinate.

Prevention of neural tube defects Recommendations of an expert advisory group of the Department of Health include the advice that:

> To prevent *recurrence of neural tube defect* (in a child of a man or woman with spina bifida or if there is a history of neural tube defect in a previous child) adolescent girls who wish to become pregnant (or who are at risk of becoming pregnant) should be advised to take folic acid supplements at a dose of 5 mg daily (reduced to 4 mg daily if a suitable preparation becomes available); supplementation should continue until week 12 of pregnancy. Those receiving antiepileptic therapy need individual counselling by their doctor before starting folic acid.
>
> To prevent *first occurrence of neural tube defect* folic acid should be taken as a medicinal or food supplement at a dose of 400 micrograms daily before conception and during the first 12 weeks of pregnancy. Those who have not been taking supplements and who suspect they are pregnant should start at once and continue until week 12 of pregnancy.

There is **no** justification for prescribing multiple-ingredient vitamin preparations containing vitamin B_{12} or folic acid.

HYDROXOCOBALAMIN

Cautions should not be given before diagnosis fully established but see also notes above; **interactions** Appendix 1 (hydroxocobalamin)

Side-effects itching, exanthema; fever, chills, hot flushes; nausea, dizziness; initial hypokalaemia; rarely acneform and bullous eruptions; anaphylaxis

Licensed use licensed for use in children (age not specified by manufacturers); not licensed for use in inborn errors of metabolism

Indication and dose

Macrocytic anaemia without neurological involvement
- **By intramuscular injection**

Child 1 month–18 years initially 250 micrograms–1 mg 3 times a week for 2 weeks then 250 micrograms once weekly until blood count normal, then 1 mg every 3 months

Macrocytic anaemia with neurological involvement
- **By intramuscular injection**

Child 1 month–18 years initially 1 mg on alternate days until no further improvement, then 1 mg every 2 months

Prophylaxis of macrocytic anaemias associated with vitamin-B_{12} deficiency
- **By intramuscular injection**

Child 1 month–18 years 1 mg every 2–3 months

Leber's optic atrophy
- **By intramuscular injection**

initially 1 mg daily for 2 weeks, then 1 mg twice weekly until no further improvement, thereafter 1 mg every 1–3 months

Congenital transcobalamin II deficiency
- **By intramuscular injection**

Neonate 1 mg 3 times a week, reduce after 1 year to 1 mg once weekly or as appropriate

Child 1 month–18 years 1 mg 3 times a week, reduce after 1 year to 1 mg once weekly or as appropriate

Methylmalonic acidaemia and homocystinuria
- **By intramuscular injection**

Child 1 month–18 years initially 1 mg daily for 5–7 days, reduce according to response to maintenance dose of up to 1 mg once or twice weekly

Methylmalonic acidaemia, maintenance once intramuscular response established
- **By mouth**

Child 1 month–18 years 5–10 mg once or twice weekly

Note Some children do not respond to the oral route

Hydroxocobalamin (Non-proprietary) PoM

Injection, hydroxocobalamin 1 mg/mL. Net price 1-mL amp = £2.46

Brands include *Cobalin-H®* NHS, *Neo-Cytamen®* NHS

Injection, hydroxocobalamin 2.5 mg/mL, 2 mL

Available from specialist importing companies

Administration injection may be given orally; it will not have prolonged effect via this route

Note The BP directs that when Vitamin B_{12} injection is prescribed or demanded hydroxocobalamin injection shall be dispensed or supplied

Powder available from specialist importing companies

FOLIC ACID

Cautions should never be given alone for vitamin-B_{12} deficiency states (may precipitate subacute combined degeneration of the spinal cord); **interactions**: Appendix 1 (folates)

Side-effects rarely gastrointestinal disturbances

Licensed use unlicensed for limiting methotrexate toxicity

Indication and dose

Folate supplementation in neonates (see notes above)
- **By mouth**

Neonate 50 micrograms once daily or 500 micrograms once weekly

Megaloblastic anaemia due to folate deficiency
- **By mouth**

Neonate initially 500 micrograms/kg once daily for up to 4 months; maintenance 500 micrograms/kg every 1–7 days

Child 1 month–1 year initially 500 micrograms/kg once daily (max. 5 mg) for up to 4 months; maintenance 500 micrograms/kg (max. 5 mg) every 1–7 days

Child 1–18 years 5 mg daily for 4 months; maintenance 5 mg every 1–7 days

Haemolytic anaemia; metabolic disorders
- **By mouth**

Child 1 month–12 years 2.5–5 mg once daily

Child 12–18 years 5–10 mg once daily

Prophylaxis of folate deficiency in dialysis
- **By mouth**

Child 1 month–12 years 250 microgram/kg (max. 10 mg) once daily

Child 12–18 years 5-10 mg once daily

Prevention of methotrexate side-effects in juvenile idiopathic arthritis
- **By mouth**

Child 2–18 years 1 mg daily or 5 mg once or twice weekly, adjusted according to local guidelines

FOLIC ACID (*continued*)

[1]**Folic Acid** (Non-proprietary) PoM
Tablets, folic acid 400 micrograms, net price 90-tab pack = £2.24; 5 mg, 28-tab pack = £1.10

Syrup, folic acid 2.5 mg/5 mL, net price 150 mL = £9.16; 400 micrograms/5 mL, 150 mL = £1.40
Brands include *Folicare*®, *Lexpec*® (sugar-free)

1. Can be sold to the public provided daily doses do not exceed 500 micrograms; brands include *Preconceive*®

9.1.3 Drugs used in hypoplastic, haemolytic, and renal anaemias

Anabolic steroids (see BNF, section 6.4.3), pyridoxine, antilymphocyte immunoglobulin, and various corticosteroids are used in hypoplastic and haemolytic anaemias.

Antilymphocyte globulin given intravenously through a central line over 12–18 hours each day for 5 days produces a response in about 50% of cases of acquired *aplastic anaemia*; the response rate may be increased when ciclosporin is given as well. Severe reactions are common in the first 2 days and profound immunosuppression can occur; antilymphocyte globulin should be given under specialist supervision with appropriate resuscitation facilities. Alternatively, oxymetholone tablets (available on named-patient basis from Cambridge) may be used in aplastic anaemia at a dose of 1–5 mg/kg daily for 3 to 6 months.

It is unlikely that dietary deficit of **pyridoxine** (section 9.6.2) produces clinically relevant haematological effects. However, certain forms of *sideroblastic anaemia* respond to pharmacological doses, possibly reflecting its role as a co-enzyme during haemoglobin synthesis. Pyridoxine is indicated in both *idiopathic acquired* and *hereditary sideroblastic anaemias*. Although complete cures have not been reported, some increase in haemoglobin may occur with high doses. *Reversible sideroblastic anaemias* respond to treatment of the underlying cause but pyridoxine is indicated in pregnancy, haemolytic anaemias, or during isoniazid treatment.

Corticosteroids (section 6.3) have an important place in the management of haematological disorders including *autoimmune haemolytic anaemia*, *idiopathic thrombocytopenias* (section 9.1.4) and *neutropenias*, and *major transfusion reactions*. They are also used in chemotherapy schedules for many types of *lymphoma*, *lymphoid leukaemias*, and *paraproteinaemias*, including *multiple myeloma*.

Erythropoietin

Epoetin (recombinant human erythropoietin) is used for the anaemia associated with erythropoietin deficiency in chronic renal failure. The clinical efficacy of epoetin alfa and epoetin beta is similar.

Epoetin beta is also used for the prevention of anaemia in preterm neonates of low birth-weight; a therapeutic response may take several weeks. Only unpreserved formulations should be used as other preparations may contain benzyl alcohol.

There is insufficient information to support the use of epoetin in children with leukaemia or in those receiving cancer chemotherapy.

Darbepoetin is a glycosylated derivative of epoetin which persists longer in the body and may be administered less frequently than epoetin.

Other factors which contribute to the anaemia of chronic renal failure such as iron or folate deficiency should be corrected before treatment and monitored during therapy. Supplemental iron may improve the response in resistant patients and in preterm neonates (see section 9.1.1.1). Aluminium toxicity, concurrent infection or other inflammatory disease may impair the response to erythropoietin.

> **CSM advice**
> There have been very rare reports of pure red cell aplasia in patients treated with epoetin alfa. The CSM has advised that in patients developing epoetin alfa failure with a diagnosis of pure red cell aplasia, treatment with epoetin alfa must be discontinued and testing for erythropoietin antibodies considered. Patients who develop pure red cell aplasia should **not** be switched to another erythropoietin.

DARBEPOETIN ALFA

Cautions see Epoetin; sickle-cell anaemia; **interactions:** Appendix 1 (epoetin)

Hepatic impairment manufacturer advises caution

Pregnancy no evidence of harm in *animal* studies but caution advised

Contra-indications see Epoetin

Breast-feeding manufacturer advises avoid—no information available

Side-effects see Epoetin; also, peripheral oedema, injection-site pain; isolated reports of pure red cell aplasia (discontinue therapy)—see also CSM advice above

Indication and dose

Anaemia associated with chronic renal failure in children on dialysis

- **By intravenous or subcutaneous injection**

Child 11–18 years initially 450 nanograms/kg once weekly adjusted according to response by approx. 25% of initial dose at intervals of at least 4 weeks; maintenance dose (when haemoglobin concentration of at least 11 g/100 mL achieved) given once weekly *or* once every 2 weeks

Anaemia associated with chronic renal failure in children not on dialysis

- **By intravenous or subcutaneous injection**

Child 11–18 years *by subcutaneous or intravenous injection*, initially 450 nanograms/kg once weekly *or by subcutaneous injection*, initially 750 nanograms/kg once every 2 weeks; adjusted according to response by approx. 25% of initial dose at intervals of at least 4 weeks; maintenance dose (when haemoglobin concentration of at least 11 g/100 mL achieved), given once weekly *or* once every 2 weeks *or* once every month

Note Reduce dose by 25–50% if haemoglobin rise exceeds 2.5 g/100 mL per month; suspend if haemoglobin exceeds 14 g/100 mL until it falls below 13 g/100 mL and then restart with dose at 25% below previous dose. When changing route give same dose then adjust according to weekly or fortnightly haemoglobin measurements. Adjust doses at 2-week intervals during maintenance treatment

Aranesp® (Amgen) ▼ PoM

Injection, prefilled syringe, darbepoetin alfa, 25 micrograms/mL, net price 0.4 mL (10 micrograms) = £15.59; 40 micrograms/mL, 0.375 mL (15 micrograms) = £23.38, 0.5 mL (20 micrograms) = £31.17; 100 micrograms/mL, 0.3 mL (30 micrograms) = £46.76, 0.4 mL (40 micrograms) = £62.34, 0.5 mL (50 micrograms) = £77.93; 200 micrograms/mL, 0.3 mL (60 micrograms) = £93.51, 0.4 mL (80 micrograms) = £124.68, 0.5 mL (100 micrograms) = £155.85; 500 micrograms/mL, 0.3 mL (150 micrograms) = £233.78, 0.6 mL (300 micrograms) = £467.55, 1 mL (500 micrograms) = £779.25

Aranesp® SureClick (Amgen) ▼ PoM

Injection, prefilled disposable injection device, darbepoetin alfa, 40 micrograms/mL, net price 0.5 mL (20 micrograms) = £31.17; 100 micrograms/mL, net price 0.4 mL (40 micrograms) = £62.34; 200 micrograms/mL, net price 0.3 mL (60 micrograms) = £93.51, 0.4mL (80 micrograms) = £124.68, 0.5 mL (100 micrograms) = £155.85; 500 microgams/mL, net price 0.3 mL (150 micrograms) = £233.78, 0.6 mL (300 micrograms) = £467.55, 1 mL (500 micrograms) = £779.25

EPOETIN ALFA and BETA
(Recombinant human erythropoietins)

Note Although epoetin alfa and beta are clinically indistinguishable the prescriber must specify which is required

Cautions inadequately treated or poorly controlled blood pressure (monitor closely blood pressure, reticulocyte counts, haemoglobin, and electrolytes), interrupt treatment if blood pressure uncontrolled; sudden stabbing migraine-like pain is warning of hypertensive crisis; sickle-cell disease (lower target haemoglobin concentration may be appropriate), exclude other causes of anaemia (e.g. folic acid or vitamin B_{12} deficiency) and give iron supplements if necessary (see also notes above); ischaemic vascular disease; thrombocytosis (monitor platelet count for first 8 weeks); epilepsy; malignant disease; increase in heparin dose may be needed; risk of thrombosis may be increased when used for anaemia before orthopaedic surgery—avoid in cardiovascular disease including cerebrovascular accident; **interactions:** Appendix 1 (epoetin)

Hepatic impairment manufacturers advise caution in chronic impairment

Pregnancy no evidence of harm; benefits probably outweigh risks of anaemia and blood transfusion

Breast-feeding unlikely to be present in milk; effect on infant minimal

Contra-indications pure red cell aplasia following erythropoietin (see also CSM advice above); uncontrolled hypertension; avoid injections containing benzyl alcohol in neonates (see under preparations, below)

Side-effects dose-dependent increase in blood pressure or aggravation of hypertension; in isolated patients with normal or low blood pressure, hypertensive crisis with encephalopathy-like symptoms and generalised tonic-clonic seizures requiring immediate medical attention; dose-dependent increase in platelet count (but thrombocytosis rare) regressing during treatment; influenza-like symptoms (may be reduced if intravenous injection given over 5 minutes); shunt thrombosis especially if tendency to hypotension or arteriovenous shunt complications; isolated reports of hyperkalaemia, skin reactions; very rarely sudden loss of response because of pure red cell aplasia, particularly following subcutaneous administration in patients with chronic renal failure (discontinue erythropoietin therapy)—see also CSM advice above

Licensed use *Eprex®* not licensed for subcutaneous use in children

EPOETIN ALFA and BETA (*continued*)

Indication and dose

Aimed at increasing haemoglobin concentration at rate not exceeding 2 g/100 mL/month to stable level of 9.5–11 g/100 mL see under preparations, below

Epoetin alfa

Eprex® (Janssen-Cilag) PoM

Injection, epoetin alfa 40 000 units/mL, net price 1-mL (40 000-unit) vial = £318.44

Injection, prefilled syringe, epoetin alfa, net price 1000 units = £7.96; 2000 units = £15.92; 3000 units = £23.88; 4000 units = £31.84; 5000 units = £39.81; 6000 units = £47.77; 8000 units = £63.69; 10 000 units = £79.61. An auto-injector device is available for use with 10 000-units prefilled syringes

Dose

Anaemia associated with chronic renal failure in children on dialysis

- **By intravenous injection over 1–5 minutes**

  Child 1 month–18years initially 50 units/kg 3 times weekly adjusted according to response in steps of 25 units/kg 3 times weekly at intervals of at least 4 weeks until desired haemoglobin concentration achieved; then adjust according to response at 1–2 week intervals

  Usual maintenance dose: body-weight under 10 kg 75–150 units/kg 3 times weekly, body-weight 10–30 kg 60–150 units/kg 3 times weekly, body-weight 30–60 kg 30–100 units/kg 3 times weekly, body-weight over 60 kg 75–300 units/kg weekly (as a single dose or in divided doses)

Safe Practice Subcutaneous injection **contra-indicated** in children with chronic renal failure

Epoetin beta

NeoRecormon® (Roche) PoM

Injection, prefilled syringe, epoetin beta, net price 500 units = £3.90; 1000 units = £7.79; 2000 units = £15.59; 3000 units = £23.38; 4000 units = £31.17; 5000 units = £38.97; 6000 units = £46.76; 10 000 units = £77.93; 20 000 units = £155.87; 30 000 units = £233.81

Excipients: include phenylalanine up to 300 micrograms/syringe (section 9.4.1)

Multidose injection, powder for reconstitution, epoetin beta, net price 50 000-unit vial = £419.01; 100 000-unit vial = £838.01 (both with solvent)

Excipients: include phenylalanine up to 5 mg/vial (section 9.4.1), benzyl alcohol (avoid in neonates, see Excipients p. 3)

Note Avoid contact of reconstituted injection with glass; use only plastic materials

Reco-Pen, (for subcutaneous use), double-chamber cartridges (containing epoetin beta and solvent), net price 10 000-unit cartridge = £77.93; 20 000-unit cartridge = £155.87; 60 000-unit cartridge = £467.61; for use with *Reco-Pen* injection device and needles (both available free from Roche)

Excipients: include phenylalanine up to 500 micrograms/cartridge (section 9.4.1), benzyl alcohol (avoid in neonates, see Excipients, p. 3)

Dose

Anaemia associated with chronic renal failure in dialysis patients, symptomatic anaemia of renal origin in patients not yet on dialysis

- **By subcutaneous injection**

  Child 1 month–18 years initially 20 units/kg 3 times weekly for 4 weeks, increased according to response at intervals of 4 weeks in steps of 20 units/kg/dose (60 units/kg/week) total weekly dose may be divided into daily doses; maintenance dose (when desired haemoglobin concentration achieved), initially reduce dose by half then adjust according to response at intervals of 1–2 weeks; max. 720 units/kg weekly

- **By intravenous injection over 2 minutes**

  Child 1 month–18 years initially 40 units/kg 3 times weekly for 4 weeks, increased according to response to 80 units/kg 3 times weekly with further increases if needed at intervals of 4 weeks in steps of 20 units/kg 3 times weekly; maintenance dose (when desired haemoglobin concentration achieved), initially reduce dose by half then adjust according to response at intervals of 1–2 weeks; max. 720 units/kg weekly

Prevention of anaemias of prematurity in neonates with birth-weight of 0.75–1.5 kg and gestational age under 34 weeks

- **By subcutaneous injection (of single-dose, unpreserved injection)**

  Neonate 250 units/kg 3 times weekly preferably starting within 3 days of birth and continued for 6 weeks

Sickle-cell disease

Sickle-cell disease is caused by a structural abnormality of haemoglobin resulting in deformed, less flexible red blood cells. Acute complications in the more severe forms include *sickle-cell crisis*, where infarction of the microvasculature and blood supply to organs results in severe pain. Sickle-cell crisis requires hospitalisation, intravenous fluids, analgesia (section 4.7) and treatment of any concurrent infection. Chronic complications include skin ulceration, renal failure and increased susceptibility to infection. Pneumococcal vaccine (section 14.4), haemophilus influenzae type b vaccine (section 14.4), and prophylactic penicillin (Table 2, section 5.1) reduce the risk of infection.

In some forms of sickle-cell disease varying degrees of haemolytic anaemia are present accompanied by increased erythropoiesis. This may increase folate requirements and folate supplementation may be necessary (section 9.1.2).

Hydroxycarbamide (hydroxyurea) may reduce the rate of crises and the need for blood transfusions [unlicensed indication]. Beneficial effects may not become evident for several months and the long-term consequences remain to be determined. Myelosuppression, nausea, and skin reactions are the most common adverse effects.

HYDROXYCARBAMIDE

(Hydroxyurea)

Cautions see section 8.1 and notes above

Renal impairment reduce dose by 50% in severe renal impairment

Side-effects see section 8.1 and notes above

Licensed use not licensed for use in children

Indication and dose

Sickle-cell disease

- By mouth

Child 1–18 years 10–20 mg/kg once daily, increased every 12 weeks in steps of 5 mg/kg daily according to response (max. dose 35 mg/kg daily)

Hydroxycarbamide (Non-proprietary) PoM

Capsules, hydroxycarbamide 500 mg, net price 20 = £2.39

Available from Medac

Capsules, 100 mg, 250 mg

Available from specialist importing companies

Hydrea® (Squibb) PoM

Capsules, pink/green, hydroxycarbamide 500 mg. Net price 20 = £2.39

Extemporaneous formulations available see Extemporaneous Preparations, p. 8

Iron overload

Severe tissue iron overload may occur in aplastic and other refractory anaemias, mainly as the result of repeated blood transfusions. It is a particular problem in refractory anaemias with hyperplastic bone marrow, especially *thalassaemia major*, where excessive iron absorption from the gut and inappropriate iron therapy may add to the tissue siderosis.

Iron overload associated with haemochromatosis may be treated with repeated venesection. Venesection may also be used for patients who have received multiple transfusions and whose bone marrow has recovered. Where venesection is contra-indicated, and in thalassaemia, the long-term administration of the iron chelating compound **desferrioxamine mesilate** is useful. Subcutaneous infusions of desferrioxamine are given over 8–12 hours, 3–7 times a week; the dose should reflect the degree of iron overload. The initial dose should not exceed 30 mg/kg. For established overload the dose is usually between 20 and 50 mg/kg daily. Desferrioxamine (up to 2 g per unit of blood) may also be given at the time of blood transfusion, provided that the desferrioxamine is **not** added to the blood and is **not** given through the same line as the blood (but the two may be given through the same cannula).

Iron excretion induced by desferrioxamine is enhanced by administration of ascorbic acid (vitamin C, section 9.6.3) in a dose of 100–200 mg daily; it should be given separately from food since it also enhances iron absorption. Ascorbic acid should not be given to children with cardiac dysfunction; in children with normal cardiac function ascorbic acid should be introduced 1 month after starting desferrioxamine.

Infusion of desferrioxamine may be used to treat *aluminium overload* in dialysis patients; theoretically 100 mg of desferrioxamine binds with 4.1 mg of aluminium.

Deferiprone, an oral iron chelator, is licensed for the treatment of iron overload in children over 6 years of age with thalassaemia major in whom desferrioxamine is contra-indicated or is not tolerated. Blood dyscrasias, particularly agranulocytosis, have been reported with deferiprone.

DEFERIPRONE

Cautions monitor neutrophil count weekly and discontinue treatment if neutropenia develops

Blood disorders Patients or their carers should be told how to recognise signs of neutropenia and advised to seek immediate medical attention if symptoms such as fever or sore throat develop

Contra-indications

Hepatic impairment manufacturer advises monitor liver function—interrupt treatment if persistent elevation in serum alanine aminotransferase

Renal impairment manufacturer advises caution—no information available

Pregnancy manufacturer advises avoid before intended conception and during pregnancy—teratogenic and embryotoxic in *animal* studies; contraception advised in girls of child-bearing potential

Breast-feeding manufacturer advises avoid—no information available

Side-effects gastro-intestinal disturbances; red-brown urine discoloration; arthropathy; neutropenia, agranulocytosis

Licensed use see notes above

Indication and dose

Iron overload in thalassaemia major

- By mouth

Child 6-18 years 25 mg/kg 3 times daily (max. 100 mg/kg daily)

DEFERIPRONE (*continued*)

Ferriprox® (Swedish Orphan) PoM
Tablets, f/c, scored, deferiprone 500 mg, net price 100-tab pack = £152.39. Label: 14, counselling, blood disorders
Extemporaneous formulation available see guidance notes for details

DESFERRIOXAMINE MESILATE

(Deferoxamine Mesilate)

Cautions eye and ear examinations before treatment and at 3-month intervals during treatment; monitor body-weight and height in children at 3-month intervals—risk of growth restriction with excessive doses; aluminium-related encephalopathy (may exacerbate neurological dysfunction); **interactions:** Appendix 1 (desferrioxamine)

Pregnancy teratogenic in *animal* studies, manufacturer advises use only if potential benefit outweighs risk

Breast-feeding manufacturer advises use only if potential benefit outweighs risk—no information available

Side-effects hypotension (especially when given too rapidly by intravenous injection), disturbances of hearing and vision (including lens opacity and retinopathy); injection site reactions, gastro-intestinal disturbances, asthma, fever, headache, arthralgia and myalgia; very rarely anaphylaxis, acute respiratory distress syndrome, neurological disturbances (including dizziness, neuropathy and paraesthesia), Yersinia and mucormycosis infections, rash, renal impairment, and blood dyscrasias

Indication and dose

Chronic iron overload see notes above

Aluminium overload in dialysis patients
- **By intravenous infusion**
  Child 1 month–18 years 5 mg/kg once weekly

Iron poisoning
see Emergency Treatment of Poisoning, p. 41

Administration For *intravenous* or *subcutaneous infusion*, reconstitute powder with Water for Injection to a concentration of 100 mg/mL; dilute with Glucose 5% *or* Sodium Chloride 0.9%. In *haemodialysis* or *haemofiltration* administer over the last hour of dialysis (may be given via the dialysis fistula). *Intraperitoneal*: may be added to dialysis fluid. In CAPD give prior to the last exchange of the day.
Note For full details and warnings relating to administration, consult product literature

Desferrioxamine mesilate (Non-proprietary) PoM
Injection, powder for reconstitution, desferrioxamine mesilate, net price 500-mg vial = £4.26; 2-g vial = £17.05

Desferal® (Novartis) PoM
Injection, powder for reconstitution, desferrioxamine mesilate, net price 500-mg vial = £4.44, 2-g vial = £17.77

9.1.4 Drugs used in platelet disorders

Idiopathic thrombocytopenic purpura Acute idiopathic thrombocytopenic purpura is usually self-limiting in children. A corticosteroid such as prednisolone (p. 427) is sometimes used if idiopathic thrombocytopenic purpura does not resolve spontaneously or if it is associated with severe cutaneous symptoms or mucous membrane bleeding; corticosteroid treatment should not be continued longer than 14 days regardless of the response.

Immunoglobulin preparations (section 14.5) may be used in idiopathic thrombocytopenic purpura or where a temporary rapid rise in platelets is needed, as in pregnancy or pre-operatively; they are often used in preference to a corticosteroid. Anti-D immunoglobulin is licensed for the management of idiopathic thrombocytopenic purpura.

Other therapy that has been tried under specialist supervision in refractory idiopathic thrombocytopenic purpura includes azathioprine (section 8.2.1), cyclophosphamide (section 8.1.1), vincristine (section 8.1.4), and ciclosporin (section 8.2.2). Rituximab is used in specialist centres but experience of its use in children is limited. For patients with chronic severe thrombocytopenia refractory to other therapy, tranexamic acid (section 2.11) may be given to reduce the severity of haemorrhage.

Splenectomy is considered in chronic thrombocytopenic purpura if a satisfactory platelet count is not achieved with regular immunoglobulin infusions, if there is a relapse on withdrawing or reducing the dose of corticosteroid and if other therapies are considered inappropriate.

Thrombocythaemia **Anagrelide** reduces platelets in primary thrombocythaemia and in thrombocythaemia secondary to myeloproliferative disorders.

ANAGRELIDE

Cautions cardiac disease; assess cardiac function before and during treatment; concomitant aspirin in patients with a history of haemorrhage or severely raised platelet count; monitor full blood count (monitor platelet count every 2 days for 1 week, then weekly until maintenance dose established), liver function, serum creatinine, and urea; **interactions:** Appendix 1 (anagrelide)

Skilled tasks Dizziness may affect performance of skilled tasks (e.g. driving)

Hepatic impairment manufacturer advises caution in mild hepatic impairment; avoid in moderate to severe impairment

Renal impairment manufacturer advises avoid if creatinine clearance less than 50 mL/minute/1.73 m^2

Contra-indications

Pregnancy manufacturer advises avoid (toxicity in *animal* studies)

Breast-feeding manufacturer advises avoid—no information available

Side-effects gastro-intestinal disturbances; palpitation, tachycardia, fluid retention; headache, dizziness, fatigue; anaemia; rash; *less commonly* pancreatitis, gastro-intestinal haemorrhage, congestive heart failure, hypertension, arrhythmias, syncope, chest pain, dyspnoea, sleep disturbances, paraesthesia, hypoaesthesia, depression, confusion, amnesia, fever, weight changes, impotence, blood disorders, myalgia, arthralgia, epistaxis, dry mouth, alopecia, skin discoloration, and pruritus; *rarely* gastritis, colitis, postural hypotension, myocardial infarction, vasodilatation, pulmonary infiltrates, impaired co-ordination, dysarthria, asthenia, tinnitus, renal failure, nocturia, visual disturbances, and gingival bleeding

Licensed use not licensed for use in children

Indication and dose

Primary thrombocythaemia in at risk children who have not responded adequately to other therapy or who are intolerant of it (initiated under specialist supervision)

- **By mouth**

  Child 7–18 years initially 500 micrograms daily adjusted according to response in steps of 500 micrograms daily at weekly intervals to max. 10 mg daily (max. single dose 2.5 mg); usual dose range 1–3 mg daily in divided doses

Xagrid® (Shire) ▼ PoM

Capsules, anagrelide (as hydrochloride), 500 micrograms, net price 100-cap pack= £337.14. Counselling, skilled tasks, see above

9 Nutrition and blood

9.1.5 G6PD deficiency

Glucose 6-phosphate dehydrogenase (G6PD) deficiency is highly prevalent in individuals originating from most parts of Africa, from most parts of Asia, from Oceania, and from Southern Europe; it can also occur, rarely, in any other individuals.

Individuals with G6PD deficiency are susceptible to developing acute haemolytic anaemia on taking a number of common drugs. They are also susceptible to developing acute haemolytic anaemia upon ingestion of fava beans (broad beans, *Vicia faba*); this is termed *favism* and can be more severe in children or when the fresh fava beans are eaten raw.

When prescribing drugs for children with G6PD deficiency, the following three points should be kept in mind:

- G6PD deficiency is genetically heterogeneous; susceptibility to the haemolytic risk from drugs varies; thus, a drug found to be safe in some G6PD-deficient individuals may not be equally safe in others;
- manufacturers do not routinely test drugs for their effects in G6PD-deficient individuals;
- the risk and severity of haemolysis is almost always dose-related.

The lists below should be read with these points in mind. Ideally, information about G6PD deficiency should be available before prescribing a drug listed below. However, in the absence of this information, the possibility of haemolysis should be considered, especially if the child belongs to a group in which G6PD deficiency is common.

A very few G6PD-deficient individuals with chronic non-spherocytic haemolytic anaemia have haemolysis even in the absence of an exogenous trigger. These children must be regarded as being at high risk of severe exacerbation of haemolysis following administration of any of the drugs listed below.

Drugs with *definite* risk of haemolysis in most G6PD-deficient individuals

Dapsone and other sulphones (higher doses for dermatitis herpetiformis more likely to cause problems)

Methylthioninium chloride (methylene blue)

Niridazole [not on UK market]

Nitrofurantoin

Pamaquin [not on UK market]

Primaquine (30 mg weekly for 8 weeks has been found to be without undue harmful effects in African and Asian people, see section 5.4.1)

Quinolones (including ciprofloxacin, moxifloxacin, nalidixic acid, norfloxacin, and ofloxacin)

Sulphonamides (including co-trimoxazole; some sulphonamides, e.g. sulfadiazine, have been tested and found not to be haemolytic in many G6PD-deficient individuals)

Drugs with *possible* risk of haemolysis in some G6PD-deficient individuals

Aspirin (acceptable up to a dose of at least 1 g daily in most G6PD-deficient individuals)

Chloroquine (acceptable in acute malaria)

Menadione, water-soluble derivatives (e.g. menadiol sodium phosphate)

Probenecid [not on UK market]

Quinidine (acceptable in acute malaria)

Quinine (acceptable in acute malaria)

Note Naphthalene in mothballs also causes haemolysis in individuals with G6PD-deficiency.

9.1.6 Drugs used in neutropenia

Recombinant human granulocyte-colony stimulating factor (rhG-CSF) stimulates the production of neutrophils and may reduce the duration of chemotherapy-induced neutropenia and thereby reduce the incidence of associated sepsis; there is as yet no evidence that it improves overall survival. **Filgrastim** (unglycosylated rhG-CSF) and **lenograstim** (glycosylated rhG-CSF) have similar effects; both have been used in a variety of clinical settings, including cytotoxic-induced neutropenia, and neutropenia following bone marrow transplantation, but they do not have any clear-cut routine indications. In congenital neutropenia filgrastim usually elevates the neutrophil count with appropriate clinical response. Prolonged use may be associated with an increased risk of myeloid malignancy.

Treatment with recombinant human growth factors should only be prescribed by those experienced in their use.

Neonatal neutropenia Filgrastim and lenograstim have been used to abolish sepsis-induced neutropenia in preterm neonates. The majority of studies have used filgrastim. The effects on survival and long-term outcome are unclear. Prophylactic use in preterm neonates is under evaluation.

Cautions Granulocyte-colony stimulating factors should be used with caution during pregnancy and breast-feeding. Blood counts (including differential white cell count and platelet count) should be monitored.

Side-effects Side-effects of granulocyte-colony stimulating factors include gastro-intestinal disturbances (including nausea, vomiting, and diarrhoea), anorexia, headache, asthenia, fever, musculoskeletal pain, bone pain, rash, alopecia, injection-site reactions, and leucocytosis. Less frequent side-effects include chest pain, hypersensitivity reactions (including anaphylaxis and bronchospasm) and arthralgia. There have been reports of pulmonary infiltrates leading to acute respiratory distress syndrome.

FILGRASTIM

(Recombinant human granulocyte-colony stimulating factor, G-CSF)

Cautions see notes above; also reduced myeloid precursors; regular morphological and cytogenetic bone-marrow examinations recommended in severe congenital neutropenia (possible risk of myelodysplastic syndromes or leukaemia); secondary acute myeloid leukaemia, sickle-cell disease; monitor spleen size (risk of rupture);

FILGRASTIM (*continued*)

osteoporotic bone disease (monitor bone density if given for more than 6 months); **interactions:** Appendix 1 (filgrastim)

Contra-indications severe congenital neutropenia (Kostman's syndrome) with abnormal cytogenetics

Side-effects see notes above; also splenic enlargement, hepatomegaly, transient hypotension, epistaxis, urinary abnormalities (including dysuria, proteinuria, and haematuria), osteoporosis, exacerbation of rheumatoid arthritis, cutaneous vasculitis, thrombocytopenia, anaemia, transient decrease in blood glucose, raised uric acid

Licensed use not licensed for treatment of glycogen storage disease or in neonates

Indication and dose

Cytotoxic-induced neutropenia
- **Preferably by subcutaneous injection or by intravenous infusion (over 30 minutes)**

Child 1 month–18 years 5 micrograms/kg daily started not less than 24 hours after cytotoxic chemotherapy, continued until neutrophil count in normal range, usually for up to 14 days (up to 38 days in acute myeloid leukaemia)

Myeloablative therapy followed by bone-marrow transplantation
- **By intravenous infusion over 30 minutes or over 24 hours or by subcutaneous infusion over 24 hours**

Child 1 month–18 years 10 micrograms/kg daily, started not less than 24 hours following cytotoxic chemotherapy (and within 24 hours of bone-marrow infusion), then adjusted according to absolute neutrophil count (consult product literature and local protocol)

Mobilisation of peripheral blood progenitor cells for autologous infusion, used alone
- **By subcutaneous injection or by subcutaneous infusion over 24 hours**

Child 1 month–18 years 10 micrograms/kg daily for 5–7 days

Mobilisation of peripheral blood progenitor cells for autologous infusion following adjunctive myelosuppressive chemotherapy (to improve yield)
- **By subcutaneous injection**

Child 1 month–18 years 5 micrograms/kg daily, started the day after completion of chemotherapy and continued until neutrophil count in normal range; for timing of leucopheresis consult product literature

Mobilisation of peripheral blood progenitor cells in normal donors for allogeneic infusion
- **By subcutaneous injection**

Child over 16 years 10 micrograms/kg daily for 4–5 days; for timing of leucopheresis consult product literature

Severe chronic neutropenia
- **By subcutaneous injection**

Child 1 month–18 years in severe congenital neutropenia, initially 12 micrograms/kg daily in single or divided doses (initially 5 micrograms/kg daily in idiopathic or cyclic neutropenia), adjusted according to response (consult product literature and local protocol)

Persistent neutropenia in HIV infection
- **By subcutaneous injection**

Child 1 month–18 years initially 1 microgram/kg daily, increased as necessary until absolute neutrophil count in normal range (usual max. 4 micrograms/kg daily), then adjusted to maintain absolute neutrophil count in normal range (consult product literature)

Neonatal neutropenia
- **By subcutaneous injection**

Neonate 10 micrograms/kg daily, discontinue if white cell count exceeds 50×10^9/litre

Glycogen storage disease types 1b and 1c
- **By subcutaneous injection**

5 micrograms/kg daily, adjusted as necessary

Administration For *subcutaneous* or *intravenous injection* or *infusion*, dilute with Glucose 5% to a concentration of not less than 15 micrograms/mL (concentration of 100 micrograms/mL adequate for subcutaneous use in neonates); to dilute to a concentration of 2–15 micrograms/mL, add albumin solution (human serum albumin) to produce a final albumin solution of 2 mg/mL; not compatible with sodium chloride solutions

Neupogen® (Amgen) PoM

Injection, filgrastim 30 million units (300 micrograms)/mL; net price 1-mL vial = £68.41

Injection (Singleject®), filgrastim 60 million units (600 micrograms)/mL, net price 0.5-mL prefilled syringe = £68.41; 96 million units (960 micrograms)/mL, 0.5-mL prefilled syringe = £109.11

LENOGRASTIM

(Recombinant human granulocyte-colony stimulating factor, rHuG-CSF)

Cautions see notes above; also pre-malignant myeloid conditions; reduced myeloid precursors; sickle-cell disease; monitor spleen size (risk of rupture)

Side-effects see notes above; also splenic rupture, cutaneous vasculitis, Sweet's syndrome, toxic epidermal necrolysis

Licensed use licensed in children over 2 years following bone-marrow transplant

9 Nutrition and blood

LENOGRASTIM (*continued*)

Indication and dose

Following bone-marrow transplantation
- **By intravenous infusion over 30 minutes**

Child 2–18 years 150 micrograms/m² daily started the day after transplantation, continued until neutrophil count stable in acceptable range (max. 28 days)

Cytotoxic-induced neutropenia
- **By subcutaneous injection**

Child 2–18 years 150 micrograms/m² daily started the day after completion of chemotherapy, continued until neutrophil count stable in acceptable range (max. 28 days)

Mobilisation of peripheral blood progenitor cells, used alone
- **By subcutaneous injection**

Child 2–18 years 10 micrograms/kg daily for 4–6 days (5–6 days in healthy donors)

Mobilisation of peripheral blood progenitor cells following adjunctive myelosuppressive chemotherapy (to improve yield)
- **By subcutaneous injection**

Child 2–18 years 150 micrograms/m² daily, started the day after completion of chemotherapy and continued until neutrophil count in acceptable range; for timing of leucopheresis consult product literature

Administration For *intravenous infusion*, dilute reconstituted solution to a concentration of not less than 2 micrograms/mL (*Granocyte-13*) or 2.5 micrograms/mL (*Granocyte-34*) with Sodium Chloride 0.9%

Granocyte® (Chugai) PoM
Injection, powder for reconstitution, lenograstim, net price 13.4 million-unit (105-microgram) vial = £42.00; 33.6 million-unit (263-microgram) vial = £67.95 (both with 1-mL prefilled syringe water for injections)

9.2 Fluids and electrolytes

The following tables give a selection of useful electrolyte values:

Electrolyte concentrations—intravenous fluids

Intravenous infusion	Millimoles per litre				
	Na^+	K^+	HCO_3^-	Cl^-	Ca^{2+}
Normal plasma values	142	4.5	26	103	2.5
Sodium Chloride 0.9%	150	—	—	150	—
Compound Sodium Lactate (Hartmann's)	131	5	29	111	2
Sodium Chloride 0.45% and Glucose 5%	75	—	—	75	—
Potassium Chloride 0.15% and Glucose 5%	—	20	—	20	—
Potassium Chloride 0.15% and Sodium Chloride 0.9%	150	20	—	170	—
Potassium Chloride 0.3% and Glucose 5%	—	40	—	40	—
Potassium Chloride 0.3% and Sodium Chloride 0.9%	150	40	—	190	—
To correct metabolic acidosis					
Sodium Bicarbonate 1.26%	150	—	150	—	—
Sodium Bicarbonate 8.4% for cardiac arrest	1000	—	1000	—	—
Sodium Lactate (m/6)	167	—	167	—	—

Electrolyte content—gastro-intestinal secretions

Type of fluid	Millimoles per litre				
	H^+	Na^+	K^+	HCO_3^-	Cl^-
Gastric	40–60	20–80	5–20	—	100–150
Biliary	—	120–140	5–15	30–50	80–120
Pancreatic	—	120–140	5–15	70–110	40–80
Small bowel	—	120–140	5–15	20–40	90–130

Faeces, vomit, or aspiration should be saved and analysed where possible if abnormal losses are suspected; where this is impracticable the approximations above may be helpful in planning replacement therapy

9.2.1 Oral preparations for fluid and electrolyte imbalance

Sodium and potassium salts, which may be given by mouth to prevent deficiencies or to treat established deficiencies of mild or moderate degree, are discussed in this section. Oral preparations for removing excess potassium and preparations for oral rehydration therapy are also included here. Oral bicarbonate, for metabolic acidosis, is also described in this section.

For reference to calcium, magnesium, and phosphate, see section 9.5.

9.2.1.1 Oral potassium

Compensation for potassium loss is especially necessary:

- in children in whom secondary hyperaldosteronism occurs, e.g. renal artery stenosis, renal tubule disorder, the nephrotic syndrome, and severe heart failure;
- in children with excessive losses of potassium in the faeces, e.g. chronic diarrhoea associated with intestinal malabsorption or laxative abuse;
- in those taking digoxin or anti-arrhythmic drugs, where potassium depletion may induce arrhythmias.

Measures to compensate for potassium loss may be required during long-term administration of drugs known to induce potassium loss (e.g. corticosteroids). Potassium supplements are **seldom required** with the small doses of diuretics given to treat hypertension; **potassium-sparing diuretics** (rather than potassium supplements) are recommended for prevention of hypokalaemia due to diuretics such as furosemide (frusemide) or the thiazides when these are given to eliminate oedema.

Dosage If potassium salts are used for the *prevention of hypokalaemia*, then doses of potassium chloride 1–2 mmol/kg (usual max. 50 mmol potassium) daily by mouth are suitable in patients taking a normal diet. *Smaller doses* must be used if there is *renal insufficiency* otherwise there is **danger of hyperkalaemia**. Potassium salts cause nausea and vomiting therefore poor compliance is a major limitation to their effectiveness (small divided doses may minimise gastric irritation); where appropriate, potassium-sparing diuretics are preferable (see also above). When there is *established potassium depletion* larger doses may be necessary, the quantity depending on the severity of any continuing potassium loss (monitoring of plasma-potassium concentration and specialist advice would be required). Potassium depletion is frequently associated with chloride depletion and with metabolic alkalosis, and these disorders require correction.

Administration Potassium salts are preferably given as a liquid (or effervescent) preparation, rather than modified-release tablets; they should be given as the chloride (the use of effervescent potassium tablets BPC 1968 should be restricted to *hyperchloraemic states*, section 9.2.1.3). Potassium chloride solutions suitable for use by mouth in neonates are available as manufactured specials; they should be used with care because they can damage the gastric mucosa and they are hypertonic.

Salt substitutes. A number of salt substitutes which contain significant amounts of potassium chloride are readily available as health food products (e.g. *LoSalt*® and *Ruthmol*®). These should not be used by patients with renal failure as potassium intoxication may result.

POTASSIUM CHLORIDE

Cautions intestinal stricture, history of peptic ulcer, hiatus hernia (for sustained-release preparations); **important**: special hazard if given with drugs liable to raise plasma potassium concentration such as potassium-sparing diuretics, ACE inhibitors, or ciclosporin, for other **interactions**: Appendix 1 (potassium salts)

Contra-indications plasma potassium concentrations above 5 mmol/litre

Renal impairment avoid routine use in moderate impairment—high risk of hyperkalaemia

Side-effects nausea and vomiting (severe symptoms may indicate obstruction), oesophageal or small bowel ulceration

POTASSIUM CHLORIDE (*continued*)

Indication and dose

Potassium depletion
• By mouth

Neonate 0.5–1 mmol/kg K^+ twice daily (total daily dose may alternatively be given in 3 divided doses), adjusted to plasma-potassium concentration

Child 1 month–18 years 0.5–1 mmol/kg K^+ twice daily (total daily dose may alternatively be given in 3 divided doses), adjusted to plasma-potassium concentration

Note Do not confuse Effervescent Potassium Tablets BPC 1968 (section 9.2.1.3) with effervescent potassium chloride tablets. Effervescent Potassium Tablets BPC 1968 do not contain chloride ions and their use should be restricted to hyperchloraemic states (section 9.2.1.3). Effervescent Potassium Chloride Tablets BP are usually available in two strengths, one containing 6.7 mmol each of K^+ and Cl^- (corresponding to *Kloref®*), the other containing 12 mmol K^+ and 8 mmol Cl^- (corresponding to *Sando-K®*). Generic prescriptions must specify the strength required.

Kay-Cee-L® (Geistlich)
Syrup, red, sugar-free, potassium chloride 7.5% (1 mmol/mL each of K^+ and Cl^-). Net price 500 mL = £3.74. Label: 21

Kloref® (Alpharma)
Tablets, effervescent, betaine hydrochloride, potassium benzoate, bicarbonate, and chloride, equivalent to potassium chloride 500 mg (6.7 mmol each of K^+ and Cl^-). Net price 50 = £2.71. Label: 13, 21
Note May be difficult to obtain

Sando-K® (HK Pharma)
Tablets, effervescent, potassium bicarbonate and chloride equivalent to potassium 470 mg (12 mmol of K^+) and chloride 285 mg (8 mmol of Cl^-). Net price 20 = £1.53. Label: 13, 21

Modified-release preparations

Avoid unless effervescent tablets or liquid preparations inappropriate

Slow-K® (Alliance)
Tablets, m/r, orange, s/c, potassium chloride 600 mg (8 mmol each of K^+ and Cl^-). Net price 20 = 54p. Label: 25, 27, counselling, swallow whole with fluid during meals while sitting or standing

Potassium removal

Ion-exchange resins may be used to remove excess potassium in *mild hyperkalaemia* or in *moderate hyperkalaemia* when there are no ECG changes. Calcium polystyrene sulphonate is preferred unless plasma-calcium concentrations are high.

Severe hyperkalaemia calls for urgent treatment with intravenous infusion of **soluble insulin** (0.3–0.6 units/kg/hour in neonates and 0.05–0.2 units/kg/hour in children over 1 month) with **glucose** 0.5–1 g/kg/hour (5–10 mL/kg of glucose 10%). If insulin cannot be used, **salbutamol** (section 3.1.1.1) can be given by intravenous infusion but it has a slower onset of action and may be less effective for reducing plasma-potassium concentration.

Calcium gluconate (section 9.5.1.1) is given by slow intravenous injection to manage cardiac excitability caused by hyperkalaemia.

POLYSTYRENE SULPHONATE RESINS

Cautions impaction of resin with excessive dosage or inadequate dilution; monitor for electrolyte disturbances (stop if plasma-potassium concentration below 5 mmol/litre); pregnancy and breast-feeding; sodium-containing resin in congestive heart failure, hypertension, renal impairment, and oedema; **interactions:** Appendix 1 (sodium polystyrene sulphonate)

Contra-indications obstructive bowel disease; oral administration or reduced gut motility in neonates; avoid calcium-containing resin in hyperparathyroidism, multiple myeloma, sarcoidosis, or metastatic carcinoma

Side-effects rectal ulceration following rectal administration; colonic necrosis reported following enemas containing sorbitol; sodium retention, hypercalcaemia, gastric irritation, anorexia, nausea and vomiting, constipation (discontinue treatment—avoid magnesium-containing laxatives), diarrhoea; calcium-containing resin may cause hypercalcaemia (in dialysed patients and occasionally in those with renal impairment), hypomagnesaemia

Licensed use licensed for use in children

Indication and dose

Hyperkalaemia associated with anuria or severe oliguria, and in dialysis patients
• By mouth

Neonate not recommended

Child 1 month–18 years 125–250 mg/kg (max. 15 g) 3–4 times daily

9 Nutrition and blood

POLYSTYRENE SULPHONATE RESINS (*continued*)

• **By rectum**

Neonate 125–250 mg/kg repeated as necessary every 6–8 hours. Irrigate colon to remove resin after 6–12 hours

Child 1 month–18 years 125–250 mg/kg repeated as necessary every 6–8 hours. Irrigate colon to remove resin after 6–12 hours

Administration By mouth: administer in water or as a paste—do not give with fruit squash, which has a high potassium content.
By rectum: mix 1 g of resin with 5–10 mL of a methylcellulose solution. Water may be used but retention is more difficult.

Calcium Resonium® (Sanofi-Synthelabo)
Powder, buff, calcium polystyrene sulphonate. Net price 300 g = £47.55. Label: 13

Resonium A® (Sanofi-Synthelabo)
Powder, buff, sodium polystyrene sulphonate. Net price 454 g = £58.53. Label: 13

9.2.1.2 Oral sodium and water

Sodium chloride is indicated in states of sodium depletion. In preterm neonates in the first few weeks of life and in chronic conditions associated with mild or moderate degrees of sodium depletion, e.g. in salt-losing bowel or renal disease, oral supplements of sodium chloride (section 9.2.1.3) may be sufficient. Sodium chloride solutions suitable for use by mouth in neonates are available as manufactured specials; they should be used with care because they are hypertonic. Supplementation with sodium chloride may be required to replace losses in children with cystic fibrosis particularly in warm weather.

SODIUM CHLORIDE

Indication and dose

See also section 9.2.2

Sodium supplementation in neonates
• **By mouth**

Preterm neonate 2 mmol/100 mL of formula feed or 3–4 mmol/100 mL of breast milk, consult dietician

Sodium replacement
• **By mouth**

Child 1 month–18 years According to requirements, generally 1–2 mmol/kg daily in divided doses, higher doses may be needed in severe depletion

Chronic renal loss
• **By mouth**

Child 1 month–18 years 1–2 mmol/kg daily in divided doses, adjusted according to requirements

Slow Sodium® (HK Pharma)
Tablets, m/r, sodium chloride 600 mg (approx. 10 mmol each of Na^+ and Cl^-). Net price 100-tab pack = £6.05. Label: 25
Capsules available from specials manufacturers.

Extemporaneous formulations available see Extemporaneous Preparations, p. 8

Oral rehydration therapy (ORT)

Diarrhoea in children is usually self-limiting, however, in children under 6 months of age, and more particularly in those under 3 months, symptoms of dehydration may be less obvious and there is a risk of rapid and severe deterioration. Intestinal absorption of sodium and water is enhanced by glucose (and other carbohydrates). Replacement of fluid and electrolytes lost through diarrhoea can therefore be achieved by giving solutions containing sodium, potassium, and glucose or another carbohydrate such as rice starch.

Oral rehydration solutions should:

- enhance the absorption of water and electrolytes;
- replace the electrolyte deficit adequately and safely;
- contain an alkalinising agent to counter acidosis;
- be slightly hypo-osmolar (about 250 mmol/litre) to prevent the possible induction of osmotic diarrhoea;
- be simple to use in hospital and at home;
- be palatable and acceptable, especially to children;
- be readily available.

9 Nutrition and blood

It is the policy of the World Health Organization (WHO) to promote a single oral rehydration solution but to use it flexibly (e.g. by giving extra water between drinks of oral rehydration solution to moderately dehydrated infants).

Oral rehydration solutions used in the UK are lower in sodium (50–60 mmol/litre) than the WHO formulation since, in general, patients suffer less severe sodium loss.

Rehydration should be rapid over 3 to 4 hours (except in hypernatraemic dehydration in which case rehydration should occur more slowly over 12 hours). The patient should be reassessed after initial rehydration and if still dehydrated rapid fluid replacement should continue.

Once rehydration is complete further dehydration is prevented by encouraging the patient to drink normal volumes of an appropriate fluid and by replacing continuing losses with an oral rehydration solution; in infants, breast-feeding or formula feeds should be offered between oral rehydration drinks.

For intravenous rehydration see section 9.2.2.

ORAL REHYDRATION SALTS (ORS)

Indication and dose

Fluid and electrolyte loss in diarrhoea see notes above

- **By mouth**

Child 1 month–1 year 1–1½ times usual feed volume

Child 1–12 years 200 mL after every loose motion

Child 12–18 years 200–400 mL after every loose motion

UK formulations

Note After reconstitution any unused solution should be discarded no later than 1 hour after preparation unless stored in a refrigerator when it may be kept for up to 24 hours.

Dioralyte® (Sanofi-Aventis)

Effervescent tablets, sodium chloride 117 mg, sodium bicarbonate 336 mg, potassium chloride 186 mg, citric acid anhydrous 384 mg, anhydrous glucose 1.62 g. Net price 10-tab pack (black currant- or citrus-flavoured) = £1.42

Dose

Reconstitute 2 tablets with 200 mL of water (only for children over 1 year)

Note Ten tablets when reconstituted with 1 litre of water provide Na^+ 60 mmol, K^+ 25 mmol, Cl^- 45 mmol, citrate 20 mmol, and glucose 90 mmol

Oral powder, sodium chloride 470 mg, potassium chloride 300 mg, disodium hydrogen citrate 530 mg, glucose 3.56 g/sachet, net price 6-sachet pack = £2.02, 20-sachet pack (black currant- or citrus-flavoured or natural) = £6.19

Dose

Reconstitute one sachet with 200 mL of water (freshly boiled and cooled for infants)

Note Five sachets reconstituted with 1 litre of water provide Na^+ 60 mmol, K^+ 20 mmol, Cl^- 60 mmol, citrate 10 mmol, and glucose 90 mmol

Dioralyte® Relief (Sanofi-Aventis)

Oral powder, sodium chloride 350 mg, potassium chloride 300 mg, sodium citrate 580 mg, cooked rice powder 6 g/sachet, net price 6-sachet pack (apricot-, black currant- or raspberry-flavoured) = £2.26, 20-sachet pack (apricot-flavoured) = £7.42

Dose

Reconstitute one sachet with 200 mL of water (freshly boiled and cooled for infants)

Note Five sachets when reconstituted with 1 litre of water provide Na^+ 60 mmol, K^+ 20 mmol, Cl^- 50 mmol and citrate 10 mmol; contains aspartame (section 9.4.1)

Electrolade® (Thornton & Ross)

Oral powder, sodium chloride 236 mg, potassium chloride 300 mg, sodium bicarbonate 500 mg, anhydrous glucose 4 g/sachet (banana-, black currant-, lemon and lime-, or orange-flavoured). Net price 6-sachet (plain or multiflavoured) pack = £1.33, 20-sachet (single- or multiflavoured) pack = £4.99

Dose

Reconstitute one sachet with 200 mL of water (freshly boiled and cooled for infants)

Note Five sachets when reconstituted with 1 litre of water provide Na^+ 50 mmol, K^+ 20 mmol, Cl^- 40 mmol, HCO_3^- 30 mmol, and glucose 111 mmol

Rapolyte® (KoGEN)

Oral powder, sodium chloride 350 mg, potassium chloride 300 mg, sodium citrate 600 mg, anhydrous glucose 4 g, net price 20-sachet pack (black currant- or raspberry-flavoured) = £4.28

Dose

Reconstitute one sachet with 200 mL of water (freshly boiled and cooled for infants)

Note Five sachets when reconstituted with 1 litre of water provide Na^+ 60 mmol, K^+ 20 mmol, Cl^- 50 mmol, citrate 10 mmol, and glucose 110 mmol

WHO formulation

Oral Rehydration Salts (Non-proprietary)

Oral powder, sodium chloride 2.6 g, potassium chloride 1.5 g, sodium citrate 2.9 g, anhydrous glucose 13.5 g. To be dissolved in sufficient water to produce 1 litre (providing Na^+ 75 mmol, K^+ 20 mmol, Cl^- 65 mmol, citrate 10 mmol, glucose 75 mmol/litre)

Note Recommended by the WHO and the United Nations Children's Fund but not commonly used in the UK

9.2.1.3 Oral bicarbonate

Sodium bicarbonate is given by mouth for *chronic acidotic states* such as uraemic acidosis or renal tubular acidosis. The dose for correction of metabolic acidosis is not predictable and the response must be assessed. For severe metabolic acidosis, sodium bicarbonate can be given intravenously (section 9.2.2).

Sodium bicarbonate may also be used to increase the pH of the urine (see also section 7.4.3).

Sodium supplements may increase blood pressure or cause fluid retention and pulmonary oedema in those at risk; hypokalaemia may be exacerbated.

Sodium bicarbonate may affect the stability or absorption of other drugs if administered at the same time. If possible, allow 1–2 hours before administering other drugs orally.

Where *hyperchloraemic acidosis* is associated with potassium deficiency, as in some renal tubular and gastro-intestinal disorders it may be appropriate to give oral **potassium bicarbonate**, although acute or severe deficiency should be managed by intravenous therapy.

SODIUM BICARBONATE

Cautions see notes above; avoid in respiratory acidosis; **interactions**: Appendix 1 (antacids)

Indication and dose

Renal acidosis
- By mouth

Neonate 1–2 mmol/kg daily in divided doses

Child 1 month–2 years 1–2 mmol/kg daily in divided doses

Child 2–18 years 70 mmol/m^2 daily in divided doses

Sodium Bicarbonate (Non-proprietary)

Capsules, sodium bicarbonate 500 mg (approx. 6 mmol each of Na^+ and HCO_3^-). Net price 20 = £5.36

Tablets, sodium bicarbonate 600 mg, net price 100 tabs = £2.48

Important Oral solutions of sodium bicarbonate are required occasionally; these need to be obtained on special order and the strength of sodium bicarbonate should be stated on the prescription

POTASSIUM BICARBONATE

Cautions cardiac disease, **interactions**: Appendix 1 (potassium salts)

Renal impairment avoid routine use in moderate impairment; high risk of hyperkalaemia

Contra-indications hypochloraemia; plasma potassium concentration above 5 mmol/litre

Side-effects nausea and vomiting

Potassium Tablets, Effervescent (Non-proprietary)

Effervescent tablets, potassium bicarbonate 500 mg, potassium acid tartrate 300 mg, each tablet providing 6.5 mmol of K^+. To be dissolved in water before administration. Net price 56 = £6.03. Label: 13, 21

Note These tablets do not contain chloride; for effervescent tablets containing potassium and chloride, see under Potassium Chloride, section 9.2.1.1

9.2.2 Parenteral preparations for fluid and electrolyte imbalance

9.2.2.1 Electrolytes and water

Solutions of electrolytes are given intravenously, to meet normal fluid and electrolyte requirements or to replenish substantial deficits or continuing losses when it is not possible or desirable to use the oral route. When intravenous administration is not possible, fluid (as sodium chloride 0.9% or glucose 5%) can also be given subcutaneously by hypodermoclysis.

In an individual patient the nature and severity of the electrolyte imbalance must be assessed from the history and clinical and biochemical examination. Sodium, potassium, chloride, magnesium, phosphate, and water depletion can occur singly and in combination with or without disturbances of acid-base balance; for reference to the use of magnesium and phosphates, see section 9.5.

Isotonic solutions may be infused safely into a peripheral vein. Solutions more concentrated than plasma, for example 15% glucose are best given through an indwelling catheter positioned in a large vein.

Maintenance fluid requirements are usually derived from the relationship that exists between body-weight and metabolic rate; the figures in the table below may be used as a guide outside the neonatal period. The glucose requirement is that needed to minimise gluconeogenesis from amino acids obtained as substrate from muscle breakdown.

It is usual to meet these requirements by using a standard solution of sodium chloride and glucose. Solutions containing 20 mmol/litre of potassium chloride meet usual potassium requirements when given in the suggested volumes; adjustments may be needed if there is an inability to excrete fluids or electrolytes, excessive renal loss or continuing extra-renal losses. The exact requirements depend upon the nature of the clinical situation and types of losses incurred; see Caution on dilutional hyponatraemia below.

Fluid requirements for children over 1 month:

Body-weight	24-hour fluid requirement
Under 10 kg	100 mL/kg
10–20 kg	100 mL/kg for the first 10 kg + 50 mL/kg for each 1 kg body-weight over 10 kg
Over 20 kg	100 mL/kg for the first 10 kg + 50 mL/kg for each 1 kg body-weight between 10–20 kg + 20 mL/kg for each 1 kg body-weight over 20 kg (max. 2 litres in females, 2.5 litres in males)

Note The baseline fluid requirement shown above should be adjusted to take account of factors that reduce water loss (e.g. increased antidiuretic hormone, renal failure, hypothermia, and high ambient humidity) or increase water loss (e.g. pyrexia or burns)

Caution During parenteral hydration, fluids and electrolytes should be monitored closely and any disturbance corrected by slow infusion of an appropriate solution. The volume of fluid infused should take into account the possibility of reduced fluid loss owing to increased antidiuretic hormone and factors such as renal failure, hypothermia, and high humidity.

Dilutional hyponatraemia is a rare but potentially fatal risk of parenteral hydration. It may be caused by inappropriate use of fluids such as sodium chloride 0.18% and glucose 4% intravenous infusion, especially in the postoperative period when antidiuretic hormone secretion is increased. Dilutional hyponatraemia is characterized by a rapid fall in plasma-sodium concentration leading to cerebral oedema and seizures; any child with severe hyponatraemia or rapidly changing plasma-sodium concentration should be referred urgently to paediatric high dependency facilities.

Replacement therapy: initial intravenous replacement fluid is generally required if the child is over 10% dehydrated, or if 5–10% dehydrated and oral or enteral rehydration is not tolerated or possible. Oral rehydration is adequate, if tolerated, in the majority of those less than 10% dehydrated. Subsequent fluid and electrolyte requirements are determined by clinical assessment of fluid balance.

Neonates Neonates lose water through the skin and nose, particularly if preterm or if the skin is damaged. The minimum basic fluid requirement for a neonate with normal renal function is 100–120 mL/kg/day and is generally provided as 10% glucose. Continuous infusion of drugs in 10% glucose limits unnecessary water intake. This requirement is modified following fluid balance and electrolyte monitoring and reduced in renal impairment. Some preterm neonates may require up to 180 mL/kg daily after the first 48 hours. Restricting water intake in the first few days of life has been advocated to aid the normal intravascular volume changes that occur after birth. The evidence for the benefit of this approach is limited and the risk of hypoglycaemia must be considered. Local guidelines for fluid management in the neonatal period should be consulted.

Intravenous sodium

Sodium chloride in isotonic (0.9%) solution provides the most important extracellular ions in near physiological concentration and is indicated in *sodium depletion*.

Intravenous sodium is commonly given as a component of maintenance and replacement therapy. It may be given as sodium chloride 0.9% for initial treatment of acute fluid loss and to replace ongoing gastro-intestinal losses from the upper gastro-intestinal tract. For maintenance and replacement therapy it is usually given in combination with other electrolytes and glucose. Sodium chloride solutions should be used cautiously in renal insufficiency, cardiac failure, cardio-respiratory diseases, hepatic cirrhosis and in children receiving glucocorticoids as sodium overload may easily occur. Conversely, hyponatraemia with serious consequences may occur if maintenance and replacement fluids do not meet sodium requirements (see Caution, dilutional hyponatraemia, above).

Chronic hyponatraemia should ideally be corrected by fluid restriction. However, if sodium chloride is required, the deficit should be corrected slowly to avoid the risk of osmotic demyelination syndrome; the rise in plasma-sodium concentration should be no more than 10 mmol/litre in 24 hours.

Sodium chloride and glucose solutions are indicated when there is combined *water and sodium depletion*. A 1:1 mixture of isotonic sodium chloride and 5% glucose allows some of the water (free of sodium) to enter body cells which suffer most from dehydration while the sodium salt with a volume of water determined by the normal plasma Na^+ remains extracellular. Maintenance fluid should accurately reflect daily requirements and close monitoring is required to avoid fluid and electrolyte imbalance. Illness or injury increase the secretion of anti-diuretic hormone and therefore the ability to excrete excess water may be impaired. Injudicious use of solutions such as sodium chloride 0.18% and glucose 4% may also cause dilutional hyponatraemia especially in children (see Caution on dilutional hyponatraemia, above); if necessary, guidance should be sought from a clinician experienced in the management of fluid and electrolytes.

Combined sodium, potassium, chloride, and water depletion may occur, for example, with severe diarrhoea or persistent vomiting; replacement is carried out with sodium chloride intravenous infusion 0.9% and glucose intravenous infusion 5% with potassium as appropriate.

Compound sodium lactate (Hartmann's solution) can be used instead of isotonic sodium chloride solution during surgery or in the initial management of the injured or wounded.

Neonates The sodium requirement for most healthy neonates is 3 mmol/kg daily. Preterm neonates, particularly below 30 weeks gestation, may require up to 6 mmol/kg daily. *Hyponatraemia* may be caused by excessive renal loss of sodium; it may also be dilutional and restriction of fluid intake may be appropriate. Sodium supplementation is likely to be required if the serum sodium concentration is significantly reduced.

Hypernatraemia may also occur due to the limited ability of the immature kidney to excrete sodium. Severe hypernatraemia can cause permanent brain damage. Sodium in drug preparations, delivered via continuous infusions, or in infusions to maintain the patency of intravascular or umbilical lines, can result in significant amounts of sodium being delivered,(e.g. 1 mL/hour of 0.9% sodium chloride infused over 24 hours is equivalent to 3.6 mmol/day of sodium).

SODIUM CHLORIDE

Cautions restrict intake in impaired renal function, cardiac failure, hypertension, peripheral and pulmonary oedema, toxaemia of pregnancy; see also notes above

Side-effects administration of large doses may give rise to sodium accumulation and oedema

Indication and dose

Electrolyte imbalance see notes above, also section 9.2.1.2

Sodium Chloride (Non-proprietary) PoM

Intravenous infusion, usual strength sodium chloride 0.9% (9 g, 150 mmol each of Na^+ and Cl^-/litre), this strength being supplied when normal saline for injection is requested. Net price 2-mL amp = 24p; 5-mL amp = 33p; 10-mL amp = 36p; 20-mL amp = £1.04; 50-mL amp = £2.01

In hospitals, 500- and 1000-mL packs, and sometimes other sizes, are available

Note The term 'normal saline' should **not** be used to describe sodium chloride intravenous infusion 0.9%; the

SODIUM CHLORIDE (*continued*)

term 'physiological saline' is acceptable but it is preferable to give the composition (i.e. sodium chloride intravenous infusion 0.9%).

With other ingredients

Note See above for warning on hyponatraemia

Sodium Chloride and Glucose (Non-proprietary) PoM
Intravenous infusion, sodium chloride 0.18% (Na^+ and Cl^- each 30 mmol/litre), glucose 4%
In hospitals, usually 500-mL packs and sometimes other sizes are available

Intravenous infusion, sodium chloride 0.45% (Na^+ and Cl^- each 75 mmol/litre), glucose 5%
In hospitals, usually 500-mL packs and sometimes other sizes are available

Intravenous infusion, sodium chloride 0.9% (Na^+ and Cl^- each 150 mmol/litre), glucose 5%
In hospitals, usually 500-mL packs and sometimes other sizes are available

Ringer's Solution (Non-proprietary) PoM
Calcium chloride (dihydrate) 322 micrograms, potassium chloride 300 micrograms, sodium chloride 8.6 mg/mL, providing the following ions (in mmol/litre), Ca^{2+} 2.2, K^+ 4, Na^+ 147, Cl^- 156
In hospitals, 500- and 1000-mL packs, and sometimes other sizes, are available

Sodium Lactate, Compound (Non-proprietary) PoM
(Hartmann's Solution; Ringer-Lactate Solution)
Intravenous infusion, sodium chloride 0.6%, sodium lactate 0.25%, potassium chloride 0.04%, calcium chloride 0.027% (containing Na^+ 131 mmol, K^+ 5 mmol, Ca^{2+} 2 mmol, HCO_3^- (as lactate) 29 mmol, Cl^- 111 mmol/litre)
In hospitals, 500- and 1000-mL packs, and sometimes other sizes, are available

Intravenous glucose

Glucose solutions are mainly used to replace body-water deficits and should be given alone only when there is no significant loss of electrolytes. Water depletion (dehydration) tends to occur when losses are not matched by a comparable intake, as for example may occur in coma or dysphagia.

Water loss rarely exceeds electrolyte losses but this can occur in fevers, hyperthyroidism, and in uncommon water-losing renal states such as diabetes insipidus or hypercalcaemia. The volume of glucose solution needed to replace deficits varies with the severity of the disorder; the rate of infusion should be adjusted to return the plasma-sodium concentration to normal over 48 hours.

Glucose solutions are also given with insulin for the emergency management of *hyperkalaemia* (see p. 501). They are also given, after correction of hyperglycaemia, during treatment of diabetic ketoacidosis, when they must be accompanied by continuous insulin infusion (section 6.1.3).

Injections containing more than 10% glucose can be irritant and should be given into a central venous line; however, solutions containing up to 12.5% may be administered for a short period into a peripheral line.

GLUCOSE
(Dextrose Monohydrate)

Note Glucose BP is the monohydrate but Glucose Intravenous Infusion BP is a sterile solution of anhydrous glucose or glucose monohydrate, potency being expressed in terms of anhydrous glucose

Side-effects glucose injections especially if hypertonic may have a low pH and may cause venous irritation and thrombophlebitis

Indication and dose

Fluid replacement see notes above

Provision of energy see section 9.3

Hypoglycaemia see section 6.1.4

Glucose (Non-proprietary) PoM
Intravenous infusion, glucose or anhydrous glucose (potency expressed in terms of anhydrous glucose), usual strengths 5% (50 mg/mL) and 10% (100 mg/mL); 25% solution, net price 25-mL amp = £2.21; 50% solution[1], 25-mL amp = £3.80, 50-mL amp = £1.63
In hospitals, 500- and 1000-mL packs, and sometimes other sizes and strengths, are available; also available *Min-I-Jet® Glucose*, 50% in 50-mL disposable syringe[1]

1. PoM restriction does not apply where administration is for saving life in emergency

Intravenous potassium

Potassium chloride and sodium chloride intravenous infusion is the initial treatment for the correction of *severe hypokalaemia* and when sufficient potassium cannot be taken by mouth. Ready-mixed infusion solutions should be used when possible (see under Safe Practice below); the concentration of potassium should not exceed 40 mmol/litre. Potassium infusions should be given slowly over at least 2–3 hours and at a rate not exceeding 0.2 mmol/kg/hour with specialist advice and ECG monitoring in difficult cases. Higher concentrations of potassium chloride or faster infusion rates may be given in very severe depletion, but require specialist advice.

Repeated measurements of plasma-potassium concentration are necessary to determine whether further infusions are required and to avoid the development of hyperkalaemia, which is especially likely in renal impairment.

Initial potassium replacement therapy should **not** involve glucose infusions, because glucose may cause a further decrease in the plasma-potassium concentration.

> Safe Practice
> Potassium overdose can be fatal. Ready-mixed infusion solutions containing potassium should be used. Exceptionally, if potassium chloride concentrate is used for preparing an infusion, the infusion solution should be **thoroughly mixed**. Local policies on avoiding inadvertent use of potassium chloride concentrate should be followed.

POTASSIUM CHLORIDE

Cautions for intravenous infusion the concentration of solution should not usually exceed 3 g (40 mmol)/litre; specialist advice and ECG monitoring (see notes above); **interactions:** Appendix 1 (potassium salts)

Renal impairment see notes above

Side-effects rapid infusion toxic to heart

Indication and dose

Electrolyte imbalance see also oral potassium supplements, section 9.2.1.1

- **By slow intravenous infusion**

depending on the deficit or the daily maintenance requirements, see also notes above

Neonate 1–2 mmol/kg daily

Child 1 month–18 years 1–2 mmol/kg daily

Administration see notes above

Potassium Chloride and Glucose (Non-proprietary) PoM

Intravenous infusion, usual strengths potassium chloride 0.3% (3 g, 40 mmol each of K^+ and Cl^-/litre) or 0.15% (1.5 g, 20 mmol each of K^+ and Cl^-/litre) with 5% of anhydrous glucose

In hospitals, 500- and 1000-mL packs, and sometimes other sizes, are available

Potassium Chloride and Sodium Chloride (Non-proprietary) PoM

Intravenous infusion, usual strength potassium chloride 0.15% (1.5 g/litre) with sodium chloride 0.9% (9 g/litre), containing K^+ 20 mmol, Na^+ 150 mmol, and Cl^- 170 mmol/litre

In hospitals, 500- and 1000-mL packs, and sometimes other sizes, are available

Potassium Chloride, Sodium Chloride, and Glucose (Non-proprietary) PoM

Intravenous infusion, sodium chloride 0.45% (4.5 g, Na^+ 75 mmol/litre) with 5% of anhydrous glucose and usually sufficient potassium chloride to provide K^+ 10–40 mmol/litre (to be specified by the prescriber)

In hospitals, 500- and 1000-mL packs, and sometimes other sizes are available

Potassium Chloride (Non-proprietary) PoM

Sterile concentrate, potassium chloride 15% (150 mg, approximately 2 mmol each of K^+ and Cl^-/mL). Net price 10-mL amp = 48p

Solutions containing 10 and 20% of potassium chloride are also available in both 5- and 10-mL ampoules

> Important Must be diluted with **not less** than 50 times its volume of Sodium Chloride 0.9% or other suitable diluent and **mixed well**; see Safe Practice, above

Bicarbonate and lactate

Sodium bicarbonate is used to control severe *metabolic acidosis* (as in renal failure). Since this condition is usually attended by sodium depletion, it is reasonable to correct this first by the administration of sodium chloride 0.9% intravenous infusion, provided the kidneys are not primarily affected and the degree of acidosis is not so severe as to impair renal function. In these circumstances, sodium chloride 0.9% alone is usually effective as it restores the ability of the kidneys to generate bicarbonate. In renal acidosis or in severe metabolic acidosis of any origin (for example blood pH < 7.1) sodium bicarbonate (1.26%) may be infused with isotonic sodium chloride when the acidosis remains unresponsive to correction of anoxia or fluid depletion. In severe shock due, for example, to cardiac arrest (see section 2.7), metabolic acidosis may develop without sodium depletion; in these circumstances sodium bicarbonate is best given intravenously in a small volume of hypertonic solution, such as 8.4%; plasma pH should be monitored.

Sodium lactate intravenous infusion is obsolete in metabolic acidosis, and carries the risk of producing lactic acidosis, particularly in seriously ill patients with poor tissue perfusion or impaired hepatic function.

Trometamol (tris-hydroxymethyl aminomethane, THAM), an organic buffer, corrects metabolic acidosis by causing an increase in urinary pH and an osmotic diuresis. It is indicated when sodium bicarbonate is unsuitable as in carbon dioxide retention, hypernatraemia or renal impairment. Respiratory support may be required as trometamol induces respiratory depression. It is also used during cardiac bypass surgery and, very rarely, in cardiac arrest. Trometamol [unlicensed] is available as 3.6% or 7.2% solution, and should be used as 3.6% solution when given intravenously.

SODIUM BICARBONATE

Indication and dose

Metabolic acidosis
- **By slow intravenous injection of a strong solution (up to 8.4%), or by continuous intravenous infusion of a weaker solution (usually 1.26%)**

an amount appropriate to the body base deficit (see notes above)

Renal hyperkalaemia
- **By slow intravenous injection**

Neonate 1 mmol/kg daily

Child 1 month–18 years 1 mmol/kg daily

Sodium Bicarbonate PoM

Intravenous infusion, usual strength sodium bicarbonate 1.26% (12.6 g, 150 mmol each of Na^+ and HCO_3^-/litre); various other strengths available

In hospitals, 500- and 1000-mL packs, and sometimes other sizes, are available

Administration For *peripheral infusion* dilute 8.4% solution at least 1 in 10; for *central line infusion* dilute 1 in 5 with Glucose 5% or 10% *or* Sodium Chloride 0.9%. Extravasation can cause severe tissue damage

Min-I-Jet® Sodium Bicarbonate (Celltech) PoM

Intravenous injection, sodium bicarbonate in disposable syringe, net price 4.2%, 10 mL = £5.29; 8.4%, 10 mL = £5.71, 50 mL = £7.75

SODIUM LACTATE

Indication and dose

See notes above

Sodium Lactate (Non-proprietary) PoM

Intravenous infusion, sodium lactate M/6, contains the following ions (in mmol/litre), Na^+ 167, HCO_3^- (as lactate) 167

Trometamol

(Tris-hydroxymethyl aminomethane, THAM)

Cautions extravasation can cause severe tissue damage

Renal impairment use with caution, may cause hyperkalaemia

Pregnancy little information available, hypoglycaemia may harm fetus

Breast-feeding no information available

Contra-indications anuria; chronic respiratory acidosis

Side-effects respiratory depression; hypoglycaemia; hyperkalaemia in renal impairment; liver necrosis reported following administration via umbilical vein in neonates

Licensed use unlicensed preparation

Indication and dose

Correction of metabolic acidosis
- **By intravenous infusion**

Preterm neonate 0.5–0.6 mmol/kg × base deficit, correct half base deficit initially then re-calculate; max. dose 10 mmol/kg in 12 hours

Neonate 0.4 mmol/kg × base deficit, correct half base deficit initially then re-calculate; max. dose 10 mmol/kg in 12 hours

Child 1 month–12 years 0.3 mmol/kg × base deficit, correct half base deficit initially then re-calculate; max. dose 10 mmol/kg in 12 hours

Child 12–18 years 0.25–0.3 mmol/kg × base deficit, correct half base deficit initially then re-calculate; max. dose 10 mmol/kg in 12 hours

Administration Dilute to at least 3.6% solution with Glucose 5% *or* Water for Injections. Do not exceed an infusion rate of 5 mmol/kg/hour. In fluid restriction 7.2% solution may be administered undiluted via central venous catheter

Note 1 mL of 7.2% solution (2 mL of 3.6% solution) ≡ 1 mmol of bicarbonate

Preparations

5 mL and 10 mL ampoules of 3.6% and 7.2% solution are available from several NHS manufacturing units

Water

Water for Injections PoM

Net price 1-mL amp = 18p; 2-mL amp = 17p; 5-mL amp = 28p; 10-mL amp = 31p; 20-mL amp = 55p; 50-mL amp = £1.91; 100-mL vial= 23p

9.2.2.2 Plasma and plasma substitutes

Albumin solutions, prepared from whole blood, contain soluble proteins and electrolytes but no clotting factors, blood group antibodies, or plasma cholinesterases; they may be given without regard to the recipient's blood group.

Albumin should usually be used after the acute phase of illness, to correct a plasma-volume deficit in patients with salt and water retention and oedema; hypoalbuminaemia itself is not an appropriate indication. The use of albumin solutions in acute plasma or blood loss may be wasteful; plasma substitutes are more appropriate. Concentrated albumin solutions may also be used to obtain a diuresis in hypoalbuminaemic patients (e.g. in nephrotic syndrome).

Recent evidence does not support the previous view that the use of albumin increases mortality.

> Plasma and plasma substitutes are often used in very ill children whose condition is unstable. Therefore, close monitoring is required and fluid and electrolyte therapy should be adjusted according to the child's condition at all times.

ALBUMIN SOLUTION

(Human Albumin Solution)

A solution containing protein derived from plasma, serum, or normal placentas; at least 95% of the protein is albumin. The solution may be isotonic (containing 4–5% protein) or concentrated (containing 15–25% protein).

Cautions history of cardiac or circulatory disease (administer slowly to avoid rapid rise in blood pressure and cardiac failure, and monitor cardiovascular and respiratory function); increased capillary permeability; correct dehydration when administering concentrated solution

Contra-indications cardiac failure; severe anaemia

Side-effects hypersensitivity reactions (including anaphylaxis) with nausea, vomiting, increased salivation, fever, tachycardia, hypotension and chills reported

Indication and dose

See under preparations, below

Isotonic solutions

Indications: acute or sub-acute loss of plasma volume e.g. in burns, pancreatitis, trauma, and complications of surgery; plasma exchange

Available as: *Human Albumin Solution 4.5%* (50-, 100-, 250- and 400-mL bottles—Baxter Bioscience); *Human Albumin Solution 5%* (100-, 250- and 500-mL bottles—Grifols); *ALBA® 4.5%* (100- and 400-mL bottles—SNBTS); *Albutein® 5%* (250- and 500-mL bottles—Grifols); *Octalbin® 5%* (100- and 200-mL bottles—Octapharm); *Zenalb® 4.5%* (50-, 100-, 250-, and 500-mL bottles—BPL)

Concentrated solutions (20–25%)

Indications: severe hypoalbuminaemia associated with low plasma volume and generalised oedema where salt and water restriction with plasma volume expansion are required; adjunct in the treatment of hyperbilirubinaemia by exchange transfusion in the newborn; paracentesis of large volume ascites associated with portal hypertension

Available as: *Human Albumin Solution 20%* (50- and 100-mL vials—Baxter Bioscience); *Human Albumin Solution 20%* (50- and 100-mL bottles—Grifols); *ALBA® 20%* (50-mL vials—SNBTS); *Albutein® 20%* (50- and 100-mL bottles—Grifols); *Albutein® 25%* (20-, 50-, and 100-mL vials—Grifols); *Octalbin® 20%* (50- and 100-mL bottles—Octapharm); *Zenalb® 20%* (50- and 100-mL bottles—BPL)

Plasma substitutes

Dextrans, **gelatin**, and the etherified starches, **hexastarch**, **hydroxyethyl starch** and **pentastarch** are macromolecular substances which are metabolised slowly; they may be used at the outset to expand and maintain blood volume in shock arising from conditions such as burns or septicaemia. Plasma substitutes may be used as an immediate short-term measure to treat haemorrhage until blood is available. They are rarely needed when shock is due to sodium and water depletion because, in these circumstances, the shock responds to water and electrolyte repletion. See also section 2.7.1 for the management of shock.

Plasma substitutes should **not** be used to maintain plasma volume in conditions such as burns or peritonitis where there is loss of plasma protein, water and electrolytes over periods of several days or weeks. In these situations, plasma or plasma protein fractions containing large amounts of albumin should be given.

Large volumes of *some* plasma substitutes can increase the risk of bleeding through depletion of coagulation factors; however, the risk is reduced if a substitute such as hexastarch is used.

Dextran 70 by intravenous infusion is used predominantly for volume expansion. Dextran 40 intravenous infusion is used in an attempt to improve peripheral blood flow in ischaemic disease of the limbs. Dextrans 40 and 70 have also been used in the prophylaxis of thromboembolism but are now rarely used for this purpose.

Dextrans may interfere with blood group cross-matching or biochemical measurements and these should be carried out before infusion is begun.

Plasma and plasma substitutes are often used in very ill children whose condition is unstable. Therefore, close monitoring is required and fluid and electrolyte therapy should be adjusted according to the child's condition at all times.

The use of plasma substitutes in children requires specialist supervision due to the risk of fluid overload; use is best restricted to an intensive care setting.

Cautions Plasma substitutes should be used with caution in cardiac disease, liver disease, or renal impairment; urine output should be monitored. Care should be taken to avoid haematocrit concentration from falling below 25–30% and the child should be monitored for hypersensitivity reactions.

Side-effects Hypersensitivity reactions may occur including, rarely, severe anaphylactoid reactions. Transient increase in bleeding time may occur.

DEXTRAN 40

Dextrans of weight average molecular weight about '40 000'

Cautions see notes above; can interfere with some laboratory tests (see also above); correct dehydration beforehand, give adequate fluids during therapy and, where possible, monitor central venous pressure

Pregnancy avoid—reports of anaphylaxis in mother causing fetal anoxia, neurological damage and death

Side-effects see notes above

Indication and dose

Conditions associated with peripheral local slowing of the blood flow; prophylaxis of post-surgical thromboembolic disease (but see notes above)

- **By intravenous infusion**
  according to the child's condition (see notes above)

Dextran 40® (Baxter) PoM
Intravenous infusion, dextran 40 intravenous infusion in glucose intravenous infusion 5% or in sodium chloride intravenous infusion 0.9%. Net price 500-mL bag (both) = £4.56

DEXTRAN 70

Dextrans of weight average molecular weight about '70 000'

Cautions see notes above; can interfere with some laboratory tests (see also above); where possible, monitor central venous pressure

Pregnancy avoid—reports of anaphylaxis in mother causing fetal anoxia, neurological damage and death

Side-effects see notes above

Indication and dose

Short-term blood volume expansion; prophylaxis of post-surgical thromboembolic disease (but see notes above)

- **By intravenous infusion**
  after moderate to severe haemorrhage or in the shock phase of burn injury (initial 48 hours), according to the child's condition; total dosage should not exceed 20 mL/kg

Dextran 70® (Baxter) PoM
Intravenous infusion, dextran 70 intravenous infusion in glucose intravenous infusion 5% or in sodium chloride intravenous infusion 0.9%. Net price 500-mL bag (both) = £4.56

Hypertonic solution

RescueFlow® (Vitaline) PoM
Intravenous infusion, dextran 70 intravenous infusion 6% in sodium chloride intravenous infusion 7.5%. Net price 250-mL bag = £28.50

Cautions see notes above; severe hyperglycaemia and hyperosmolality

GELATIN

Note The gelatin is partially degraded

Cautions see notes above

Side-effects see notes above

Indication and dose

Low blood volume in hypovolaemic shock, burns and cardiopulmonary bypass
- **By intravenous infusion**
  initially 10–20 mL/kg of a 3.5–4% solution (see notes above)

Gelofusine® (Braun) PoM
Intravenous infusion, succinylated gelatin (modified fluid gelatin, average molecular weight 30 000) 40 g (4%), Na^+ 154 mmol, Cl^- 124 mmol/litre, net price 500-mL *Ecobag®* = £4.63, 1-litre *Ecobag®* = £9.45
Contains traces of calcium

Haemaccel® (Syner-Med) PoM
Intravenous infusion, polygeline (gelatin derivative, average molecular weight 30 000) 35 g (3.5%), Na^+ 145 mmol, K^+ 5.1 mmol, Ca^{2+} 6.25 mmol, Cl^- 145 mmol/litre, net price 500-mL bottle = £5.00

Volplex® (Cambridge) PoM
Intravenous infusion, succinylated gelatin (modified fluid gelatin, average molecular weight 30 000) 40 g (4%), Na^+ 154 mmol, Cl^- 125 mmol/litre, net price 500-mL bag = £5.05

ETHERIFIED STARCH

A starch composed of more than 90% of amylopectin that has been etherified with hydroxyethyl groups; hetastarch has a higher degree of etherification than pentastarch

Cautions see notes above

Side-effects see notes above; also pruritus, raised serum amylase

Indication and dose

Low blood volume
- **By intravenous infusion**
  according to the child's condition (see notes above)

Hexastarch

eloHAES® (Fresenius Kabi) PoM
Intravenous infusion, hexastarch (weight average molecular weight 200 000) 6% in sodium chloride intravenous infusion 0.9%. Net price 500-mL *Steriflex®* bag = £12.50

Pentastarch

HAES-steril® (Fresenius Kabi) PoM
Intravenous infusion, pentastarch (weight average molecular weight 200 000), net price (both in sodium chloride intravenous infusion 0.9%) 6%, 500 mL = £10.50; 10%, 500 mL = £16.50

Hemohes® (Braun) PoM
Intravenous infusion, pentastarch (weight average molecular weight 200 000), net price (both in sodium chloride intravenous infusion 0.9%) 6%, 500 mL = £12.50; 10%, 500 mL = £16.50

Tetrastarch

Voluven® (Fresenius Kabi) PoM
Intravenous infusion, hydroxyethyl starch (weight average molecular weight 130 000) 6% in sodium chloride intravenous infusion 0.9%, net price 500-mL bag = £12.50

Hypertonic solution

HyperHAES® (Fresenius Kabi) PoM
Intravenous infusion, hydroxyethyl starch (weight average molecular weight 200 000) 6% in sodium chloride intravenous infusion 7.2%, net price 250-mL bag = £28.00
Cautions see notes above; also diabetes

9.3 Intravenous nutrition

When adequate feeding through the alimentary tract is not possible, nutrients may be given by intravenous infusion. This may be in addition to oral or enteral tube feeding—**supplemental parenteral nutrition**, or may be the sole source of nutrition—**total parenteral nutrition** (TPN). Complete enteral starvation is undesirable and total parenteral nutrition is a last resort.

Indications for parenteral nutrition include prematurity; severe or prolonged disorders of the gastro-intestinal tract; preparation of undernourished patients for surgery, chemotherapy, or radiation therapy; major surgery, trauma, or burns; prolonged coma or inability to eat; and some patients with renal or hepatic failure. The composition of proprietary preparations used in children is given in the table below.

Proprietary infusion fluids for parenteral feeding

Preparation	Nitrogen g/litre	Energy[1] kJ/litre	Electrolytes mmol/litre					Other components/litre
			K^+	Mg^{2+}	Na^+	$Acet^-$	Cl^-	
ClinOleic 20% (Baxter) Net price 100 mL = £6.28; 250 mL = £10.08; 500 mL = £13.88		8360						purified olive and soya oil 200 g, glycerol 22.5 g, egg phosphatides 12 g
Glamin (Fresenius Kabi) Net price 250 mL = £14.16; 500 mL = £26.38	22.4					62		
Intralipid 10% (Fresenius Kabi) Net price 100 mL = £4.70; 500 mL = £10.30		4600						soya oil 100 g, glycerol 22 g, purified egg phospholipids 12 g, phosphate 15 mmol
Intralipid 20% (Fresenius Kabi) Net price 100 mL = £7.05; 250 mL = £11.60; 500 mL = £15.45		8400						soya oil 200 g, glycerol 22 g, purified egg phospholipids 12 g, phosphate 15 mmol
Intralipid 30% (Fresenius Kabi) Net price 333 mL = £17.30		12600						soya oil 300 g, glycerol 16.7 g, purified egg phospholipids 12 g, phosphate 15 mmol
Ivelip 10% (Baxter) Net price 500 mL = £9.08		4600						soya oil 100 g, glycerol 25 g
Ivelip 20% (Baxter) Net price 100 mL = £6.28; 500 mL = £13.88		8400						soya oil 200 g, glycerol 25 g
Lipofundin MCT/LCT 10% (Braun) Net price 100 mL = £7.70; 500 mL = £12.90		4430						soya oil 50 g, medium chain triglycerides 50 g
Lipofundin MCT/LCT 20% (Braun) Net price 100 mL = £12.51; 250 mL = £11.30; 500 mL = £19.18		8000						soya oil 100 g, medium chain triglycerides 100 g
Primene 10% (Baxter)[2] Net price 100 mL = £5.78, 250 mL = £7.92	15						19	
Synthamin 9 (Baxter) Net price 500 mL = £6.66; 1000 mL = £12.34	9.1		60	5	70	100	70	acid phosphate 30 mmol
Synthamin 9 EF (electrolyte-free) (Baxter) Net price 500 mL = £6.66; 1000 mL = £12.34	9.1					44	22	
Vamin 9 (Fresenius Kabi) Net price 500 mL = £7.30; 1000 mL = £12.55	9.4		20	1.5	50		50	Ca^{2+} 2.5 mmol
Vamin 9 Glucose (Fresenius Kabi) Net price 100 mL = £3.80; 500 mL = £7.70; 1000 mL = £13.40	9.4	1700	20	1.5	50		50	Ca^{2+} 2.5 mmol, anhydrous glucose 100 g
Vaminolact (Fresenius Kabi) Net price 100 mL = £4.20; 500 mL = £9.70	9.3							

1. Excludes protein- or amino acid-derived energy
Note. 1000 kcal = 4200 kJ; 1000 kJ= 238.8 kcal. All entries are PoM
2. For use in neonates and children only
Note. 1000 kcal = 4200 kJ; = 238.8 kcal. All entries are PoM

Parenteral nutrition requires the use of a solution containing amino acids, glucose, lipids, electrolytes, trace elements, and vitamins. This is now commonly provided by the pharmacy in the form of an amino-acid, glucose, electrolyte bag and a separate lipid infusion or, in older children a single 'all-in-one' bag. If the patient is able to take small amounts by mouth, vitamins may be given orally.

The nutrition solution is infused through a central venous catheter inserted under full surgical precautions. Alternatively infusion through a peripheral vein may be used for supplementary as well as total parenteral nutrition, depending on the availability of peripheral veins; factors prolonging cannula life and preventing thrombophlebitis include the use of soft polyurethane paediatric cannulas and use of nutritional solutions of low osmolality and neutral pH. Nutritional fluids should be given by a dedicated intravenous line; if not possible, compatibility with any drugs or fluids should be checked as precipitation of components may occur. Extravasation of parenteral nutrition solution can cause severe tissue damage and injury; the infusion site should be regularly monitored.

Before starting intravenous nutrition the patient should be clinically stable and renal function and acid-base status should be assessed. Appropriate biochemical tests should have been carried out beforehand and serious deficits corrected. Nutritional and electrolyte status must be monitored throughout treatment. The nutritional components of parenteral nutrition regimens are usually increased gradually over a number of days to prevent metabolic complications and to allow metabolic adaptation to the infused nutrients. The solutions are usually infused over 24 hours but this may be gradually reduced if long-term nutrition is required. Home parenteral nutrition is usually infused over 12 hours overnight.

Complications of long-term parenteral nutrition include gall bladder sludging, gall stones, cholestasis and abnormal liver function tests. For details of the prevention and management of parenteral nutrition complications, specialist literature should be consulted.

Protein (nitrogen) is given as mixtures of essential and non-essential synthetic L-amino acids. Ideally, all essential amino acids should be included with a wide variety of non-essential ones to provide sufficient nitrogen together with electrolytes (see also section 9.2.2). Solutions vary in their composition of amino acids; they often contain an energy source (usually glucose) and electrolytes. Solutions for use in neonates and children under 1 year of age are based on the amino acid profile of umbilical cord blood (*Primene®*) or breast milk (*Vaminolact®*) and contain amino acids that are essential in this age group; these amino acids may not be present in sufficient quantities in preparations designed for older children and adults.

Energy requirements must be met if amino acids are to be utilised for tissue maintenance. An appropriate energy to protein ratio is essential and requirements will vary depending on the child's age and condition. A mixture of carbohydrate and fat energy sources (usually 30–50% as fat) gives better utilisation of amino acids than glucose alone.

Glucose is the preferred source of carbohydrate, but frequent monitoring of blood glucose is required particularly during initiation and build-up of the regimen; insulin may be necessary. Glucose above a concentration of 12.5% must be infused through a central venous catheter to avoid thrombosis; the maximum concentration of glucose that should normally be infused in fluid restricted children is 20–25%.

In parenteral nutrition regimens, it is necessary to provide adequate phosphate in order to allow phosphorylation of glucose. Neonates, particularly preterm neonates, and young children also require phosphorus and calcium to ensure adequate bone mineralisation. The compatibility and solubility of calcium and phosphorus salts is complex and unpredictable; precipitation is a risk and specialist pharmacy advice should be sought.

Fat (lipid) emulsions have the advantages of a high energy to fluid volume ratio, neutral pH, and iso-osmolarity with plasma, and provide essential fatty acids. Several days of adaptation may be required to attain maximal utilisation. Reactions include occasional febrile episodes (usually only with 20% emulsions) and rare anaphylactic responses. Interference with biochemical measurements such as those for blood gases and calcium may occur if samples are taken before fat has been cleared. Regular monitoring of plasma cholesterol and triglyceride is necessary to ensure clearance from the plasma, particularly in conditions where fat metabolism may be disturbed e.g. infection. Emulsions containing 20% or 30% fat should be used in neonates as they are cleared more efficiently. **Additives may only be mixed with fat emulsions where compatibility is known.**

Electrolytes are usually provided as the chloride salts of potassium and sodium. Acetate salts can be used to reduce the amount of chloride infused; hyperchloraemic acidosis or hypochloraemic alkalosis can occur in preterm neonates or children with renal impairment.

> **Administration**. Because of the complex requirements relating to parenteral nutrition full details relating to administration have been omitted. In all cases *specialist pharmacy advice, product literature and other specialist literature should be consulted.*

Supplementary preparations

> Compatibility with the infusion solution must be ascertained before adding supplementary preparations.

Addiphos® (Fresenius Kabi) PoM
Solution, sterile, phosphate 40 mmol, K^+ 30 mmol, Na^+ 30 mmol/20 mL. For addition to *Vamin®* solutions and glucose intravenous infusions. Net price 20-mL vial = £1.44

Additrace® (Fresenius Kabi) PoM
Solution, trace elements for addition to *Vamin®* solutions and glucose intravenous infusions, traces of Fe^{3+}, Zn^{2+}, Mn^{2+}, Cu^{2+}, Cr^{3+}, Se^{4+}, Mo^{6+}, F^-, I^-. For children over 40 kg. Net price 10-mL amp = £2.18

Cernevit® (Baxter) PoM
Solution, *dl*-alpha tocopherol 11.2 units, ascorbic acid 125 mg, biotin 69 micrograms, colecalciferol 220 units, cyanocobalamin 6 micrograms, folic acid 414 micrograms, glycine 250 mg, nicotinamide 46 mg, pantothenic acid (as dexpanthenol) 17.25 mg, pyridoxine hydrochloride 5.5 mg, retinol (as palmitate) 3500 units, riboflavin (as dihydrated sodium phosphate) 4.14 mg, thiamine (as cocarboxylase tetrahydrate) 3.51 mg. Dissolve in 5 mL water for injections. Net price per vial = £2.90

Decan® (Baxter) PoM
Solution, trace elements for addition to infusion solutions, Fe^{2+}, Zn^{2+}, Cu^{2+}, Mn^{2+}, F^-, Co^{2+} I^-, Se^{4+}, Mo^{6+}, Cr^{3+}. For children over 40 kg. Net price 40-mL vial = £2.00

Dipeptiven® (Fresenius Kabi) PoM
Solution, *N*(2)-L-alanyl-L-glutamine 200 mg/mL (providing L-alanine 82 mg, L-glutamine 134.6 mg). For addition to infusion solutions containing amino acids. Net price 50 mL = £15.90, 100 mL = £29.60

Dose

> **Amino acid supplement for hypercatabolic or hypermetabolic states**
> 300–400 mg/kg daily; max. 400 mg/kg daily, dose not to exceed 20% of total amino acid intake

Glycophos® Sterile Concentrate (Fresenius Kabi) PoM
Solution, sterile, phosphate 20 mmol, Na^+ 40 mmol/20 mL. For addition to *Vamin®* and *Vaminolact®* solutions, and glucose intravenous infusions. Net price 20-mL vial = £4.25

Peditrace® (Fresenius Kabi) PoM
Solution, trace elements for addition to *Vaminolact®*, *Vamin® 14 Electrolyte-Free* solutions and glucose intravenous infusions, traces of Zn^{2+}, Cu^{2+}, Mn^{2+}, Se^{4+}, F^-, I^-. For use in neonates (when kidney function established, usually second day of life), infants, and children. Net price 10-mL vial = £3.88

Cautions reduced biliary excretion especially in cholestatic liver disease or in markedly reduced urinary excretion (careful biochemical monitoring required); total parenteral nutrition exceeding 1 month (measure serum manganese concentration and check liver function before commencing treatment and regularly during treatment)—discontinue if manganese concentration raised or if cholestasis develops

Solivito N® (Fresenius Kabi) PoM
Solution, powder for reconstitution, biotin 60 micrograms, cyanocobalamin 5 micrograms, folic acid 400 micrograms, glycine 300 mg, nicotinamide 40 mg, pyridoxine hydrochloride 4.9 mg, riboflavin sodium phosphate 4.9 mg, sodium ascorbate 113 mg, sodium pantothenate 16.5 mg, thiamine mononitrate 3.1 mg. Dissolve in water for injections or glucose intravenous infusion for adding to glucose intravenous infusion or *Intralipid®*; dissolve in *Vitlipid N®* or *Intralipid®* for adding to *Intralipid®* only. Net price per vial = £2.19

Vitlipid N® (Fresenius Kabi) PoM
Emulsion, adult, vitamin A 330 units, ergocalciferol 20 units, *dl*-alpha tocopherol 1 unit, phytomenadione 15 micrograms/mL. For addition to *Intralipid®*. For adults and children over 11 years. Net price 10-mL amp = £2.19

Emulsion, infant, vitamin A 230 units, ergocalciferol 40 units, *dl*-alpha tocopherol 0.7 unit, phytomenadione 20 micrograms/mL. For addition to *Intralipid®*. Net price 10-mL amp = £2.19

9.4 Oral nutrition

9.4.1 Foods for special diets

These are preparations that have been modified to eliminate a particular constituent from a food or are nutrient mixtures formulated as substitutes for the food. They are for children who either cannot tolerate or cannot metabolise certain common constituents of food.

> **ACBS.** In certain clinical conditions some foods may have the characteristics of drugs and the Advisory Committee on Borderline Substances advises as to the circumstances in which such foods may be regarded as drugs and so can be prescribed in the NHS. Prescriptions for these foods issued in accordance with the advice of this committee and endorsed 'ACBS' will normally not be investigated. The preparations most commonly used in children are listed. See Appendix 2 for details of these foods and a listing by clinical condition (consult Drug Tariff for late amendments).

Coeliac disease Coeliac disease, which results from an intolerance to gluten, is managed by completely eliminating gluten from the diet.

Phenylketonuria Phenylketonuria (phenylalaninaemia, PKU), which results from the inability to metabolise phenylalanine, is managed by restricting its dietary intake to a small amount sufficient for tissue building and repair. Some forms of phenylketonuria are caused by a deficiency of tetrahydrobiopterin; treatment involves oral supplementation of tetrahydrobiopterin. In some severe cases, the addition of the neurotransmitter precursors levodopa (L-dopa, section 4.9.1) and 5-hydroxytryptophan is also necessary.

Aspartame (as a sweetener in some foods and medicines) contributes to the phenylalanine intake and may affect control of phenylketonuria. If alternatives are unavailable, children with phenylketonuria should not be denied access to appropriate medication; the amount of aspartame can be taken in to account in the management of the condition. Where the presence of aspartame is specified in the product literature this is indicated against the preparation.

TETRAHYDROBIOPTERIN

Cautions

Renal impairment use with caution—accumulation of metabolites

Pregnancy crosses the placenta; use only if benefit outweighs risk

Breast-feeding present in milk, effects unknown

Side-effects diarrhoea, urinary frequency, disturbed sleep

Licensed use not licensed in the UK

Indication and dose

Monotherapy in tetrahydrobiopterin-sensitive phenylketonuria

Child 1 month–18 years 10 mg/kg twice daily (total daily dose may alternatively be given in 3 divided doses), adjusted according to response

In combination with neurotransmitter precursors for tetrahydrobiopterin-sensitive phenylketonuria

Child 1 month–2 years initially 250–750 micrograms/kg 4 times daily (total daily dose may alternatively be given in 3 divided doses), adjusted according to response; max. 7 mg/kg daily

Child 2–18 years initially 250–750 micrograms/kg 4 times daily (total daily dose may alternatively be given in 3 divided doses), adjusted according to response; usual max. 10 mg/kg daily

Tetrahydrobiopterin (Non-proprietary)
Tablets, tetrahydrobiopterin 10 mg and 50 mg
Available from specialist importing companies

9.4.2 Enteral nutrition

Children have higher nutrient requirements per kg body-weight, different metabolic rates, and physiological responses compared to adults. They have low nutritional stores and are particularly vulnerable to growth and nutritional problems during critical periods of development. Major illness, operations, or trauma impose increased metabolic demands and can rapidly exhaust nutritional reserves.

Every effort should be made to optimise oral food intake before beginning enteral tube feeding; this may include change of posture, special seating, feeding equipment, oral desensitisation, food texture changes, thickening of liquids, increasing energy density of food, treatment of reflux or oesophagitis, as well as using age-specific nutritional supplements.

Enteral tube feeding has a role in both short-term rehabilitation and long-term nutritional management in paediatrics. It can be used as supportive therapy, in which the enteral feed supplies a proportion of the needed nutrients, or as primary therapy, in which the enteral feed delivers all the necessary nutrients. Most children receiving tube feeds should be encouraged to take oral food and drink. Tube feeding should be considered in the following situations:

- unsafe swallowing and aspiration;
- inability to consume at least 60% of energy needs by mouth;
- total feeding time of more than 4 hours per day;
- weight loss or no weight gain for a period of 3 months (less for younger children and infants);
- weight for height (or length) less than 2nd percentile for age and sex.

There are a number of nutritionally complete foods available and their use reduces an otherwise heavy workload in hospital or in the home. Most contain protein derived from milk or soya. Some contain protein hydrolysates or free amino acids and are only appropriate for patients who have diminished ability to break down protein, as may be the case in inflammatory bowel disease or pancreatic insufficiency.

Even when nutritionally complete feeds are being given it may be important to monitor water and electrolyte balance. Extra minerals (e.g. magnesium and zinc) may be needed in patients where gastro-intestinal secretions are being lost. Additional vitamins may also be needed. Regular haematological and biochemical tests may be needed particularly in the unstable child.

Choosing the best formula for children depends on several factors including: nutritional requirements, gastro-intestinal function, underlying disease, nutrient restrictions, age, and feed characteristics (nutritional composition, viscosity, osmolality, availability and cost). Children have special requirements and in many situations liquid feeds prepared for adults are totally unsuitable and should not be given. Expert advice from a dietician should be sought.

Some feeds are supplemented with vitamin K; for drug interactions of vitamin K see **interactions:** Appendix 1 (vitamins).

Complete enteral feeds **Child 0–12 months**. Term infants with normal gastro-intestinal function are given either breast milk or normal infant formula during the first year of life. The average intake is between 150 mL and 200 mL/kg/day. Infant milk formulas are based on whey or casein dominant protein, lactose with or without maltodextrin, amylose, vegetable oil and milk fat. The composition of all normal and soya infant formulas have to meet The Infant Formula and Follow-on Formula Regulations 1995, which enact the European Community Regulations 91/321/EC; the composition of other enteral and specialist feeds has to meet the Commission Directive (1999/21/EC) on Dietary Foods for Special Medical Purposes.

An infant who is inadequately growing, may be given a high-energy feed, which contains 9–11% of energy derived from protein. Alternatively, energy supplements may be added to normal infant formula to achieve a higher energy content (but this will reduce the protein to energy ratio) or the normal infant formula concentration may be slightly increased from the norm of around 13% up to 17%. Care should be taken not to present an osmotic load of more than 500 milliosmols/kg water to the normal functioning gut, otherwise osmotic diarrhoea will result. Concentrating or supplementing feeds should not be attempted without the advice of a paediatric dietician.

Child 1–6 years (8–20 kg). Nutritionally complete, ready-to-use feeds containing 0.75 kcal/mL, 1.0 kcal/mL and 1.5 kcal/mL are available based on caseinates, maltodextrin and vegetable oils (with or without added medium chain triglyceride (MCT) oil or fibre); they contain residual lactose. They are well tolerated and effective in improving nutritional status in this age group. They are administered at a rate of 85–110 mL/kg/day depending on age, weight, condition and nutritional requirements. Although originally designed for 1–6 year old (8–20 kg) children, some products have had ACBS extensions for children weighing up to 30 kg (approx. 10 years of age). Enteral feeds formulated for younger children are low in sodium and potassium; electrolyte intake and biochemical status should be monitored. Intake of micronutrients may also be low in older children taking small feed volumes. The fibre content of 1.0 kcal/mL feeds varies between 0.5 g–0.75g/100 kcal. There is little data on their efficacy but fibre-enriched feeds may be helpful for children with chronic constipation or diarrhoea.

Child 7–12 years. Nutritionally complete 1.0 kcal/mL and 1.5 kcal/mL ready-to-use feeds formulated for 7–12 year olds are available. They are also based on caseinates, maltodextrin and vegetable oils (with or without fibre) and contain residual lactose only. Depending on age, weight, clinical condition and nutritional requirements they may be given at a rate of 50–70 mL/kg/day.

Child 13 years and over. As there are no standard enteral feeds formulated for this age group, 1.0 kcal/mL and 1.5 kcal/mL adult formulations are used. The intake of protein, electrolytes, vitamins, and trace minerals should be carefully assessed and monitored.

Note Adult feeds containing more than 6.0 g/100 mL protein or 2 g/100 mL fibre should be used with caution and expert advice.

Specialised formula It is essential that any infant or child who is intolerant of breast milk or normal infant formula, or whose condition requires nutrient-specific adaptation, is prescribed a nutritionally complete replacement formula in adequate volume. In the first 4 months of life, a volume of 150–200 mL/kg/day is recommended. After 6 months, should the formula still be required, a volume of 600 mL/day should be maintained, in addition to solids.

Products for cow's milk protein intolerance or lactose intolerance. There are a number of infant formulas formulated for cow's milk protein intolerance or lactose intolerance. If the intake of these formulas is low, it may be necessary to supplement with calcium, and a vitamin and mineral supplement.

Soya-based infant formula has a high phytoestrogen content and this may be a long-term reproductive health risk. The Chief Medical Officer has advised that soya-based infant formulas should not be used as the first choice for the management of infants with proven cow's milk sensitivity, lactose intolerance, galactokinase deficiency and galactosaemia. Most UK paediatricians with expertise in inherited metabolic disease still advocate soya-based formulations for infants with galactosaemia as there are concerns about the residual lactose content of low lactose formulas and protein hydrolysates based on cow's milk protein.

Low lactose formulations, based on whole cow's milk protein, are unsuitable for infants with cow's milk protein intolerance. Liquid soya milks purchased from supermarkets and health food stores are not nutritionally complete and should never be used for infants under 1 year of age.

Protein hydrolysate formulas. These formulas, based on casein, whey, meat and soya, are suitable for infants with disaccharide or whole protein intolerance. Some of the formulations contain a significant proportion of their fat source in the form of medium chain triglyceride (MCT) oil and are prescribable for indications where amino acids or peptides are necessary in conjunction with MCT oil. There is only one peptide-based feed for children over 1 year of age (*Pepdite 1+*®). All the other peptide-based formulas are formulated for adults and when used for children the intake of electrolytes, vitamins and minerals should be carefully assessed and modified to meet the child's nutritional requirements; they have a high osmolality when given at recommended dilution and need gradual and careful introduction.

Elemental (amino acid based formula). *Neocate*® is the only nutritionally complete elemental formula for infants. There is some evidence to demonstrate that growth while on this formula is satisfactory. *Neocate*® *Advance* is the only elemental formula based on L-amino acids specifically produced for young children. Adult elemental formula may be used for children over 6 years; the intake of electrolytes, vitamins and minerals should be carefully assessed and modified to meet the nutritional requirements of children. They have a high osmolality when given at recommended dilution and need gradual and careful introduction.

Modular feeds. Modular feeds are based on individual protein, fat, carbohydrate, vitamin and mineral components or modules which can be combined to meet the specific needs of a child. Modular feeds are used when nutritionally complete specialised formula are not tolerated, or if the fluid and nutrient requirements change e.g. in gastro-intestinal, renal or liver disease. The main advantage of modular feeds is their flexibility; disadvantages include their complexity and preparation difficulties. Modular feeds should not be used without the supervision of a paediatric dietician.

Miscellaneous formula. A number of highly specialised formulas are available where nutrients have been modified to meet the specific requirements in various clinical conditions such as renal and liver diseases. When using these formulas, monitoring of growth and biochemistry should be undertaken at regular intervals.

Feed thickeners **Carob based thickeners** may be used to thicken feeds for infants under 1 year. Breast-fed infants can be given the thickener mixed to a paste prior to feeds.

Starched based thickeners can be used to thicken liquids and feeds for children over 1 year of age.

Pre-thickened formula is a casein-based infant formula, which contains small quantities of pre-gelatinized starch and is recommended primarily for infants with mild gastro-oesophageal reflux. Pre-thickened formula is prepared in the same way as normal infant formula and flows through a standard teat. The feeds do not thicken on standing but thicken in the stomach when exposed to acid pH.

Dietary supplements for oral use Three types of prescribable fortified dietary supplements are available: fortified milk shakes providing 1.0–1.5 kcal/mL, fortified non-milk tasting supplements and fortified desserts. The daily quantity recommended is age-dependent and the following is a useful guide: 1–2 years, 200 kcal (840 kJ); 3–5 years, 400 kcal (1680 kJ); 6–11 years, 600 kcal (2520 kJ); and over 12 years, 800 kcal (3360 kJ). Adult supplements containing 1.5 kcal/mL are high in protein and should not be used for children under 3 years of age. Many supplements are high in sugar or maltodextrin; care should be taken to prevent prolonged contact with teeth. Ideally supplements should be administered after meals or at bedtime so as not to affect appetite.

Other dietary supplements A number of dietary supplements based on carbohydrates, fat or protein are available to enhance the nutrient density of feeds and diet, or are used as the components of modular feeds. Details are shown in Appendix 2. Careful attention to dental hygiene is necessary in children receiving carbohydrate-based supplements.

Products for metabolic disease There is a large range of disease-specific infant formulas and amino acid supplements for metabolic diseases; some are nutritionally incomplete and supplementation with vitamins and other nutrients may be necessary. Many of the product names are similar and to prevent metabolic complications it is important the correct supplement is supplied.

Preparations
See Appendix 2

9.5 Minerals

See section 9.1.1 for iron salts.

9.5.1 Calcium and magnesium

9.5.1.1 Calcium supplements

Calcium supplements are usually only required where dietary calcium intake is deficient. This dietary requirement varies with age and is relatively greater in childhood, pregnancy, and lactation, due to an increased demand.

Hypocalcaemia may be caused by vitamin D deficiency (section 9.6.4), impaired metabolism, a failure of secretion (hypoparathyroidism), or resistance to parathyroid hormone (pseudohypoparathyroidism).

Mild asymptomatic hypocalcaemia may be managed with oral calcium supplements. Severe symptomatic hypocalcaemia requires an intravenous infusion of calcium gluconate 10% over 5 to 10 minutes, repeating the dose if symptoms persist; in exceptional cases it may be necessary to maintain a continuous calcium infusion over a day or more. Intravenous calcium gluconate can also be used immediately to temporarily reduce the toxic effects of *hyperkalaemia*.

Persistent hypocalcaemia requires oral calcium supplements and either a vitamin D analogue (alfacalcidol or calcitriol) for hypoparathyroidism and pseudohypoparathyroidism or natural vitamin D (calciferol) if due to vitamin D deficiency (section 9.6.4). It is important to monitor plasma and urinary calcium during long-term maintenance therapy.

Neonates Hypocalcaemia is common in the first few days of life, particularly following birth asphyxia or respiratory distress. Late onset at 4–10 days after birth may be secondary to vitamin D deficiency, hypoparathyroidism or hypomagnesaemia and may be associated with seizures.

CALCIUM SALTS

Cautions sarcoidosis; history of nephrolithiasis; avoid calcium chloride in respiratory acidosis or respiratory failure; **interactions**: Appendix 1 (antacids, calcium salts)

Renal impairment use with caution, risk of hypercalcaemia and renal calculi

Contra-indications conditions associated with hypercalcaemia and hypercalciuria (e.g. some forms of malignant disease)

Side-effects gastro-intestinal disturbances, constipation; bradycardia, arrhythmias; with injection, peripheral vasodilatation, fall in blood pressure, injection-site reactions, severe tissue damage with extravasation

Indication and dose

See notes above; calcium deficiency
- **By mouth**

Neonate 0.25 mmol/kg 4 times a day, adjusted to response

Child 1 month–4 years 0.25 mmol/kg 4 times a day, adjusted to response

Child 5–12 years 0.2 mmol/kg 4 times a day, adjusted to response

Child 12–18 years 10 mmol 4 times a day, adjusted to response

Acute hypocalcaemia, urgent correction; hyperkalaemia (prevention of arrhythmias)
- **By slow intravenous injection over 5–10 minutes**

Neonate 0.11 mmol/kg (0.5 mL/kg of calcium gluconate 10%) as a single dose. [Some units use a dose of 0.46 mmol/kg (2 mL/kg calcium gluconate 10%) for hypocalcaemia in line with US practice]

Child 1 month–18 years 0.11 mmol/kg (0.5 mL/kg calcium gluconate 10%), max 4.5 mmol (20 mL calcium gluconate 10%)

CALCIUM SALTS (*continued*)

Acute hypocalcaemia, maintenance
- **By continuous intravenous infusion**

Neonate 0.5 mmol/kg daily over 24 hours, adjusted to response, use oral route as soon as possible due to risk of extravasation

Child 1 month–2 years 1 mmol/kg daily (usual max 8.8 mmol) over 24 hours, use oral route as soon as possible due to risk of extravasation

Child 2–18 years 8.8 mmol over 24 hours, use oral route as soon as possible due to risk of extravasation

Oral preparations

Calcium Gluconate (Non-proprietary)
Tablets, calcium gluconate 600 mg (calcium 53.4 mg or Ca^{2+} 1.35 mmol), net price 20 = £1.43. Label: 24

Effervescent tablets, calcium gluconate 1 g (calcium 89 mg or Ca^{2+} 2.25 mmol), net price 28-tab pack = £4.62. Label: 13
Note Each tablet usually contains 4.46 mmol Na^+

Calcium Lactate (Non-proprietary)
Tablets, calcium lactate 300 mg (calcium 39 mg or Ca^{2+} 1 mmol), net price 20 = 72p

Adcal® (Strakan)
Chewable tablets, calcium carbonate 1.5 g (calcium 600 mg or Ca^{2+} 15 mmol), net price 100-tab pack = £7.25. Label: 24

Cacit® (Procter & Gamble Pharm.)
Tablets, effervescent, pink, calcium carbonate 1.25 g, providing calcium citrate when dispersed in water (calcium 500 mg or Ca^{2+} 12.6 mmol), net price 76-tab pack = £16.72. Label: 13

Calcichew® (Shire)
Tablets (chewable), gluten-free, calcium carbonate 1.25 g (calcium 500 mg or Ca^{2+} 12.6 mmol), net price 100-tab pack = £9.33

Forte tablets (chewable), scored, gluten-free, calcium carbonate 2.5 g (calcium 1 g or Ca^{2+} 25 mmol), net price 60-tab pack = £13.16. Label: 24
Excipients: include aspartame (section 9.4.1)

Calcium-500 (Martindale)
Tablets, pink, f/c, calcium carbonate 1.25 g (calcium 500 mg or Ca^{2+} 12.5 mmol). Net price 100-tab pack = £9.46. Label: 25

Calcium-Sandoz® (Alliance)
Syrup, calcium glubionate 1.09 g, calcium lactobionate 727 mg (calcium 108.3 mg or Ca^{2+} 2.7 mmol)/5 mL. Net price 300 mL = £3.39
Note Avoid in galactosaemia

Sandocal® (Novartis Consumer Health)
Sandocal-400 tablets, effervescent, calcium lactate gluconate 930 mg, calcium carbonate 700 mg, anhydrous citric acid 1.189 g, providing calcium 400 mg (Ca^{2+} 10 mmol). Net price 5 × 20-tab pack = £6.87. Label: 13
Excipients: include aspartame (section 9.4.1)

Sandocal-1000 tablets, effervescent, calcium lactate gluconate 2.327 g, calcium carbonate 1.75 g, anhydrous citric acid 2.973 g providing 1 g calcium (Ca^{2+} 25 mmol). Net price 3 × 10-tab pack = £6.17. Label: 13
Excipients: include aspartame (section 9.4.1)

Parenteral preparations

Calcium Gluconate (Non-proprietary) PoM
Injection, calcium gluconate 10% (calcium 8.9 mg or Ca^{2+} 220 micromol)/mL. Net price 10-mL amp = 60p
Administration For *intravenous infusion* dilute to at least 0.045 mmol/mL with glucose 5% or 10% or sodium chloride 0.9%. Maximum administration rate 0.045 mmol/kg/hour (or in neonates max. 0.02 mmol/minute). May be given more concentrated via a central venous line. May be used undiluted (10% calcium gluconate) in emergencies. Avoid extravasation; should not be given by intramuscular injection. Incompatible with sodium bicarbonate and phosphate solutions.

Calcium Chloride (Non-proprietary) PoM
Injection, calcium chloride (as calcium chloride dihydrate 10% 27.3 mg or Ca^{2+} 680 micromol/mL). Net price 10-mL disposable syringe = £4.42
Brands include *Minijet® Calcium Chloride 10%*

Injection, calcium chloride (as calcium chloride dihydrate 13.4%) 100 mg/mL (calcium 36 mg or Ca^{2+} 910 micromol/mL). Net price 10–mL amp = £14.94

With vitamin D

Section 9.6.4

9.5.1.2 Hypercalcaemia and hypercalciuria

Severe hypercalcaemia Severe hypercalcaemia calls for urgent treatment before detailed investigation of the cause. Dehydration should be corrected first with intravenous infusion of **sodium chloride 0.9%**. Drugs (such as thiazides and vitamin D compounds) which promote hypercalcaemia, should be discontinued and dietary calcium should be restricted.

If *severe hypercalcaemia persists* drugs which inhibit mobilisation of calcium from the skeleton may be required. The **bisphosphonates** are useful and disodium pamidronate (section 6.6.2) is probably the most effective.

Corticosteroids (section 6.3) are widely given, but may only be useful where hypercalcaemia is due to sarcoidosis or vitamin D intoxication; they often take several days to achieve the desired effect.

Calcitonin (section 6.6.1) is relatively non-toxic but is expensive and its effect can wear off after a few days despite continued use; it is rarely effective where bisphosphonates have failed to reduce serum calcium adequately.

After treatment of severe hypercalcaemia the underlying cause must be established. *Further treatment* is governed by the same principles as for initial therapy. Salt and water depletion and drugs promoting hypercalcaemia should be avoided; oral administration of a bisphosphonate may be useful. Parathyroidectomy may be indicated for hyperparathyroidism.

Hypercalciuria Hypercalciuria should be investigated for an underlying cause, which should be treated. Reducing dietary calcium intake may be beneficial but severe restriction of calcium intake has not proved beneficial and may even be harmful.

9.5.1.3 Magnesium

Magnesium is an essential constituent of many enzyme systems, particularly those involved in energy generation; the largest stores are in the skeleton.

Magnesium salts are not well absorbed from the gastro-intestinal tract, which explains the use of magnesium sulphate (section 1.6.4) as an osmotic laxative.

Magnesium is excreted mainly by the kidneys and is therefore retained in renal failure, but significant *hypermagnesaemia* (causing muscle weakness and arrhythmias) is rare.

Hypomagnesaemia Since magnesium is secreted in large amounts in the gastro-intestinal fluid, excessive losses in diarrhoea, stoma or fistula are the most common causes of *hypomagnesaemia*; deficiency may also occur as a result of treatment with certain drugs. Hypomagnesaemia often causes secondary hypocalcaemia (with which it may be confused), particularly in neonates, and also hypokalaemia and hyponatraemia.

Symptomatic *hypomagnesaemia* is associated with a deficit of 0.5–1 mmol/kg. Magnesium is given initially by intravenous infusion or by intramuscular injection of **magnesium sulphate**; the intramuscular injection is painful. Plasma magnesium concentration should be measured to determine the rate and duration of infusion and the dose should be reduced in renal impairment. To prevent *recurrence of the deficit*, magnesium may be given by mouth in divided doses. For maintenance (e.g. in intravenous nutrition), parenteral doses of magnesium are of the order of 0.2–0.4 mmol/kg (usual max. 20 mmol) Mg^{2+} daily.

Arrhythmias Magnesium sulphate has also been recommended for the emergency treatment of *serious arrhythmias*, especially in the presence of hypokalaemia (when hypomagnesaemia may also be present) and when salvos of rapid ventricular tachycardia show the characteristic twisting wave front known as *torsades de pointes* (see also section 2.3.1).

9 Nutrition and blood

MAGNESIUM SULPHATE

Cautions see notes above; in severe hypomagnesaemia administer initially via controlled infusion device (preferably syringe pump); monitor blood pressure, respiratory rate, urinary output and for signs of overdosage (loss of patellar reflexes, weakness, nausea, sensation of warmth, flushing, drowsiness, double vision, and slurred speech); **interactions**: Appendix 1 (magnesium, parenteral)

Renal impairment avoid or reduce dose in moderate renal impairment; risk of toxicity

Pregnancy sufficient may cross the placenta in mothers treated with high doses e.g. in pre-eclampsia, causing hypotonia and respiratory depression in newborns

Breast-feeding present in breast milk; may cause diarrhoea in breast-fed babies

Side-effects generally associated with hypermagnesaemia, nausea, vomiting, thirst, flushing of skin, hypotension, arrhythmias, coma, respiratory depression, drowsiness, confusion, loss of tendon reflexes, muscle weakness

Licensed use 20% injection licensed for use in children. Other strengths unlicensed

Indication and dose

(See also notes above)

Neonatal hypocalcaemia
- **By deep intramuscular injection or intravenous infusion**

Neonate 0.4 mmol/kg Mg^{2+} (100 mg/kg magnesium sulphate) 12 hourly for 2–3 doses

MAGNESIUM SULPHATE (*continued*)

Hypomagnesaemia
- **By intravenous injection over at least 10 minutes**

Neonate 0.4 mmol/kg Mg^{2+} (100 mg/kg magnesium sulphate) 6–12 hourly as necessary

Child 1 month–12 years 0.2 mmol/kg Mg^{2+} (50 mg/kg magnesium sulphate) 12 hourly as necessary

Child 12–18 years 4 mmol Mg^{2+} (1 g magnesium sulphate) 12 hourly as necessary

Acute severe asthma section 3.1

Persistent pulmonary hypertension section 2.5.1

Torsades de pointes (consult local guidelines)
- **By intravenous injection over 10–15 minutes**

Child 1 month–18 years 0.1–0.2 mmol/kg (25–50 mg/kg magnesium sulphate); max. 8 mmol (2 g magnesium sulphate); dose repeated once if necessary

Administration Dilute to 10% (100 mg in 1 mL) with Glucose 5 *or* 10%, Sodium Chloride 0.45 *or* 0.9% *or* Glucose and Sodium Chloride combinations. Up to 20% solution may be given in fluid restriction. Rate of administration should not exceed 10 mg/kg/minute of magnesium sulphate

Note Magnesium sulphate 1 g equivalent to Mg^{2+} approx. 4 mmol

Magnesium Sulphate (Non-proprietary) PoM
Injection, magnesium sulphate 20% (Mg^{2+} approx. 0.8 mmol/mL), net price 20-mL (4-g) amp = £2.75; 50% (Mg^{2+} approx. 2 mmol/mL), 2-mL (1-g) amp = £2.59, 4-mL (2-g) prefilled syringe = £6.50; 5-mL (2.5-g) amp = £2.50, 10-mL (5-g) amp = £3.35; 10-mL (5-g) prefilled syringe = £4.95
Brands include *Min-I-Jet® Magnesium Sulphate 50%*

MAGNESIUM-L-ASPARTATE

Cautions see under Magnesium Sulphate

Renal impairment use with caution; avoid in severe impairment

Side-effects diarrhoea; see also under Magnesium Sulphate

Licensed use classified as a Food for Special Medical Purposes for use in children over 2 years

Indication and dose

Hypomagnesaemia
- **By mouth**

Child 1 month–2 years initially 0.2 mmol/kg of Mg^{2+} 3 times daily dissolved in water, dose adjusted as required

Child 2–10 years half a sachet (5 mmol Mg^{2+}) daily dissolved in 100 mL of water, dose adjusted as required

Child 10–18 years one sachet (10 mmol Mg^{2+}) daily dissolved in 200 mL of water, dose adjusted as required

Magnaspartate® (KoRa)
Oral powder, magnesium-L-aspartate 6.5 g (10 mmol Mg^{2+})/sachet
Excipients: include sucrose

MAGNESIUM GLYCEROPHOSPHATE

Cautions see under Magnesium Sulphate

Renal impairment use with caution; avoid in severe impairment

Side-effects diarrhoea; see also under Magnesium Sulphate

Licensed use unlicensed preparation

Indication and dose

Hypomagnesaemia
- **By mouth**

Child 1 month–12 years initially 0.2 mmol/kg Mg^{2+} 3 times daily, dose adjusted as required

Child 12–18 years initially 4–8 mmol Mg^{2+} 3 times daily, dose adjusted as required

Administration tablets may be dispersed in water

Magnesium Glycerophosphate (Non-proprietary)
Tablets, magnesium glycerophosphate 97 mg (4 mmol Mg^{2+})
Available as a manufactured special from specialist importing company

Extemporaneous formulations available see Extemporaneous Preparations, p. 8

9.5.2 Phosphorus

9.5.2.1 Phosphate supplements

Oral phosphate supplements may be required in addition to vitamin D in children with hypophosphataemic vitamin D-resistant rickets (section 9.6.4). Diarrhoea is a common side-effect and should prompt a reduction in dosage.

Phosphate infusion is occasionally needed in phosphate deficiency arising from use of parenteral nutrition deficient in phosphate supplements; phosphate depletion also occurs in severe diabetic ketoacidosis. It is difficult to provide detailed guidelines for the treatment of *severe hypophosphatemia* because the extent of total body deficits and response to therapy are difficult to predict. High doses of phosphate may result in a transient serum elevation followed by redistribution into intracellular compartments or bone tissue; excessive doses may cause hypocalcaemia and metastatic calcification. It is essential to monitor plasma concentrations of calcium, phosphate, potassium and other electrolytes. It is recommended that severe hypophosphataemia be treated intravenously as large doses of oral phosphate may cause diarrhoea; intestinal absorption may be unreliable and dose adjustment may be necessary.

Phosphate is not the first choice for the treatment of hypercalcaemia because of the risk of precipitation of calcium phosphate in the kidney and other tissues. If used, the child should be well hydrated and electrolytes monitored.

Neonates Phosphate deficiency may occur in very low-birthweight infants and may compromise bone growth if not corrected. Parenterally fed infants may be at risk of phosphate deficiency due to the limited solubility of phosphate. Some units routinely supplement expressed breast milk with phosphate, although the effect on the osmolality of the milk should be considered.

9 Nutrition and blood

PHOSPHATE

Cautions see notes above, also cardiac disease, diabetes mellitus, dehydration; avoid extravasation with parenteral forms, severe tissue necrosis; sodium and potassium concentrations of preparations

Renal impairment reduce dose in renal impairment, monitor closely

Contra-indications hyperphosphataemia

Side-effects nausea, diarrhoea; hypotension, oedema; hypocalcaemia; acute renal failure; phlebitis; tissue necrosis on extravasation

Indication and dose

Hypophosphataemia, including hypophosphataemic rickets and osteomalacia (see notes above)

- **By mouth**

Neonate 1 mmol/kg daily in 1–2 divided doses, or as a supplement in breast milk

Child 1 month–18 years 2–3 mmol/kg (max. 97 mmol) phosphate daily in 2–4 divided doses, adjusted as necessary

Administration Caution, solubility in breast milk is limited to 1.2 mmol in 100 mL if calcium also added, contact pharmacy department for details

- **By intravenous infusion (see administration below)**

Neonate 1 mmol/kg phosphate daily, adjusted as necessary

Child 1 month–2 years 0.7 mmol/kg phosphate daily, adjusted as necessary

Child 2–18 years 0.4 mmol/kg phosphate daily, adjusted as necessary

Administration Dilute injection to 0.1 mmol phosphate in 1 mL with sodium chloride 0.9%/0.45% or glucose 5%/10%. Administration rate should not exceed 0.05 mmol/kg/hour. In emergencies in intensive care may increase rate to 0.5 mmol/kg/hour via central line only

Oral

Phosphate-Sandoz® (HK Pharma)

Tablets, effervescent, anhydrous sodium acid phosphate 1.936 g, sodium bicarbonate 350 mg, potassium bicarbonate 315 mg, equivalent to phosphorus 500 mg (phosphate 16.1 mmol), sodium 468.8 mg (Na^+ 20.4 mmol), potassium 123 mg (K^+ 3.1 mmol). Net price 20 = £3.29. Label: 13

Extemporaneous formulations available see Extemporaneous Preparations, p. 8

Various strengths and salts available, caution electrolyte load

Injection

Phosphates (Fresenius Kabi) PoM

Intravenous infusion, phosphates (providing PO_4^{3-} 100 mmol/litre), net price 500 mL (*Polyfusor®*) = £3.75.

Potassium acid phosphate (Non-proprietary) PoM

Injection, 13.6% (1 mmol/mL phosphate, 1 mmol/mL potassium) 10 mL ampoule

PHOSPHATE (*continued*)

Dipotassium hydrogen phosphate (Non-proprietary) PoM

Injection, 17.42% (1 mmol/mL phosphate and 2 mmol/mL potassium) 10 mL ampoule

Disodium hydrogen phosphate (Non-proprietary) PoM

Injection, 17.42% (0.6 mmol/mL phosphate and 1.2 mmol/mL sodium) 10 mL ampoule

9.5.2.2 Phosphate-binding agents

Aluminium-containing and calcium-containing preparations are used as phosphate-binding agents in the management of hyperphosphataemia complicating renal failure. Calcium-containing phosphate-binding agents are preferred in children but are contra-indicated in hypercalcaemia or hypercalciuria. Phosphate-binding agents which contain aluminium may increase plasma aluminium in dialysis patients.

Sevelamer is licensed for the treatment of hyperphosphataemia in adults on haemodialysis. Although experience is limited in children sevelamer may be useful when hypercalcaemia prevents the use of calcium carbonate.

ALUMINIUM HYDROXIDE

Cautions hyperaluminaemia; porphyria (section 9.8.2); see also notes above; **interactions:** Appendix 1 (antacids)

Side-effects see section 1.1.1

Dose

Hyperphosphataemia
- By mouth

Child 5–12 years 1–2 capsules 3–4 times daily, adjusted as necessary

Child 12–18 years 1–5 capsules 3–4 times daily, adjusted as necessary

Alu-Cap® (3M)

Capsules, green/red, dried aluminium hydroxide 475 mg (low Na^+). Net price 120-cap pack = £3.75

CALCIUM SALTS

Cautions see notes above; **interactions:** Appendix 1 (antacids, calcium salts)

Side-effects hypercalcaemia

Indication and dose

Phosphate binding in renal failure and hyperphosphataemia (see notes above)
- By mouth

Child 1 month–1 year 120 mg calcium carbonate 3–4 times daily with feeds, adjusted as necessary

Child 1–6 years 300 mg calcium carbonate 3–4 times daily prior to or with meals, adjusted as necessary

Child 6–12 years 600 mg calcium carbonate 3–4 times daily prior to or with meals, adjusted as necessary

Child 12–18 years 1.25 g calcium carbonate 3–4 times daily prior to or with meals, adjusted as necessary

Adcal®

Section 9.5.1.1

Calcichew®

Section 9.5.1.1

Calcium-500

Section 9.5.1.1

Phosex® (Vitaline)

Tablets, yellow, calcium acetate 1 g (calcium 250 mg or Ca^{2+} 6.2 mmol), net price 180-tab pack = £19.79. Label: 25

Dose

Phosphate-binding agent (with meals) in renal failure, according to the requirements of the patient

Extemporaneous formulations available see Extemporaneous Preparations, p. 8

SEVELAMER

Cautions gastro-intestinal disorders

Pregnancy manufacturer advises use only if potential benefit outweighs risk

Breast-feeding manufacturer advises use only if potential benefit outweighs risk

Contra-indications bowel obstruction

Licensed use not licensed for use in children

Indication and dose

Hyperphosphataemia in patients on haemodialysis (limited information in children)
- By mouth

Child 12–18 years initially 0.8–1.6 g 3 times daily with meals, then adjusted according to plasma-phosphate concentration

Renagel® (Genzyme) PoM

Tablets, f/c, sevelamer 800 mg, net price 180-tab pack = £122.76. Label: 25, with meals

9.5.3 Fluoride

Availability of adequate fluoride confers significant resistance to dental caries. It is now considered that the topical action of fluoride on enamel and plaque is more important than the systemic effect.

Where the fluoride content of the drinking water is less than 700 micrograms per litre (0.7 parts per million), daily administration of fluoride tablets or drops is a suitable means of supplementation. Systemic fluoride supplements should not be prescribed without reference to the fluoride content of the local water supply. Infants need not receive fluoride supplements until the age of 6 months.

Dentifrices which incorporate sodium fluoride or monofluorophosphate are also a convenient source of fluoride.

Individuals who are either particularly caries prone or medically compromised may be given additional protection by use of fluoride rinses or by application of fluoride gels. Rinses may be used daily or weekly; daily use of a less concentrated rinse is more effective than weekly use of a more concentrated one. High-strength gels must be applied on a regular basis under professional supervision; extreme caution is necessary to prevent the child from swallowing any excess. Less concentrated gels are available for home use. Varnishes are also available and are particularly valuable for young or disabled children since they adhere to the teeth and set in the presence of moisture.

Fluoride mouthwash, oral drops, tablets, and toothpaste are prescribable on form FP10D (GP14 in Scotland, WP10D in Wales; for details see preparations below).

There are also arrangements for health authorities to supply fluoride tablets in the course of pre-school dental schemes, and they may also be supplied in school dental schemes.

Fluoride gels are not prescribable on form FP10D (GP14 in Scotland, WP10D in Wales).

FLUORIDES

Note Sodium fluoride 2.2 mg provides approx. 1 mg fluoride ion

Contra-indications not for areas where drinking water is fluoridated

Side-effects occasional white flecks on teeth with recommended doses; rarely yellowish-brown discoloration if recommended doses are exceeded

Indication and dose

Prophylaxis of dental caries—see notes above

Note Dose expressed as fluoride ion (F^-):

Water content less than F^- 300 micrograms/litre (0.3 parts per million)

- **By mouth**

Child 6 months–3 years F^- 250 micrograms daily

Child 3–6 years F^- 500 micrograms daily

Child 6 years and over F^- 1 mg daily

Water content between F^- 300 and 700 micrograms/litre (0.3–0.7 parts per million)

Child 3–6 years F^- 250 micrograms daily

Child 6 years and over F^- 500 micrograms daily

Water content above F^- 700 micrograms/litre (0.7 parts per million), supplements not advised

Note These doses reflect the recommendations of the British Dental Association, the British Society of Paediatric Dentistry and the British Association for the Study of Community Dentistry (*Br Dent J* 1997; **182**: 6–7)

Tablets

Counselling Tablets should be sucked or dissolved in the mouth and taken preferably in the evening

There are arrangements for health authorities to supply fluoride tablets in the course of pre-school dental schemes, and they may also be supplied in school dental schemes.

En-De-Kay® (Manx)

Fluotabs 3–6 years, orange-flavoured, scored, sodium fluoride 1.1 mg (F^- 500 micrograms). Net price 200-tab pack = £1.80

Fluotabs 6+ years, orange-flavoured, scored, sodium fluoride 2.2 mg (F^- 1 mg). Net price 200-tab pack = £1.80

Dental prescribing on NHS May be prescribed as Sodium Fluoride Tablets

Fluor-a-day® (Dental Health)

Tablets, buff, sodium fluoride 1.1 mg (F^- 500 micrograms), net price 200-tab pack = £1.91; 2.2 mg (F^- 1 mg), 200-tab pack = £1.91

Dental prescribing on NHS May be prescribed as Sodium Fluoride Tablets

FluoriGard® (Colgate-Palmolive)

Tablets 0.5, purple, grape-flavoured, scored, sodium fluoride 1.1 mg (F^- 500 micrograms). Net price 200-tab pack = £1.91

Tablets 1.0, orange, orange-flavoured, scored, sodium fluoride 2.2 mg (F^- 1 mg). Net price 200-tab pack = £1.91

Dental prescribing on NHS May be prescribed as Sodium Fluoride Tablets

FLUORIDES (*continued*)

Oral drops

Note Fluoride supplements not considered necessary below 6 months of age (see notes above)

En-De-Kay® (Manx)

Fluodrops® (= paediatric drops), sugar-free, sodium fluoride 550 micrograms (F^- 250 micrograms)/0.15 mL. Net price 60 mL = £1.82

Dental prescribing on NHS Corresponds to Sodium Fluoride Oral Drops DPF 0.37% equivalent to sodium fluoride 80 micrograms (F^- 36 micrograms)/drop

Mouthwashes

Rinse mouth for 1 minute and spit out

Counselling Avoid eating, drinking, or rinsing mouth for 15 minutes after use

Duraphat® (Colgate-Palmolive)

Weekly dental rinse (= mouthwash), blue, sodium fluoride 0.2%. Net price 150 mL = £2.42. Counselling, see above

Dose

Child 6 years and over for *weekly* use, rinse with 10 mL

Dental prescribing on NHS May be prescribed as Sodium Fluoride Mouthwash 0.2%

En-De-Kay® (Manx)

Daily fluoride mouthrinse (= mouthwash), blue, sodium fluoride 0.05%. Net price 250 mL = £1.51

Dose

Child 6 years and over for *daily* use, rinse with 10 mL

Dental prescribing on NHS May be prescribed as Sodium Fluoride Mouthwash 0.05%

Fluorinse PoM (= mouthwash), red, sodium fluoride 2%. Net price 100 mL = £3.97. Counselling, see above

Dose

Child 8 years and over for *daily* use, dilute 5 drops to 10 mL of water; for *weekly* use, dilute 20 drops to 10 mL

Dental prescribing on NHS May be prescribed as Sodium Fluoride Mouthwash 2%

FluoriGard® (Colgate-Palmolive)

Daily dental rinse (= mouthwash), blue, sodium fluoride 0.05%. Net price 500 mL = £3.11. Counselling, see above

Dose

Child 6 years and over for *daily* use, rinse with 10 mL

Dental prescribing on NHS May be prescribed as Sodium Fluoride Mouthwash 0.05%

Gels

FluoriGard® (Colgate-Palmolive)

Gel-Kam (= gel), stannous fluoride 0.4% in glycerol basis. Net price 100 mL = £3.05. Counselling, see below

Dose

Child over 3 years for *daily* use, using a toothbrush, apply on to all tooth surfaces

Counselling Swish between teeth for 1 minute before spitting out. Avoid eating, drinking, or rinsing mouth for at least 30 minutes after use

Toothpastes

Duraphat® (Colgate-Palmolive) PoM

Toothpaste, sodium fluoride 0.619%. Net price 75 mL = £2.86. Counselling, see below

Dose

Child over 10 years apply 1 cm twice daily using a toothbrush

Counselling Brush teeth for 1 minute before spitting out. Avoid drinking or rinsing mouth for 30 minutes after use

Dental prescribing on NHS May be prescribed as Sodium Fluoride Toothpaste 0.619%

9.5.4 Zinc

Zinc supplements should be given only when there is good evidence of deficiency (hypoproteinaemia spuriously lowers plasma-zinc concentration) or in zinc-losing conditions. Zinc deficiency can occur as a result of inadequate diet or malabsorption; excessive loss of zinc can occur in trauma, burns and protein-losing conditions. A zinc supplement is given until clinical improvement occurs but it may need to be continued in severe malabsorption, metabolic disease or in zinc-losing states. Zinc is used in the treatment of Wilson's disease (section 9.8.1) and acrodermatitis enteropathica, a rare inherited abnormality of zinc absorption.

Total parenteral nutrition regimens usually include trace amounts of zinc (section 9.3). If necessary, further zinc can be added to some intravenous feeding regimens.

ZINC SULPHATE

Cautions interactions: Appendix 1 (zinc)

Renal impairment accumulation may occur in acute renal failure

Pregnancy crosses placenta, risk theoretically minimal but no information available

Breast-feeding present in breast milk, risk theoretically minimal but no information available

Side-effects abdominal pain, dyspepsia, nausea, vomiting, diarrhoea, gastric irritation, gastritis; irritability, headache, lethargy

Licensed use *Solvazinc®* not licensed in Wilson's disease or acrodermatitis enteropathica

ZINC SULPHATE (*continued*)

Solvazinc® (KoGEN)
Effervescent tablets, yellow-white, zinc sulphate monohydrate 125 mg (45 mg zinc). Net price 30 = £4.32. Label: 13, 21

Dose

Zinc deficiency (see notes above)
- By mouth

Neonate 1 mg/kg elemental zinc daily

Child under 10 kg half a tablet daily in water after food, adjusted as necessary

Child 10–30 kg half a tablet 1–3 times daily in water after food, adjusted as necessary

Child over 30 kg 1 tablet 1–3 times daily in water after food, adjusted as necessary

Acrodermatitis enteropathica
- By mouth

Neonate 0.5–1 mg/kg elemental zinc twice daily (total daily dose may alternatively be given in 3 divided doses), adjusted as necessary

Child 1 month–18 years 0.5–1 mg/kg elemental zinc twice daily (total daily dose may alternatively be given in 3 divided doses), adjusted as necessary

Administration *Solvazinc®* tablet may be dispersed in 4.5 mL water to give a solution of 10 mg elemental zinc in 1 mL

9.6 Vitamins

Vitamins are used for the prevention and treatment of specific deficiency states or where the diet is known to be inadequate; they may be prescribed in the NHS to prevent or treat deficiency but not as dietary supplements. Except for iron-deficiency anaemia, a primary vitamin or mineral deficiency due to simple dietary inadequacy is rare in the developed world. Some children may be at risk of developing deficiencies because of an inadequate intake, impaired vitamin synthesis or malabsorption in disease states such as cystic fibrosis and Crohn's disease.

The use of vitamins as general 'pick-me-ups' is of unproven value and the 'fad' for mega-vitamin therapy with water-soluble vitamins, such as ascorbic acid and pyridoxine, is unscientific and can be harmful. Many vitamin supplements are described as 'multivitamin' but few contain the whole range of essential vitamins and many contain relatively high amounts of vitamins A and D. Care should be taken to ensure the correct dose is not exceeded.

Dietary reference values for vitamins are available in the Department of Health publication:

Dietary Reference Values for Food Energy and Nutrients for the United Kingdom: Report of the Panel on Dietary Reference Values of the Committee on Medical Aspects of Food Policy. *Report on Health and Social Subjects 41*. London: HMSO, 1991

Dental patients Most patients who develop a nutritional deficiency despite an adequate intake of vitamins have malabsorption and if this is suspected the patient should be referred to a medical practitioner.

It is unjustifiable to treat stomatitis or glossitis with mixtures of vitamin preparations; this delays diagnosis and correct treatment.

9.6.1 Vitamin A

Deficiency of vitamin A (retinol) is associated with ocular defects (particularly xerophthalmia) and an increased susceptibility to infections, but deficiency is rare in the UK (even in disorders of fat absorption).

Vitamin A supplementation may be required in children with liver disease, particularly cholestatic liver disease, due to the malabsorption of fat soluble vitamins. In those with complete biliary obstruction an intramuscular dose once a month may be appropriate.

Treatment is sometimes initiated with very high doses of vitamin A and the child should be monitored closely; very high doses are associated with acute toxicity.

Preterm neonates have low plasma concentrations of vitamin A and are usually given vitamin A supplements, often as part of an oral multivitamin preparation (section 9.6.7) once enteral feeding has been established.

Massive overdose can cause rough skin, dry hair, an enlarged liver, and a raised erythrocyte sedimentation rate and raised serum calcium and serum alkaline phosphatase concentrations.

Pregnancy In view of evidence suggesting that high levels of vitamin A may cause birth defects, women who are (or may become) pregnant are advised not to take vitamin A supplements (including tablets and fish-liver oil drops), except on the advice of a doctor or an antenatal clinic; nor should they eat liver or products such as liver paté or liver sausage.

VITAMIN A

(Retinol)

Cautions see notes above; **interactions**: Appendix 1 (vitamins)

Pregnancy teratogenic; see notes above

Breast-feeding toxicity likely if mother taking high doses

Side-effects see notes above

Licensed use preparations containing only vitamin A are not licensed

Indication and dose

See also notes above

Vitamin A deficiency
- **By mouth**

Neonate 5000 units daily

Child 1 month–1 year 5000 units daily with or after food

Child 1–18 years 10 000 units daily with or after food

Note Higher doses may be used initially for treatment of severe deficiency

Prevention of deficiency in complete biliary obstruction
- **By intramuscular injection**

Neonate 50 000 units once a month

Child 1 month–1 year 50 000 units once a month

Arovit® (Non-proprietary)
Oral solution, vitamin A 150 000 units/mL
Available from specialist importing companies

Aquasol-A® (Non-proprietary)
Injection, vitamin A (as palmitate) 50 000 units/mL, 2-mL amp
Available from specialist importing companies

VITAMINS A and D

Cautions see notes above and section 9.6.4; prolonged excessive ingestion of vitamins A and D can lead to hypervitaminosis; **interactions**: Appendix 1 (vitamins)

Pregnancy see notes above

Side-effects see notes above and section 9.6.4

Licensed use not licensed in children under 6 months of age

Indication and dose

See notes above and section 9.6.4

Prevention of vitamin A and D deficiency see individual preparations for dose information

Vitamins A and D (Non-proprietary)
Capsules, vitamin A 4000 units, vitamin D 400 units. Net price 20 = 64p
Dose
Child 1–18 years 1 capsule daily

Halycitrol® (LAB)
Emulsion, vitamin A 4600 units, vitamin D 380 units/5 mL
Dose
Child 1–6 months 2.5 mL daily
Child 6 months–18 years 5 mL daily

9.6.2 Vitamin B group

Deficiency of the B vitamins, other than deficiency of vitamin B_{12} (section 9.1.2), is rare in the UK and is usually treated by preparations containing thiamine (B_1), riboflavin (B_2), and nicotinamide, which is used in preference to nicotinic acid, as it does not cause vasodilatation. Other members (or substances traditionally classified as members) of the vitamin B complex such as aminobenzoic acid, biotin, choline, inositol, and pantothenic acid or panthenol may be included in vitamin B preparations but there is no evidence of their value as supplements; however they can be used in the management of certain metabolic disorders (section 9.8). Anaphylaxis has been reported with parenteral B vitamins (see CSM advice, below).

As with other vitamins of the B group, pyridoxine (B_6) deficiency is rare, but it may occur during isoniazid therapy (section 5.1.9) or penicillamine treatment in Wilson's disease (section 9.8.1) and is characterised by peripheral neuritis. High doses of pyridoxine are given in some metabolic disorders, such as hyperoxaluria, cystathioninuria and homocystinuria; folic acid supplementation may also be beneficial in these disorders (section 9.1.2). Pyridoxine is also used in sideroblastic anaemia (section 9.1.3). Rarely, seizures in the neonatal period or during infancy respond to pyridoxine treatment; pyridoxine should be tried in all cases of early-onset intractable seizures and status epilepticus. Pyridoxine has been tried for a wide variety of other disorders, but there is little sound evidence to support the claims of efficacy, and overdosage induces toxic effects.

A number of mitochondrial disorders may respond to treatment with certain B vitamins but these disorders require specialist management. Thiamine is used in the treatment of maple syrup urine disease, mitochondrial respiratory chain defects and, together with riboflavin, in the treatment of congenital lactic acidosis; riboflavin is also used in glutaric acidaemias and cytochrome oxidase deficiencies; biotin (section 9.8.1) is used in carboxylase defects.

Nicotinic acid inhibits the synthesis of cholesterol and triglyceride (section 2.12). Folic acid and vitamin B_{12} are used in the treatment of megaloblastic anaemia (section 9.1.2). Folinic acid (available as calcium folinate) is used in association with cytotoxic therapy (section 8.1).

RIBOFLAVIN

(Riboflavine, vitamin B_2)

Cautions see notes above

Pregnancy crosses the placenta but no adverse effects reported, information at high doses limited

Breast-feeding present in breast milk but no adverse effects reported, information at high doses limited

Side-effects bright yellow urine

Licensed use not licensed in children

Indication and dose

See also notes above

Metabolic diseases
- **By mouth**

Neonate 50 mg 1–2 times daily, adjusted according to response

Child 1 month–18 years 50–100 mg 1–2 times daily, adjusted according to response, up to 400 mg daily has been used

Riboflavin (Non-proprietary)
Tablets, 10 mg, 50 mg and 100 mg
Available from specialist importing companies

Capsules, 50 mg
Available as health food supplement

Oral vitamin B complex preparations
See below

THIAMINE

(Vitamin B_1)

CSM advice
Since potentially serious allergic adverse reactions may occur during, or shortly after, parenteral administration, the CSM has recommended that:

1. Use be restricted to patients in whom parenteral treatment is essential;
2. Intravenous injections should be administered slowly (over 10 minutes);
3. Facilities for treating anaphylaxis should be available when administered.

Cautions anaphylactic shock may occasionally follow injection (see CSM advice above)

Contra-indications

Breast-feeding severely thiamine-deficient mothers should avoid breast-feeding as toxic methyl-glyoxal present in milk

Side-effects hypersensitivity reactions to injection

Licensed use not licensed in children

Indication and dose

See also notes above

Maple syrup urine disease
- **By mouth**

Neonate 5 mg/kg daily; adjusted as necessary

Child 1 month–18 years 5 mg/kg daily adjusted as necessary

Metabolic disorders including congenital lactic acidosis
- **By mouth or by intravenous injection over 10 minutes**

Neonate 50–200 mg once daily (total dose may alternatively be given in 2–3 divided doses), adjusted as necessary

Child 1 month–18 years 100–300 mg once daily (total dose may alternatively be given in 2–3 divided doses), adjusted as necessary; up to 2 g daily may be necessary in those under 12 years of age or 4 g in older children

Thiamine (Non-proprietary)
Tablets, thiamine hydrochloride 50 mg, net price 20 = 80p; 100 mg, 20 = £1.23
Brands include *Benerva*® (NHS)

THIAMINE (*continued*)

Injection, 50 mg/mL, 2-mL vial; 100 mg/mL, 2-mL vial

Injection (intramuscular), 100 mg/mL, 5-mL vial

Available from specialist importing companies

Note Some preparations may contain phenol as a preservative

Oral vitamin B complex preparations

See below

PYRIDOXINE HYDROCHLORIDE

(Vitamin B_6)

Cautions see notes above; risk of cardiovascular collapse with intravenous injection; **interactions**: Appendix 1 (vitamins)

Side-effects sensory neuropathy reported with high doses given for extended periods

Licensed use not licensed for use in children

Indication and dose

See also notes above

Metabolic diseases including cystathioninuria, homocystinuria and Wilson's disease
- By mouth

Neonate 50–100 mg 1–2 times daily

Child 1 month–18 years 50–250 mg 1–2 times daily

Treatment of isoniazid-induced neuropathy
- By mouth

Neonate 5–10 mg daily

Child 1 month–12 years 10–20 mg 2–3 times daily

Child 12–18 years 30–50 mg 2–3 times daily

Prevention of isoniazid-induced neuropathy
- By mouth

Neonate 5 mg daily

Child 1 month–12 years 5–10 mg daily

Child 12–18 years 10 mg daily

Pyridoxine-dependent seizures
- **By intravenous injection or by mouth**

Neonate initial test dose 50–100 mg by intravenous injection, may be repeated; if responsive followed by an oral maintenance dose of 50–100mg once daily, adjusted as necessary

Child 1 month–12 years initial test dose 50–100 mg daily; if responsive followed by an oral dose of 20–50 mg 1–2 times daily, adjusted as necessary; doses up to 30 mg/kg or 1 g daily have been used

Pyridoxine (Non-proprietary)

Tablets, pyridoxine hydrochloride 10 mg, net price 20 = 34p; 20 mg, 20 = 34p; 50 mg, 20 = 38p

Injection, 25 mg/mL, 2 mL vial

Available as a manufactured special from Martindale Pharmaceuticals

Extemporaneous formulations available see Extemporaneous Preparations, p. 8

Injections of vitamins B and C

See under Thiamine

NICOTINAMIDE

Indication and dose

See notes above, Acne vulgaris see section 13.6.1

Nicotinamide (Non-proprietary)

Tablets, nicotinamide 50 mg. Net price 20 = £1.37

Injections of vitamins B and C

See under Thiamine

Oral vitamin B complex preparations

Note Other multivitamin preparations are in section 9.6.7.

Vitamin B Tablets, Compound

Tablets, nicotinamide 15 mg, riboflavin 1 mg, thiamine hydrochloride 1 mg. Net price 20 = 7p

Vitamin B Tablets, Compound, Strong

Tablets, brown, f/c or s/c, nicotinamide 20 mg, pyridoxine hydrochloride 2 mg, riboflavin 2 mg, thiamine hydrochloride 5 mg. Net price 28-tab pack = £1.11p

Dental prescribing on the NHS Vitamin B Tablets, Compound Strong may be prescribed

Vigranon B® (Wallace Mfg) NHS

Syrup, thiamine hydrochloride 5 mg, riboflavin 2 mg, nicotinamide 20 mg, pyridoxine hydrochloride 2 mg, panthenol 3 mg/5 mL. Net price 150 mL = £2.41

Dose

Treatment of deficiency
- By mouth

Child 1 month–1 year 5 mL 3 times daily

Child 1–12 years 10 mL 3 times daily

Child 12–18 years 10–15mL 3times daily

Prophylaxis of deficiency
- By mouth

Child 1 month–1 year 5 mL once daily

Child 1–12 years 5 mL twice daily

Child 12–18 years 5 mL 3 times daily

9 Nutrition and blood

9.6.3 Vitamin C

(Ascorbic acid)

Vitamin C therapy is essential in scurvy, but less florid manifestations of vitamin C deficiency have been reported. Vitamin C is used to enhance the excretion of iron one month after starting desferrioxamine therapy (section 9.1.3); it is given separately from food as it also enhances iron absorption. Vitamin C is also used in the treatment of some inherited metabolic disorders, particularly mitochondrial disorders; specialist management of these conditions is required.

Severe scurvy causes gingival swelling and bleeding margins as well as petechiae on the skin. This is, however, exceedingly rare and a child with these signs is more likely to have leukaemia. Investigation should not be delayed by a trial period of vitamin treatment.

Claims that vitamin C ameliorates colds or promotes wound healing have not been proved.

ASCORBIC ACID

(Vitamin C)

Contra-indications hyperoxaluria

Side-effects nausea, diarrhoea; headache, fatigue; hyperoxaluria

Licensed use not licensed for metabolic disorders

Indication and dose

Treatment of scurvy
- By mouth

Child 1 month–4 years 125–250 mg daily in 1–2 divided doses

Child 4–12 years 250–500 mg daily in 1–2 divided doses

Child 12–18 years 500 mg–1 g daily in 1–2 divided doses

Adjunct to desferrioxamine (see notes above)
- By mouth

Child 1 month–18 years 100–200 mg daily 1 hour before food

Metabolic disorders (tyrosinaemia type III; transient tyrosinaemia of the newborn; glutathione synthase deficiency; Hawkinsinuria)
- By mouth

Neonate 50–200 mg daily, adjusted as necessary

Child 1 month–18 years 200–400 mg daily in 1–2 divided doses, adjusted as necessary; up to 1 g daily may be required

Ascorbic Acid (Non-proprietary)

Tablets, ascorbic acid 50 mg, net price 20 = 84p; 100 mg, 20 = 18p; 200 mg, 20 = 22p; 500 mg (label: 24), 20 = £1.49

Excipients: may include aspartame

Brands include *Redoxon®* NHS

Dental prescribing on the NHS Ascorbic Acid Tablets may be prescribed

Injection, ascorbic acid 100 mg/mL. Net price 5-mL amp = £2.51

Excipients: include metabisulphite

Available from UCB Pharma

9.6.4 Vitamin D

Note The term Vitamin D is used for a range of compounds including ergocalciferol (calciferol, vitamin D_2), colecalciferol (vitamin D_3), dihydrotachysterol, alfacalcidol (1α-hydroxycholecalciferol), and calcitriol (1,25-dihydroxycholecalciferol).

Nutritional deficiency of vitamin D is uncommon, but may occur in certain ethnic groups, and rarely in association with malabsorption. The amount of vitamin D required in infancy is related to the stores built up *in-utero* and subsequent exposure to sunlight. The amount of vitamin D in breast milk varies and some breast-fed babies, particularly if preterm or born to vitamin D deficient mothers, may become deficient. Most formula milk and supplement feeds contain adequate vitamin D to prevent deficiency.

Simple vitamin D deficiency can be prevented by oral supplementation of 200–400 units of ergocalciferol (calciferol, vitamin D_2) daily, using multi-vitamin drops (section 9.6.7), manufactured 'special' solutions, or as calcium and ergocalciferol tablets (although the calcium is unnecessary); excessive supplementation may cause hypercalcaemia.

Inadequate bone mineralisation can be caused by a deficiency, or a lack of action of vitamin D or its active metabolite. In childhood this causes bowing and distortion of bones (rickets); initial high doses of vitamin D should be reduced after a few weeks, as there is a significant risk of hypercalcaemia (see caution below).

Poor bone mineralisation in neonates and young children may also be due to inadequate intake of phosphate or calcium particularly during long-term parenteral nutrition—supplementation with phosphate (section 9.5.2.1) or calcium (section 9.5.1.1) may be required.

Hypophosphataemic rickets occurs due to abnormal phosphate excretion; treatment with high doses of oral phosphate (section 9.5.2.1), and hydroxylated (activated) forms of vitamin D allow bone mineralisation and optimise growth.

Nutritional deficiency of vitamin D is best treated with colecalciferol or ergocalciferol. Vitamin D deficiency caused by *intestinal malabsorption* or *chronic liver disease* usually requires vitamin D in pharmacological doses, such as **ergocalciferol** in doses of up to 40 000 units daily; the hypocalcaemia of *hypoparathyroidism* often requires higher doses in order to achieve normocalcaemia and alfacalcidol is generally preferred.

Vitamin D supplementation is often given in combination with calcium supplements for persistent hypocalcaemia in neonates, and in chronic renal disease.

Vitamin D requires hydroxylation, by the kidney and liver, to its active form therefore the hydroxylated derivatives **alfacalcidol** or **calcitriol** should be prescribed if patients with *severe liver or renal impairment* require vitamin D therapy. Alfacalcidol is generally preferred in children as there is more experience of its use and appropriate formulations are available. Calcitriol is unlicensed for use in children and is generally reserved for those with severe liver disease.

Important. All patients receiving pharmacological doses of vitamin D should have the plasma-calcium concentration checked at intervals (initially weekly) and whenever nausea or vomiting are present. Breast milk from women taking pharmacological doses of vitamin D may cause hypercalcaemia if given to an infant.

ERGOCALCIFEROL

(Calciferol, Vitamin D_2)

Cautions monitor plasma calcium in patients receiving high doses and in renal impairment; **interactions**: Appendix 1 (vitamins)

Pregnancy avoid excessive supplementation

Breast-feeding avoid excessive supplementation, monitor serum-calcium concentration in child

Contra-indications hypercalcaemia; metastatic calcification

Renal impairment avoid in severe impairment

Side-effects symptoms of overdosage include anorexia, lassitude, nausea and vomiting, diarrhoea, weight loss, polyuria, sweating, headache, thirst, vertigo, and raised concentrations of calcium and phosphate in plasma and urine

Indication and dose

See also notes above

Nutritional vitamin-D deficiency rickets
- **By mouth**

Child 1–6 months 3000 units daily, adjusted as necessary

Child 6 months–12 years 6000 units daily, adjusted as necessary

Child 12–18 years 10 000 units daily, adjusted as necessary

Nutritional or physiological supplement; prevention of rickets
- **By mouth**

Neonate 200–400 units daily

Child 1 month–18 years 400–600 units daily

Vitamin D deficiency in intestinal malabsorption or in chronic liver disease
- **By mouth or by intramuscular injection**

Child 1–12 years 10 000–25 000 units daily, adjusted as necessary

Child 12–18 years 10 000–40 000 units daily, adjusted as necessary

Pharmacological strengths

(see notes above)

The BP directs that when calciferol is prescribed or demanded, colecalciferol or ergocalciferol should be dispensed or supplied

Ergocalciferol (Non-proprietary)

Tablets, ergocalciferol 250 micrograms (10 000 units), net price 20 = £4.31; 1.25 mg (50 000 units) may also be available

Note When the strength of the tablets ordered or prescribed is not clear, the intention of the prescriber or purchaser with respect to the strength (expressed in micrograms or milligrams per tablet) should be ascertained.

Solution ergocalciferol 3000 units/mL

Excipients: may include peanut oil

Available from specials manufacturers

Injection, colecalciferol or ergocalciferol, 7.5 mg (300 000 units)/mL in oil. Net price 1-mL amp = £5.92, 2-mL amp = £7.07

Daily supplements

Note There is no plain vitamin D tablet available for treating simple deficiency (see notes above). Alternatives include vitamins capsules (see section 9.6.7), preparations of vitamins A and D (see section 9.6.1), and calcium and ergocalciferol tablets (see below).

Calcium and Ergocalciferol (Non-proprietary)
(Calcium and Vitamin D)

Tablets, calcium lactate 300 mg, calcium phosphate 150 mg (calcium 97 mg or Ca^{2+} 2.4 mmol), ergocalciferol 10 micrograms (400 units). Net price 28-tab pack = £1.43. Counselling, crush before administration or may be chewed

Adcal-D_3® (Strakan)

Tablets (chewable), calcium carbonate 1.5 g (calcium 600 mg or Ca^{2+} 15.1 mmol), colecalciferol 10 micrograms (400 units), net price 100-tab pack = £7.25. Label: 24

ERGOCALCIFEROL (*continued*)

Cacit® D3 (Procter & Gamble Pharm.)
Granules, effervescent, calcium carbonate 1.25 g (calcium 500 mg or Ca^{2+} 12.6 mmol), colecalciferol 11 micrograms (440 units)/sachet. Net price 30-sachet pack = £5.75. Label: 13

Calceos® (KoGEN)
Tablets (chewable), calcium carbonate 1.25 g (calcium 500 mg or Ca^{2+} 12.6 mmol), colecalciferol 10 micrograms (400 units). Net price 60-tab pack = £4.74. Label: 24

Calcichew® D3 (Shire)
Tablets (chewable), gluten-free, calcium carbonate 1.25 g (calcium 500 mg or Ca^{2+} 12.6 mmol), colecalciferol 5 micrograms (200 units). Net price 100-tab pack = £15.02. Label: 24
Excipients: include aspartame (section 9.4.1)

Calcichew® D3 Forte (Shire)
Tablets (chewable), gluten-free, calcium carbonate 1.25 g (calcium 500 mg or Ca^{2+} 12.6 mmol), colecalciferol 10 micrograms (400 units). Net price 100-tab pack = £7.50. Label: 24
Excipients: include aspartame (section 9.4.1)

Calfovit D3® (Trinity) PoM
Powder, calcium phosphate 3.1 g (calcium 1.2 g or Ca^{2+} 30 mmol), colecalciferol 20 micrograms (800 units), net price 30-sachet pack = £4.32. Label: 13, 21

ALFACALCIDOL
(1α-Hydroxycholecalciferol)

Cautions see under Ergocalciferol

Contra-indications see under Ergocalciferol

Side-effects see under Ergocalciferol

Licensed use *AlfaD®* not licensed for use in children under 20 kg

Indication and dose

See also notes above

Hypophosphataemic rickets; persistent hypocalcaemia due to hypoparathyroidism or pseudohypoparathyroidism
- **By mouth or by intravenous injection**

Child 1 month–12 years 25–50 nanograms/kg (max. 1 microgram) once daily, adjusted as necessary

Child 12–18 years 1 microgram once daily, adjusted as necessary

Persistent neonatal hypocalcaemia
- **By mouth or by intravenous injection**

Neonate 50–100 nanograms/kg once daily, adjusted as necessary (up to 2 micrograms/kg daily may be needed in resistant cases)

Prevention of vitamin D deficiency in renal or cholestatic liver disease
- **By mouth or by intravenous injection**

Neonate 20 nanograms/kg once daily, adjusted as necessary

Child 1 month–12 years, body-weight under 20 kg 15–30 nanograms/kg (max. 500 nanograms) once daily; **body-weight over 20 kg** 250–500 nanograms once daily, adjusted as necessary

Child 12–18 years 250–500 nanograms once daily, adjusted as necessary

Alfacalcidol (Non-proprietary) PoM
Capsules, alfacalcidol 250 nanograms, net price 30-cap pack = £4.78; 500 nanograms 30-cap pack = £8.19; 1 microgram 30-cap pack = £11.49

One-Alpha® (LEO) PoM
Capsules, alfacalcidol 250 nanograms (white), net price 30-cap pack = £3.37; 500 nanograms (red), 30-cap pack = £6.27; 1 microgram (brown), 30-cap pack = £8.75
Excipients: include sesame oil

Oral drops, sugar-free, alfacalcidol 2 micrograms/mL (1 drop contains approx. 100 nanograms), net price 10 mL = £24.18
Excipients: include alcohol
Note The concentration of alfacalcidol in *One-Alpha® drops* is **10 times greater** than that of the former presentation *One-Alpha® solution.*

Injection, alfacalcidol 2 micrograms/mL, net price 0.5-mL amp = £2.16, 1-mL amp = £4.11
Note Contains propylene glycol and should be used with caution in small preterm neonates

CALCITRIOL
(1,25-Dihydroxycholecalciferol)

Cautions see under Ergocalciferol; monitor plasma calcium, phosphate, and creatinine during dosage titration

Contra-indications see under Ergocalciferol

Side-effects see under Ergocalciferol

Licensed use not licensed for use in children

Indication and dose

See also notes above

Vitamin D dependent rickets; hypophosphataemic rickets; persistent hypocalcaemia due to hypoparathyroidism or pseudo-hypoparathyroidism (limited experience)
- **By mouth**

Child 1 month–12 years initially 15 nanograms/kg (max. 250 nanograms) once daily, increased if necessary in steps of 5 nanograms/kg daily (max. 250 nanograms) every 2–4 weeks

Child 12–18 years initially 250 nanograms once daily increased if necessary in steps of 5 nanograms/kg daily (max. 250 nanograms step) every 2–4 weeks; usual dose 0.5–1 microgram daily

CALCITRIOL (*continued*)

Hypocalcaemia in dialysis patients (limited experience)
- **By intravenous injection**

Child 12–18 years initially 250–500 nanograms (approx. 10 nanograms/kg) 3 times a week, increased if necessary in steps of 2–5 nanograms/kg every 2–4 weeks; usual dose 0.5–3 micrograms 3 times a week

Administration *Oral*: injection may be given orally or contents of capsule administered by syringe; capsules contain approx. 0.168 mL of fluid.
Intravenous: injection may be given via catheter after dialysis

Calcitriol (Non-proprietary) PoM
Capsules, calcitriol 250 nanograms, net price 30-cap pack = £6.18; 500 nanograms, 30-cap pack = £11.05

Rocaltrol® (Roche) PoM
Capsules, calcitriol 250 nanograms (red/white), net price 20 = £3.83; 500 nanograms (red), 20 = £6.85

Calcijex® (Abbott) PoM
Injection, calcitriol 1 microgram/mL, net price 1-mL amp = £5.14; 2 micrograms/mL, 1-mL amp = £10.28

COLECALCIFEROL
(Cholecalciferol, vitamin D_3)

Cautions see under Ergocalciferol
Contra-indications see under Ergocalciferol
Side-effects see under Ergocalciferol

Indication and dose

See under Ergocalciferol—alternative to Ergocalciferol in calciferol tablets and injection, see Pharmacological Strengths

Extemporaneous formulations available see Extemporaneous Preparations, p. 8

9.6.5 Vitamin E
(Tocopherols)

The daily requirement of vitamin E has not been well defined. Vitamin E supplements are given to children with fat malabsorption such as in cystic fibrosis and cholestatic liver disease. In children with abetalipoproteinaemia abnormally low vitamin E concentrations may occur in association with neuromuscular problems; this usually responds to high doses of vitamin E. Some neonatal units still administer a single intramuscular dose of vitamin E at birth to preterm neonates to reduce the risk of complications; no trials of long-term outcome have been carried out.

Vitamin E has been tried for various other conditions but there is little scientific evidence of its value.

ALPHA TOCOPHERYL ACETATE

Cautions predisposition to thrombosis; increased risk of necrotising enterocolitis in preterm neonates (see administration)
Pregnancy avoid high doses in first trimester
Breast-feeding excreted in breast milk, minimal risk although caution with large doses

Side-effects diarrhoea and abdominal pain, particularly with high doses

Indication and dose

Vitamin E deficiency
- **By mouth**

Neonate 10 mg/kg once daily

Child 1 month–18 years 2–10 mg/kg daily, up to 20 mg/kg has been used

Supplementation in cystic fibrosis
- **By mouth (with food and pancreatic enzymes)**

Child 1 month–1 year 50 mg once daily, adjusted as necessary

Child 1–12 years 100 mg once daily, adjusted as necessary

Child 12–18 years 200 mg once daily, adjusted as necessary

Vitamin E deficiency in cholestatic liver disease
- **By mouth**

Child 1 month–12 years initially 100 mg daily, adjusted according to response; up to 200 mg/kg daily may be required

Child 12–18 years initially 200 mg daily, adjusted according to response; up to 200 mg/kg daily may be required

Severe liver disease or biliary obstruction
- **By intramuscular injection**

Neonate 10 mg/kg once or twice a month

Child 1 month–18 years 10 mg/kg (max. 100 mg) once a month

Abetalipoproteinaemia
- **By mouth**

Neonate 100 mg/kg once daily

Child 1 month–18 years 50–100 mg/kg once daily

▢ **ALPHA TOCOPHERYL ACETATE (*continued*)**

Vitamin E Suspension (Cambridge)
Suspension, alpha tocopheryl acetate 100 mg/mL. Net price 100 mL = £17.23
Excipients: include sucrose
Administration consider dilution in neonates due to high osmolality (see Cautions)

Note Tablets containing tocopheryl acetate 100 mg are available on a named-patient basis from Bell and Croyden (*Ephynal®*)

Vitamin E Injection (Roche)
Injection tocopheryl acetate 50 mg/mL, 2-mL ampoule
Available from specialist importing companies

9.6.6 Vitamin K

Vitamin K is necessary for the production of blood clotting factors and proteins necessary for the normal calcification of bone.

Because vitamin K is fat soluble, children with fat malabsorption, especially in biliary obstruction or hepatic disease, may become deficient. For oral administration to prevent vitamin-K deficiency in malabsorption syndromes, a water-soluble preparation, **menadiol sodium phosphate** (see Contra-indications below) must be used.

Oral coumarin anticoagulants act by interfering with vitamin-K metabolism in the hepatic cells and their effects can be antagonised by giving vitamin K (see also section 2.8.2).

Vitamin K-deficiency bleeding Neonates are relatively deficient in vitamin K and those who do not receive supplements are at risk of serious bleeds (haemorrhagic disease), including intracranial bleeding. The Chief Medical Officer and the Chief Nursing Officer have recommended that all newborn babies should receive vitamin K to prevent vitamin-K deficiency bleeding (haemorrhagic disease of the newborn). Local protocols may vary and an appropriate regimen should be selected after discussion with parents in the antenatal period.

Vitamin K (as phytomenadione) 1 mg may be given by a single intramuscular injection at birth; this prevents vitamin-K deficiency bleeding in virtually all babies; preterm neonates may be given 400 micrograms/kg (max. 1 mg). The intravenous route is preferred in preterm neonates of very low birth-weight but it does not provide the prolonged protection of the intramuscular injection, and any babies receiving intravenous vitamin K should be given subsequent oral doses, as described below.

Babies considered at particular risk of vitamin-K deficiency bleeding should receive intramuscular vitamin K at birth; this includes those experiencing birth asphyxia or bleeding problems, those born to mothers with liver disease or taking enzyme inducing anticonvulsant drugs (carbamazepine, phenobarbital, phenytoin), rifampicin or warfarin. In infants with cholestatic disease, vitamin K must be given either intramuscularly or intravenously because oral absorption is likely to be impaired.

Alternatively, in healthy babies who are not at particular risk of bleeding disorders, vitamin K may be given by mouth, and arrangements must be in place to ensure the appropriate regimen is followed. Two doses of a colloidal (mixed micelle) preparation of phytomenadione 2 mg should be given in the first week, the first dose being given at birth. For exclusively breast-fed babies, a third dose of phytomenadione 2 mg is given at 1 month of age; the third dose is omitted in formula-fed babies because formula feeds contain vitamin K.

MENADIOL SODIUM PHOSPHATE

Cautions G6PD deficiency (section 9.1.5) and vitamin E deficiency (risk of haemolysis); **interactions:** Appendix 1 (vitamins)

Contra-indications neonates and infants, late pregnancy

Indication and dose

See notes above

Supplementation in vitamin-K malabsorption
- By mouth

Child 1–12 years 5–10 mg daily, adjusted as necessary

Child 12–18 years 10–20 mg daily, adjusted as necessary

9 Nutrition and blood

MENADIOL SODIUM PHOSPHATE (*continued*)

Menadiol Phosphate (Cambridge)
Tablets, menadiol sodium phosphate equivalent to 10 mg of menadiol phosphate. Net price 100-tab pack = £37.34

Extemporaneous formulations available see Extemporaneous Preparations, p. 8

PHYTOMENADIONE
(Vitamin K_1)

Cautions intravenous injections should be given very slowly—risk of vascular collapse (see also below); **interactions**: Appendix 1 (vitamins)

Indication and dose

Neonatal prophylaxis of vitamin-K deficiency bleeding see notes above

Neonatal hypoprothrombinaemia or vitamin-K deficiency bleeding
- By intravenous injection

Neonate 1 mg repeated 8 hourly if necessary

Neonatal biliary atresia and liver disease
- By mouth

Neonate 1 mg daily

Reversal of coumarin anticoagulation when continued anticoagulation required or if no significant bleeding (section 2.8.2)—seek specialist advice
- By intravenous injection

Child 1 month–18 years 15–30 micrograms/kg (max. 1 mg) as a single dose, repeated as necessary

Reversal of coumarin anticoagulation when anticoagulation not required or if significant bleeding; treatment of haemorrhage associated with vitamin-K deficiency (section 2.8.2)—seek specialist advice
- By intravenous injection

Child 1 month–18 years 250–300 micrograms/kg (max. 10 mg) as a single dose

Konakion® (Roche) PoM
Tablets, s/c, phytomenadione 10 mg, net price 10-tab pack = £1.65. To be chewed or allowed to dissolve slowly in the mouth (Label: 24)

Colloidal formulation

Konakion® MM (Roche) PoM
Injection, phytomenadione 10 mg/mL in a mixed micelles vehicle. Net price 1-mL amp = 40p
Excipients: include glycocholic acid 54.6 mg/amp, lecithin
Cautions reduce dose in liver impairment (glycocholic acid may displace bilirubin); reports of anaphylactoid reactions
Administration *Konakion® MM* may be administered by slow intravenous injection or by intravenous infusion in glucose 5%; **not** for intramuscular injection

Konakion® MM Paediatric (Roche) ▼ PoM
Injection, phytomenadione 10 mg/mL in a mixed micelles vehicle. Net price 0.2-mL amp = £1.00
Excipients: include glycocholic acid 10.9 mg/amp, lecithin
Cautions parenteral administration in premature infants of less than 2.5 kg (increased risk of kernicterus)
Administration *Konakion® MM Paediatric* may be administered *by mouth* or *by intramuscular injection* or *by intravenous injection*. May be diluted with glucose 5% infusion for intravenous use

9.6.7 Multivitamin preparations

Multivitamin supplements are used in children with vitamin deficiencies and also in malabsorption conditions such as cystic fibrosis or liver disease. To avoid potential toxicity, the content of all vitamin preparations, particularly vitamin A, should be considered when used together with other supplements. Supplementation is not required if nutrient enriched feeds are used; consult a dietician for further advice.

MULTIVITAMIN PREPARATIONS

Cautions see individual vitamins; vitamin A concentration of preparations varies

Contra-indications see individual vitamins

Side-effects see individual vitamins

Licensed use *Dalivit®* not licensed for use in children under 6 weeks

Indication and dose

Prevention of deficiency
- By mouth

Neonate 0.3 mL daily

Child 1 month–1 year 0.3 mL daily

Child 1–18 years 0.6 mL daily *or* 1–2 capsules daily

Cystic fibrosis: prevention of deficiency
- By mouth

Child 1 month–1 year 0.6 mL daily

Child 1–18 years 1–1.2 mL daily *or* 2–3 capsules daily

MULTIVITAMIN PREPARATIONS (*continued*)

Vitamins

Capsules, ascorbic acid 15 mg, nicotinamide 7.5 mg, riboflavin 500 micrograms, thiamine hydrochloride 1 mg, vitamin A 2500 units, vitamin D 300 units. Net price 20 = 22p

Abidec® (Chefaro UK)

Drops, vitamins A, B group, C, and D. Net price 25 mL (with dropper) = £1.84

Note Contains 1333 units of vitamin A (as palmitate) per 0.6 mL dose

Excipients: include arachis (peanut) oil and sucrose

Dalivit® (LPC)

Oral drops, vitamins A, B group, C, and D, net price 25 mL = £1.60, 50 mL = £2.85

Note Contains 5000 units of vitamin A (as palmitate) per 0.6 mL dose

Excipients: include sucrose

Vitamin and mineral supplements and adjuncts to synthetic diets

Forceval® (Alliance)

Capsules, brown/red, vitamins (ascorbic acid 60 mg, biotin 100 micrograms, cyanocobalamin 3 micrograms, folic acid 400 micrograms, nicotinamide 18 mg, pantothenic acid 4 mg, pyridoxine 2 mg, riboflavin 1.6 mg, thiamine 1.2 mg, vitamin A 2500 units, vitamin D_2 400 units, vitamin E 10 mg, minerals and trace elements (calcium 100 mg, chromium 200 micrograms, copper 2 mg, iodine 140 micrograms, iron 12 mg, magnesium 30 mg, manganese 3 mg, molybdenum 250 micrograms, phosphorus 77 mg, potassium 4 mg, selenium 50 micrograms, zinc 15 mg). Net price 30-cap pack = £4.94, 45-cap pack = £6.47; 90-cap pack = £11.93

Dose

Vitamin and mineral deficiency and as adjunct in synthetic diets
- **Child 12–18 years** 1 capsule daily

Junior capsules, brown, vitamins (ascorbic acid 25 mg, biotin 50 micrograms, cyanocobalamin 2 micrograms, folic acid 100 micrograms, nicotinamide 7.5 mg, pantothenic acid 2 mg, pyridoxine 1 mg, riboflavin 1 mg, thiamine 1.5 mg, vitamin A 1250 units, vitamin D_2 200 units, vitamin E 5 mg, vitamin K_1 25 micrograms), minerals and trace elements (chromium 50 micrograms, copper 1 mg, iodine 75 micrograms, iron 5 mg, magnesium 1 mg, manganese 1.25 mg, molybdenum 50 micrograms, selenium 25 micrograms, zinc 5 mg). Net price 30-cap pack = £3.52, 60-cap pack = £6.69

Dose

Vitamin and mineral deficiency and as adjunct in synthetic diets
- **Child 5–12 years** 2 capsules daily

Ketovite® (Paines & Byrne)

Tablets (PoM), yellow, ascorbic acid 16.6 mg, riboflavin 1 mg, thiamine hydrochloride 1 mg, pyridoxine hydrochloride 330 micrograms, nicotinamide 3.3 mg, calcium pantothenate 1.16 mg, alpha tocopheryl acetate 5 mg, inositol 50 mg, biotin 170 micrograms, folic acid 250 micrograms, acetomenaphthone 500 micrograms. Net price 100-tab pack = £4.17

Dose

Prevention of vitamin deficiency in disorders of carbohydrate or amino-acid metabolism and adjunct in restricted, specialised, or synthetic diets
- **Child 1 month–18 years** 1 tablet 3 times daily; dose adjusted according to condition, diet or age; use with *Ketovite® Liquid* for complete vitamin supplementation

Administration may be crushed immediately before use

Liquid, pink, sugar-free, vitamin A 2500 units, ergocalciferol 400 units, choline chloride 150 mg, cyanocobalamin 12.5 micrograms/5 mL. Net price 150-mL pack = £2.70

Dose

Prevention of vitamin deficiency in disorders of carbohydrate or amino-acid metabolism and adjunct in restricted, specialised, or synthetic diets
- **Child 1 month–18 years** 5 mL daily; dose adjusted according to condition, diet or age; use with *Ketovite® Tablets* for complete vitamin supplementation

Administration may be mixed with milk, cereal or fruit juice

9.7 Bitters and tonics

Classification not included in *BNF for Children*

9.8 Metabolic disorders

This section covers drugs used in metabolic disorders and not readily classified elsewhere.

9.8.1 Drugs used in metabolic disorders

Metabolic disorders should be managed under the guidance of a specialist. As many preparations are unlicensed and may be difficult to obtain, arrangements for continued prescribing and supply should be made in primary care.

General advice on the use of medicines in metabolic disorders can be obtained from

Alder Hey Children's Hospital
Medicines Information Centre
Tel: (0151) 252 5381

and

Great Ormond Street Hospital for Children
Pharmacy
Tel: (020) 7405 9200

Wilson's disease

Penicillamine is used in Wilson's disease (hepatolenticular degeneration) to aid the elimination of copper ions. See below for other indications. Children who are hypersensitive to penicillin may react rarely to penicillamine.

Trientine is used for the treatment of Wilson's disease only, in patients intolerant of penicillamine; it is **not** an alternative to penicillamine in other diseases such as cystinuria. Penicillamine-induced systemic lupus erythematosus may not resolve on transfer to trientine.

Zinc prevents the absorption of copper in Wilson's disease. Symptomatic patients should be treated initially with a chelating agent because zinc has a slow onset of action. When transferring from chelating treatment to zinc maintenance therapy, chelating treatment should be co-administered for 2–3 weeks until zinc produces its maximal effect.

PENICILLAMINE

Cautions concomitant nephrotoxic drugs (increased risk of toxicity); monitor urine for proteinuria; monitor blood and platelet count regularly (see below); **interactions:** Appendix 1 (penicillamine)

Renal impairment reduce dose and monitor renal function in mild impairment; avoid in moderate to severe impairment

Pregnancy fetal abnormalities reported rarely; avoid if possible

Breast-feeding manufacturer advises avoid unless potential benefit outweighs risk—no information available

Blood counts and urine tests Consider withdrawal if platelet count falls below 120 000/mm³ or white blood cells below 2500/mm³ or if 3 successive falls within reference range (can restart at reduced dose when counts return to within reference range but permanent withdrawal necessary if recurrence of leucopenia or thrombocytopenia)

Counselling Warn child and carer to tell doctor immediately if sore throat, fever, infection, non-specific illness, unexplained bleeding and bruising, purpura, mouth ulcers, or rashes develop

Contra-indications lupus erythematosus

Side-effects initially nausea, anorexia, fever, and skin reactions; taste loss (mineral supplements not recommended); blood disorders including thrombocytopenia, leucopenia, agranulocytosis and aplastic anaemia; proteinuria, rarely haematuria (withdraw immediately); haemolytic anaemia, nephrotic syndrome, lupus erythematosus-like syndrome, myasthenia gravis-like syndrome, polymyositis (rarely with cardiac involvement), dermatomyositis, mouth ulcers, stomatitis, alopecia, bronchiolitis and pneumonitis, pemphigus, Goodpasture's syndrome, and Stevens-Johnson syndrome also reported; male and female breast enlargement reported; in non-rheumatoid conditions rheumatoid arthritis-like syndrome also reported; late rashes (consider withdrawing treatment)

Indication and dose

Wilson's disease
- **By mouth**

Child 1 month–12 years 2.5 mg/kg twice daily before food, increased at 1–2 week intervals to 10 mg/kg twice daily

Child 12–18 years 0.75–1 g twice daily before food, max. 2 g daily for 1 year; usual maintenance dose 0.75–1 g daily

Cystinuria
- **By mouth**

Child 1 month–12 years 5–10 mg/kg twice daily before food, adjusted to maintain urinary cystine below 200 mg/litre; maintain adequate fluid intake

Child 12–18 years 0.5–1.5 g twice daily before food, adjusted to maintain urinary cystine below 200 mg/litre; maintain adequate fluid intake

Lead poisoning see Emergency Treatment of Poisoning, p. 44

Penicillamine (Non-proprietary) PoM
Tablets, penicillamine 125 mg, net price 20 = £1.96; 250 mg, 20 = £3.41. Label: 6, 22, counselling, blood disorder symptoms (see above)

Distamine® (Alliance) PoM
Tablets, all f/c, penicillamine 125 mg, net price 20 = £1.96; 250 mg, 20 = £3.41. Label: 6, 22, counselling, blood disorder symptoms (see above)

TRIENTINE DIHYDROCHLORIDE

Cautions see notes above; **interactions:** Appendix 1 (trientine)

Pregnancy teratogenic in *animal* studies—use only if benefit outweighs risk; monitor maternal and neonatal serum-copper concentrations

Side-effects nausea, rash; rarely anaemia

Indication and dose

Wilson's disease in patients intolerant of penicillamine

- By mouth

Child 2–12 years 0.6–1.5 g daily in 2–4 divided doses before food, adjusted according to response; reduce dose and increase frequency if nausea is a problem

Child 12–18 years 1.2–2.4 g daily in 2–4 divided doses before food, adjusted according to response; reduce dose and increase frequency if nausea is a problem

Trientine Dihydrochloride (Univar) PoM

Capsules, trientine dihydrochloride 300 mg. Label: 6, 22

Note The CSM has requested that in addition to the usual CSM reporting request, special records should also be kept by the pharmacist

ZINC ACETATE

Cautions portal hypertension (risk of hepatic decompensation when switching from chelating agent); monitor full blood count and serum cholesterol; **interactions:** Appendix 1 (zinc)

Pregnancy usual dose 25 mg 3 times daily adjusted according to plasma-copper concentration and urinary copper excretion

Contra-indications breast-feeding

Side-effects gastric irritation (usually transient; may be reduced if first dose taken mid-morning or with a little protein); *less commonly* sideroblastic anaemia and leucopenia

Indication and dose

Wilson's disease

Note dose expressed as elemental zinc

- By mouth

Child 1–6 years 25 mg twice daily

Child 6–16 years body-weight under 57 kg, 25 mg 3 times daily; body-weight 57 kg or over, 50 mg 3 times daily

Child 16–18 years 50 mg 3 times daily

Wilzin® (Orphan Europe) ▼ PoM

Capsules, zinc (as acetate) 25 mg (blue), net price 250-cap pack = £123.00; 50 mg (orange), 250-cap pack = £233.00. Label: 23

Administration capsules may be opened and the contents mixed with water

Carnitine deficiency

Carnitine is available for the management of primary carnitine deficiency due to inborn errors of metabolism or of secondary deficiency in haemodialysis patients.

Carnitine is also used in the treatment of some organic acidaemias; however, use in fatty acid oxidation is controversial.

CARNITINE

Cautions diabetes mellitus

Renal impairment accumulation may occur; monitoring of free and acyl carnitine in blood and urine recommended

Pregnancy appropriate to use; no evidence of teratogenicity in *animal* studies

Side-effects nausea, vomiting, abdominal pain, diarrhoea, fishy body odour; side-effects may be dose-related—monitor tolerance during first week and after any dose increase

Licensed use not licensed in children for secondary deficiency

Indication and dose

Primary deficiency, organic acidaemias and fatty acid oxidation disorders

- By mouth

Neonate 50 mg/kg twice daily, higher doses up to 200 mg/kg daily occasionally required

Child 1 month–18 years 50 mg/kg twice daily, higher doses up to 200 mg/kg daily or 3 g daily occasionally required

- By intravenous infusion

Neonate initially 100 mg/kg over 30 minutes followed by a continuous infusion of 4 mg/kg/hour

Child 1month–18 years initially 100 mg/kg over 30 minutes followed by a continuous infusion of 4mg/kg/hour

- By slow intravenous injection over 5–10 minutes

Neonate 100 mg/kg/daily in 2–4 divided doses

Child 1 month–18 years 100 mg/kg/daily in 2–4 divided doses

CARNITINE (*continued*)

Secondary deficiency in dialysis patients
- **By slow intravenous injection**

Child 1–18 years 20 mg/kg after each dialysis session, adjusted according to serum carnitine concentration

Administration for *intravenous infusion*, dilute injection with Sodium Chloride 0.9%, or Glucose 5% or 10%.

Carnitor® (Shire) PoM
Oral liquid, L-carnitine 100 mg/mL (10%), net price 10 × 10-mL (1-g) single-dose bottle = £35.00

Paediatric solution, L-carnitine 300 mg/mL (30%), net price 20 mL = £21.00
Excipients: include sorbitol and sucrose

Injection, L-carnitine 200 mg/mL, net price 5-mL amp = £11.90

Fabry's disease

Agalsidase beta, an enzyme produced by recombinant DNA technology, is licensed for long-term enzyme replacement therapy in Fabry's disease (a lysosomal storage disorder caused by deficiency of α-galactosidase).

AGALSIDASE BETA

Cautions interactions: Appendix 1 (agalsidase beta)

Pregnancy manufacturer advises avoid unless essential—no information available

Breast-feeding manufacturer advises avoid unless essential—no information available

Hypersensitivity reactions Hypersensitivity reactions common, calling for use of antihistamine, antipyretic and corticosteroid; consult product literature for details

Side-effects nausea, vomiting, oedema, hypertension, hypersensitivity reactions, fever, headache, tremor, myalgia, injection-site pain; commonly abdominal pain, bradycardia, tachycardia, palpitation, fatigue, drowsiness, paraesthesia, dizziness, anaemia, proteinuria, visual disturbances, and abnormal tear secretion

Indication and dose

Fabry's disease (specialist use only)
- **By intravenous infusion**

Child 16–18 years 1 mg/kg every 2 weeks

Administration for *intravenous infusion* reconstitute initially with Water for Injections (5 mg in 1.1 mL, 35 mg in 7.2 mL) to produce a solution containing 5 mg/mL; dilute requisite dose to 500 mL with Sodium Chloride 0.9% and give over at least 2 hours.

Fabrazyme (Genzyme) PoM
Intravenous infusion, powder for reconstitution, agalsidase beta, net price 5-mg vial = £325.50; 35-mg vial = £2269.20

Gaucher's disease

Imiglucerase, an enzyme produced by recombinant DNA technology, is administered as enzyme replacement therapy in Gaucher's disease, a familial disorder affecting principally the liver, spleen, bone marrow, and lymph nodes.

Miglustat, an inhibitor of glucosylceramide synthase, is licensed in adults for the treatment of mild to moderate type I Gaucher's disease in patients for whom imiglucerase is unsuitable; it is given by mouth.

IMIGLUCERASE

Cautions monitor for imiglucerase antibodies; when stabilised, monitor all parameters and response to treatment at intervals of 6–12 months

Pregnancy manufacturer advises use only if potential benefit outweighs risk—no information available

Breast-feeding no information available

Side-effects hypersensitivity reactions (including urticaria, angioedema, hypotension, flushing, tachycardia); *less commonly* nausea, vomiting, diarrhoea, abdominal cramps, fatigue, injection site reactions, headache, dizziness, fever

Indication and dose

Gaucher's disease type I (specialist use only)
- **By intravenous infusion over 1–2 hours**

Neonate 60 units/kg once every 2 weeks, adjusted according to response

Child 1 month–18 years 60 units/kg once every 2 weeks, adjusted according to response

Gaucher's disease type III (specialist use only)
- **By intravenous infusion over 1–2 hours**

Neonate 120 units/kg once every 2 weeks, adjusted according to response

Child 1 month–18 years 120 units/kg once every 2 weeks, adjusted according to response

Administration For *intravenous infusion*, dilute to a concentration of 0.2–0.4 units/mL with Sodium Chloride 0.9% or 0.45% infusion; max. infusion rate 1 unit/kg/minute

Cerezyme® (Genzyme) PoM
Intravenous infusion, powder for reconstitution, imiglucerase, net price 200-unit vial = £553.35; 400-unit vial = £1106.70

Mucopolysaccharidosis I

Laronidase, an enzyme produced by recombinant DNA technology, is licensed for long-term replacement therapy in the treatment of non-neurological manifestations of mucopolysaccharidosis I, a lysosomal storage disorder caused by deficiency of α-L- iduronidase.

LARONIDASE

Cautions interactions: Appendix 1 (laronidase)

Pregnancy manufacturer advises avoid unless essential—no information available

Breast-feeding manufacturer advises avoid—no information available

Infusion-related reactions Infusion-related reactions very common, calling for use of antihistamine and antipyretic; recurrent reactions may require corticosteroid; consult product literature for details

Side-effects flushing, musculoskeletal pain, rash, headache, abdominal pain

Indication and dose

Non-neurological manifestations of mucopolysaccharidosis I (specialist use only)

Child 5–18 years 100 units/kg once weekly

Administration for *intravenous infusion* dilute with Sodium Chloride 0.9%; body-weight under 20 kg, dilute to 100 mL, body-weight over 20 kg dilute to 250 mL; give through in-line filter (0.22 micron) initially at a rate of 2 units/kg/hour then increase gradually every 15 minutes to max. 43 units/kg/hour

Aldurazyme (Genzyme) PoM

Concentrate for intravenous infusion, laronidase 100 units/mL, net price 5-mL vial = £460.35

Urea cycle disorders

Sodium benzoate and **sodium phenylbutyrate** are used in the management of urea cycle disorders. Both, either singly or in combination, are indicated as adjunctive therapy in all patients with neonatal-onset disease and in those with late-onset disease who have a history of hyperammonaemic encephalopathy. Sodium benzoate is also used in non-ketotic hyperglycinaemia. In anuric states dialysis is necessary to treat hyperammonaemia.

Gastro-intestinal side-effects of sodium benzoate or sodium phenylbutyrate may be reduced by giving smaller doses more frequently. The preparations contain significant amounts of sodium; therefore, they should be used with caution in children with congestive heart failure, renal insufficiency and clinical conditions involving sodium retention with oedema.

The long-term management of urea cycle disorders includes oral maintenance treatment with sodium benzoate and sodium phenylbutyrate combined with a low protein diet and other drugs such as arginine or citrulline, depending on the specific disorder.

Carglumic acid is licensed for the treatment of hyperammonaemia due to *N*-acetylglutamate synthase deficiency.

ARGININE

Cautions monitor plasma pH and chloride

Contra-indications not to be used in the treatment of arginase deficiency

Pregnancy no information available

Breast-feeding no information available

Side-effects intravenous injection only: nausea, vomiting; flushing, hypotension; headache, numbness; hyperchloraemic metabolic acidosis; irritation at injection-site

Licensed use injection and tablets not licensed in children; powder licensed for urea cycle disorders in children

Indication and dose

Carbamylphosphate synthetase deficiency, ornithine carbamyl transferase deficiency; acute hyperammonaemia (specialist use only)

- **By intravenous infusion**

Neonate initially 200 mg/kg over 90 minutes followed by 8 mg/kg/hour

Child 1 month–18 years initially 200 mg/kg over 90 minutes followed by 8 mg/kg/hour

Maintenance treatment of hyperammonaemia (specialist use only)

- **By mouth**

Neonate 100 mg/kg/daily in 3–4 divided doses

Child 1 month–18 years 100 mg/kg/daily in 3–4 divided doses

9 Nutrition and blood

ARGININE (*continued*)

Citrullinaemia, arginosuccinic aciduria; acute hyperammonaemia (specialist use only)
- **By intravenous infusion**

Neonate initially 600 mg/kg over 90 minutes followed by 25 mg/kg/hour

Child 1 month–18 years initially 600 mg/kg over 90 minutes followed by 25 mg/kg/hour

Maintenance treatment of hyperammonaemia (specialist use only)
- **By mouth**

Neonate 100–175 mg/kg 3–4 times daily, with food, adjusted according to response

Child 1 month–18 years 100–175 mg/kg 3–4 times daily, with food, adjusted according to response

L-Arginine (Non-proprietary)

Tablets, L-arginine (as hydrochloride) 500 mg,

Oral solution, L-arginine (as hydrochloride) 50 mg/mL

Available as a manufactured special from Special Products Ltd, see guidance on unlicensed drugs, p. 7

Powder, L-arginine (as hydrochloride), net price 100 g = £8.39

Available from SHS

Prescribe as a borderline substance (ACBS). For use as a supplement in urea cycle disorders other than arginase deficiency, such as hyperammonaemia types I and II, citrullinaemia, arginosuccinic aciduria, and deficiency of N-acetyl glutamate synthetase

Injection, L-arginine (as hydrochloride) 500 mg/mL, 10-mL ampoules; 100 mg/mL, 200-mL amp

Available as a manufactured special from Special Products Ltd, see guidance on unlicensed drugs, p. 7

Note Other strengths may be available locally as manufactured specials

Administration dilute to a concentration of 20 mg/mL with Sodium Chloride 0.9% or 0.45%, *or* Glucose 5% or 10%; max. concentration 100 mg/mL; may be given orally

CARGLUMIC ACID

Cautions

Pregnancy manufacturer advises avoid unless essential—no information available

Breast-feeding manufacturer advises avoid unless essential—no information available

Side-effects raised transaminases, sweating

Indication and dose

N-acetyl glutamate synthase deficiency (initiated under specialist supervision)
- **By mouth**

Neonate 100 mg/kg daily in 2–4 divided doses adjusted according to response; usual max. 250 mg/kg daily

Child 1 month–18 years 100 mg/kg daily in 2–4 divided doses adjusted according to response; usual max. 250 mg/kg daily

Carbaglu® (Orphan Europe) ▼ PoM

Dispersible tablets, carglumic acid 200 mg, net price 15-tab pack = £679.00, 60-tab pack = £2685.00. Label: 13

CITRULLINE

Cautions

Pregnancy no information available

Breast-feeding no information available

Indication and dose

Carbamyl phosphate synthase deficiency, ornithine carbamyl transferase deficiency
- **By mouth**

Neonate 150 mg/kg daily in 3–4 divided doses, adjusted according to response

Child 1 month–18 years 150 mg/kg daily in 3–4 divided doses, adjusted according to response

Citrulline Powder (Non-proprietary)

Powder, L-citrulline, net price 100 g = £122.20

Available as a manufactured special from SHS, see guidance on unlicensed drugs p. 7

Administration May be mixed with other drinks or taken as a paste

SODIUM BENZOATE

Cautions see notes above; neonates (risk of kernicterus and increased side-effects)

Pregnancy no information available

Breast-feeding no information available

Side-effects nausea, vomiting, anorexia; irritability, lethargy, coma

Licensed use not licensed for use in children

Indication and dose

Acute hyperammonaemia due to urea cycle disorders (specialist use only)
- **By intravenous infusion**

Neonate initially 250 mg/kg over 90 minutes followed by 20 mg/kg/hour, adjusted according to response

Child 1 month–18 years initially 250 mg/kg over 90 minutes followed by 20 mg/kg/hour, adjusted according to response

SODIUM BENZOATE (*continued*)

Maintenance treatment of hyperammonaemia due to urea cycle disorders; non-ketotic hyperglycinaemia (specialist use only)

- By mouth

Neonate 50–150 mg/kg 3–4 times daily, with food, adjusted according to response

Child 1 month–18 years 50–150 mg/kg 3–4 times daily, with food, adjusted according to response

Administration for administration *by mouth*, oral solution or powder may be administered in fruit drinks; less soluble in acidic drinks

Sodium Benzoate (Non-proprietary) PoM

Tablets, sodium benzoate 500 mg

Available as a manufactured special from Special Products Ltd, see guidance on unlicensed drugs p. 7

Capsules, sodium benzoate 50 mg; 250 mg; 400 mg; 500 mg

Available as a manufactured special, see guidance on unlicensed drugs p. 7

Oral solution, sodium benzoate 100 mg/mL; 200 mg/mL; 300 mg/mL when reconstituted with water

Available as a manufactured special, see guidance on unlicensed drugs p. 7

Powder

Available as a manufactured special, see guidance on unlicensed drugs p. 7

Injection, sodium benzoate 200 mg/mL, 5-mL amp

Note Contains Na^+ 1.4 mmol /mL

Available as a manufactured special, see guidance on unlicensed drugs p. 7

Administration for *intravenous infusion*, dilute to a concentration of 20 mg/mL with Sodium Chloride 0.9% or 0.45%, *or* Glucose 5% or 10%; max. concentration 50 mg/mL

SODIUM PHENYLBUTYRATE

Cautions congestive heart failure, hepatic and renal impairment

Contra-indications

Pregnancy avoid

Breast-feeding avoid

Side-effects amenorrhoea and irregular menstrual cycles, decreased appetite, body odour, taste disturbances; less commonly nausea, vomiting, abdominal pain, peptic ulcer, pancreatitis, rectal bleeding, arrhythmia, oedema, syncope, depression, headache, rash, weight gain, renal tubular acidosis, aplastic anaemia, ecchymoses

Indication and dose

Acute hyperammonaemia due to urea cycle disorders (specialist use only)

- By continuous intravenous infusion

Neonate initially 250 mg/kg over 90 minutes followed by 20 mg/kg/hour adjusted according to response

Child 1 month–18 years initially 250 mg/kg over 90 minutes followed by 20 mg/kg/hour adjusted according to response

Maintenance treatment of hyperammonaemia due to urea cycle disorders (specialist use only)

- By mouth

Neonate 75–150 mg/kg 3–4 times daily, with food

Child 1 month–18 years 75–150 mg/kg 3–4 times daily, with food (max. 20 g daily)

Administration Oral dose may be mixed with fruit drinks, milk, or feeds

Sodium Phenylbutyrate (Non-proprietary) PoM

Injection, sodium phenylbutyratein 200 mg/mL, 5-mL amp

Note Contains Na^+ 1.1 mmol /mL

Available as a manufactured special from Martindale or Special Products Ltd, see guidance on unlicensed drugs p. 7

Administration for *intravenous infusion*, dilute to a concentration of 20 mg/mL (max. 50 mg/mL) with Glucose 5% or 10%

Ammonaps® (Orphan Europe) PoM

Tablets, sodium phenylbutyrate 500 mg. Contains Na^+ 2.7 mmol/tablet. Net price 250-tab pack = £493.00

Granules, sodium phenylbutyrate 940 mg/g. Contains Na^+ 5.4 mmol/g. Net price 266-g pack = £860.00

Note Granules should be mixed with food before taking

Nephropathic cystinosis

Mercaptamine (cysteamine) is available for the treatment of nephropathic cystinosis. The oral dose is increased over several weeks to avoid intolerance.

Mercaptamine eye drops are used in the management of ocular symptoms arising from the deposition of cystine crystals in the eye.

Phosphocysteamine is a pro-drug of mercaptamine; it is available from specialist centres only, as a powder or specially manufactured capsule. Mercaptamine does not contain phosphate, therefore, if transferring from phosphocysteamine to mercaptamine phosphate supplements may need to be initiated or adjusted. Mercaptamine 1 mg is approximately equivalent to 3 mg of phosphocysteamine.

Both mercaptamine and phosphocysteamine have a very unpleasant taste and smell, which can affect compliance.

All patients receiving mercaptamine and phosphocysteamine should be registered (contact local specialist centre for details).

> Safe Practice
> Mercaptamine has been confused with mercaptopurine; care must be taken to ensure the correct drug is prescribed and dispensed.

MERCAPTAMINE
(Cysteamine)

Cautions leucocyte-cystine concentration and haematological monitoring required—consult product literature; dose of phosphate supplement may need to be adjusted

Contra-indications hypersensitivity to mercaptamine or penicillamine

Pregnancy avoid

Breast-feeding avoid

Side-effects breath and body odour, nausea, vomiting, diarrhoea, anorexia, lethargy, fever, rash; also reported dehydration, hypertension, abdominal discomfort, gastroenteritis, drowsiness, encephalopathy, headache, nervousness, depression; anaemia, leucopenia, rarely gastro-intestinal ulceration and bleeding, seizures, hallucinations, urticaria, interstitial nephritis

Licensed use eye drops not licensed

Indication and dose

Nephropathic cystinosis (specialist use only)
- By mouth

Neonate initially 2–3 mg/kg 4 times daily, increased over 4–6 weeks to 12.5 mg/kg 4 times daily

Child 1 month–12 years or under 50 kg initially 2–3 mg/kg 4 times daily, increased over 4–6 weeks to 12.5 mg/kg 4 times daily

Child 12–18 years or over 50 kg initially 100 mg 4 times daily, increased over 4–6 weeks to 500 mg 4 times daily

Cystagon® (Orphan Europe) PoM

Capsules, mercaptamine (as bitartrate) 50 mg, net price 100-cap pack = £44.00; 150 mg, 100-cap pack = £125.00

Note For child under 6 years at risk of aspiration, capsules can be opened and contents sprinkled on food (at a temperature suitable for eating); avoid adding to acidic drinks (e.g. orange juice)

Eye drops

Mercaptamine (Non-proprietary)

Eye drops, mercaptamine 0.11%, 10 mL

Available as a manufactured special, see guidance on unlicensed drugs p. 7

Other metabolic disorders

Other metabolic disorders and the drugs used in their management include:

Amino acid disorders: maple syrup urine disease (thiamine section 9.6.2); tyrosinaemia type III, hawkinsinuria (Vitamin C, section 9.6.3); tyrosinaemia type I (nitisinone).

Mitochondrial disorders: isolated carboxylase defects, defects of biotin metabolism (biotin, see below); mitochondrial myopathies (ubidecarenone); congenital lactic acidosis (riboflavine and thiamine, section 9.6.2); respiratory chain defects (thiamine, section 9.6.2); pyruvate dehydrogenase defects (sodium dichloroacetate)

Homocystinuria and defects in cobalamin metabolism: betaine, pyridoxine (section 9.6.2), hydroxocobalamin (section 9.1.2)

Tetrahydrofolate reductase deficiency: (betaine, folic acid section 9.1.2)

BETAINE

Cautions

Pregnancy no information available

Breast-feeding no information available

Side-effects nausea, diarrhoea; rarely cerebral oedema (withdraw treatment)

Indication and dose

Homocystinuria; tetrahydrofolate reductase deficiency
- By mouth

Neonate 50 mg/kg twice daily, dose and frequency adjusted according to response

Child 1 month–18 years 50 mg/kg twice daily, dose and frequency adjusted according to response

Betaine (Non-proprietary) PoM

Powder (for oral solution), betaine anhydrous 500 mg/mL when reconstituted.

Available as a manufactured special from Special Products Ltd, see guidance on unlicensed drugs p. 7

Tablets, betaine anhydrous 500 mg

Available as a manufactured special from specialist importing company

Powder, betaine anhydrous 1 g in 1 level scoop

BIOTIN

(Vitamin H)

Cautions

Pregnancy no information available

Breast-feeding no information available

Indication and dose

Isolated carboxylase defects

- **By mouth or by slow intravenous injection**

Neonate 5 mg once daily, adjusted according to response; usual maintenance 10–50 mg daily, higher doses may be required

Child 1 month–18 years 10 mg once daily, adjusted according to response; usual maintenance 10–50 mg daily but up to 100 mg daily may be required

Defects of biotin metabolism

- **By mouth or by slow intravenous injection**

Neonate 10 mg once daily adjusted according to response; usual maintenance 5–20 mg daily but higher doses may be required

Child 1 month–18 years 10 mg once daily adjusted according to response; usual maintenance 5–20 mg daily but higher doses may be required

Biotin (Non-proprietary) PoM

Tablets, biotin 5 mg, 20-tab pack

Injection, biotin 5 mg/mL

Available from specialist importing company or via Roche

Administration tablets may be crushed and mixed with food or drink

NITISINONE

(NTBC)

Cautions

Pregnancy no information available

Breast-feeding no information available

Side-effects leucopenia, thrombocytopenia, hypoglycaemia

Indication and dose

Tyrosinaemia type I

- **By mouth**

Child 1 month–18 years initially 500 micrograms/kg twice daily, adjusted according to response; up to 2 mg/kg daily may be required

Nitisinone (Non-proprietary) PoM

Capsules, Nitisinone 2 mg, 5 mg, 10 mg

Available from Orphan Europe on a named patient basis

SODIUM DICHLOROACETATE

Cautions

Pregnancy no information available

Breast-feeding no information available

Side-effects polyneuropathy on prolonged use; abnormal oxalate metabolism; metabolic acidosis

Indication and dose

Pyruvate dehydrogenase defects

- **By mouth**

Neonate initially 12.5 mg/kg 4 times daily, adjusted according to response; up to 200 mg/kg daily may be required

Child 1 month–18 years initially 12.5 mg/kg 4 times daily, adjusted according to response; up to 200 mg/kg daily may be required

Sodium dichloroacetate (Non-proprietary) PoM

Powder (for oral solution), sodium dichloroacetate 50 mg/mL when reconstituted with water

Available as a manufactured special from Special Products Ltd, see guidance on unlicensed drugs, p. 7

UBIDECARENONE

(Ubiquinone, Co-enzyme Q10)

Cautions may reduce insulin requirement in diabetes mellitus; **interactions**: Appendix 1 (ubidecarenone)

Hepatic impairment reduce dose in moderate and severe liver disease

Side-effects nausea, diarrhoea, heartburn; rarely headache, irritability, agitation, dizziness

Licensed use not licensed for the treatment of mitochondrial disorders

Indication and dose

Mitochondrial disorders

- **By mouth**

Neonate initially 5 mg once or twice daily with food, adjusted according to response, up to 200 mg daily may be required

Child 1 month–18 years initially 5 mg once or twice daily with food, adjusted according to response, up to 300 mg daily may be required

Ubidecarenone (Non-proprietary) PoM

Oral solution ubidecarenone 50 mg/10mL

Tablets, ubidecarenone 10 mg

Capsules, ubidecarenone 10 mg, 30 mg

Available from specialist health food suppliers

9.8.2 Acute porphyrias

The acute porphyrias (acute intermittent porphyria, variegate porphyria, hereditary coproporphyria and 5-aminolaevulinic acid dehydratase deficiency porphyria) are hereditary disorders of haem biosynthesis; they have a prevalence of about 1 in 10 000 of the population.

Great care must be taken when prescribing for patients with acute porphyria since many drugs can induce acute porphyric crises. Since acute porphyrias are hereditary, relatives of affected individuals should be screened and advised about the potential danger of certain drugs.

Treatment of serious or life-threatening conditions should not be withheld from patients with acute porphyria. Where there is no safe alternative, urinary porphobilinogen excretion should be measured regularly; if it increases or symptoms occur, the drug can be withdrawn and the acute attack treated.

Haem arginate is administered by short intravenous infusion as haem replacement in moderate, severe or unremitting acute porphyria crises.

Supplies of haem arginate may be obtained outside office hours from the on-call pharmacist at:

St. James' University Hospital, Leeds
Tel: (0113) 243 3144 or
Tel: (0113) 283 7010

St Thomas' Hospital, London
Tel: (020) 7188 7188

HAEM ARGINATE

(Human hemin)

Cautions

Pregnancy manufacturer advises avoid unless essential

Breast-feeding manufacturer advises avoid unless essential—no information available

Side-effects rarely hypersensitivity reactions and fever; pain and thrombophlebitis at injection site

Indication and dose

Acute porphyrias (acute intermittent porphyria, porphyria variegata, hereditary coproporphyria)

- **By intravenous infusion**

Child 1 month–18 years 3 mg/kg once daily (max. 250 mg daily) for 4 days; if response inadequate, repeat 4-day course with close biochemical monitoring

Normosang® (Orphan Europe) ▼ PoM

Concentrate for intravenous infusion, haem arginate 25 mg/mL, net price 10-mL amp = £281.25

Administration administer over at least 30 minutes diluted in sodium chloride 0.9%; max. concentration 2.5 mg/mL

Drugs unsafe for use in acute porphyrias

The following list contains drugs on the UK market that have been classified as 'unsafe' in porphyria because they have been shown to be porphyrinogenic in animals or *in vitro*, or have been associated with acute attacks in patients. Absence of a drug from the following lists does not necessarily imply that the drug is safe. For many drugs no information about porphyria is available.

Further information may be obtained from www.porphyria-europe.com and also from:

Welsh Medicines Information Centre
University Hospital of Wales
Cardiff, CF14 4XW.
Tel: (029) 2074 2979/3877

Note Quite modest changes in chemical structure can lead to changes in porphyrinogenicity but where possible general statements have been made about groups of drugs; these should be checked first

Unsafe drug groups (check first)

Amphetamines
Anabolic Steroids
Antidepressants[1]
Antihistamines[2]
Barbiturates[3]
Contraceptives, hormonal[4]
Ergot Derivatives[5]
Gold Salts
Hormone Replacement Therapy[4]
Progestogens[4]
Statins[6]
Sulphonamides[7]
Sulphonylureas[8]

Unsafe drugs (check groups above first)

Aceclofenac
Alcohol
Amiodarone
Baclofen
Bromocriptine
Busulfan
Cabergoline
Carbamazepine
Carisoprodol
Chloral Hydrate [9]
Chlorambucil
Chloramphenicol
Chloroform[10]
Clindamycin
Clonidine
Cocaine
Colistin
Cyclophosphamide[11]
Cycloserine
Danazol
Dapsone
Dexfenfluramine
Dextropropoxyphene
Diazepam[12]
Diclofenac
Doxycycline
Econazole
Erythromycin
Etamsylate
Ethosuximide
Etomidate
Fenfluramine
Flupentixol
Griseofulvin
Halothane
Hydralazine
Hyoscine
Indinavir
Indapamide
Isometheptene Mucate
Isoniazid
Ketamine
Ketoconazole
Ketorolac
Lidocaine (lignocaine)[13]
Mebeverine
Mefenamic Acid[11]
Meprobamate
Methyldopa
Metoclopramide[11]
Metolazone
Metronidazole[11]
Metyrapone
Miconazole
Mifepristone
Minoxidil [11]
Nalidixic Acid
Nifedipine
Nitrofurantoin
Orphenadrine
Oxcarbazepine
Oxybutynin
Oxycodone
Oxytetracycline
Pentazocine[14]
Pentoxifylline (oxpentifylline)
Phenoxybenzamine
Phenytoin
Pivmecillinam
Porfimer
Probenecid
Pyrazinamide
Rifabutin [15]
Rifampicin [15]
Ritonavir
Simvastatin
Spironolactone
Sulfinpyrazone
Sulpiride
Tamoxifen
Temoporfin
Theophylline[16]
Tiagabine
Tinidazole
Topiramate
Triclofos[9]
Trimethoprim
Valproate[12]
Verapamil
Xipamide
Zuclopenthixol

1. Includes tricyclic (and related) and MAOIs; fluoxetine thought to be safe.
2. Chlorphenamine, ketotifen, loratadine, and alimemazine (trimeprazine) thought to be safe.
3. Includes primidone and thiopental.
4. Progestogens are more porphyrinogenic than oestrogens; oestrogens may be safe at least in replacement doses. Progestogens should be avoided whenever possible by all young women susceptible to acute porphyria; however, where non-hormonal contraception is inappropriate, progestogens may be used with extreme caution if the potential benefit outweighs risk. The risk of an acute attack is greatest in young women who have had a previous attack. Long-acting progestogen preparations should never be used in those at risk of acute porphyria.
5. Includes ergometrine (oxytocin probably safe), lisuride and pergolide.
6. Rosuvastatin thought to be safe.
7. Includes co-trimoxazole and sulfasalazine.
8. Glipizide is thought to be safe.
9. Although evidence of hazard is uncertain, manufacturer advises avoid.
10. Small amounts in medicines probably safe.
11. May be used with caution if safer alternative not available.
12. Status epilepticus has been treated successfully with intravenous diazepam.
13. For local anaesthesia, bupivacaine, lidocaine (lignocaine), and prilocaine are thought to be safe.
14. Buprenorphine, codeine, diamorphine, dihydrocodeine, fentanyl, morphine, and pethidine are thought to be safe.
15. Rifamycins have been used in a few patients without evidence of harm—use with caution if safer alternative not available.
16. Includes aminophylline.

10 Musculoskeletal and joint diseases

This chapter includes advice on the drug management of the following:

For treatment of septic arthritis see section 5.1, table 1.

10.1 Drugs used in rheumatic diseases

Juvenile idiopathic arthritis and other inflammatory disorders

Rheumatic diseases generally require symptomatic treatment to relieve pain, swelling, and stiffness, together with treatment to control and suppress disease activity. Treatment of juvenile idiopathic arthritis may involve non-steroidal anti-inflammatory drugs (NSAIDs) (section 10.1.1); a disease modifying antirheumatic drug (DMARD) (section 10.1.3), usually methotrexate or etanercept; and intra-articular, intravenous, or oral corticosteroids (section 10.1.2).

Soft-tissue and musculoskeletal disorders

The management of children with soft-tissue injuries and strains, and musculoskeletal disorders, may include temporary rest together with the local application of heat or cold, local massage and physiotherapy. For pain relief paracetamol (section 4.7.1) is often adequate and should be used first. Alternatively, the lowest effective dose of a NSAID may be used. If pain relief with either drug is inadequate, both paracetamol (in a full dose appropriate for the child) and a NSAID may be required.

10.1.1 Non-steroidal anti-inflammatory drugs

In *single doses* non-steroidal anti-inflammatory drugs (NSAIDs) have analgesic activity comparable to that of paracetamol (section 4.7.1), but paracetamol is preferred.

In regular *full dosage* NSAIDs have both a lasting analgesic and an anti-inflammatory effect which makes them particularly useful for the treatment of continuous or regular pain associated with inflammation.

Choice Differences in anti-inflammatory activity between different NSAIDs are small, but there is considerable variation in individual patient tolerance and response. A large proportion of children will respond to any NSAID; of the others, those who do not respond to one may well respond to another. Pain relief starts soon after taking the first dose and a full analgesic effect should normally be obtained within a week, whereas an anti-inflammatory effect may not be achieved (or may not be clinically assessable) for up to 3 weeks. In juvenile idiopathic arthritis, NSAIDs may take 4–12 weeks to be effective. If appropriate responses are not obtained within these times, another NSAID should be tried.

Differences exist between NSAIDs in the incidence and type of side-effects, and in the availability of appropriate formulations.

NSAIDs vary in their selectivity for inhibiting different types of cyclo-oxygenase; selective inhibition of cyclo-oxygenase-2 improves gastro-intestinal tolerance. However, in children gastro-intestinal symptoms are rare in those taking NSAIDs for short periods. The role of selective inhibitors of cyclo-oxygenase-2 is undetermined in children and in the light of emerging concerns about cardiovascular safety they should be used in preference to non-selective NSAIDs **only** when specifically indicated (i.e. for patients who are at a particularly high risk of developing gastroduodenal ulcer, perforation, or bleeding).

Ibuprofen and **naproxen** are propionic acid derivatives used in children.

Ibuprofen combines anti-inflammatory, analgesic, and antipyretic properties. It has fewer side-effects than other NSAIDs but its anti-inflammatory properties are weaker.

Naproxen combines good efficacy with a low incidence of side-effects.

Diclofenac, **indometacin**, **mefenamic acid**, and **piroxicam** have properties similar to those of propionic acid derivatives:

Diclofenac has actions and side-effects similar to those of naproxen.

Indometacin (indomethacin) has an action equal to or superior to that of naproxen, but with a high incidence of side-effects including headaches, dizziness, and gastro-intestinal disturbances. It is rarely used in children and should be reserved for when other NSAIDs have been unsuccessful.

Mefenamic acid has minor anti-inflammatory properties. Occasionally, it has been associated with diarrhoea and haemolytic anaemia which require discontinuation of treatment.

Piroxicam is as effective as naproxen and has a prolonged duration of action which permits once-daily administration. It has more gastro-intestinal side-effects than ibuprofen.

Meloxicam is a selective inhibitor of cyclo-oxygenase-2. Its use may be considered in adolescents intolerant to other NSAIDs.
For the role of aspirin in children see section 2.9.

Dental and orofacial pain Most mild to moderate dental pain and inflammation is effectively relieved by **ibuprofen**. Ibuprofen causes gastro-intestinal irritation, but in an appraisal of the relative safety of 7 non-selective NSAIDs the CSM has assessed it to have the lowest risk of serious gastro-intestinal side-effects (see below).

For further information on the management of dental and orofacial pain, see p. 235.

Cautions and contra-indications NSAIDs should be used with caution in children with a history of hypersensitivity to any NSAID—which includes those in whom attacks of asthma, angioedema, urticaria or rhinitis have been precipitated by any NSAID. NSAIDs should also be used with caution during pregnancy (see below) and breast-feeding (see individual drug monographs), and in coagulation defects. Caution may also be required in children with allergic disorders.

In patients with renal, cardiac, or hepatic impairment caution is required since the use of NSAIDs may result in deterioration of renal function (see also under Side-effects below); the dose should be kept as **low as possible** and renal function should be **monitored**. In mild renal impairment the lowest effective dose should be used and renal function monitored; sodium and water retention may occur, as may deterioration in renal function possibly leading to renal failure. In moderate to severe renal impairment NSAIDs should be avoided if possible.

Most manufacturers advise avoiding NSAIDs during pregnancy or avoiding them unless the potential benefit outweighs risk. Ibuprofen and diclofenac are generally considered safe during the first and second trimesters. In the third trimester, NSAIDs are associated with a risk of closure of fetal ductus arteriosus and possibly persistent pulmonary hypertension of the newborn; also, labour may be delayed and its duration may be increased.

NSAIDs are generally contra-indicated if there is active or previous gastro-intestinal ulceration or bleeding; however, some children may require NSAIDs for effective relief of pain and stiffness, and prophylaxis and treatment of NSAID-associated peptic ulcers may be necessary (see section 1.3).

For **interactions** of NSAIDs, see Appendix 1 (NSAIDs).

Side-effects The side-effects of NSAIDs vary in severity and frequency. Gastro-intestinal discomfort, nausea, diarrhoea, and occasionally bleeding and ulceration may occur. Children appear to tolerate NSAIDs better than adults and gastro-intestinal side-effects are less common; use of gastroprotective drugs such as ranitidine and omeprazole may not be necessary. Other side-effects include hypersensitivity reactions (particularly rashes, angioedema, and bronchospasm), headache, dizziness, nervousness, depression, drowsiness, insomnia, vertigo, hearing disturbances such as tinnitus, photosensitivity, and haematuria. Blood disorders have also occurred. Fluid retention may occur; blood pressure may be raised. Renal failure may be provoked by NSAIDs especially in patients with pre-existing renal impairment (**important**, see also under Cautions above). Rarely, papillary necrosis or interstitial fibrosis associated with NSAIDs may lead to renal failure. Hepatic damage, alveolitis, pulmonary eosinophilia, pancreatitis, eye changes, Stevens-Johnson syndrome and toxic epidermal necrolysis are other rare side-effects. Induction of or exacerbation of colitis has been reported. Aseptic meningitis has been reported rarely with NSAIDs; patients with connective tissue disorders such as systemic lupus erythematosus may be especially susceptible.

Overdosage: see Emergency Treatment of Poisoning, p. 35.

IBUPROFEN

Cautions see notes above; **interactions:** Appendix 1 (NSAIDs)

Hepatic impairment increased risk of gastro-intestinal bleeding and can cause fluid retention; avoid in severe liver disease

Breast-feeding amount too small to be harmful, but some manufacturers advise avoid

Contra-indications see notes above

Side-effects see notes above; **overdosage:** see Emergency Treatment of Poisoning, p. 35

Licensed use not licensed for use in children under 3 months or body-weight under 5 kg

Indication and dose

Mild to moderate pain, pain and inflammation of soft-tissue injuries, pyrexia

- By mouth

Child 1–3 months and body-weight over 5 kg 5 mg/kg 3–4 times daily preferably after food; in severe conditions and body-weight over 5 kg max. 30 mg/kg daily in 3–4 divided doses

Child 3–6 months and body-weight over 5 kg 50 mg 3 times daily preferably after food; in severe conditions up to 30 mg/kg daily in 3–4 divided doses

Child 6 months–1 year 50 mg 3–4 times daily preferably after food; in severe conditions up to 30 mg/kg daily in 3–4 divided doses

Child 1–4 years 100 mg 3 times daily preferably after food; in severe conditions up to 30 mg/kg daily in 3–4 divided doses

Child 4–7 years 150 mg 3 times daily preferably after food; in severe conditions up to 30 mg/kg in 3–4 divided doses; max. 2.4 g daily

Child 7–10 years 200 mg 3 times daily preferably after food; in severe conditions up to 30 mg/kg in 3–4 divided doses; max. 2.4 g daily

IBUPROFEN (*continued*)

Child 10–12 years 300 mg 3 times daily preferably after food; in severe conditions up to 30 mg/kg in 3–4 divided doses; max. 2.4 g daily

Child 12–18 years 200–400 mg 3–4 times daily preferably after food; increased if necessary to max. 2.4 g daily

Pain and inflammation in rheumatic disease including juvenile idiopathic arthritis
- **By mouth**

Child 3 months–18 years (and body-weight over 5 kg) 10 mg/kg 3–4 times daily preferably after food; in systemic juvenile idiopathic arthritis up to 60 mg/kg daily in 4–6 divided doses

Post-immunisation pyrexia in infants
- **By mouth**

Child 2–3 months 50 mg as a single dose

Closure of patent ductus arteriosus in neonates see section 2.14

Ibuprofen (Non-proprietary) PoM

Tablets, coated, ibuprofen 200 mg, net price 84-tab pack = £2.12; 400 mg, 84-tab pack = £2.66; 600 mg, 84-tab pack = £4.10. Label: 21
Brands include *Arthrofen®*, *Ebufac®*, *Rimafen®*

Oral suspension, ibuprofen 100 mg/5 mL, net price 100 mL = £2.15, 150 mL = £2.71, 500 mL = £8.88. Label: 21
Note Sugar-free versions are available and can be ordered by specifying 'sugar-free' on the prescription
Brands include *Calprofen®*, *Fenpaed®*, *Galprofen®*, *Nurofen® for Children*, *Orbifen® for Children*

Dental prescribing on NHS Ibuprofen Tablets and Ibuprofen Oral Suspension Sugar-free may be prescribed

Brufen® (Abbott) PoM

Tablets, all magenta, ibuprofen 200 mg (s/c), net price 20 = 82p; 400 mg (s/c), 20 = £1.63; 600 mg (f/c), 20 = £2.45. Label: 21

Syrup, orange, ibuprofen 100 mg/5 mL. Net price 500 mL = £8.07. Label: 21

Granules, effervescent, ibuprofen 600 mg/sachet. Net price 20-sachet pack = £6.80. Label: 13, 21
Note Contains sodium approx. 9 mmol/sachet

Preparations on sale to the public

Many preparations on sale to the public contain **ibuprofen**. To identify the active ingredients in such preparations consult the product literature or manufacturer.
Note The correct proprietary name should be ascertained—many products have very similar names but different active ingredients.

Modified release

Brufen Retard® (Abbott) PoM

Tablets, m/r, f/c, ibuprofen 800 mg, net price 56-tab pack = £6.74. Label: 25, 27

Fenbid® (Goldshield) PoM

Spansule® (= capsule m/r), maroon/pink, enclosing off-white pellets, ibuprofen 300 mg. Net price 120-cap pack = £9.64. Label: 25

DICLOFENAC SODIUM

Cautions see notes above; **interactions:** Appendix 1 (NSAIDs)

Hepatic impairment increased risk of gastro-intestinal bleeding and fluid retention; avoid in severe liver disease

Breast-feeding amount too small to be harmful

Contra-indications see notes above; porphyria (section 9.8.2)

Intravenous use Additional contra-indications include concomitant NSAID or anticoagulant use (including low-dose heparin), history of haemorrhagic diathesis, history of confirmed or suspected cerebrovascular bleeding, operations with high risk of haemorrhage, history of asthma, moderate or severe renal impairment, hypovolaemia, dehydration

Rectal route Additional contra-indications include ulcerative or acute inflammatory conditions of the anus, rectum, or sigmoid colon

Side-effects see notes above; suppositories may cause rectal irritation; injection site reactions

Licensed use licensed for *oral* (25 mg e/c tablets only) and *rectal* (12.5 mg and 25 mg suppositories only) use in children 1–12 years for bone pain and inflammation associated with juvenile idiopathic arthritis; licensed for *rectal* (12.5 mg and 25 mg suppositories only) use in children 6–12 years for postoperative pain; diclofenac potassium tablets not licensed for use in children under 14 years; *injection* not licensed for use in children

Indication and dose

Mild to moderate pain, pyrexia, relief of pain and inflammation in soft-tissue disorders
- **By mouth or by rectum**

Child 6 months–18 years 0.3–1 mg/kg 3 times daily (max. total dose 150 mg daily)

- **By intravenous infusion or deep intramuscular injection into gluteal muscle**

Child 2–18 years 0.3–1 mg/kg once or twice daily (for max. 2 days; total daily dose not to exceed 150 mg daily)

Postoperative pain
- **By rectum**

Child 6–18 years 1–2 mg/kg (max. 150 mg) daily in 2–3 divided doses for max. 4 days

Pain and inflammation in rheumatic disease including juvenile idiopathic arthritis
- **By mouth**

Child 6 months–18 years 3–5 mg/kg daily in 3–4 divided doses (max. total dose 150 mg daily)

DICLOFENAC SODIUM (*continued*)

Administration for *intravenous infusion*, dilute 75 mg with 100–500 mL Glucose 5% *or* Sodium Chloride 0.9% (previously buffered with 0.5 mL Sodium Bicarbonate 8.4% solution *or* with 1 mL Sodium Bicarbonate 4.2% solution); give over 30–120 minutes

Diclofenac Sodium (Non-proprietary) PoM

Tablets, both e/c, diclofenac sodium 25 mg, net price 84-tab pack = £1.52; 50 mg, 84-tab pack = £2.14. Label: 5, 25

Note Other brands include *Acoflam®*, *Defenac®*, *Dicloflex®*, *Diclovol®*, *Diclozip®*, *Fenactol®*, *Flamrase®*, *Lofensaid®*, *Volraman®*

Suppositories, diclofenac sodium 100 mg, net price 10 = £3.04

Brands include *Econac®*

Injection, diclofenac sodium 25 mg/mL. Net price 3-mL amp = 74p

Note Licensed for intramuscular use

Voltarol® (Novartis) PoM

Tablets, both e/c, diclofenac sodium 25 mg (yellow), net price 84-tab pack = £3.67; 50 mg (brown), 84-tab pack = £5.71. Label: 5, 25

Dispersible tablets, sugar-free, pink, diclofenac, equivalent to diclofenac sodium 50 mg, net price 21-tab pack = £5.63. Label: 13, 21

Injection, diclofenac sodium 25 mg/mL. Net price 3-mL amp = 83p

Excipients: include benzyl alcohol (see Excipients, p. 3)

Suppositories, diclofenac sodium 12.5 mg, net price 10 = 71p; 25 mg, 10 = £1.26; 50 mg, 10 = £2.07; 100 mg, 10 = £3.70

Emulgel® gel, section 10.3.2

Diclofenac potassium

Voltarol® Rapid (Novartis) PoM

Tablets, s/c, diclofenac potassium 25 mg (red), net price 28-tab pack = £3.67; 50 mg (brown), 28-tab pack = £7.03

Dose

Rheumatic disease, musculoskeletal disorders, postoperative pain

Child 14–18 years 75–100 mg daily in 2–3 divided doses

Modified release

Diclomax SR® (Provalis) PoM

Capsules, m/r, yellow, diclofenac sodium 75 mg. Net price 56-cap pack = £13.01. Label: 21, 25

Diclomax Retard® (Provalis) PoM

Capsules, m/r, diclofenac sodium 100 mg. Net price 28-tab pack = £9.36. Label: 21, 25

Motifene® 75 mg (Sankyo) PoM

Capsules, e/c, m/r, diclofenac sodium 75 mg (enclosing e/c pellets containing diclofenac sodium 25 mg and m/r pellets containing diclofenac sodium 50 mg). Net price 56-cap pack = £8.00. Label: 25

Voltarol® 75 mg SR (Novartis) PoM

Tablets, m/r, pink, diclofenac sodium 75 mg. Net price 28-tab pack = £8.08; 56-tab pack = £16.15. Label: 21, 25

Note Other brands of modified-release tablets containing diclofenac sodium 75 mg include *Acoflam® 75 SR, Defenac® SR, Dexomon® 75 SR, Dicloflex® 75 SR, Diclovol® SR, Fenactol® 75 mg SR, Flamatak® 75 MR, Flamrase® SR, Flexotard® MR 75, Rheumatac® Retard 75, Rhumalgan® CR, Slofenac® SR, Volsaid® Retard 75*

Voltarol® Retard (Novartis) PoM

Tablets, m/r, red, diclofenac sodium 100 mg. Net price 28-tab pack = £11.84. Label: 21, 25

Note Other brands of modified-release tablets containing diclofenac sodium 100 mg include *Acoflam® Retard, Defenac® Retard, Dexomon® Retard 100, Dicloflex® Retard, Diclovol® Retard, Fenactol® Retard 100 mg, Flamatak® 100 MR, Flamrase® SR, Rhumalgan® CR, Slofenac® SR, Volsaid® Retard 100*

INDOMETACIN
(Indomethacin)

Cautions see notes above; also epilepsy, psychiatric disturbances; during prolonged therapy ophthalmic and blood examinations particularly advisable; avoid rectal administration in proctitis and haemorrhoids; **interactions**: Appendix 1 (NSAIDs)

Skilled tasks Dizziness may affect performance of skilled tasks (e.g. driving)

Hepatic impairment increased risk of gastro-intestinal bleeding and can cause fluid retention; avoid in severe liver disease

Breast-feeding amount probably too small to be harmful—manufacturer advises avoid

Contra-indications see notes above

Side-effects see notes above; frequently gastro-intestinal disturbances (including diarrhoea), headache, dizziness, and light-headedness; also gastro-intestinal ulceration and bleeding; rarely, drowsiness, confusion, insomnia, convulsions, psychiatric disturbances, depression, syncope, blood disorders (particularly thrombocytopenia), hypertension, hyperglycaemia, blurred vision, corneal deposits, peripheral neuropathy, and intestinal strictures; suppositories may cause rectal irritation and occasional bleeding

Licensed use not licensed for use in children

Indication and dose

Relief of pain and inflammation in rheumatic diseases including juvenile idiopathic arthritis

- By mouth

Child 1 month –18 years 0.5–1 mg/kg twice daily; higher doses may be used under specialist supervision

Closure of patent ductus arteriosus in premature babies section 2.14

INDOMETACIN (*continued*)

Indometacin (Non-proprietary) PoM
Capsules, indometacin 25 mg, net price 20 = £1.26; 50 mg, 20 = £1.06. Label: 21, counselling, driving, see above
Brands include *Rimacid®*

Suppositories, indometacin 100 mg. Net price 10 = £1.20. Counselling, driving, see above

Suspension, available as manufactured special and from specialist importing companies

Modified release

Indometacin m/r preparations PoM
Capsules, m/r, indometacin 75 mg. Label: 21, 25, counselling, driving, see above
Brands include *Indolar SR®*, *Indomax 75 SR®*, *Pardelprin®*, *Rheumacin LA®*, *Slo-Indo®*

MEFENAMIC ACID

Cautions see notes above; porphyria (section 9.8.2); **interactions:** Appendix 1 (NSAIDs)

Hepatic impairment increased risk of gastro-intestinal bleeding and can cause fluid retention; avoid in severe liver disease

Breast-feeding amount too small to be harmful but manufacturer advises avoid

Contra-indications see notes above; inflammatory bowel disease

Side-effects see notes above; drowsiness; diarrhoea or rashes (withdraw treatment); thrombocytopenia, haemolytic anaemia (positive Coombs' test), and aplastic anaemia reported; convulsions in overdosage

Licensed use in children over 6 months for relief of pain and inflammation associated with juvenile idiopathic arthritis, postoperative analgesia, mild to moderate pain; in children over 12 for primary dysmenorrhoea and menorrhagia

Indication and dose

Relief of pain and inflammation associated with juvenile idiopathic arthritis, postoperative analgesia, mild to moderate pain —not recommended so no dose stated

Acute pain including dysmenorrhoea, menorrhagia
- By mouth

Child 12–18 years 500 mg 3 times daily for not longer than 7 days

Mefenamic Acid (Non-proprietary) PoM
Capsules, mefenamic acid 250 mg. Net price 20 = 72p. Label: 21

Tablets, mefenamic acid 500 mg, net price 28-tab pack = £2.93. Label: 21

MELOXICAM

Cautions see notes above; **interactions:** Appendix 1 (NSAIDs)

Hepatic impairment increased risk of gastro-intestinal bleeding and can cause fluid retention; avoid in severe liver disease

Breast-feeding no information available—manufacturer advises avoid

Contra-indications see notes above; renal failure (unless receiving dialysis); severe heart failure

Side-effects see notes above

Licensed use in children over 15 for pain and inflammation in rheumatic disease and ankylosing spondylitis

Indication and dose

Relief of pain and inflammation in juvenile idiopathic arthritis and other musculoskeletal disorders in adolescents intolerant to other NSAIDs
- By mouth

Child 12–18 years and body-weight under 50 kg 7.5 mg once daily

Child 12–18 years and body-weight over 50 kg 15 mg once daily

Meloxicam (Non-proprietary) PoM
Tablets, meloxicam 7.5 mg, net-price 30-tab pack = £8.95; 15 mg, 30-tab pack = £11.95

Mobic® (Boehringer Ingelheim) PoM
Tablets, both yellow, scored, meloxicam 7.5 mg, net price 30-tab pack = £9.30; 15 mg, 30-tab pack = £12.93. Label: 21

NAPROXEN

Cautions see notes above; **interactions:** Appendix 1 (NSAIDs)

Hepatic impairment increased risk of gastro-intestinal bleeding and can cause fluid retention; avoid in severe liver disease

Breast-feeding amount too small to be harmful but manufacturer advises avoid

Contra-indications see notes above

Side-effects see notes above

Licensed use children over 5 years—juvenile idiopathic arthritis; children over 16 years—pain and inflammation in rheumatic disease and other musculoskeletal disorders, dysmenorrhoea

NAPROXEN (*continued*)

Indication and dose

Juvenile idiopathic arthritis, pain and inflammation in rheumatic disease and other musculoskeletal disorders, dysmenorrhoea

- By mouth

Child 1 month–18 years 5–10 mg/kg twice daily; in severe disease, 10–15 mg/kg twice daily for short-term use only. (max. 1 g daily)

Naproxen (Non-proprietary) PoM

Tablets, naproxen 250 mg, net price 28-tab pack = 46p; 500 mg, 28-tab pack = £1.60. Label: 21

Brands include *Arthroxen®*

Tablets, e/c, naproxen 250 mg, net price 56-tab pack = £4.15; 375 mg, 56-tab pack = £6.83; 500 mg, 56-tab pack = £8.15. Label: 5, 25

Suspension, available from specialist importing companies

Naprosyn® (Roche) PoM

Tablets, all scored, naproxen 250 mg (buff), net price 56-tab pack = £4.55; 500 mg (buff), 56-tab pack = £9.09. Label: 21

Tablets, e/c, (*Naprosyn EC®*), naproxen 250 mg, net price 56-tab pack = £4.55; 375 mg, 56-tab pack = £6.82; 500 mg, 56-tab pack = £9.09. Label: 5, 25

Synflex® (Roche) PoM

Tablets, blue, naproxen sodium 275 mg. Net price 60-tab pack = £7.54. Label: 21

Note 275 mg naproxen sodium ≡ 250 mg naproxen

PIROXICAM

Cautions see notes above; avoid in porphyria (section 9.8.2); **interactions:** Appendix 1 (NSAIDs)

Hepatic impairment increased risk of gastro-intestinal bleeding and can cause fluid retention; avoid in severe liver disease

Breast-feeding amount too small to be harmful

Contra-indications see notes above

Side-effects see notes above; pain at injection site (occasionally tissue damage)

Licensed use dispersible tablets only for treatment of juvenile idiopathic arthritis in children over 6 years

Indication and dose

Relief of bone pain and inflammation in juvenile idiopathic arthritis and musculoskeletal disorders

- By mouth

Child 6–18 years and body-weight under 15 kg 5 mg daily

Child 6–18 years and body-weight 16–25 kg 10 mg daily

Child 6–18 years and body-weight 26–45 kg 15 mg daily

Child 6–18 years and body-weight over 46 kg 20 mg daily

Piroxicam (Non-proprietary) PoM

Capsules, piroxicam 10 mg, net price 56-cap pack = £4.40; 20 mg, 28-cap pack = £3.58. Label: 21

Dispersible tablets, piroxicam 10 mg, net price 56-tab pack = £9.33; 20 mg, 28-tab pack = £12.48. Label: 13, 21

Feldene® (Pfizer) PoM

Capsules, piroxicam 10 mg (maroon/blue), net price 56-cap pack = £7.20; 20 mg (maroon), 28-cap pack = £7.20. Label: 21

Tablets, (*Feldene Melt®*), piroxicam 20 mg, net price 28-tab pack = £9.83. Label: 10, patient information leaflet, 21

Excipients: include aspartame equivalent to phenylalanine 140 micrograms/tablet (section 9.4.1)

Note Tablets may be halved [unlicensed] to give 10-mg dose; tablet placed on tongue and allowed to dissolve or may be swallowed

Dispersible tablets, piroxicam 10 mg (scored), net price 56-tab pack = £11.70; 20 mg, 28-tab pack = £11.70. Label: 13, 21

Brexidol® (Trinity) PoM

Tablets, yellow, scored, piroxicam (as betadex) 20 mg, net price 30-tab pack = £12.22. Label: 21

10.1.2 Corticosteroids

10.1.2.1 Systemic corticosteroids

The general actions and uses of the corticosteroids are described in section 6.3. In children with rheumatic diseases corticosteroids should be reserved for specific indications (e.g. when other anti-inflammatory drugs are unsuccessful) and should be used only under the supervision of a specialist.

Systemic corticosteroids may be considered for the management of juvenile idiopathic arthritis in systemic disease or when several joints are affected. Systemic corticosteroids may also be considered in severe, possibly life-threatening conditions such as systemic lupus erythematosus, systemic vasculitis, juvenile dermatomyositis, Behçet disease, and polyarticular joint disease.

In severe conditions, short courses ('pulses') of high-dose intravenous methylprednisolone or a pulsed oral corticosteroid may be particularly effective for providing rapid relief, and has fewer long-term adverse effects than continuous treatment.

Corticosteroid doses should be reduced with care because relapse may occur if the reduction is too rapid. If complete discontinuation of corticosteroids is not possible, consideration should be given to alternate day (or alternate high-dose, low-dose) administration; on days when no corticosteroid is given, or a lower dose is given, an additional dose of a NSAID may be helpful. In some conditions, alternative treatment using an antimalarial may be appropriate, or concomitant use of corticosteroid sparing-drugs, such as azathioprine and cyclophosphamide may prove useful; in less severe conditions treatment with a NSAID alone may be adequate.

Administration of corticosteroids may result in suppression of growth and may affect the development of puberty. The risk of corticosteroid-induced osteoporosis should be considered for those on long-term corticosteroid treatment (section 6.6); corticosteroids may also increase the risk of osteopenia in those unable to exercise. For the disadvantages of corticosteroid treatment see section 6.3.2.

10.1.2.2 Local corticosteroid injections

Corticosteroids are injected locally for an anti-inflammatory effect. In inflammatory conditions of the joints, including juvenile idiopathic arthritis, they are given by *intra-articular injection* as an adjunct to long-term therapy to reduce swelling and deformity in one or a few joints. Aseptic precautions (e.g. a no-touch technique) are essential, as is a clinician skilled in the technique; infected areas should be avoided and general anaesthesia, or local anaesthesia, or conscious sedation should be used. Occasionally an acute inflammatory reaction develops after an intra-articular or soft-tissue injection of a corticosteroid. This may be a reaction to the microcrystalline suspension of the corticosteroid used, but must be distinguished from sepsis introduced into the injection site.

Triamcinolone hexacetonide is preferred for intra-articular injection because it is almost insoluble and has a long-acting (depot) effect. Triamcinolone acetonide and methylprednisolone may also be considered for intra-articular injection into larger joints, whilst hydrocortisone acetate should be reserved for smaller joints or for soft-tissue injections. Flushing has been reported with intra-articular corticosteroid injections. Intra-articular injections may affect the hyaline cartilage and each joint should usually be treated no more than 3–4 times in one year.

A smaller amount of corticosteroid may also be injected directly into soft tissues for the relief of inflammation in conditions such as *tennis* or *golfer's elbow* or *compression neuropathies*. In *tendinitis*, injections should be made into the tendon sheath and not directly into the tendon (due to the absence of a true tendon sheath, the Achilles tendon should not be injected). A soluble preparation (e.g. containing betamethasone or dexamethasone sodium phosphate) is preferred for injection into the carpal tunnel.

Corticosteroid injections are also injected into soft tissues for the treatment of skin lesions (see section 13.4).

LOCAL CORTICOSTEROID INJECTIONS

Cautions see notes above and consult product literature; see also section 6.3.2

Contra-indications see notes above and consult product literature

Side-effects see notes above and consult product literature

Licensed use hydrocortisone acetate for intra-articular injection; triamcinolone acetonide for intra-articular injection in children over 6 years; methylprednisolone acetate for intra-articular injection

Indication and dose

See under preparations

LOCAL CORTICOSTEROID INJECTIONS (*continued*)

Hydrocortisone acetate

Hydrocortistab® (Sovereign) PoM
Injection, (aqueous suspension), hydrocortisone acetate 25 mg/mL. Net price 1-mL amp = £4.77

Dose

- **By intra-articular or intrasynovial injection** (for details consult product literature)
  Child 1 month–12 years 5–30 mg according to size of child and joint
  Child 12–18 years 5–50 mg according to size of child and joint
  Note Where appropriate may be repeated at intervals of 21 days; not more than 3 joints should be treated on any one day

Methylprednisolone acetate

Depo-Medrone® (Pharmacia) PoM
Injection (aqueous suspension), methylprednisolone acetate 40 mg/mL. Net price 1-mL vial = £2.87; 2-mL vial = £5.15; 3-mL vial = £7.47

Depo-Medrone® with Lidocaine (Pharmacia) PoM
Injection (aqueous suspension), methylprednisolone acetate 40 mg, lidocaine hydrochloride 10 mg/mL. Net price 1-mL vial = £3.28; 2-mL vial = £5.88

Triamcinolone hexacetonide

Available on a named patient basis from specialist import companies.

Triamcinolone acetonide

Adcortyl® Intra-articular/Intradermal (Squibb) PoM
Injection (aqueous suspension), triamcinolone acetonide 10 mg/mL. Net price 1-mL amp = £1.02; 5-mL vial = £4.14

Dose

- **By intra-articular injection or intrasynovial injection** (for details consult product literature)
  Child 1–18 years 500 micrograms/kg for smaller joints, max. 20 mg for small joints and max. 10 mg for finger and toe joints; 1 mg/kg for larger joints (max. 40 mg), may be repeated for relapse

Kenalog® Intra-articular/Intramuscular (Squibb) PoM
Injection (aqueous suspension), triamcinolone acetonide 40 mg/mL, net price 1-mL vial = £1.70; 1-mL prefilled syringe = £2.11; 2-mL prefilled syringe = £3.66
Note Intramuscular needle with prefilled syringe should be replaced for intra-articular injection

Dose

- **By intra-articular or intrasynovial injection** (for details consult product literature)
  Child 1–18 years 1 mg/kg for larger joints (max. 40 mg), 500 micrograms/kg for smaller joints, max. 20 mg for small joints and max. 10 mg for finger and toe joints; may be repeated for relapse

10.1.3 Drugs which suppress the rheumatic disease process

Certain drugs such as methotrexate, etanercept, and sulfasalazine may suppress the disease process in *juvenile idiopathic arthritis*; these drugs are known as disease-modifying antirheumatic drugs (DMARDs). In children, disease-modifying antirheumatic drugs should generally be used under specialist supervision.

Some children with *juvenile idiopathic arthritis* (juvenile chronic arthritis) do not require disease-modifying antirheumatic drugs. Methotrexate is effective in juvenile idiopathic arthritis; sulfasalazine is an alternative but should be avoided in systemic-onset juvenile idiopathic arthritis. Gold and penicillamine are no longer used. For the role of etanercept in polyarticular-course juvenile idiopathic arthritis, see p. 560.

Unlike NSAIDs, disease modifying anti-rheumatic drugs can affect the progression of disease but they require 4–6 months of treatment for a full therapeutic response. If one of these drugs does not lead to objective benefit within 6 months of initiating treatment or 3 months after maximum treatment, it should be discontinued and a different drug tried. Response to a disease-modifying antirheumatic drug may allow the dose of the NSAID to be reduced.

Disease-modifying antirheumatic drugs may improve not only the symptoms and signs of inflammatory joint disease but also extra-articular manifestations such as vasculitis. They reduce the erythrocyte sedimentation rate and C-reactive protein.

Antimalarials

The antimalarial **hydroxychloroquine** is rarely used to treat juvenile idiopathic arthritis. Hydroxychloroquine may also be useful for systemic or discoid lupus erythematosus, particularly involving cutaneous and joint manifestations; and in sarcoidosis.

Retinopathy (see below) occurs rarely provided that the recommended doses are not exceeded.

Mepacrine is sometimes used in discoid lupus erythematosus [unlicensed].

Cautions Hydroxychloroquine should be used with caution in hepatic impairment and in renal impairment (see hydroxychloroquine sulphate, below). Children with rheumatic disease, including those receiving hydroxychloroquine, may be susceptible to the development of uveitis; routine slit-lamp examination should be considered, as should establishing a screening protocol with local ophthalmologists.

It is not necessary to withdraw an antimalarial during pregnancy if the rheumatic disease is well controlled. Hydroxychloroquine is present in breast milk and breast-feeding should be avoided when it is used to treat rheumatic disease.

Hydroxychloroquine should be used with caution in neurological disorders (especially in those with a history of epilepsy), in severe gastro-intestinal disorders, in G6PD deficiency (section 9.1.5), and in porphyria. Hydroxychloroquine may exacerbate psoriasis and aggravate myasthenia gravis. Concurrent use of hepatotoxic drugs should be avoided; other **interactions**: Appendix 1 (chloroquine and hydroxychloroquine).

Note To avoid excessive dosage in obese children, the dose of hydroxychloroquine and chloroquine should be calculated on the basis of lean body weight; ocular toxicity is unlikely with doses under 5–6.5 mg/kg or max. 400 mg daily.

Side-effects The side-effects of hydroxychloroquine include gastro-intestinal disturbances, headache and skin reactions (rashes, pruritus); those occurring less frequently include ECG changes, convulsions, visual changes, retinal damage (see above), keratopathy, ototoxicity, hair depigmentation, hair loss, and discoloration of skin, nails, and mucous membranes. Side-effects that occur rarely include blood disorders (including thrombocytopenia, agranulocytosis, and aplastic anaemia), mental changes (including emotional disturbances and psychosis), myopathy (including cardiomyopathy and neuromyopathy), acute generalised exanthematous pustulosis, exfoliative dermatitis, Stevens-Johnson syndrome, photosensitivity, and hepatic damage. **Important**: very toxic in overdosage—immediate advice from poisons centres essential (see also p. 39).

HYDROXYCHLOROQUINE SULPHATE

Cautions see notes above

Renal impairment creatinine clearance 10-50 ml/minute/1.73m², reduce dose on prolonged use; creatinine clearance less than 10 mL/minute/1.73m², avoid

Pregnancy manufacturer advises avoid but see also notes above

Breast-feeding avoid—risk of toxicity in infant

Side-effects see notes above

Licensed use Juvenile idiopathic arthritis, systemic and discoid lupus erythematosus, dermatological conditions caused or aggravated by sunlight

Indication and dose

Juvenile idiopathic arthritis, systemic and discoid lupus erythematosus, dermatological conditions caused or aggravated by sunlight
- **By mouth**

Child 1 month–18 years 5–6.5 mg/kg (max. 400 mg) once daily

Plaquenil® (Sanofi-Synthelabo) PoM

Tablets, f/c, hydroxychloroquine sulphate 200 mg. Net price 60-tab pack = £4.55. Label: 5, 21

Extemporaneous formulations available see Extemporaneous Preparations, p. 8

Drugs affecting the immune response

Methotrexate, given as a once weekly dose, is the disease-modifying antirheumatic drug of choice in the treatment of juvenile idiopathic arthritis and also has a role in juvenile dermatomyositis, vasculitis, uveitis, systemic lupus erythromatosus, localised scleroderma, and sarcoidosis. For these indications it is given by the intramuscular, subcutaneous, or oral routes. Absorption from intramuscular or subcutaneous routes may be more predictable than from the oral route; if the oral route is ineffective subcutaneous administration is generally preferred. Regular full blood counts (including differential white cell count and platelet count), renal and liver-function tests are required. Folic acid may reduce mucosal or gastro-intestinal side-effects of methotrexate. The dosage regimen for folic acid has not been established—in children over 2 years a dose of 5 mg weekly may be given, usually at least 24 hours after the dose of methotrexate.

Azathioprine may be used in children for vasculitis which has failed to respond to other treatments, for the management of severe cases of *systemic lupus erythe-*

matosus and other connective tissue disorders, in conjunction with corticosteroids for patients with severe or progressive renal disease, and in cases of *polymyositis* which are resistant to corticosteroids. Azathioprine has a corticosteroid-sparing effect in patients whose corticosteroid requirements are excessive.

Ciclosporin (cyclosporin) is rarely used in juvenile idiopathic arthritis, connective tissue diseases, vasculitis, and uveitis; it may be considered if the condition has failed to respond to other treatments.

AZATHIOPRINE

Cautions see section 8.2.1

Contra-indications see section 8.2.1

Side-effects see section 8.2.1

Licensed use treatment of auto-immune conditions usually when corticosteroid therapy alone inadequate; see also section 8.2.1

Indication and dose

Inflammatory arthritis, vasculitis, auto-immune conditions usually when corticosteroid therapy alone has proved inadequate

- **By mouth**

  Child 1 month–18 years initially 1 mg/kg daily, adjusted according to response to max. 3 mg/kg daily (consider withdrawal if no improvement within 3 months)

Preparations
Section 8.2.1

METHOTREXATE

Cautions section 8.1.3; see advice below (blood count, gastro-intestinal, liver, and pulmonary toxicity); extreme caution in blood disorders (avoid if severe); risk of accumulation in pleural effusion or ascites—drain before treatment; full blood count and liver function tests before starting treatment repeated fortnightly for at least the first 4 weeks and at this frequency after any change in dose until therapy stabilised, thereafter monthly; regular renal function tests are also necessary; children or their carers should report all symptoms and signs suggestive of infection, especially sore throat; treatment with folinic acid (as calcium folinate, section 8.1) may be required in acute toxicity; porphyria (section 9.8.2); **interactions:**see below and Appendix 1 (methotrexate)

Blood count Haematopoietic suppression may occur abruptly; factors likely to increase toxicity include renal impairment and concomitant administration of another anti-folate drug. Any profound drop in white cell or platelet count calls for immediate withdrawal of methotrexate and introduction of supportive therapy

Gastrointestinal toxicity Withdraw treatment if stomatitis develops—may be first sign of gastro-intestinal toxicity

Liver toxicity Persistent 2-fold rise in liver transaminases may necessitate dose reduction or rarely discontinuation; abrupt withdrawal should be avoided as this can lead to disease flare

Pulmonary toxicity Acute pulmonary toxicity is rare in children treated for juvenile idiopathic arthritis, but children and carers should seek medical attention if dyspnoea, cough or fever develops; discontinue if pneumonitis suspected.

NSAIDs Children and carers should be advised to avoid self-medication with over-the-counter ibuprofen

Hepatic impairment dose-related toxicity—avoid in non-malignant conditions

Contra-indications see section 8.1.3 and cautions above

Side-effects section 8.1.3; chronic pulmonary fibrosis; blood dyscrasias (including fatalities); liver cirrhosis

Licensed use not licensed in children for non-malignant conditions

Indication and dose

Juvenile idiopathic arthritis, juvenile dermatomyositis, vasculitis, uveitis, systemic lupus erythematosis, localised scleroderma, sarcoidosis

- **By mouth, subcutaneous injection, or intramuscular injection**

  Child 1 month–18 years 10–15 mg/m² once weekly initially, increased if necessary to max. 25 mg/m² once weekly

Important Note that the above dose is a **weekly** dose. The CSM has received reports of prescription and dispensing errors including fatalities. Attention should be paid to the **strength** of methotrexate tablets prescribed and the **frequency** of dosing.

Methotrexate (Non-proprietary) PoM

Tablets, yellow, methotrexate 2.5 mg, net price 28-tab pack = £3.27. Counselling, dose, NSAIDs
Brands include *Maxtrex®*

Tablets, yellow, methotrexate 10 mg, net price 20 (Mayne) = £11.01; (Pharmacia, *Maxtrex®*) = £9.03. Counselling, dose, NSAIDs

Suspension, available as a manufactured special

Parenteral preparations
Section 8.1.3

Cytokine inhibitors

Cytokine inhibitors should be used under specialist supervision.

Adalimumab, **etanercept**, and **infliximab** inhibit the activity of tumour necrosis factor.

> NICE guidance (etanercept for juvenile idiopathic arthritis).
> NICE has recommended (March 2002) the use of etanercept in children aged 4–17 years with active polyarticular-course juvenile idiopathic arthritis who have not responded adequately to methotrexate or who are intolerant of it. Etanercept should be used under specialist supervision according to the guidelines of the British Society for Paediatric and Adolescent Rheumatology [previously the British Paediatric Rheumatology Group].
>
> Etanercept should be withdrawn if severe side-effects develop or if there is no response after 6 months or if the initial response is not maintained. A decision to continue therapy beyond 2 years should be based on disease activity and clinical effectiveness in individual cases.
>
> Prescribers of etanercept and infliximab should register consenting patients with the Biologics Registry of the British Society for Paediatric and Adolescent Rheumatology [previously the British Paediatric Rheumatology Group].

Adalimumab, etanercept, and infliximab have been associated with infections, sometimes severe, including tuberculosis and septicaemia. Other side-effects include nausea, abdominal pain, worsening heart failure, hypersensitivity reactions (including angioedema, bronchospasm, urticaria, and anaphylaxis), fever, headache, depression, lupus erythematosus-like syndrome, pruritus, injection-site reactions, and blood disorders (including anaemia, leucopenia, thrombocytopenia, pancytopenia, aplastic anaemia).

ETANERCEPT

Cautions predisposition to infection (avoid if predisposition to septicaemia); significant exposure to herpes zoster virus—interrupt treatment and consider varicella–zoster immunoglobulin; heart failure (risk of exacerbation); demyelinating CNS disorders (risk of exacerbation); history of blood disorders; **interactions:** Appendix 1 (etanercept)

Tuberculosis Children should be evaluated for tuberculosis before treatment. Active tuberculosis should be treated with standard treatment (section 5.1.9) for at least 2 months before starting etanercept. Children who have previously received adequate treatment for tuberculosis can start etanercept but should be monitored every 3 months for possible recurrence. In those without active tuberculosis but who were previously not treated adequately, chemoprophylaxis should ideally be completed before starting etanercept. Children and their carers should be advised to seek medical attention if symptoms suggestive of tuberculosis (e.g. persistent cough, weight loss, and fever) develop

Blood disorders Children and their carers should be advised to seek medical attention if symptoms suggestive of blood disorders (such as fever, sore throat, bruising, or bleeding) develop.

Contra-indications active infection

Pregnancy manufacturer advises avoid—no information available

Breast-feeding manufacturer advises avoid—no information available

Side-effects see under Cytokine Inhibitors above; also vomiting, oesophagitis, cholecystitis, pancreatitis, gastro-intestinal haemorrhage, myocardial or cerebral ischaemia, venous thromboembolism, hypotension, hypertension, dyspnoea, demyelinating disorders, seizures, bone fracture, renal impairment, polymyositis, bursitis, lymphadenopathy

Licensed use Polyarticular-course juvenile idiopathic arthritis in children aged 4–17 years who have had an inadequate response to methotrexate or who cannot tolerate it

Indication and dose

Polyarticular-course juvenile idiopathic arthritis

- **By subcutaneous injection**

Child 4–17 years 400 micrograms/kg twice weekly (max. 25 mg twice weekly)

Enbrel (Wyeth) ▼ PoM

Injection, powder for reconstitution, etanercept, net price 25-mg vial = £89.38

Sulfasalazine

Sulfasalazine (sulphasalazine) has a beneficial effect in suppressing the inflammatory activity associated with some forms of juvenile idiopathic arthritis; it is generally not used in systemic-onset disease. Sulfasalazine may cause haematological abnormalities including leucopenia, neutropenia, and thrombocytopenia and close monitoring of full blood counts (including differential white cell count and platelet count) is necessary initially, and at monthly intervals during the first 3 months (liver-function tests also being performed at monthly intervals for the first 3 months). Although the manufacturer recommends renal function tests, evidence of practical value is unsatisfactory. For use of sulfasalazine also see section 1.5, aminosalicylates.

SULFASALAZINE
(Sulphasalazine)

Cautions see section 1.5 and notes above

Contra-indications see section 1.5

Side-effects see section 1.5 and notes above

Licensed use see section 1.5; unlicensed in juvenile idiopathic arthritis

Indication and dose

Juvenile idiopathic arthritis (see also notes above)

- By mouth

Child 2–18 years initially 5 mg/kg twice daily for 1 week, then 10 mg/kg twice daily for 1 week, then 20 mg/kg twice daily for 1 week, maintenance dose 20–25 mg/kg twice daily; **Child 2–12 years** max. 2 g daily, **Child 12–18 years** max. 3 g daily

Preparations
see section 1.5

10.1.4 Cytotoxic-induced hyperuricaemia

This section is not included in BNF for Children. For the role of allopurinol and rasburicase in the prophylaxis of hyperuricaemia associated with cancer chemotherapy and in enzyme disorders causing increased serum urate see section 8.1. The management of gout in adolescents requires specialist supervision.

10.2 Drugs used in neuromuscular disorders

10.2.1 Drugs which enhance neuromuscular transmission

Anticholinesterases are used as first-line treatment in *ocular myasthenia gravis* and as an adjunct to immunosuppressant therapy for *generalised myasthenia gravis*.

Corticosteroids are used when anticholinesterases do not control symptoms completely. A second-line immunosuppressant such as azathioprine is frequently used to reduce the dose of corticosteroid.

Plasmapheresis or infusion of intravenous immunoglobulin [unlicensed indication] may induce temporary remission in severe relapses, particularly where bulbar or respiratory function is compromised or before thymectomy.

Anticholinesterases

Anticholinesterase drugs enhance neuromuscular transmission in voluntary and involuntary muscle in myasthenia gravis. They prolong the action of acetylcholine by inhibiting the action of the enzyme acetylcholinesterase. Excessive dosage of these drugs may impair neuromuscular transmission and precipitate 'cholinergic crises' by causing a depolarising block. This may be difficult to distinguish from a worsening myasthenic state.

Muscarinic side-effects of anticholinesterases include increased sweating, salivary and gastric secretion, also increased gastro-intestinal and uterine motility, and bradycardia. These parasympathomimetic effects are antagonised by atropine.

Edrophonium has a very brief action and it is therefore used mainly for the diagnosis of myasthenia gravis. However, such testing should be performed only by those experienced in its use; other means of establishing the diagnosis are available. A single test-dose usually causes substantial improvement in muscle power (lasting about 5 minutes) in patients with the disease (if respiration already impaired, *only* in conjunction with someone skilled at intubation).

Edrophonium can also be used to determine whether a patient with myasthenia is receiving inadequate or excessive treatment with cholinergic drugs. If treatment is excessive an injection of edrophonium will either have no effect or will intensify symptoms (if respiration already impaired, *only* in conjunction with someone skilled at intubation). Conversely, transient improvement may be seen if the patient is being inadequately treated. The test is best performed just before the next dose of anticholinesterase.

Neostigmine produces a therapeutic effect for up to 4 hours. Its pronounced muscarinic action is a disadvantage, and simultaneous administration of an antimuscarinic drug such as atropine or propantheline may be required to prevent colic, excessive salivation, or diarrhoea. In severe disease neostigmine may be given every 2 hours. In infants, neostigmine by either subcutaneous or intramuscular injection is preferred for the short-term management of myasthenia.

Pyridostigmine is less powerful and slower in action than neostigmine but it has a longer duration of action. It is preferable to neostigmine because of its smoother action and the need for less frequent dosage. It is particularly preferred in patients whose muscles are weak on waking. It has a comparatively mild gastro-intestinal effect but an antimuscarinic drug may still be required. It is inadvisable to use excessive doses because acetylcholine receptor down regulation may occur. Immunosuppressant therapy may be considered if high doses of pyridostigmine are needed.

Neostigmine and edrophonium are also used to reverse the actions of the non-depolarising muscle relaxants (section 15.1.6).

NEOSTIGMINE

Cautions asthma (*extreme* caution), bradycardia, arrhythmias, recent myocardial infarction, epilepsy, hypotension, parkinsonism, vagotonia, peptic ulceration, hyperthyroidism, renal impairment; atropine or other antidote to muscarinic effects may be necessary (particularly when neostigmine is given by injection), but not given routinely because it may mask signs of overdosage; **interactions:** Appendix 1 (parasympathomimetics)

Pregnancy manufacturer advises use only if potential benefit outweighs risk

Breast-feeding amount probably too small to be harmful; monitor infant

Contra-indications intestinal or urinary obstruction

Side-effects nausea, vomiting, increased salivation, diarrhoea, abdominal cramps (more marked with higher doses); signs of overdosage include bronchoconstriction, increased bronchial secretions, lacrimation, excessive sweating, involuntary defaecation and micturition, miosis, nystagmus, bradycardia, heart block, arrhythmias, hypotension, agitation, excessive dreaming, and weakness eventually leading to fasciculation and paralysis

Licensed use licensed for use in infants and children for treatment of myasthenia gravis

Indication and dose

Treatment of myasthenia gravis

- **By mouth (as neostigmine bromide)**

Neonate initially 1–2 mg, then 1–5 mg every 4 hours, give 30 minutes before feeds

Child up to 6 years initially 7.5 mg repeated at suitable intervals throughout the day, total daily dose 15–90 mg

Child 6–12 years initially 15 mg repeated at suitable intervals throughout the day, total daily dose 15–90 mg

Child 12–18 years initially 15–30 mg repeated at suitable intervals throughout the day, total daily dose 75–300 mg (but max. most can tolerate is 180 mg daily)

- **By subcutaneous or intramuscular injection (as neostigmine metilsulfate)**

Neonate initially 100 micrograms by intramuscular injection, followed by 50–250 micrograms every 4 hours, 30 minutes before feeds

Child 1 month–12 years 200–500 micrograms repeated at suitable intervals throughout the day

Child 12–18 years 1–2.5 mg repeated at suitable intervals throughout the day

Neostigmine (Non-proprietary) PoM

Tablets, scored, neostigmine bromide 15 mg. Net price 20 = £4.24

Injection, neostigmine metilsulfate 2.5 mg/mL. Net price 1-mL amp = 58p

EDROPHONIUM CHLORIDE

Cautions see under Neostigmine; have resuscitation facilities; *extreme* caution in respiratory distress (see notes above) and in asthma

Note Severe cholinergic reactions can be counteracted by injection of atropine sulphate (which should always be available)

Contra-indications see under Neostigmine

Side-effects see under Neostigmine

Licensed use in children over 1 year as a diagnostic test for myasthenia gravis

Indication and dose

Diagnostic test for myasthenia gravis

• By intravenous injection

Child 1 month–12 years 20 micrograms/kg followed after 30 seconds (if no adverse reaction has occurred) by 80 micrograms/kg

Child 12–18 years 2 mg followed after 30 seconds (if no adverse reaction has occurred) by 8 mg

Detection of overdosage or underdosage of cholinergic drugs

• By intravenous injection

Child 1 month–12 years 20 micrograms/kg (preferably just before next dose of anticholinesterase, see notes above)

Child 12–18 years 2 mg (preferably just before next dose of anticholinesterase, see notes above)

Edrophonium (Cambridge) PoM

Injection, edrophonium chloride 10 mg/mL. Net price 1-mL amp = £4.76

PYRIDOSTIGMINE BROMIDE

Cautions see under Neostigmine; weaker muscarinic action

Contra-indications see under Neostigmine

Side-effects see under Neostigmine

Licensed use for children of all ages for treatment of myasthenia gravis

Indication and dose

Treatment of myasthenia gravis

• By mouth

Neonate initially 1–1.5 mg/kg, increased gradually to max. 10 mg, repeated throughout the day, give 30–60 minutes before feeds

Child 1 month–6 years initially 30 mg, repeated throughout the day; usual total daily dose 30–360 mg

Child 6–12 years initially 60 mg, repeated throughout the day; usual total daily dose 30–360 mg

Child 12–18 years 30–120 mg, repeated throughout the day; usual total daily dose 0.3–1.2 g (but consider immunosuppressant therapy if total daily dose exceeds 360 mg, down-regulation of acetylcholine receptors possible if total daily dose exceeds 450 mg; see notes above)

Mestinon® (Valeant) PoM

Tablets, scored, pyridostigmine bromide 60 mg. Net price 20 = £4.81

Extemporaneous formulations available see Extemporaneous Preparations, p. 8

Immunosuppressant therapy

A course of **corticosteroids** (section 6.3) is an established treatment in severe cases of myasthenia gravis and may be particularly useful when antibodies to the acetylcholine receptor are present in high titre. Short courses of high-dose ('pulsed') methylprednisolone followed by maintenance therapy with oral corticosteroids may also be useful.

Corticosteroid treatment is usually initiated under specialist supervision. For disadvantages of corticosteroid treatment, see section 6.3.2. Transient but very serious worsening of symptoms can occur in the first 2–3 weeks, especially if the corticosteroid is started at a high dose. Once remission has occurred (usually after 2–6 months), the dose of prednisolone should be reduced slowly to the minimum effective dose.

10.2.2 Skeletal muscle relaxants

Drugs described below are used for the relief of chronic muscle spasm or spasticity associated with neurological damage; they are not indicated for spasm associated with minor injuries. They act principally on the central nervous system with the exception of dantrolene which has a peripheral site of action. They differ in action from the muscle relaxants used in anaesthesia (section 15.1.5) which block transmission at the neuromuscular junction.

The underlying cause of spasticity should be treated and any aggravating factors (e.g. pressure sores, infection) remedied. Skeletal muscle relaxants are effective in most forms of spasticity except the rare alpha variety. The major disadvantage of treatment with these drugs is that reduction in muscle tone can cause a loss of splinting action of the spastic leg and trunk muscles and sometimes lead to an increase in disability.

Dantrolene acts directly on skeletal muscle and produces fewer central adverse effects. It is generally used in resistant cases. The dose should be increased slowly.

Baclofen inhibits transmission at spinal level and also depresses the central nervous system. The dose should be increased slowly to avoid the major side-effects of sedation and muscular hypotonia (other adverse events are uncommon).

Diazepam has undoubted efficacy in some children. Sedation and, occasionally, extensor hypotonus are disadvantages. Other benzodiazepines also have muscle-relaxant properties.

BACLOFEN

Cautions psychiatric illness, respiratory impairment, epilepsy; history of peptic ulcer; diabetes; hypertonic bladder sphincter; avoid abrupt withdrawal (risk of hyperactive state, may exacerbate spasticity, and precipitate autonomic dysfunction including hyperthermia, psychiatric reactions and convulsions, see also under Withdrawal below); porphyria (section 9.8.2); **interactions:** Appendix 1 (muscle relaxants)

Withdrawal CSM has advised that serious side-effects can occur on abrupt withdrawal; to minimise risk, discontinue by gradual dose reduction over at least 1–2 weeks (longer if symptoms occur)

Skilled tasks Drowsiness may affect performance of skilled tasks (e.g. driving); effects of alcohol enhanced

Renal impairment mild, use smaller doses; excreted by kidney

Pregnancy manufacturer advises use only if potential benefit outweighs risk (toxicity in *animal* studies)

Breast-feeding amount too small to be harmful

Contra-indications peptic ulceration

Side-effects frequently sedation, drowsiness, muscular hypotonia, nausea, urinary disturbances; occasionally lassitude, confusion, speech disturbance, dizziness, ataxia, hallucinations, nightmares, headache, euphoria, insomnia, depression, anxiety, agitation, tremor, nystagmus, paraesthesias, seizures, myalgia, fever, respiratory or cardiovascular depression, hypotension, dry mouth, gastro-intestinal disturbances, sexual dysfunction, visual disorders, rash, pruritus, urticaria, hyperhidrosis, angioedema; rarely taste alterations, blood sugar changes, and paradoxical increase in spasticity

Licensed use oral use in children over 1 year for chronic severe spasticity resulting from disorders such as multiple sclerosis or traumatic partial section of spinal cord; intrathecal use in children for spasticity of cerebral origin only

Indication and dose

Chronic severe spasticity of voluntary muscle
- By mouth

Child 1–10 years 0.75–2 mg/kg daily *or* 2.5 mg 4 times daily increased gradually according to age to maintenance: **Child 1–2 years** 10–20 mg daily in divided doses, **Child 2–6 years** 20–30 mg daily in divided doses, **Child 6–10 years** 30–60 mg daily in divided doses

Child 10–18 years 5 mg 3 times daily increased gradually; max. 2.5 mg/kg *or* 100 mg daily

Severe chronic spasticity unresponsive to oral antispastic drugs (or oral therapy not tolerated), as alternative to ablative neurosurgical procedures—specialist use only
- By intrathecal injection

Child 4–18 years (spasticity of cerebral origin only) initial *test dose* 25 micrograms over at least 1 minute via catheter or lumbar puncture, increased in 25-microgram steps (not more often than every 24 hours) to max. 100 micrograms to determine appropriate dose *then dose-titration phase*, most often using infusion pump (implanted into chest wall or abdominal wall tissues) to establish *appropriate maintenance dose* (ranging from 24 micrograms to 1.2 mg daily in children under 12 years or 1.4 mg daily for those over 12 years) retaining some spasticity to avoid sensation of paralysis

Safe Practice Consult product literature for details on dose testing and titration—important to monitor patients closely in appropriately equipped and staffed environment during screening and immediately after pump implantation, and to have resuscitation equipment available for immediate use

Baclofen (Non-proprietary) PoM

Tablets, baclofen 10 mg, net price 28-tab pack = 74p, 84-tab pack = £2.60. Label: 2, 8

Brands include *Baclospas®*

Oral solution, baclofen 5 mg/5 mL, net price 300 mL = £7.95. Label: 2, 8

Brands include *Lyflex®* (sugar-free)

Lioresal® (Novartis) PoM

Tablets, scored, baclofen 10 mg. Net price 84-tab pack = £10.84. Label: 2, 8

Excipients: include gluten

Liquid, sugar-free, raspberry–flavoured, baclofen 5 mg/5 mL. Net price 300 mL = £8.95. Label: 2, 8

By intrathecal injection

Lioresal® (Novartis) PoM

Intrathecal injection, baclofen, 50 micrograms/mL, net price 1-mL amp (for test dose) = £2.74; 500 micrograms/mL, 20-mL amp (for use with implantable pump) = £60.77; 2 mg/mL, 5-mL amp (for use with implantable pump) = £60.77

DANTROLENE SODIUM

Cautions impaired cardiac and pulmonary function; test liver function before and at intervals during therapy; therapeutic effect may take a few weeks to develop but if treatment is ineffective it should be discontinued after 4–6 weeks. Avoid when spasticity is useful, for example, locomotion; **interactions:** Appendix 1 (muscle relaxants).

Skilled tasks Drowsiness may affect performance of skilled tasks (e.g. driving); effects of alcohol enhanced

Breast-feeding present in milk—manufacturer advises avoid

Contra-indications hepatic impairment (may cause severe liver damage); acute muscle spasm

Pregnancy avoid use in chronic spasticity—embryotoxic in *animal* studies

Side-effects transient drowsiness, dizziness, weakness, malaise, fatigue, diarrhoea (withdraw if severe, discontinue treatment if recurs on re-introduction), anorexia, nausea, headache, rash; less frequently constipation, dysphagia, speech and visual disturbances, confusion, nervousness, insomnia, depression, seizures, chills, fever, increased urinary frequency; rarely, tachycardia, erratic blood pressure, dyspnoea, haematuria, possible crystalluria, urinary incontinence or retention, pleural effusion, pericarditis, dose-related hepatotoxicity (occasionally fatal)

Licensed use not licensed for use in children

Indication and dose

Chronic severe spasticity of voluntary muscle
- **By mouth**

Child 5–12 years initially 500 micrograms/kg once daily; after 7 days increase to 500 micrograms/kg/dose 3 times daily; every 7 days increase by further 500 micrograms/kg/dose until satisfactory response; max. 2 mg/kg 3–4 times daily (max. total daily dose 400 mg)

Child 12–18 years initially 25 mg once daily; increase to 3 times daily after 7 days; every 7 days increase by further 500 micrograms/kg/dose until satisfactory response; max. 2 mg/kg 3–4 times daily (max. total daily dose 400 mg)

Dantrium® (Procter & Gamble Pharm.) PoM
Capsules, both orange/brown, dantrolene sodium 25 mg, net price 20 = £2.46; 100 mg, 20 = £8.61. Label: 2

DIAZEPAM

Cautions see section 4.1.2; special precautions for intravenous injection (section 4.8.2)

Contra-indications see section 4.1.2

Side-effects see section 4.1.2; also hypotonia

Licensed use muscle spasm of varied aetiology, including tetanus; other indications (section 4.1.2, section 4.8.2, section 15.1.4.1)

Indication and dose

Muscle spasm in cerebral spasticity or in postoperative skeletal muscle spasm
- **By mouth**

Child 1–12 months initially 250 microgram/kg twice daily

Child 1–5 years initially 2.5 mg twice daily

Child 5–12 years initially 5 mg twice daily

Child 12–18 years initially 10 mg twice daily; max. total daily dose 40 mg

Tetanus
- **By intravenous injection**

Child 1 month–18 years 100–300 micrograms/kg repeated every 1–4 hours

- **By intravenous infusion (or by nasoduodenal tube)**

Child 1 month–18 years 3–10 mg/kg over 24 hours, adjusted according to response

Administration for *continuous intravenous infusion* of diazepam emulsion, dilute to a concentration of max. 400 micrograms/mL with Glucose 5% or 10%; max. 6 hours between addition and completion of infusion; diazepam adsorbed by plastics of infusion bags and giving sets

For *continuous intravenous infusion* of diazepam solution, dilute to a concentration of max. 50 micrograms/mL with Glucose 5% or Sodium Chloride 0.9%; diazepam adsorbed by plastics of infusion bags and giving sets

Oral preparations
Section 4.1.2

Parenteral preparations
Section 4.8.2

10.3 Drugs for the relief of soft-tissue inflammation

Extravasation

Local guidelines for the management of extravasation should be followed where they exist or specialist advice sought.

Extravasation injury follows leakage of drugs or intravenous fluids from the veins or inadvertent administration into the subcutaneous or subdermal tissue. It must be dealt with **promptly** to prevent tissue necrosis.

Acidic or alkaline preparations and those with an osmolarity greater than that of plasma can cause extravasation injury, and excipients including alcohol and polyethylene glycol have also been implicated. Cytotoxic drugs commonly cause extravasation injury. Very young children are at increased risk. Those receiving anticoagulants are more likely to lose blood into surrounding tissues if extravasation occurs whilst those receiving sedatives or analgesics may not notice the early signs or symptoms of extravasation.

Prevention of extravasation Precautions should be taken to avoid extravasation; ideally, drugs liable to cause extravasation injury should be given through a central line and children receiving repeated doses of hazardous drugs peripherally should have the cannula resited at regular intervals. Attention should be paid to the manufacturers' recommendations for administration. Placing a glyceryl trinitrate patch or using glyceryl trinitrate ointment distal to the cannula may improve the patency of the vessel in children with small veins or in those whose veins are prone to collapse.

Children or their carers should be asked to report any pain or burning at the site of injection immediately.

Management of extravasation If extravasation is suspected the infusion should be stopped immediately but the cannula should not be removed until after an attempt has been made to aspirate the area (through the cannula) in order to remove as much of the drug as possible. Aspiration is sometimes possible if the extravasation presents with a raised bleb or blister at the injection site and is surrounded by hardened tissue, but it is often unsuccessful if the tissue is soft or soggy. Corticosteroids are usually given to treat inflammation, although there is little evidence to support their use in extravasation. Hydrocortisone or dexamethasone (section 6.3.2) may be given either locally by subcutaneous injection or intravenously at a site distant from the injury. Antihistamines (section 3.4.1) and analgesics (section 4.7) may be required for symptom relief.

The management of extravasation beyond these measures is not well standardised and calls for specialist advice. Treatment depends on the nature of the offending substance; one approach is to localise and neutralise the substance whereas another is to spread and dilute it. The first method may be appropriate following extravasation of vesicant drugs and involves administration of an antidote (if available) and the application of cold compresses 3–4 times a day (consult specialist literature for details of specific antidotes). Spreading and diluting the offending substance involves infiltrating the area with physiological saline, applying warm compresses, elevating the affected limb, and administering hyaluronidase. A saline flush-out technique (involving flushing the subcutaneous tissue with physiological saline) may be effective but requires specialist advice. Hyaluronidase should **not** be administered following extravasation of vesicant drugs (unless it is either specifically indicated or used in the saline flush-out technique).

10.3.1 Enzymes

Classification not included in BNF for Children.

10.3.2 Rubefacients and other topical antirheumatics

Classification not included in BNF for Children.

11 Eye

11.1 Administration of drugs to the eye

Drugs are most commonly administered to the eye by topical application as eye drops or eye ointments. Where a higher drug concentration is required within the eye, a local injection may be necessary.

Eye-drop dispenser devices are available to aid the instillation of eye drops from plastic bottles especially by the visually impaired or otherwise physically limited patients; they may be useful in children in whom normal application is difficult. Eye-drop dispensers are for use with plastic eye-drop bottles, for repeat use by individual patients.

Eye drops and eye ointments Eye drops are generally instilled into the pocket formed by gently pulling down the lower eyelid and keeping the eye closed for as long as possible after application; in neonates and infants it may be more appropriate to administer the drop in the inner angle of the open eye. One drop is all that is needed. A small amount of eye ointment is applied similarly; the ointment melts rapidly and blinking helps to spread it.

When two different eye-drop preparations are used at the same time of day, dilution and overflow may occur when one immediately follows the other. The carer or child should therefore leave an interval of at least 5 minutes between the two. Eye ointment should be applied after drops. Both drops and ointment may cause transient blurred vision.

Systemic effects may arise from absorption of drugs into the general circulation from conjunctival vessels or from the nasal mucosa after the excess preparation has drained down through the tear ducts. The extent of systemic absorption following ocular administration is highly variable; nasal drainage of drugs is associated with eye drops much more often than with eye ointments.

For warnings relating to eye drops and contact lenses, see section 11.9.

Eye lotions These are solutions for the irrigation of the conjunctival sac. They act mechanically to flush out irritants or foreign bodies as a first-aid treatment. Sterile sodium chloride 0.9% solution (section 11.8.1) is usually used. Clean water will suffice in an emergency.

Other preparations Subconjunctival injection may be used to administer anti-infective drugs, mydriatics, or corticosteroids for conditions not responding to topical therapy. The drug diffuses through the cornea and sclera to the anterior and posterior chambers and vitreous humour. However, because the dose-volume is limited, this route is suitable only for drugs which are readily soluble.

Drugs such as antimicrobials and corticosteroids may be administered systemically to treat an eye condition.

Preservatives and sensitisers Information on preservatives and on substances identified as skin sensitisers (see section 13.1.3) is provided under preparation entries.

11.2 Control of microbial contamination

Preparations for the eye should be sterile when issued. Eye drops in multiple-application containers include a preservative but care should nevertheless be taken to avoid contamination of the contents during use.

Eye drops in multiple-application containers for *home use* should not be used for more than 4 weeks after first opening (unless otherwise stated).

Eye drops for use in *hospital wards* are normally discarded 1 week after first opening (24 hours if preservative-free). Individual containers should be provided for each child, and for each eye if there are special concerns about contamination. Containers used before an operation should be discarded at the time of the operation and fresh containers supplied. A fresh supply should also be provided upon discharge from hospital; in specialist ophthalmology units it may be acceptable to issue eye-drop bottles that have been dispensed to the patient on the day of discharge

In *out-patient departments* single-application packs should preferably be used; if multiple-application packs are used, they should be discarded at the end of each day. In clinics for eye diseases and in accident and emergency departments, where the dangers of infection are high, single-application packs should be used; if a multiple-application pack is used, it should be discarded after single use.

Diagnostic dyes (e.g. fluorescein) should be used only from single-application packs.

In *eye surgery* single-application containers should be used if possible; if a multiple-application pack is used, it should be discarded after single use. Preparations used during intra-ocular procedures and others that may penetrate into the anterior chamber must be isotonic and without preservatives and buffered if necessary to a neutral pH. Specially formulated fluids should be used for intra-ocular surgery; large volume intravenous infusion preparations are not suitable for this purpose. For all surgical procedures, a previously unopened container is used for each patient.

11.3 Anti-infective eye preparations

Eye infections Most acute superficial eye infections can be treated topically. Blepharitis and conjunctivitis are often caused by staphylococci; keratitis and endophthalmitis may be bacterial, viral, or fungal.

Bacterial *blepharitis* is treated by lid hygiene and application of an antibacterial eye ointment to the conjunctival sac or to the lid margins. Systemic treatment may occasionally be required and is usually undertaken after culturing organisms from the lid margin and determining their antimicrobial sensitivity; antibacterials may be required for 3 months or longer.

Most cases of acute bacterial conjunctivitis are self-limiting; where treatment is appropriate, antibacterial eye drops or an eye ointment are used. A poor response might indicate viral or allergic conjunctivitis.

Corneal ulcer and *keratitis* require specialist treatment and may call for subconjunctival or systemic administration of antimicrobials.

Endophthalmitis is a medical emergency which also calls for specialist management and often requires parenteral, subconjunctival, or intra-ocular administration of antimicrobials.

For reference to the treatment of *crab lice of the eyelashes*, see section 13.10.4

11.3.1 Antibacterials

Bacterial infections are generally treated topically with eye drops and eye ointments. Systemic administration is sometimes appropriate in blepharitis. In intra-ocular infection, a variety of routes (intracorneal, intravitreal and systemic) may be used.

Chloramphenicol has a broad spectrum of activity and is the drug of choice for *superficial eye infections*. Chloramphenicol eye drops are well tolerated and the recommendation that chloramphenicol eye drops should be avoided because of an increased risk of aplastic anaemia is not well founded.

Other antibacterials with a broad spectrum of activity include the quinolones, **ciprofloxacin** and **ofloxacin**; **framycetin**, **gentamicin**, and **neomycin** are also active against a wide variety of bacteria. Gentamicin, ciprofloxacin, ofloxacin and **polymyxin B** are effective for infections caused by *Pseudomonas aeruginosa*.

Ciprofloxacin eye drops are licensed for *corneal ulcers*; intensive application (especially in the first 2 days) is required throughout the day and night.

Trachoma, which results from chronic infection with *Chlamydia trachomatis*, can be treated with **azithromycin** by mouth [unlicensed indication].

Fusidic acid is useful for staphylococcal infections.

Propamidine isetionate is of little value in bacterial infections but is specific for the rare but potentially devastating condition of *acanthamoeba keratitis* (see also section 11.9).

Other antibacterial eye drops may be prepared aseptically in a specialist manufacturing unit from material supplied for injection, see section 11.8

Neonates Antibacterial eye drops are used to treat acute bacterial conjunctivitis in neonates (ophthalmia neonatorum); where possible the causative micro-organism should be identified. **Chloramphenicol** or **neomycin** eye drops are used to treat mild conjunctivitis; more serious infections also require a systemic antibacterial. Failure to respond to initial treatment requires further investigation; chlamydial infection should be considered.

Gonococcal eye infections are treated with a single-dose of **ceftriaxone**. *Chlamydial eye infections* should be managed with oral **erythromycin**. **Gentamicin** eye drops together with appropriate systemic antibacterials are used in the treatment of *pseudomonal eye infections*; high-strength gentamicin eye drops (1.5%) [unlicensed] are available for severe infections.

With corticosteroids Many antibacterial preparations also incorporate a corticosteroid but such mixtures should **not** be used unless a patient is under close specialist supervision. In particular they should not be prescribed for undiagnosed 'red eye' which is sometimes caused by the herpes simplex virus and may be difficult to diagnose (section 11.4).

Administration Antibacterial eye preparations are usually administered as follows.

Eye drops. Apply 1 drop at least every 2 hours in severe infection then reduce frequency as infection is controlled and continue for 48 hours after healing. For less severe infection 3–4 times daily is generally sufficient.

Eye ointment. Apply *either* at night (if eye drops used during the day) *or* 3–4 times daily (if eye ointment used alone).

CHLORAMPHENICOL

Side-effects transient stinging; see also notes above

Indication and dose

See notes above

[1]**Chloramphenicol** (Non-proprietary) PoM
Eye drops, chloramphenicol 0.5%. Net price 10 mL = £1.43

Eye ointment, chloramphenicol 1%. Net price 4 g = £1.59

1. Chloramphenicol 0.5% eye drops can be sold to the public (in max. pack size 10 mL) for treatment of acute bacterial conjunctivitis in adults and children over 2 years; max. duration of treatment 5 days; proprietary brands on sale to the public include *Optrex Infected Eyes®*

Chloromycetin® (Goldshield) PoM
Redidrops (= eye drops), chloramphenicol 0.5%. Net price 5 mL = £1.65; 10 mL = £2.01
Excipients: include phenylmercuric acetate

Ophthalmic ointment (= eye ointment), chloramphenicol 1%. Net price 4 g = £2.01

Single use

Minims® Chloramphenicol (Chauvin) PoM
Eye drops, chloramphenicol 0.5%. Net price 20 × 0.5 mL = £4.92

CIPROFLOXACIN

Cautions not recommended for children under 1 year

Pregnancy Manufacturer advises caution

Breast-feeding Manufacturer advises caution but unlikely to appear in milk

Side-effects local burning and itching; lid margin crusting; hyperaemia; taste disturbances; corneal staining, keratitis, lid oedema, lacrimation, photophobia, corneal infiltrates; nausea and visual disturbances reported

Licensed use not licensed for use in children under 1 year

Indication and dose

Superficial bacterial infections
see notes above

Corneal ulcer
Apply eye drops throughout day and night, day 1 apply every 15 minutes for 6 hours then every 30 minutes, day 2 apply every hour, days 3–14 apply every 4 hours (max. duration of treatment 21 days)

Apply eye ointment throughout day and night; apply 1.25 cm ointment every 1–2 hours for 2 days then every 4 hours for next 12 days

Ciloxan® (Alcon) PoM
Ophthalmic solution (= eye drops), ciprofloxacin (as hydrochloride) 0.3%. Net price 5 mL = £4.94
Excipients: include benzalkonium chloride

Eye ointment, ciprofloxacin (as hydrochloride) 0.3%. Net price 3.5 g = £5.49

FRAMYCETIN SULPHATE

Indication and dose

See notes above

Soframycin® (Sanofi-Aventis) PoM
Eye drops, framycetin sulphate 0.5%. Net price 10 mL = £4.30
Excipients: include benzalkonium chloride

FUSIDIC ACID

Indication and dose

See under preparation below

Fucithalmic® (Leo) PoM
Eye drops, m/r, fusidic acid 1% in gel basis (liquifies on contact with eye). Net price 5 g = £2.09
Excipients: include benzalkonium chloride, disodium edetate

Dose

Apply twice daily

GENTAMICIN

Indication and dose

See notes above

Genticin® (Roche) PoM
Drops (for ear or eye), gentamicin 0.3% (as sulphate). Net price 10 mL = £1.78
Excipients: include benzalkonium chloride

Gentamicin (Non-proprietary) PoM
Eye drops, gentamicin 1.5%, 10 mL, available as a manufactured special from Moorfields Eye Hospital

Single use

Minims® Gentamicin Sulphate (Chauvin) PoM
Eye drops, gentamicin 0.3% (as sulphate). Net price 20 × 0.5 mL = £5.75

NEOMYCIN SULPHATE

Licensed use *Neosporin*® not licensed for use in children under 2 years

Indication and dose

See notes above and under preparations below

Neomycin (Non-proprietary) PoM

Eye drops, neomycin sulphate 0.5% (3500 units/mL). Net price 10 mL = £3.11

Eye ointment, neomycin sulphate 0.5% (3500 units/g). Net price 3 g = £2.44

With other antibacterials

Neosporin® (PLIVA) PoM

Eye drops, gramicidin 25 units, neomycin sulphate 1700 units, polymyxin B sulphate 5000 units/mL. Net price 5 mL = £4.86

Excipients: include thiomersal

Dose

Apply 2–4 times daily or more frequently if required

With hydrocortisone

Section 12.1.1

OFLOXACIN

Cautions not to be used for more than 10 days

Pregnancy manufacturer advises use only if benefit outweighs risk; systemic quinolones have caused arthropathy in animal studies

Breast-feeding manufacturer advises avoid

Side-effects local irritation including photophobia; dizziness, numbness, nausea and headache reported

Indication and dose

See notes above

Exocin® (Allergan) PoM

Ophthalmic solution (= eye drops), ofloxacin 0.3%. Net price 5 mL = £2.17

Excipients: include benzalkonium chloride

POLYMYXIN B SULPHATE

Indication and dose

See notes above

With other antibacterials

Polyfax® (PLIVA) PoM

Eye ointment, polymyxin B sulphate 10 000 units, bacitracin zinc 500 units/g. Net price 4 g = £3.26

Polytrim® (PLIVA) PoM

Eye drops, trimethoprim 0.1%, polymyxin B sulphate 10 000 units/mL. Net price 5 mL = £3.05

Excipients: include benzalkonium chloride

Eye ointment, trimethoprim 0.5%, polymyxin B sulphate 10 000 units/g. Net price 4 g = £2.90

PROPAMIDINE ISETIONATE

Indication and dose

See notes above and under preparations below

Brolene® (Aventis Pharma)

Eye drops, propamidine isetionate 0.1%. Net price 10 mL = £2.73

Excipients: include benzalkonium chloride

Dose

Local treatment of infections (but see notes above) apply 4 times daily

Note Eye drops containing propamidine isetionate 0.1% also available from Typharm (*Golden Eye Drops*)

Eye ointment, dibromopropamidine isetionate 0.15%. Net price 5 g = £2.85

Dose

Local treatment of infections (but see notes above) apply 1–2 times daily

Note Eye ointment containing dibromopropamidine isetionate 0.15% also available from Typharm (*Golden Eye Ointment*)

11.3.2 Antifungals

Fungal infections of the cornea are rare. Orbital mycosis is rarer, and when it occurs it is usually because of a direct spread of infection from the paranasal sinuses. Debility or immunosuppression may encourage fungal proliferation. The spread of infection through blood occasionally produces a metastatic endophthalmitis.

Many different fungi are capable of producing ocular infection; they may be identified by appropriate laboratory procedures.

Antifungal preparations for the eye are not generally available. Treatment is normally carried out at specialist centres, but requests for information about supplies of preparations not available commercially should be addressed to the local Health Authority (or equivalent in Scotland or Northern Ireland), or to the nearest hospital ophthalmology unit, or to Moorfields Eye Hospital, City Road, London EC1V 2PD (tel. (020) 7253 3411).

11.3.3 Antivirals

Herpes simplex infections producing, for example, dendritic corneal ulcer can be treated with **aciclovir**. **Ganciclovir** eye drops are licensed in adults for the treatment of acute herpetic keratitis.

For systemic treatment of CMV retinitis, see section 5.3.

ACICLOVIR
(Acyclovir)

Side-effects local irritation and inflammation reported

Indication and dose

Local treatment of herpes simplex infections
: Apply 5 times daily (continue for at least 3 days after complete healing)

Zovirax® (GSK) PoM
: Eye ointment, aciclovir 3%. Net price 4.5 g = £9.92

Tablets, see section 5.3.2.1

Injection, see section 5.3.2.1

Cream, see section 13.10.3

GANCICLOVIR

Cautions

Pregnancy manufacturer advises use only if benefit outweighs risk—systemic ganciclovir teratogenic in *animal* studies

Breast-feeding manufacturer advises use only if benefit outweighs risk—no information available

Side-effects ocular irritation, visual disturbances; superficial punctate keratitis

Licensed use not licensed for use in children

Indication and dose

Acute herpetic keratitis
: Apply 5 times daily until complete corneal re-epithelialisation, then 3 times daily for 7 days (usual duration of treatment 21 days)

Virgan® (Chauvin) PoM
: Eye drops, ganciclovir 0.15 % in gel basis, net price 5 g = £10.64

Excipients: include benzalkonium chloride

11.4 Corticosteroids and other anti-inflammatory preparations

11.4.1 Corticosteroids

Corticosteroids administered locally (as eye drops, eye ointments or subconjunctival injection) or by mouth have an important place in treating anterior segment inflammation, including that which results from surgery.

Topical corticosteroids should normally only be used under expert supervision; three main dangers are associated with their use:

- a 'red eye', where the diagnosis is unconfirmed, may be due to herpes simplex virus, and a corticosteroid may aggravate the condition, leading to corneal ulceration, with possible damage to vision and even loss of the eye. Bacterial, fungal and amoebic infections pose a similar hazard;
- 'steroid glaucoma' may follow the use of corticosteroid eye preparations in susceptible individuals;
- a 'steroid cataract' may follow prolonged use.

Other side-effects include thinning of the cornea and sclera. Prolonged use in neonates and infants may cause adrenal suppression.

Products combining a corticosteroid with an antimicrobial are used after occular surgery to reduce inflammation and prevent infection: use of combination products is otherwise rarely justified.

Systemic corticosteroids (section 6.3.2) may be useful for ocular conditions. The risk of producing a 'steroid cataract' increases with the dose and duration of corticosteroid use.

BETAMETHASONE

Cautions see notes above

Side-effects see notes above

Indication and dose

Local treatment of inflammation (short-term)
Apply eye drops every 1–2 hours until controlled then reduce frequency; eye ointment 2–4 times daily or at night when used with eye drops

Betnesol® (Celltech) PoM
Drops (for ear, eye, or nose), betamethasone sodium phosphate 0.1%. Net price 10 mL = £2.32
Excipients: include benzalkonium chloride, disodium edetate

Eye ointment, betamethasone sodium phosphate 0.1%. Net price 3 g = £1.41

Vista-Methasone® (Martindale) PoM
Drops (for ear, eye, or nose), betamethasone sodium phosphate 0.1%. Net price 5 mL = £1.02; 10 mL = £1.16
Excipients: include benzalkonium chloride

With neomycin

Betnesol-N® (Celltech) PoM
Drops (for ear, eye, or nose), see section 12.1.1

Eye ointment, betamethasone sodium phosphate 0.1%, neomycin sulphate 0.5%. Net price 3 g = £1.28
Note May be difficult to obtain

Vista-Methasone N® (Martindale) PoM
Drops (for ear, eye, or nose), see section 12.1.1

DEXAMETHASONE

Cautions see notes above

Side-effects see notes above

Indication and dose

Local treatment of inflammation (short-term)
Apply eye drops 4–6 times daily; severe conditions every 30–60 minutes until controlled then reduce frequency

Maxidex® (Alcon) PoM
Eye drops, dexamethasone 0.1%, hypromellose 0.5%. Net price 5 mL = £1.49; 10 mL = £2.95
Excipients: include benzalkonium chloride, disodium edetate, polysorbate 80

Single use

Minims® Dexamethasone (Chauvin) PoM
Eye drops, dexamethasone sodium phosphate 0.1%. Net price 20 × 0.5 mL = £6.95
Excipients: include disodium edetate

With antibacterials

Maxitrol® (Alcon) PoM
Eye drops, dexamethasone 0.1%, hypromellose 0.5%, neomycin 0.35% (as sulphate), polymyxin B sulphate 6000 units/mL. Net price 5 mL = £1.77
Excipients: include benzalkonium chloride, polysorbate 20

Eye ointment, dexamethasone 0.1%, neomycin 0.35% (as sulphate), polymyxin B sulphate 6000 units/g. Net price 3.5 g = £1.52
Excipients: include hydroxybenzoates (parabens), wool fat

Sofradex® (Sanofi-Aventis) PoM
Drops (for ear or eye), see section 12.1.1

FLUOROMETHOLONE

Cautions see notes above

Side-effects see notes above

Licensed use not licensed for use in children under 2 years

Indication and dose

Local treatment of inflammation (short-term)
Apply 2–4 times daily (initially every hour for 24–48 hours then reduce frequency)

FML® (Allergan) PoM
Ophthalmic suspension (= eye drops), fluorometholone 0.1%, polyvinyl alcohol (*Liquifilm®*) 1.4%. Net price 5 mL = £1.71; 10 mL = £2.95
Excipients: include benzalkonium chloride, disodium edetate, polysorbate 80

HYDROCORTISONE ACETATE

Cautions see notes above

Side-effects see notes above

Indication and dose

Local treatment of inflammation (short-term)
Apply eye drops 4 times daily; apply eye ointment twice daily or at night

Hydrocortisone (Non-proprietary) PoM
Eye drops, hydrocortisone acetate 1%. Net price 10 mL = £3.21

Eye ointment, hydrocortisone acetate 0.5%, net price 3 g = £2.40; 1%, 3 g = £2.42; 2.5%, 3 g = £2.44

With neomycin

Neo-Cortef® (PLIVA) PoM
Ointment (for ear or eye), see section 12.1.1
Note May be difficult to obtain

PREDNISOLONE

Cautions see notes above

Side-effects see notes above

Indication and dose

Local treatment of inflammation (short-term)
Apply every 1–2 hours until controlled then reduce frequency

Pred Forte® (Allergan) PoM
Eye drops, prednisolone acetate 1%. Net price 5 mL = £1.52; 10 mL = £3.05
Excipients: include benzalkonium chloride, disodium edetate, polysorbate 80

Dose

Apply 2–4 times daily

Predsol® (Celltech) PoM
Drops (for ear or eye), prednisolone sodium phosphate 0.5%. Net price 10 mL = £2.00
Excipients: include benzalkonium chloride, disodium edetate

Single use

Minims® Prednisolone Sodium Phosphate (Chauvin) PoM
Eye drops, prednisolone sodium phosphate 0.5%. Net price 20 × 0.5 mL = £5.75
Excipients: include disodium edetate

With neomycin

Predsol-N® (Celltech) PoM
Drops (for ear or eye), see section 12.1.1

11 Eye

11.4.2 Other anti-inflammatory preparations

Topical preparations of **antihistamines** such as eye drops containing **antazoline** (with xylometazoline as *Otrivine-Antistin®*), **azelastine**, **epinastine**, **ketotifen**, and **olopatadine** may be used for allergic conjunctivitis.

Sodium cromoglicate (sodium cromoglycate) and **nedocromil sodium** eye drops may be useful for vernal keratoconjunctivitis and other allergic forms of conjunctivitis.

Lodoxamide eye drops are used for allergic conjunctival conditions including seasonal allergic conjunctivitis.

Emedastine eye drops are licensed for seasonal allergic conjunctivitis.

ANTAZOLINE SULPHATE

Indication and dose

Allergic conjunctivitis see under preparations below

Otrivine-Antistin® (Novartis Consumer Health)
Eye drops, antazoline sulphate 0.5%, xylometazoline hydrochloride 0.05%. Net price 10 mL = £2.35
Excipients: include benzalkonium chloride, disodium edetate

Dose

Child 5–18 years apply 2–3 times daily

Note Xylometazoline is a sympathomimetic; it should be avoided in angle-closure glaucoma; absorption of antazoline and xylometazoline may result in systemic side-effects and the possibility of interaction with other drugs, see Appendix 1 (antihistamines and sympathomimetics)

AZELASTINE HYDROCHLORIDE

Side-effects mild transient irritation; bitter taste reported

Indication and dose

Allergic conjunctivitis, seasonal allergic conjunctivitis
Child 4–18 years apply twice daily, increased if necessary to 4 times daily

AZELASTINE HYDROCHLORIDE (*continued*)

Perennial conjunctivitis

Child 12–18 years apply twice daily, increased if necessary to 4 times daily; max. duration of treatment 6 weeks

[1]**Optilast®** (Viatris) PoM

Eye drops, azelastine hydrochloride 0.05%. Net price 8 mL = £6.40

Excipients: include benzalkonium chloride, disodium edetate

1. Azelastine 0.05% eye drops can be sold to the public (in max. pack size of 6 mL) for treatment of seasonal and perennial allergic conjunctivitis in children over 12 years; proprietary brands on sale to the public include *Aller-eze®*

EMEDASTINE

Side-effects transient burning or stinging; blurred vision, local oedema, keratitis, irritation, dry eye, lacrimation, corneal infiltrates (discontinue) and staining; photophobia; headache, and rhinitis occasionally reported

Indication and dose

Seasonal allergic conjunctivitis

Child 3–18 years apply twice daily

Emadine® (Alcon) PoM

Eye drops, emedastine 0.05% (as difumarate), net price 5 mL = £7.69

Excipients: include benzalkonium chloride

EPINASTINE HYDROCHLORIDE

Side-effects burning; less commonly dry mouth, taste disturbance; nasal irritation, rhinitis; headache, blepharoptosis, conjunctival oedema and hyperaemia, dry eye, local irritation, photophobia, visual disturbance; pruritus

Indication and dose

Seasonal allergic conjunctivitis

Child 12–18 years apply twice daily; max. duration of treatment 8 weeks

Relestat® (Allergan) PoM

Eye drops, epinastine hydrochloride 500 micrograms/mL, net price 5 mL = £14.50

Excipients: include benzalkonium chloride, disodium edetate

KETOTIFEN

Side-effects transient burning or stinging, punctate corneal epithelial erosion; less commonly dry eye, subconjunctival haemmorhage, photophobia; headache, drowsiness, skin reactions, and dry mouth also reported

Indication and dose

Seasonal allergic conjunctivitis

Child 3–18 years apply twice daily

Zaditen® (Novartis) PoM

Eye drops, ketotifen (as fumarate) 250 micrograms/mL, net price 5 mL = £9.75

Excipients: include benzalkonium chloride

LODOXAMIDE

Side-effects mild transient burning, stinging, itching, and lacrimation; flushing and dizziness reported

Indication and dose

Allergic conjunctivitis

Child 4–18 years apply 4 times daily

[1]**Alomide®** (Alcon) PoM

Ophthalmic solution (= eye drops), lodoxamide 0.1% (as trometamol). Net price 10 mL = £5.48

Excipients: include benzalkonium chloride, disodium edetate

1. Lodoxamide 0.1% eye drops can be sold to the public for treatment of allergic conjunctivitis in children over 4 years; proprietary brands on sale to the public include *Alomide Allergy®*

NEDOCROMIL SODIUM

Side-effects transient burning and stinging; distinctive taste reported

Indication and dose

Seasonal and perennial allergic conjunctivitis

Child 6–18 years apply twice daily increased if necessary to 4 times daily; max. 12 weeks treatment for seasonal allergic conjunctivitis

Vernal keratoconjunctivitis

Child 6–18 years apply 4 times daily

Rapitil® (Aventis Pharma) PoM

Eye drops, nedocromil sodium 2%. Net price 5 mL = £5.12

Excipients: include benzalkonium chloride, disodium edetate

OLOPATADINE

Side-effects local irritation; less commonly keratitis, dry eye, local oedema, photophobia; headache, asthenia, dizziness; dry nose also reported

Indication and dose

Seasonal allergic conjunctivitis

Child 3–18 years apply twice daily; max. duration of treatment 4 months

Opatanol® (Alcon) ▼ PoM
Eye drops, olopatadine (as hydrochloride) 1 mg/mL, net price 5 mL = £4.11
Excipients: include benzalkonium chloride

SODIUM CROMOGLICATE

(Sodium cromoglycate)

Side-effects transient burning and stinging

Indication and dose

Allergic conjunctivitis, vernal keratoconjunctivitis

apply eye drops 4 times daily

[1]**Sodium Cromoglicate** (Non-proprietary) PoM
Eye drops, sodium cromoglicate 2%. Net price 13.5 mL = £3.08
Brands include *Hay-Crom® Aqueous, Opticrom® Aqueous, Vividrin®*)

1. Sodium cromoglicate 2% eye drops can be sold to the public (in max. pack size of 10 mL) for treatment of acute seasonal and perennial allergic conjunctivitis; proprietary brands on sale to the public include *Boots Hayfever Relief, Clariteyes®, Opticrom® Allergy, Optrex® Allergy,* and *Vivicrom®*

11.5 Mydriatics and cycloplegics

Antimuscarinics dilate the pupil and paralyse the ciliary muscle; they vary in potency and duration of action.

Short-acting, relatively weak mydriatics, such as **tropicamide** 0.5% (action lasts for 4–6 hours), facilitate the examination of the fundus of the eye. **Cyclopentolate** 1% (action up to 24 hours) or **atropine** are preferable for producing cycloplegia for refraction in young children as tropicamide may be inadequate; tropicamide may be preferred in neonates. Atropine ointment 1% is sometimes preferred for children under 5 years because the ointment formulation reduces systemic absorption. Atropine, which has a longer duration of action (up to 7 days), is also used for the treatment of anterior uveitis mainly to prevent posterior synechiae, often in combination with phenylephrine eye drops. **Homatropine** 1% is also used in the treatment of anterior segment inflammation, and may be preferred for its shorter duration of action. **Phenylephrine** 2.5% is used for mydriasis in diagnostic or therapeutic procedures; mydriasis occurs within 60–90 minutes and lasts up to 5–7 hours. Phenylephrine 10% drops are contra-indicated in children owing to the risk of systemic effects.

Cautions and contra-indications Darkly pigmented irides are more resistant to pupillary dilatation and caution should be exercised to avoid overdosage. Mydriasis may precipitate acute angle-closure glaucoma in the very few children who are predisposed to the condition because of a shallow anterior chamber. Atropine, cyclopentolate and homatropine should be used with caution in children under 3 months owing to the possible association between cycloplegia and the development of amblyopia; also, neonates are at increased risk of systemic toxicity.

Skilled tasks Children may not be able to undertake skilled tasks for 1–2 hours after mydriasis.

Side-effects Ocular side-effects of mydriatics and cycloplegics include transient stinging and raised intra-ocular pressure; on prolonged administration, local irritation, hyperaemia, oedema and conjunctivitis may occur. Contact dermatitis (conjunctivitis) is not uncommon with the antimuscarinic mydriatic drugs, especially atropine.

Toxic systemic reactions to atropine and cyclopentolate may occur in neonates and children; see section 1.2 for systemic side-effects of antimuscarinic drugs.

Antimuscarinics

ATROPINE SULPHATE

Cautions risk of systemic effects with eye drops in infants under 3 months—eye ointment preferred; see also notes above

Side-effects see notes above

Licensed use not licensed for use in children under 3 months for refraction; not licensed for use in children for uveitis

Indication and dose

Cycloplegia

Child 3 months–18 years apply drops or ointment twice daily for 3 days before procedure

Anterior uveitis

Child 2–18 years 1 drop up to 4 times daily

Atropine (Non-proprietary) PoM

Eye drops, atropine sulphate 0.5%, net price 10 mL = £2.32; 1%, 10 mL = 91p

Eye ointment, atropine sulphate 1%. Net price 3 g = £2.96

Isopto Atropine® (Alcon) PoM

Eye drops, atropine sulphate 1%, hypromellose 0.5%. Net price 5 mL = 99p

Excipients: include benzalkonium chloride

Single use

Minims® Atropine Sulphate (Chauvin) PoM

Eye drops, atropine sulphate 1%. Net price 20 × 0.5 mL = £4.92

CYCLOPENTOLATE HYDROCHLORIDE

Cautions see notes above

Side-effects see notes above

Licensed use not licensed for use in children under 3 months

Indication and dose

See notes above

Cycloplegia

Child 3 months–12 years 1 drop of 1% eye drops 30–60 minutes before examination

Child 12–18 years 1 drop of 0.5% eye drops 30–60 minutes before examination

Uveitis

Child 3 months–18 years 1 drop of 0.5% eye drops (1% for deeply pigmented eyes) 2–4 times daily

Mydrilate® (Intrapharm) PoM

Eye drops, cyclopentolate hydrochloride 0.5%, net price 5 mL = 97p; 1%, 5 mL = £1.19

Excipients: include benzalkonium chloride

Single use

Minims® Cyclopentolate Hydrochloride (Chauvin) PoM

Eye drops, cyclopentolate hydrochloride 0.5 and 1%. Net price 20 × 0.5 mL (both) = £4.92

HOMATROPINE HYDROBROMIDE

Cautions see notes above

Side-effects see notes above

Licensed use not licensed for use in children under 3 months

Indication and dose

See notes above

Child 3 months–2 years (0.5% only) 1 drop daily or on alternate days adjusted according to response

Child 2–18 years 1 drop twice daily adjusted according to response

Homatropine (Non-proprietary) PoM

Eye drops, homatropine hydrobromide 1%, net price 10 mL = £2.14; 2%, 10 mL = £2.26

Available without preservatives as manufactured specials from Moorfields Eye Hospital

Eye drops, homatropine 0.125 and 0.5%, 10 mL, available as a manufactured special from Moorfields Eye Hospital

Excipients: include chlorhexidine

TROPICAMIDE

Cautions see notes above

Side-effects see notes above

Indication and dose

See notes above

Funduscopy

Neonate and child apply 0.5% eye drops 20 minutes before examination

Mydriacyl® (Alcon) PoM

Eye drops, tropicamide 0.5%, net price 5 mL = £1.36; 1%, 5 mL = £1.68

Excipients: include benzalkonium chloride, disodium edetate

Single use

Minims® Tropicamide (Chauvin) PoM

Eye drops, tropicamide 0.5 and 1%. Net price 20 × 0.5 mL (both) = £5.75

Sympathomimetics

PHENYLEPHRINE HYDROCHLORIDE

Cautions cardiovascular disease (avoid or use 2.5% strength only); tachycardia; hyperthyroidism; diabetes; see also notes above

Contra-indications angle-closure glaucoma; 10% drops in neonates and children

Side-effects eye pain and stinging; blurred vision, photophobia; systemic effects include arrhythmias, hypertension, coronary artery spasm

Indication and dose

Mydriasis see notes above

Single use

Minims® Phenylephrine Hydrochloride (Chauvin)
Eye drops, phenylephrine hydrochloride 2.5%, net price 20 × 0.5 mL = £5.75
Excipients: include disodium edetate, sodium metabisulphite

11.6 Treatment of glaucoma

Glaucoma describes a group of disorders characterised by a loss of visual field associated with cupping of the optic disc and optic nerve damage. While glaucoma is generally associated with raised intra-ocular pressure, it can occur when the intra-ocular pressure is within the normal range.

Primary open-angle glaucoma (chronic simple glaucoma; wide-angle glaucoma), results from obstruction in the trabecular meshwork. The condition is often asymptomatic and the child may present with significant visual field loss. *Primary angle closure glaucoma* (acute closed-angle glaucoma, narrow angle glaucoma) results from blockage of aqueous humour flow into the anterior chamber and is a medical emergency.

Glaucoma is rare in children and should always be managed by a specialist. Drugs which reduce intra-ocular pressure by a variety of mechanisms are available for managing glaucoma. A topical beta-blocker or a prostaglandin analogue may be used. It may be necessary to combine these drugs or add others such as miotics, sympathomimetics and carbonic anhydrase inhibitors to control intra-ocular pressure.

For urgent reduction of intra-ocular pressure and before surgery, mannitol 20% (up to 500 mL) is given by slow intravenous infusion until the intra-ocular pressure has been satisfactorily reduced (see section 2.2.5). Acetazolamide by intravenous injection may also be used for the emergency management of raised intra-ocular pressure.

Standard antiglaucoma therapy is used if supplementary treatment is required after iridotomy, iridectomy or a drainage operation in either primary open-angle or acute closed-angle glaucoma.

Beta-blockers

Topical application of a beta-blocker to the eye reduces intra-ocular pressure effectively in *primary open-angle glaucoma*, probably by reducing the rate of production of aqueous humour. Administration by mouth also reduces intra-ocular pressure but this route is not used since side-effects may be troublesome.

Cautions, contra-indications and side-effects Systemic absorption may follow topical application therefore eye drops containing a beta-blocker are contra-indicated in bradycardia, heart block, or uncontrolled heart failure. **Important:** avoid in asthma, see CSM advice below. Consider also other cautions, contra-indications and side-effects of beta-blockers (p. 110). Local side-effects of eye drops include ocular stinging, burning, pain, itching, erythema, dry eyes and allergic reactions including anaphylaxis and blepharoconjunctivitis; occasionally corneal disorders have been reported.

CSM advice. The CSM has advised that beta-blockers, even those with apparent cardioselectivity, should not be used in patients with asthma or a history of obstructive airways disease, unless no alternative treatment is available. In such cases the risk of inducing bronchospasm should be appreciated and appropriate precautions taken.

Interactions Since systemic absorption may follow topical application the possibility of interactions, in particular with drugs such as verapamil, should be borne in mind. See also Appendix 1 (beta-blockers).

BETAXOLOL HYDROCHLORIDE

Cautions see notes above
Contra-indications see notes above
Side-effects see notes above
Licensed use not licensed for use in children
Indication and dose

See notes above
Apply twice daily

Betoptic® (Alcon) PoM
Ophthalmic solution (= eye drops), betaxolol (as hydrochloride) 0.5%, net price 5 mL = £2.00
Excipients: include benzalkonium chloride, disodium edetate

Ophthalmic suspension (= eye drops), m/r, betaxolol (as hydrochloride) 0.25%, net price 5 mL = £2.80
Excipients: include benzalkonium chloride, disodium edetate

Unit dose eye drop suspension, m/r, betaxolol (as hydrochloride) 0.25%, net price 50 × 0.25 mL = £14.49

CARTEOLOL HYDROCHLORIDE

Cautions see notes above
Contra-indications see notes above
Side-effects see notes above
Licensed use not licensed for use in children
Indication and dose

See notes above
Apply twice daily

Teoptic® (Novartis) PoM
Eye drops, carteolol hydrochloride 1%, net price 5 mL = £4.60; 2%, 5 mL = £5.40
Excipients: include benzalkonium chloride

LEVOBUNOLOL HYDROCHLORIDE

Cautions see notes above
Contra-indications see notes above
Side-effects see notes above; anterior uveitis occasionally reported
Licensed use not licensed for use in children
Indication and dose

See notes above
Apply once or twice daily

Levobunolol (Non-proprietary) PoM
Eye drops, levobunolol hydrochloride 0.5%. Net price 5 mL = £2.28

Betagan® (Allergan) PoM
Eye drops, levobunolol hydrochloride 0.5%, polyvinyl alcohol (*Liquifilm®*) 1.4%. Net price 5-mL = £2.85
Excipients: include benzalkonium chloride, disodium edetate, sodium metabisulphite

Unit dose eye drops, levobunolol hydrochloride 0.5%, polyvinyl alcohol (*Liquifilm®*) 1.4%. Net price 30 × 0.4 mL = £9.98
Excipients: include disodium edetate

TIMOLOL MALEATE

Cautions see notes above
Contra-indications see notes above
Side-effects see notes above
Licensed use not licensed for use in children
Indication and dose

See notes above
Apply twice daily; long-acting preparations, see under preparations below

Timolol (Non-proprietary) PoM
Eye drops, timolol (as maleate) 0.25%, net price 5 mL = £1.75; 0.5%, 5 mL = £1.69

Timoptol® (MSD) PoM
Eye drops, in *Ocumeter®* metered-dose unit, timolol (as maleate) 0.25%, net price 5 mL = £3.12; 0.5%, 5 mL = £3.12
Excipients: include benzalkonium chloride

Unit dose eye drops, timolol (as maleate) 0.25%, net price 30 × 0.2 mL = £8.45; 0.5%, 30 × 0.2 mL = £9.65

Once-daily preparations

Nyogel® (Novartis) PoM
Eye gel (= eye drops), timolol (as maleate) 0.1%, net price 5 g = £2.85
Excipients: include benzalkonium chloride
Dose

Child 12–18 years apply once daily

Timoptol®-LA (MSD) PoM
Ophthalmic gel-forming solution (= eye drops), timolol (as maleate) 0.25%, net price 2.5 mL = £3.12; 0.5%, 2.5 mL = £3.12
Excipients: include benzododecinium bromide
Dose

Apply eye drops once daily

With dorzolamide

See under Dorzolamide

Prostaglandin analogues

Latanoprost and **travoprost** are prostaglandin analogues which increase uveoscleral outflow; **bimatoprost** is a related drug. They are used to reduce intra-ocular pressure in ocular hypertension or in open-angle glaucoma. They are not licensed for use in children. Children receiving prostaglandin analogues should be managed by a specialist and monitored for any changes to eye coloration since an increase in the brown pigment in the iris may occur; particular care is required in those with mixed coloured irides and those receiving treatment to one eye only.

Sympathomimetics

Dipivefrine is a pro-drug of adrenaline. It is claimed to pass more rapidly than adrenaline through the cornea and is then converted to the active form. Adrenaline (epinephrine) probably acts both by reducing the rate of production of aqueous humour and by increasing the outflow through the trabecular meshwork. It is contra-indicated in angle-closure glaucoma because it is a mydriatic, unless an iridectomy has been carried out. Side-effects include severe smarting and redness of the eye; adrenaline should be used with caution in children with hypertension and heart disease..

Apraclonidine (section 11.8.2) is an alpha$_2$-adrenoceptor stimulant. Eye drops containing apraclonidine 0.5% are used for a short period to delay laser treatment or surgery for glaucoma in patients not adequately controlled by another drug; eye drops containing 1% are used for control of intra-ocular pressure after anterior segment laser surgery.

DIPIVEFRINE HYDROCHLORIDE

Contra-indications see notes above

Side-effects see notes above

Licensed use not licensed for use in children

Indication and dose

See notes above
Apply twice daily

Propine® (Allergan) PoM

Eye drops, dipivefrine hydrochloride 0.1%, net price 5 mL = £3.81, 10 mL = £4.77

Excipients: include benzalkonium chloride, disodium edetate

Carbonic anhydrase inhibitors and systemic drugs

The **carbonic anhydrase inhibitors**, acetazolamide, brinzolamide and dorzolamide, reduce intra-ocular pressure by reducing aqueous humour production. Systemic use of acetazolamide also produces weak diuresis.

Acetazolamide is given by mouth or, rarely in children, by intravenous injection (intramuscular injections are painful because of the alkaline pH of the solution). It is used as an adjunct to other treatment for reducing intra-ocular pressure. Acetazolamide is a sulphonamide; blood disorders, rashes and other sulphonamide-related side-effects occur occasionally. It is not generally recommended for long-term use; electrolyte disturbances and metabolic acidosis that occur may be corrected by administering potassium bicarbonate (as effervescent potassium tablets, section 9.2.1.3).

Dorzolamide and **brinzolamide** are topical carbonic anhydrase inhibitors. They are unlicensed in children but are used in those resistant to beta-blockers or those in whom beta-blockers are contra-indicated. They are used alone or as an adjunct to a topical beta-blocker. Systemic absorption may rarely give rise to sulphonamide-like side-effects and may require discontinuation if severe.

The **osmotic diuretics**, intravenous hypertonic **mannitol** (section 2.2.5), or **glycerol** by mouth, are useful short-term ocular hypotensive drugs.

ACETAZOLAMIDE

Cautions not generally recommended for prolonged use but if given monitor blood count and plasma electrolyte concentration; pulmonary obstruction (risk of acidosis); avoid extravasation at injection site (risk of necrosis); **interactions:** Appendix 1 (diuretics)

Pregnancy manufacturer advises avoid, especially in first trimester (toxicity in *animal* studies)

Breast-feeding amount too small to be harmful

Contra-indications hypokalaemia, hyponatraemia, hyperchloraemic acidosis; sulphonamide hypersensitivity

Renal impairment avoid in even mild impairment

Hepatic impairment avoid in severe impairment

Side-effects nausea, vomiting, diarrhoea, taste disturbance; loss of appetite, paraesthesia, flushing, headache, dizziness, fatigue, irritability, depression; thirst, polyuria; metabolic acidosis and electrolyte disturbances on long-term therapy; occasionally, drowsiness, confusion, hearing disturbances, urticaria, melaena, glycosuria, haematuria, abnormal liver function, renal calculi, blood disorders including agranulocytosis and thrombocytopenia, rashes including Stevens-Johnson syndrome and toxic epidermal necrolysis; rarely, photosensitivity, liver damage, flaccid paralysis, convulsions; transient myopia reported

Licensed use not licensed for use in children for treatment of glaucoma

Indication and dose

Reduction of intra-ocular pressure in open-angle glaucoma, secondary glaucoma, peri-operatively in angle closure glaucoma
- **By mouth or by intravenous injection**

Child 1 month–12 years 5 mg/kg 2–4 times daily, adjusted according to response, max. 750 mg daily

Child 12–18 years 250 mg 2–4 times daily

Epilepsy
- **By mouth or slow intravenous injection**

Neonate initially 2.5 mg/kg 2–3 times daily, followed by 5–7 mg/kg 2–3 times daily (maintenance dose)

Child 1 month–12 years initially 2.5 mg/kg 2–3 times daily, followed by 5–7 mg/kg 2–3 times daily, max. 750 mg daily (maintenance dose)

Child 12–18 years 250 mg 2–4 times daily, max. 1 g daily

Raised intracranial pressure
- **By mouth or slow intravenous injection**

Child 1 month–12 years initially 8 mg/kg 3 times daily, increased as necessary to max. 100 mg/kg daily

Diamox® (Goldshield) PoM

Tablets, acetazolamide 250 mg. Net price 112-tab pack = £12.68. Label: 3

Sodium Parenteral (= injection), powder for reconstitution, acetazolamide (as sodium salt). Net price 500-mg vial = £14.76

Diamox® SR (Goldshield) PoM

Capsules, m/r, two-tone orange, enclosing orange f/c pellets, acetazolamide 250 mg. Net price 28-cap pack = £11.55. Label: 3, 25

Dose

Child 12–18 years glaucoma, 1–2 capsules daily

Extemporaneous formulations available see Extemporaneous Preparations, p. 8

BRINZOLAMIDE

Cautions interactions: Appendix 1 (brinzolamide)

Hepatic impairment manufacturer advises caution—no information available

Pregnancy manufacturer advises avoid unless essential—embryotoxic in *animal* studies

Contra-indications hyperchloraemic acidosis

Renal impairment avoid if creatinine clearance less than 30 mL/minute/1.73 m^2

Breast-feeding manufacturer advises avoid—no information available

Side-effects local irritation, taste disturbance; less commonly nausea, dyspepsia, dry mouth, chest pain, epistaxis, haemoptysis, dyspnoea, rhinitis, pharyngitis, bronchitis, paraesthesia, depression, dizziness, headache, dermatitis, alopecia, corneal erosion

Licensed use not licensed for use in children

Indication and dose

Adjunct to beta-blockers or used alone in raised intra-ocular pressure in ocular hypertension and in open-angle glaucoma if beta-blocker alone inadequate or inappropriate

Apply twice daily increased to 3 times daily if necessary

Azopt® (Alcon) PoM

Eye drops, brinzolamide 10 mg/mL, net price 5 mL = £6.90

Excipients: include benzalkonium chloride, disodium edetate

DORZOLAMIDE

Cautions systemic absorption follows topical application; history of renal calculi; chronic corneal defects, history of intra-ocular surgery; **interactions**: Appendix 1 (dorzolamide)

Hepatic impairment manufacturer advises caution—no information available

Contra-indications hyperchloraemic acidosis

Renal impairment avoid if creatinine clearance less than 30 mL/minute/1.73 m² and in neonates and infants with immature renal tubules—risk of metabolic acidosis

Pregnancy manufacturer advises avoid—embryotoxic in *animal* studies

Breast-feeding manufacturer advises avoid—no information available

Side-effects ocular burning, stinging and itching, blurred vision, lacrimation, conjunctivitis, superficial punctate keratitis, eyelid inflammation and crusting, anterior uveitis, transient myopia, corneal oedema, iridocyclitis; headache, dizziness, paraesthesia, asthenia, sinusitis, rhinitis, nausea; metabolic acidosis in neonates and children; hypersensitivity reactions (including urticaria, angioedema, bronchospasm); bitter taste, epistaxis, urolithiasis

Licensed use not licensed for use in children

Indication and dose

Raised intra-ocular pressure in ocular hypertension, open-angle glaucoma, pseudo-exfoliative glaucoma *either* as adjunct to beta-blocker *or* used alone in patients unresponsive to beta-blockers or if beta-blockers contra-indicated

Used alone, apply 3 times daily; with topical beta-blocker, apply twice daily

Trusopt® (MSD) PoM

Ophthalmic solution (= eye drops), dorzolamide (as hydrochloride) 2%, net price 5 mL = £6.33

Excipients: include benzalkonium chloride

With timolol

For cautions, contra-indications, and side-effects of timolol, see section 11.6, Beta-blockers

Cosopt® (MSD) PoM

Ophthalmic solution (= eye drops), dorzolamide (as hydrochloride) 2%, timolol (as maleate) 0.5%, net price 5 mL = £10.05

Excipients: include benzalkonium chloride

Dose

Raised intra-ocular pressure in open-angle glaucoma, or pseudoexfoliative glaucoma when beta-blockers alone not adequate

Apply twice daily

Miotics

Pilocarpine is a miotic used in the management of raised intra-ocular pressure. The small pupil is an unfortunate side-effect of these drugs (except when pilocarpine is used temporarily before an operation for angle-closure glaucoma). Miotics act by opening up the inefficient drainage channels in the trabecular meshwork which may be occluded by contraction or spasm of the ciliary muscle.

Cautions A darkly pigmented iris may require higher concentration of the miotic or more frequent administration and care should be taken to avoid overdosage. Retinal detachment has occurred in susceptible individuals and those with retinal disease; therefore fundus examination is advised before starting treatment with a miotic. Care is also required in conjunctival or corneal damage. Intra-ocular pressure and visual fields should be monitored in those with chronic simple glaucoma and those receiving long-term treatment with a miotic. Miotics should be used with caution in cardiac disease, hypertension, asthma, peptic ulceration and urinary-tract obstruction.

Counselling Blurred vision may affect performance of skilled tasks (e.g. driving) particularly at night or in reduced lighting

Contra-indications Miotics are contra-indicated in conditions where pupillary constriction is undesirable such as acute iritis, anterior uveitis and some forms of secondary glaucoma. They should be avoided in acute inflammatory disease of the anterior segment.

Side-effects Ciliary spasm leads to headache and browache which may be more severe in the initial 2–4 weeks of treatment. Ocular side-effects include burning, itching, smarting, blurred vision, conjunctival vascular congestion, myopia, lens changes with chronic use, vitreous haemorrhage, and pupillary block. Systemic side-effects are rare following application to the eye.

PILOCARPINE

Cautions see notes above

Contra-indications see notes above

Side-effects see notes above

Licensed use not licensed for use in children

Indication and dose

See also notes above

Raised intra-ocular pressure in ocular hypertension and open-angle glaucoma
Child 1 month–2 years 1 drop of 0.5% or 1% solution 3 times daily
Child 2–18 years 1 drop 4 times daily

Pre-operatively in goniotomy and trabeculotomy
Child 1 month–18 years apply 1% or 2% solution once daily

Dry mouth (section 12.3.5)

Pilocarpine Hydrochloride (Non-proprietary) PoM
Eye drops, pilocarpine hydrochloride 0.5%, net price 10 mL = £1.39; 1%, 10 mL = £2.29; 2%, 10 mL = £2.09; 3%, 10 mL = £1.44; 4%, 10 mL = £2.83

Single use

Minims® Pilocarpine Nitrate (Chauvin) PoM
Eye drops, pilocarpine nitrate 2 and 4%, net price 20 × 0.5 mL (both) = £4.92

11.7 Local anaesthetics

Oxybuprocaine and **tetracaine** (amethocaine) are widely used topical local anaesthetics. **Proxymetacaine** causes less initial stinging and is particularly useful for children. Oxybuprocaine or a combined preparation of lidocaine (lignocaine) and fluorescein is used for tonometry. Tetracaine produces more profound anaesthesia and is suitable for use before minor surgical procedures, such as the removal of corneal sutures. It has a temporary disruptive effect on the corneal epithelium. **Lidocaine**, with or without adrenaline (epinephrine), is injected into the eyelids for minor surgery, while retrobulbar or peribulbar injections are used for surgery of the globe itself. Local anaesthetics should never be used for the management of ocular symptoms.

Caution Lidocaine, proxymetacaine and tetracaine should be avoided in preterm neonates because of the immaturity of the metabolising enzyme system.

LIDOCAINE HYDROCHLORIDE
(Lignocaine hydrochloride)

Contra-indications avoid in preterm neonates

Indication and dose

Local anaesthetic
Use as required

Minims® Lignocaine and Fluorescein (Chauvin) PoM
Eye drops, lidocaine hydrochloride 4%, fluorescein sodium 0.25%. Net price 20 × 0.5 mL = £6.93

OXYBUPROCAINE HYDROCHLORIDE

Indication and dose

Local anaesthetic
Use as required

Minims® Benoxinate (Oxybuprocaine) Hydrochloride (Chauvin) PoM
Eye drops, oxybuprocaine hydrochloride 0.4%. Net price 20 × 0.5 mL = £4.92

PROXYMETACAINE HYDROCHLORIDE

Contra-indications avoid in preterm neonates

Indication and dose

Local anaesthetic
Use as required

Minims® Proxymetacaine (Chauvin) PoM
Eye drops, proxymetacaine hydrochloride 0.5%. Net price 20 × 0.5 mL = £6.95

With fluorescein

Minims® Proxymetacaine and Fluorescein (Chauvin) PoM
Eye drops, proxymetacaine hydrochloride 0.5%, fluorescein sodium 0.25%. Net price 20 × 0.5 mL = £7.95

TETRACAINE HYDROCHLORIDE
(Amethocaine hydrochloride)

Contra-indications avoid in preterm neonates

Indication and dose

Local anaesthetic
Use as required

Minims® Amethocaine Hydrochloride (Chauvin) PoM
Eye drops, tetracaine hydrochloride 0.5 and 1%. Net price 20 × 0.5 mL (both) = £5.75

11.8 Miscellaneous ophthalmic preparations

Certain eye drops, e.g. amphotericin, ceftazidime, cefuroxime, colistin, desferrioxamine, dexamethasone, gentamicin and vancomycin may be prepared aseptically in a specialist manufacturing unit from material supplied for injection.

Preparations may also be available from Moorfields Eye Hospital as manufactured specials.

11.8.1 Tear deficiency, ocular lubricants, and astringents

Chronic soreness of the eyes associated with reduced or abnormal tear secretion (e.g. in Sjögren's syndrome) often responds to tear replacement therapy. The severity of the condition and the child's preference will often guide the choice of preparation.

Hypromellose is the traditional choice of treatment for tear deficiency. It may need to be instilled frequently (e.g. hourly) for adequate relief. Ocular surface mucin is often abnormal in tear deficiency and the combination of hypromellose with a mucolytic such as **acetylcysteine** can be helpful.

The ability of **carbomers** to cling to the eye surface may help reduce frequency of application to 4 times daily.

Polyvinyl alcohol increases the persistence of the tear film and is useful when the ocular surface mucin is reduced.

Sodium chloride 0.9% drops are sometimes useful in tear deficiency, and can be used as 'comfort drops' by contact lens wearers, and to facilitate lens removal. Special presentations of sodium chloride 0.9% and other irrigation solutions are used routinely for intra-ocular surgery and in first-aid for removal of harmful substances.

Eye ointments containing a **paraffin** may be used to lubricate the eye surface, especially in cases of recurrent corneal epithelial erosion. They may cause temporary visual disturbance and are best suited for application before sleep. Ointments should not be used during contact lens wear.

ACETYLCYSTEINE

Indication and dose

Tear deficiency, impaired or abnormal mucus production
Apply 3–4 times daily

Ilube® (Alcon) PoM
Eye drops, acetylcysteine 5%, hypromellose 0.35%. Net price 10 mL = £4.63
Excipients: include benzalkonium chloride, disodium edetate

CARBOMERS
(Polyacrylic acid)

Synthetic high molecular weight polymers of acrylic acid cross-linked with either allyl ethers of sucrose or allyl ethers of pentaerithrityl

Licensed use some preparations not licensed for use in children

Indication and dose

Dry eyes including keratoconjunctivitis sicca, unstable tear film
Apply 3–4 times daily or as required

GelTears® (Chauvin)
Gel (= eye drops), carbomer 980 (polyacrylic acid) 0.2%, net price 10 g = £2.80
Excipients: include benzalkonium chloride

Liposic® (Bausch & Lomb)
Gel (= eye drops), carbomer 980 (polyacrylic acid) 0.2%, net price 10 g = £2.96
Excipients: include cetrimide

CARBOMERS (*continued*)

Viscotears® (Novartis Ophthalmics)
Liquid gel (= eye drops), carbomer 980 (polyacrylic acid) 0.2%, net price 10 g = £3.12
Excipients: include cetrimide, disodium edetate

Liquid gel (= eye drops), carbomer 980 (polyacrylic acid) 0.2%, net price 30 × 0.6-mL single-dose units = £5.75

CARMELLOSE SODIUM

Indication and dose

Dry eye conditions
Apply as required

Celluvisc® (Allergan)
Eye drops, carmellose sodium 1%, net price 30 × 0.4 mL = £5.75, 60 × 0.4 mL = £10.99

HYDROXYETHYLCELLULOSE

Indication and dose

Tear deficiency
Apply as required

Minims® Artificial Tears (Chauvin)
Eye drops, hydroxyethylcellulose 0.44%, sodium chloride 0.35%. Net price 20 × 0.5 mL = £5.75

HYPROMELLOSE

Indication and dose

Tear deficiency
Apply as required
Note The Royal Pharmaceutical Society of Great Britain has stated that where it is not possible to ascertain the strength of hypromellose prescribed, the prescriber should be contacted to clarify the strength intended.

Hypromellose (Non-proprietary)
Eye drops, hypromellose 0.3%, net price 10 mL = 75p

Isopto Alkaline® (Alcon)
Eye drops, hypromellose 1%, net price 10 mL = 99p
Excipients: include benzalkonium chloride

Isopto Plain® (Alcon)
Eye drops, hypromellose 0.5%, net price 10 mL = 85p
Excipients: include benzalkonium chloride

Tears Naturale® (Alcon)
Eye drops, dextran '70' 0.1%, hypromellose 0.3%, net price 15 mL = £1.68
Excipients: include benzalkonium chloride, disodium edetate

Single use
Artelac® SDU (Pharma-Global)
Eye drops, hypromellose 0.32%, net price 30 × 0.5 mL = £11.88

LIQUID PARAFFIN

Indication and dose

Dry eye conditions
Apply as required

Lacri-Lube® (Allergan)
Eye ointment, white soft paraffin 57.3%, liquid paraffin 42.5%, wool alcohols 0.2%. Net price 3.5 g = £1.90, 5 g = £2.47

Lubri-Tears® (Alcon)
Eye ointment, white soft paraffin 60%, liquid paraffin 30%, wool fat 10%. Net price 5 g = £2.29

PARAFFIN, YELLOW, SOFT

Indication and dose

See notes above
Apply 2 hourly as required

Simple Eye Ointment
Ointment, liquid paraffin 10%, wool fat 10%, in yellow soft paraffin. Net price 4 g = £2.68

POLYVINYL ALCOHOL

Indication and dose

Tear deficiency
Apply as required

Liquifilm Tears® (Allergan)
Ophthalmic solution (= eye drops), polyvinyl alcohol 1.4%. Net price 15 mL = £1.61
Excipients: include benzalkonium chloride, disodium edetate

Ophthalmic solution (= eye drops), polyvinyl alcohol 1.4%, povidone 0.6%. Net price 30 × 0.4 mL = £5.35

Sno Tears® (Chauvin)
Eye drops, polyvinyl alcohol 1.4%. Net price 10 mL = £1.06
Excipients: include benzalkonium chloride, disodium edetate

SODIUM CHLORIDE

Indication and dose

Irrigation, including first-aid removal of harmful substances
Use as required

Sodium Chloride 0.9% Solutions
See section 13.11.1

Balanced Salt Solution
Solution (sterile), sodium chloride 0.64%, sodium acetate 0.39%, sodium citrate 0.17%, calcium chloride 0.048%, magnesium chloride 0.03%, potassium chloride 0.075%
For intra-ocular or topical irrigation during surgical procedures
Brands include *Iocare*®

Single use

Minims® Saline (Chauvin)
Eye drops, sodium chloride 0.9%. Net price 20 × 0.5 mL = £4.92

11.8.2 Ocular diagnostic and peri-operative preparations and photodynamic treatment

Ocular diagnostic preparations

Fluorescein sodium and **rose bengal** are used in diagnostic procedures and for locating damaged areas of the cornea due to injury or disease. Rose bengal is more efficient for the diagnosis of conjunctival epithelial damage but it often stings excessively unless a local anaesthetic is instilled beforehand.

FLUORESCEIN SODIUM

Indication and dose

Detection of lesions and foreign bodies
sufficient to stain damaged areas

Minims® Fluorescein Sodium (Chauvin)
Eye drops, fluorescein sodium 1 or 2%. Net price 20 × 0.5 mL (both) = £4.92

With local anaesthetic
Section 11.7

ROSE BENGAL

Indication and dose

Detection of lesions and foreign bodies
sufficient to stain damaged areas

Minims® Rose Bengal (Chauvin)
Eye drops, rose bengal 1%. Net price 20 × 0.5 mL = £5.75

Ocular peri-operative drugs

Drugs used to prepare the eye for surgery and drugs that are injected into the anterior chamber at the time of surgery are included here.

Sodium hyaluronate is used during surgical procedures on the eye.

Apraclonidine, an alpha$_2$-adrenoceptor stimulant, reduces intra-ocular pressure possibly by reducing the production of aqueous humour. It is used for short-term treatment only.

Balanced Salt Solution is used routinely in intra-ocular surgery (section 11.8.1).

ACETYLCHOLINE CHLORIDE

Licensed use not licensed for use in children

Indication and dose

Cataract surgery, penetrating keratoplasty, iridectomy, other anterior segment surgery requiring rapid complete miosis
consult product literature

Miochol-E® (Novartis) PoM
Solution for intra-ocular irrigation, acetylcholine chloride 1%, mannitol 3% when reconstituted. Net price 2 mL-vial = £9.10

APRACLONIDINE

Note Apraclonidine is a derivative of clonidine

Cautions history of angina, severe coronary insufficiency, recent myocardial infarction, heart failure, cerebrovascular disease, vasovagal attack, chronic renal failure; depression; pregnancy and breast-feeding; monitor intra-ocular pressure and visual fields; loss of effect may occur over time; suspend treatment if reduction in vision occurs in end-stage glaucoma; monitor for excessive reduction in intra-ocular pressure following peri-operative use; **interactions:** Appendix 1 (alpha$_2$-adrenoceptor stimulants)

Skilled tasks Drowsiness may affect performance of skilled tasks (e.g. driving)

Contra-indications history of severe or unstable and uncontrolled cardiovascular disease

Side-effects dry mouth, taste disturbance; hyperaemia, ocular pruritus, discomfort and lacrimation (withdraw if ocular intolerance including oedema of lids and conjunctiva); headache, asthenia, dry nose; lid retraction, conjunctival blanching and mydriasis reported after peri-operative use; since absorption may follow topical application systemic effects (see Clonidine Hydrochloride, section 2.5.2) may occur

Licensed use 0.5% drops not licensed for use in children under 12 years; 1% drops not licensed for use in children

Indication and dose

See under preparations below

Iopidine® (Alcon) PoM

Ophthalmic solution (= eye drops), apraclonidine 1% (as hydrochloride). Net price 12 × 2 single use 0.25-mL units = £81.90

Dose

Control or prevention of postoperative elevation of intra-ocular pressure after anterior segment laser surgery

apply 1 drop 1 hour before laser procedure then 1 drop immediately after completion of procedure

Ophthalmic solution (= eye drops), apraclonidine 0.5% (as hydrochloride). Net price 5 mL = £11.45

Excipients: include benzalkonium chloride

Dose

Short-term adjunctive treatment of chronic glaucoma in patients not adequately controlled by another drug (see note below)

Child 12–18 years apply 1 drop 3 times daily usually for max. 1 month

Note May not provide additional benefit if patient already using two drugs that suppress the production of aqueous humour

DICLOFENAC SODIUM

Licensed use not licensed for use in children

Indication and dose

Inhibition of intra-operative miosis during cataract surgery (but does not possess intrinsic mydriatic properties), postoperative inflammation in cataract surgery, strabismus surgery, argon laser trabeculoplasty

consult product literature

Voltarol® Ophtha Multidose (Novartis) PoM

Eye drops, diclofenac sodium 0.1%, net price 5 mL = £6.68

Excipients: include benzalkonium chloride, disodium edetate, propylene glycol

Single use

Voltarol® Ophtha (Novartis) PoM

Eye drops, diclofenac sodium 0.1%. Net price pack of 5 single-dose units = £4.00, 40 single-dose units = £32.00

FLURBIPROFEN SODIUM

Licensed use not licensed for use in children

Indication and dose

Inhibition of intra-operative miosis (but does not possess intrinsic mydriatic properties), control of postoperative and post-laser trabeculoplasty inflammation (if corticosteroids contra-indicated)

consult product literature

Ocufen® (Allergan) PoM

Ophthalmic solution (= eye drops), flurbiprofen sodium 0.03%, polyvinyl alcohol (*Liquifilm®*) 1.4%. Net price 40 × 0.4 mL = £37.15

KETOROLAC TROMETAMOL

Licensed use not licensed for use in children

Indication and dose

Prophylaxis and reduction of inflammation and associated symptoms following ocular surgery

consult product literature

Acular® (Allergan) PoM

Eye drops, ketorolac trometamol 0.5%. Net price 5 mL = £5.00

Excipients: include benzalkonium chloride, disodium edetate

11.9 Contact lenses

Note Some recommendations in this section involve non-licensed indications.

For cosmetic reasons some children and adolescents prefer to wear contact lenses rather than spectacles; contact lenses are also sometimes required for medical indications. Visual defects are corrected by either rigid ('hard' or gas permeable) lenses or soft (hydrogel) lenses; soft lenses are the most popular type, because they are the most comfortable, though they may not give the best vision. Lenses should usually be worn for a specified number of hours each day. Continuous (extended) wear involves much greater risks to eye health and is not recommended except where medically indicated.

Contact lenses require meticulous care. Poor compliance with directions for use, and with daily cleaning and disinfection, may result in complications which include ulcerative keratitis, conjunctival problems (such as purulent or papillary conjunctivitis). One-day disposable lenses, which are worn only once and therefore require no maintenance or storage, are becoming increasingly popular.

Acanthamoeba keratitis, a sight-threatening condition, is associated with ineffective lens cleaning and disinfection or the use of contaminated lens cases. The condition is especially associated with the use of soft lenses (including frequently replaced lenses). Acanthamoeba keratitis requires urgent treatment by specialists with intensive use of polihexanide (polyhexamethylene biguanide), propamidine isetionate, chlorhexidine and neomycin drops, sometimes in combination.

Contact lenses and drug treatment Special care is required in prescribing eye preparations for contact lens users. Some drugs and preservatives in eye preparations can accumulate in hydrogel lenses and may cause adverse reactions. Therefore, unless medically indicated, the lenses should be removed before instillation and not worn during the period of treatment. Alternatively, unpreserved drops can be used. Eye drops may, however, be instilled over rigid corneal contact lenses. Ointment preparations should never be used in conjunction with contact lens wear; oily eye drops should also be avoided.

Many drugs given systemically can also have adverse effects on contact lens wear. These include oral contraceptives (particularly those with a higher oestrogen content), drugs which reduce blink rate (e.g. anxiolytics, hypnotics, antihistamines, and muscle relaxants), drugs which reduce lacrimation (e.g. antihistamines, antimuscarinics, phenothiazines and related drugs, some beta-blockers, diuretics, and tricyclic antidepressants), and drugs which increase lacrimation (including ephedrine and hydralazine). Other drugs that may affect contact lens wear are isotretinoin (may cause conjunctival inflammation), aspirin (salicylic acid appears in tears and may be absorbed by contact lenses—leading to irritation), and rifampicin and sulfasalazine (may discolour lenses).

12 Ear, nose, and oropharynx

This chapter includes advice on the drug management of the following:

allergic rhinitis, p. 595
nasal polyps, p. 595
oropharyngeal infections, p. 604
periodontitis, p. 602

12.1 Drugs acting on the ear

12.1.1 Otitis externa
12.1.2 Otitis media
12.1.3 Removal of ear wax

12.1.1 Otitis externa

Otitis externa is an inflammatory reaction of the lining of the ear canal usually associated with an underlying seborrhoeic dermatitis or eczema; it is important to exclude an underlying chronic otitis media before treatment is commenced. Many cases recover after thorough cleansing of the external ear canal by suction or dry mopping.

A frequent problem in resistant cases is the difficulty in applying lotions and ointments satisfactorily to the relatively inaccessible affected skin. The most effective method is to introduce a ribbon gauze dressing or sponge wick soaked with **corticosteroid** ear drops or with an astringent such as **aluminium acetate** solution. When this is not practical, the ear should be gently cleansed with a probe covered in cotton wool and the patient encouraged to lie with the affected ear uppermost for ten minutes after the canal has been filled with a liberal quantity of the appropriate solution.

Secondary infection in otitis externa may be of bacterial, fungal, or viral origin. If infection is present, a topical anti-infective which is not used systemically (such as **neomycin** or **clioquinol**) may be used, but for only about a week because excessive use may result in fungal infections that are difficult to treat. Sensitivity to the anti-infective or solvent may occur and resistance to antibacterials is a possibility with prolonged use. **Aluminium acetate** ear drops are also effective against bacterial infection and inflammation of the ear. **Chloramphenicol** may be used, but the ear drops contain propylene glycol and cause sensitivity in about 10% of patients. Solutions containing an anti-infective and a corticosteroid (such as *Locorten-Vioform*®) are used for treating children when infection is present with inflammation and eczema. **Clotrimazole** 1% solution is used topically to treat fungal infection in otitis externa.

In view of reports of ototoxicity in patients with a perforated tympanic membrane (eardrum), the CSM has stated that treatment with a topical aminoglycoside antibiotic is contra-indicated in those with a tympanic perforation. However, many specialists do use these drops cautiously in the presence of a perforation in children with otitis media (section 12.1.2) and where other measures have failed for otitis externa.

A solution of **acetic acid** 2% acts as an antifungal and antibacterial in the external ear canal and may be used to treat mild otitis externa. More severe cases require treatment with an anti-inflammatory preparation with or without an anti-infective drug. A proprietary preparation containing acetic acid 2% (*EarCalm*® spray) is on sale to the public for children over 12 years.

Acute infection may cause severe pain and should be treated with a systemic antibacterial (Table 1, section 5.1) and an analgesic such as **paracetamol** (section 4.7.1) or **ibuprofen** (section 10.1.1). When a resistant staphylococcal infection (a boil) is present in the external auditory canal, oral **flucloxacillin** (section 5.1.1.2) is the drug of choice; oral **ciprofloxacin** (section 5.1.12) or a systemic aminoglycoside may be needed for pseudomonal infections, particularly in children with diabetes or compromised immunity.

The skin of the pinna adjacent to the ear canal is often affected by eczema. A topical corticosteroid (section 13.4) cream or ointment is then required, but prolonged use should be avoided.

Administration To administer ear drops, lay the child down with the head turned to one side; for an infant pull the earlobe back and down, for an older child pull the earlobe back and up.

Astringent preparations

ALUMINIUM ACETATE

Licensed use not licensed

Indication and dose

Inflammation in otitis externa (see notes above)
Insert into meatus or apply on a ribbon gauze dressing or sponge wick which should be kept saturated with the ear drops

Aluminium Acetate (Non-proprietary)
Ear drops 13%, aluminium sulphate 2.25 g, calcium carbonate 1 g, tartaric acid 450 mg, acetic acid (33%) 2.5 mL, purified water 7.5 mL
Available as manufactured special

Ear drops 8%, dilute 8 parts aluminium acetate ear drops (13%) with 5 parts purified water. Must be freshly prepared

Anti-inflammatory preparations

BETAMETHASONE SODIUM PHOSPHATE

Cautions avoid prolonged use

Contra-indications untreated infection

Side-effects local sensitivity reactions

Licensed use licensed for use in children (age range not specified by manufacturers)

Indication and dose

Eczematous inflammation in otitis externa (see notes above); for dose, see under preparations

Eye section 11.4.1

Nose section 12.2.1 and section 12.2.3

Betnesol® (Celltech) PoM
Drops (for ear, eye, or nose), betamethasone sodium phosphate 0.1%. Net price 10 mL = £2.32
Excipients: include benzalkonium chloride, disodium edetate

Dose

Ear, instil 2–3 drops every 2–3 hours; reduce frequency when relief obtained

BETAMETHASONE SODIUM PHOSPHATE (*continued*)

Vista-Methasone® (Martindale) PoM
Drops (for ear, eye, or nose), betamethasone sodium phosphate 0.1%. Net price 5 mL = £1.10; 10 mL = £1.25
Excipients: include benzalkonium chloride, disodium edetate

Dose

Ear, instil 2–3 drops every 3–4 hours; reduce frequency when relief obtained

Vista-Methasone N® (Martindale) PoM
Drops (for ear, eye, or nose), betamethasone sodium phosphate 0.1%, neomycin sulphate 0.5%. Net price 5 mL = £1.09; 10 mL = £1.20
Excipients: include thiomersal

Dose

Ear, instil 2–3 drops every 3–4 hours; reduce frequency when relief obtained

With antibacterial

Betnesol-N® (Celltech) PoM
Drops (for ear, eye, or nose), betamethasone sodium phosphate 0.1%, neomycin sulphate 0.5%. Net price 10 mL = £2.39
Excipients: include benzalkonium chloride, disodium edetate

Dose

Ear, instil 2–3 drops 3–4 times daily

DEXAMETHASONE

Cautions avoid prolonged use

Contra-indications untreated infection

Side-effects local sensitivity reactions

Licensed use licensed for use in children (age range not specified by manufacturers)

Indication and dose

Eczematous inflammation in otitis externa (see notes above); for dose, see under preparations

With antibacterial

Otomize® (GSK Consumer Healthcare) PoM
Ear spray, dexamethasone 0.1%, neomycin sulphate 3250 units/mL, glacial acetic acid 2%. Net price 5-mL pump-action aerosol unit = £4.24
Excipients: include hydroxybenzoates (parabens)

Dose

Ear, apply 1 metered spray into the ear 3 times daily

Sofradex® (Sanofi-Aventis) PoM
Drops (for ear or eye), dexamethasone (as sodium metasulphobenzoate) 0.05%, framycetin sulphate 0.5%, gramicidin 0.005%. Net price 10 mL = £4.85
Excipients: include polysorbate 80

Dose

Ear, instil 2–3 drops 3–4 times daily; *eye*, section 11.4.1

FLUMETASONE PIVALATE
(Flumethasone Pivalate)

Cautions avoid prolonged use

Contra-indications untreated infection; perforated tympanic membrane

Side-effects local sensitivity reactions

Indication and dose

Eczematous inflammation in otitis externa (see notes above); for dose, see under preparation

With antibacterial

Locorten-Vioform® (Amdipharm) PoM
Ear drops, flumetasone pivalate 0.02%, clioquinol 1%. Net price 7.5 mL = £1.47

Contra-indications iodine sensitivity

Dose

Child 2–18 years instil 2–3 drops into the ear twice daily for up to 7–10 days

Note Clioquinol stains skin and clothing

HYDROCORTISONE

Cautions avoid prolonged use

Contra-indications untreated infection

Side-effects local sensitivity reactions

Licensed use *Otosporin®* not licensed for use in children under 3 years; *other preparations* licensed for use in children (age range not specified by manufacturers)

Indication and dose

Eczematous inflammation in otitis externa (see notes above); for dose, see under preparations

With antibacterial

Gentisone® HC (Roche) PoM
Ear drops, hydrocortisone acetate 1%, gentamicin 0.3% (as sulphate). Net price 10 mL = £3.69
Excipients: include benzalkonium chloride, disodium edetate

Dose

Ear, instil 2–4 drops 3–4 times daily and at night

HYDROCORTISONE (*continued*)

Neo-Cortef® (PLIVA) PoM
Ointment (for ear or eye), hydrocortisone acetate 1.5%, neomycin sulphate 0.5%. Net price 3.9 g = £1.53
Excipients: include wool fat

Dose

Ear, apply 1–2 times daily; *eye*, section 11.4.1

Note May be difficult to obtain

Otosporin® (GSK) PoM
Ear drops, hydrocortisone 1%, neomycin sulphate 3400 units, polymyxin B sulphate 10 000 units/mL. Net price 5 mL = £2.00; 10 mL = £4.00
Excipients: include cetostearyl alcohol, hydroxybenzoates (parabens), polysorbate 20

Dose

Child 3–18 years instil 3 drops into the ear 3–4 times daily

PREDNISOLONE SODIUM PHOSPHATE

Cautions avoid prolonged use

Contra-indications untreated infection

Side-effects local sensitivity reactions

Licensed use licensed for use in children (age range not specified by manufacturers)

Indication and dose

Eczematous inflammation in otitis externa (see notes above); for dose, see under preparations

Eye section 11.4.1

Predsol® (Celltech) PoM
Drops (for ear or eye), prednisolone sodium phosphate 0.5%. Net price 10 mL = £2.00
Excipients: include benzalkonium chloride, disodium edetate

Dose

Ear, instil 2–3 drops every 2–3 hours; reduce frequency when relief obtained

With antibacterial

Predsol-N® (Celltech) PoM
Drops (for ear or eye), prednisolone sodium phosphate 0.5%, neomycin sulphate 0.5%. Net price 10 mL = £2.36
Excipients: include benzalkonium chloride, disodium edetate

Dose

Ear, instil 2–3 drops 3–4 times daily

TRIAMCINOLONE ACETONIDE

Cautions avoid prolonged use

Contra-indications untreated infection

Side-effects local sensitivity reactions

Indication and dose

Eczematous inflammation in otitis externa (see notes above); for dose, see under preparation

With antibacterial

Tri-Adcortyl Otic® (Squibb) PoM
Ear ointment, triamcinolone acetonide 0.1%, gramicidin 0.025%, neomycin 0.25% (as sulphate), nystatin 100 000 units/g in *Plastibase®*. Net price 10 g = £1.58

Dose

Child 1–18 years apply into the ear 2–3 times daily

Anti-infective preparations

CHLORAMPHENICOL

Cautions avoid prolonged use (see notes above)

Side-effects high incidence of sensitivity reactions to vehicle

Licensed use licensed for use in children (age range not specified by manufacturers)

Indication and dose

Bacterial infection in otitis externa (but see notes above); for dose, see under preparation

Chloramphenicol (Non-proprietary) PoM
Ear drops, chloramphenicol in propylene glycol, net price 5%, 10 mL = £1.47; 10%, 10 mL = £1.40
Excipients: include propylene glycol

Dose

Ear, instil 2–3 drops 2–3 times daily

CLOTRIMAZOLE

Side-effects occasional local irritation or sensitivity

Licensed use licensed for use in children (age range not specified by manufacturer)

Indication and dose

Fungal infection in otitis externa (see notes above); for dose, see under preparation

Canesten® (Bayer Consumer Care)
Solution, clotrimazole 1% in polyethylene glycol 400 (macrogol 400). Net price 20 mL = £2.43

Dose

Ear, apply 2–3 times daily continuing for at least 14 days after disappearance of infection

FRAMYCETIN SULPHATE

Cautions see under Gentamicin

Contra-indications perforated tympanic membrane (see notes above)

Side-effects local sensitivity

Indication and dose

Bacterial infection in otitis externa (see notes above)

Eye section 11.3.1

With corticosteroid

Sofradex®

see Dexamethasone, p. 591

GENTAMICIN

Cautions avoid prolonged use (see notes above)

Contra-indications perforated tympanic membrane (but see also notes above and section 12.1.2)

Side-effects local sensitivity

Licensed use licensed for use in children (age range not specified by manufacturer)

Indication and dose

Bacterial infection in otitis externa (see notes above); for dose, see under preparations

Genticin® (Roche) PoM

Drops (for ear or eye), gentamicin 0.3% (as sulphate). Net price 10 mL = £1.91

Excipients: include benzalkonium chloride

Dose

Ear, instil 2–3 drops 3–4 times daily and at night; *eye*, section 11.3.1

With corticosteroid

Gentisone® HC

see Hydrocortisone, p. 591

NEOMYCIN SULPHATE

Cautions avoid prolonged use (see notes above)

Contra-indications perforated tympanic membrane (see notes above)

Side-effects local sensitivity

Indication and dose

Bacterial infection in otitis externa (see notes above) ;

With corticosteroid

Betnesol-N® PoM

see Betamethasone, p. 591

Neo-Cortef® PoM

see Hydrocortisone, p. 591

Otomize®

see Dexamethasone, p. 591

Otosporin®

see Hydrocortisone, p. 592

Predsol-N®

see Prednisolone, p. 592

Tri-Adcortyl Otic® PoM

see Triamcinolone, p. 592

Vista-Methasone N® PoM

see Betamethasone, p. 590

Other aural preparations

Choline salicylate is a mild analgesic but it is of doubtful value when applied topically.

Audax® (SSL) NHS

Ear drops, choline salicylate 21.6%, glycerol 12.6%. Net price 10 mL = £2.62

Excipients: include propylene glycol

Note Audax® is licensed for use in children (age range not specified by manufacturer)

12.1.2 Otitis media

Acute otitis media Acute otitis media is the commonest cause of severe aural pain in young children and may occur with even minor upper respiratory tract infections. Children diagnosed with acute otitis media should not be prescribed antibacterials routinely as many infections, especially those accompanying coryza, are caused by viruses. Most uncomplicated cases resolve without antibacterial treatment and a **simple analgesic**, such as paracetamol, may be sufficient. In children without systemic features, a systemic antibacterial (Table 1, section 5.1) may be started after 72 hours if there is no improvement, or earlier if there is deterioration. Following spontaneous perforation of the tympanic membrane, the majority of children improve rapidly without treatment; if there is no improvement a systemic antibacterial should be given. Topical antibacterial treatment of acute otitis media is ineffective and there is no place for ear drops containing a local anaesthetic.

In *recurrent acute otitis media* a systemic antibacterial (Table 1, section 5.1) should be given at the first sign of an upper respiratory-tract infection. A full course of a systemic antibacterial is required if otitis media recurs.

Otitis media with effusion Otitis media with effusion ('glue ear') occurs in about 10% of children and in 90% of children with cleft palates. Antimicrobials, corticosteroids, decongestants, and antihistamines have little place in the routine management of otitis media with effusion. If 'glue ear' persists for more than a month or two, the child should be referred for assessment and follow up because of the risk of long-term hearing impairment which can delay language development. Untreated or resistant glue ear may be responsible for some types of *chronic otitis media.*

Chronic otitis media Opportunistic organisms are often present in the debris, keratin, and necrotic bone of the middle ear and mastoid in children with chronic otitis media. The mainstay of treatment is thorough cleansing with aural microsuction, which may completely resolve long-standing infection. Cleansing may be followed by topical treatment as for otitis externa (section 12.1.1); this is particularly beneficial for discharging ears or infections of the mastoid cavity. Acute exacerbations of chronic infection may require treatment with an oral antibacterial (Table 1, section 5.1); a swab should be taken to identify infecting organisms and antibacterial sensitivity. Parenteral antibacterial treatment is required if *Pseudomonas aeruginosa* or *Proteus spp.* are present.

The CSM has stated that topical treatment with ototoxic antibacterials is contra-indicated in the presence of a perforation (section 12.1.1). However, many specialists use ear drops containing **aminoglycosides** (e.g. neomycin) or **polymyxins** if the otitis media has failed to settle with systemic antibacterials; it is considered that the pus in the middle ear associated with otitis media carries a higher risk of ototoxicity than the drops themselves. **Ciprofloxacin** or **ofloxacin** ear drops (available from specialist importing companies) or eye drops used in the ear [unlicensed indication] are an effective alternative to aminoglycoside ear drops for chronic otitis media in patients with perforation of the tympanic membrane.

12.1.3 Removal of ear wax

Ear wax (cerumen) is a normal bodily secretion which provides a protective film on the meatal skin and need only be removed if it causes hearing loss or interferes with a proper view of the ear drum. Irrigation of the ear canal is generally best avoided in young children and in children with a history of recurrent otitis externa, a history of ear-drum perforation, previous ear surgery, or unilateral deafness.

Ear wax causing discomfort or impaired hearing may be softened with simple remedies such as **olive oil** ear drops or **almond oil** ear drops; **sodium bicarbonate** ear drops are also effective but may cause dryness of the ear canal. If the wax is hard and impacted the drops may be used twice daily for a few days before syringing or cleansing with aural microsuction. The child should lie with the affected ear uppermost for 5 to 10 minutes after a generous amount of the softening remedy has been introduced into the ear. Proprietary preparations containing organic solvents can irritate the meatal skin, and in most cases the simple remedies indicated above are just as effective and less likely to cause irritation. Docusate sodium or urea hydrogen peroxide are ingredients in a number of proprietary preparations for softening ear wax.

For administration of ear drops, see p. 590.

Almond Oil (Non-proprietary)
Ear drops, almond oil in a suitable container
Allow to warm to room temperature before use

Olive Oil (Non-proprietary)
Ear drops, olive oil in a suitable container
Allow to warm to room temperature before use

Sodium Bicarbonate (Non-proprietary)
Ear drops, sodium bicarbonate 5%, net price 10 mL = £1.25

Cerumol® (LAB)
Ear drops, chlorobutanol 5%, paradichlorobenzene 2%, arachis (peanut) oil 57.3%. Net price 11 mL = £1.60

Exterol® (Dermal)
Ear drops, urea–hydrogen peroxide complex 5% in glycerol. Net price 8 mL = £1.83

Molcer® (Wallace Mfg)
Ear drops, docusate sodium 5%. Net price 15 mL = £1.90
Excipients: include propylene glycol

Otex® (DDD)
Ear drops, urea–hydrogen peroxide 5%. Net price 8 mL = £2.64

Waxsol® (Norgine)
Ear drops, docusate sodium 0.5%. Net price 10 mL = £1.26

12.2 Drugs acting on the nose

Rhinitis is often self-limiting but bacterial sinusitis may require treatment with antibacterials (Table 1, section 5.1). Many nasal preparations contain sympathomimetic drugs (section 12.2.2) which can give rise to rebound congestion (*rhinitis medicamentosa*) and may damage the nasal cilia. **Sodium chloride 0.9%** solution may be used as a douche or 'sniff' following endonasal surgery.

Administration To administer nasal drops, lay the child face-upward with the neck extended, instil the drops, then sit the child up and tilt the head forward.

Nasal polyps Short-term use of corticosteroid nasal drops helps to shrink nasal polyps; to be effective, the drops must be administered with the child in the 'head down' position. A short course of a systemic corticosteroid (section 6.3.2) may be required initially to shrink large polyps. A corticosteroid nasal spray can be used to maintain the reduction in swelling and also for the initial treatment of small polyps.

12.2.1 Drugs used in nasal allergy

Mild allergic rhinitis is controlled by **antihistamines** (see also section 3.4.1) or topical **nasal corticosteroids**; systemic nasal decongestants (section 3.10) are not recommended for use in children. Topical nasal decongestants can be used for a short period to relieve congestion and allow penetration of a topical nasal corticosteroid.

More persistent symptoms can be relieved by topical nasal **corticosteroids** and **cromoglicate**; the topical **antihistamine**, azelastine, is useful for controlling breakthrough symptoms in allergic rhinitis. Azelastine is less effective than nasal corticosteroids, but probably more effective than sodium cromoglicate. Intranasal preparations for rhinitis have little effect on allergic conjunctivitis—a topical ophthalmic solution (section 11.4.2) may be needed as well. In seasonal allergic rhinitis (e.g. hay fever), treatment should begin 2 to 3 weeks before the season commences and may have to be continued for several months; continuous long-term treatment may be required in perennial rhinitis.

Children with disabling symptoms of seasonal rhinitis (e.g. students taking important examinations), may be treated with oral **corticosteroids** (section 6.3.2) for short periods. Oral corticosteroids may also be used at the beginning of a course of treatment with a corticosteroid spray to relieve severe mucosal oedema and allow the spray to penetrate the nasal mucosa.

Sometimes allergic rhinitis is accompanied by vasomotor rhinitis. In this situation, the addition of topical nasal **ipratropium bromide** (section 12.2.2) can reduce watery rhinorrhoea.

Pregnancy If a pregnant woman cannot tolerate the symptoms of allergic rhinitis, treatment with nasal beclometasone or sodium cromoglicate may be considered

Antihistamines

AZELASTINE HYDROCHLORIDE

Side-effects irritation of nasal mucosa; bitter taste (if applied incorrectly)

Indication and dose

Treatment of allergic rhinitis for dose, see under preparation

[1]**Rhinolast®** (Viatris) PoM

Nasal spray, azelastine hydrochloride 140 micrograms (0.14 mL)/metered spray. Net price 22 mL (with metered pump) = £11.09

Excipients: include sodium edetate

Dose

Child 5–18 years apply 140 micrograms (1 spray) into each nostril twice daily

1. Can be sold to the public for nasal administration in aqueous form for the treatment of seasonal allergic rhinitis or perennial allergic rhinitis in children over 5 years, subject to max. single dose of 140 micrograms per nostril, max. daily dose of 280 micrograms per nostril, and a pack size limit of 36 doses

Corticosteroids

Nasal preparations containing corticosteroids have a useful role in the prophylaxis and treatment of allergic rhinitis (see notes above).

Cautions Corticosteroid nasal preparations should be avoided in the presence of untreated nasal infections, and also after nasal surgery (until healing has occurred); they should also be avoided in pulmonary tuberculosis. Systemic absorption may follow nasal administration particularly if high doses are used or if treatment is prolonged; for cautions and side-effects of systemic corticosteroids, see section 6.3.2. The risk of systemic effects may be greater with nasal drops than with nasal sprays; drops are administered incorrectly more often than sprays. The CSM recommends that the height of children receiving prolonged treatment with nasal corticosteroids is monitored; if growth is slowed, referral to a paediatrician should be considered.

Side-effects Local side-effects include dryness, irritation of nose and throat, epistaxis and rarely ulceration; nasal septal perforation (usually following nasal surgery) and raised intra-ocular pressure or glaucoma may also occur rarely. Headache, smell and taste disturbances may also occur. Hypersensitivity reactions, including bronchospasm, have been reported.

BECLOMETASONE DIPROPIONATE

(Beclomethasone Dipropionate)

Cautions see notes above

Side-effects see notes above

Indication and dose

Prophylaxis and treatment of allergic and vasomotor rhinitis

Child 6–18 years apply 100 micrograms (2 sprays) into each nostril twice daily; max. total 400 micrograms (8 sprays) daily; when symptoms controlled, dose reduced to 50 micrograms (1 spray) into each nostril twice daily

Beclometasone (Non-proprietary) PoM

Nasal spray, beclometasone dipropionate 50 micrograms/metered spray. Net price 200-spray unit = £3.49

Brands include *Nasobec Aqueous®*

Beconase® (A&H) PoM

Nasal spray (aqueous suspension), beclometasone dipropionate 50 micrograms/metered spray. Net price 200-spray unit with applicator = £2.19

Excipients: include benzalkonium chloride, polysorbate 80

BETAMETHASONE SODIUM PHOSPHATE

Cautions see notes above

Side-effects see notes above

Licensed use licensed for use in children (age range not specified by manufacturer)

Indication and dose

Non-infected inflammatory conditions of nose for dose, see under preparations

Eye section 11.4.1

Ear section 12.1.1

Betnesol® (Celltech) PoM
Drops (for ear, eye, or nose), betamethasone sodium phosphate 0.1%, net price 10 mL = £2.32
Excipients: include benzalkonium chloride, disodium edetate

Dose

Nose, instil 2–3 drops into each nostril 2–3 times daily

Vista-Methasone® (Martindale) PoM
Drops (for ear, eye, or nose), betamethasone sodium phosphate 0.1%. Net price 5 mL = £1.02, 10 mL = £1.16
Excipients: include benzalkonium chloride, disodium edetate

Dose

Nose, instil 2–3 drops into each nostril twice daily

BUDESONIDE

Cautions see notes above; **interactions**: Appendix 1 (corticosteroids)

Side-effects see notes above

Indication and dose

See under preparations

Budesonide (Non-proprietary) PoM
Nasal spray, budesonide 100 micrograms/metered spray, net price 100-spray unit = £5.85

Dose

Prophylaxis and treatment of allergic and vasomotor rhinitis
Child 12–18 years apply 200 micrograms (2 sprays) into each nostril once daily in the morning *or* 100 micrograms (1 spray) into each nostril twice daily; when control achieved reduce to 100 micrograms (1 spray) into each nostril once daily

Nasal polyps
Child 12–18 years apply 100 micrograms (1 spray) into each nostril twice daily for up to 3 months

Rhinocort Aqua® (AstraZeneca) PoM
Nasal spray, budesonide 64 micrograms/metered spray. Net price 120-spray unit = £4.49
Excipients: include disodium edetate, polysorbate 80, potassium sorbate

Dose

Rhinitis
Child 12–18 years apply 128 micrograms (2 sprays) into each nostril once daily in the morning *or* 64 micrograms (1 spray) into each nostril twice daily; when control achieved reduce to 64 micrograms (1 spray) into each nostril once daily; max. duration of treatment 3 months

Nasal polyps
Child 12–18 years apply 64 micrograms (1 spray) into each nostril twice daily for up to 3 months

DEXAMETHASONE ISONICOTINATE

Cautions see notes above; avoid contact with eyes

Side-effects see notes above

Indication and dose

See under preparation

With sympathomimetic
For cautions and side-effects of sympathomimetics see Ephedrine Hydrochloride, section 12.2.2

Dexa-Rhinaspray Duo® (Boehringer Ingelheim) PoM
Nasal spray, dexamethasone isonicotinate 20 micrograms, tramazoline hydrochloride 120 micrograms/metered spray. Net price 110-dose unit = £2.15
Excipients: include benzalkonium chloride, polysorbate 80

Dose

Treatment of allergic rhinitis
Child 5–12 years apply 1 spray into each nostril up to twice daily; max. duration 14 days
Child 12–18 years apply 1 spray into each nostril 2–3 times daily, max. 6 times daily; max. duration 14 days

FLUNISOLIDE

Cautions see notes above

Side-effects see notes above

Indication and dose

Prophylaxis and treatment of allergic rhinitis
Child 5–14 years initially 25 micrograms (1 spray) into each nostril up to 3 times daily then reduced for maintenance
Child 14–18 years 50 micrograms (2 sprays) into each nostril twice daily, increased if necessary to max. 3 times daily then reduced for maintenance

Syntaris® (IVAX) PoM
Aqueous nasal spray, flunisolide 25 micrograms/metered spray. Net price 240-spray unit with pump and applicator = £5.05
Excipients: include benzalkonium chloride, butylated hydroxytoluene, disodium edetate, polysorbate 20, propylene glycol

FLUTICASONE PROPIONATE

Cautions see notes above; **interactions:** Appendix 1 (corticosteroids)

Side-effects see notes above

Indication and dose

Prophylaxis and treatment of allergic rhinitis

CHILD 4–12 years apply 50 micrograms (1 spray) into each nostril once daily, preferably in the morning, increased to max. twice daily if required

Child 12–18 years apply 100 micrograms (2 sprays) into each nostril once daily, preferably in the morning, increased to max. twice daily if required; when control achieved reduce to 50 micrograms (1 spray) into each nostril once daily

Nasal polyps see *Flixonase Nasule®* below

Flixonase® (A&H) PoM

Aqueous nasal spray, fluticasone propionate 50 micrograms/metered spray. Net price 150-spray unit with applicator = £11.69

Excipients: include benzalkonium chloride, polysorbate 80

Flixonase Nasule® (A&H) PoM

Nasal drops, fluticasone propionate 400 micrograms/unit dose, net price 28 × 0.4-mL units = £13.76

Excipients: include polysorbate 20

Dose

Nasal polyps

Child 16–18 years instil 200 micrograms (approx. 6 drops) into each nostril once or twice daily; consider alternative treatment if no improvement after 4–6 weeks

Nasofan® (IVAX) PoM

Aqueous nasal spray, fluticasone propionate 50 micrograms/metered spray. Net price 150-spray unit = £10.52

Excipients: include benzalkonium chloride, polysorbate 80

MOMETASONE FUROATE

Cautions see notes above

Side-effects see notes above

Indication and dose

See under preparation

Nasonex® (Schering-Plough) PoM

Nasal spray, mometasone furoate 50 micrograms/metered spray. Net price 140-spray unit = £7.83

Excipients: include benzalkonium chloride, polysorbate 80

Dose

Prophylaxis and treatment of allergic rhinitis

Child 6–12 years apply 50 micrograms (1 spray) into each nostril once daily

Child 12–18 years apply 100 micrograms (2 sprays) into each nostril once daily, increased if necessary to max. 200 micrograms (4 sprays) into each nostril once daily; when control achieved reduce to 50 micrograms (1 spray) into each nostril once daily

TRIAMCINOLONE ACETONIDE

Cautions see notes above

Side-effects see notes above

Indication and dose

Treatment of allergic rhinitis

Child 6–12 years apply 55 micrograms (1 spray) into each nostril once daily, increased if necessary to 110 micrograms (2 sprays) into each nostril once daily; when control achieved reduce to 55 micrograms (1 spray) into each nostril once daily; max. duration of treatment 3 months

Child 12–18 years apply 110 micrograms (2 sprays) into each nostril once daily; when control achieved, reduce to 55 micrograms (1 spray) into each nostril once daily

Nasacort® (Aventis Pharma) PoM

Aqueous nasal spray, triamcinolone acetonide 55 micrograms/metered spray. Net price 120-spray unit = £7.39

Excipients: include benzalkonium chloride, disodium edetate, polysorbate 80

Cromoglicate

SODIUM CROMOGLICATE

(Sodium Cromoglycate)

Side-effects local irritation; rarely transient bronchospasm

Licensed use licensed for use in children (age range not specified by manufacturers)

Indication and dose

Prophylaxis of allergic rhinitis for dose, see under preparations

SODIUM CROMOGLICATE (*continued*)

Rynacrom® (Sanofi-Aventis)
4% aqueous nasal spray, sodium cromoglicate 4% (5.2 mg/spray). Net price 22 mL with pump = £17.76
Excipients: include benzalkonium chloride, disodium edetate

Dose

Nose, apply 1 spray into each nostril 2–4 times daily

Vividrin® (Pharma-Global)
Nasal spray, sodium cromoglicate 2%. Net price 15 mL = £8.56
Excipients: include benzalkonium chloride, edetic acid, polysorbate 80

Dose

Nose, apply 1 spray into each nostril 4–6 times daily

12.2.2 Topical nasal decongestants

Topical nasal decongestants containing sympathomimetics can cause rebound congestion (*rhinitis medicamentosa*) following prolonged use (more than 7 days), and are therefore of limited value in the treatment of nasal congestion.

Sodium chloride 0.9% given as nasal drops may relieve nasal congestion by helping to liquefy mucous secretions in children with rhinitis. In infants, 1–2 drops of sodium chloride 0.9% solution in each nostril before feeds will help relieve congestion and allow more effective suckling.

Ephedrine nasal drops is the least likely of the sympathomimetic nasal decongestants to cause rebound congestion and can provide relief for several hours. The more potent sympathomimetic drugs **oxymetazoline** and **xylometazoline** are more likely to cause a rebound effect.

Non-allergic watery rhinorrhoea often responds well to treatment with the antimuscarinic **ipratropium bromide**.

Corticosteroid nasal drops produce shrinkage of nasal polyps (section 12.2).

Inhalation of **warm moist air** is useful in the treatment of symptoms of acute nasal congestion in infants and children, but the use of boiling water for steam inhalation is dangerous for children and should **not** be recommended. Volatile substances (section 3.8) such as menthol and eucalyptus may encourage the use of warm moist air.

Recurrent, persistent bleeding may respond to the use of a sympathomimetic nasal spray; if infection is present, chlorhexidine and neomycin (*Naseptin®*) cream (section 12.2.3) may be effective.

Systemic nasal decongestants—see section 3.10.

Sinusitis and oral pain Sinusitis affecting the maxillary antrum can cause pain in the upper jaw. Where this is associated with blockage of the opening from the sinus into the nasal cavity, it may be helpful to relieve the congestion with inhalation of warm moist air (section 3.8) or with **ephedrine nasal drops** (see above). For antibacterial treatment of sinusitis, see Table 1, section 5.1.

Sympathomimetics

EPHEDRINE HYDROCHLORIDE

Cautions avoid excessive or prolonged use; caution in infants under 3 months (no good evidence of value—if irritation occurs might narrow nasal passage); **interactions**: Appendix 1 (sympathomimetics)

Side-effects local irritation, nausea, headache; after excessive use tolerance with diminished effect, rebound congestion; cardiovascular effects also reported

Licensed use not licensed for use in children under 3 months

Indication and dose

Nasal congestion (see notes above)
Child 1–3 months instil 1–2 drops (0.25% strength) into each nostril 3–4 times daily, 15 minutes before feeds (for max. 7 days)
Child 3 months–18 years instil 1–2 drops (0.5% strength) into each nostril 3–4 times daily (for max. 7 days)

Ephedrine (Non-proprietary)
Nasal drops, ephedrine hydrochloride 0.5%, net price 10 mL = £1.33; 1%, 10 mL = £1.39
Note Ephedrine 0.25% nasal solution is prepared by diluting ephedrine 0.5% solution with sodium chloride 0.9% solution. Discard diluted solution after 1 week. The BP directs that if no strength is specified 0.5% drops should be supplied
Dental prescribing on NHS Ephedrine nasal drops may be prescribed

XYLOMETAZOLINE HYDROCHLORIDE

Cautions see under Ephedrine Hydrochloride and notes above

Side-effects see under Ephedrine Hydrochloride and notes above

Indication and dose

Nasal congestion for dose, see under preparations

Xylometazoline (Non-proprietary)

Nasal drops, xylometazoline hydrochloride 0.1%, net price 10 mL = £1.91

Dose

Child 12–18 years instil 2–3 drops into each nostril 2–3 times daily when required; max. duration 7 days

Brands include *Otradrops*®, *Otrivine*® (NHS)

Paediatric nasal drops, xylometazoline hydrochloride 0.05%, net price 10 mL = £1.59

Dose

Child 3 months–12 years instil 1–2 drops into each nostril 1–2 times daily when required (on doctor's advice only under 2 years); max. duration 7 days

Brands include *Otradrops*®, *Otrivine*® (NHS), *Tixycolds*®

Nasal spray, xylometazoline hydrochloride 0.1%, net price 10 mL = £1.91

Dose

Child 12–18 years apply 1 spray into each nostril 2–3 times daily when required; max. duration 7 days

Brands include *Otraspray*®, *Otrivine*® (NHS)

Antimuscarinic

IPRATROPIUM BROMIDE

Cautions see section 3.1.2; avoid spraying near eyes

Side-effects epistaxis, nasal dryness, and irritation; less frequently nausea, headache, and pharyngitis; *very rarely* antimuscarinic effects such as gastro-intestinal motility disturbances, palpitations, and urinary retention

Indication and dose

Rhinorrhoea associated with allergic and non-allergic rhinitis
Child 12–18 years apply 42 micrograms (2 sprays) into each nostril 2–3 times daily

Asthma and reversible airways obstruction section 3.1.2

Rinatec® (Boehringer Ingelheim) (PoM)

Nasal spray 0.03%, ipratropium bromide 21 micrograms/metered spray. Net price 180-dose unit = £4.55

Excipients: include benzalkonium chloride, disodium edetate

12.2.3 Nasal preparations for infection

There is **no** evidence that topical anti-infective nasal preparations have any therapeutic value in rhinitis or sinusitis; for elimination of nasal staphylococci, see below. Acute complications such as periorbital cellulitis require hospital treatment. For systemic treatment of sinusitis, see Table 1, section 5.1.

Betnesol-N® (Celltech) (PoM)

Drops (for ear, eye, or nose), betamethasone sodium phosphate 0.1%, neomycin sulphate 0.5%. Net price 10 mL = £2.39

Excipients: include benzalkonium chloride, disodium edetate

Dose

Nose, instil 2–3 drops into each nostril 2–3 times daily

Note *Betnesol-N*® licensed for use in children (age range not specified by manufacturer)

Vista-Methasone N® (Martindale) (PoM)

Drops (for ear, eye, or nose), betamethasone sodium phosphate 0.1%, neomycin sulphate 0.5%. Net price 5 mL = £1.09, 10 mL = £1.20

Excipients: include thiomersal

Dose

Nose, instil 2–3 drops into each nostril twice daily

Note *Vista-Methasone N*® licensed for use in children (age range not specified by manufacturer)

Nasal staphylococci

Elimination of organisms such as staphylococci from the nasal vestibule can be achieved by the use of a cream containing **chlorhexidine** and **neomycin** (*Naseptin*®), but re-colonisation frequently occurs. Coagulase-positive staphylococci are present in the noses of 40% of the population. A nasal ointment containing **mupirocin** is also available; it should probably be held in reserve for resistant infections. In hospitals or in care establishments, mupirocin nasal ointment should be reserved for the *eradication* (in both patients and staff) of nasal carriage of meticillin-resistant *Staphylococcus aureus* (MRSA). The ointment should be applied 3 times daily for 5 days and a sample taken 2 days after treatment to confirm eradication. The course may be repeated if the sample is positive (and the throat is not colonised). To avoid the development of resistance, the treatment course should not exceed 7 days and the course should not be repeated on more than one occasion. If the MRSA strain is mupirocin-resistant or does not respond after 2 courses, consider alternative products such as chlorhexidine and neomycin cream. For eradication of MRSA also consult local infection control policy. See section 13.10.1 for treatment of MRSA-infected open wounds. See section 5.1.1.2 for *treatment* of children with MRSA-positive throat swabs or systemic MRSA infection.

Bactroban Nasal® (GSK) PoM
Nasal ointment, mupirocin 2% (as calcium salt) in white soft paraffin basis. Net price 3 g = £5.80

Dose

For eradication of nasal carriage of staphylococci, including meticillin-resistant *Staphylococcus aureus* (MRSA)
apply 2–3 times daily to the inner surface of each nostril (see notes above)

Naseptin® (Alliance) PoM
Cream, chlorhexidine hydrochloride 0.1%, neomycin sulphate 0.5%, net price 15 g = £1.58
Excipients: include arachis (peanut) oil, cetostearyl alcohol

Dose

For eradication of nasal carriage of staphylococci
apply to nostrils 4 times daily for 10 days

For preventing nasal carriage of staphylococci
apply to nostrils twice daily

12.3 Drugs acting on the oropharynx

12.3.1 Drugs for oral ulceration and inflammation

Ulceration of the oral mucosa may be caused by trauma (physical or chemical), recurrent aphthous ulcers, infections, carcinoma, dermatological disorders, nutritional deficiencies, gastro-intestinal disease, haematopoietic disorders, and drug therapy. It is important to establish the diagnosis in each case as the majority of these lesions require specific management in addition to local treatment. Children with an unexplained mouth ulcer of more than 3 weeks' duration require urgent referral to hospital to exclude oral cancer. Local treatment aims at protecting the ulcerated area, at relieving pain or reducing inflammation, or at controlling secondary infection.

Simple mouthwashes A **saline** mouthwash (section 12.3.4) may relieve the pain of traumatic ulceration. The mouthwash is made up with warm water and used at frequent intervals until the discomfort and swelling subsides.

Antiseptic mouthwashes Secondary bacterial infection may be a feature of any mucosal ulceration; it can increase discomfort and delay healing. Use of a **chlorhexidine** or **povidone–iodine** mouthwash (section 12.3.4) is often beneficial and may accelerate healing of recurrent aphthous ulcers.

Mechanical protection **Carmellose gelatin paste** may relieve some discomfort arising from ulceration by protecting the ulcer site. The paste adheres to dry mucosa, but is difficult to apply effectively to some parts of the mouth. *Gelclair®* is available for the management of oral lesions; it forms a film of povidone and sodium hyaluronate on the lesion.

Corticosteroids Topical corticosteroid therapy may be used for some forms of oral ulceration; for aphthous ulcers it is most effective if applied in the 'prodromal' phase. Thrush or other types of candidiasis are recognised complications of corticosteroid treatment.

Hydrocortisone oromucosal tablets are useful in recurrent aphthous ulcers and erosive lichenoid lesions.

Triamcinolone dental paste is formulated to keep the corticosteroid in contact with the mucosa for long enough to permit penetration of the lesion, but may be difficult to apply properly.

Beclometasone dipropionate inhaler (p. 178) 50–100 micrograms sprayed twice daily on the oral mucosa is used to manage oral ulceration [unlicensed indication]. Alternatively, **betamethasone** soluble tablets (p. 428) dissolved in water, may be used as a mouthwash to treat oral ulceration.
Systemic corticosteroid therapy (section 6.3.2) is reserved for severe conditions such as pemphigus vulgaris.

Local analgesics Local analgesics have a limited role in the management of oral ulceration. When applied topically their action is of a relatively short duration and analgesia cannot be maintained continuously throughout the day. When local anaesthetics are used in the mouth care must be taken not to produce anaesthesia of the pharynx before meals as this might lead to choking.

Benzydamine mouthwash or spray may be useful in palliating the discomfort associated with a variety of ulcerative conditions. It has also been found to be effective in reducing the discomfort of tonsillectomy and post-irradiation mucositis. Some children may find the full-strength mouthwash causes some stinging and, for them, it should be diluted with an equal volume of water.

Flurbiprofen lozenges are licensed for the relief of sore throat in adolescents.

Choline salicylate dental gel has some analgesic action and may provide relief for recurrent aphthous ulcers. Benefit in teething may merely be due to pressure of application (comparable with biting a teething ring); excessive use of choline salicylate dental gel can lead to salicylate poisoning.

Periodontitis Low-dose **doxycycline** (*Periostat*®) is licensed as an adjunct to scaling and root planing for the treatment of periodontitis in children over 12 years; a low dose of doxycycline reduces collagenase activity without inhibiting bacteria associated with periodontitis. For anti-infectives used in the treatment of destructive (refractory) forms of periodontal disease, see section 12.3.2 and Table 1, section 5.1. For mouthwashes used for oral hygiene and plaque inhibition, see section 12.3.4.

BENZYDAMINE HYDROCHLORIDE

Side-effects occasional numbness or stinging; rarely hypersensitivity reactions

Licensed use *Difflam*® *Spray* licensed for use in children (age range not specified by manufacturer)

Indication and dose

Painful inflammatory conditions of oropharynx for dose, see under preparations

Difflam® (3M)

Oral rinse, green, benzydamine hydrochloride 0.15%, net price 200 mL (*Difflam*® *Sore Throat Rinse*) = £2.63; 300 mL = £4.01

Dose

Child 12–18 years rinse or gargle, using 15 mL (diluted with water if stinging occurs) every 1½–3 hours as required, usually for not more than 7 days

Dental prescribing on NHS May be prescribed as Benzydamine Mouthwash 0.15%

Spray, benzydamine hydrochloride 0.15%. Net price 30-mL unit = £3.17

Dose

Child under 6 years 1 puff per 4 kg body-weight to max. 4 puffs onto affected area every 1½–3 hours

Child 6–12 years 4 puffs onto affected area every 1½–3 hours

Child 12–18 years 4–8 puffs onto affected area every 1½–3 hours

Dental prescribing on NHS May be prescribed as Benzydamine Oromucosal Spray 0.15%

CARMELLOSE SODIUM

Licensed use licensed for use in children (age range not specified by manufacturer)

Indication and dose

Mechanical protection of oral and perioral lesions for dose, see under preparation

Orabase® (ConvaTec)
Protective paste (= oral paste), carmellose sodium 16.7%, pectin 16.7%, gelatin 16.7%, in *Plastibase®*. Net price 30 g = £1.94; 100 g = £4.32

Dose

Apply a thin layer when necessary after meals

Dental prescribing on NHS May be prescribed as Carmellose Gelatin Paste

CORTICOSTEROIDS

Contra-indications untreated oral infection; manufacturer of triamcinolone contra-indicates use on tuberculous and viral lesions

Side-effects occasional exacerbation of local infection; thrush or other candidal infections

Licensed use *Adcortyl in Orabase®* licensed for use in children (age range not specified by manufacturer); *Corlan® Pellets* licensed for use in children (under 12 years—on medical advice only)

Indication and dose

Oral and perioral lesions for dose, see under preparations

[1]Adcortyl in Orabase® (Squibb) PoM
Oral paste, triamcinolone acetonide 0.1% in adhesive basis. Net price 10 g = £1.27

Dose

Apply a thin layer 2–4 times daily for max. 5 days; do not rub in

Dental prescribing on NHS May be prescribed as Triamcinolone Dental Paste

1. A 5-g tube (*Adcortyl in Orabase® for Mouth Ulcers*) is on sale to the public for the treatment of common mouth ulcers for max. 5 days

Corlan® (Celltech)
Pellets (= oromucosal tablets), hydrocortisone 2.5 mg (as sodium succinate). Net price 20 = £2.54

Dose

1 lozenge 4 times daily, allowed to dissolve slowly in the mouth in contact with the ulcer

Dental prescribing on NHS May be prescribed as Hydrocortisone Oromucosal Tablets

DOXYCYCLINE

Cautions section 5.1.3; monitor for superficial fungal infection, particularly if predisposition to oral candidiasis

Contra-indications section 5.1.3

Side-effects section 5.1.3; fungal superinfection

Indication and dose

See under preparations

Oral herpes section 12.3.2

Other indications section 5.1.3

Periostat® (Alliance) PoM
Tablets, f/c, doxycycline (as hyclate) 20 mg, net price 56-tab pack = £16.50. Label: 6, 11, 27, counselling, posture

Dose

Periodontitis (as an adjunct to gingival scaling and root planing)
Child 12–18 years 20 mg twice daily for 3 months

Counselling Tablets should be swallowed whole with plenty of fluid, while sitting or standing
Dental prescribing on NHS May be prescribed as Doxycycline Tablets 20 mg

Local application

For severe recurrent aphthous ulceration, the contents of a 100 mg doxycycline capsule can be stirred into a small amount of water then rinsed around the mouth for 2–3 minutes 4 times daily usually for 3 days; it should preferably not be swallowed [unlicensed indication].

Note Doxycycline stains teeth; avoid in children under 12 years of age

FLURBIPROFEN

Cautions see section 10.1.1

Contra-indications see section 10.1.1

Side-effects taste disturbance, mouth ulcers (move lozenge around mouth); see also section 10.1.1

Indication and dose

Relief of sore throat for dose, see under preparation

Strefen® (Crookes)
Lozenges, flurbiprofen 8.75 mg, net price 16 = £2.08

Dose

Child 12–18 years allow 1 lozenge to dissolve slowly in the mouth every 3–6 hours, max. 5 lozenges in 24 hours, for max. 3 days

SALICYLATES

Cautions frequent application, especially in children, may give rise to salicylate poisoning

Note CSM warning on aspirin and Reye's syndrome does not apply to non-aspirin salicylates or to topical preparations such as teething gels

Indication and dose

Mild oral and perioral lesions for dose, see under preparations

Choline salicylate

Choline Salicylate Dental Gel, BP

Oral gel, choline salicylate 8.7% in a flavoured gel basis, net price 15 g = £1.79

Brands include *Bonjela®* (sugar-free)

Dose

Child 4 months–12 years apply ¼-inch of gel not more often than every 3 hours; max. 6 applications daily

Child 12–18 years apply ½-inch of gel with gentle massage not more often than every 3 hours

Dental prescribing on NHS Choline Salicylate Dental Gel may be prescribed

Salicylic acid

Pyralvex® (Norgine)

Oral paint, brown, rhubarb extract (anthraquinone glycosides 0.5%), salicylic acid 1%. Net price 10 mL with brush = £1.69

Dose

Child 12–18 years apply 3–4 times daily

12.3.2 Oropharyngeal anti-infective drugs

Sore throat is usually a self-limiting condition often caused by viral infection which does not benefit from anti-infective treatment. Adequate analgesia may be all that is required. Systemic **antibacterials** (Table 1, section 5.1) should only be used in severe cases where there is concern for the child's overall clinical condition. Acute ulcerative gingivitis (Vincent's infection) requires treatment with oral **metronidazole** (section 5.1.11).

Benzydamine (section 12.3.1) may be beneficial in relieving pain and dysphagia in children, especially after tonsillectomy or the use of a nasogastric tube.

Oropharyngeal viral infections

Children with varicella–zoster infection often develop painful lesions in the mouth and throat. **Benzydamine** (section 12.3.1) may be used to provide local analgesia. **Chlorhexidine** mouthwash or gel (section 12.3.4) will control plaque accumulation if toothbrushing is painful and will also help to control secondary infection in general.

In severe herpetic stomatitis systemic **aciclovir** or **valaciclovir** (section 5.3.2.1) may be used for oral lesions associated with herpes zoster. Aciclovir and valaciclovir are also used to prevent frequently recurring herpes simplex lesions of the mouth particularly when associated with the initiation of erythema multiforme. For the treatment of labial herpes simplex infections, see section 13.10.3.

Herpes infections of the mouth in children aged over 12 years may also respond to rinsing the mouth with **doxycycline** (section 12.3.1).

Oropharyngeal fungal infections

Fungal infections of the mouth are usually caused by *Candida* spp. (candidiasis or candidosis). Different types of oropharyngeal candidiasis are managed as follows:

Thrush Acute pseudomembranous candidiasis (thrush), is classically an acute infection but one which may persist for months in patients receiving inhaled corticosteroids, cytotoxics or broad-spectrum antibacterials. Thrush is also associated with serious systemic disease associated with reduced immunity such as leukaemia, other malignancies, and HIV infection. The predisposing cause should be dealt with. When associated with corticosteroid inhalers, rinsing the mouth with water (or cleaning a child's teeth) immediately after using the inhaler may avoid the problem. Treatment with **nystatin**, **amphotericin**, or **miconazole** may be needed. **Fluconazole** (section 5.2) is effective for unresponsive infections or if a topical antifungal drug cannot be used.

Acute erythematous candidiasis Acute erythematous (atrophic) candidiasis is a relatively uncommon condition associated with corticosteroid and broad-spectrum antibacterial use and with HIV disease. It is usually treated with **fluconazole** (section 5.2).

Angular cheilitis Angular cheilitis (angular stomatitis) is characterised by soreness, erythema and fissuring at the angles of the mouth. It may represent a nutritional deficiency or it may be related to orofacial granulomatosis or HIV infection. Both yeasts (*Candida* spp.) and bacteria (*Staphylococcus aureus* and beta-haemolytic streptococci) are commonly involved as interacting, infective factors. While the underlying cause is being identified and treated, it is often helpful to apply **miconazole** and **hydrocortisone** cream or ointment (see p. 624), **nystatin** ointment (see p. 661), or **sodium fusidate** ointment (p. 657).

Immunocompromised patients For advice on prevention of fungal infections in immunocompromised children see p. 347.

Drugs used in oropharyngeal candidiasis **Amphotericin** and **nystatin** are not absorbed from the gastro-intestinal tract and are applied locally (as lozenges or suspension) to the mouth for treating local fungal infections. Nystatin ointment is available for use on perioral lesions (p. 661). **Miconazole** is used by local application (as an oral gel) in the mouth but it is also absorbed to the extent that potential interactions need to be considered. Miconazole may be more effective than amphotericin or nystatin for some types of candidiasis, particularly chronic hyperplastic candidiasis or chronic mucocutaneous candidiasis (chronic thrush). Miconazole also has some activity against Gram-positive bacteria including streptococci and staphylococci. **Fluconazole** and **itraconazole** (section 5.2) are absorbed when taken by mouth; they are used for oropharyngeal candidiasis that does not respond to topical therapy.

In neonates, nystatin and amphotericin oral suspension are used for the prevention of candidiasis; nystatin is also used for the treatment of oropharyngeal candidiasis. To prevent re-infection it is important to ensure that the mother's breast nipples and the teats of feeding bottles are cleaned adequately.

If candidal infection fails to respond after 1 to 2 weeks of treatment with antifungal drugs the child should be sent for investigation to eliminate the possibility of underlying disease. Persistent infection may also be caused by re-infection from the genito-urinary or gastro-intestinal tract.

For the role of antiseptic mouthwashes in the prevention of oral candidiasis in immunocompromised children, see section 12.3.4.

AMPHOTERICIN

Side-effects mild gastro-intestinal disturbances reported

Licensed use *suspension* not licensed for use in children under 1 month for the treatment of candidiasis; *lozenges* not licensed for use in children

Indication and dose

Oral and perioral fungal infections for doses, see under preparations

Intestinal candidiasis section 5.2

Fungilin® (Squibb) PoM

Lozenges, yellow, amphotericin 10 mg. Net price 60-lozenge pack = £3.67. Label: 9, 24, counselling, after food

Dose

Allow 1 lozenge to dissolve slowly in the mouth 4 times daily for 10–15 days (continued for 48 hours after lesions have resolved); increase to 8 daily if infection severe

Dental prescribing on NHS May be prescribed as Amphotericin Lozenges

Oral suspension, yellow, sugar-free, amphotericin 100 mg/mL. Net price 12 mL with pipette = £2.15. Label: 9, counselling, use of pipette, hold in mouth, after food

Dose

Prophylaxis against oral candidiasis

Neonate 1 mL once daily

Treatment of oral candidiasis

Child 1 month–18 years place 1 mL in the mouth after food and retain near lesions 4 times daily for 14 days (continued for 48 hours after lesions have resolved)

Dental prescribing on NHS May be prescribed as Amphotericin Oral Suspension

MICONAZOLE

Cautions avoid in porphyria (section 9.8.2); **interactions**: Appendix 1 (antifungals, imidazole)

Pregnancy manufacturer advises avoid unless essential

Breast-feeding manufacturer advises caution—no information available

Contra-indications

Hepatic impairment avoid

Side-effects nausea and vomiting, diarrhoea (with long-term treatment); rarely allergic reactions; isolated reports of hepatitis

Licensed use not licensed for use in neonates

Indication and dose

See under preparation

Intestinal fungal infections section 5.2

[1]**Daktarin**® (Janssen-Cilag) PoM
Oral gel, sugar-free, orange-flavoured, miconazole 24 mg/mL (20 mg/g). Net price 15-g tube = £2.45, 80-g tube = £4.75. Label: 9, counselling, hold in mouth, after food

Dose

Prevention and treatment of oral fungal infections

Neonate 1 mL in the mouth after feed 2–4 times daily

Child 1 month–2 years 2.5 mL in the mouth after food and retain near lesions twice daily

Child 2–6 years 5 mL in the mouth after food and retain near lesions twice daily

Child 6–12 years 5 mL in the mouth after food and retain near lesions 4 times daily

Child 12–18 years 5–10 mL in the mouth after food and retain near lesions 4 times daily

Note Treatment should be continued for 48 hours after lesions have healed

Localised lesions

Child 6–18 years smear small amount on affected area with clean finger 4 times daily for 5–7 days (orthodontic appliances should be removed at night and brushed with gel)

Dental prescribing on NHS May be prescribed as Miconazole Oromucosal Gel

1. 15-g tube can be sold to the public

NYSTATIN

Side-effects oral irritation and sensitisation, nausea reported; see also section 5.2

Licensed use *pastilles* licensed for use in children (age range not specified by manufacturer); *suspension* not licensed for use in neonates for the treatment of candidiasis; licensed for use in neonates for prophylaxis as once daily dose

Indication and dose

Oral and perioral fungal infections

Neonate *prophylaxis*, 100 000 units 3 times daily after feeds; *treatment* 100 000 units 4 times daily after feeds

Child 1 month–18 years *prophylaxis* and *treatment*, 100 000 units 4 times daily after food

Note Treatment is usually given for 7 days, and continued for 48 hours after lesions have healed. Immunocompromised children may require higher doses (e.g. 500 000 units 4 times daily)

Intestinal fungal infections section 5.2

Vaginal infections section 7.2.2

Skin infections section 13.10.2

Nystan® (Squibb) PoM
Pastilles, yellow/brown, nystatin 100 000 units. Net price 28-pastille pack = £3.24. Label: 9, 24, counselling, after food
Dental prescribing on NHS May be prescribed as Nystatin Pastilles

Oral suspension, yellow, nystatin 100 000 units/mL. Net price 30 mL with pipette = £2.05. Label: 9, counselling, use of pipette, hold in mouth, after food
Dental prescribing on NHS May be prescribed as Nystatin Oral Suspension

12.3.3 Lozenges and sprays

There is no convincing evidence that antiseptic lozenges and sprays have a beneficial action and they sometimes irritate and cause sore tongue and sore lips. Some preparations also contain local anaesthetics which relieve pain but may cause sensitisation.

12.3.4 Mouthwashes and gargles

Superficial infections of the mouth are often helped by warm mouthwashes which have a mechanical cleansing effect and cause some local hyperaemia. However, to be effective, they must be used frequently and vigorously. Mouthwashes may not be suitable for children under 7 years (risk of the solution being swallowed); the mouthwash or dental gel may be applied using a cotton bud.

A warm saline mouthwash is ideal for its cleansing effect and can be prepared either by dissolving half a teaspoonful of salt in a glassful of warm water or by diluting **compound sodium chloride mouthwash** with an equal volume of warm water. **Mouthwash solution-tablets** containing thymol are used to remove unpleasant tastes.

Mouthwashes containing an oxidising agent, such as **hydrogen peroxide**, may be useful in the treatment of acute ulcerative gingivitis (Vincent's infection). Hydrogen peroxide solution has also a mechanical cleansing effect arising from frothing when in contact with oral debris, but in concentrations greater than 1.5% may cause ulceration and tissue damage.

Chlorhexidine is an effective antiseptic which has the advantage of inhibiting plaque formation on the teeth. It does not, however, completely control plaque deposition and is not a substitute for effective toothbrushing. Moreover, chlorhexidine preparations do not penetrate significantly into stagnation areas and are therefore of little value in the control of dental caries or of periodontal disease once pocketing has developed. Chlorhexidine preparations are of little value in the control of acute necrotising ulcerative gingivitis. With prolonged use, chlorhexidine causes reversible brown staining of teeth and tongue. Chlorhexidine may be incompatible with some ingredients in toothpaste, causing an unpleasant taste in the mouth; allow at least 30 minutes between using the mouthwash and toothpaste.

Chlorhexidine can be used as a mouthwash, spray or gel for secondary infection in mucosal ulceration and for controlling gingivitis, as an adjunct to other oral hygiene measures. These preparations may also be used instead of toothbrushing where there is a painful periodontal condition (e.g. primary herpetic stomatitis) or if the child has a haemorrhagic disorder, or is disabled. Chlorhexidine mouthwash is used in the prevention of oral candidiasis in immunocompromised patients. It is also used to prevent bacteraemia in children undergoing dental procedures requiring antibacterial prophylaxis (Table 2, section 5.1). Chlorhexidine mouthwash reduces the incidence of alveolar osteitis following tooth extraction.

Povidone–iodine mouthwash is licensed for oral mucosal infections but does not inhibit plaque accumulation. It should not be used for longer than 14 days because a significant amount of iodine is absorbed. As with chlorhexidine, povidone–iodine mouthwash is of little value in the control of acute necrotising ulcerative gingivitis.

CHLORHEXIDINE GLUCONATE

Side-effects mucosal irritation (if desquamation occurs, discontinue treatment or dilute mouthwash with an equal volume of water); taste disturbance; reversible brown staining of teeth, and of silicate or composite restorations; tongue discoloration; parotid gland swelling reported

Note Chlorhexidine gluconate may be incompatible with some ingredients in toothpaste; leave an interval of at least 30 minutes between using mouthwash and toothpaste

Licensed use licensed for use in children (age range not specified by manufacturer)

Indication and dose

See under preparations below

Chlorhexidine (Non-proprietary)

Mouthwash, chlorhexidine gluconate 0.2%, net price 300 mL = £1.86

Dose

Oral hygiene and plaque inhibition

rinse mouth with 10 mL for about 1 minute twice daily

Prophylaxis of endocarditis for dental procedures (as adjunct to antibacterial prophylaxis)

Table 2, section 5.1

Dental prescribing on NHS Chlorhexidine Mouthwash may be prescribed

Chlorohex® (Colgate-Palmolive)

Chlorohex 1200® mouthwash, chlorhexidine gluconate 0.12% (mint-flavoured). Net price 300 mL = £2.20

Dose

Oral hygiene and plaque inhibition

rinse mouth with 15 mL for about 30 seconds twice daily

Corsodyl® (GSK Consumer Healthcare)

Dental gel, chlorhexidine gluconate 1%. Net price 50 g = £1.21

Dose

Oral hygiene and plaque inhibition and gingivitis

brush on the teeth once or twice daily

Oral candidiasis and management of aphthous ulcers

apply to affected areas once or twice daily

Prophylaxis of endocarditis for dental procedures (as adjunct to antibacterial prophylaxis)

Table 2, section 5.1

Dental prescribing on NHS May be prescribed as Chlorhexidine Gluconate Gel 1%

Mouthwash, chlorhexidine gluconate 0.2%. Net price 300 mL (original or mint) = £1.81, 600 mL (mint) = £3.62

Dose

Oral hygiene and plaque inhibition, oral candidiasis, gingivitis, and management of aphthous ulcers
rinse mouth with 10 mL for about 1 minute twice daily

Prophylaxis of endocarditis for dental procedures (as adjunct to antibacterial prophylaxis)
Table 2, section 5.1

Oral spray, chlorhexidine gluconate 0.2% (mint-flavoured). Net price 60 mL = £4.10

Dose

Oral hygiene and plaque inhibition, oral candidiasis, gingivitis, and management of aphthous ulcers
apply as required to tooth, gingival, or ulcer surfaces using up to 12 actuations (approx. 0.14 mL/actuation) twice daily

Dental prescribing on NHS May be prescribed as Chlorhexidine Oral Spray

With chlorobutanol

Eludril® (Fabre)
Mouthwash or gargle, chlorhexidine gluconate 0.1%, chlorobutanol 0.5% (mint-flavoured), net price 90 mL = £1.22, 250 mL = £2.56, 500 mL = £4.64

Dose

Oral hygiene and plaque inhibition
Use 10–15 mL (diluted with warm water in measuring cup provided) 2–3 times daily

HEXETIDINE

Side-effects local irritation; *very rarely* taste disturbance and transient anaesthesia

Indication and dose

Oral hygiene for dose, see preparation below

Oraldene® (Warner Lambert)
Mouthwash or gargle, red, hexetidine 0.1%. Net price 100 mL = £1.31; 200 mL = £2.02

Dose

Child 6–18 years use 15 mL (undiluted) 2–3 times daily

HYDROGEN PEROXIDE

Side-effects reversible hypertrophy of the papillae of the tongue on prolonged use

Indication and dose

Oral hygiene (see notes above); for dose, see under preparations

Hydrogen Peroxide Mouthwash, BP
Mouthwash, consists of Hydrogen Peroxide Solution 6% (= approx. 20 volume) BP

Dose

Rinse the mouth for 2–3 minutes with 15 mL diluted in half a tumblerful of warm water 2–3 times daily (see notes above)

Dental prescribing on NHS Hydrogen Peroxide Mouthwash may be prescribed

Peroxyl® (Colgate-Palmolive)
Mouthwash, hydrogen peroxide 1.5%, net price 300 mL = £2.81

Dose

Child 6–18 years, rinse the mouth with 10 mL for about 1 minute 3 times daily (after meals and at bedtime) for max. 7 days

POVIDONE–IODINE

Cautions see notes above

Pregnancy absorbed iodine may affect the fetal thyroid—avoid regular use of iodine-containing mouthwash

Breast-feeding absorbed iodine present in milk—avoid regular use of iodine-containing mouthwash

Contra-indications avoid regular use in children with thyroid disorders or those receiving lithium therapy

Side-effects idiosyncratic mucosal irritation and hypersensitivity reactions; may interfere with thyroid-function tests and with tests for occult blood

Indication and dose

Oral hygiene for dose, see preparation below

Skin disinfection, section 13.11.4

Betadine® (Medlock)
Mouthwash or gargle, amber, povidone–iodine 1%. Net price 250 mL = £1.12

Dose

Child 6–18 years up to 10 mL undiluted or diluted with an equal quantity of warm water for up to 30 seconds up to 4 times daily for up to 14 days

SODIUM CHLORIDE

Indication and dose

Oral hygiene (see notes above); for dose, see under preparation

Sodium Chloride Mouthwash, Compound, BP
Mouthwash, sodium bicarbonate 1%, sodium chloride 1.5% in a suitable vehicle with a peppermint flavour

Dose

Extemporaneous preparations should be prepared according to the following formula: sodium chloride 1.5 g, sodium bicarbonate 1 g, concentrated peppermint emulsion 2.5 mL, double-strength chloroform water 50 mL, water to 100 mL

To be diluted with an equal volume of warm water

Dental prescribing on NHS Compound Sodium Chloride Mouthwash may be prescribed

THYMOL

Indication and dose

Oral hygiene (see notes above); for dose, see under preparation

Mouthwash Solution-tablets
Consist of tablets which may contain antimicrobial, colouring, and flavouring agents in a suitable soluble effervescent basis to make a mouthwash suitable for dental purposes.

Dose

Dissolve 1 tablet in a tumblerful of warm water

Note Mouthwash Solution-tablets may contain ingredients such as thymol
Dental prescribing on NHS Mouthwash Solution-tablets may be prescribed

12.3.5 Treatment of dry mouth

Dry mouth (xerostomia) may be caused by drugs with antimuscarinic (anticholinergic) side-effects (e.g. antispasmodics and sedating antihistamines), by irradiation of the head and neck region or by damage to or disease of the salivary glands. Children with a persistently dry mouth may develop a burning or scalded sensation and have poor oral hygiene; they may develop dental caries, periodontal disease, and oral infections (particularly candidiasis). Dry mouth may be relieved in many patients by simple measures such as frequent sips of cool drinks or sucking pieces of ice or sugar-free fruit pastilles. Sugar-free chewing gum stimulates salivation in patients with residual salivary function.

Artificial saliva can provide useful relief of dry mouth. A properly balanced artificial saliva should be of a neutral pH and contain electrolytes (including fluoride) to correspond approximately to the composition of saliva. The pH of some artificial saliva products may be inappropriate.

Local treatment

Artificial saliva products with **ACBS approval** may be prescribed for children with dry mouth as a result of having (or having undergone) radiotherapy, or sicca syndrome. SST tablets and *Salinum*® liquid may also be prescribed on the NHS.

AS Saliva Orthana® (AS Pharma)
Oral spray, gastric mucin (porcine) 3.5%, xylitol 2%, sodium fluoride 4.2 mg/litre, with preservatives and flavouring agents. Net price 50-mL bottle = £4.25; 450-mL refill = £29.69

Dose

(ACBS) spray 2–3 times onto oral and pharyngeal mucosa, when required

Lozenges, mucin 65 mg, xylitol 59 mg, in a sorbitol basis. Net price 45-lozenge pack = £3.02
Note *AS Saliva Orthana®* lozenges do not contain fluoride
Dental prescribing on NHS *AS Saliva Orthana®* Oral Spray and Lozenges may be prescribed

Glandosane® (Fresenius Kabi)
Aerosol spray, carmellose sodium 500 mg, sorbitol 1.5 g, potassium chloride 60 mg, sodium chloride 42.2 mg, magnesium chloride 2.6 mg, calcium chloride 7.3 mg, and dipotassium hydrogen phosphate 17.1 mg/50 g. Net price 50-mL unit (neutral, lemon or peppermint flavoured) = £4.48

Dose

(ACBS) spray onto oral and pharyngeal mucosa as required

Dental prescribing on NHS *Glandosane®* Aerosol Spray may be prescribed

Luborant® (Goldshield)
Oral spray, pink, sorbitol 1.8 g, carmellose sodium (sodium carboxymethylcellulose) 390 mg, dibasic potassium phosphate 48.23 mg, potassium chloride 37.5 mg, monobasic potassium phosphate 21.97 mg, calcium chloride 9.972 mg, magnesium chloride 3.528 mg, sodium fluoride 258 micr-

ograms/60 mL, with preservatives and colouring agents. Net price 60-mL unit = £3.96

Dose

Saliva deficiency

2–3 sprays onto oral mucosa up to 4 times daily, or as directed

Note May be difficult to obtain

Dental prescribing on NHS *Luborant*® Oral Spray may be prescribed as Artificial Saliva

Biotène Oralbalance® (Anglian)

Saliva replacement gel, lactoperoxidase, lactoferrin, lysozyme, glucose oxidase, xylitol in a gel basis, net price 50-g tube = £4.10; 24 × 12.4 mL tube = £30.40 (for hospital use)

Dose

(ACBS) apply to gums and tongue as required

Note Avoid use with toothpastes containing detergents (including foaming agents)

Dental prescribing on NHS *Biotène Oralbalance*® Saliva Replacement Gel may be prescribed

BioXtra® (Molar)

Gel, lactoperoxidase, lactoferrin, lysozyme, whey colostrum, xylitol and other ingredients, net price 40-mL tube = £2.25

Dose

(ACBS) apply to oral mucosa as required

Dental prescribing on NHS *BioXtra*® Gel may be prescribed

Salinum® (Crawford)

Liquid sugar free, linseed extract (containing polysaccharides), with dipotassium phosphate buffer and preservatives, net price 300-mL bottle = £13.50

Dose

Symptomatic treatment of dry mouth

approx. 2 mL rinsed around the mouth and then swallowed, when required

Saliveze® (KoGEN)

Oral spray, carmellose sodium (sodium carboxymethylcellulose), calcium chloride, magnesium chloride, potassium chloride, sodium chloride, and dibasic sodium phosphate. Net price 50-mL bottle (mint-flavoured) = £3.50

Dose

(ACBS) 1 spray onto oral mucosa as required

Dental prescribing on NHS *Saliveze*® Oral Spray may be prescribed

Salivix® (Provalis)

Pastilles, sugar-free, reddish-amber, acacia, malic acid and other ingredients. Net price 50-pastille pack = £2.86

Dose

(ACBS) suck 1 pastille when required

Dental prescribing on NHS *Salivix*® Pastilles may be prescribed

SST (Medac)

Tablets, sugar-free, citric acid, malic acid and other ingredients in a sorbitol base, net price 100-tab pack = £4.86

Dose

Symptomatic treatment of dry mouth in patients with impaired salivary gland function and patent salivary ducts

allow 1 tablet to dissolve slowly in the mouth when required

13 Skin

This chapter includes advice on the drug management of the following:
nappy rash, p. 618
rosacea, p. 641
photodamage, p. 652
dermatophytoses, p. 658
pityriasis versicolor, p. 659
candidiasis, p. 659
scabies, p. 664
head lice, p. 664
crab lice, p. 665

13.1 Management of skin conditions

When prescribing topical preparations for the treatment of skin conditions in children, the site of application, the condition being treated, and the child's (and carer's) preference for a particular vehicle all need to be taken into consideration.

Neonates Caution is required when prescribing topical preparations for neonates—their large body surface area in relation to body mass increases susceptibility to toxicity from systemic absorption of substances applied to the skin. Topical preparations containing potentially sensitising substances such as corticosteroids, aminoglycosides, iodine, and parasiticidal drugs should be avoided. Preparations containing alcohol should be avoided because they can dehydrate the skin, cause pain if applied to raw areas, and the alcohol can cause necrosis.

In *preterm neonates*, the skin is more fragile and offers a poor barrier, especially in the first fortnight after birth. Preterm infants, especially if below 32 weeks postmenstrual age, may also require special measures to maintain skin hydration.

13.1.1 Vehicles

The vehicle in topical preparations for the skin affects the degree of hydration, has a mild anti-inflammatory effect, and aids the penetration of the active drug. Therefore, the active drug as well as the vehicle should be chosen on the basis of their suitability for the child's skin condition.

Applications are usually viscous solutions, emulsions, or suspensions for application to the skin (including the scalp) or nails.

Collodions are painted on the skin and allowed to dry to leave a flexible film over the site of application.

Creams are emulsions of oil and water and are generally well absorbed into the skin. They may contain an antimicrobial preservative unless the active ingredient or basis is intrinsically bactericidal and fungicidal. Generally, creams are cosmetically more acceptable than ointments because they are less greasy and easier to apply.

Gels consist of active ingredients in suitable hydrophilic or hydrophobic bases; they generally have a high water content. Gels are particularly suitable for application to the face and scalp.

Lotions have a cooling effect and may be preferred to ointments or creams for application over a hairy area. Lotions in alcoholic basis can sting if used on broken skin. *Shake lotions* (such as calamine lotion) contain insoluble powders which leave a deposit on the skin surface.

Ointments are greasy preparations which are normally anhydrous and insoluble in water, and are more occlusive than creams. They are particularly suitable for chronic, dry lesions. The most commonly used ointment bases consist of soft paraffin or a combination of soft, liquid and hard paraffin. Some ointment bases have both *hydrophilic* and *lipophilic* properties; they may have occlusive properties on the skin surface, encourage hydration, and also be miscible with water; they often have a mild anti-inflammatory effect. *Water-soluble ointments* contain macrogols which are freely soluble in water and are therefore readily washed off; they have a limited but useful role where ready removal is desirable.

Pastes are stiff preparations containing a high proportion of finely powdered solids such as zinc oxide and starch suspended in an ointment. They are used for circumscribed lesions such as those which occur in lichen simplex, chronic eczema, or psoriasis. They are less occlusive than ointments and can be used to protect inflamed, lichenified, or excoriated skin.

Dusting powders are used only rarely. They reduce friction between opposing skin surfaces. Dusting powders should not be applied to moist areas because they can cake and abrade the skin. Talc is a lubricant but it does not absorb moisture whereas starch is less lubricant but absorbs water.

Dilution The BP directs that creams and ointments should **not** normally be diluted but that should dilution be necessary care should be taken, in particular, to prevent microbial contamination. The appropriate diluent should be used and heating should be avoided during mixing; excessive dilution may affect the stability of some creams. Diluted creams should normally be used within 2 weeks of their preparation.

13.1.2 Suitable quantities for prescribing

Suitable quantities of dermatological preparations:

Suitable quantities of dermatological preparations to be prescribed for specific areas of the body

Area of the body	Creams and Ointments	Lotions
Face	15–30 g	100 mL
Both hands	25–50 g	200 mL
Scalp	50–100 g	200 mL
Both arms or both legs	100–200 g	200 mL
Trunk	400 g	500 mL
Groins and genitalia	15–25 g	100 mL

The amounts shown above are usually suitable for children 12–18 years for twice daily application for 1 week; smaller quantities will be required for children under 12 years. These recommendations **do not apply** to corticosteroid preparations.

13.1.3 Excipients and sensitisation

Excipients in topical products rarely cause problems. If a patch test indicates allergy to an excipient, then products containing the substance should be avoided (see also Anaphylaxis p. 189). The following excipients in topical preparations may rarely be associated with sensitisation; the presence of these excipients is indicated in the entries for topical products.

- Beeswax
- Benzyl alcohol
- Butylated hydroxyanisole
- Butylated hydroxytoluene
- Cetostearyl alcohol (including cetyl and stearyl alcohol)
- Chlorocresol
- Edetic acid (EDTA)
- Ethylenediamine
- Fragrances
- Hydroxybenzoates (parabens)
- Imidurea
- Isopropyl palmitate
- *N*-(3-Chloroallyl)hexaminium chloride (quaternium 15)
- Polysorbates
- Propylene glycol
- Sodium metabisulphite
- Sorbic acid
- Wool fat and related substances including lanolin[1]

1. Purified versions of wool fat have reduced the problem

13.2 Emollient and barrier preparations

Borderline substances The preparations marked 'ACBS' are regarded as drugs when prescribed in accordance with the advice of the Advisory Committee on Borderline Substances for the clinical conditions listed. Prescriptions issued in accordance with this advice and endorsed 'ACBS' will normally not be investigated. See Appendix 2 for listing by clinical condition.

13.2.1 Emollients

Emollients hydrate the skin, soften the skin, act as barrier to water and external irritants, and are indicated for all dry or scaling disorders. Their effects are short-lived and they should be applied frequently even after improvement occurs. They are useful in dry and eczematous disorders, and to a lesser extent in psoriasis (section 13.5.2); they should be applied immediately after washing or bathing to maximise the effect of skin hydration. Light emollients such as **aqueous cream** are suitable for many dry skin conditions but more greasy preparations such as **white soft paraffin**, **emulsifying ointment**, and **liquid and white soft paraffin ointment** are often more effective. The severity of the condition, the child's (or carer's) preference and the site of application will often guide the choice of emollient. Some ingredients may rarely cause sensitisation (section 13.1.3) and this should be suspected if an eczematous reaction occurs.

Preparations such as **aqueous cream** and **emulsifying ointment** can be used as soap substitutes; the preparation is rubbed on the skin before rinsing off completely. The addition of a bath oil (section 13.2.1.1) may also be helpful.

In the *neonate,* a preservative-free paraffin-based emollient hydrates the skin without affecting the normal skin flora; substances such as olive oil are also used. The development of blisters (epidermolysis bullosa) or ichthyosis may be alleviated by applying liquid and white soft paraffin ointment while awaiting dermatological investigation.

Preparations containing an antibacterial should be avoided unless infection is present (section 13.10.1) or is a frequent complication of the dry skin condition.

Urea is a keratin softener used in the treatment of dry, scaling conditions. It is occasionally used with other topical agents such as corticosteroids to enhance penetration.

Non-proprietary emollient preparations

Aqueous Cream, BP
Cream, emulsifying ointment 30%, [1]phenoxyethanol 1% in freshly boiled and cooled purified water, net price 100 g = 50p
Excipients: include cetostearyl alcohol

1. The BP permits use of alternative antimicrobials provided their identity and concentration are stated on the label

Emulsifying Ointment, BP
Ointment, emulsifying wax 30%, white soft paraffin 50%, liquid paraffin 20%, net price 100 g = 57p
Excipients: include cetostearyl alcohol

Hydrous Ointment, BP
Ointment, (oily cream), dried magnesium sulphate 0.5%, phenoxyethanol 1%, wool alcohols ointment 50%, in freshly boiled and cooled purified water, net price 100 g = 40p

Liquid and White Soft Paraffin Ointment, NPF
Ointment, liquid paraffin 50%, white soft paraffin 50%, net price 250 g = £3.24

Paraffin, White Soft, BP
White petroleum jelly, net price 100 g = 52p

Paraffin, Yellow Soft, BP
Yellow petroleum jelly, net price 100 g = 33p

Proprietary emollient preparations

Aveeno® (J&J)
Cream, colloidal oatmeal in emollient basis, net price 100 mL = £3.78
Excipients: include benzyl alcohol, cetyl alcohol, isopropyl palmitate
ACBS: For endogenous and exogenous eczema, xeroderma, and ichthyosis

Lotion, colloidal oatmeal in emollient basis, net price 400-mL pump pack = £6.42
Excipients: include benzyl alcohol, cetyl alcohol, isopropyl palmitate
ACBS: as for *Aveeno® Cream*

Cetraben® (Genus)
Emollient cream, white soft paraffin 13.2%, light liquid paraffin 10.5%, net price 50 g = £1.17, 125 g = £2.38, 500-g pump pack = £5.61
Excipients: include cetostearyl alcohol, hydroxybenzoates (parabens)

Decubal® Clinic (Alpharma)
Cream, isopropyl myristate 17%, glycerol 8.5%, wool fat 6%, dimeticone 5%, net price 50 g = £1.02, 100 g = £1.98
Excipients: include cetyl alcohol, polysorbates, sorbic acid, wool fat

Dermamist® (Astellas)
Spray application, white soft paraffin 10% in a basis containing liquid paraffin, fractionated coconut oil, net price 250-mL pressurised aerosol unit = £9.22
Excipients: none as listed in section 13.1.3
Note Flammable

Diprobase® (Schering-Plough)
Cream, cetomacrogol 2.25%, cetostearyl alcohol 7.2%, liquid paraffin 6%, white soft paraffin 15%, water-miscible basis used for *Diprosone®* cream, net price 50 g = £1.43; 500-g dispenser = £6.15
Excipients: include cetostearyl alcohol, chlorocresol

Ointment, liquid paraffin 5%, white soft paraffin 95%, basis used for *Diprosone®* ointment, net price 50 g = £1.54
Excipients: none as listed in section 13.1.3

Doublebase® (Dermal)
Gel, isopropyl myristate 15%, liquid paraffin 15%, net price 100 g = £2.77, 500 g = £6.09
Excipients: none as listed in section 13.1.3

Drapolene®
Section 13.2.2

E45® (Crookes)
Cream, light liquid paraffin 12.6%, white soft paraffin 14.5%, hypoallergenic hydrous wool fat (hypoallergenic lanolin) 1% in self-emulsifying monostearin, net price 50 g = £1.18, 125 g = £2.39, 350 g = £4.14, 500-g pump pack = £6.20
Excipients: include cetyl alcohol, hydroxybenzoates (parabens)

Emollient Wash Cream, soap substitute, zinc oxide 5% in an emollient basis, net price 250-mL pump pack = £2.95
Excipients: none as listed in section 13.1.3
ACBS: for endogenous and exogenous eczema, xeroderma, and ichthyosis

Lotion, light liquid paraffin 4%, cetomacrogol, white soft paraffin 10%, hypoallergenic anhydrous wool fat (hypoallergenic lanolin) 1% in glyceryl monostearate, net price 200 mL = £2.40, 500-mL pump pack = £4.50
Excipients: include isopropyl palmitate, hydroxybenzoates (parabens), benzyl alcohol
ACBS: for symptomatic relief of dry skin conditions, such as those associated with atopic eczema and contact dermatitis

Epaderm® (Medlock)
Ointment, emulsifying wax 30%, yellow soft paraffin 30%, liquid paraffin 40%, net price 125 g = £3.48, 500 g = £5.90
Excipients: include cetostearyl alcohol

Gammaderm® (Linderma)
Cream, evening primrose oil 20%, net price 50 g = £2.83, 250 g = £8.20
Excipients: include beeswax, hydroxybenzoates (parabens), propylene glycol
Cautions epilepsy (but hazard unlikely with topical preparations)

Hewletts® (Kestrel)
Cream, hydrous wool fat 4%, zinc oxide 8%, arachis (peanut) oil, oleic acid, white soft paraffin, net price 35 g = £1.43, 400 g = £6.69
Excipients: include fragrance

Hydromol® (Ferndale)
Cream, sodium pidolate 2.5%, net price 50 g = £2.04, 100 g = £3.80, 500 g = £12.60
Excipients: include cetostearyl alcohol, hydroxybenzoates (parabens)

Ointment, yellow soft paraffin 30%, emulsifying wax 30%, net price 125 g = £2.79, 500 g = £4.74
Excipients: include cetostearyl alcohol

Kamillosan® (Goldshield)
Ointment, chamomile extracts 10.5% in a basis containing wool fat, net price 50 g = £2.50, 100 g = £5.00
Excipients: include beeswax, cetostearyl alcohol, hydroxybenzoates (parabens)

Keri® (Bristol-Myers Squibb)
Lotion, mineral oil 16%, with lanolin oil, net price 190-mL pump pack = £3.56, 380-mL pump pack = £5.81
Excipients: include fragrance, hydroxybenzoates (parabens), *N*-(3-chloroallyl)hexaminium chloride (quaternium 15), propylene glycol

Lipobase® (Astellas)
Cream, fatty cream basis used for *Locoid Lipocream®*, net price 50 g = £2.08
Excipients: include cetostearyl alcohol, hydroxybenzoates (parabens)
For dry skin conditions, also for use during treatment with topical corticosteroid and as diluent for *Locoid Lipocream®*

Neutrogena® Dermatological Cream (J&J)
Cream, glycerol 40% in an emollient basis, net price 100 g = £3.77
Excipients: include cetostearyl alcohol, hydroxybenzoates (parabens)

Oilatum® (Stiefel)
Cream, light liquid paraffin 6%, white soft paraffin 15%, net price 40 g = £1.79, 150 g = £3.38
Excipients: include benzyl alcohol, cetostearyl alcohol

Shower emollient (gel), light liquid paraffin 70%, net price 150 g = £5.15
Excipients: include fragrance

Ultrabase® (Schering Health)
Cream, water-miscible, containing liquid paraffin and white soft paraffin, net price 50 g = 89p, 500-g dispenser = £6.44
Excipients: include fragrance, hydroxybenzoates (parabens), disodium edetate, stearyl alcohol

Unguentum M® (Crookes)
Cream, containing saturated neutral oil, liquid paraffin, white soft paraffin, net price 50 g = £1.59, 100 g = £3.13, 200-mL dispenser = £6.19, 500 g = £9.55
Excipients: include cetostearyl alcohol, polysorbate 40, propylene glycol, sorbic acid

Vaseline Dermacare® (Elida Fabergé)
Cream, dimeticone 1%, white soft paraffin 15%, net price 150 mL = £2.11
Excipients: include hydroxybenzoates (parabens)
ACBS: for endogenous and exogenous eczema, xeroderma, and ichthyosis

Lotion, dimeticone 1%, liquid paraffin 4%, white soft paraffin 5% in an emollient basis, net price 75 mL = 78p, 200 mL = £1.49
Excipients: include disodium edetate, hydroxybenzoates (parabens), wool fat
ACBS: as for *Vaseline Dermacare® Cream*

Zerobase® (Zeroderma)
Cream, liquid paraffin 11%, net price 500 g dispenser = £5.99
Excipients: include cetostearyl alcohol, chlorocresol

Preparations containing urea

Aquadrate® (Alliance)
Cream, urea 10%, net price 30 g = £1.37, 100 g = £3.64
Excipients: none as listed in section 13.1.3

Dose
Apply thinly and rub into area when required

Balneum® Plus (Crookes)
Cream, urea 5%, lauromacrogols 3%, net price 100 g = £5.58, 175-g pump pack = £7.81, 500-g pump pack = £19.50
Excipients: include benzyl alcohol, polysorbates

Dose
Apply twice daily

Calmurid® (Galderma)
Cream, urea 10%, lactic acid 5%, net price 100 g = £6.84, 500-g dispenser = £25.78
Excipients: none as listed in section 13.1.3

Dose
Apply a thick layer for 3–5 minutes, massage into area, and remove excess, usually twice daily. Use half-strength cream for 1 week if stinging occurs

Note Can be diluted with aqueous cream (life of diluted cream 14 days)

E45® Itch Relief Cream (Crookes)
Cream, urea 5%, macrogol lauryl ether 3%, net price 50 g = £2.16, 100 g = £3.47
Excipients: include benzyl alcohol, polysorbates

Dose
Apply twice daily

Eucerin® (Beiersdorf)
Cream, urea 10%, net price 50 mL = £5.85, 150 mL = £9.23
Excipients: include benzyl alcohol, isopropyl palmitate, wool fat

Dose
Apply thinly and rub into area twice daily

Lotion, urea 10%, net price 250 mL = £7.69
Excipients: include benzyl alcohol, isopropyl palmitate

Dose
Apply sparingly and rub into area twice daily

Nutraplus® (Galderma)
Cream, urea 10%, net price 100 g = £4.37
Excipients: include hydroxybenzoates (parabens), propylene glycol

Dose
Apply 2–3 times daily

With antimicrobials

Dermol® (Dermal)
Cream, benzalkonium chloride 0.1%, chlorhexidine hydrochloride 0.1%, isopropyl myristate 10%, liquid paraffin 10%, net price 100-g tube = £3.22, 500-g bottle = £7.45
Excipients: include cetostearyl alcohol

Dose
Apply to skin or use as soap substitute

Dermol® 500 Lotion, benzalkonium chloride 0.1%, chlorhexidine hydrochloride 0.1%, liquid paraffin 2.5%, isopropyl myristate 2.5%, net price 500-mL dispenser = £6.31
Excipients: include cetostearyl alcohol

Dose
Apply to skin or use as soap substitute

Dermol® 200 Shower Emollient, benzalkonium chloride 0.1%, chlorhexidine hydrochloride 0.1%, liquid paraffin 2.5%, isopropyl myristate 2.5%, net price 200 mL = £3.71
Excipients: include cetostearyl alcohol

Dose
Apply to skin or use as soap substitute

13.2.1.1 Emollient bath additives

Bath emollient additives should be added to bath water; some can be applied to wet skin undiluted and rinsed off. Hydration may be improved by soaking in the bath for 10–20 minutes. In dry skin conditions soap should be avoided (see section 13.2.1 for soap substitutes).

The quantities of bath additives recommended for older children are suitable for an adult-size bath. Proportionately less should be used for a child-size bath or a washbasin; recommended bath additive quantities for younger children reflect this.

Note These preparations make skin and surfaces slippery—particular care is needed when bathing a child.

Alpha Keri Bath® (Bristol-Myers Squibb)
Bath oil, liquid paraffin 91.7%, oil-soluble fraction of wool fat 3%, net price 240 mL = £3.45, 480 mL = £6.43
Excipients: include fragrance

Dose
Neonate add 5 mL to bath water or apply to wet skin and rinse

Child 1 month–2 years add 5 mL to bath water or apply to wet skin and rinse

Child 2–18 years add 10–20 mL to bath water or apply to wet skin and rinse

Aveeno® (J&J)
Aveeno® Bath oil, colloidal oatmeal, white oat fraction in emollient basis, net price 250 mL = £4.28
Excipients: include beeswax, fragrance
ACBS: for endogenous and exogenous eczema, xeroderma, and ichthyosis

Dose
Child 2–18 years add 30 mL to bath water

Aveeno Colloidal® Bath additive, oatmeal, white oat fraction in emollient basis, net price 10 × 50-g sachets = £7.33
Excipients: none as listed in section 13.1.3
ACBS: as for Aveeno® Bath oil

Dose

Neonate add ½ sachetful to bath water

Child 1 month–2 years add ½ sachetful to bath water

Child 2–18 years add 1 sachetful to bath water

Balneum® (Crookes)

Balneum® bath oil, soya oil 84.75%, net price 200 mL = £2.79, 500 mL = £6.06, 1 litre = £11.70
Excipients: include butylated hydroxytoluene, propylene glycol, fragrance

Dose

Neonate add 5–15 mL to bath water; do not use undiluted

Child 1 month–2 years add 5–15 mL to bath water; do not use undiluted

Child 2–18 years add 20–60 mL to bath water; do not use undiluted

Balneum Plus® bath oil, soya oil 82.95%, mixed lauromacrogols 15%, net price 500 mL = £7.50
Excipients: include butylated hydroxytoluene, propylene glycol, fragrance

Dose

Neonate add 5 mL to bath water or apply to wet skin and rinse

Child 1 month–2 years add 5 mL to bath water or apply to wet skin and rinse

Child 2–18 years add 10–20 mL to bath water or apply to wet skin and rinse

Cetraben® (Sankyo)

Emollient bath additive, light liquid paraffin 82.8%, net price 500 mL = £5.25

Dose

Neonate add ½ capful to bath water or apply to wet skin and rinse

Child 1 month–12 years add ½–1 capful to bath water or apply to wet skin and rinse

Child 12–18 years add 1–2 capfuls to bath water or apply to wet skin and rinse

Dermalo® (Dermal)

Bath emollient, acetylated wool alcohols 5%, liquid paraffin 65%, net price 500 mL = £3.60
Excipients: none as listed in section 13.1.3

Dose

Neonate add 5 mL to bath water or apply to wet skin and rinse

Child 1 month–12 years add 5–10 mL to bath water or apply to wet skin and rinse

Child 12–18 years add 15–20 mL to bath water or apply to wet skin and rinse

Diprobath® (Schering-Plough)

Bath additive, isopropyl myristate 39%, light liquid paraffin 46%, net price 500 mL = £6.97
Excipients: none as listed in section 13.1.3

Dose

Neonate add 5 mL to bath water; do not use undiluted

Child 1 month–12 years add 10 mL to bath water; do not use undiluted

Child 12–18 years add 25–50 mL to bath water; do not use undiluted

E45® (Crookes)

Emollient bath oil, cetyl dimeticone 5%, liquid paraffin 91%, net price 250 mL = £2.95, 500 mL = £4.70
Excipients: none as listed in section 13.1.3
ACBS: for endogenous and exogenous eczema, xeroderma, and ichthyosis

Dose

Neonate add 5 mL to bath water or apply to wet skin and rinse

Child 1 month–12 years add 5–10 mL to bath water or apply to wet skin and rinse

Child 12–18 years add 15 mL to bath water or apply to wet skin and rinse

Emollient Medicinal Bath Oil (Ashbourne)

Emollient bath oil, liquid paraffin 65%, acetylated wool alcohols 5%, net price 250 mL = £2.75, 500 mL = £5.46

Dose

Neonate add 5 mL to bath water; do not use undiluted

Child 1 month–12 years add 5–10 mL to bath water; do not use undiluted

Child 12–18 years add 15–20 mL to bath water; do not use undiluted

Hydromol Emollient® (Ferndale)

Bath additive, isopropyl myristate 13%, light liquid paraffin 37.8%, net price 350 mL = £3.80, 500 mL = £5.14, 1 litre = £9.00
Excipients: none as listed in section 13.1.3

Dose

Neonate add ½ capful to bath water or apply to wet skin and rinse

Child 1 month–12 years add ½–2 capfuls to bath water or apply to wet skin and rinse

Child 12–18 years add 1–3 capfuls to bath water or apply to wet skin and rinse

Imuderm® (Goldshield)

Bath oil, almond oil 30%, light liquid paraffin 69.6%, net price 250 mL = £3.75
Excipients: include butylated hydroxyanisole

Dose

Neonate add 7.5 mL to bath water or rub into dry skin until absorbed

Child 1 month–12 years add 7.5–15 mL to bath water or rub into dry skin until absorbed

Child 12–18 years add 15–30 mL to bath water or rub into dry skin until absorbed

Oilatum® (Stiefel)

Oilatum® Emollient bath additive (emulsion), acetylated wool alcohols 5%, liquid paraffin 63.4%, net price 250 mL = £2.75, 500 mL = £4.57
Excipients: include isopropyl palmitate, fragrance

Dose

Neonate add ½ capful to bath water or apply to wet skin and rinse

Child 1 month–12 years add ½–2 capfuls to bath water or apply to wet skin and rinse

Child 12–18 years add 1–3 capfuls to bath water or apply to wet skin and rinse

Oilatum® Fragrance Free Junior bath additive, light liquid paraffin 63.4%, net price 250 mL = £3.25, 500 mL = £5.75, 1 litre = £11.50
Excipients: include wool fat, isopropyl palmitate

Dose

Neonate add ½ capful to bath water or apply to wet skin and rinse

Child 1 month–12 years add ½–2 capfuls to bath water or apply to wet skin and rinse

Child 12–18 years add 1–3 capfuls to bath water or apply to wet skin and rinse

◢With antimicrobials

Dermol® (Dermal)
Dermol® 600 Bath Emollient, benzalkonium chloride 0.5%, liquid paraffin 25%, isopropyl myristate 25%, net price 600 mL = £7.90
Excipients: include polysorbate 60

Dose

Child 1 month–2 years add 5–15 mL to bath water; do not use undiluted

Child 2–18 years add 15–30 mL to bath water; do not use undiluted

Emulsiderm® (Dermal)
Liquid emulsion, liquid paraffin 25%, isopropyl myristate 25%, benzalkonium chloride 0.5%, net price 300 mL (with 15-mL measure) = £4.03, 1 litre (with 30-mL measure) = £12.55
Excipients: include polysorbate 60

Dose

Child 1 month–2 years add 5–10 mL to bath water or rub into dry skin until absorbed

Child 2–18 years add 10–30 mL to bath water or rub into dry skin until absorbed

Oilatum® (Stiefel)
Oilatum® Plus bath additive, benzalkonium chloride 6%, triclosan 2%, light liquid paraffin 52.5%, net price 500 mL = £6.98, 1 litre = £13.59
Excipients: include wool fat, isopropyl palmitate

Dose

Child 6 months–1 year add 1 mL to bath water; do not use undiluted

Child 1–18 years add 1–2 capfuls to bath water; do not use undiluted

◢With tar

Section 13.5.2

13.2.2 Barrier preparations

Barrier preparations often contain water-repellent substances such as **dimeticone** (dimethicone), natural oils, and paraffins, to help protect the skin from abrasion and irritation; they are used to protect intact skin around stomas and pressure sores, and as a barrier against nappy rash. In neonates, barrier preparations which do not contain potentially sensitising excipients (section 13.1.3) may be preferred. Where the skin has broken down, barrier preparations have a limited role in protecting adjacent skin. **Zinc ointments** or barrier creams with zinc oxide or titanium salts, are used to aid healing of uninfected, excoriated skin.

Nappy rash (dermatitis) The first line of treatment is to ensure that nappies are changed frequently and that tightly fitting water-proof pants are avoided. The rash may clear when left exposed to the air and a barrier preparation may be helpful. If the rash is associated with a yeast or fungal infection, an antifungal cream such as clotrimazole cream (section 13.10.2) is useful. A mild corticosteroid such as hydrocortisone 1% is useful in moderate to severe inflammation, but it should be avoided in neonates. The barrier preparation is applied after the corticosteroid preparation to prevent further damage. Hydrocortisone may be used in combination with antifungal and antibacterial drugs (section 13.4) if there is considerable inflammation, erosion, and infection. Preparations containing hydrocortisone should be applied for no more than a week; the occlusive effect of nappies and water-proof pants may increase absorption of corticosteroid (for cautions, see section 13.4).

◢Non-proprietary barrier preparations

Zinc Cream, BP
Cream, zinc oxide 32%, arachis (peanut) oil 32%, calcium hydroxide 0.045%, oleic acid 0.5%, wool fat 8%, in freshly boiled and cooled purified water, net price 50 g = 50p

Zinc Ointment, BP
Ointment, zinc oxide 15%, in Simple Ointment BP 1988 (which contains wool fat 5%, hard paraffin 5%, cetostearyl alcohol 5%, white soft paraffin 85%), net price 25 g = 16p

Zinc and Castor Oil Ointment, BP
Ointment, zinc oxide 7.5%, castor oil 50%, arachis (peanut) oil 30.5%, white beeswax 10%, cetostearyl alcohol 2%, net price 25 g = 14p

◢Proprietary barrier preparations

Conotrane® (Astellas)
Cream, benzalkonium chloride 0.1%, dimeticone 22%, net price 100 g = 74p, 500 g = £3.51
Excipients: include cetostearyl alcohol, fragrance

Drapolene® (Warner Lambert)
Cream, benzalkonium chloride 0.01%, cetrimide 0.2% in a basis containing white soft paraffin, cetyl alcohol and wool fat, net price 100 g = £1.43, 200 g = £2.38, 350 g = £3.66
Excipients: include cetyl alcohol, chlorocresol, wool fat

Medicaid® (LPC)
Cream, cetrimide 0.5% in a basis containing light liquid paraffin, white soft paraffin, cetostearyl alcohol, glyceryl monostearate, net price 50 g = £1.69
Excipients: include cetostearyl alcohol, fragrance, hydroxybenzoates (parabens), wool fat

Metanium® (Ransom)
Ointment, titanium dioxide 20%, titanium peroxide 5%, titanium salicylate 3% in a basis containing dimeticone, light liquid paraffin, white soft paraffin, and benzoin tincture, net price 30 g = £2.01
Excipients: none as listed in section 13.1.3

Morhulin® (Thornton & Ross)
Ointment, cod-liver oil 11.4%, zinc oxide 38%, in a basis containing liquid paraffin and yellow soft paraffin, net price 50 g = £1.62
Excipients: include wool fat derivative

Siopel® (Centrapharm)
Barrier cream, dimeticone '1000' 10%, cetrimide 0.3%, arachis (peanut) oil, net price 50 g = £1.66
Excipients: include butylated hydroxytoluene, cetostearyl alcohol, hydroxybenzoates (parabens)

Sprilon® (Ayrton Saunders)
Spray application, dimeticone 1.04%, zinc oxide 12.5%, in a basis containing wool alcohols, cetostearyl alcohol, dextran, white soft paraffin, liquid paraffin, propellants, net price 115-g pressurised aerosol unit = £3.54
Excipients: include cetostearyl alcohol, hydroxybenzoates (parabens), wool fat
Note Flammable

Sudocrem® (Forest)
Cream, benzyl alcohol 0.39%, benzyl benzoate 1.01%, benzyl cinnamate 0.15%, hydrous wool fat (hypoallergenic lanolin) 4%, zinc oxide 15.25%, net price 30 g = £1.01, 60 g = £1.07, 125 g = £1.62, 250 g = £2.75, 400 g = £3.88
Excipients: include beeswax (synthetic), propylene glycol, fragrance

Vasogen® (Forest)
Barrier cream, dimeticone 20%, calamine 1.5%, zinc oxide 7.5%, net price 50 g = 80p, 100 g = £1.36
Excipients: include hydroxybenzoates (parabens), wool fat

13.3 Topical antipruritics

Pruritus may be caused by systemic disease (such as drug hypersensitivity, obstructive jaundice, endocrine disease, and certain malignant diseases), skin disease (e.g. eczema, psoriasis, urticaria, and scabies) or as a side-effect of opioid analgesics. Where possible the underlying cause should be treated. For the treatment of pruritus in palliative care, see Prescribing in Palliative Care p. 27. Pruritus caused by cholestasis generally requires a bile acid sequestrant (section 1.9.2).

An **emollient** (section 13.2.1) may be of value where the pruritus is associated with dry skin. Preparations containing **calamine** or **crotamiton** are sometimes used but are of uncertain value.

A topical preparation containing **doxepin 5%** is licensed for the relief of pruritus in eczema in children over 12 years; it can cause drowsiness and there may be a risk of sensitisation.

Topical antihistamines and local anaesthetics (section 15.2) are only marginally effective and may occasionally cause sensitisation. For *insect stings* and *insect bites*, a short course of a topical corticosteroid is appropriate. Short treatment with a **sedating antihistamine** (section 3.4.1) may help in insect stings and in intractable pruritus where sedation is desirable. Insect stings and bites should not be treated with calamine preparations.

In *pruritus ani*, the underlying cause such as faecal soiling, eczema, psoriasis, or helminth infection should be treated; for preparations used to relieve pruritus ani, see section 1.7.

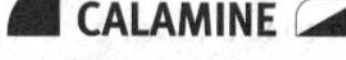

CALAMINE

Indication and dose
Pruritus but see notes above

Calamine (Non-proprietary)
Aqueous cream, calamine 4%, zinc oxide 3%, liquid paraffin 20%, self-emulsifying glyceryl monostearate 5%, cetomacrogol emulsifying wax 5%, phe-

CALAMINE (*continued*)

noxyethanol 0.5%, freshly boiled and cooled purified water 62.5%, net price 100 mL = 59p

Lotion (= cutaneous suspension), calamine 15%, zinc oxide 5%, glycerol 5%, bentonite 3%, sodium citrate 0.5%, liquefied phenol 0.5%, in freshly boiled and cooled purified water, net price 200 mL = 63p

Oily lotion (BP 1980), calamine 5%, arachis (peanut) oil 50%, oleic acid 0.5%, wool fat 1%, in calcium hydroxide solution, net price 200 mL = £1.57

CROTAMITON

Cautions avoid use near eyes and broken skin; use on doctor's advice for children under 3 years

Contra-indications acute exudative dermatoses

Indication and dose

Pruritus but see notes above
Apply 2–3 times daily (for pruritus after scabies in children under 3 years apply once daily only)

Eurax® (Novartis Consumer Health)
Cream, crotamiton 10%, net price 30 g = £2.27, 100 g = £3.95
Excipients: include beeswax, fragrance, hydroxybenzoates (parabens), stearyl alcohol

Lotion, crotamiton 10%, net price 100 mL = £2.99
Excipients: include cetyl alcohol, fragrance, propylene glycol, sorbic acid, stearyl alcohol

DOXEPIN HYDROCHLORIDE

Cautions glaucoma, urinary retention, severe liver impairment, mania; avoid application to large areas; **interactions:** Appendix 1 (antidepressants, tricyclic)
Driving Drowsiness may affect performance of skilled tasks (e.g. driving); effects of alcohol enhanced

Pregnancy manufacturer advises use only if potential benefit outweighs risk

Breast-feeding manufacturer advises use only if potential benefit outweighs risk

Side-effects drowsiness; local burning, stinging, irritation, tingling and rash; dry mouth and other systemic side-effects reported (section 4.3.1)

Indication and dose

Pruritus in eczema
Child 12–18 years apply thinly 3–4 times daily; usual max. 3 g per application; usual total max. 12 g daily; coverage should be less than 10% of body surface area

Xepin® (CHS) PoM
Cream, doxepin hydrochloride 5%, net price 30 g = £11.70. Label: 2, 10, patient information leaflet
Excipients: include benzyl alcohol

13.4 Topical corticosteroids

Topical corticosteroids are used for the treatment of inflammatory conditions of the skin (other than those arising from an infection) particularly eczema (section 13.5.1), contact dermatitis, insect stings (p. 47), and eczema of scabies (section 13.10.4). Corticosteroids suppress the inflammatory reaction during use; they are not curative and on discontinuation a rebound exacerbation of the condition may occur. They are generally used to relieve symptoms and suppress signs of the disorder when other measures such as emollients are ineffective.

Children, especially infants, are particularly susceptible to side-effects. However, concern about the safety of topical corticosteroids in children should not result in the child being undertreated. The aim is to control the condition as well as possible; inadequate treatment will perpetuate the condition. Carers of young children should be advised that treatment should **not** necessarily be reserved to 'treat only the worst areas' and they may need to be advised that patient information leaflets may contain inappropriate advice for the child's condition.

In an acute flare-up of atopic eczema, it may be appropriate to use more potent formulations of topical corticosteroids for a short period to regain control of the condition. Continuous daily application of a mild corticosteroid such as hydrocortisone 1% is equivalent to a potent corticosteroid such as betamethasone 0.1% applied intermittently.

Topical corticosteroids are of no value in the treatment of *urticaria*; they may worsen ulcerated or secondarily infected lesions. They should not be used indiscriminately in *pruritus* (where they will only benefit if inflammation is causing the itch) and are **not** recommended for *acne vulgaris*.

Systemic or potent topical corticosteroids should be avoided or given only under specialist supervision in *psoriasis* because, although they may suppress the psoriasis in the short term, relapse or vigorous rebound occurs on withdrawal (sometimes precipitating severe pustular psoriasis). Topical use of potent corticosteroids on widespread psoriasis can lead to systemic as well as to local side-effects. It is reasonable, however, to prescribe a mild to moderate topical corticosteroid for a short period (2–4 weeks) for *flexural* and *facial psoriasis*. In the case of scalp psoriasis it is reasonable to use a more potent corticosteroid such as betamethasone or fluocinonide (see below for cautions in psoriasis).

In general, the most potent topical corticosteroids should be reserved for recalcitrant dermatoses such as *chronic discoid lupus erythematosus*, *lichen simplex chronicus*, *hypertrophic lichen planus*, and *palmoplantar pustulosis*. Potent corticosteroids should generally be avoided on the face and skin flexures, but specialists occasionally prescribe them for these areas in certain circumstances.

When topical treatment has failed, intralesional corticosteroid injections (section 10.1.2.2) may be used. These are more effective than the very potent topical corticosteroid preparations and should be reserved for severe cases where there are localised lesions such as *keloid scars*, *hypertrophic lichen planus*, or *localised alopecia areata*.

Choice Water-miscible corticosteroid *creams* are suitable for moist or weeping lesions whereas *ointments* are generally chosen for dry, lichenified or scaly lesions or where a more occlusive effect is required. *Lotions* may be useful when minimal application to a large or hair-bearing area is required or for the treatment of exudative lesions. *Occlusive polythene or hydrocolloid dressings, disposable nappies, and tight-fitting plastic pants* increase absorption, but also increase the risk of side-effects; they are therefore used only under supervision on a short-term basis for areas of very thick skin (such as the palms and soles). The inclusion of urea or salicylic acid also increases the penetration of the corticosteroid.

'Wet-wrap bandaging' (section 13.5.1) increases absorption into the skin, but should be initiated only by a dermatologist and application supervised by a healthcare professional trained in the technique.

In the *BNF for Children* topical corticosteroids for the skin are categorised as 'mild', 'moderately potent', 'potent' or 'very potent' (see p. 623); the **least potent** preparation which is effective should be chosen but dilution should be avoided whenever possible.

For infants under 1 year, hydrocortisone is the only corticosteroid recommended for use; more potent corticosteroids are **contra-indicated**. For children over 1 year moderately potent and potent topical corticosteroids should be used with great care and for short periods (1–2 weeks) only. *Very potent* corticosteroids should be prescribed only on the advice of a dermatologist.

Appropriate topical corticosteroids for specific conditions are:

- *insect bites and stings*—mild corticosteroid such as hydrocortisone 1% cream;
- *severely inflamed nappy rash* in infant over 1 month (section 13.2.2)—mild corticosteroid such as hydrocortisone 0.5 or 1% for 5–7 days (combined with antimicrobial if infected);
- *mild to moderate eczema, flexural and facial eczema or psoriasis*—mild corticosteroid such as hydrocortisone 1%;
- *severe eczema on the trunk and limbs* in children over 1 year—moderately potent or potent corticosteroid for 1–2 weeks only, switching to a less potent preparation as the condition improves;
- *eczema affecting area with thickened skin* (e.g. soles of feet)—potent topical corticosteroid in combination with urea or salicylic acid (to increase penetration of corticosteroid).

Perioral lesions **Hydrocortisone** cream 1% can be used for up to 7 days to treat uninfected inflammatory lesions on the lips and on the skin surrounding the mouth. **Hydrocortisone and miconazole** cream or ointment is useful where infection by susceptible organisms and inflammation co-exist, particularly for initial treatment (up to 7 days) e.g. in angular cheilitis (see also p. 605). Organisms susceptible to miconazole include *Candida* spp. and many Gram-positive bacteria including streptococci and staphylococci.

Cautions Avoid prolonged use of a topical corticosteroid particularly on the face (and keep away from eyes). Use potent or very potent corticosteroids under specialist supervision; extreme caution is required in dermatoses of infancy including nappy rash—treatment should be limited to 5–7 days.

Psoriasis The use of potent or very potent corticosteroids in psoriasis can result in rebound relapse, development of generalised pustular psoriasis, and local and systemic toxicity, see notes above.

Contra-indications Topical corticosteroids are contra-indicated in untreated bacterial, fungal, or viral skin lesions, in acne, and in perioral dermatitis; potent corticosteroids are contra-indicated in widespread plaque psoriasis (see notes above).

Side-effects *Mild* and *moderately potent* topical corticosteroids are associated with few side-effects but particular care is required when treating neonates and infants, and in the use of *potent* and *very potent* corticosteroids. Absorption through the skin can rarely cause adrenal suppression and even Cushing's syndrome (section 6.3.2), depending on the area of the body being treated and the duration of treatment. Absorption of corticosteroid is greatest from severely inflamed skin, thin skin (especially on the face or genital area), from flexural sites (e.g. axillae groins), and in infants where skin surface area is higher in relation to body-weight; absorption is increased by occlusion.

Local side-effects include: spread and worsening of untreated infection; thinning of the skin which may be restored over a period after stopping treatment but the original structure may never return; irreversible striae atrophicae and telangiectasia; contact dermatitis; perioral dermatitis; acne, or worsening of acne or acne rosacea; mild depigmentation which may be reversible; hypertrichosis also reported.

Children and their carers should be reassured that side effects such as skin thinning and systemic effects rarely occur when topical corticosteroids are used appropriately.

> Safe Practice
> In order to minimise the side-effects of a topical corticosteroid, it is important to apply it **thinly** to affected areas **only**, no more frequently than **twice daily**, and to use the least potent formulation which is fully effective.

Application Topical corticosteroid preparations should be applied no more frequently than twice daily; once daily is often sufficient.

Topical corticosteroids are spread thinly on the skin; the length of cream or ointment expelled from a tube may be used to specify the quantity to be applied to a given area of skin. This length can be measured in terms of a *fingertip unit* (the distance from the tip of the adult index finger to the first crease). One fingertip unit (approximately 500 mg) is sufficient to cover an area that is twice that of the flat adult palm.

Mixing topical preparations on the skin should be avoided where possible; at least 30 minutes should elapse between application of different preparations. The practice of using an emollient immediately before a topical corticosteroid is inappropriate.

Compound preparations The advantages of including other substances (such as antibacterials or antifungals) with corticosteroids in topical preparations are uncertain, but such combinations may have a place where inflammatory skin conditions are associated with bacterial or fungal infection, such as infected eczema. In these cases the antimicrobial drug should be chosen according to the sensitivity of the infecting organism and used regularly for a short period (typically twice daily for 1 week). Longer use increases the likelihood of resistance and of sensitisation.

Topical corticosteroid potencies

Potency of a topical corticosteroid preparation depends upon the formulation as well as the corticosteroid. Therefore, proprietary names are shown below.

Mild

Hydrocortisone 0.1–2.5%, *Dioderm, Efcortelan, Mildison*

Mild with antimicrobials *Canesten HC, Daktacort, Econacort, Fucidin H, Nystaform-HC, Synalar 1 in 10 Dilution, Timodine, Vioform-Hydrocortisone*

Mild with crotamiton *Eurax-Hydrocortisone*

Moderate

Betnovate-RD, Eumovate, Haelan, Modrasone, Synalar 1 in 4 Dilution, Ultralanum Plain

Moderate with antimicrobials *Trimovate*

Moderate with urea *Alphaderm, Calmurid HC*

Potent

Betamethasone valerate 0.1%, *Betacap, Bettamousse, Betnovate, Cutivate, Diprosone, Elocon, Locoid, Locoid Crelo, Metosyn, Nerisone, Propaderm, Synalar*

Potent with antimicrobials *Aureocort, Betnovate-C, Betnovate-N, FuciBET, Locoid C, Lotriderm, Synalar C, Synalar N, Tri-Adcortyl*

Potent with salicylic acid *Diprosalic*

Very potent

Dermovate, Halciderm Topical, Nerisone Forte

Very potent with antimicrobials *Dermovate-NN*

HYDROCORTISONE

Cautions see notes above

Contra-indications see notes above

Side-effects see notes above

Indication and dose

Mild inflammatory skin disorders such as eczemas (but for over-the-counter preparations, see below)
Apply thinly 1–2 times daily

Nappy rash see notes above and section 13.2.2

Over-the-counter hydrocortisone preparations

Skin creams and ointments containing hydrocortisone (alone or with other ingredients) can be sold to the public for the treatment of allergic contact dermatitis, irritant dermatitis, insect bite reactions and mild to moderate eczema in children over 10 years, to be applied sparingly over the affected area 1–2 times daily for max. 1 week. Over-the-counter hydrocortisone preparations should not be sold without medical advice for children under 10 years or for pregnant women; they should **not** be sold for application to the face, anogenital region, broken or infected skin (including cold sores, acne, and athlete's foot).

Hydrocortisone (Non-proprietary) PoM

Cream, hydrocortisone 0.5%, net price, 15 g = 97p, 30 g = £1.52; 1%, 15 g = £1.41. Label: 28. Potency: mild

Dental prescribing on NHS Hydrocortisone Cream 1% 15 g may be prescribed

Ointment, hydrocortisone 0.5%, net price 15 g = £1.21, 30 g = £1.82; 1%, 15 g = £1.28. Label: 28. Potency: mild

When hydrocortisone cream or ointment is prescribed and no strength is stated, the 1% strength should be supplied

Proprietary hydrocortisone preparations

Dioderm® (Dermal) PoM

Cream, hydrocortisone 0.1%, net price 30 g = £2.50. Label: 28. Potency: mild

Excipients: include cetostearyl alcohol, propylene glycol

Note Although this contains only 0.1% hydrocortisone, the formulation is designed to provide a clinical activity comparable to that of Hydrocortisone Cream 1% BP

Efcortelan® (GSK) PoM

Cream, hydrocortisone 0.5%, net price, 30 g = 61p; 1%, 30 g = 75p. Label: 28. Potency: mild

Excipients: include cetostearyl alcohol, chlorocresol

Ointment, hydrocortisone 0.5%, net price, 30 g = 61p; 1%, 30 g = 75p; 2.5%, 30 g = £1.70. Label: 28. Potency: mild

Excipients: none as listed in section 13.1.3

Mildison® (Astellas) PoM

Lipocream, hydrocortisone 1%, net price 30 g = £2.45. Label: 28. Potency: mild

Excipients: include cetostearyl alcohol, hydroxybenzoates (parabens)

HYDROCORTISONE (*continued*)

Compound preparations

Compound preparations with coal tar see section 13.5.2

Alphaderm® (Alliance) PoM

Cream, hydrocortisone 1%, urea 10%, net price 30 g = £1.98; 100 g = £5.86. Label: 28. Potency: moderate

Excipients: none as listed in section 13.1.3

Calmurid HC® (Galderma) PoM

Cream, hydrocortisone 1%, urea 10%, lactic acid 5%, net price 30 g = £2.80, 50 g = £4.67. Label: 28. Potency: moderate

Excipients: none as listed in section 13.1.3

Note Manufacturer advises dilute to half-strength with aqueous cream for 1 week if stinging occurs then transfer to undiluted preparation (but see section 13.1.1 for advice to avoid dilution where possible)

[1]**Eurax-Hydrocortisone®** (Novartis Consumer Health) PoM

Cream, hydrocortisone 0.25%, crotamiton 10%, net price 30 g = 87p. Label: 28. Potency: mild

Excipients: include fragrance, hydroxybenzoates (parabens), propylene glycol, stearyl alcohol

1. A 15-g tube is on sale to the public for treatment of contact dermatitis and insect bites in children 10–18 years.

With antimicrobials

See notes above for comment on compound preparations

[1]**Canesten HC®** (Bayer Consumer Care) PoM

Cream, hydrocortisone 1%, clotrimazole 1%, net price 30 g = £2.15. Label: 28. Potency: mild

Excipients: include benzyl alcohol, cetostearyl alcohol

1. A 15-g tube is on sale to the public for the treatment of athlete's foot and fungal infection of skin folds with associated inflammation in children 10–18 years.

[1]**Daktacort®** (Janssen-Cilag) PoM

Cream, hydrocortisone 1%, miconazole nitrate 2%, net price 30 g = £2.13. Label: 28. Potency: mild

Excipients: include butylated hydroxyanisole, disodium edetate

Ointment, hydrocortisone 1%, miconazole nitrate 2%, net price 30 g = £2.14. Label: 28. Potency: mild

Excipients: none as listed in section 13.1.3

Dental prescribing on NHS May be prescribed as Hydrocortisone and Miconazole Cream or Ointment for max. 7 days

1. A 15-g tube is on sale to the public for the treatment of athlete's foot and candidal intertrigo in children 10–18 years

Econacort® (Squibb) PoM

Cream, hydrocortisone 1%, econazole nitrate 1%, net price 30 g = £2.25. Label: 28. Potency: mild

Excipients: include butylated hydroxyanisole

Fucidin H® (Leo) PoM

Cream, hydrocortisone acetate 1%, fusidic acid 2%, net price 30 g = £5.30, 60 g = £10.60. Label: 28. Potency: mild

Excipients: include butylated hydroxyanisole, cetyl alcohol, potassium sorbate

Ointment, hydrocortisone acetate 1%, sodium fusidate 2%, net price 30 g = £3.26, 60 g = £6.53. Label: 28. Potency: mild

Excipients: include cetyl alcohol, wool fat

Nystaform-HC® (Typharm) PoM

Cream, hydrocortisone 0.5%, nystatin 100 000 units/g, chlorhexidine hydrochloride 1%, net price 30 g = £2.66. Label: 28. Potency: mild

Excipients: include benzyl alcohol, cetostearyl alcohol, polysorbate '60'

Ointment, hydrocortisone 1%, nystatin 100 000 units/g, chlorhexidine acetate 1%, net price 30 g = £2.66. Label: 28. Potency: mild

Excipients: none as listed in section 13.1.3

Timodine® (R&C) PoM

Cream, hydrocortisone 0.5%, nystatin 100 000 units/g, benzalkonium chloride solution 0.2%, dimeticone '350' 10%, net price 30 g = £2.38. Label: 28. Potency: mild

Excipients: include butylated hydroxyanisole, cetostearyl alcohol, hydroxybenzoates (parabens), sodium metabisulphite, sorbic acid

Vioform-Hydrocortisone® (Novartis Consumer Health) PoM

Cream, hydrocortisone 1%, clioquinol 3%, net price 30 g = £1.46. Label: 28. Potency: mild

Excipients: include cetostearyl alcohol

Ointment, hydrocortisone 1%, clioquinol 3%, net price 30 g = £1.46. Label: 28. Potency: mild

Excipients: none as listed in section 13.1.3

Note Stains clothing

HYDROCORTISONE BUTYRATE

Cautions see under Hydrocortisone and notes above

Contra-indications see notes above

Side-effects see notes above

Indication and dose

Severe inflammatory skin disorders such as eczemas unresponsive to less potent corticosteroids, psoriasis see notes above

Child 1–18 years apply thinly 1–2 times daily

Locoid® (Astellas) PoM

Cream, hydrocortisone butyrate 0.1%, net price 30 g = £2.29, 100 g = £7.05. Label: 28. Potency: potent

Excipients: include cetostearyl alcohol, hydroxybenzoates (parabens)

Lipocream, hydrocortisone butyrate 0.1%, net price 30 g = £2.41, 100 g = £7.38. Label: 28. Potency: potent

Excipients: include cetostearyl alcohol, hydroxybenzoates (parabens)

Note For bland cream basis see *Lipobase®*, section 13.2.1

HYDROCORTISONE BUTYRATE (*continued*)

Ointment, hydrocortisone butyrate 0.1%, net price 30 g = £2.29, 100 g = £7.05. Label: 28. Potency: potent
Excipients: none as listed in section 13.1.3

Scalp lotion, hydrocortisone butyrate 0.1%, in an aqueous isopropyl alcohol basis, net price 100 mL = £9.76. Label: 15, 28. Potency: potent
Excipients: none as listed in section 13.1.3

Locoid Crelo® (Astellas) PoM
Lotion (topical emulsion), hydrocortisone butyrate 0.1% in a water-miscible basis, net price 100 g (with applicator nozzle) = £8.44. Label: 28. Potency: potent
Excipients: include butylated hydroxytoluene, cetostearyl alcohol, hydroxybenzoates (parabens), propylene glycol

With antimicrobials
See notes above for comment on compound preparations

Locoid C® (Astellas) PoM
Cream, hydrocortisone butyrate 0.1%, chlorquinaldol 3%, net price 30 g = £3.00. Label: 28. Potency: potent
Excipients: include cetostearyl alcohol
Note Stains clothing and can darken skin and hair

Ointment, ingredients as for cream, in a greasy basis, net price 30 g = £3.00. Label: 28. Potency: potent
Excipients: none as listed in section 13.1.3
Note Stains clothing and can darken skin and hair

ALCLOMETASONE DIPROPIONATE

Cautions see under Hydrocortisone and notes above

Contra-indications see notes above

Side-effects see notes above

Licensed use licensed for use in children (age range not specified by manufacturer)

Indication and dose

Inflammatory skin disorders such as eczemas
Apply thinly 1–2 times daily

Modrasone® (PLIVA) PoM
Cream, alclometasone dipropionate 0.05%, net price 50 g = £2.68. Label: 28. Potency: moderate
Excipients: include cetostearyl alcohol, chlorocresol, propylene glycol

Ointment, alclometasone dipropionate 0.05%, net price 50 g = £2.68. Label: 28. Potency: moderate
Excipients: include beeswax, propylene glycol

BECLOMETASONE DIPROPIONATE
(Beclomethasone dipropionate)

Cautions see under Hydrocortisone and notes above

Contra-indications see notes above

Side-effects see notes above

Licensed use not licensed for use in children under 1 year

Indication and dose

Severe inflammatory skin disorders such as eczemas unresponsive to less potent corticosteroids, psoriasis see notes above
Apply thinly 1–2 times daily

Propaderm® (GSK) PoM
Cream, beclometasone dipropionate 0.025%, net price 30 g = £1.77. Label: 28. Potency: potent
Excipients: include cetostearyl alcohol, chlorocresol

Ointment, beclometasone dipropionate 0.025%, net price 30 g = £1.77. Label: 28. Potency: potent
Excipients: include propylene glycol

BETAMETHASONE ESTERS

Cautions see under Hydrocortisone and notes above; use of more than 100 g per week of 0.1% preparation likely to cause adrenal suppression

Contra-indications see notes above

Side-effects see notes above

Licensed use *Bettamousse®* not licensed for use in children under 6 years, *Betnovate-N®* not licensed for use in children under 2 years, *Lotriderm®* not licensed for use in children under 12 years; *all other preparations* licensed for use in children (age range not specified by manufacturer)

Indication and dose

Severe inflammatory skin disorders such as eczemas unresponsive to less potent corticosteroids, psoriasis see notes above
Apply thinly 1–2 times daily

Betamethasone Valerate (Non-proprietary) PoM
Cream, betamethasone (as valerate) 0.1%, net price 30 g = £1.43. Label: 28. Potency: potent

Ointment, betamethasone (as valerate) 0.1%, net price 30 g = £1.68. Label: 28. Potency: potent

Betacap® (Dermal) PoM
Scalp application, betamethasone (as valerate) 0.1% in a water-miscible basis containing coconut oil derivative, net price 100 mL = £3.92. Label: 15, 28. Potency: potent
Excipients: none as listed in section 13.1.3

Betnovate® (GSK) PoM
Cream, betamethasone (as valerate) 0.1% in a water-miscible basis, net price 30 g = £1.43, 100 g = £4.05. Label: 28. Potency: potent
Excipients: include cetostearyl alcohol, chlorocresol

BETAMETHASONE ESTERS (*continued*)

Ointment, betamethasone (as valerate) 0.1% in an anhydrous paraffin basis, net price 30 g = £1.43, 100 g = £4.05. Label: 28. Potency: potent
Excipients: none as listed in section 13.1.3

Lotion, betamethasone (as valerate) 0.1%, net price 100 mL = £4.86. Label: 28. Potency: potent
Excipients: include cetostearyl alcohol, hydroxybenzoates (parabens)

Scalp application, betamethasone (as valerate) 0.1% in a water-miscible basis, net price 100 mL = £5.30. Label: 15, 28. Potency: potent
Excipients: none as listed in section 13.1.3

Betnovate-RD® (GSK) PoM

Cream, betamethasone (as valerate) 0.025% in a water-miscible basis (1 in 4 dilution of *Betnovate®* cream), net price 100 g = £3.34. Label: 28. Potency: moderate
Excipients: include cetostearyl alcohol, chlorocresol

Ointment, betamethasone (as valerate) 0.025% in an anhydrous paraffin basis (1 in 4 dilution of *Betnovate®* ointment), net price 100 g = £3.34. Label: 28. Potency: moderate
Excipients: none as listed in section 13.1.3

Bettamousse® (Celltech) PoM

Foam (= scalp application), betamethasone valerate 0.12% (≡ betamethasone 0.1%), net price 100 g = £9.75. Label: 28. Potency: potent
Excipients: include cetyl alcohol, polysorbate 60, propylene glycol, stearyl alcohol
Note Flammable

Diprosone® (Schering-Plough) PoM

Cream, betamethasone (as dipropionate) 0.05%, net price 30 g = £2.24, 100 g = £6.36. Label: 28. Potency: potent
Excipients: include cetostearyl alcohol, chlorocresol

Ointment, betamethasone (as dipropionate) 0.05%, net price 30 g = £2.24, 100 g = £6.36. Label: 28. Potency: potent
Excipients: none as listed in section 13.1.3

Lotion, betamethasone (as dipropionate) 0.05%, net price 30 mL = £2.83, 100 mL = £8.10. Label: 28. Potency: potent
Excipients: none as listed in section 13.1.3

With salicylic acid

See notes above for comment on compound preparations

Diprosalic® (Schering-Plough) PoM

Ointment, betamethasone (as dipropionate) 0.05%, salicylic acid 3%, net price 30 g = £3.30, 100 g = £9.50. Label: 28. Potency: potent
Excipients: none as listed in section 13.1.3

Dose

Apply thinly 1–2 times daily; max. 60 g per week

Scalp application, betamethasone (as dipropionate) 0.05%, salicylic acid 2%, in an alcoholic basis, net price 100 mL = £10.50. Label: 28. Potency: potent
Excipients: include disodium edetate

Dose

Apply a few drops 1–2 times daily

With antimicrobials

See notes above for comment on compound preparations

Betnovate-C® (GSK) PoM

Cream, betamethasone (as valerate) 0.1%, clioquinol 3%, net price 30 g = £1.76. Label: 28. Potency: potent
Excipients: include cetostearyl alcohol, chlorocresol
Note Stains clothing

Ointment, betamethasone (as valerate) 0.1%, clioquinol 3%, net price 30 g = £1.76. Label: 28. Potency: potent
Excipients: none as listed in section 13.1.3
Note Stains clothing

Betnovate-N® (GSK) PoM

Cream, betamethasone (as valerate) 0.1%, neomycin sulphate 0.5%, net price 30 g = £1.76, 100 g = £4.88. Label: 28. Potency: potent
Excipients: include cetostearyl alcohol, chlorocresol

Ointment, betamethasone (as valerate) 0.1%, neomycin sulphate 0.5%, net price 30 g = £1.76, 100 g = £4.88. Label: 28. Potency: potent
Excipients: none as listed in section 13.1.3

FuciBET® (Leo) PoM

Cream, betamethasone (as valerate) 0.1%, fusidic acid 2%, net price 30 g = £5.62, 60 g = £11.23. Label: 28. Potency: potent
Excipients: include cetostearyl alcohol, chlorocresol

Lotriderm® (PLIVA) PoM

Cream, betamethasone dipropionate 0.064% (≡ betamethasone 0.05%), clotrimazole 1%, net price 30 g = £6.34. Label: 28. Potency: potent
Excipients: include benzyl alcohol, cetostearyl alcohol, propylene glycol

CLOBETASOL PROPIONATE

Cautions see under Hydrocortisone and notes above

Contra-indications see notes above

Side-effects see notes above

Licensed use *Dermovate®* not licensed for use in children under 1 year, *Dermovate NN®* not licensed for use in children under 2 years

Indication and dose

Short-term treatment only of severe resistant inflammatory skin disorders such as recalcitrant eczemas unresponsive to less potent corticosteroids, psoriasis see notes above

Apply thinly 1–2 times daily for up to 4 weeks; max. 50 g of 0.05% preparation per week

13 Skin

CLOBETASOL PROPIONATE (*continued*)

Dermovate® (GSK) PoM
Cream, clobetasol propionate 0.05%, net price 30 g = £2.86, 100 g = £8.39. Label: 28. Potency: very potent
Excipients: include beeswax (or beeswax substitute), cetostearyl alcohol, chlorocresol, propylene glycol

Ointment, clobetasol propionate 0.05%, net price 30 g = £2.86, 100 g = £8.39. Label: 28. Potency: very potent
Excipients: include propylene glycol

Scalp application, clobetasol propionate 0.05%, in a thickened alcoholic basis, net price 30 mL = £3.26, 100 mL = £11.06. Label: 15, 28. Potency: very potent
Excipients: none as listed in section 13.1.3

With antimicrobials
See notes above for comment on compound preparations

Dermovate-NN® (GSK) PoM
Cream, clobetasol propionate 0.05%, neomycin sulphate 0.5%, nystatin 100 000 units/g, net price 30 g = £3.91. Label: 28. Potency: very potent
Excipients: include arachis (peanut) oil, beeswax substitute

CLOBETASONE BUTYRATE

Cautions see under Hydrocortisone and notes above

Contra-indications see notes above

Side-effects see notes above

Licensed use licensed for use in children (age range not specified by manufacturer)

Indication and dose

Eczemas and dermatitis of all types; maintenance between courses of more potent corticosteroids
Apply thinly 1–2 times daily

[1]**Eumovate®** (GSK) PoM
Cream, clobetasone butyrate 0.05%, net price 30 g = £1.97, 100 g = £5.77. Label: 28. Potency: moderate
Excipients: include beeswax substitute, cetostearyl alcohol, chlorocresol

Ointment, clobetasone butyrate 0.05%, net price 30 g = £1.97, 100 g = £5.77. Label: 28. Potency: moderate
Excipients: none as listed in section 13.1.3

1. Cream can be sold to the public for short-term symptomatic treatment and control of patches of eczema and dermatitis (but not seborrhoeic dermatitis) in children over 12 years provided pack does not contain more than 15 g

With antimicrobials
See notes above for comment on compound preparations

Trimovate® (GSK) PoM
Cream, clobetasone butyrate 0.05%, oxytetracycline 3% (as calcium salt), nystatin 100 000 units/g, net price 30 g = £3.49. Label: 28. Potency: moderate
Excipients: include cetostearyl alcohol, chlorocresol, sodium metabisulphite
Note Stains clothing

DIFLUCORTOLONE VALERATE

Cautions see under Hydrocortisone and notes above

Contra-indications see notes above

Side-effects see notes above

Licensed use *Nerisone®* licensed for use in children (age range not specified by manufacturer); *Nerisone Forte®* not licensed for use in children under 4 years

Indication and dose

Severe inflammatory skin disorders such as eczemas unresponsive to less potent corticosteroids; high strength (0.3%), short-term treatment of severe exacerbations, psoriasis see notes above
Apply thinly 1–2 times daily for up to 4 weeks (0.1% preparations) or 2 weeks (0.3% preparations), reducing strength as condition responds; max. 60 g of 0.3% per week

Nerisone® (Meadow) PoM
Cream, diflucortolone valerate 0.1%, net price 30 g = £1.59. Label: 28. Potency: potent
Excipients: include disodium edetate, hydroxybenzoates (parabens), stearyl alcohol

Oily cream, diflucortolone valerate 0.1%, net price 30 g = £2.56. Label: 28. Potency: potent
Excipients: include beeswax

Ointment, diflucortolone valerate 0.1%, net price 30 g = £1.59. Label: 28. Potency: potent
Excipients: none as listed in section 13.1.3

Nerisone Forte® (Meadow) PoM
Oily cream, diflucortolone valerate 0.3%, net price 15 g = £2.09. Label: 28. Potency: very potent
Excipients: include beeswax

Ointment, diflucortolone valerate 0.3%, net price 15 g = £2.09. Label: 28. Potency: very potent
Excipients: none as listed in section 13.1.3

FLUDROXYCORTIDE
(Flurandrenolone)

Cautions see under Hydrocortisone and notes above

Contra-indications see notes above

Side-effects see notes above

Licensed use licensed for use in children (age range not specified by manufacturer)

FLUDROXYCORTIDE (*continued*)

Indication and dose

Inflammatory skin disorders such as eczemas
Apply thinly 1–2 times daily

Haelan® (Typharm) PoM
Cream, fludroxycortide 0.0125%, net price 60 g = £3.26. Label: 28. Potency: moderate
Excipients: include cetyl alcohol, propylene glycol

Ointment, fludroxycortide 0.0125%, net price 60 g = £3.26. Label: 28. Potency: moderate
Excipients: include beeswax, cetyl alcohol, polysorbate

Tape, polythene adhesive film impregnated with fludroxycortide 4 micrograms / cm^2, net price 7.5 cm × 50 cm = £9.27, 7.5 cm × 200 cm = £24.95

Dose

Chronic localised recalcitrant dermatoses (but not acute or weeping)
Cut tape to fit lesion, apply to clean, dry skin shorn of hair, usually for 12 hours daily

FLUOCINOLONE ACETONIDE

Cautions see under Hydrocortisone and notes above

Contra-indications see notes above

Side-effects see notes above

Licensed use not licensed for use in children under 1 year

Indication and dose

Severe inflammatory skin disorders such as eczemas, psoriasis see notes above
Apply thinly 1–2 times daily, reducing strength as condition responds

Synalar® (GP Pharma) PoM
Cream, fluocinolone acetonide 0.025%, net price 30 g = £2.26, 100 g = £6.42. Label: 28. Potency: potent
Excipients: include benzyl alcohol, cetostearyl alcohol, polysorbates, propylene glycol

Gel, fluocinolone acetonide 0.025%, net price 30 g = £3.34. For use on scalp and other hairy areas. Label: 28. Potency: potent
Excipients: include hydroxybenzoates (parabens), propylene glycol

Ointment, fluocinolone acetonide 0.025%, net price 30 g = £2.26, 100 g = £6.42. Label: 28. Potency: potent
Excipients: include propylene glycol, wool fat

Synalar 1 in 4 Dilution® (GP Pharma) PoM
Cream, fluocinolone acetonide 0.00625%, net price 50 g = £2.64. Label: 28. Potency: moderate
Excipients: include benzyl alcohol, cetostearyl alcohol, polysorbates, propylene glycol

Ointment, fluocinolone acetonide 0.00625%, net price 50 g = £2.64. Label: 28. Potency: moderate
Excipients: include propylene glycol, wool fat

Synalar 1 in 10 Dilution® (GP Pharma) PoM
Cream, fluocinolone acetonide 0.0025%, net price 50 g = £2.50. Label: 28. Potency: mild
Excipients: include benzyl alcohol, cetostearyl alcohol, polysorbates, propylene glycol

With antibacterials

See notes above for comment on compound preparations

Synalar C® (GP Pharma) PoM
Cream, fluocinolone acetonide 0.025%, clioquinol 3%, net price 15 g = £1.46. Label: 28. Potency: potent
Excipients: include cetostearyl alcohol, disodium edetate, hydroxybenzoates (parabens), polysorbates, propylene glycol

Ointment, ingredients as for cream, net price 15 g = £1.46. Label: 28. Potency: potent.
Note stains clothing
Excipients: include propylene glycol, wool fat

Synalar N® (GP Pharma) PoM
Cream, fluocinolone acetonide 0.025%, neomycin sulphate 0.5%, net price 30 g = £2.38. Label: 28. Potency: potent
Excipients: include cetostearyl alcohol, hydroxybenzoates (parabens), polysorbates, propylene glycol

Ointment, ingredients as for cream, in a greasy basis, net price 30 g = £2.38. Label: 28. Potency: potent
Excipients: include propylene glycol, wool fat

FLUOCINONIDE

Cautions see under Hydrocortisone and notes above

Contra-indications see notes above

Side-effects see notes above

Licensed use not licensed for use in children under 1 year

Indication and dose

Severe inflammatory skin disorders such as eczemas unresponsive to less potent corticosteroids, psoriasis see notes above
Apply thinly 1–2 times daily

Metosyn® (GP Pharma) PoM
FAPG cream, fluocinonide 0.05%, net price 25 g = £1.98, 100 g = £6.68. Label: 28. Potency: potent
Excipients: include propylene glycol

Ointment, fluocinonide 0.05%, net price 25 g = £1.76, 100 g = £6.59. Label: 28. Potency: potent
Excipients: include propylene glycol, wool fat

FLUOCORTOLONE

Cautions see under Hydrocortisone and notes above

Contra-indications see notes above

Side-effects see notes above

Licensed use licensed for use in children (age range not specified by manufacturer)

Indication and dose

Severe inflammatory skin disorders such as eczemas unresponsive to less potent corticosteroids, psoriasis see notes above
Apply thinly 1–2 times daily

Ultralanum Plain® (Meadow) PoM
Cream, fluocortolone caproate 0.25%, fluocortolone pivalate 0.25%, net price 50 g = £2.95. Label: 28. Potency: moderate
Excipients: include disodium edetate, fragrance, hydroxybenzoates (parabens), stearyl alcohol

Ointment, fluocortolone 0.25%, fluocortolone caproate 0.25%, net price 50 g = £2.95. Label: 28. Potency: moderate
Excipients: include wool fat, fragrance

FLUTICASONE PROPIONATE

Cautions see under Hydrocortisone and notes above

Contra-indications see notes above

Side-effects see notes above

Licensed use not licensed for use in children under 1 year

Indication and dose

Inflammatory skin disorders such as dermatitis and eczemas unresponsive to less potent corticosteroids, psoriasis see notes above
Apply thinly 1–2 times daily

Cutivate® (GSK) PoM
Cream, fluticasone propionate 0.05%, net price 15 g = £2.41, 50 g = £7.11. Label: 28. Potency: potent
Excipients: include cetostearyl alcohol, imidurea, propylene glycol

Ointment, fluticasone propionate 0.005%, net price 15 g = £2.41, 50 g = £7.11. Label: 28. Potency: potent
Excipients: include propylene glycol

HALCINONIDE

Cautions see under Hydrocortisone and notes above

Contra-indications see notes above

Side-effects see notes above

Licensed use licensed for use in children (age range not specified by manufacturer)

Indication and dose

Short-term treatment only of severe resistant inflammatory skin disorders such as recalcitrant eczemas unresponsive to less potent corticosteroids, psoriasis see notes above
Apply thinly 1–2 times daily

Halciderm Topical® (Squibb) PoM
Cream, halcinonide 0.1%, net price 30 g = £3.16. Label: 28. Potency: very potent
Excipients: include propylene glycol

MOMETASONE FUROATE

Cautions see under Hydrocortisone and notes above

Contra-indications see notes above

Side-effects see notes above

Licensed use licensed for use in children (age range not specified by manufacturer)

Indication and dose

Severe inflammatory skin disorders such as eczemas unresponsive to less potent corticosteroids, psoriasis see notes above
Apply thinly once daily (to scalp in case of lotion)

Elocon® (Schering-Plough) PoM
Cream, mometasone furoate 0.1%, net price 30 g = £4.54, 100 g = £13.07. Label: 28. Potency: potent
Excipients: include stearyl alcohol

Ointment, mometasone furoate 0.1%, net price 30 g = £4.54, 100 g = £13.07. Label: 28. Potency: potent
Excipients: none as listed in section 13.1.3

Scalp lotion, mometasone furoate 0.1% in an aqueous isopropyl alcohol basis, net price 30 mL = £4.54. Label: 28. Potency: potent
Excipients: include propylene glycol

TRIAMCINOLONE ACETONIDE

Cautions see under Hydrocortisone and notes above

Contra-indications see notes above

Side-effects see notes above

Licensed use *Aureocort*® not licensed for use in children under 8 years; *Tri-Adcortyl*® not licensed for use in children under 1 year

Indication and dose

Severe inflammatory skin disorders such as eczemas unresponsive to less potent corticosteroids, psoriasis see notes above
Apply thinly 1–2 times daily

With antimicrobials

See notes above for comment on compound preparations

Aureocort® (Lederle) PoM
Ointment, triamcinolone acetonide 0.1%, chlortetracycline hydrochloride 3%, in an anhydrous greasy basis containing wool fat and white soft paraffin, net price 15 g = £2.70. Label: 28. Potency: potent
Excipients: include wool fat
Note Stains clothing

Tri-Adcortyl® (Squibb) PoM
Cream, triamcinolone acetonide 0.1%, gramicidin 0.025%, neomycin (as sulphate) 0.25%, nystatin 100 000 units/g, net price 30 g = £3.15. Label: 28. Potency: potent
Excipients: include benzyl alcohol, ethylenediamine, propylene glycol, fragrance

Ointment, triamcinolone acetonide 0.1%, gramicidin 0.025%, neomycin (as sulphate) 0.25%, nystatin 100 000 units/g, net price 30 g = £3.15. Label: 28. Potency: potent
Excipients: none as listed in section 13.1.3
Note Not recommended owing to presence of ethylenediamine in the cream and also because combination of antibacterial with antifungal not considered useful in either the cream or ointment

13.5 Preparations for eczema and psoriasis

13.5.1 Preparations for eczema

The main types of eczema (dermatitis) in children are atopic, irritant and allergic contact; different types may co-exist. *Atopic eczema* is the most common type and it usually involves dry skin as well as infection and lichenification caused by scratching and rubbing. *Seborrhoeic dermatitis* (see below) is also common in children.

Management of eczema involves the removal or treatment of contributory factors; known or suspected irritants and contact allergens should be avoided. Rarely, ingredients in topical medicinal products may sensitise the skin (section 13.1.3); active ingredients together with excipients that have been associated with skin sensitisation are included with details for individual skin preparations.

Skin dryness and the consequent irritant eczema requires **emollients** (section 13.2.1). applied regularly and liberally to the affected area; this may be supplemented with bath or shower emollients. The use of emollients should continue even if the eczema improves or if other treatment is being used.

Topical corticosteroids (section 13.4) are also required in the management of eczema; the potency of the corticosteroid should be appropriate to the severity and site of the condition. Mild corticosteroids are generally used on the face and on flexures; the more potent corticosteroids are generally required for use on lichenified areas of eczema or for severe eczema on the scalp, limbs, and trunk. Treatment should be reviewed regularly, especially if a potent corticosteroid is required.

Bandages (including those containing **zinc** and **ichthammol**) are sometimes applied over topical corticosteroids to treat eczema of the limbs. Wet elasticated viscose stockinette is used for 'wet-wrap' bandaging over topical corticosteroids to cool the skin and relieve itching but there is an increased risk of infection and excessive absorption of the corticosteroid; 'wet-wrap' bandaging should be used under specialist supervision.

Infection Bacterial infection (commonly with *Staphylococcus aureus* and occasionally with *Streptococcus pyogenes*) can exacerbate eczema. A topical antibacterial such as fusidic acid (section 13.10.1) may be used for small areas of mild infection; treatment should be limited to a short course (typically 1 week) to reduce the risk of drug resistance or skin sensitisation. Associated eczema is treated simultaneously with a moderately potent or potent topical corticosteroid which can be combined with an antimicrobial such as clioquinol.

Eczema involving moderate to severe, widespread, or recurrent infection requires the use of a systemic antibacterial (section 5.1, table 1) that is active against the infecting organism. Preparations that combine an antiseptic with an emollient application (section 13.2.1) and with a bath emollient (section 13.2.1.1) may also be used; antiseptic shampoos (section 13.9) may be used on the scalp.

Intertriginous eczema commonly involves candida and bacteria; it is best treated with a mild or moderately potent topical corticosteroid combined with a suitable antimicrobial drug. For the treatment of nappy rash, see section 13.2.2.

Widespread *herpes simplex infection* may complicate atopic eczema (eczema herpeticum) and treatment under specialist supervision with a systemic antiviral drug (section 5.3.2.1) is indicated. Secondary bacterial infection often exacerbates eczema herpeticum.

The management of *seborrhoeic dermatitis* is described below.

Management of other features of eczema *Lichenification,* which results from repeated scratching is treated initially with a potent corticosteroid. Bandages containing **ichthammol** (to reduce pruritus) and other substances such as **zinc oxide** may be applied over the corticosteroid. **Coal tar** (section 13.5.2) and ichthammol can be useful in some cases of *chronic eczema. Discoid eczema,* with thickened plaques in chronic atopic eczema, is usually treated with a topical antiseptic preparation, a potent topical corticosteroid, and paste bandages containing zinc oxide and ichthammol.

A systemic **antihistamine** (section 3.4.1) may be of some value in relieving the *itch* of atopic eczema, usually because of their sedating effect. A sedating antihistamine used at night may help the child fall asleep but a large dose may be needed and drowsiness may persist on the following day.

Exudative ('*weeping*') *eczema* requires a potent corticosteroid initially; infection may also be present and require specific treatment (see above). **Potassium permanganate** solution (1 in 10 000) can be used as a soak in exudating eczema for its antiseptic and astringent effect; treatment should be stopped when exudation stops.

Severe refractory eczema is best managed under specialist supervision; it may require phototherapy, systemic corticosteroids (section 6.3.2), or other drugs acting on the immune system (e.g. tacrolimus and pimecrolimus, section 13.5.3).

Seborrhoeic dermatitis *Seborrhoeic dermatitis* (*seborrhoeic eczema*) is associated with species of the yeast *Malassezia* and affects the scalp, paranasal areas, and eyebrows.

Shampoos active against the yeast (including those containing ketoconazole and coal tar, section 13.9) and combinations of mild corticosteroids with suitable antimicrobials (section 13.4) are used to treat seborrhoeic dermatitis.

Infantile seborrhoeic dermatitis affects particularly the body folds, nappy area and scalp. It is treated with emollients and mild corticosteroids with suitable antimicrobials. Infantile seborrhoeic dermatitis affecting the scalp (*cradle cap*) is treated by hydrating the scalp using natural oils and the use of mild shampoo (section 13.9).

ICHTHAMMOL

Side-effects skin irritation

Licensed use no information available

Indication and dose

Chronic lichenified eczema
Apply 1–3 times daily

Ichthammol Ointment, BP 1980
Ointment, ichthammol 10%, yellow soft paraffin 45%, wool fat 45%, net price 25 g = 53p

Zinc and Ichthammol Cream, BP
Cream, ichthammol 5%, cetostearyl alcohol 3%, wool fat 10%, in zinc cream, net price 100 g = 79p

ICHTHAMMOL (*continued*)

Zinc Paste and Ichthammol Bandage, BP 1993
Cotton fabric, plain weave, impregnated with suitable paste containing zinc oxide and ichthammol; requires additional bandaging. Net price 6 m × 7.5 cm = £3.24 (SSL—*Icthaband®* (15/2%), *excipients: include* hydroxybenzoates; S&N Hlth—*Ichthopaste®* (6/2%)
Excipients: none as listed in section 13.1.3

Medicated bandages

Zinc paste bandages are also used with **coal tar** or **ichthammol** in chronic lichenified skin conditions such as chronic eczema (ichthammol often being preferred since its action is considered to be milder). They are also used with **calamine** in milder eczematous skin conditions (but the inclusion of **clioquinol** may lead to irritation in susceptible children).

Zinc Paste Bandage, BP 1993
Cotton fabric, plain weave, impregnated with suitable paste containing zinc oxide; requires additional bandaging. Net price 6 m × 7.5 cm = £3.28 (SSL—*Steripaste®* (15%), *excipients: include* polysorbate 80); £3.23 (SSL—*Zincaband®* (15%), *excipients: include* hydroxybenzoates); £3.37 (S&N Hlth—*Viscopaste PB7®* (10%) *excipients: include* hydroxybenzoates)

Zinc Paste and Calamine Bandage
(Drug Tariff specification 5). Cotton fabric, plain weave, impregnated with suitable paste containing calamine and zinc oxide; requires additional bandaging. Net price 6 m × 7.5 cm = £3.33 (SSL—*Calaband®*)

Zinc Paste, Calamine, and Clioquinol Bandage, BP 1993
Cotton fabric, plain weave, impregnated with suitable paste containing calamine, clioquinol, and zinc oxide; requires additional bandaging. Net price 6 m × 7.5 cm = £3.33 (SSL—*Quinaband®* *excipients: include* hydroxybenzoates)

13.5.2 Preparations for psoriasis

Psoriasis is characterised by epidermal thickening and scaling. It commonly affects extensor surfaces and the scalp. For mild psoriasis, reassurance and treatment with an emollient may be all that is necessary. *Guttate psoriasis* is a distinctive form of psoriasis that characteristically occurs in children and young adults, often following a streptococcal throat infection or tonsillitis.

Occasionally psoriasis is provoked or exacerbated by drugs such as lithium, chloroquine and hydroxychloroquine, beta-blockers, non-steroidal anti-inflammatory drugs, and ACE inhibitors. Psoriasis may not occur until the drug has been taken for weeks or months.

Emollients (section 13.2.1), in addition to their effects on dryness, scaling and cracking, may have an antiproliferative effect in psoriasis. They are particularly useful in *inflammatory psoriasis* and in *chronic stable plaque psoriasis.*

For *chronic stable plaque psoriasis* on extensor surfaces of trunk and limbs preparations containing **coal tar** are moderately effective, but the smell is unacceptable to some children. **Vitamin D** and its analogues are effective and cosmetically acceptable alternatives to preparations containing coal tar or dithranol. **Dithranol** is the most effective topical antipsoriatic agent but it irritates and stains the skin and it should be used only under specialist supervision. Adverse effects of dithranol are minimised by using a 'short-contact technique' (see below) and by starting with low concentration preparations. **Tazarotene**, a topical retinoid for the treatment of mild to moderate plaque psoriasis, is not recommended for use in children under 18 years. These medications can irritate the skin particularly in the flexures and they are not suitable for the more inflammatory forms of psoriasis; their use should be suspended during an inflammatory phase of psoriasis. The efficacy and the irritancy of each substance varies between patients. If a substance irritates significantly, it should be stopped or the concentration reduced; if it is tolerated, its effects should be assessed after 4 to 6 weeks and treatment continued if it is effective.

Widespread *unstable psoriasis* of erythrodermic or generalised pustular type requires urgent specialist assessment. Initial topical treatment should be limited to using emollients frequently and generously. More localised acute or subacute *inflammatory psoriasis* with hot, spreading or itchy lesions, should be treated topically with emollients or with a corticosteroid of moderate potency.

Scalp psoriasis is usually scaly, and the scale may be thick and adherent. This requires softening with an emollient ointment, cream, or oil and usually combined with **salicylic acid** as a keratolytic.

Some preparations for psoriasis affecting the scalp combine salicylic acid with coal tar or **sulphur**. The preparation should be applied generously and left on for at least an hour, often more conveniently overnight, before washing it off. If a corticosteroid lotion or gel is required (e.g. for itch), it can be used in the morning.

Calcipotriol and **tacalcitol** are analogues of vitamin D that affect cell division and differentiation. **Calcitriol** is an active form of vitamin D. Vitamin D and its analogues do not smell or stain and they may be more acceptable than tar or dithranol products. Of the vitamin D analogues, tacalcitol and calcitriol are less likely to irritate.

Coal tar has anti-inflammatory properties that are useful in chronic plaque psoriasis; it also has antiscaling properties. Contact of coal tar products with normal skin is not normally harmful and preparations containing coal tar can be used for widespread small lesions; however, irritation, contact allergy, and sterile folliculitis can occur. Preparations containing up to 6% coal tar may be used on children 1 month to 2 years; preparations containing coal tar 10% may be used on children over 2 years with more severe psoriasis. For shampoo preparations containing coal tar, see section 13.9.

Dithranol is effective for chronic plaque psoriasis. Its major disadvantages are irritation (for which individual susceptibility varies) and staining of skin and of clothing. It should be applied to chronic extensor plaques only, carefully avoiding normal skin. Dithranol is not generally suitable for widespread small lesions nor should it be used in the flexures or on the face. Treatment should be started with a low concentration such as dithranol 0.1%, and the strength increased gradually every few days up to 3%, according to tolerance. Proprietary preparations are more suitable for home use; they are usually washed off after 20–30 minutes ('short contact' technique). Specialist nurses may apply intensive treatment with dithranol paste which is covered by stockinette dressings and usually retained overnight. Dithranol should be discontinued if even a low concentration causes acute inflammation; continued use can result in the psoriasis becoming unstable. When applying dithranol, hands should be protected by gloves or they should be washed thoroughly afterwards.

A topical **corticosteroid** (section 13.4) is not generally suitable as the sole treatment of extensive chronic plaque psoriasis; any early improvement is not usually maintained and there is a risk of the condition deteriorating or of precipitating an unstable form of psoriasis (e.g. erythrodermic psoriasis or generalised pustular psoriasis). However, it may be appropriate to treat psoriasis in specific sites such as the face and flexures usually with a mild corticosteroid, and psoriasis of the scalp, palms and soles with a potent corticosteroid.

Combining the use of a corticosteroid with another specific topical treatment may be beneficial in chronic plaque psoriasis; the drugs may be used separately at different times of the day or used together in a single formulation. *Eczema* co-existing with psoriasis may be treated with a corticosteroid, or coal tar, or both. Systemic or potent topical corticosteroids should be avoided or used only under specialist supervision; although corticosteroids may suppress psoriasis in the short term, relapse or vigorous rebound occurs on withdrawal.

Phototherapy **Phototherapy** is available in specialist centres under the supervision of a dermatologist. **Ultraviolet B** (UVB) radiation is usually effective for *chronic stable psoriasis* and for *guttate psoriasis*. It may be considered for children with moderately severe psoriasis in whom topical treatment has failed, but it may irritate inflammatory psoriasis. The use of phototherapy and photochemotherapy in children is limited by concerns over carcinogenicity and premature ageing.

Photochemotherapy combining long-wave ultraviolet A radiation with a psoralen (PUVA) is available in specialist centres under the supervision of a dermatologist. The psoralen, which enhances the effect of irradiation, is administered either by mouth or topically. PUVA is effective in most forms of psoriasis, including the *localised palmoplantar pustular psoriasis*. Early adverse effects include phototoxicity and pruritus. Higher cumulative doses exaggerate skin ageing, increase the risk of dysplastic and neoplastic skin lesions especially squamous cancer, and pose a theoretical risk of cataracts.

Phototherapy combined with coal tar, dithranol, vitamin D or vitamin D analogues allows reduction of the cumulative dose of phototherapy required to treat psoriasis.

Systemic treatment Systemic treatment is required for severe, resistant, unstable or complicated forms of psoriasis, and it should be initiated only under specialist supervision. Systemic drugs for psoriasis include acitretin and drugs that act on the immune system (section 13.5.3).

Acitretin, a metabolite of etretinate, is a retinoid (vitamin A derivative); it is prescribed by specialists. The main indication of acitretin is severe psoriasis resistant to other forms of therapy. It is also used in disorders of keratinisation such as severe *Darier's disease* (keratosis follicularis), and some forms of *ichthyosis.* Although a minority of cases of psoriasis respond well to acitretin alone, it is only moderately effective in many cases; toxicity and relapse when treatment is stopped are limiting factors. A therapeutic effect occurs after 2 to 4 weeks and the maximum benefit after 4 to 6 weeks or longer; in children with severe ichthyosis, long-term treatment may be necessary. Topical preparations containing keratolytics should normally be stopped before administration of acitretin. Liberal use of emollients should be encouraged and topical corticosteroids may be continued if necessary.

Apart from teratogenicity, acitretin is the least toxic systemic treatment for psoriasis; in women with a potential for child-bearing, the possibility of pregnancy must be excluded before treatment and pregnancy must be avoided during treatment and for a period of 2 years afterwards. Common side effects derive from its widespread but reversible effects on epithelia, such as dry and cracking lips, dry skin and mucosal surfaces, hair thinning, paronychia, and soft and sticky palms and soles. Liver function and blood-lipid concentration should be monitored before starting treatment, after 1 month, and then 3-monthly during treatment.

Topical preparations for psoriasis

Vitamin D and analogues

Calcipotriol, **calcitriol**, and **tacalcitol** are used for the management of *plaque psoriasis.* They should be avoided by those with calcium metabolism disorders, and used with caution in *generalised pustular* or *erythrodermic exfoliative psoriasis* (enhanced risk of hypercalcaemia). Local skin reactions (itching, erythema, burning, paraesthesia, dermatitis) are common. Hands should be washed thoroughly after application to avoid inadvertent transfer to other body areas. Aggravation of psoriasis has also been reported.

CALCIPOTRIOL

Cautions see notes above; avoid use on face; if used with UV treatment apply at least 2 hours before UV exposure

Pregnancy manufacturer advises avoid if possible

Breast-feeding no information available

Contra-indications see notes above

Side-effects see notes above; also photosensitivity; rarely facial or perioral dermatitis, skin atrophy

Licensed use *Dovonex® Scalp Solution* and *Dovobet®* not licensed for use in children

Indication and dose

Plaque psoriasis

Child 6–18 years apply cream or ointment twice daily; 6–12 years max. 50 g weekly (less with scalp solution, see below); over 12 years max. 75 g weekly

Note Patient information leaflets for *Dovonex®* cream and ointment advise liberal application (but note max. recommended weekly dose, above)

Dovonex® (Leo) PoM

Cream, calcipotriol 50 micrograms/g, net price 60 g = £13.04, 120 g = £26.07

Excipients: include cetostearyl alcohol, disodium edetate

Ointment, calcipotriol 50 micrograms/g, net price 60 g = £12.02, 120 g = £26.07

Excipients: include disodium edetate, propylene glycol

Scalp solution, calcipotriol 50 micrograms/mL, net price 60 mL = £13.04, 120 mL = £26.07

Excipients: include propylene glycol

Dose

Scalp psoriasis (specialist use only)

apply to scalp twice daily; max. 60 mL weekly (less when used with cream or ointment, see below)

Note When preparations used together max. total calcipotriol 5 mg in any one week (e.g. scalp solution 60 mL with cream or ointment 30 g *or* cream or ointment 60 g with scalp solution 30 mL)

With betamethasone

For cautions, contra-indications, side-effects, and for comment on the limited role of corticosteroids in psoriasis, see section 13.4.

Dovobet® (Leo) PoM

Ointment, betamethasone 0.05% (as dipropionate), calcipotriol 50 micrograms/g, net price 60 g = £35.00. Label: 28

Excipients: none as listed in section 13.1.3

Dose

Initial treatment of stable plaque psoriasis (specialist use only)

apply once daily to max. 30% of body surface for up to 4 weeks; max. 15 g daily, max. 100 g weekly

CALCITRIOL

Cautions see notes above

Hepatic impairment avoid in severe liver disease

Renal impairment avoid in severe renal impairment

Pregnancy avoid; use in restricted amounts if clearly necessary (significant systemic absorption); monitor urine and plasma-calcium concentration

Breast-feeding manufacturer advises avoid

Contra-indications see notes above; do not apply under occlusion

Side-effects see notes above

Indication and dose

Mild to moderate plaque psoriasis

Child 12–18 years apply twice daily; not more than 35% of body surface to be treated daily, max. 30 g daily

Silkis® (Galderma) ▼ PoM

Ointment, calcitriol 3 micrograms/g, net price 30 g = £5.76, 100 g = £16.34

Excipients: none as listed in section 13.1.3

TACALCITOL

Cautions see notes above; avoid eyes; monitor plasma-calcium concentration if risk of hypercalcaemia or in renal impairment; if used in conjunction with UV treatment, UV radiation should be given in the morning and tacalcitol applied at bedtime

Pregnancy avoid if possible

Breast-feeding no information on presence in milk; avoid application to breast area

Contra-indications see notes above

Side-effects see notes above

Indication and dose

Plaque psoriasis

Child 12–18 years apply daily preferably at bedtime; max. 10 g daily

Curatoderm® (Crookes) PoM

Ointment, tacalcitol (as monohydrate) 4 micrograms/g, net price 30 g = £15.09, 60 g = £26.06, 100 g = £34.75

Excipients: none as listed in section 13.1.3

Tars

TARS

Cautions avoid eyes, mucosa, genital or rectal areas, and broken or inflamed skin; use suitable chemical protection gloves for extemporaneous preparation

Pregnancy no adverse effects reported

Breast-feeding no adverse effects reported

Contra-indications not for use in sore, acute, or pustular psoriasis or in presence of infection

Side-effects skin irritation and acne-like eruptions, photosensitivity; stains skin, hair, and fabric

Indication and dose

Psoriasis and occasionally chronic atopic eczema

Apply 1–3 times daily starting with low-strength preparations; proprietary preparations, see individual entries below

Note For shampoo preparations see section 13.9

Non-proprietary preparations

May be difficult to obtain—some patients may find newer proprietary preparations more acceptable

Coal Tar Paste, BP

Paste, strong coal tar solution 7.5%, in compound zinc paste

Zinc and Coal Tar Paste, BP

Paste, zinc oxide 6%, coal tar 6%, emulsifying wax 5%, starch 38%, yellow soft paraffin 45%

Excipients: include cetostearyl alcohol

Proprietary preparations

Carbo-Dome® (Sandoz)

Cream, coal tar solution 10%, in a water-miscible basis, net price 30 g = £4.77, 100 g = £16.38

Excipients: include beeswax, hydroxybenzoates (parabens)

Dose

Psoriasis

apply to skin 2–3 times daily

Clinitar® (CHS)

Cream, coal tar extract 1%, net price 100 g = £10.99

Excipients: include cetostearyl alcohol, isopropyl palmitate, propylene glycol

Dose

Psoriasis and eczema

apply to skin 1–2 times daily

Cocois® (Celltech)

Scalp ointment, coal tar solution 12%, salicylic acid 2%, precipitated sulphur 4%, in a coconut oil emollient basis, net price 40 g (with applicator nozzle) = £6.65, 100 g = £12.30

Excipients: include cetostearyl alcohol

Dose

Scaly scalp disorders including psoriasis, eczema, seborrhoeic dermatitis and dandruff

Child 6–18 years apply to scalp once weekly as necessary (if severe use daily for first 3–7 days), shampoo off after 1 hour

TARS (*continued*)

Exorex® (Forest)
Lotion, prepared coal tar 1% in an emollient basis, net price 100 mL = £8.11, 250 mL = £16.24
Excipients: include hydroxybenzoates (parabens), polysorbate 80

Dose

Psoriasis
apply to skin or scalp 2–3 times daily; product may be diluted with a few drops of water before applying

Psoriderm® (Dermal)
Cream, coal tar 6%, lecithin 0.4%, net price 225 mL = £9.85
Excipients: include isopropyl palmitate, propylene glycol

Dose

Psoriasis
apply to skin or scalp 1–2 times daily

Scalp lotion—section 13.9

Sebco® (Centrapharm)
Scalp ointment, coal tar solution 12%, salicylic acid 2%, precipitated sulphur 4%, in a coconut oil emollient basis, net price 40 g = £4.54, 100 g = £8.52
Excipients: include cetostearyl alcohol

Dose

Scaly scalp disorders including psoriasis, eczema, seborrhoeic dermatitis and dandruff
Child 6–12 years medical supervision required
Child 12–18 years apply to scalp as necessary (if severe use daily for first 3–7 days), shampoo off after 1 hour

Bath preparations

Coal Tar Solution, BP
Solution, coal tar 20%, polysorbate '80' 5%, in alcohol (96%), net price 100 mL = 95p
Excipients: include polysorbates

Dose

Use 100 mL in an adult-size bath, and proportionally less for a child's bath

Note Strong Coal Tar Solution BP contains coal tar 40%

Pinetarsol® (Crawford)
Bath oil, tar 2.3% in a light liquid paraffin basis, net price 200 mL = £4.75, 500 mL = £7.95
Excipients: include fragrance

Dose

Eczema and psoriasis use 15–30 mL in adult-size bath *or* apply directly to wet skin and rinse after a few minutes; can be used as a soap substitute

Gel, tar 1.6%, net price 100 g = £4.95

Dose

Eczema and psoriasis apply directly to wet skin and rinse after a few minutes; can be used as a soap substitute

Solution, tar 2.3%, net price 200 mL = £4.45, 500 mL = £7.45

Dose

Eczema and psoriasis use 15–30 mL in adult-size bath *or* dilute 15 mL with 3 litres of water and apply to affected areas *or* apply solution directly to wet skin and rinse after a few minutes; can be used as a soap substitute

Polytar Emollient® (Stiefel)
Bath additive, coal tar solution 2.5%, arachis (peanut) oil extract of coal tar 7.5%, tar 7.5%, cade oil 7.5%, liquid paraffin 35%, net price 500 mL = £5.78
Excipients: include isopropyl palmitate

Dose

Psoriasis, eczema, atopic and pruritic dermatoses
use 2–4 capfuls (15–30 mL) in adult-size bath and proportionally less for a child's bath; soak for 20 minutes

Psoriderm® (Dermal)
Bath emulsion, coal tar 40%, net price 200 mL = £2.87
Excipients: include polysorbate 20

Dose

Psoriasis
use 30 mL in adult-size bath, and proportionally less for a child's bath; soak for 5 minutes

With corticosteroids

Alphosyl HC® (GSK Consumer Healthcare) PoM
Cream, coal tar extract 5%, hydrocortisone 0.5%, allantoin 2%, net price 100 g = £3.54. Label: 28. Potency: mild
Excipients: include beeswax, cetyl alcohol, hydroxybenzoates (parabens), isopropyl palmitate, wool fat

Dose

Psoriasis
Child 5–18 years apply thinly 1–2 times daily

Dithranol

DITHRANOL
(Anthralin)

Cautions avoid use near eyes and sensitive areas of skin; see also notes above

Pregnancy no adverse effects reported

Breast-feeding no adverse effects reported

Contra-indications hypersensitivity; acute and pustular psoriasis

Side-effects local burning sensation and irritation; stains skin, hair, and fabrics

Licensed use *Dithrocream®*, licensed for use in children (age range not specified by manufacturer); *Micanol®*, licensed for use in children, but not recommended for infants or young children (age range not specified by manufacturer); *Psorin®*, age range not specified by manufacturer

DITHRANOL (*continued*)

Indication and dose

Subacute and chronic psoriasis

see notes above and under preparations

Note Some of these dithranol preparations also contain coal tar or salicylic acid—for cautions and side-effects see under Coal Tar (above) or under Salicylic Acid

Non-proprietary preparations

[1]**Dithranol Ointment, BP** PoM

Ointment, dithranol, in yellow soft paraffin; usual strengths 0.1–2%. Part of basis may be replaced by hard paraffin if a stiffer preparation is required. Label: 28

1. PoM if dithranol content more than 1%, otherwise may be sold to the public

Dithranol Paste, BP

Paste, dithranol in zinc and salicylic acid (Lassar's) paste. Usual strengths 0.1–1% of dithranol. Label: 28

Proprietary preparations

Dithrocream® (Dermal)

Cream, dithranol 0.1%, net price 50 g = £3.94; 0.25%, 50 g = £4.23; 0.5%, 50 g = £4.87; 1%, 50 g = £5.67; PoM 2%, 50 g = £7.10. Label: 28

Excipients: include cetostearyl alcohol, chlorocresol

Dose

For application to skin or scalp; 0.1–0.5% suitable for overnight treatment, 1–2% for max. 1 hour

Micanol® (GP Pharma)

Cream, dithranol 1% in a lipid-stabilised basis, net price 50 g = £10.37; PoM 3%, 50 g = £12.92. Label: 28

Excipients: none as listed in section 13.1.3

Dose

1% Cream for application to skin, for up to 30 minutes, if necessary 3% cream may be used under medical supervision; apply to scalp for up to 30 minutes

Note At the end of contact time use plenty of lukewarm (not hot) water to rinse off cream; soap may be used *after* the cream has been rinsed off

Psorin® (LPC)

Ointment, dithranol 0.11%, coal tar 1%, salicylic acid 1.6%, net price 50 g = £8.20, 100 g = £16.35. Label: 28

Excipients: include beeswax, wool fat

Dose

For application to skin up to twice daily

Scalp gel, dithranol 0.25%, salicylic acid 1.6% in gel basis containing methyl salicylate, net price 50 g = £6.25. Label: 28

Excipients: none as listed in section 13.1.3

Dose

For application to scalp, initially apply on alternate days for 10–20 minutes; may be increased to daily application for max. 1 hour and then wash off

Salicylic acid

SALICYLIC ACID

For coal tar preparations containing salicylic acid, see under Coal Tar p. 635; for dithranol preparations containing salicylic acid see under Dithranol, above

Cautions see notes above; avoid broken or inflamed skin

Salicylate toxicity Salicylate toxicity may occur particularly if applied on large areas of skin or on neonatal skin

Side-effects sensitivity, excessive drying, irritation, systemic effects after widespread use (see under Cautions)

Indication and dose

Hyperkeratotic skin disorders see under preparation

Acne section 13.6.1

Warts and calluses section 13.7

Scalp conditions section 13.9

Fungal nail infections section 13.10.2

Zinc and Salicylic Acid Paste, BP

Paste, (Lassar's Paste), zinc oxide 24%, salicylic acid 2%, starch 24%, white soft paraffin 50%, net price 25 g = 17p

Dose

Child 1 month–18 years apply twice daily

Oral retinoids for psoriasis

ACITRETIN

Note Acitretin is a metabolite of etretinate

Cautions in children use only in exceptional circumstances (premature epiphyseal closure reported); exclude pregnancy before starting (test for pregnancy within 2 weeks before treatment and monthly thereafter; start treatment on day 2 or 3 of menstrual cycle)—women (including those with history of infertility) should avoid pregnancy for at least 1 month before, during, and for at least 2 years after treatment; patients should avoid concomitant tetracycline or methotrexate, high doses of vitamin A (more than

ACITRETIN (*continued*)

4000–5000 units daily) and use of keratolytics, and should not donate blood during or for at least 1 year after stopping therapy (teratogenic risk); check liver function at start, after 1 month, then every 3 months; monitor plasma lipids; diabetes (can alter glucose tolerance—initial frequent blood glucose checks); radiographic assessment on long-term treatment; investigate atypical musculoskeletal symptoms; avoid excessive exposure to sunlight and unsupervised use of sunlamps; **interactions:** Appendix 1 (retinoids)

Contra-indications hyperlipidaemia

Hepatic impairment avoid—further impairment may occur

Renal impairment avoid even in mild impairment—increased risk of toxicity

Pregnancy teratogenic; effective contraception must be used (see Cautions above)

Breast-feeding avoid

Side-effects dryness of mucous membranes (sometimes erosion), of skin (sometimes scaling, thinning, erythema especially of face, and pruritus), and of conjunctiva (sometimes conjunctivitis and decreased tolerance of contact lenses); sticky skin, dermatitis; other side-effects reported include palmoplantar exfoliation, epistaxis, epidermal and nail fragility, oedema, paronychia, granulomatous lesions, bullous eruptions, reversible hair thinning and alopecia, myalgia and arthralgia, occasional nausea, headache, malaise, drowsiness, rhinitis, sweating, taste disturbance, and gingivitis; benign intracranial hypertension (discontinue if severe headache, vomiting, diarrhoea, abdominal pain, and visual disturbance occur; **avoid** concomitant tetracyclines); photosensitivity, corneal ulceration, raised liver enzymes, rarely jaundice and hepatitis (**avoid** concomitant methotrexate); raised triglycerides; decreased night vision reported; skeletal hyperostosis and extraosseous calcification reported following long-term administration of etretinate (and premature epiphyseal closure in children, see Cautions)

Indication and dose

Harlequin ichthyosis (under expert supervision only)

- **By mouth**

Neonate 500 micrograms/kg once daily with food or milk (occasionally up to 1 mg/kg daily) with careful monitoring of musculoskeletal development

Severe extensive psoriasis resistant to other forms of therapy, palmoplantar pustular psoriasis, severe congenital ichthyosis, severe Darier's disease (keratosis follicularis) (all under expert supervision **only**)

- **By mouth**

Child 1 month–12 years 500 micrograms/kg once daily with food or milk (occasionally up to 1 mg/kg daily) to max. 35 mg daily with careful monitoring of musculoskeletal development (max. continuous treatment duration 6 months)

Child 12–18 years initially 25–30 mg daily (Darier's disease 10 mg daily) for 2–4 weeks, then adjusted according to response, usual range 25–50 mg daily (max. 75 mg daily) for further 6–8 weeks (in Darier's disease and ichthyosis not more than 50 mg daily for up to 6 months)

Neotigason® (Roche) PoM

Capsules, acitretin 10 mg (brown/white), net price 60-cap pack = £25.25; 25 mg (brown/yellow), 60-cap pack = £58.59. Label: 10, patient information leaflet, 21

Extemporaneous formulations available see Extemporaneous Preparations, p. 8

13.5.3 Drugs affecting the immune response

Drugs affecting the immune response are used for eczema or psoriasis.

Systemic treatment Systemic drugs acting on the immune system are generally used by **specialists** in a hospital setting.

Ciclosporin (cyclosporin) by mouth can be used for *severe psoriasis* and for *severe eczema*. **Azathioprine** (section 8.2.1) or **mycophenolate mofetil** (section 8.2.1) are also used for severe refractory eczema in children.

Methotrexate may be used for *severe resistant psoriasis*, the dose is given **once weekly**, and adjusted according to severity of the condition and haematological and biochemical measurements. Folic acid may be given to reduce the possibility of methotrexate toxicity.

For *severe psoriasis* refractory to at least two systemic treatments and photochemotherapy or if other treatments are not tolerated, **efalizumab**, which inhibits T-cell activation and is licensed in adults for moderate and severe *chronic plaque psoriasis*, or the cytokine inhibitors **etanercept** and **infliximab** (section 10.1.3; not licensed for use in children) may be used; etanercept and infliximab are also licensed for *psoriatic arthritis* in adults.

13 Skin

Topical preparations **Pimecrolimus** by topical application is licensed for *mild to moderate atopic eczema* for short-term use to treat signs and symptoms and for intermittent use to prevent flares. **Tacrolimus** is licensed for topical use in *moderate to severe atopic eczema.* Both are drugs whose long-term safety and place in therapy is still being evaluated and they should not usually be considered first-line treatment unless there is a specific reason to avoid or reduce the use of topical corticosteroids.

For the role of topical corticosteroids in eczema see section 13.5.1 and for comment on their limited role in psoriasis see section 13.4. Systemic corticosteroids (section 6.3.2) may be used in *severe* refractory eczema.

NICE guidance (tacrolimus and pimecrolimus for atopic eczema)
NICE has recommended (August 2004) that topical pimecrolimus and tacrolimus are options for atopic eczema not controlled by maximal topical corticosteroid treatment or if there is a risk of important corticosteroid side-effects (particularly skin atrophy).

Topical pimecrolimus is recommended for moderate atopic eczema on the face and neck of children aged 2–16 years and topical tacrolimus is recommended for moderate to severe atopic eczema in children over 2 years. Pimecrolimus and tacrolimus should be used within their licensed indications.

CICLOSPORIN
(Cyclosporin)

Cautions see section 8.2.2

Additional cautions in atopic dermatitis and psoriasis *Contra-indicated* in abnormal renal function, hypertension not under control (see also below), infections not under control, and malignancy (see also below). Dermatological and physical examination, including blood pressure and renal function measurements required at least twice before starting; discontinue if hypertension develops that cannot be controlled by dose reduction or antihypertensive therapy; avoid excessive exposure to sunlight and use of UVB or PUVA; *in atopic dermatitis,* also allow herpes simplex infections to clear before starting (if they occur during treatment withdraw if severe); *Staphylococcus aureus* skin infections not absolute contra-indication providing controlled (but avoid erythromycin unless no other alternative—see also **interactions**: Appendix 1 (ciclosporin)); monitor serum creatinine every 2 weeks during treatment; *in psoriasis,* also exclude malignancies (including those of skin and cervix) before starting (biopsy any lesions not typical of psoriasis) and treat patients with malignant or pre-malignant conditions of skin only after appropriate treatment (and if no other option); monitor serum creatinine every 2 weeks for first 3 months then every 2 months (monthly if dose more than 2.5 mg/kg daily), reducing dose by 25–50% if increases more than 30% above baseline (even if within normal range) and discontinuing if reduction not successful within 1 month; also discontinue if lymphoproliferative disorder develops

Side-effects see section 8.2.2

Licensed use licensed for use in children 16–18 years for atopic eczema (dermatitis)

Indication and dose

Short-term treatment (usually max. 8 weeks but may be used for longer by specialists) of severe atopic dermatitis where conventional therapy ineffective or inappropriate

- **By mouth, administered in accordance with expert advice**

  Child 1 month–18 years initially 1.25 mg/kg twice daily, if good initial response not achieved within 2 weeks, increase rapidly to max. 2.5 mg/kg twice daily; initial dose of 2.5 mg/kg twice daily if very severe

Severe psoriasis where conventional therapy ineffective or inappropriate

- **By mouth, administered in accordance with expert advice**

  Child 1 month–18 years initially 1.25 mg/kg twice daily, increased gradually to max. 2.5 mg/kg twice daily if no improvement within 1 month (discontinue if response still insufficient after 6 weeks); initial dose of 2.5 mg/kg twice daily justified if condition requires rapid improvement

  Important For preparations and counselling and for advice on conversion between the preparations, see section 8.2.2

Transplantation and graft-versus-host disease section 8.2.2

Preparations
Section 8.2.2

METHOTREXATE

Cautions see section 8.1.3, also photosensitivity—psoriasis lesions aggravated by UV radiation (skin ulceration reported)

Contra-indications see section 8.1.3

Side-effects see section 8.1.3

Licensed use not licensed for use in children with psoriasis

METHOTREXATE (continued)

Indication and dose

Severe uncontrolled psoriasis unresponsive to conventional therapy (specialist use only)
- **By mouth**

  Child 2–18 years initially 200 micrograms/kg (max. 10 mg) once **weekly** increased according to response to 400 micrograms/kg (max. 25 mg) once **weekly**

Important Note that the above dose is a **weekly** dose. The CSM has received reports of prescription and dispensing errors including fatalities. Attention should be paid to the **strength** of methotrexate tablets prescribed and the **frequency** of dosing.

Malignant disease section 8.1.3

Rheumatoid arthritis section 10.1.3

Preparations
Section 10.1.3

PIMECROLIMUS

Cautions UV light (avoid excessive exposure to sunlight and sunlamps), avoid other topical treatments except emollients at treatment site; alcohol consumption (risk of facial flushing and skin irritation)

Contra-indications contact with eyes and mucous membranes, application under occlusion, infection at treatment site; congenital epidermal barrier defects; generalised erythroderma

Side-effects burning sensation, pruritus, erythema, skin infections (including folliculitis and *less commonly* impetigo, herpes simplex and zoster, molluscum contagiosum); *rarely* papilloma, local reactions including pain, paraesthesia, peeling, dryness, oedema, and worsening of eczema; skin malignancy reported

Indication and dose

Acute treatment of mild to moderate atopic eczema (including flares) see NICE guidance above

Child 2–18 years apply twice daily until symptoms resolve

Elidel® (Novartis) ▼ PoM

Cream, pimecrolimus 1%, net price 30 g = £19.69, 60 g = £37.41, 100 g = £59.07. Label: 4, 28

Excipients: include benzyl alcohol, cetyl alcohol, propylene glycol, stearyl alcohol

TACROLIMUS

Cautions infection at treatment site, UV light (avoid excessive exposure to sunlight and sunlamps); alcohol consumption (risk of facial flushing and skin irritation)

Contra-indications avoid contact with eyes and mucous membranes, application under occlusion; congenital epidermal barrier defects; generalised erythroderma

Pregnancy avoid; manufacturer advises toxicity in *animal* studies following systemic administration

Breast-feeding avoid—present in milk following systemic administration

Side-effects application-site reactions including rash, irritation, pain and paraesthesia; herpes simplex infection, Kaposi's varicelliform eruption; *less commonly* acne; acne rosacea also reported; skin malignancy reported

Indication and dose

Moderate to severe atopic eczema unresponsive to conventional therapy (prescribed by physicians experienced in treating atopic eczema)

Child 2–16 years initially apply 0.03% ointment thinly twice daily for up to 3 weeks then reduce to once daily until lesion clears

Child 16–18 years initially apply 0.1% ointment thinly twice daily until lesion clears (consider other treatment options if no improvement after 2 weeks); reduce to once daily or switch to 0.03% ointment if clinical condition allows

Other indications section 8.2.2

Protopic (Astellas) ▼ PoM

Ointment, tacrolimus (as monohydrate) 0.03%, net price 30 g = £19.44, 60 g = £36.94; 0.1%, 30 g = £21.60, 60 g = £41.04. Label: 4, 11, 28

Excipients: include beeswax

13.6 Acne and rosacea

Acne vulgaris Acne vulgaris commonly affects children around puberty and occasionally affects infants. Treatment of acne should be commenced early to prevent scarring; lesions may worsen before improving. The choice of treatment depends on age, severity, and whether the acne is predominantly inflammatory or comedonal.

13 Skin

Mild to moderate acne is generally treated with topical preparations (section 13.6.1). **Benzoyl peroxide** is suitable for mild acne with superficial inflammation; a topical **retinoid** is used when acne is predominantly comedonal. Topical antibacterials are probably no more effective than benzoyl peroxide and may promote the emergence of resistant organisms.

For *moderate to severe inflammatory acne* or where topical preparations are not tolerated or are ineffective or where application to the site is difficult, systemic treatment (section 13.6.2) with oral antibacterials may be effective. **Co-cyprindiol** (cyproterone acetate with ethinylestradiol) has anti-androgenic properties and may be useful in young women with acne refractory to other treatments.

Severe acne, acne unresponsive to prolonged courses of oral antibacterials, acne with scarring, or acne associated with psychological problems calls for early referral to a consultant dermatologist who may prescribe oral **isotretinoin** (section 13.6.2).

Neonatal and infantile acne Inflammatory papules, pustules, and occasionally comedones may develop at birth or within the first month; most neonates with acne do not require treatment. Acne developing at 3–6 months of age may be more severe and persistent; lesions are usually confined to the face. Topical preparations containing **benzoyl peroxide** (at the lowest strength possible to avoid irritation), **azelaic acid**, **adapalene**, or **tretinoin** may be used if treatment for infantile acne is necessary. In infants with inflammatory acne, oral **erythromycin** (section 5.1.5) is used because topical antibacterials are not well tolerated. Tetracyclines are **contra-indicated** in children under 12 years.

Rosacea The adult form of rosacea rarely occurs in children. Persistent or repeated use of potent topical corticosteroids may cause periorificial rosacea (steroid acne). The pustules and papules of rosacea may be treated for at least 6 weeks with a topical **metronidazole** preparation (section 13.10.1.2) or a systemic antibacterial such as **erythromycin** (section 5.1.5) and **oxytetracycline** (section 5.1.3) for a child over 12 years.

13.6.1 Topical preparations for acne

Topical preparations are effective in mild to moderate acne, but may cause irritation. Significant comedonal acne responds well to topical retinoids, whereas both comedones and inflamed lesions respond well to benzoyl peroxide, azelaic acid, or the retinoid-like drug adapalene. Alternatively, topical application of an antibacterial such as erythromycin or clindamycin may be effective for inflammatory acne. If topical preparations prove inadequate oral preparations may be needed (section 13.6.2). The choice of product and formulation (gel, solution, lotion, or cream) is largely determined by skin type, patient preference, and previous usage of acne products.

Benzoyl peroxide and azelaic acid

Benzoyl peroxide is effective in mild to moderate acne. Both comedones and inflamed lesions respond well to benzoyl peroxide. The lower concentrations seem to be as effective as higher concentrations in reducing inflammation. It is usual to start with a lower strength and to increase the concentration of benzoyl peroxide gradually. Adverse effects include local skin irritation, particularly when therapy is initiated, but the scaling and redness often subside with a reduction in benzoyl peroxide concentration, frequency, and area of application. If the acne does not respond after 2 months then use of a topical antibacterial should be considered.

Azelaic acid has antimicrobial and anticomedonal properties. It may be used as an alternative to benzoyl peroxide or to a topical retinoid for treating mild to moderate comedonal acne, particularly of the face; it is less likely to cause local irritation than benzoyl peroxide.

BENZOYL PEROXIDE

Cautions avoid contact with eyes, mouth, and mucous membranes; may bleach fabrics and hair; avoid excessive exposure to sunlight

Side-effects skin irritation (reduce frequency or suspend use until irritation subsides and re-introduce at reduced frequency)

Licensed use *Quinoderm*® is licensed for use in children; *all other preparations*, not licensed for use in treatment of infantile acne

Indication and dose

Acne vulgaris

Child 12–18 years apply 1–2 times daily preferably after washing with soap and water, start treatment with lower-strength preparations
Note May bleach clothing

Infantile acne

Neonate apply 1–2 times daily; start treatment with lower-strength preparations

Child 1 month–2 years apply 1–2 times daily; start treatment with lower-strength preparations

Brevoxyl® (Stiefel)
Cream, benzoyl peroxide 4% in an aqueous basis, net price 40 g = £3.30
Excipients: include cetyl alcohol, fragrance, stearyl alcohol

PanOxyl® (Stiefel)
Aquagel (= aqueous gel), benzoyl peroxide 2.5%, net price 40 g = £1.76; 5%, 40 g = £1.92; 10%, 40 g = £2.07
Excipients: include propylene glycol

Cream, benzoyl peroxide 5% in a non-greasy basis, net price 40 g = £1.51
Excipients: include isopropyl palmitate, propylene glycol

Gel, benzoyl peroxide 5% in an aqueous alcoholic basis, net price 40 g = £1.51; 10%, 40 g = £1.69
Excipients: include fragrance

Wash, benzoyl peroxide 10% in a detergent basis, net price 150 mL = £4.00
Excipients: include imidurea

With antimicrobials

Benzamycin® (Schwarz) PoM
Gel, pack for reconstitution, providing erythromycin 3% and benzoyl peroxide 5% in an alcoholic basis, net price per pack to provide 46.6 g = £15.62
Excipients: none as listed in section 13.1.3

Dose

Acne vulgaris

apply twice daily (very fair skin, initially once daily at night)

Duac® **Once Daily** (Stiefel) PoM
Gel, benzoyl peroxide 5%, clindamycin 1% (as phosphate) in an aqueous basis, net price 25 g = £9.95, 50 g = £19.90
Excipients: include disodium edetate

Dose

Acne vulgaris

apply once daily in the evening

Quinoderm® (Ferndale)
Cream, benzoyl peroxide 5%, potassium hydroxyquinoline sulphate 0.5%, in an astringent vanishing-cream basis, net price 50 g = £2.21
Excipients: include cetostearyl alcohol, edetic acid (EDTA)

Cream, benzoyl peroxide 10%, potassium hydroxyquinoline sulphate 0.5%, in an astringent vanishing-cream basis, net price 25 g = £1.30, 50 g = £2.49
Excipients: include cetostearyl alcohol, edetic acid (EDTA)

Dose

Infantile acne, acne vulgaris, acneform eruptions, impetigo, folliculitis

apply 2–3 times daily

AZELAIC ACID

Cautions avoid contact with eyes

Pregnancy no evidence of risk in *animal studies*—manufacturer advises avoid

Breast-feeding negligible amount in milk—manufacturer advises avoid

Side-effects local irritation (reduce frequency or discontinue use temporarily); rarely photosensitisation

Licensed use not licensed for use in infantile acne

Indication and dose

See under preparation

Skinoren® (Schering Health) PoM
Cream, azelaic acid 20%, net price 30 g = £3.74
Excipients: include propylene glycol

Dose

Acne vulgaris, infantile acne

apply twice daily (sensitive skin, once daily for first week). Extended treatment may be required but manufacturer advises period of treatment should not exceed 6 months

Topical antibacterials for acne

In the treatment of mild to moderate inflammatory acne, topical antibacterials may be no more effective than topical benzoyl peroxide or tretinoin. Topical antibacterials are probably best reserved for children who wish to avoid oral antibacterials or who cannot tolerate them.

Topical preparations of **erythromycin** and **clindamycin** may be used to treat *inflamed lesions* in mild to moderate acne when topical benzoyl peroxide or tretinoin is ineffective or poorly tolerated. Topical preparations of **tetracycline** may be effective. Topical benzoyl peroxide, azelaic acid, or retinoids used in combination with an antibacterial (topical or systemic) may be more effective than an antibacterial used alone. Topical antibacterials can produce mild irritation of the skin, and on rare occasions cause sensitisation.

Antibacterial resistance of *Propionibacterium acnes* is increasing; there is cross-resistance between erythromycin and clindamycin. To avoid development of resistance:

- when possible use non-antibiotic antimicrobials (such as benzoyl peroxide or azelaic acid);
- avoid concomitant treatment with different oral and topical antibacterials;
- if a particular antibacterial is effective, use it for repeat courses if needed (short intervening courses of benzoyl peroxide or azelaic acid may eliminate any resistant propionibacteria);
- do not continue treatment for longer than necessary (but treatment with a topical preparation should be continued for at least 6 months)

ANTIBACTERIALS

Cautions some manufacturers advise preparations containing alcohol are not suitable for use with benzoyl peroxide

Indication and dose

Acne vulgaris for dose, see under preparations

Benzamycin® (PoM)
See under Benzoyl Peroxide above

Dalacin T® (Pharmacia) (PoM)
Topical solution, clindamycin 1% (as phosphate), in an aqueous alcoholic basis, net price (both with applicator) 30 mL = £4.34, 50 mL = £7.23
Excipients: include propylene glycol

Dose

Apply twice daily

Lotion, clindamycin 1% (as phosphate) in an aqueous basis, net price 30 mL = £5.08, 50 mL = £8.47
Excipients: include cetostearyl alcohol, hydroxybenzoates (parabens)

Dose

Apply twice daily

Stiemycin® (Stiefel) (PoM)
Solution, erythromycin 2% in an alcoholic basis, net price 50 mL = £8.00
Excipients: include propylene glycol

Dose

Apply twice daily

Topicycline® (Shire) (PoM)
Solution, powder for reconstitution, tetracycline hydrochloride, 4-epitetracycline hydrochloride, providing tetracycline hydrochloride 2.2 mg/mL when reconstituted with solvent containing *n*-decyl methyl sulphoxide and citric acid in 40% alcohol. Net price per pack of powder and solvent to provide 70 mL = £6.15
Excipients: none as listed in section 13.1.3

Dose

Apply twice daily

Zindaclin® (Crawford) (PoM)
Gel, clindamycin 1% (as phosphate), net price 30 g = £8.66
Excipients: include propylene glycol

Dose

Child 12–18 years apply once daily

Zineryt® (Astellas) (PoM)
Topical solution, powder for reconstitution, erythromycin 40 mg, zinc acetate 12 mg/mL when reconstituted with solvent containing ethanol, net price per pack of powder and solvent to provide 30 mL = £7.71, 90 mL = £22.24
Excipients: none as listed in section 13.1.3

Dose

Child 13–18 years apply twice daily

Topical retinoids and related preparations for acne

Topical preparations of **tretinoin** and its isomer **isotretinoin** are useful in treating comedonal acne; some redness and skin peeling might occur initially but settles with time. Several months of treatment may be needed to achieve an optimal response and the treatment should be continued until no new lesions develop.

Topical **isotretinoin** is used to treat non-inflammatory and inflammatory lesions in patients with mild to moderate acne vulgaris. **Tretinoin** is used under specialist supervision to treat infantile acne, see Neonatal and Infantile Acne, p. 641.

Adapalene, a retinoid-like drug, is used for mild to moderate acne vulgaris and may also be used to treat infantile acne. It is less irritant than topical retinoids.

Cautions Topical retinoids should be avoided in severe acne involving large areas. Contact with eyes, nostrils, mouth and mucous membranes, eczematous, broken or sunburned skin should be avoided. Topical retinoids should be used with caution on sensitive areas such as the neck, and accumulation in angles of the nose should be avoided. Exposure to UV light (including sunlight, solariums) should be avoided; if sun exposure is unavoidable, an appropriate sunscreen (section 13.8.1) or protective clothing should be used. Use of retinoids with abrasive cleaners, comedogenic or astringent cosmetics should be avoided. Allow peeling (e.g. resulting from use of benzoyl peroxide) to subside before using a topical retinoid; alternating a preparation that causes peeling with a topical retinoid may give rise to contact dermatitis (reduce frequency of retinoid application).

Contra-indications Tretinoin is contra-indicated in children with personal or familial history of cutaneous epithelioma. Topical retinoids are contra-indicated in **pregnancy**; females of child-bearing age should take adequate contraceptive precautions.

Side-effects Local reactions include burning, erythema, stinging, pruritus, dry or peeling skin (discontinue if severe). Increased sensitivity to UVB light or sunlight occurs. Temporary changes of skin pigmentation have been reported. Eye irritation and oedema, and blistering or crusting of skin have been reported rarely.

ADAPALENE

Cautions see notes above

Contra-indications see notes above

Side-effects see notes above

Licensed use not licensed for use in infantile acne

Indication and dose

Infantile acne

Neonate apply thinly once daily at night

Child 1 month–2 years apply thinly once daily at night

Mild to moderate acne vulgaris

Apply thinly once daily before retiring

Differin® (Galderma) PoM

Cream, adapalene 0.1%, net price 45 g = £11.40

Excipients: include disodium edetate, hydroxybenzoates (parabens)

Gel, adapalene 0.1%, net price 45 g = £11.40

Excipients: include disodium edetate, hydroxybenzoates (parabens), propylene glycol

TRETINOIN

Note Tretinoin is the acid form of vitamin A

Cautions see notes above

Contra-indications see notes above

Side-effects see notes above

Licensed use *Retin-A®* not licensed for use in infantile acne

Indication and dose

See under preparations below

Malignant disease (section 8.1.5)

Retin-A® (Janssen-Cilag) PoM

Cream, tretinoin 0.025%, net price 60 g = £5.73

Excipients: include butylated hydroxytoluene, sorbic acid, stearyl alcohol

Dose

Acne vulgaris, particularly for dry or fair skin

apply thinly 1–2 times daily

Infantile acne

apply thinly 1–2 times daily

Gel, tretinoin 0.01%, net price 60 g = £5.73; 0.025%, 60 g = £5.73

Excipients: include butylated hydroxytoluene

Dose

Acne vulgaris, particularly that associated with oily skin

apply thinly 1–2 times daily

Lotion, tretinoin 0.025%, net price 100 mL = £6.59

Excipients: include butylated hydroxytoluene

Dose

Acne vulgaris and other keratotic conditions, particularly for very oily skin

apply thinly 1–2 times daily

With antibacterial

Aknemycin Plus® (Crookes) PoM

Solution, tretinoin 0.025%, erythromycin 4% in an alcoholic basis, net price 25 mL = £7.94

Dose

Acne (all forms), particularly that associated with oily skin

apply thinly 1–2 times daily

Excipients: none as listed in section 13.1.3

ISOTRETINOIN

Note Isotretinoin is an isomer of tretinoin

Important For **indications, cautions, contra-indications** and **side-effects** of isotretinoin **when given by mouth**, see p. 647

Cautions (*topical application* **only**) see notes above

Contra-indications (*topical application* **only**) see notes above

Indication and dose

Acne vulgaris
apply thinly 1–2 times daily

Isotrex® (Stiefel) PoM
Gel, isotretinoin 0.05%, net price 30 g = £6.18
Excipients: include butylated hydroxytoluene

With antibacterial

Isotrexin® (Stiefel) PoM
Gel, isotretinoin 0.05%, erythromycin 2% in ethanolic basis, net price 30 g = £7.78
Excipients: include butylated hydroxytoluene

Other topical preparations for acne

Salicylic acid is available in various preparations for sale direct to the public for the treatment of mild acne. Other products are more suitable for acne; salicylic acid is used mainly for its keratolytic effect.

Preparations containing **sulphur** and **abrasive agents** are not considered beneficial in acne.

Topical **corticosteroids** should **not** be used in acne.

A topical preparation of **nicotinamide** is available for inflammatory acne.

NICOTINAMIDE

Cautions avoid contact with eyes and mucous membranes (including nose and mouth); reduce frequency of application if excessive dryness, irritation or peeling

Side-effects dryness of skin; also pruritus, erythema, burning and irritation

Licensed use licensed for use in children (age range not specified by manufacturer)

Indication and dose

Inflammatory acne vulgaris see under preparations below

Nicam® (Dermal)
Gel, nicotinamide 4%, net price 60 g = £7.42
Excipients: none as listed in section 13.1.3

Dose

Apply twice daily; reduce to once daily or on alternate days if irritation occurs

SALICYLIC ACID

Cautions risk of significant systemic absorption in neonates; avoid contact with mouth, eyes, mucous membranes; systemic effects after excessive use

Side-effects local irritation

Licensed use licensed for use in children (age range not specified by manufacturer)

Indication and dose

Acne vulgaris see under preparation below

Psoriasis section 13.5.2

Warts and calluses section 13.7

Fungal nail infections section 13.10.2

Acnisal® (Alliance)
Topical solution, salicylic acid 2% in a detergent and emollient basis, net price 177 mL = £4.03.
Excipients: include benzyl alcohol

Dose

Apply up to 3 times daily

13.6.2 Oral preparations for acne

Oral antibacterials for acne

Oral antibacterials may be used in *moderate to severe inflammatory acne* when topical treatment is not adequately effective or is inappropriate. Concomitant anticomedonal treatment with topical benzoyl peroxide or azelaic acid may also be required (section 13.6.1).

In children over 12 years either **oxytetracycline** or **tetracycline** (section 5.1.3) is usually given for acne in a dose of 500 mg twice daily. If there is no improvement after the first 3 months another oral antibacterial should be used. Maximum improvement usually occurs after 4 to 6 months but in more severe cases treatment may need to be continued for 2 years or longer.

Doxycycline and **minocycline** (section 5.1.3) are alternatives to tetracycline in children over 12 years. Doxycycline may be used in a dose of 100 mg daily. Minocycline offers less likelihood of bacterial resistance but may sometimes cause irreversible pigmentation and a lupus-like syndrome; it is given in a dose of 100 mg once daily *or* 50 mg twice daily.

Erythromycin (section 5.1.5) in a dose of 500 mg twice daily for children over 12 years is an alternative for the management of moderate to severe acne with inflamed lesions, but propionibacteria strains resistant to erythromycin are becoming widespread and this may explain poor response. Infants with acne requiring oral treatment with erythromycin should be given 250 mg once daily *or* 125 mg twice daily; in cases of erythromycin-resistant *P. acnes* in infants, oral isotretinoin may be used on the advice of a consultant dermatologist.

Concomitant use of different topical and systemic antibacterials is undesirable owing to the increased likelihood of the development of bacterial resistance.

Hormone treatment for acne

Co-cyprindiol (cyproterone acetate with ethinylestradiol) contains an anti-androgen. It is no more effective than an oral broad-spectrum antibacterial but is useful in women who also wish to receive oral contraception.

Improvement of acne with co-cyprindiol probably occurs because of decreased sebum secretion which is under androgen control. Some women with moderately severe hirsutism may also benefit because hair growth is also androgen-dependent. Contra-indications of co-cyprindiol include pregnancy and a predisposition to thrombosis.

CSM advice

Venous thromboembolism occurs more frequently in women taking co-cyprindiol than those taking a low-dose combined oral contraceptive. The CSM has reminded prescribers that co-cyprindiol is licensed for use in women with severe acne which has not responded to oral antibacterials and for moderately severe hirsutism; it should not be used solely for contraception. It is contra-indicated in those with a personal or close family history of venous thromboembolism. Women with severe acne or hirsutism may have an inherently increased risk of cardiovascular disease.

CO-CYPRINDIOL

A mixture of cyproterone acetate and ethinylestradiol in the mass proportions 2000 parts to 35 parts, respectively

Cautions see under Combined Hormonal Contraceptives, BNF section 7.3.1

Contra-indications see under Combined Hormonal Contraceptives, BNF section 7.3.1

Side-effects see under Combined Hormonal Contraceptives, BNF section 7.3.1

Licensed use licensed for use in females of child-bearing age

Indication and dose

Severe acne in women refractory to prolonged oral antibacterial therapy (but see notes above)

Moderately severe hirsutism

- **By mouth**

1 tablet daily for 21 days starting on day 1 of menstrual cycle and repeated after a 7-day interval, usually for several months; withdraw when acne or hirsutism completely resolved (repeat courses may be given if recurrence)

Co-cyprindiol (Non-proprietary) PoM

Tablets, co-cyprindiol 2000/35 (cyproterone acetate 2 mg, ethinylestradiol 35 micrograms), net price 21-tab pack = £3.70

Brands include *Acnocin®*, *Cicafem®*, *Diva®*

Dianette® (Schering Health) PoM

Tablets, beige, s/c, co-cyprindiol 2000/35 (cyproterone acetate 2 mg, ethinylestradiol 35 micrograms), net price 21-tab pack = £3.11

Oral retinoid for acne

The retinoid **isotretinoin** (*Roaccutane®*) reduces sebum secretion. It is used for the systemic treatment of nodulo-cystic and conglobate acne, severe acne, acne with scarring, or for acne which has not responded to an adequate course of a systemic antibacterial.

Isotretinoin is a toxic drug that should be prescribed **only** by, or under the supervision of, a consultant dermatologist. It is given for at least 16 weeks; repeat courses are not normally required.

Side-effects of isotretinoin include severe dryness of the skin and mucous membranes, nose bleeds, and joint pains. The drug is **teratogenic** and must **not** be given to females of child-bearing age unless they practise effective contraception and then only after detailed assessment and explanation by the physician. They must also be registered with a pregnancy prevention programme (see under Cautions below).

Although a causal link between isotretinoin use and psychiatric changes (including suicidal ideation) has not been established, the possibility should be considered before initiating treatment; if psychiatric changes occur during treatment, isotretinoin should be stopped, the prescriber informed, and specialist psychiatric advice should be sought.

ISOTRETINOIN

Note Isotretinoin is an isomer of tretinoin

Cautions avoid blood donation during treatment and for at least 1 month after treatment; history of depression—monitor all patients for depression; measure hepatic function and serum lipids before treatment, 1 month after starting and then every 3 months (reduce dose or discontinue if transaminase or serum lipids persistently raised); discontinue if uncontrolled hypertriglyceridaemia or pancreatitis; diabetes; dry eye syndrome (associated with risk of keratitis); avoid keratolytics; **interactions:** Appendix 1 (retinoids)

Counselling Warn patient to avoid wax epilation (risk of epidermal stripping), dermabrasion, and laser skin treatments (risk of scarring) during treatment and for at least 6 months after stopping; patient should avoid exposure to UV light (including sunlight) and use sunscreen and emolient (including lip balm) preparations from the start of treatment

Renal impairment in severe renal impairment start with 10 mg daily and increase if necessary to max. 1 mg/kg daily

Contra-indications hypervitaminosis A, hyperlipidaemia

Hepatic impairment avoid—further impairment may occur

Pregnancy (**important teratogenic risk**) exclude pregnancy before starting (perform pregnancy test 2–3 days before expected menstruation, start treatment on day 2 or 3 of menstrual cycle)—effective contraception must be practised at least 1 month before, during, and for at least 1 month after treatment (see also notes above)

Breast-feeding avoid

Side-effects dryness of skin (with dermatitis, scaling, thinning, erythema, pruritus), epidermal fragility (trauma may cause blistering), dryness of lips (sometimes cheilitis), dryness of eyes (with blepharitis and conjunctivitis), dryness of pharyngeal mucosa (with epistaxis), headache, myalgia and arthralgia, raised plasma concentration of triglycerides, of glucose, of serum transaminases, and of cholesterol (risk of pancreatitis if triglycerides above 8 g/litre), haematuria and proteinuria, thrombocytopenia, thrombocytosis, neutropenia and anaemia; *rarely* irreversible mood changes (depression, suicidal ideation, aggressive behaviour, anxiety)—expert referral required, exacerbation of acne, acne fulminans, allergic skin reactions, and hypersensitivity, alopecia; *very rarely* nausea, inflammatory bowel disease, diarrhoea (discontinue if severe) benign intracranial hypertension (avoid concomitant tetracyclines) convulsions, malaise, drowsiness, lymphadenopathy, increased sweating, hyperuricaemia, raised serum creatinine concentration and glomerulonephritis, hepatitis, tendonitis, bone changes (including reduced bone density, early epiphyseal closure, and skeletal hyperstosis following long-term administration), visual disturbances (papilloedema, corneal opacities, cataracts, decreased night vision, photophobia, blurred vision, colour blindness)—expert referral required and consider withdrawal, decreased tolerance to contact lenses and keratitis, impaired hearing, Gram-positive infections of skin and mucous membranes, allergic vasculitis and granulomatous lesions, paronychia, hirsutism, nail dystrophy, skin hyperpigmentation, photosensitivity

Indication and dose

Acne vulgaris under supervision of consultant dermatologist, see notes above

- **By mouth**

  Child 12–18 years 500 micrograms/kg once daily increased if necessay to 1 mg/kg (in 1–2 divided doses) for 16–24 weeks (8 weeks if failure or relapse after first course); max. cumulative dose 150 mg/kg per course

Isotretinoin (Non-proprietary) PoM

Capsules, isotretinoin 5 mg, net price 56-cap pack = £15.00; 20 mg, 56-cap pack = £40.00. Label: 10, patient information leaflet, 11, 21

Roaccutane® (Roche) PoM

Capsules, isotretinoin 5 mg (red-violet/white), net price 30-cap pack = £9.08; 20 mg (red-violet/white), 30-cap pack = £25.02. Label: 10, patient information card, 11, 21

Excipients: include arachis (peanut) oil

13.7 Preparations for warts and calluses

Warts (verruca vulgaris) are common, benign, self-limiting, and usually asymptomatic. They are caused by a human papillomavirus, which most frequently affects the hands, feet (plantar warts), and the anogenital region (see below); treatment usually relies on local tissue destruction and is required only if the warts are painful, unsightly, persistent, or cause distress. In immunocompromised children, warts may be more difficult to eradicate.

Preparations of **salicylic acid, formaldehyde, gluteraldehyde** or **silver nitrate** are used for the removal of warts on hands and feet. **Salicylic acid** is a useful keratolytic which may be considered first-line in the treatment of warts; it is also suitable for the removal of *corns and calluses.* Preparations of salicylic acid in a collodion basis are available but some children may develop an allergy to colophony in the formulation; collodion should be avoided in children allergic to elastic adhesive plaster. An ointment combining **salicylic acid** with **podophyllum resin** (*Posalfilin*®) is available for treating plantar warts. Cryotherapy causes pain, swelling, and blistering and may be no more effective than topical salicylic acid in the treatment of warts.

SALICYLIC ACID

Cautions significant peripheral neuropathy, patients with diabetes at risk of neuropathic ulcers; protect surrounding skin and avoid broken skin; not suitable for application to face, anogenital region, or large areas

Side-effects skin irritation, see notes above

Licensed use not licensed for use in children under 2 years

Indication and dose

Warts on hands and feet (plantar)

for dose, see under preparations; apply carefully to wart and protect surrounding skin (e.g. with soft paraffin or specially designed plaster); rub wart surface gently with file or pumice stone once weekly; treatment may need to be continued for up to 3 months

Psoriasis section 13.5.2

Acne section 13.6.1

Fungal nail infections section 13.10.2

Cuplex® (Crawford)
Gel, salicylic acid 11%, lactic acid 4%, in a collodion basis, net price 5 g = £2.23. Label: 15

Dose

Apply twice daily

Note Contains colophony (see notes above)

Duofilm® (Stiefel)
Paint, salicylic acid 16.7%, lactic acid 16.7%, in flexible collodion, net price 15 mL (with applicator) = £1.74. Label: 15

Dose

Apply daily

Occlusal® (Alliance)
Cutaneous solution, salicylic acid 26% in polyacrylic solution, net price 10 mL (with applicator) = £3.39. Label: 15

Dose

Apply daily

Salactol® (Dermal)
Paint, salicylic acid 16.7%, lactic acid 16.7%, in flexible collodion, net price 10 mL (with applicator) = £1.79. Label: 15

Dose

Apply daily

Note contains colophony (see notes above)

Salatac® (Dermal)
Gel, salicylic acid 12%, lactic acid 4% in a collodion basis, net price 8 g (with applicator) = £3.12. Label: 15

Dose

Apply daily

Verrugon® (Pickles)
Ointment, salicylic acid 50% in a paraffin basis, net price 6 g = £2.83

Dose

Apply daily

With podophyllum

Posalfilin® (Norgine)
Ointment, podophyllum resin 20%, salicylic acid 25%, net price 10 g = £3.51

Dose

Plantar warts

apply daily

Note Owing to the salicylic acid content, not suitable for anogenital warts; owing to the podophyllum content also contra-indicated in pregnancy and breast-feeding

FORMALDEHYDE

Cautions see under Salicylic Acid

Side-effects see under Salicylic Acid

Licensed use licensed for use in children (age range not specified by manufacturer)

Indication and dose

Warts, particularly plantar warts for dose see preparation below

Veracur® (Typharm)

Gel, formaldehyde 0.75% in a water-miscible gel basis, net price 15 g = £2.41.

Dose

Apply twice daily

GLUTARALDEHYDE

Cautions protect surrounding skin; not for application to face, mucosa, or anogenital areas

Side-effects rashes, skin irritation (discontinue if severe); stains skin brown

Licensed use licensed for use in children (age range not specified by manufacturer)

Indication and dose

Warts, particularly plantar warts
apply twice daily

Glutarol® (Dermal)

Solution (= application), glutaraldehyde 10%, net price 10 mL (with applicator) = £2.17

SILVER NITRATE

Cautions protect surrounding skin and avoid broken skin; not suitable for application to face, anogenital region, or large areas

Side-effects chemical burns on surrounding skin; stains skin and fabric

Licensed use no age range specified by manufacturer

Indication and dose

Common warts and verrucas
apply moistened caustic pencil tip for 1–2 minutes; repeat after 24 hours up to max. 3 applications for warts *or* max. 6 applications for verrucas
Instructions in proprietary packs generally incorporate advice to remove dead skin before use by gentle filing and to cover with adhesive dressing after application

Umbilical granulomas
apply moistened caustic pencil tip for 1–2 minutes while protecting surrounding skin with soft paraffin

Silver nitrate (Non-proprietary)

Caustic pencil, tip containing silver nitrate 40%, potassium nitrate 60%, net price = 91p
Available from Bray

AVOCA® (Bray)

Caustic pencil, tip containing silver nitrate 95%, potassium nitrate 5%, net price, treatment pack (including emery file, 6 adhesive dressings and protector pads) = £1.89.

Anogenital warts

Anogenital warts (condylomata acuminata) in children are often asymptomatic and require only a simple barrier preparation. If treatment is required it should be carried out under the supervision of a hospital specialist. Persistent warts on genital skin may require treatment with cryotherapy or other forms of physical ablation under general anaesthesia.

Podophyllotoxin (the major active ingredient of podophyllum), or **imiquimod** are used to treat external anogenital warts; these preparations can cause considerable irritation of the treated area and are therefore suitable only for children who are able to cooperate with the treatment.

Severe systemic toxicity including gastro-intestinal, renal, haematological, and CNS effects may occur with excessive application of podophyllum.

Pregnant women should be warned of the risk of fetal toxicity and teratogenicity of podophyllum when handling preparations.

IMIQUIMOD

Cautions avoid normal skin, inflamed skin and open wounds; not suitable for internal genital warts; uncircumcised males (risk of phimosis or stricture of foreskin)

Side-effects local reactions including itching, pain, erythema, erosion, oedema, and excoriation; less commonly local ulceration and scab-

IMIQUIMOD (*continued*)

bing; permanent hypopigmentation or hyperpigmentation reported

Licensed use not licensed for use in children

Indication and dose

External genital and perianal warts (for use under specialist supervision only)

Apply thinly 3 times a week at night until lesions resolve (max. 16 weeks)

Important Should be rubbed in and allowed to stay on the treated area for 6–10 hours then washed off with mild soap and water (uncircumcised males treating warts under foreskin should wash the area daily). The cream should be washed off before sexual contact

Aldara® (3M) PoM

Cream, imiquimod 5%, net price 12-sachet pack = £51.32. Label: 10, patient information leaflet

Excipients: include benzyl alcohol, cetyl alcohol, hydroxybenzoates (parabens), polysorbate 60, stearyl alcohol

Condoms: may damage latex condoms and diaphragms

PODOPHYLLUM

Cautions see notes above; avoid normal skin and open wounds; keep away from face; very irritant to eyes; **important**: see also warnings below

Contra-indications

Pregnancy avoid—neonatal death and teratogenesis have been reported

Breast-feeding avoid

Side-effects see notes above

Licensed use not licensed for use in children

Indication and dose

See under preparations (for use under specialist supervision only)

Podophyllin Paint, Compound, BP (Non-proprietary) PoM

(podophyllum resin 15% in compound benzoin tincture), podophyllum resin 1.5 g, compound benzoin tincture to 10 mL; 5 mL to be dispensed unless otherwise directed. Label: 15

Dose

External genital warts

Child 2–18 years (see notes above) applied weekly in genitourinary clinic (or at a general practitioner's surgery by trained nurses after screening for other sexually transmitted diseases)

Important Should be allowed to stay on the treated area for not longer than 6 hours and then washed off. Care should be taken to avoid splashing the surrounding skin during application (which must be covered with soft paraffin as a protection). Where there are a large number of warts only a few should be treated at any one time as **severe toxicity** caused by absorption of podophyllin has been reported

Podophyllotoxin

Condyline® (Ardern) PoM

Solution, podophyllotoxin 0.5% in alcoholic basis, net price 3.5 mL (with applicators) = £14.49. Label: 15

Dose

Condylomata acuminata affecting the penis or the female external genitalia

Child 2–18 years (see notes above) apply twice daily for 3 consecutive days; treatment may be repeated at weekly intervals if necessary for a total of five 3-day treatment courses; direct medical supervision for lesions in the female and for lesions greater than 4 cm^2 in the male; max. 50 single applications ('loops') per session (consult product literature)

Warticon® (Stiefel) PoM

Cream, podophyllotoxin 0.15%, net price 5 g (with mirror) = £15.46

Excipients: include butylated hydroxyanisole, cetyl alcohol, hydroxybenzoates (parabens), sorbic acid, stearyl alcohol

Dose

Condylomata acuminata affecting the penis or the female external genitalia

Child 2–18 years (see notes above) apply twice daily for 3 consecutive days; treatment may be repeated at weekly intervals if necessary for a total of four 3-day treatment courses; direct medical supervision for lesions greater than 4 cm^2

Solution, blue, podophyllotoxin 0.5% in alcoholic basis, net price 3 mL (with applicators— *Warticon®* [for men]; with applicators and mirror—*Warticon Fem®* [for women]) = £12.88. Label: 15

Dose

Condylomata acuminata affecting the penis or the female external genitalia

Child 2–18 years (see notes above) apply twice daily for 3 consecutive days; treatment may be repeated at weekly intervals if necessary for a total of four 3-day treatment courses; direct medical supervision for lesions greater than 4 cm^2; max. 50 single applications ('loops') per session (consult product literature)

13.8 Sunscreens and camouflagers

13.8.1 Sunscreen preparations

Solar ultraviolet irradiation can be harmful to the skin. It is responsible for disorders such as *polymorphic light eruption, solar urticaria*, and it provokes the various *cutaneous porphyrias*. It also provokes (or at least aggravates) skin lesions of *lupus erythematosus* and may aggravate some other *dermatoses*. Sunlight may also cause photosensitivity in children taking some drugs such as demeclocycline, phenothiazines, or amiodarone. All these conditions (as well as *sunburn*) may occur after relatively short periods of exposure to the sun. Solar ultraviolet irradiation may provoke attacks of recurrent herpes labialis (but it is not known whether the effect of sunlight exposure is local or systemic).

The effects of exposure over longer periods include *ageing changes* and more importantly the initiation of *skin cancer*.

Sunburn is caused by medium wavelength solar radiation (UVB), and *photosensitivity reactions* and *photodermatoses* by the longer wavelengths (UVA). Both UVA and UVB contribute to long-term *photodamage* and to the pathogenesis of *skin cancer*.

Sunscreen preparations contain substances that protect the skin against UVB and hence against sunburn, but they are no substitute for covering the skin and avoiding sunlight. Protective clothing and sun avoidance (rather than the use of sunscreen preparations) is recommended for newborn babies and infants under 6 months.

The sun protection factor (SPF, usually indicated in the preparation title) provides guidance on the degree of protection offered against UVB; it indicates the multiples of protection provided against burning, compared with unprotected skin; for example, an SPF of 8 should enable a child to remain 8 times longer in the sun without burning. However, in practice users do not apply sufficient sunscreen product and the protection is lower than that found in experimental studies. Sunscreen preparations do not prevent long-term damage associated with UVA, which might not become apparent for 10 to 20 years. Preparations that contain reflective substances, such as titanium dioxide, provide the most effective protection against UVA. Some products use a star rating system to indicate the protection against UVA relative to protection against UVB. Four stars indicate that the product offers balanced UVA and UVB protection; products with 3, 2, or 1 star rating indicate progressively less protection against UVA. However, the usefulness of the star rating system remains controversial.

Sunscreen preparations may rarely cause allergic reactions.

> For optimum photoprotection, sunscreen preparations should be applied **thickly** and **frequently** (approximately 2 hourly). In photodermatoses, they should be used from spring to autumn. As maximum protection from sunlight is desirable, preparations with the highest SPF should be prescribed.

Borderline substances The preparations marked 'ACBS' cannot be prescribed on the NHS except for skin protection against ultraviolet radiation in abnormal cutaneous photosensitivity resulting from genetic disorders or photodermatoses, including vitiligo and those resulting from radiotherapy; chronic or recurrent herpes simplex labialis. Preparations with SPF less than 15 are not prescribable.

Delph® (Fenton)

Lotion, (UVA and UVB protection; UVB-SPF 15), ethylhexyl *p*-methoxycinnamate 7.5%, oxybenzone 3%, titanium dioxide 0.6%, net price 200 mL = £1.99. ACBS
Excipients: include cetostearyl alcohol, fragrance, hydroxybenzoates (parabens), imidurea

Lotion, (UVA and UVB protection; UVB-SPF 20), ethylhexyl *p*-methoxycinnamate 7.5%, oxybenzone 3%, titanium dioxide 1.6%, net price 200 mL = £1.99. ACBS
Excipients: include cetostearyl alcohol, fragrance, hydroxybenzoates (parabens), imidurea

Lotion, (UVA and UVB protection; UVB-SPF 25), avobenzone 4%, ethylhexyl *p*-methoxycinnamate 3.5%, titanium dioxide 2.1%, oxybenzone 1.3%, net price 200 mL = £2.85. ACBS
Excipients: include cetostearyl alcohol, fragrance, hydroxybenzoates (parabens), imidurea

Lotion, (UVA and UVB protection; UVB-SPF 30), ethylhexyl *p*-methoxycinnamate 4.8%, avobenzone 4%, titanium dioxide 2.5%, oxybenzone 1.5%, net price 200 mL = £2.85. ACBS
Excipients: include cetostearyl alcohol, fragrance, hydroxybenzoates (parabens), imidurea

E45 Sun® (Crookes)

Reflective Sunscreen (UVA and UVB protection; UVB-SPF 25), waterproof, titanium dioxide 3.6%, zinc oxide 13.9%, net price 150 mL = £6.56. ACBS
Excipients: include hydroxybenzoates (parabens), isopropyl palmitate

Reflective Sunscreen (UVA and UVB protection; UVB-SPF 50), waterproof, titanium dioxide 6.4%, zinc oxide 16%, net price 150 mL = £7.09. ACBS
Excipients: include hydroxybenzoates (parabens), isopropyl palmitate

RoC Sante Soleil® (J&J)
Cream (UVA and UVB protection; UVB-SPF 25), containing avobenzone 2%, ethylhexyl *p*-methoxycinnamate 7.5%, titanium dioxide 5.5%, net price 50 mL = £4.06. ACBS
Excipients: include beeswax, cetostearyl alcohol, disodium EDTA, hydroxybenzoates (parabens)

SpectraBan® (Stiefel)
Lotion (UVB protection; UVB-SPF 25), aminobenzoic acid 5%, padimate-O 3.2%, in an alcoholic basis, net price 150 mL = £3.45. ACBS
Excipients: include fragrance
Note Flammable; stains clothing

Ultra lotion (UVA and UVB protection; UVB-SPF 28), water resistant, avobenzone 2%, oxybenzone 3%, padimate-O 8%, titanium dioxide 2%, net price 150 mL = £5.45. ACBS
Excipients: include benzyl alcohol, disodium edetate, sorbic acid, fragrance

Sunsense® Ultra (Typharm)
Lotion (UVA and UVB protection; UVB-SPF 60), ethylhexyl *p*-methoxycinnamate 7.5% oxybenzone 3%, titanium dioxide 3.5%, net price 50-mL bottle with roll-on applicator = £3.11, 125 mL = £5.10. ACBS
Excipients: include butylated hydroxytoluene, cetyl alcohol, fragrance, hydroxybenzoates (parabens), propylene glycol

Uvistat® (LPC)
Cream (UVA and UVB protection; UVB-SPF 22 but marketed as 'factor 20'), water-resistant, ethylhexyl *p*-methoxycinnamate 7%, avobenzone 4%, titanium dioxide 4.5%, net price 125 g = £5.10. ACBS
Excipients: include disodium edetate, fragrance, hydroxybenzoates (parabens)

Ultrablock cream (UVA and UVB protection; UVB-SPF 30), water-resistant, ethylhexyl *p*-methoxycinnamate 7.5%, avobenzone 4%, titanium dioxide 6.5%, net price 125 g = £5.10. ACBS
Excipients: include disodium edetate, fragrance, hydroxybenzoates (parabens)

Photodamage

Actinic keratoses occur very rarely in healthy children; *actinic cheilitis* may occur on the lips of adolescents following excessive sun exposure.

Diclofenac gel (*Solaraze®*) and **fluorouracil** cream are licensed for the treatment of actinic keratoses but they are not licensed for use in children.

In children with photosensitivity disorders, such as erythropoietic protoporphyria, specialists may use **betacarotene, mepacrine, chloroquine** or **hydroxychloroquine** (section 10.1.3) to reduce skin reactions.

13 Skin

BETACAROTENE

Note Betacarotene is a precursor to vitamin A

Cautions monitor vitamin A intake; **interactions:** Appendix 1 (vitamins)

Renal impairment use with caution

Pregnancy partially converted to vitamin A, but does not give rise to abnormally high serum concentration; manufacturer advises use only if potential benefit outweighs risk

Breast-feeding use with caution, present in milk

Contra-indications

Hepatic impairment avoid

Side-effects loose stools; yellow discoloration of skin; *rarely*, bruising, arthralgia

Licensed use not licensed for use in UK

Indication and dose

Management of photosensitivity reactions in erythropoietic protoporphyria (specialist use only)

- By mouth

Child 1–5 years 60–90 mg daily in single or divided doses

Child 5–9 years 90–120 mg daily in single or divided doses

Child 9–12 years 120–150 mg daily in single or divided doses

Child 12–16 years 150–180 mg daily in single or divided doses

Child 16–18 years 180–300 mg daily in single or divided doses

Note Protection not total—avoid strong sunlight and use sunscreen preparations; generally 2–6 weeks of treatment (resulting in yellow coloration of palms and soles) necessary before increasing exposure to sunlight; dose should be adjusted according to level of exposure to sunlight

Betacarotene (Non-proprietary)
Capsules, 15 mg, 25 mg are available via specialist importing company. Label: 21

13.8.2 Camouflagers

Disfigurement of the skin can be very distressing and may have a marked psychological effect, especially in children. Cosmetic preparations may be used to camouflage unsightly scars, skin deformities, and pigment abnormalities, such as vitiligo and birthmarks.

Opaque cover foundation or cream is used to mask skin pigment abnormalities; careful application using a combination of dark- and light-coloured cover creams set with powder helps to minimise the appearance of skin deformities.

Borderline substances The preparations marked 'ACBS' cannot be prescribed on the NHS for postoperative scars and other deformities except as adjunctive therapy in the relief of emotional disturbances due to disfiguring skin disease, such as vitiligo.

Covermark® (Epiderm)
Classic foundation (masking cream), net price 15 mL (10 shades) = £10.75. ACBS
Excipients: include beeswax, hydroxybenzoates (parabens), fragrance

Finishing powder, net price 60 g = £10.55. ACBS
Excipients: include beeswax, hydroxybenzoates (parabens), fragrance

Dermacolor® (Fox)
Camouflage creme, (100 shades), net price 25 g = £8.10. ACBS
Excipients: include beeswax, butylated hydroxytoluene, fragrance, propylene glycol, stearyl alcohol, wool fat

Fixing powder, (7 shades), net price 60 g = £6.55. ACBS
Excipients: include fragrance

Keromask® (Network)
Masking cream, (2 shades), net price 15 mL = £5.67. ACBS
Excipients: include butylated hydroxyanisole, hydroxybenzoates (parabens), wool fat, propylene glycol

Finishing powder, net price 20 g = £5.67. ACBS
Excipients: include butylated hydroxytoluene, hydroxybenzoates (parabens)

Veil® (Blake)
Cover cream, (20 shades), net price 19 g = £8.23, 44 g = £13.90, 70 g = £18.44. ACBS
Excipients: include hydroxybenzoates (parabens), wool fat derivative

Finishing powder, translucent, net price 35 g = £8.79. ACBS
Excipients: include butylated hydroxyanisole, hydroxybenzoates (parabens)

13.9 Shampoos and other preparations for scalp conditions

The detergent action of shampoo removes grease (sebum) from hair. Prepubertal children produce very little grease and require shampoo less frequently than adults. Shampoos can be used as vehicles for medicinal products, but their usefulness is limited by the short time the product is in contact with the scalp and by their irritant nature.

Oils and ointments are very useful for scaly, dry scalp conditions; if a greasy appearance is cosmetically unacceptable, the preparation may be applied at night and washed out in the morning. Alcohol-based lotions are rarely used in children; alcohol causes painful stinging on broken skin and the fumes may exacerbate asthma.

Itchy, inflammatory, eczematous scalp conditions may be relieved by a simple emollient oil such as **coconut oil** or **arachis oil (ground nut oil** or **peanut oil**—best avoided in children under 5 years). In more severe cases a topical **corticosteroid** (section 13.4) may be required. Preparations containing **coal tar** are used for the common scaly scalp conditions of childhood including seborrhoeic dermatitis, dandruff (a mild form of seborrhoeic dermatitis), and psoriasis (section 13.5.2); **salicylic acid** is used as a keratolytic in some scalp preparations.

Shampoos containing antimicrobials such as **selenium sulphide** or **ketoconazole** are used for seborrhoeic dermatitis and dandruff in which yeast infection has been implicated, and for tinea capitis (ringworm of the scalp, section 13.10.2). Bacterial infection affecting the scalp—usually secondary to eczema, head lice, or ringworm, may be treated with shampoos containing antimicrobials such as **pyrithione zinc**, **cetrimide**, or **povidone–iodine**.

In neonates and infants, *cradle cap* (which is also a form of seborrhoeic eczema) may be treated by massaging **coconut oil** or **olive oil** into the scalp; a bland emollient such as **emulsifying ointment** may be rubbed onto the affected area once or twice daily before bathing and a mild shampoo used.

Shampoos

[1]**Ketoconazole** (Non-proprietary) PoM
Cream—section 13.10.2

Shampoo, ketoconazole 2%, net price 120 mL = £3.89
Excipients: include imidurea
Brands include *Dandrazol® 2% Shampoo, Nizoral®*

Dose

Seborrhoeic dermatitis and dandruff
treatment, apply twice weekly for 2–4 weeks; prophylaxis, apply once every 1–2 weeks

Pityriasis versicolor
treatment, apply once daily for max. 5 days; prophylaxis, apply once daily for up to 3 days before sun exposure; leave preparation on for 3–5 minutes before rinsing

1. Can be sold to the public for the prevention and treatment of dandruff and seborrhoeic dermatitis of the scalp as a shampoo formulation containing ketoconazole max. 2%, in a pack containing max. 120 mL and labelled to show a max. frequency of application of once every 3 days; brands on sale to the public include *Dandrazol® Antidandruff 2% Shampoo, Nizoral® Dandruff Shampoo*, and *Nizoral® Anti-Dandruff Shampoo*

13 Skin

Alphosyl 2 in 1® (GSK Consumer Healthcare)
Shampoo, alcoholic coal tar extract 5%, net price 125 mL = £1.81, 250 mL = £3.43
Excipients: include hydroxybenzoates (parabens), fragrance

Dose

Dandruff
use once or twice weekly as necessary

Psoriasis, seborrhoeic dermatitis, scaling and itching
use every 2–3 days

Betadine® (Medlock)
Skin disinfectants—section 13.11.4

Shampoo, povidone–iodine 4%, in a surfactant solution, net price 250 mL = £2.32
Excipients: include fragrance

Dose

Seborrhoeic scalp conditions associated with excessive dandruff, pruritus, scaling, exudation and erythema, infected scalp lesions (recurrent furunculosis, infective folliculitis, impetigo)
Child 2–18 years apply 1–2 times weekly

Cautions; Contra-indications; Side-effects: see section 13.11.4, Povidone–Iodine

Capasal® (Dermal)
Shampoo, coal tar 1%, coconut oil 1%, salicylic acid 0.5%, net price 250 mL = £4.91
Excipients: none as listed in section 13.1.3

Dose

Scaly scalp disorders including psoriasis, seborrhoeic dermatitis, dandruff, and cradle cap
apply daily as necessary

Ceanel Concentrate® (Ferndale)
Shampoo, cetrimide 10%, undecenoic acid 1%, phenylethyl alcohol 7.5%, net price 150 mL = £3.40, 500 mL = £9.80
Excipients: none as listed in section 13.1.3

Dose

Scalp psoriasis, seborrhoeic dermatitis, dandruff
apply 3 times in first week then twice weekly

Clinitar® (CHS)
Shampoo, coal tar extract 2%, net price 100 g = £2.50
Excipients: include polysorbates, fragrance

Dose

Scalp psoriasis, seborrhoeic dermatitis, and dandruff
apply up to 3 times weekly

Meted® (Alliance)
Shampoo, salicylic acid 3%, sulphur 5%, net price 120 mL = £3.80
Excipients: include fragrance

Dose

Scaly scalp disorders including psoriasis, seborrhoeic dermatitis, and dandruff
apply at least twice weekly

Pentrax® (Alliance)
Shampoo, coal tar 4.3%, net price 120 mL = £3.80
Excipients: none as listed in section 13.1.3

Dose

Scaly scalp disorders including psoriasis, seborrhoeic dermatitis, and dandruff
apply at least twice weekly

Polytar AF® (Stiefel)
Shampoo, arachis (peanut) oil extract of coal tar 0.3%, cade oil 0.3%, coal tar solution 0.1%, pine tar 0.3%, pyrithione zinc 1%, net price 150 mL = £3.91
Excipients: include fragrance, imidurea

Dose

Scaly scalp disorders including psoriasis, seborrhoeic dermatitis, and dandruff
apply 2–3 times weekly for at least 3 weeks

Psoriderm® (Dermal)
Scalp lotion (= shampoo), coal tar 2.5%, lecithin 0.3%, net price 250 mL = £4.96
Excipients: include disodium edetate

Dose

Scalp psoriasis
use as necessary

Selsun® (Abbott)
Shampoo, selenium sulphide 2.5%, net price 50 mL = £1.44, 100 mL = £1.96, 150 mL = £2.75
Excipients: include fragrance

Dose

Seborrhoeic dermatitis and dandruff
Child 5–18 years apply twice weekly for 2 weeks then once weekly for 2 weeks and then as necessary

Pityriasis versicolor [unlicensed indication]
Child 5–18 years dilute shampoo with water and apply to affected area, leave on for at least 30 minutes; apply 2–7 times over a two-week period; repeat course as necessary

Cautions avoid using 48 hours before or after applying hair colouring, straightening or waving preparations

T/Gel® (Neutrogena)
Shampoo, coal tar extract 2%, net price 125 mL = £3.18, 250 mL = £4.78
Excipients: include fragrance, hydroxybenzoates (parabens), imidurea, tetrasodium edetate

Dose

Scalp psoriasis, seborrhoeic dermatitis, dandruff
apply as necessary

Other scalp preparations

Cocois®
Section 13.5.2

Polytar® (Stiefel)
Liquid, arachis (peanut) oil extract of coal tar 0.3%, cade oil 0.3%, coal tar solution 0.1%, oleyl alcohol 1%, tar 0.3%, net price 250 mL = £2.23
Excipients: include fragrance, imidurea, polysorbate 80

Dose

Scalp disorders including psoriasis, seborrhoea, eczema, pruritus, and dandruff
apply 1–2 times weekly

Polytar Plus® (Stiefel)
Liquid, ingredients as *Polytar®* liquid with hydrolysed animal protein 3%, net price 500 mL = £3.91
Excipients: include fragrance, imidurea, polysorbate 80

Dose

Scalp disorders including psoriasis, seborrhoea, eczema, pruritus, and dandruff
apply 1–2 times weekly

13.10 Anti-infective skin preparations

13.10.1 Antibacterial preparations

Topical antibacterial preparations are used to treat localised bacterial skin infections caused by Gram-positive organisms (particularly by staphylococci or streptococci). Systemic antibacterial treatment (Table 1, section 5.1) is more appropriate for deep-seated skin infections.

Problems associated with the use of topical antibacterials include bacterial resistance and contact sensitisation. In order to minimise the development of resistance, antibacterials used systemically (e.g. fusidic acid) should not generally be chosen for topical use. **Neomycin** applied topically may cause sensitisation and cross-sensitivity with other aminoglycoside antibacterials such as gentamicin may occur. Topical antibacterials applied over large areas can cause systemic toxicity; ototoxicity with neomycin and with polymyxins is a particular risk for neonates and children with renal impairment.

Superficial bacterial infection of the skin may be treated with a topical antiseptic such as **povidine–iodine** (section 13.11.4) which also softens crusts.

Bacterial infections such as *impetigo* and *folliculitis* may be treated with a short course of a topical antibacterial such as **mupirocin** or **fusidic acid**.

For extensive or long-standing impetigo, an oral antibacterial such as **flucloxacillin** (or **erythromycin** in children with penicillin-allergy), should be used. A mild antiseptic such as **povidine–iodine** may help to soften crusts and clear exudate. Mild antiseptics may be useful in reducing the spread of infection, but there is little evidence to support the use of topical antiseptics alone in the treatment of impetigo.

Cellulitis, a rapidly spreading deeply seated inflammation of the skin and subcutaneous tissue, requires systemic antibacterial treatment (see Table 1, section 5.1); it often involves staphylococcal infection. Lower leg infections or infections spreading around wounds are almost always cellulitis. *Erysipelas,* a superficial infection with clearly defined edges (and often affecting the face), is also treated with a systemic antibacterial (see Table 1, section 5.1); it usually involves streptococcal infection.

Mupirocin is not related to any other antibacterial in use; it is effective for skin infections, particularly those due to Gram-positive organisms but it is not indicated for pseudomonal infection. Although *Staphylococcus aureus* strains with low-level resistance to mupirocin are emerging, it is generally useful in infections resistant to other antibacterials. To avoid the development of resistance, mupirocin or fusidic acid should not be used for longer than 10 days and local microbiology advice should be sought before using it in hospital. In the presence of mupirocin-resistant MRSA infection, a polymyxin or an antiseptic like povidone–iodine, chlorhexidine, and alcohol can be used; their use should be discussed with the local microbiologist.

Mupirocin ointment contains macrogol; extensive absorption of macrogol through the mucous membranes or through application to thin or damaged skin may result in renal toxicity, especially in neonates. Mupirocin nasal ointment is formulated in a paraffin base and may be more suitable for the treatment of MRSA-infected open wound in neonates.

Metronidazole gel is used topically in children to reduce the odour associated with anaerobic infections and for the treatment of periorificial rosacea (section 13.6); oral metronidazole (section 5.1.11) is used to treat wounds infected with anaerobic bacteria.

Silver sulfadiazine (silver sulphadiazine) is licensed for the prevention and treatment of infection in burns but the use of appropriate dressings may be more effective. Systemic effects may occur following extensive application of silver sulfadiazine; its use is not recommended in neonates.

13.10.1.1 Antibacterial preparations only used topically

MUPIROCIN

Side-effects local reactions including urticaria, pruritus, burning sensation, rash

Licensed use *Bactroban® ointment* licensed for use in children (age range not specified by manufacturer). *Bactroban* cream not recommended for use in child under 1 year

Indication and dose

Bacterial skin infections (see also notes above)
Child 1 month–18 years apply up to 3 times daily for up to 10 days

Bactroban® (GSK) PoM
Cream, mupirocin (as mupirocin calcium) 2%, net price 15 g = £4.38
Excipients: include benzyl alcohol, cetyl alcohol, stearyl alcohol

Ointment, mupirocin 2%, net price 15 g = £4.38
Excipients: none as listed in section 13.1.3

Note Contains macrogol and manufacturer advises caution in renal impairment; may sting

Nasal ointment—section 12.2.3

NEOMYCIN SULPHATE

Cautions large areas—if large areas of skin are being treated ototoxicity may be a hazard in children, particularly in those with renal impairment

Contra-indications neonates

Side-effects sensitisation (see also notes above)

Licensed use *Neomycin Cream BPC*—no information available; *Cicatrin®*, licensed for use in children 2–18 years; *Graneodin®*, licensed for use in children (age range not specified by manufacturer)

Indication and dose

Bacterial skin infections see under preparations

Neomycin Cream BPC PoM
Cream, neomycin sulphate 0.5%, cetomacrogol emulsifying ointment 30%, chlorocresol 0.1%, disodium edetate 0.01%, in freshly boiled and cooled purified water, net price 15 g = £2.17
Excipients: include cetostearyl alcohol, edetic acid (EDTA)

Dose

Apply up to 3 times daily (short-term use)

Cicatrin® (GSK) PoM
Cream, neomycin sulphate 3300 units, bacitracin zinc 250 units, cysteine 2 mg, glycine 10 mg, threonine 1 mg/g, net price 15 g = 92p, 30 g = £1.84
Excipients: include wool fat derivative, polysorbates

Dose

Superficial bacterial infection of skin
apply up to 3 times daily (short-term use)

Dusting powder, neomycin sulphate 3300 units, bacitracin zinc 250 units, cysteine 2 mg, glycine 10 mg, threonine 1 mg/g, net price 15 g = 92p, 50 g = £3.07
Excipients: none as listed in section 13.1.3

Dose

Superficial bacterial infection of skin
Child 2–18 years apply up to 3 times daily (short-term use)

Graneodin® (Squibb) PoM
Ointment, neomycin sulphate 0.25% (1625 units), gramicidin 0.025%, net price 25 g = £1.37
Excipients: none as listed in section 13.1.3

Dose

Superficial bacterial infection of skin
apply 2–4 times daily (for max. 7 days)

POLYMYXINS

(Includes colistin sulphate and polymyxin B sulphate)

Cautions large areas—if large areas of skin are being treated nephrotoxicity and neurotoxicity may be a hazard, particularly in children with renal impairment

Side-effects sensitisation (see also notes above)

Licensed use licensed for use in children (age range not specified by manufacturer)

Indication and dose

Bacterial skin infections see under preparation

Polyfax® (PLIVA) PoM
Ointment, polymyxin B sulphate 10 000 units, bacitracin zinc 500 units/g, net price 4 g = £3.26, 20 g = £4.62
Excipients: none as listed in section 13.1.3

Dose

Apply twice daily or more frequently if required

SILVER SULFADIAZINE

(Silver sulphadiazine)

Cautions G6PD deficiency; may inactivate enzymatic debriding agents—concomitant use may be inappropriate; **interactions**: Appendix 1 (sulphonamides)

Hepatic impairment severe, use with caution (see Large Areas, below)

Renal impairment severe, use with caution (see Large Areas, below)

Pregnancy avoid in third trimester, risk of neonatal haemolysis and methaemoglobinaemia

Breast-feeding small risk of kernicterus in jaundiced neonates and of haemolysis in G6PD deficient infant

Large areas Plasma-sulfadiazine concentrations may approach therapeutic levels with *side-effects* and *interactions* as for sulphonamides (see section 5.1.8) if large areas of skin are treated. Owing to the association of sulphonamides with severe blood and skin disorders treatment should be stopped immediately if blood disorders or rashes develop—but leucopenia developing 2–3 days after starting treatment of burns patients is reported usually to be self-limiting and silver sulfadiazine need not usually be discontinued provided blood counts are monitored carefully to ensure return to baseline within a few days. Argyria may also occur if large areas of skin are treated (or if application is prolonged).

Contra-indications sensitivity to sulphonamides; neonates

Side-effects allergic reactions including burning, itching and rashes; argyria reported following prolonged use; leucopenia reported (monitor blood count)

Licensed use no age range specified by manufacturer but see contra-indications, above

Indication and dose

Prophylaxis and treatment of infection in burn wounds, for conservative management of finger-tip injuries see under preparation below

Adjunct to short-term treatment of infection in pressure sores, adjunct to prophylaxis of infection in skin graft donor sites and extensive abrasions consult product literature for details

Flamazine® (S&N Hlth.) PoM

Cream, silver sulfadiazine 1%, net price 20 g = £2.91, 50 g = £3.85, 250 g = £10.32, 500 g = £18.27

Excipients: include cetyl alcohol, polysorbates, propylene glycol

Dose

Burns

Child 1 month–18 years apply daily or more frequently if very exudative

Finger-tip injuries

Child 1 month–18 years apply every 2–3 days

Note apply with sterile applicator

13.10.1.2 Antibacterial preparations also used systemically

Sodium fusidate is a narrow-spectrum antibacterial used for staphylococcal infections. For the role of sodium fusidate in the treatment of impetigo see p. 655.

Metronidazole is used topically for acne rosacea and to reduce the odour associated with anaerobic infections; oral metronidazole (section 5.1.11) is used to treat wounds infected with anaerobic bacteria.

Angular cheilitis An ointment containing sodium fusidate is used in the fissures of angular cheilitis when associated with staphylococcal infection. For further information on angular cheilitis, see p. 605.

FUSIDIC ACID

Cautions see notes above; avoid contact with eyes

Side-effects rarely hypersensitivity reactions

Licensed use licensed for use in children (age range not specified by manufacturer)

Indication and dose

Staphylococcal skin infections
apply 3–4 times daily, usually for up to 5 days

Penicillin-resistant staphylococcal infections
section 5.1.7

Staphylococcal eye infections
section 11.3.1

Fucidin® (Leo) PoM

Cream, fusidic acid 2%, net price 15 g = £2.00, 30 g = £3.79

Excipients: include butylated hydroxyanisole, cetyl alcohol

Ointment, sodium fusidate 2%, net price 15 g = £2.23, 30 g = £3.79

Excipients: include cetyl alcohol, wool fat

Dental prescribing on NHS May be prescribed as Sodium Fusidate ointment

METRONIDAZOLE

Cautions avoid exposure to strong sunlight or UV light

Side-effects skin irritation

Licensed use *Metrotop®* licensed for use in children (age range not specified by manufacturer); *Anabact®* licensed for use in children 12–18 years

Indication and dose

Malodorous tumours and wounds
for dose see under preparations

***Helicobacter pylori* eradication**
section 1.3

METRONIDAZOLE (*continued*)

Anaerobic infections
section 5.1.11 and section 7.2.2

Protozoal infections
section 5.4.2

Rosacea

(see also section 13.6)

Metrogel® (Galderma) PoM
Gel, metronidazole 0.75%, net price 40 g = £19.90. Label: 10, patient information leaflet
Excipients: include hydroxybenzoates (parabens), propylene glycol

Dose
Acute inflammatory exacerbations of rosacea
apply thinly twice daily

Metrosa® (Linderma) PoM
Gel, metronidazole 0.75%, net price 40 g = £19.90. Label: 10, patient information leaflet
Excipients: include propylene glycol

Dose
Acute exacerbation of rosacea
apply thinly twice daily

Noritate® (Aventis Pharma) PoM
Cream, metronidazole 1%, net price 30 g = £19.08. Label: 10, patient information leaflet
Excipients: include hydroxybenzoates (parabens)

Dose
Rosacea
apply once daily

Rozex® (Galderma) PoM
Cream, metronidazole 0.75%, net price 40 g = £15.28. Label: 10, patient information leaflet
Excipients: include benzyl alcohol, isopropyl palmitate

Gel, metronidazole 0.75%, net price 40 g = £15.28. Label: 10, patient information leaflet
Excipients: include disodium edetate, hydroxybenzoates (parabens), propylene glycol

Dose
Inflammatory papules, pustules and erythema of rosacea
apply twice daily

Zyomet® (Goldshield) PoM
Gel, metronidazole 0.75%, net price 30 g = £12.00. Label: 10, patient information leaflet
Excipients: include benzyl alcohol, disodium edetate, propylene glycol

Dose
Acute inflammatory exacerbations of rosacea
apply thinly twice daily

Malodorous tumours and skin ulcers

Anabact® (CHS) PoM
Gel, metronidazole 0.75%, net price 15 g = £4.47, 30 g = £7.89
Excipients: include hydroxybenzoates (parabens), propylene glycol

Dose
Apply to clean wound 1–2 times daily and cover with non-adherent dressing

Metrotop® (Medlock) PoM
Gel, metronidazole 0.8%, net price 15 g = £4.73, 30 g = £8.36
Excipients: none as listed in section 13.1.3

Dose
Apply to clean wound 1–2 times daily and cover (flat wounds, apply liberally; cavities, smear gel on paraffin gauze and pack loosely)

13.10.2 Antifungal preparations

Most localised fungal infections are treated with topical preparations. Systemic therapy (section 5.2) is necessary for nail or scalp infection or if the skin infection is widespread, disseminated or intractable. Specimens of scale, nail or hair should be sent for mycological examination before starting treatment, unless the diagnosis is certain.

Dermatophytoses Ringworm infection can affect the scalp (tinea capitis), body (tinea corporis), groin (tinea cruris), hand (tinea manuum), foot (tinea pedis, athlete's foot), or nail (tinea unguium, onychomycosis). Tinea capitis is a common childhood infection that requires systemic treatment with an oral antifungal (section 5.2). **Griseofulvin** (section 5.2) is used to treat microsporum infections (cat or dog ringworm). **Terbinafine** is effective in the treatment of trichophyton infections. A shampoo (section 13.9) containing **selenium sulphide** or **ketoconazole** may also be used in the early stages of treatment to reduce the risk of transmission of infection; other children in the family should also be treated with an antifungal shampoo.

Tinea corporis and tinea pedis infections in children respond to treatment with a topical **imidazole** (clotrimazole, econazole, ketoconazole, miconazole, or sulconazole) or **terbinafine** cream. Nystatin is less effective against tinea.

Compound benzoic acid ointment (Whitfield's ointment) has been used for ringworm infections but it is cosmetically less acceptable than proprietary preparations. Antifungal dusting powders are of little therapeutic value in the treatment of fungal skin infections and may cause skin irritation; they may have some role in preventing re-infection.

Tinea infection of the nail is almost always treated systemically (section 5.2); topical application of **amorolfine** or **tioconazole** may be effective for treating early onychomycosis when involvement is limited to mild distal disease in up to 2 nails. Chronic paronychia on the fingers (usually due to a candidal infection) should be treated with topical clotrimazole or nystatin, but they should be used with caution for children who suck their fingers. Chronic paronychia of the toes (usually due to dermatophyte infection) may be treated with topical terbinafine.

Pityriasis versicolor Pityriasis (tinea) versicolor may be treated with **ketoconazole** shampoo (section 13.9). Alternatively, **selenium sulphide** shampoo (section 13.9) may be used as a lotion. Topical imidazole antifungals **clotrimazole**, **econazole**, **ketoconazole**, **miconazole**, and **sulconazole** and topical **terbinafine** are alternatives but large quantities may be required.

If topical therapy fails, or if the infection is widespread, pityriasis versicolor is treated systemically with an azole antifungal (section 5.2). Relapse is common, especially in the immunocompromised.

Candidiasis Candidal skin infections may be treated with topical imidazole antifungals **clotrimazole**, **econazole**, **ketoconazole**, **miconazole**, and **sulconazole**; topical terbinafine is an alternative. Topical application of **nystatin** is also effective for candidiasis but it is ineffective against dermatophytosis. Refractory candidiasis requires systemic treatment (section 5.2) generally with a triazole such as fluconazole; systemic treatment with griseofulvin or terbinafine is **not appropriate** for refractory candidiasis. For the treatment of oral candiasis see section 12.3.2 and for the management of nappy rash see section 13.2.2.

Angular cheilitis Nystatin ointment is used in the fissures of angular cheilitis when associated with *Candida*. For further information on angular cheilitis, see p. 605.

Cautions Contact with eyes and mucous membranes should be avoided.

Side-effects Occasional local irritation and hypersensitivity reactions include mild burning sensation, erythema, and itching. Treatment should be discontinued if symptoms are severe.

Compound topical preparations Combination of an imidazole and a mild corticosteroid (such as hydrocortisone 1%) (section 13.4) may be of value in the treatment of eczematous intertrigo and, in the first few days only, of a severely inflamed patch of ringworm. Combination of a mild corticosteroid with either an imidazole or nystatin may be of use in the treatment of *intertriginous eczema* associated with candida.

AMOROLFINE

Cautions see notes above; also avoid contact with ears; pregnancy and breast-feeding

Side-effects see notes above

Licensed use not licensed for use in children under 12 years

Indication and dose

See under preparations

Loceryl® (Galderma) PoM

Cream, amorolfine (as hydrochloride) 0.25%, net price 20 g = £4.83. Label: 10, patient information leaflet

Excipients: include cetostearyl alcohol, disodium edetate

Dose

Fungal skin infections

apply once daily after cleansing in the evening for at least 2–3 weeks (up to 6 weeks for foot infection) continuing for 3–5 days after lesions have healed

Nail lacquer, amorolfine (as hydrochloride) 5%, net price 5-mL pack (with nail files, spatulas and cleansing swabs) = £21.43. Label: 10, patient information leaflet

Excipients: none as listed in section 13.1.3

Dose

Fungal nail infections

apply to infected nails 1–2 times weekly after filing and cleansing; allow to dry (approx. 3 minutes); treat finger nails for 6 months, toe nails for 9–12 months (review at intervals of 3 months); avoid nail varnish or artificial nails during treatment

Note Use with caution in child likely to suck affected digits

BENZOIC ACID

Licensed use licensed for use in children (age range not specified by manufacturer)

Indication and dose

Ringworm (tinea) but see notes above and under preparation below

Benzoic Acid Ointment, Compound, BP (Whitfield's ointment)
Ointment, benzoic acid 6%, salicylic acid 3%, in emulsifying ointment

Dose

Child 1 month–18 years apply twice daily

Excipients: include cetostearyl alcohol

CLOTRIMAZOLE

Cautions see notes above

Side-effects see notes above

Licensed use licensed for use in children (age range not specified by manufacturer)

Indication and dose

Fungal skin infections
apply 2–3 times daily

Vaginal candidiasis section 7.2.2

Otitis externa section 12.1.1

Clotrimazole (Non-proprietary)
Cream, clotrimazole 1%, net price 20 g = £2.12

[1]**Canesten®** (Bayer Consumer Care)
Cream, clotrimazole 1%, net price 20 g = £2.14, 50 g = £3.80
Excipients: include benzyl alcohol, cetostearyl alcohol, polysorbate 60

Powder, clotrimazole 1%, net price 30 g = £1.52
Excipients: none as listed in section 13.1.3

Solution, clotrimazole 1% in macrogol 400 (polyethylene glycol 400), net price 20 mL = £2.43. For hairy areas
Excipients: none as listed in section 13.1.3

Spray, clotrimazole 1%, in 30% isopropyl alcohol, net price 40-mL atomiser = £4.99. Label: 15. For large or hairy areas
Excipients: include propylene glycol

1. The brand name *Canesten® AF Once Daily* is used for bifonazole

13 Skin

ECONAZOLE NITRATE

Cautions see notes above
Side-effects see notes above
Licensed use *Ecostatin®* not licensed for use in children under 1 year; *Pevaryl®*, no age range specified by manufacturer

Indication and dose

Fungal skin infections
apply twice daily

Fungal nail infections
apply once daily under occlusive dressing

Vaginal candidiasis section 7.2.2

Ecostatin® (Squibb)
Cream, econazole nitrate 1%, net price 15 g = £1.49; 30 g = £2.75
Excipients: include butylated hydroxyanisole, fragrance

Pevaryl® (Janssen-Cilag)
Cream, econazole nitrate 1%, net price 30 g = £2.65
Excipients: include butylated hydroxyanisole, fragrance

KETOCONAZOLE

Cautions see notes above; do **not** use within 2 weeks of a potent topical corticosteroid for seborrhoeic dermatitis—risk of skin sensitisation
Side-effects see notes above

Indication and dose

Tinea pedis
apply twice daily

Other fungal infections
apply 1–2 times daily

Systemic or resistant fungal infections section 5.2

Vulval candidiasis section 7.2.2

[1]**Nizoral®** (Janssen-Cilag) PoM
[2]Cream, ketoconazole 2%, net price 30 g = £3.62
Excipients: include cetyl alcohol, polysorbates, propylene glycol, stearyl alcohol

Shampoo—section 13.9

1. A 15-g tube is available for sale to the public for the treatment of tinea pedis, tinea cruris, and candidal intertrigo
2. NHS except for seborrhoeic dermatitis and pityriasis versicolor and endorsed 'SLS'

MICONAZOLE NITRATE

Cautions see notes above

Side-effects see notes above

Licensed use Licensed for use in children (age range not specified by manufacturer)

Indication and dose

Fungal skin infections

Neonate apply twice daily continuing for 10 days after lesions have healed

Child 1 month–18 years apply twice daily continuing for 10 days after lesions have healed

Fungal nail infections
apply 1–2 times daily

Intestinal fungal infections section 5.2

Oral fungal infections section 12.3.2

Vaginal candidiasis section 7.2.2

Miconazole (Non-proprietary)
Cream, miconazole nitrate 2%, net price 20 g = £2.05, 45 g = £1.97
Brands include *Acorvio®* (*excipients: include* cetostearyl alcohol, polysorbate 40, propylene glycol)

Daktarin® (Janssen-Cilag)
Cream, miconazole nitrate 2%, net price 30 g = £1.97. Also on sale to the public as *Daktarin® Dual Action cream* for athlete's foot
Excipients: include butylated hydroxyanisole
Note A 15-g tube NHS is on sale to the public.

Powder NHS, miconazole nitrate 2%, net price 20 g = £1.81
Excipients: include none as listed in section 13.1.3

Dual Action Spray powder, miconazole nitrate 0.16%, in an aerosol basis, net price 100 g = £2.27
Excipients: none as listed in section 13.1.3

NYSTATIN

Cautions see notes above

Side-effects see notes above

Licensed use licensed for use in children (age range not specified by manufacturer)

Indication and dose

Skin infections due to *Candida* spp. for dose, see preparations below

Intestinal candidiasis section 5.2

Vaginal candidiasis section 7.2.2

Oral fungal infections section 12.3.2

Nystaform® (Typharm) PoM
Cream, nystatin 100 000 units/g, chlorhexidine hydrochloride 1%, net price 30 g = £2.62
Excipients: include benzyl alcohol, cetostearyl alcohol, polysorbate 60

Dose

Apply 2–3 times daily continuing for 7 days after lesions have healed.

Nystan® (Squibb) PoM
Cream, nystatin 100 000 units/g, net price 30 g = £2.18
Excipients: include benzyl alcohol, propylene glycol, fragrance

Dose

Apply 2–4 times daily

Ointment, nystatin 100 000 units/g, in *Plastibase®*, net price 30 g = £1.75
Excipients: none as listed in section 13.1.3

Dose

Apply 2–4 times daily

Dental prescribing on NHS May be prescribed as Nystatin Ointment

Tinaderm-M® (Schering-Plough) PoM
Cream, nystatin 100 000 units/g, tolnaftate 1%, net price 20 g = £1.83
Excipients: include butylated hydroxytoluene, cetostearyl alcohol, hydroxybenzoates (parabens), fragrance

Dose

Apply 2–3 times daily

SALICYLIC ACID

Cautions avoid broken or inflammed skin
Salicylate toxicity Salicylate toxicity may occur particularly if applied on large areas of skin

Contra-indications children under 5 years

Side-effects see notes above

Licensed use not licensed for use in children under 5 years

Indication and dose

Fungal nail infections, particularly tinea
apply twice daily
Note Use with caution in child likely to suck affected digits

Hyperkeratotic skin disorders section 13.5.2

Acne vulgaris section 13.6.1

Warts and calluses section 13.7

Phytex® (Wynlit)
Paint, salicylic acid 1.46% (total combined), tannic acid 4.89% and boric acid 3.12% (as borotannic complex), in a vehicle containing alcohol and ethyl acetate, net price 25 mL (with brush) = £1.56
Excipients: none as listed in section 13.1.3
Note Flammable

SULCONAZOLE NITRATE

Cautions see notes above

Side-effects see notes above; also blistering

Indication and dose

Fungal skin infections
apply 1–2 times daily continuing for 2–3 weeks after lesions have healed

Exelderm® (Centrapharm)
Cream, sulconazole nitrate 1%, net price 30 g = £3.00
Excipients: include cetyl alcohol, polysorbates, propylene glycol, stearyl alcohol

TERBINAFINE

Cautions avoid contact with eyes

Pregnancy manufacturer advises avoid—studies in *animals* suggest no adverse effects

Breast-feeding manufacturer advises avoid—present in milk, but less than 5% of the dose is absorbed after topical application of terbinafine

Side-effects redness, itching, or stinging; *rarely* allergic reactions (discontinue)

Licensed use not licensed for use in children

Indication and dose

Fungal skin infections

[1]**Lamisil®** (Novartis) PoM
Cream, terbinafine hydrochloride 1%, net price 15 g = £4.86, 30 g = £8.76

Dose

Apply thinly 1–2 times daily for up to 1 week in tinea pedis, 1–2 weeks in tinea corporis and tinea cruris, 2 weeks in cutaneous candidiasis and pityriasis versicolor; review after 2 weeks

Excipients: include benzyl alcohol, cetyl alcohol, polysorbate 60, stearyl alcohol

Tablets—section 5.2

1. Can be sold to the public for external use in children over 16 years for the treatment of tinea pedis and tinea cruris as a cream containing terbinafine hydrochloride max. 1% in a pack containing max. 15 g; also for the treatment of tinea pedis, tinea cruris, and tinea corporis as a spray containing terbinafine hydrochloride max. 1% in a pack containing max. 30 mL or as a gel containing terbinafine hydrochloride max. 1% in a pack containing max. 30 g

TIOCONAZOLE

Cautions see notes above

Contra-indications

Pregnancy manufacturer advises avoid

Side-effects see notes above; also local oedema, dry skin, nail discoloration, periungual inflammation, nail pain, rash, exfoliation

Licensed use licensed for use in children (age range not specified by manufacturer)

Indication and dose

Fungal nail infections
apply to nails and surrounding skin twice daily for up to 6 months (may be extended to 12 months)

Trosyl® (Pfizer) PoM
Cutaneous solution, tioconazole 28%, net price 12 mL (with applicator brush) = £27.38
Excipients: none as listed in section 13.1.3
Note Use with caution in child likely to suck affected digits

UNDECENOATES

Side-effects see notes above

Licensed use *Monphytol®* not licensed for use in children under 12 years; *Mycota®* licensed for use in children (age range not specified by manufacturer)

Indication and dose

See under preparations below

Monphytol® (LAB)
Paint, methyl undecenoate 5%, propyl undecenoate 0.7%, salicylic acid 3%, methyl salicylate 25%, propyl salicylate 5%, chlorobutanol 3%, net price 18 mL (with brush) = £1.77
Excipients: none as listed in section 13.1.3

Dose

Fungal skin and nail infections
apply twice daily

Mycota® (Thornton & Ross)
Cream, zinc undecenoate 20%, undecenoic acid 5%, net price 25 g = £1.31
Excipients: include fragrance

Dose

Treatment of athlete's foot
apply twice daily continuing for 7 days after lesions have healed

Prevention of athlete's foot
apply once daily

Powder, zinc undecenoate 20%, undecenoic acid 2%, net price 70 g = £1.87
Excipients: include fragrance

Dose

Treatment of athlete's foot
apply twice daily continuing for 7 days after lesions have healed

Skin 13

UNDECENOATES (*continued*)

Prevention of athlete's foot
apply once daily

Spray application, undecenoic acid 2.5%, dichlorophen 0.25% (pressurised aerosol pack), net price 100 mL = £2.13
Excipients: include fragrance

Dose

Treatment of athlete's foot
apply twice daily continuing for 7 days after lesions have healed

Prevention of athlete's foot
apply once daily

13.10.3 Antiviral preparations

See section 12.3.2 for drugs used in *herpetic stomatitis*, section 13.5.1 for *eczema herpeticum*, and section 11.3.3 for viral infections of the *eye*.

Aciclovir cream is used for the treatment of initial and recurrent labial and genital *herpes simplex infections* in children; treatment should begin as early as possible. Systemic treatment is necessary for buccal or vaginal infections or if cold sores recur frequently (for details of systemic use see section 5.3.2.1).

Herpes labialis **Aciclovir** cream can be used for the treatment of initial and recurrent labial herpes simplex infections (cold sores). It is best applied at the earliest possible stage, usually when prodromal changes of sensation are felt in the lip and before vesicles appear.

Penciclovir cream is also licensed for the treatment of herpes labialis; it needs to be applied more frequently than aciclovir cream. These creams should not be used in the mouth.

ACICLOVIR
(Acyclovir)

Cautions avoid contact with eyes and mucous membranes

Side-effects transient stinging or burning; occasionally erythema, itching or drying of the skin

Licensed use licensed for use in children (age range not specified by manufacturer)

Indication and dose

Herpes simplex infections
apply to lesions every 4 hours (5 times daily) for 5–10 days, starting at first sign of attack

Herpes simplex and varicella–zoster infections
section 5.3.2.1

Eye infections section 11.3.3

Aciclovir (Non-proprietary) PoM
Cream, aciclovir 5%, net price 2 g = £1.81, 10 g = £4.74
Excipients: include propylene glycol
Brands include *Zuvogen®* (*excipients* also include cetyl alcohol, propylene glycol)
Dental prescribing on NHS Aciclovir Cream may be prescribed

Zovirax® (GSK) PoM
Cream, aciclovir 5%, net price 2 g = £4.92, 10 g = £14.82
Excipients: include cetostearyl alcohol, propylene glycol

Eye ointment—section 11.3.3

Tablets—section 5.3.2.1

PENCICLOVIR

Cautions avoid contact with eyes and mucous membranes

Side-effects transient stinging, burning, numbness

Licensed use not licensed for use in children under 12 years

Vectavir® (Novartis Consumer Health) PoM
Cream, penciclovir 1%, net price 2 g = £4.20
Excipients: include cetostearyl alcohol, propylene glycol

Dose

Herpes labialis
apply to lesions every 2 hours during waking hours for 4 days, starting at first sign of attack

Dental prescribing on NHS May be prescribed as Penciclovir Cream

13 Skin

13.10.4 Parasiticidal preparations

Suitable quantities of parasiticidal preparations

Suitable quantities of parasiticidal preparations

	Skin creams	Lotions	Cream rinses
Scalp (head lice)	—	50–100 mL	50–100 mL
Body (scabies)	30–60 g	100 mL	—
Body (crab lice)	30–60 g	100 mL	—

These amounts are usually suitable for a child 12–18 years for single application

Scabies

Permethrin is effective for the treatment of *scabies* (*Sarcoptes scabiei*); **malathion** can be used if permethrin is inappropriate.

Aqueous preparations are preferable; alcoholic lotions cause irritation of excoriated skin and the genitalia.

Benzyl benzoate is an irritant and should be avoided in children; it is less effective than malathion and permethrin.

Ivermectin (available from specialist importing company), is used in combination with topical drugs, for the treatment of hyperkeratotic (crusted or 'Norwegian') scabies that does not respond to topical treatment alone.

Application Although acaricides have traditionally been applied after a hot bath, this is **not** necessary and there is even evidence that a hot bath may increase absorption into the blood, removing them from their site of action on the skin.

All members of the affected household should be treated simultaneously. Treatment should be applied to the whole body including the scalp, neck, face, and ears. Particular attention should be paid to the webs of the fingers and toes and lotion brushed under the ends of nails. Malathion and permethrin should be applied twice, one week apart. It is important to warn users to reapply treatment to the hands if they are washed. Children with hyperkeratotic scabies may require 2 or 3 applications of acaricide on consecutive days to ensure that enough penetrates the skin crusts to kill all the mites.

Itching The *itch* and *eczema* of scabies persists for some weeks after the infestation has been eliminated and treatment for pruritus and eczema (section 13.5.1) may be required. Application of **crotamiton** can be used to control itching after treatment with more effective acaricides. A topical **corticosteroid** (section 13.4) may help to reduce itch and inflammation after scabies has been treated successfully; however, persistent symptoms suggest failure of scabies eradication. Oral administration of a **sedating antihistamine** (section 3.4.1) at night may also be useful.

Head lice

Carbaryl, **malathion**, and **phenothrin** are effective against head lice (*Pediculus humanus capitis*) but lice in some districts have developed resistance; resistance to two or more parasiticidal preparations has also been reported. **Permethrin** is effective against head lice but no suitable preparation for a contact time of 12 hours exists. Careful application of **dimeticone**, which acts on the surface of head lice, is also effective. Benzyl benzoate is licensed for the treatment of head lice but it is not recommended for use in children.

Head lice infestation (pediculosis) should be treated using lotion or liquid formulations. Shampoos are diluted too much in use to be effective. Alcoholic formulations are effective but aqueous formulations are preferred in children, especially those with severe eczema or asthma. A contact time of 12 hours or overnight treatment is recommended for lotions and liquids; a 2-hour treatment is not sufficient to kill eggs.

In general, a course of treatment for head lice should be 2 applications of product 7 days apart to prevent lice emerging from any eggs that survive the first application.

The policy of rotating insecticides on a district-wide basis is now considered outmoded. To overcome the development of resistance, a mosaic strategy is required whereby, if a course of treatment fails to cure, a different insecticide is used for the next course. If a course of treatment with either permethrin or phenothrin fails, then a non-pyrethroid parasiticidal product should be used for the next course.

Wet combing methods Head lice may be mechanically removed by combing wet hair meticulously with a plastic detection comb (probably for at least 30 minutes each time) over the whole scalp at 4-day intervals for a minimum of 2 weeks; hair conditioner or vegetable oil may be used to facilitate the process. Several products are available and some are prescribable on the NHS.

Crab lice

Carbaryl [unlicensed for crab lice], **permethrin, phenothrin**, and **malathion** are effective for *crab lice* (*Pthirus pubis*); permethrin is not licensed for treatment of crab lice in children under 18 years. An aqueous preparation should be applied, allowed to dry naturally and washed off after 12 hours; a second treatment is needed after 7 days to kill lice emerging from surviving eggs. All surfaces of the body should be treated, including the scalp, neck, ears, and face (paying particular attention to the eyebrows and any beard). A different insecticide should be used if a course of treatment fails. Alcoholic lotions are not recommended (owing to irritation of excoriated skin and the genitalia).

Aqueous **malathion** lotion is effective for *crab lice of the eye lashes* [unlicensed use].

Parasiticidal preparations

Carbaryl is recommended for *head lice*; an aqueous preparation is recommended for *crab lice* (see notes above) but a suitable product is not currently licensed for this indication. In the light of experimental data in *animals* it would be prudent to consider carbaryl as a potential human carcinogen and it has been restricted to prescription only use. The Department of Health has emphasised that the risk is a theoretical one and that any risk from the intermittent use of head lice preparations is likely to be exceedingly small.

Dimeticone coats head lice and interferes with water balance in lice by preventing excretion of water; it is less active against eggs and treatment should be repeated after 7 days.

Malathion is recommended for *scabies, head lice* and *crab lice* (see notes above). The risk of systemic effects associated with 1–2 applications of malathion is considered to be very low; however, except in the treatment of hyperkeratotic scabies (see notes above), applications of lotion repeated at intervals of less than 1 week *or* application for more than 3 consecutive weeks should be **avoided** since the likelihood of eradication of lice is not increased.

Permethrin is effective for *scabies.* It is active against *head lice* but the formulation and licensed methods of application of the current products make them unsuitable for the treatment of head lice. Permethrin is also effective against *crab lice* but it is not licensed for this purpose in children under 18 years.

Phenothrin is recommended for *head lice* and *crab lice.*

CARBARYL
(Carbaril)

Cautions avoid contact with eyes; do not use on broken or secondarily infected skin; do not use more than once a week for 3 consecutive weeks; alcoholic lotions **not** recommended for pediculosis in children with severe eczema, or asthma

Side-effects skin irritation

Licensed use not licensed for use in children under 6 months except under medical supervision; not licensed for treatment of crab lice

Indication and dose

Head lice see also notes above

Rub into dry hair and scalp, allow to dry naturally, shampoo after 12 hours, and comb wet hair; repeat application after 7 days

Crab lice

Apply aqueous solution over whole body (see notes above), allow to dry naturally and wash off after 12 hours or overnight; repeat application after 7 days

CARBARYL (*continued*)

Carylderm® (SSL) PoM
Liquid, carbaryl 1% in an aqueous basis, net price 50 mL = £2.28
Excipients: include cetostearyl alcohol, hydroxybenzoates (parabens)

Lotion, carbaryl 0.5%, in an alcoholic basis, net price 50 mL = £2.28. Label: 15
Excipients: include fragrance
Note Flammable

DIMETICONE

Cautions avoid contact with eyes

Side-effects skin irritation

Licensed use not licensed for use in children under 6 months except under medical supervision

Indication and dose

Head lice
Rub into dry hair and scalp, allow to dry naturally, shampoo after 8 hours (or overnight); repeat application after 7 days

Hedrin® (Thornton & Ross)
Lotion, dimeticone 4%, net price 50 mL = £2.98, 150 mL = £6.83

MALATHION

Cautions avoid contact with eyes; do not use on broken or secondarily infected skin; do not use lotion more than once a week for 3 consecutive weeks; alcoholic lotions **not** recommended for head lice in children with severe eczema or asthma, or for scabies or crab lice (see notes above)

Side-effects skin irritation

Licensed use not licensed for use in children under 6 months except under medical supervision

Indication and dose

See notes above and under preparations

Head lice
Rub 0.5% preparation into dry hair and scalp, allow to dry naturally, remove by washing after 12 hours; repeat application after 7 days (see also notes above)

Crab lice
Apply 0.5% aqueous preparation over whole body, allow to dry naturally, wash off after 12 hours or overnight; repeat application after 7 days

Scabies
Apply 0.5% preparation over whole body, and wash off after 24 hours; if hands are washed with soap within 24 hours, they should be retreated; see also notes above; repeat application after 7 days

Note For scabies, manufacturer recommends application to the body but not necessarily to the head and neck. However, application should be extended to the scalp, neck, face, and ears

Derbac-M® (SSL)
Liquid, malathion 0.5% in an aqueous basis, net price 50 mL = £2.22, 200 mL = £5.70
Excipients: include cetostearyl alcohol, fragrance, hydroxybenzoates (parabens)
For crab lice, head lice, and scabies

Prioderm® (SSL)
Lotion, malathion 0.5%, in an alcoholic basis, net price 50 mL = £2.22, 200 mL = £5.70. Label: 15
Excipients: include fragrance
For head lice (alcoholic formulation, see notes above)

Cream shampoo NHS, malathion 1%, net price 40 g = £2.77
Excipients: include cetostearyl alcohol, fragrance, hydroxybenzoates (parabens), sodium edetate, wool fat
Note Head and crab lice, not recommended, therefore no dose stated (product too diluted in use and insufficient contact time)

Quellada M® (GSK Consumer Healthcare)
Liquid, malathion 0.5% in an aqueous basis, net price 50 mL = £1.85, 200 mL = £4.62
Excipients: include cetostearyl alcohol, fragrance, hydroxybenzoates (parabens)
For crab lice, head lice, and scabies

Cream shampoo, malathion 1%, net price 40 g = £2.18
Excipients: include cetostearyl alcohol, fragrance, hydroxybenzoates (parabens), sodium edetate, wool fat
Note Head and crab lice, not recommended, therefore no dose stated (product too diluted in use and insufficient contact time)

Suleo-M® (SSL)
Lotion, malathion 0.5%, in an alcoholic basis, net price 50 mL = £2.22, 200 mL = £5.70. Label: 15
Excipients: include fragrance
For head lice (alcoholic formulation, see notes above)

PERMETHRIN

Cautions avoid contact with eyes; do not use on broken or secondarily infected skin

Side-effects pruritus, erythema, and stinging; rarely rashes and oedema

Licensed use *Dermal Cream* (scabies), not licensed for use in children under 2 months; children aged 2 months–2 years, medical supervison required; not licensed for treatment of crab lice in children under 18 years; *Creme Rinse* (head

PERMETHRIN (*continued*)

lice) not licensed for use in children under 6 months except under medical supervision

Indication and dose

See notes above

Scabies

Apply 5% preparation over whole body including face, neck, scalp and ears; wash off after 8-12 hours; if hands washed with soap within 8 hours of application, they should be treated again with cream (see notes above); repeat application after 7 days

Note Manufacturer recommends application to the body but to exclude head and neck. However, application should be extended to the scalp, neck, face, and ears

Permethrin (Non-proprietary)

Cream, permethrin 5%, net price 30 g = £5.52

Lyclear® Creme Rinse (Chefaro UK)

Cream rinse, permethrin 1% in basis containing isopropyl alcohol 20%, net price 59 mL = £2.38, 2 × 59-mL pack = £4.32

Excipients: include cetyl alcohol

Note Head lice, not recommended, therefore no dose stated (product too diluted in use and insufficient contact time)

Lyclear® Dermal Cream (Chefaro UK)

Dermal cream, permethrin 5%, net price 30 g = £5.52. Label: 10, patient information leaflet

Excipients: include butylated hydroxytoluene, wool fat derivative

PHENOTHRIN

Cautions avoid contact with eyes; do not use on broken or secondarily infected skin; do not use more than once a week for 3 weeks at a time; alcoholic preparations **not** recommended for head lice in severe eczema, in asthma, in small children, or for crab lice (see notes above)

Side-effects skin irritation

Indication and dose

See notes above and under preparations

Full Marks® (SSL)

Liquid, phenothrin 0.5% in an aqueous basis, net price 50 mL = £2.22, 200 mL = £5.70

Excipients: include cetostearyl alcohol, fragrance, hydroxybenzoates (parabens)

Dose

Head lice

apply to dry hair, allow to dry naturally; shampoo after 12 hours or next day, comb wet hair; repeat application after 7 days

Lotion, phenothrin 0.2% in basis containing isopropyl alcohol 69.3%, net price 50 mL = £2.22, 200 mL = £5.70. Label: 15

Excipients: include fragrance

Dose

Crab lice and head lice

(alcoholic formulation, see notes above) apply to dry hair, allow to dry naturally; shampoo after 12 hours [unlicensed contact duration], comb wet hair; repeat application after 7 days

Mousse (= foam application), phenothrin 0.5% in an alcoholic basis, net price 50 g = £2.44, 150 g = £6.11. Label: 15

Excipients: include cetostearyl alcohol

Dose

Head lice

(alcoholic formulation, see notes above) apply to dry hair, shampoo after 30 minutes, comb wet hair—but product not recommended because contact time insufficient (longer contact time not recommended because of risk of irritation)

13.10.5 Preparations for minor cuts and abrasions

Cetrimide cream is used to treat minor cuts and abrasions. **Proflavine** cream may be used to treat infected wounds or burns, but has now been largely superseded by other antiseptics or suitable antibacterials.

Cetrimide Cream, BP

Cream, cetrimide 0.5% in a suitable water-miscible basis such as cetostearyl alcohol 5%, liquid paraffin 50% in freshly boiled and cooled purified water, net price 50 g = 76p

Proflavine Cream, BPC

Cream, proflavine hemisulphate 0.1%, yellow beeswax 2.5%, chlorocresol 0.1%, liquid paraffin 67.3%, freshly boiled and cooled purified water 25%, wool fat 5%, net price 100 mL = 85p

Excipients: include beeswax, wool fat

Note Stains clothing

Collodion

Flexible collodion may be used to seal minor cuts and wounds that have partially healed.

Collodion, Flexible, BP

Collodion, castor oil 2.5%, colophony 2.5% in a collodion basis, prepared by dissolving pyroxylin (10%) in a mixture of 3 volumes of ether and 1 volume of alcohol (90%), net price 10 mL = 27p. Label: 15

Contra-indications allergy to colophony in elastic adhesive plasters and tape

Skin tissue adhesive

Tissue adhesives are used for closure of minor skin wounds and for additional suture support. They should be applied by an appropriately trained healthcare professional. Skin tissue adhesives may cause skin sensitisation.

Dermabond® (Ethicon)
Topical skin adhesive, sterile, ocrilate, net price 0.5 mL = £10.18

Epiglu® (ICN)
Tissue adhesive, sterile, ethyl-2-cyanoacrylate 954.5 mg/g, polymethylmethacrylate, net price 4 × 3-g vials = £95.00 (with dispensing pipettes and pallete)

Indermil® (Tyco)
Tissue adhesive, sterile, enbucrilate, net price 5 × 500-mg units = £32.50, 20 × 500-mg units = £130.00

Histoacryl® (Braun)
Tissue adhesive, sterile, enbucrilate, net price 5 × 200-mg unit (blue) = £32.00, 10 × 200-mg unit (blue) = £67.20, 5 × 500-mg unit (clear or blue) = £34.68, 10 × 500-mg unit (blue) = £69.30

LiquiBand® (MedLogic)
Tissue adhesive, sterile, enbucrilate, net price 0.5-g amp = £5.50

13.11 Skin cleansers and antiseptics

Soap or detergent is used with water to cleanse intact skin but they can irritate infantile skin; emollient preparations such as aqueous cream or emulsifying ointment (section 13.2.1) that do not irritate the skin are best used for cleansing dry skin.

An antiseptic is used for skin that is infected or that is susceptible to recurrent infection. Detergent preparations containing **chlorhexidine**, **triclosan**, or **povidone–iodine**, which should be thoroughly rinsed off, are used. Emollients may also contain antiseptics (section 13.2.1).

Antiseptics such as **chlorhexidine** or **povidone–iodine** are used on intact skin before surgical procedures; their antiseptic effect is enhanced by an alcoholic solvent. **Cetrimide** solution may be used if a detergent effect is also required. On neonatal skin, regular use of povidone–iodine and of preparations containing alcohol should be avoided.

For irrigating ulcers or wounds, lukewarm sterile **sodium chloride 0.9% solution** is used but tap water is often appropriate.

Potassium permanganate solution 1 in 10 000, a mild antiseptic with astringent properties, can be used as a soak for exudative eczematous areas (section 13.5.1); treatment should be stopped when the skin becomes dry. Potassium permanganate can stain skin and nails especially with prolonged use.

13.11.1 Alcohols and saline

ALCOHOL

Cautions flammable; avoid broken skin; patients have suffered severe burns when diathermy has been preceded by application of alcoholic skin disinfectants

Contra-indications neonates, see section 13.1

Indication and dose

Skin preparation before injection
apply to skin as necessary

ALCOHOL (*continued*)

Industrial Methylated Spirit, BP
Solution, 19 volumes of ethanol and 1 volume approved wood naphtha, net price '66 OP' (containing 95% by volume alcohol) 100 mL = 32p; '74 OP' (containing 99% by volume alcohol) 100 mL = 32p. Label: 15

Surgical Spirit, BP
Spirit, methyl salicylate 0.5 mL, diethyl phthalate 2%, castor oil 2.5%, in industrial methylated spirit, net price 100 mL = 20p. Label: 15

SODIUM CHLORIDE

Indication and dose

See notes above

Nebuliser diluent section 3.1.5

Sodium depletion section 9.2.1.2

Electrolyte imbalance section 9.2.2.1

Eye section 11.8.1

Oral hygiene section 12.3.4

Sodium Chloride (Non-proprietary)
Solution (sterile), sodium chloride 0.9%, net price 10 × 10-mL unit = £3.60, 10 × 20-mL unit = £10.36, 10 × 30-mL unit = £3.00, 200–mL can = £2.65

Flowfusor® (Fresenius Kabi)
Solution (sterile), sodium chloride 0.9%, net price 120-mL Bellows Pack = £1.55

Irriclens® (ConvaTec)
Solution in aerosol can (sterile), sodium chloride 0.9%, net price 240-mL can = £3.00

Irripod® (C D Medical)
Solution (sterile), sodium chloride 0.9%, net price 25 × 20-mL sachet = £5.50

Miniversol® (Aguettant)
Solution (sterile), sodium chloride 0.9%, net price 30 × 45-mL unit = £15.00; 30 × 100-mL unit = £21.30

Normasol® (Medlock)
Solution (sterile), sodium chloride 0.9%, net price 25 × 25-mL sachet = £5.95; 10 × 100-mL sachet = £7.28

Stericlens® (C D Medical)
Solution in aerosol can (sterile), sodium chloride 0.9%, net price 100-mL can = £1.94, 240-mL can = £2.95

Steripod® Sodium Chloride (Medlock)
Steripod® sodium chloride 0.9% solution (sterile), sodium chloride 0.9%, net price 25 × 20-mL sachet = £6.95

13.11.2 Chlorhexidine salts

CHLORHEXIDINE

Cautions avoid contact with eyes, brain, meninges and middle ear; not for use in body cavities; alcoholic solutions not suitable before diathermy or for use on neonatal skin

Side-effects occasional sensitivity

Indication and dose

See under preparations

Bladder irrigation and catheter patency solutions see section 7.4.4

Chlorhexidine 0.05% (Baxter)
2000 Solution (sterile), pink, chlorhexidine acetate 0.05%, net price 500 mL = 72p, 1000 mL = 77p
For cleansing and disinfecting wounds and burns

Cepton® (LPC)
Skin wash (= solution), red, chlorhexidine gluconate 1%, net price 150 mL = £1.99
For use as skin wash in acne

Lotion, blue, chlorhexidine gluconate 0.1%, net price 150 mL = £1.99
For skin disinfection in acne

CX Antiseptic Dusting Powder® (Adams Hlth.)
Dusting powder, sterile, chlorhexidine acetate 1%, net price 15 g = £2.52
For skin disinfection

Hibiscrub® (SSL)
Cleansing solution, red, chlorhexidine gluconate solution 20% (≡ 4% chlorhexidine gluconate), perfumed, in a surfactant solution, net price 250 mL = £1.10, 500 mL = £1.60, 5 litres = £12.70
Excipients: include fragrance
Use instead of soap for pre-operative hand and skin preparation and for general hand and skin disinfection

Hibisol® (SSL)
Solution, chlorhexidine gluconate solution 2.5% (≡ 0.5% chlorhexidine gluconate), in isopropyl alcohol 70% with emollients, net price 500 mL = £1.70
To be used undiluted for hand and skin disinfection

CHLORHEXIDINE (*continued*)

Hibitane Obstetric® (Centrapharm)
Cream, chlorhexidine gluconate solution 5% (≡ 1% chlorhexidine gluconate), in a pourable water-miscible basis, net price 250 mL = £2.89
For use in obstetrics and gynaecology as an antiseptic and lubricant (for application to skin around vulva and perineum and to hands of midwife or doctor)

Hydrex® (Adams Hlth.)
Solution, chlorhexidine gluconate solution 2.5% (≡ chlorhexidine gluconate 0.5%), in an alcoholic solution, net price 600 mL (clear) = £1.94; 600 mL (pink) = £1.94, 200-mL spray = £1.77, 500-mL spray = £3.01; 600 mL (blue) = £2.12
For pre-operative skin disinfection
Note Flammable
Surgical scrub, chlorhexidine gluconate 4% in a surfactant solution, net price 250 mL = £1.82, 500 mL = £1.92
For pre-operative hand and skin preparation and for general hand disinfection

Unisept® (Medlock)
Solution (sterile), pink, chlorhexidine gluconate 0.05%, net price 25 × 25-mL sachet = £5.59; 10 × 100-mL sachet = £6.84
For cleansing and disinfecting wounds and burns and swabbing in obstetrics

With cetrimide

Tisept® (Medlock)
Solution (sterile), yellow, chlorhexidine gluconate 0.015%, cetrimide 0.15%, net price 25 × 25-mL sachet = £5.59; 10 × 100-mL sachet = £6.84
To be used undiluted for general skin disinfection and wound cleansing

Travasept 100® (Baxter)
Solution (sterile), yellow, chlorhexidine acetate 0.015%, cetrimide 0.15%, net price 500 mL = 72p, 1 litre = 77p
To be used undiluted in skin disinfection such as wound cleansing and obstetrics

Concentrates

Hibitane 5% Concentrate® (SSL)
Solution, red, chlorhexidine gluconate solution 25% (≡ 5% chlorhexidine gluconate), in a perfumed aqueous solution, net price 5 litres = £11.50

Dose

Pre-operative skin preparation
dilute 1 in 10 (0.5%) with alcohol 70%

General skin disinfection
dilute 1 in 100 (0.05%) with water

Note Alcoholic solutions not suitable for use before diathermy (see Alcohol, p. 668) or on neonatal skin

With cetrimide

Hibicet Hospital Concentrate® (SSL)
Solution, orange, chlorhexidine gluconate solution 7.5% (≡ chlorhexidine gluconate 1.5%), cetrimide 15%, net price 5 litres = £8.55

Dose

Skin disinfection and wound cleansing
dilute 1 in 100 (1%) to 1 in 30 with water

Pre-operative skin preparation
dilute 1 in 30 in alcohol 70%

Note Alcoholic solutions not suitable for use before diathermy (see Alcohol, p. 668) or on neonatal skin

13.11.3 Cationic surfactants and soaps

CETRIMIDE

Cautions avoid contact with eyes; avoid use in body cavities

Side-effects skin irritation and occasionally sensitisation

Indication and dose

Skin disinfection

Preparations
Ingredient of *Hibicet Hospital Concentrate®*, *Tisept®*, and *Travasept® 100*, see above

13.11.4 Iodine

POVIDONE–IODINE

Cautions broken skin (see below)

Renal impairment *severe*, avoid regular application to inflamed or broken skin or mucosa
Large open wounds The application of povidone–iodine to large wounds or severe burns may produce systemic adverse effects such as metabolic acidosis, hypernatraemia and impairment of renal function.

Contra-indications preterm neonate gestational age under 32 weeks; infants body-weight under 1.5 kg; regular use in neonates; thyroid disorders; concomitant lithium treatment

Pregnancy avoid regular use

Breast-feeding avoid

13 Skin

POVIDONE–IODINE (*continued*)

Side-effects rarely sensitivity; may interfere with thyroid function tests

Licensed use *Betadine® Dry powder spray* and *Ointment* not licensed for use in children under 2 years; all other *Betadine®* preparations licensed for use in children (age range not specified by manufacturer), but see Contra-indications above

Indication and dose

Skin disinfection for dose see under preparations below

Betadine® (Medlock)

Antiseptic paint, povidone–iodine 10% in an alcoholic solution, net price 8 mL (with applicator brush) = £1.01

Dose

Minor wounds and infections
apply undiluted twice daily

Alcoholic solution, povidone–iodine 10%, net price 500 mL = £1.91

Dose

Pre- and post-operative skin disinfection
apply undiluted

Note Flammable—caution in procedures involving hot wire cautery and diathermy; avoid use in neonates

Antiseptic solution, povidone–iodine 10% in aqueous solution, net price 500 mL = £1.75

Dose

Pre- and post-operative skin disinfection
apply undiluted

Note Not for body cavity irrigation

Dry powder spray, povidone–iodine 2.5% in a pressurised aerosol unit, net price 150-g unit = £2.79

For skin disinfection, particularly minor wounds and infections; **infant** under 2 years not recommended

Note Not for use in serous cavities

Ointment, povidone–iodine 10%, in a water-miscible basis, net price 20 g = £1.39, 80 g = £2.79

Excipients: none as listed in section 13.1.3

For skin disinfection, particularly minor wounds and infections; **infant** under 2 years not recommended

Skin cleanser solution, povidone–iodine 4%, in a surfactant basis, net price 250 mL = £2.14

Dose

retain on skin for 3–5 minutes before rinsing; repeat twice daily; **infant** under 2 years max. treatment duration 3 days

Surgical scrub, povidone–iodine 7.5%, in a non-ionic surfactant basis, net price 500 mL = £1.58

To be used as a pre-operative scrub for hands and skin

Savlon® Dry Antiseptic (Novartis Consumer Health)

Powder spray, povidone–iodine 1.14% in a pressurised aerosol unit, net price 50-mL unit = £2.39

For minor wounds

Videne® (Adams Hlth.)

Alcoholic tincture, povidone–iodine 10%, net price 500 mL = £2.35

Dose

Apply undiluted in pre-operative skin disinfection

Note Flammable—caution in procedures involving hot wire cautery and diathermy; avoid use in neonates

Antiseptic solution, povidone–iodine 10% in aqueous solution, net price 500 mL = £2.35

Dose

Apply undiluted in pre-operative skin disinfection and general antisepsis

Surgical scrub, povidone–iodine 7.5% in aqueous solution, net price 500 mL = £2.35

Dose

Use as a pre-operative scrub for hand and skin disinfection

13.11.5 Phenolics

TRICLOSAN

Cautions avoid contact with eyes

Licensed use no information available

Indication and dose

See under preparations

Aquasept® (Medlock)

Skin cleanser, blue, triclosan 2%, net price 250 mL = £1.10, 500 mL = £1.68

Excipients: include chlorocresol, propylene glycol, fragrance, tetrasodium edetate

For disinfection and pre-operative hand preparation

Manusept® (Medlock)

Antibacterial hand rub, triclosan 0.5%, isopropyl alcohol 70%, net price 250 mL = £1.07, 500 mL = £1.56

Excipients: none as listed in section 13.1.3

For disinfection and pre-operative hand preparation

Note Flammable

Ster-Zac Bath Concentrate® (Medlock)

Solution, triclosan 2%, net price 28.5 mL = 40p, 500 mL = £2.24

Dose

Prevention of cross-infection
use 28.5 mL in an adult-size bath, or 1 mL in 5 litres of water

Excipients: include trisodium edetate

13.11.6 Astringents, oxidisers, and dyes

HYDROGEN PEROXIDE

Cautions large or deep wounds; avoid on healthy skin and eyes; bleaches fabric; incompatible with products containing iodine or potassium permanganate

Licensed use licensed for use in children (age range not specified by manufacturer)

Indication and dose

Superficial bacterial skin infection see under preparation below

Crystacide® (GP Pharma)
Cream, hydrogen peroxide 1%, net price 10 g = £3.71, 25 g = £6.21

Dose

Superficial bacterial skin infection
apply 2–3 times daily for up to 3 weeks

Excipients: include edetic acid (EDTA), propylene glycol

Hioxyl®
Section 13.11.7

POTASSIUM PERMANGANATE

Cautions irritant to mucous membranes

Indication and dose

Cleansing and deodorising suppurating eczematous reactions (section 13.5.1) and wounds
for wet dressings or baths, use approx. 0.01% (1 in 10 000) solution
Note Stains skin and clothing

Potassium Permanganate Solution
Solution, potassium permanganate 0.1% (1 in 1000) in water
Note to be diluted 1 in 10 to provide a 0.01% (1 in 10 000) solution

Permitabs® (Centrapharm)
Solution tablets, for preparation of topical solution, potassium permanganate 400 mg, net price 30-tab pack = £6.22
Note 1 tablet dissolved in 4 litres of water provides a 0.01% (1 in 10 000) solution

13.11.7 Preparations for promotion of wound healing

Desloughing agents Alginate, hydrogel and hydrocolloid dressings (BNF Appendix 8) are effective at wound debridement. Sterile larvae (maggots) (*LarvE®*, Zoobiotic) are also used for managing sloughing wounds and are prescribable on the NHS. Dextranomer beads are designed for applying to sloughing ulcers but they are less effective than dressings and are rarely used nowadays.

Desloughing solutions and creams are also of little clinical value and are rarely used nowadays. Substances applied to an open area are easily absorbed and perilesional skin is easily sensitised; gravitational dermatitis may be complicated by superimposed contact sensitivity to substances such as neomycin or lanolin.

The enzyme preparation streptokinase–streptodornase, which removes slough, can provoke hypersensitivity reactions; furthermore, antibodies against streptokinase may reduce the thrombolytic effectiveness of parenteral streptokinase.

Growth factor A topical preparation of **becaplermin** (recombinant human platelet-derived growth factor) is used as an adjunct treatment of full-thickness, neuropathic, diabetic ulcers. It enhances the formulation of granulation tissue, thereby promoting wound healing.

Aserbine® (Goldshield)
Solution, benzoic acid 0.15%, malic acid 2.25%, propylene glycol 40%, salicylic acid 0.0375%, net price 500 mL = £3.61
Excipients: include fragrance

Dose

Use as wash before each application of cream (or use as wet dressing)

Hioxyl® (Ferndale)
Cream, hydrogen peroxide (stabilised) 1.5%, net price 25 g = £2.16, 100 g = £6.76
Excipients: include cetostearyl alcohol

Dose

Apply when necessary and if necessary cover with a dressing

Regranex® (Janssen-Cilag) PoM
Gel, becaplermin (recombinant human platelet-derived growth factor) 0.01%, net price 15 g = £275
Excipients: include hydroxybenzoates

Dose

Full-thickness, neuropathic, diabetic ulcers (no larger than 5 cm²)
apply thin layer daily and cover with gauze dressing moistened with physiological saline; max. duration of treatment 20 weeks (reassess if no healing after first 10 weeks)

Cautions malignant disease; avoid on sites with infection, malignancy or peripheral arteriopathy

Side-effects pain; infections including cellulitis and osteomyelitis, local reactions including erythema; *rarely* bullous eruption, oedema, and hypertrophic granulation

Note Regranex® is not licensed for use in children

Varidase Topical® (Wyeth) PoM
Powder, streptokinase 100 000 units, streptodornase 25 000 units. For preparing solutions for topical use, net price with sterile physiological saline 20 mL (combi-pack) = £10.06
Excipients: none as listed in section 13.1.3

Dose

Reconstitute with 20 mL sterile Sodium Chloride 0.9% (or Water for Injections) and apply as wet dressing 1–2 times daily; cover with semi-occlusive dressing; irrigate lesion thoroughly with Sodium Chloride 0.9% and remove loosened material before next application; also used to dissolve clots in the bladder or urinary catheters

Contra-indications active haemorrhage, severe hypertension

Side-effects infrequent allergic reactions (reduced by careful and frequent removal of exudate and thorough irrigation with physiological saline); fever, transient burning, haemorrhage, and hypersensitivity reactions including shock reported

13.12 Antiperspirants

Aluminium chloride is a potent antiperspirant used in the treatment of axillary, palmar, and plantar hyperhidrosis. Aluminium salts are also incorporated in preparations used for minor fungal skin infections associated with hyperhidrosis.

In more severe cases specialists use tap water or **glycopyrronium bromide** (as a 0.05% solution) in the iontophoretic treatment of hyperhidrosis of palms and soles.

Botulinum A toxin-haemagglutinin complex (section 4.9.3) is licensed for use intradermally for severe hyperhidrosis of the axillae unresponsive to topical antiperspirant or other antihidrotic treatment; intradermal treatment is unlikely to be tolerated by most children and should be administered under hospital specialist supervision.

ALUMINIUM SALTS

Cautions avoid contact with eyes or mucous membranes; avoid use on broken or irritated skin; do not shave axillae or use depilatories within 12 hours of application; avoid contact with clothing

Side-effects skin irritation

Licensed use licensed for use in children (age range not specified by manufacturer)

Indication and dose

Hyperhidrosis affecting axillae, hands or feet
Apply liquid formulation at night to dry skin, wash off the following morning, initially apply daily then reduce frequency as condition improves—do not bathe immediately before use

Hyperhidrosis, bromidrosis, intertrigo, and prevention of tinea pedis and related conditions
Apply powder to dry skin

Anhydrol Forte® (Dermal)
Solution (= application), aluminium chloride hexahydrate 20% in an alcoholic basis, net price 60-mL bottle with roll-on applicator = £2.62. Label: 15
Excipients: none as listed in section 13.1.3

[1]**Driclor®** (Stiefel)
Application, aluminium chloride hexahydrate 20% in an alcoholic basis, net price 60-mL bottle with roll-on applicator = £2.82. Label: 15
Excipients: none as listed in section 13.1.3
1. A 30-mL pack is on sale to the public

ZeaSORB® (Stiefel)
Dusting powder, aldioxa 0.22%, chloroxylenol 0.5%, net price 50 g = £2.15
Excipients: include fragrance

GLYCOPYRRONIUM BROMIDE

Cautions see section 15.1.3 (but poorly absorbed and systemic effects unlikely)

Contra-indications see section 15.1.3 (but poorly absorbed and systemic effects unlikely), infections affecting the treatment site

Side-effects see section 15.1.3 (but poorly absorbed and systemic effects unlikely), tingling at administration site

Licensed use licensed for use in children (age range not specified by manufacturer)

Indication and dose

Iontophoretic treatment of hyperhidrosis
consult product literature; only 1 site to be treated at a time, max. 2 sites treated in any 24 hours, treatment not to be repeated within 7 days

Other indications section 15.1.3

Robinul® (Antigen) PoM
Powder, glycopyrronium bromide, net price 3 g = £110.00

13.13 Wound management products and Elastic Hosiery

Preparations
See BNF Appendix 8

13.14 Topical circulatory preparations

These preparations are used to improve circulation in conditions such as bruising and superficial thrombophlebitis but are of little value. First aid measures such as rest, ice, compression, and elevation should be used. Topical preparations containing heparinoids should not be used on large areas of skin, broken or sensitive skin, or mucous membranes. Chilblains are best managed by avoidance of exposure to cold; neither systemic nor topical vasodilator therapy is established as being effective.

Hirudoid® (Genus)
Cream, heparinoid 0.3% in a vanishing-cream basis, net price 50 g = £1.39
Excipients: include cetostearyl alcohol, hydroxybenzoates (parabens)

Dose

Superficial thrombophlebitis, bruising, and haematoma
Child 5–18 years apply up to 4 times daily

Gel, heparinoid 0.3%, net price 50 g = £1.39
Excipients: include propylene glycol, fragrance

Dose

Superficial thrombophlebitis, bruising, and haematoma
Child 5–18 years apply up to 4 times daily

Lasonil® (Bayer Consumer Care)
Ointment, heparinoid 0.8% in white soft paraffin, net price 40 g = £1.08
Excipients: include wool fat derivative

Dose

Superficial soft-tissue injuries
Child 6–18 years apply 2–3 times daily

14 Immunological products and vaccines

14.1 Active immunity

Vaccines may consist of:

1. a *live attenuated* form of a virus (e.g. rubella or measles vaccine) or bacteria (e.g. BCG vaccine)
2. *inactivated* preparations of the virus (e.g. influenza vaccine) or bacteria, or
3. *extracts of* or *detoxified exotoxins* produced by a micro-organism (e.g. tetanus vaccine).

They stimulate production of antibodies and other components of the immune mechanism.

Live attenuated vaccines usually produce a durable immunity but not always as long-lasting as that of the natural infection. When two live virus vaccines are required (and are not available as a combined preparation) they should be given either simultaneously at different sites or separated by an interval of at least 4 weeks.

Inactivated vaccines may require a primary series of injections of vaccine to produce adequate antibody response and in most cases booster (reinforcing) injections are required; the duration of immunity varies from months to many years. Some inactivated vaccines are adsorbed onto an adjuvant (such as aluminium hydroxide) to enhance the antibody response.

> Advice in this chapter reflects that in the handbook *Immunisation against Infectious Disease* (1996), which in turn reflects the guidance of the Joint Committee on Vaccination and Immunisation (JCVI).
>
> Chapters from the handbook are available at www.dh.gov.uk
>
> The advice incorporates changes announced by the Chief Medical Officer and Health Department Updates.

Side-effects Some vaccines (e.g. poliomyelitis) produce very few reactions, while others (e.g. measles and rubella) may produce a very mild form of the disease. Some vaccines may produce discomfort at the site of injection and mild fever and malaise. Occasionally there are more serious untoward reactions and these should always be reported to the CSM. Anaphylactic reactions are very rare but can be fatal (see section 3.4.3 for management). The product literature should be consulted for full details of side-effects.

> Post-immunisation pyrexia in infants
>
> The parent should be advised that if pyrexia develops after childhood immunisation, the infant can be given a dose of paracetamol and, if necessary, a second dose given 6 hours later; ibuprofen may be used if paracetamol is unsuitable. The parent should be warned to seek medical advice if the pyrexia persists.
>
> For post-immunisation pyrexia in an infant aged 2–3 months, the dose of paracetamol is 60 mg; the dose of ibuprofen is 50 mg (on doctor's advice). An oral syringe can be obtained from any pharmacy to give the small volume required.

Contra-indications Most vaccines have some basic contra-indication to their use, and the product literature and *Immunisation against Infectious Disease* should be consulted for details. In general, vaccination should be postponed if the child is suffering from an *acute illness*. Minor illnesses without fever or systemic upset are not contra-indications. Anaphylaxis with a preceding dose of a vaccine (or vaccine component) is a contra-indication to further doses.

Hypersensitivity to egg, with evidence of previous anaphylactic reaction, contra-indicates influenza vaccine, tick-borne encephalitis vaccine, and yellow fever vaccine. Some viral vaccines contain small quantities of antibacterials; such vaccines may need to be withheld from children who are *extremely sensitive to the antibacterial*. Other excipients in vaccines may also rarely cause allergic reactions. The presence of the following excipients in vaccines and immunological products has been noted under the relevant entries:

Gelatin	Neomycin	Streptomycin
Gentamicin	Penicillins	Thiomersal
Kanamycin	Polymyxin B	

Live vaccines should not be administered routinely during pregnancy because of possible harm to the fetus but where there is a significant risk of exposure (e.g. to yellow fever), the need for vaccination usually outweighs any possible risk to the fetus. Without specialist advice, live vaccines should not be given to individuals with *impaired immune response*, whether caused by disease (for special reference to *HIV infection*, see below) or treatment with high doses of corticosteroids or other immunosuppressive drugs. They should not be given to those being treated for *malignant conditions* with chemotherapy or generalised radiotherapy[1,2]. The response to vaccines may be reduced and there is risk of generalised infection with live vaccines.

The Royal College of Paediatrics and Child Health has produced a statement, *Immunisation of the Immunocompromised Child (2002)* (available at www.rcpch.ac.uk).

The intramuscular route should not be used in children with bleeding disorders such as haemophilia or thrombocytopenia. Vaccines that are usually given by the intramuscular route may be given by subcutaneous injection in those with bleeding disorders.

Note The Department of Health has advised *against the use of jet guns* for vaccination owing to the risk of transmitting blood-borne infections, such as HIV.

Vaccines and HIV infection HIV-positive children with or without symptoms can receive the following live vaccines:

MMR (but not whilst severely immunosuppressed), varicella-zoster (but avoid if immunity significantly impaired—consult product literature);[2,3]

and the following inactivated vaccines:

cholera (oral), diphtheria, haemophilus influenzae type b, hepatitis A, hepatitis B, influenza, meningococcal, pertussis, pneumococcal, poliomyelitis[4], rabies, tetanus, typhoid (injection).

HIV-positive individuals should **not** receive:

BCG, yellow fever[5]

Note The above advice differs from that for other immunocompromised patients.

Vaccines and asplenia The following vaccines are recommended for asplenic children or those with splenic dysfunction:

haemophilus influenzae type b, meningococcal group C, pneumococcal, influenza.

For antibiotic prophylaxis in asplenia see p. 289.

1. Live vaccines should be postponed until at least 3 months after stopping corticosteroids or other immunosuppressive drugs and 6 months after stopping chemotherapy or generalised radiotherapy (at least 12 months after discontinuing immunosuppressants following bone-marrow transplantation).
2. Use of normal immunoglobulin should be considered after exposure to measles (see p. 700) and varicella–zoster immunoglobulin considered after exposure to chickenpox or herpes zoster (see p. 701).
3. The Royal College of Paediatrics and Child Health recommends that MMR is not given to a child with HIV infection whilst severely immunosuppressed.
4. Inactivated poliomyelitis vaccine is now used instead of oral poliomyelitis vaccine for routine immunisation of children.
5. If yellow fever risk is unavoidable, specialist advice should be sought.

Prematurity Children born prematurely should receive all routine immunisations based on the actual date of birth. There is no evidence that premature infants are at increased risk of adverse reactions from vaccines. Seroconversion may be unreliable in babies born earlier than 28 weeks' gestation or in babies treated with corticosteroids for chronic lung disease; consideration should be given to testing for antibodies against *Haemophilus influenzae* (type b), meningococcal C, and hepatitis B after primary immunisation.

Immunisation schedule

Vaccines for the childhood immunisation schedule should be obtained from **local health authorities** or **direct from Farillon**—not to be prescribed on FP10 (HS21 in Northern Ireland; GP10 in Scotland; WP10 in Wales).

During first year of life

Diphtheria, Tetanus, Pertussis (Acellular, Component), Poliomyelitis (Inactivated) and Haemophilus Type b Conjugate Vaccine (Adsorbed)

3 doses at intervals of 4 weeks; first dose at 2 months of age

plus

Meningococcal Group C Conjugate Vaccine

3 doses at intervals of 4 weeks; first dose at 2 months of age

BCG Vaccine (for neonates at risk only)

See section 14.4, BCG Vaccines

> Changes to the immunisation schedule to protect against pneumococcal infection and to extend protection against *Haemophilus influenzae* type b and meningococcal group C infections were announced in February 2006; further details, including the date for introducing the changes, are available from www.dh.gov.uk.

During second year of life

Measles, Mumps and Rubella Vaccine, Live (MMR)

Single dose at 12–15 months of age

Before school or nursery school entry

Adsorbed Diphtheria [low dose], **Tetanus, Pertussis (Acellular, Component) and Inactivated Poliomyelitis Vaccine**

or

Adsorbed Diphtheria, Tetanus, Pertussis (Acellular, Component) and Inactivated Poliomyelitis Vaccine

Single booster dose

Preferably allow interval of at least 3 years after completing basic course; can be given at same session as MMR Vaccine but use separate syringe and needle, and give in different limb

plus

Measles, Mumps and Rubella Vaccine, Live (MMR)

Single dose

Can be given at same session as Adsorbed Diphtheria [low dose], Tetanus, Pertussis (Acellular, Component) and Inactivated Poliomyelitis Vaccine but use separate syringe and needle, and use different limb

Before leaving school or before employment or further education

Adsorbed Diphtheria [low dose], **Tetanus and Inactivated Poliomyelitis Vaccine**

Single booster dose

During adult life

Measles, Mumps and Rubella Vaccine, Live (MMR) (for females of child-bearing age susceptible to rubella)

Single dose

Females of child-bearing age should be tested for rubella antibodies and if sero-negative offered rubella immunisation (using the MMR vaccine)—exclude pregnancy before immunisation, but see also section 14.4, Measles, Mumps and Rubella Vaccine

Adsorbed Diphtheria [low dose], **Tetanus and Inactivated Poliomyelitis Vaccine** (if not previously immunised)

3 doses at intervals of 4 weeks

Booster dose at least 1 year after primary course and again 5–10 years later maintains satisfactory level of protection

High-risk groups

For information on high-risk groups, see section 14.4 under individual vaccines

BCG Vaccines

Hepatitis A Vaccine

Hepatitis B Vaccine

Influenza Vaccine

Pneumococcal Vaccines

Tetanus Vaccines

14.2 Passive immunity

Immunity with immediate protection against certain infective organisms can be obtained by injecting preparations made from the plasma of immune individuals with adequate levels of antibody to the disease for which protection is sought (see under Immunoglobulin section 14.5). This passive immunity lasts only a few weeks; where necessary passive immunisation can be repeated.

Antibodies of human origin are usually termed *immunoglobulins*. The term *antiserum* is applied to material prepared in animals. Because of serum sickness and other allergic-type reactions that may follow injections of antisera, this therapy has been replaced wherever possible by the use of immunoglobulins. Reactions are theoretically possible after injection of human immunoglobulins but reports of such reactions are very rare.

14.3 Storage and use

Care must be taken to store all vaccines and other immunological products under the conditions recommended in the product literature, otherwise the preparation may become ineffective. **Refrigerated storage** is usually necessary; many vaccines need to be stored at 2–8°C and not allowed to freeze. Vaccines should be protected from light. Unused vaccine in multidose vials without preservative (most live virus vaccines) should be discarded within 1 hour of first use; those containing a preservative should be discarded within 3 hours or at the end of a session. Unused vaccines should be disposed of by incineration at a registered disposal contractor.

Particular attention must be paid to instructions on the use of diluents. Vaccines which are liquid suspensions or are reconstituted before use should be adequately mixed to ensure uniformity of the material to be injected.

14.4 Vaccines and antisera

Availability Anthrax and yellow fever vaccines, botulism antitoxin, diphtheria antitoxin, and snake and spider venom antitoxins are available from local designated holding centres.

For antivenom, see Emergency Treatment of Poisoning, p. 47.

Enquiries for vaccines not available commercially can also be made to:

Immunisation and Communicable Diseases Branch
Department of Health
Skipton House
80 London Road
London, SE1 6LH.
Tel: (020) 7972 1522

In Scotland information about availability of vaccines can be obtained from a Specialist in Pharmaceutical Public Health. In Wales enquiries for vaccines not commercially available should be directed to:

Welsh Medicines Information Centre
University Hospital of Wales
Cardiff, CF14 4XW.
Tel: (029) 2074 2979

and in Northern Ireland:

Regional Pharmacist (procurement co-ordination)
United Hospitals Trust Pharmacy Dept
Whiteabbey Hospital
Doagh Road
Newtownabbey, BT37 9RH.
Tel: (028) 9086 5181 ext 2386

For further details of availability, see under individual vaccines.

Anthrax vaccine

Anthrax vaccine is rarely required for children. For further information see BNF section 14.4.

BCG vaccines

BCG (Bacillus Calmette-Guérin) is a live attenuated strain derived from *Mycobacterium bovis* which stimulates the development of hypersensitivity to *M. tuberculosis*. BCG vaccine should be given intradermally by operators skilled in the technique (see below).

The expected reaction to successful BCG vaccination is induration at the site of injection followed by a local lesion which starts as a papule 2 or more weeks after vaccination; the lesion may ulcerate then subside over several weeks or months, leaving a small flat scar. A dry dressing may be used if the ulcer discharges, but air should **not** be excluded.

Serious reactions with BCG are uncommon and most often consist of prolonged ulceration or subcutaneous abscess formation due to faulty injection technique. Anaphylaxis and disseminated BCG complications, such as osteitis or osteomyelitis, are rare.

BCG is recommended for the following groups of children if BCG immunisation has not previously been carried out and they are negative for tuberculoprotein hypersensitivity:

- all neonates and infants (0–12 months) living in areas where the incidence of tuberculosis is greater than 40 per 100 000;
- neonates, infants, and children under 16 years with a parent or grandparent born in a country with an incidence of tuberculosis greater than 40 per 100 000;
- new immigrants aged under 16 who were born in, or lived for more than 3 months in a country with an incidence of tuberculosis greater than 40 per 100 000;
- contacts of those with active respiratory tuberculosis;
- children staying for more than 1 month in countries with an incidence of tuberculosis greater than 40 per 100 000 (section 14.6).

All children of 6 years and over being considered for BCG immunisation must first be given a skin test for hypersensitivity to tuberculoprotein (see under Diagnostic agents, below). A skin test is not necessary a child under 6 years provided that the child has not stayed for longer than 1 month in a country with an incidence of tuberculosis of greater than 40 per 100 000, and has not had contact with a person with tuberculosis.

BCG vaccine may be given simultaneously with another live vaccine (see also section 14.1), but if they are not given at the same time, an interval of 4 weeks should normally be allowed between them. When BCG is given to infants, there is no need to delay the primary immunisations.

See section 14.1 for general contra-indications. BCG is also contra-indicated in children with generalised septic skin conditions (in the case of eczema, a vaccination site free from lesions should be chosen).

For advice on chemoprophylaxis against tuberculosis, see section 5.1.9.

Intradermal

Bacillus Calmette-Guérin Vaccine ▼ PoM

BCG Vaccine, Dried/Tub/BCG

A freeze-dried preparation of live bacteria of a strain derived from the bacillus of Calmette and Guérin.

Dose

- **By intradermal injection**

  Neonate 0.05 mL

  Child 1 month–1 year 0.05 mL

  Child 1–18 years 0.1 mL

Available from health authorities or direct from Farillon (SSI brand, multidose vial with diluent)

Intradermal injection technique Skin is stretched between thumb and forefinger and needle (size 25G or 26G) inserted (bevel upwards) for about 3 mm into superficial layers of dermis (almost parallel with surface). Needle should be short with short bevel (can usually be seen through epidermis during insertion). Tense raised blanched bleb showing tips of hair follicles is sign of correct injection; 7 mm bleb ≡ 0.1 mL injection, 3 mm bleb ≡ 0.05 mL injection; if considerable resistance not felt, needle is too deep and should be removed and reinserted before giving more vaccine.
To be injected at insertion of deltoid muscle onto humerus (keloid formation more likely with sites higher on arm); tip of shoulder should be **avoided**.

Diagnostic agents

The *Mantoux test* is recommended for tuberculin skin testing, but no licensed preparation is currently available. Guidance for healthcare professionals is available at www.immunisation.nhs.uk.

In the Mantoux test, the diagnostic dose is given by intradermal injection of Tuberculin Purified Protein Derivative (PPD).

The *Heaf test* (involving the use of multiple-puncture apparatus) is no longer available.

Note Tuberculin testing should not be carried out within 4 weeks of receiving a live viral vaccine since response to tuberculin may be inhibited.

> **Safe use**
> The strength of tuberculin PPD in the following product may be different to the strengths of products used previously for the Mantoux test; care is required to select the correct strength

Tuberculin Purified Protein Derivative (Non-proprietary) PoM

(Tuberculin PPD)

Injection, heat-treated products of growth and lysis of appropriate *Mycobacterium* spp. 20 units/mL (2 units/0.1-mL dose) (for routine use), 1.5-mL vial; 100 units/0.1 mL (10 units/0.1 mL dose), 1.5-mL vial

Dose

Mantoux test

- **By intradermal injection**

  2 units (0.1 mL of 20 units/mL strength) for routine Mantoux test; if first test is negative and a further test is considered appropriate 10 units (0.1 mL of 100 units/mL strength)

Available on a named patient basis from Farillon (SSI brand)

Botulism antitoxin

A trivalent botulism antitoxin is available for the post-exposure prophylaxis of botulism and for the treatment of children thought to be suffering from botulism. It specifically neutralises the toxins produced by *Clostridium botulinum* types A, B, and E. It is not effective against infantile botulism as the toxin (type A) is seldom, if ever, found in the blood in this type of infection.

Hypersensitivity reactions are a problem. It is essential to read the contra-indications, warnings, and details of sensitivity tests on the package insert. Prior to treatment checks should be made regarding previous administration of any antitoxin and history of any allergic condition, e.g. asthma, hay fever, etc. All children should be tested for sensitivity (diluting the antitoxin if history of allergy).

Botulism Antitoxin PoM

A preparation containing the specific antitoxic globulins that have the power of neutralising the toxins formed by types A, B, and E of *Clostridium botulinum*.

Note The BP title Botulinum Antitoxin is not used because the preparation currently in use may have a different specification

Dose

Prophylaxis

Consult product literature

Available from local designated centres, for details see TOXBASE (requires registration) www.spib.axl.co.uk. For supplies outside working hours apply to other designated centres and, as a last resort, to Department of Health Duty Officer (Tel (020) 7210 3000).

Cholera vaccine

Cholera vaccine (oral) contains inactivated Inaba (including El-Tor biotype) and Ogawa strains of *Vibrio cholerae*, serotype O1 together with recombinant B-subunit of the cholera toxin produced in Inaba strains of *V.cholerae*, serotype O1.

Oral cholera vaccine is licensed for travellers to endemic or epidemic areas on the basis of current recommendations (see also section 14.6). Immunisation should be completed at least 1 week before potential exposure. However, there is no requirement for cholera vaccination for international travel.

Immunisation with cholera vaccine does not provide complete protection and all travellers to a country where cholera exists should be warned that scrupulous attention to food, water, and personal hygiene is **essential**.

Cautions and side-effects Food, drink, and other oral medicines should be avoided 1 hour before and after vaccination. Side-effects of oral cholera vaccine include diarrhoea, abdominal pain, headache; rarely nausea, vomiting, loss of appetite, dizziness, fever, and respiratory symptoms can also occur.

See section 14.1 for general contra-indications.

Injectable cholera vaccine provides unreliable protection and is no longer available in the UK.

Dukoral (Chiron) ▼ PoM

Oral suspension, for dilution with solution of effervescent sodium bicarbonate granules, heat- and formaldehyde-inactivated Inaba (including El-Tor biotype) and Ogawa strains of *Vibrio cholerae* bacteria and recombinant cholera toxin B-subunit produced in *V. cholerae*, net price 2-dose pack = £16.00

Dose

- **By mouth**

  Child 2–6 years 3 doses each separated by an interval of 1 week

  Child 6–18 years 2 doses separated by an interval of 1 week

Booster dose can be given after 6 months for child 2–6 years, and after 2 years for child over 6 years

Administration Consult product literature for dilution and administration

Diphtheria vaccines

Diphtheria vaccines are prepared from the toxin of *Corynebacterium diphtheriae* and adsorption on aluminium hydroxide or aluminium phosphate improves antigenicity. The vaccine stimulates the production of the protective antitoxin. Single-antigen diphtheria vaccine is not available and adsorbed diphtheria vaccine is given as a combination product containing other vaccines.

For primary immunisation *of children aged between 2 months and 10 years* vaccination is recommended usually in the form of 3 doses (separated by 1-month intervals) of **diphtheria, tetanus, pertussis (acellular, component), poliomyelitis (inactivated) and haemophilus type b conjugate vaccine (adsorbed)** (see schedule, section 14.1). In unimmunised children aged *over 10 years* the primary course comprises of 3 doses of **adsorbed diphtheria** [low dose], **tetanus and inactivated poliomyelitis vaccine**.

Important
See changes to immunisation schedule, p. 677

A booster dose should be given 3 years after the primary course. Children *under 10 years* should receive *either* **adsorbed diphtheria, tetanus, pertussis (acellular, component) and inactivated poliomyelitis vaccine** *or* **adsorbed diphtheria** [low dose], **tetanus, pertussis (acellular, component) and inactivated polio-**

myelitis vaccine. Children aged *over 10 years* should receive **adsorbed diphtheria** [low dose], **tetanus, and inactivated poliomyelitis vaccine**.

A second booster dose of adsorbed diphtheria [low dose], tetanus and inactivated poliomyelitis vaccine should be given 10 years after the previous booster dose.

Children travelling to areas with a risk of diphtheria infection should be fully immunised according to the UK schedule. If more than 10 years have lapsed since completion of the UK schedule, a dose of **adsorbed diphtheria** [low dose], **tetanus and inactivated poliomyelitis vaccine** should be administered.

Advice on the management of cases of diphtheria, carriers, contacts and outbreaks must be sought from health protection units. The immunisation history of infected children and their contacts should be determined; those who have been incompletely immunised should complete their immunisation and fully immunised individuals should receive a reinforcing dose. For advice on antibacterial treatment to prevent a secondary case of diphtheria in a non-immune child, see Table 2, section 5.1.

See section 14.1 for general contra-indications.

Diphtheria vaccines for children under 10 years

Important **Not** recommended for children *aged 10 years or over* (see Diphtheria vaccines for children over 10)

Diphtheria, Tetanus, Pertussis (Acellular, Component), Poliomyelitis (Inactivated) and Haemophilus Type b Conjugate Vaccine (Adsorbed)

Injection, suspension of diphtheria toxoid, tetanus toxoid, acellular pertussis, inactivated poliomyelitis and *Haemophilus influenzae* type b (conjugated to tetanus protein), net price 0.5-mL prefilled syringe = £19.94

Excipients: may include neomycin, polymyxin B and streptomycin

Dose

Primary immunisation
- **By intramuscular injection**
  Child 2 months–10 years 3 doses of 0.5 mL at intervals of 1 month (see schedule, section 14.1)

Available as part of childhood immunisation schedule, from health authorities or Farillon; brands include ▼*Infanrix-IPV+Hib*®, ▼*Pediacel*®

Important See changes to immunisation schedule, p. 677

Adsorbed Diphtheria, Tetanus, Pertussis (Acellular, Component) and Inactivated Poliomyelitis Vaccine

Injection, suspension of diphtheria toxoid, tetanus toxoid, acellular pertussis and inactivated poliomyelitis vaccine components adsorbed on a mineral carrier, net price 0.5-mL prefilled syringe = £17.56

Excipients: include neomycin and polymyxin B

Dose
- **By intramuscular injection**
  Child 3–10 years 0.5 mL (see schedule, section 14.1)

Available as part of childhood immunisation schedule, from health authorities or Farillon; brands include ▼ *Infanrix-IPV*®

Adsorbed Diphtheria [low dose], Tetanus, Pertussis (Acellular, Component) and Inactivated Poliomyelitis Vaccine

Injection, suspension of diphtheria toxoid [low dose], tetanus toxoid, acellular pertussis and inactivated poliomyelitis vaccine components adsorbed on a mineral carrier, net price 0.5-mL prefilled syringe = £11.98

Excipients: include neomycin, polymyxin B and streptomycin

Dose
- **By intramuscular injection**
  Child 3–10 years 0.5 mL (see schedule, section 14.1)

Available as part of childhood immunisation schedule, from health authorities or Farillon; brands include ▼*Repevax*®

Diphtheria vaccines for children over 10 years

A low dose of diphtheria toxoid is sufficient to recall immunity in older children previously immunised against diphtheria but whose immunity may have diminished with time; it is insufficient to cause serious reactions that may occur when a higher-dose vaccine is used in a child who is already immune. Preparations containing low dose diphtheria should be used for children *over 10 years*, whether for primary immunisation or for booster doses.

Adsorbed Diphtheria [low dose], Tetanus and Inactivated Poliomyelitis Vaccine

Injection, suspension of diphtheria toxoid [low dose], tetanus toxoid and inactivated poliomyelitis vaccine components adsorbed on a mineral carrier, net price 0.5-mL prefilled syringe = £6.74

Excipients: include neomycin, polymyxin B and streptomycin

Dose
- **By intramuscular injection**
  Child 10-18 years primary immunisation, 3 doses of 0.5 mL at intervals of 1 month; booster, 0.5 mL after 5 years, repeated 10 years later (see schedule, section 14.1)

Available as part of childhood schedule, from health authorities or Farillon; brands include ▼*Revaxis*®

Adsorbed Diphtheria [low dose] and Tetanus Vaccine for Adults and Adolescents PoM

DT/Vac/Ads(Adult)

Injection, suspension of diphtheria formol toxoid and tetanus formol toxoid adsorbed on a mineral carrier, net price 0.5-mL prefilled syringe = £2.48

Note Not recommended for routine use (vaccines which also protect against poliomyelitis should be used for primary immunisation and for boosters)

Brands include *Diftavax®*

Diphtheria antitoxin

Diphtheria antitoxin is used for passive immunisation. It is derived from horse serum and reactions are common after administration; resuscitation facilities should be available immediately.

It is now only used in suspected cases of diphtheria (without waiting for bacteriological confirmation); tests for hypersensitivity should be first carried out.

It is no longer used for prophylaxis because of the risk of hypersensitivity; unimmunised contacts should be promptly investigated and given antibacterial prophylaxis (section 5.1, table 2) and vaccine (see notes above).

Diphtheria Antitoxin PoM

Dip/Ser

Dose

Prophylaxis not recommended therefore no dose stated (see notes above)

Treatment of nasal diphtheria
- **By intravenous infusion**
  Child under 10 years 5000–10 000 units
  Child 10-18 years 10 000–20 000 units

Treatment of tonsillar diphtheria
- **By intravenous infusion**
  Child under 10 years 7500–12 500 units
  Child 10-18 years 15 000–25 000 units

Treatment of pharyngeal or laryngeal diphtheria
- **By intravenous infusion**
  Child under 10 years 10 000–20 000 units
  Child 10-18 years 20 000–40 000 units

Combined types of diphtheria or delayed diagnosis
- **By intravenous infusion**
  Child under 10 years 20 000–30 000 units
  Child 10–18 years 40 000–60 000 units

Severe diphtheria
- **By intravenous infusion**
  Child under 10 years 20 000–50 000 units
  Child 10–18 years 40 000–100 000 units

Available from Communicable Disease Surveillance Centre (Tel (020) 8200 6868) or in Northern Ireland from Public Health Laboratory, Belfast City Hospital (Tel (028) 9032 9241).

Haemophilus influenzae type B vaccine

Haemophilus influenzae type b (Hib) vaccine is made from capsular polysaccharide; it is conjugated with a protein such as tetanus toxoid to increase immunogenicity, especially in young children. Haemophilus influenzae type b vaccine is a component of the primary course of childhood immunisation (see schedule, section 14.1); it is combined with diphtheria, tetanus, pertussis (acellular, component) and inactivated poliomyelitis vaccine (see under Diphtheria Vaccines). For infants under 1 year, the course consists of 3 doses of a vaccine containing haemophilus influenzae type b component, with an interval of 1 month between doses. Unimmunised children over 12 months need receive only 1 dose of the vaccine, but for full protection against other diseases, 3 doses should be given of diphtheria, tetanus, pertussis (acellular, component), poliomyelitis (inactivated) and haemophilus type b conjugate vaccine (adsorbed). The risk of infection falls sharply in older children and the vaccine is not normally required for children over 10 years.

Important

See changes to immunisation schedule, p. 677

Haemophilus influenzae type b vaccine may be given to those over 10 years who are considered to be at increased risk of invasive *H. influenzae* type b disease (such as those with sickle-cell disease and those receiving treatment for malignancy). Also, children over 1 year with asplenia or splenic dysfunction, irrespective of age or the time lapsed since splenectomy, should receive a single dose of haemophilus influenzae type b vaccine; infants under 1 year should be given 3 doses. Children vaccinated in infancy who have had a splenectomy or develop splenic dysfunction should receive a single booster dose of haemophilus influenzae type b vaccine after the age of 1 year. For elective splenectomy, the vaccine should ideally be given at least 2 weeks before surgery.

Side-effects of haemophilus influenzae type b vaccine include fever, restlessness, prolonged crying, loss of appetite, vomiting, diarrhoea; hypersensitivity reactions (including anaphylaxis) and collapse have been reported.

See section 14.1 for general contra-indications.

Single component

Hiberix® (GSK) PoM

Injection, powder for reconstitution, capsular polysaccharide of *Haemophilus influenzae* type b (conjugated to tetanus protein), net price single-dose vial = £8.97

Dose

- **By intramuscular injection**

  Child 2 months–18 years at risk because of asplenia (and where combination vaccination not required—see notes above), 0.5 mL

Combined vaccines

See also Diphtheria vaccines

Menitorix® (GSK) ▼ PoM

Injection, powder for reconstitution, capsular polysaccharide of *Haemophilus influenzae* type b and capsular polysaccharide of *Nerisseria meningitidis* group C (both conjugated to tetanus protein), net price single dose vial (with syringe containing 0.5 mL diluent) = £39.87

Dose

- **By intramuscular injection**

  Child 2 months–2 years 0.5 mL

  Note This vaccine combination will form part of the childhood immunisation schedule to be introduced in 2006–7, see p. 677

Important See changes to immunisation schedule, p. 677

Hepatitis A vaccine

Hepatitis A vaccine is prepared from formaldehyde-inactivated hepatitis A virus grown in human diploid cells.

Immunisation is recommended for:

- residents of homes for those with severe learning difficulties;
- children with haemophilia treated with plasma-derived clotting factors;
- children with severe liver disease;
- children travelling to high-risk areas (see p. 703);
- adolescents who are at risk due to their sexual behaviour;
- parenteral drug abusers.

Immunisation should be considered for:

- children with chronic liver disease including chronic hepatitis B or chronic hepatitis C;
- prevention of secondary cases in close contacts of confirmed cases of hepatitis A, within 7 days of onset of disease in the primary case.

Side-effects of hepatitis A vaccine, usually mild, include transient soreness, erythema, and induration at the injection site. Less common effects include fever, malaise, fatigue, headache, nausea, diarrhoea, and loss of appetite; arthralgia, myalgia, and, generalised rashes are occasionally reported.

See section 14.1 for general contra-indications.

Single component

Avaxim® (Sanofi Pasteur) PoM

Injection, suspension of formaldehyde-inactivated hepatitis A virus (GBM grown in human diploid cells) 320 antigen units/mL adsorbed onto aluminium hydroxide, net price 0.5-mL prefilled syringe = £19.19

Excipients: include neomycin

Dose

- **By intramuscular injection** (see note below)

  Child 16–18 years 0.5 mL as a single dose; booster dose 0.5 mL 6–12 months after initial dose; further booster doses, 0.5 mL every 10 years

  Note Booster dose may be delayed by up to 3 years if not given after recommended interval following primary dose with *Avaxim®*. The deltoid region is the preferred site of injection. The subcutaneous route may be used for children with bleeding disorders

14 Immunological products and vaccines

Epaxal® (MASTA) PoM

Injection, suspension of formaldehyde-inactivated hepatitis A virus (RG-SB grown in human diploid cells) at least 48 units/mL, net price 0.5-mL prefilled syringe = £23.81

Dose

- **By intramuscular injection** (see note below)

  Child 1–18 years 0.5 mL as a single dose; booster dose 0.5 mL 6–12 months after initial dose (1–6 months if splenectomised)

  Note Booster dose may be delayed by up to 4 years if not given after recommended interval following primary dose. The deltoid region is the preferred site of injection. The subcutaneous route may be used for children with bleeding disorders

Safe Practice *Epaxal®* contains influenza virus haemagglutinin grown in the allantoic cavity of chick embryos, therefore contra-indicated in those hypersensitive to eggs or chicken protein.

Havrix Monodose® (GSK) PoM

Injection, suspension of formaldehyde-inactivated hepatitis A virus (HM 175 grown in human diploid cells) 1440 ELISA units/mL adsorbed onto aluminium hydroxide, net price 1-mL prefilled syringe = £22.14, 0.5-mL (720 ELISA units) prefilled syringe (*Havrix Junior Monodose®*) = £16.77

Excipients: include neomycin

Dose

- **By intramuscular injection** (see note below)

  Child 1–15 years 0.5 mL as a single dose; booster dose 0.5 mL 6–12 months after initial dose

  Child 16–18 years 1 mL as a single dose; booster dose 1 mL 6–12 months after initial dose

  Note Booster dose may be delayed by up to 3 years if not given after recommended interval following primary dose with *Havrix Monodose®*. The deltoid region is the preferred site of injection. The subcutaneous route may be used for children with bleeding disorders

Vaqta® Paediatric (Sanofi Pasteur) PoM

Injection, suspension of formaldehyde-inactivated hepatitis A virus (grown in human diploid cells) 50 antigen units/mL adsorbed onto hydroxyphosphate sulphate, net price 0.5-mL vial = £14.55

Excipients: include neomycin

Dose

- **By intramuscular injection** (see note below)

  Child 1–18 years 0.5 mL as a single dose; booster dose 0.5 mL 6–18 months after initial dose

  Note The deltoid region is the preferred site of injection. The subcutaneous route may be used for children with bleeding disorders

◢With hepatitis B vaccine

Twinrix® (GSK) PoM

Injection, inactivated hepatitis A virus 720 ELISA units and recombinant (DNA) hepatitis B surface antigen 20 micrograms/mL adsorbed onto aluminium hydroxide and aluminium phosphate, net price 1-mL prefilled syringe (*Twinrix® Adult*) = £27.76, 0.5-mL prefilled syringe (*Twinrix® Paediatric*) = £20.79

Excipients: include neomycin and thiomersal

Dose

- **By intramuscular injection** (see note below)

  Child 1–15 years primary course 3 doses of 0.5 mL, the second 1 month and the third 6 months after first dose

  Child 16–18 years primary course, 3 doses of 1 mL, the second 1 month and the third 6 months after first dose

  Accelerated schedule (e.g. for travellers departing within 1 month) for child over 16 years, second dose given 7 days after first dose, third dose after further 14 days and fourth dose after 12 months

Note Primary course should be completed with *Twinrix®* (single component vaccines given at appropriate intervals may be used for booster dose); the deltoid region is the preferred site of injection in older children; anterolateral thigh is the preferred site in infants; not to be injected into the buttock (vaccine efficacy reduced); subcutaneous route used for children with bleeding disorders (but immune response may be reduced).

Important *Twinrix®* **not** recommended for post-exposure prophylaxis following percutaneous (needle-stick), ocular or mucous membrane exposure to hepatitis B virus.

◢With typhoid vaccine

Hepatyrix® (GSK) PoM

Injection, suspension of inactivated hepatitis A virus (grown in human diploid cells) 1440 ELISA units/mL adsorbed onto aluminium hydroxide, combined with typhoid vaccine containing 25 micrograms/mL virulence polysaccharide antigen of *Salmonella typhi*, net price 1-mL prefilled syringe = £32.08

Excipients: include neomycin

Dose

- **By intramuscular injection** (see note below)

  Child 15-18 years 1 mL as a single dose; booster doses, see under single component hepatitis A vaccine and under polysaccharide typhoid vaccine

  Note The deltoid region is the preferred site of injection. The subcutaneous route may be used for children with bleeding disorders

ViATIM® (Sanofi Pasteur) PoM

Injection, suspension of inactivated hepatitis A virus (grown in human diploid cells) 160 antigen units/mL adsorbed onto aluminium hydroxide, combined with typhoid vaccine containing 25 micrograms/mL virulence polysaccharide antigen of *Salmonella typhi*, net price 1-mL prefilled syringe = £30.22

Dose

- **By intramuscular injection** (see note below)

  Child 16-18 years 1 mL as a single dose; booster doses, see under single component hepatitis A vaccine and under polysaccharide typhoid vaccine

  Note The deltoid region is the preferred site of injection. The subcutaneous route may be used for children with bleeding disorders

Hepatitis B vaccine

Hepatitis B vaccine contains inactivated hepatitis B virus surface antigen (HBsAg) adsorbed on aluminium hydroxide adjuvant. It is made biosynthetically using recombinant DNA technology. The vaccine is used in individuals at high risk of contracting hepatitis B.

In the UK, high-risk groups include:

- parenteral drug abusers and their household contacts;
- adolescents who are at risk from their sexual behaviour,
- close family contacts of a case or carrier;
- babies whose mothers have had hepatitis B during pregnancy *or* are positive for hepatitis B surface antigen (regardless of e-antigen markers); hepatitis B vaccination is started immediately on delivery and *hepatitis B immunoglobulin* (see p. 701) given at the same time (but preferably at a different site). Babies whose mothers are positive for hepatitis B surface antigen and for e-antigen antibody should receive the vaccine only (but babies weighing 1.5 kg or less should receive the immunoglobulin regardless of the mother's e-antigen antibody status);
- children with haemophilia, those receiving regular blood transfusions or blood products, and carers responsible for the administration of such products;
- children with chronic renal failure including those on haemodialysis. Children receiving haemodialysis should be monitored for antibodies annually and re-immunised if necessary. Home carers (of dialysis patients) who are negative for hepatitis B surface antigen should be vaccinated;
- children with chronic liver disease;
- patients of day-care or residential accommodation for those with severe learning difficulties;
- children in custodial institutions;
- children travelling to areas of high or intermediate prevalence who are at increased risk or who plan to remain there for lengthy periods (see p. 703);
- families adopting children from countries with a high or intermediate prevalence of hepatitis B;
- foster carers.

Immunisation may take up to 6 months to confer adequate protection; the duration of immunity is not known precisely, but a single booster 5 years after the primary course may be sufficient to maintain immunity for those who continue to be at risk.

More detailed guidance is given in the memorandum *Immunisation against Infectious Disease*. Immunisation does not eliminate the need for commonsense precautions for avoiding the risk of infection from known carriers by the routes of infection which have been clearly established, consult *Guidance for Clinical Health Care Workers: Protection against Infection with Blood-borne Viruses* (available at www.dh.gov.uk). Accidental inoculation of hepatitis B virus-infected blood into a wound, incision, needle-prick, or abrasion may lead to infection, whereas it is unlikely that indirect exposure to a carrier will do so.

Specific **hepatitis B immunoglobulin** ('HBIG') is available for use with the vaccine in those accidentally inoculated and in neonates at special risk of infection (section 14.5).

A combined hepatitis A and hepatitis B vaccine is also available.

See section 14.1 for general contra-indications.

Single component

Engerix B® (GSK) PoM

Injection, suspension of hepatitis B surface antigen (rby, prepared from yeast cells by recombinant DNA technique) 20 micrograms/mL adsorbed onto aluminium hydroxide, net price 0.5-mL (paediatric) vial = £9.16, 0.5-mL (paediatric) prefilled syringe = £9.67, 1-mL vial = £12.34, 1-mL prefilled syringe = £12.99

Excipients: include thiomersal

Dose

- **By intramuscular injection** (see note below)

Neonate (except if born to hepatitis B surface antigen-positive mother, see below), 3 doses of 10 micrograms, second dose 1 month and third dose 6 months after first dose

Child 1 month–15 years 3 doses of 10 micrograms, second dose 1 month and third dose 6 months after first dose; if compliance likely to be low in child 10-15 years increase dose to 20 micrograms

Child 15–18 years 3 doses of 20 micrograms, second dose 1 month and third dose 6 months after first dose

Accelerated schedule may be used with third dose 2 months after first dose and fourth dose at 12 months in all age groups; *exceptionally* (e.g. for travellers departing within 1 month) children over 15 years can be given second dose 7 days after first dose, third dose after further 14 days and fourth dose after 12 months

Infant born to hepatitis B surface antigen-positive mother
- **By intramuscular injection**
  (see note below)

Neonate 4 doses of 10 micrograms, first dose at birth with hepatitis B immunoglobulin injection (separate site) the second 1 month, the third 2 months and the fourth 12 months after first dose

Chronic haemodialysis patients
- **By intramuscular injection**
  (see note below)

Child 15–18 years 4 doses of 40 micrograms, the second 1 month, the third 2 months and the fourth 6 months after the first dose; immunisation schedule and booster doses may need to be adjusted in those with low antibody concentration

Note Deltoid muscle is preferred site of injection in older children; anterolateral thigh is preferred site in neonates, infants and young children; not to be injected into the buttock (vaccine efficacy reduced); subcutaneous route used for children with bleeding disorders

Fendrix® (GSK) ▼ PoM
Injection, suspension of hepatitis B surface antigen (prepared from yeast cells by recombinant DNA technique) 40 micrograms/mL adsorbed onto aluminium phosphate, net price 0.5-mL prefilled syringe = £38.10

Dose

Renal insufficiency patients (including pre-haemodialysis and haemodialysis patients)
- **By intramuscular injection**
  (see note below)

Child 15–18 years 4 doses of 20 micrograms, the second 1 month, the third 2 months and the fourth 6 months after the first dose; immunisation schedule and booster doses may need to be adjusted in those with low antibody concentration

Note Deltoid muscle is preferred site of injection; not to be injected into the buttock (vaccine efficacy reduced); subcutaneous route used for children with bleeding disorders

HBvaxPRO® (Sanofi Pasteur) PoM
Injection, suspension of hepatitis B surface antigen (prepared from yeast cells by recombinant DNA technique) 10 micrograms/mL adsorbed onto aluminium hydroxyphosphate sulphate, net price 0.5-mL (5-microgram) vial = £9.02, 1-mL (10-microgram) vial = £12.00; 40 micrograms/mL, 1-mL (40-microgram) vial = £29.30

Dose
- **By intramuscular injection**
  (see note below)

Neonate (except if born to hepatitis B surface antigen-positive mother, see below), 3 doses of 5 micrograms, second dose 1 month and third dose 6 months after first dose

Child 1 month–16 years 3 doses of 5 micrograms, second dose 1 month and third dose 6 months after first dose

Child 16–18 years 3 doses of 10 micrograms, second dose 1 month and third dose 6 months after first dose

Accelerated schedule (all ages) third dose 2 months after first dose and fourth dose at 12 months

Booster doses may be required in immunocompromised patients with low antibody concentration

Infant born to hepatitis B surface antigen-positive mother (see also notes above)
- **By intramuscular injection**
  (see note below)

Neonate 5 micrograms, first dose at birth with hepatitis B immunoglobulin injection (separate site), the second 1 month, the third 2 months and the fourth 12 months after the first dose

Chronic haemodialysis patients
- **By intramuscular injection**
  (see note below)

Child 16–18 years 3 doses of 40 micrograms, second dose 1 month and third dose 6 months after first dose; booster doses may be required in those with low antibody concentration

Note Deltoid muscle is preferred site of injection in older children; anterolateral thigh is preferred site in neonates and infants; not to be injected into the buttock (vaccine efficacy reduced); subcutaneous route used for children with bleeding disorders

With hepatitis A vaccine

See Hepatitis A Vaccine

Influenza vaccine

While most viruses are antigenically stable, the influenza viruses A and B (especially A) are constantly altering their antigenic structure as indicated by changes in the haemagglutinins (H) and neuraminidases (N) on the surface of the viruses. It is essential that influenza vaccines in use contain the H and N components of the prevalent strain or strains. Every year the World Health Organization recommends which strains should be included.

The recommended strains are grown in the allantoic cavity of chick embryos (therefore **contra-indicated** in those with anaphylactic hypersensitivity to eggs).

Since **influenza vaccines** will not control epidemics they are recommended *only for persons at high risk*. Annual immunisation is strongly recommended for children (including infants that were preterm or low birth-weight) aged over 6 months with the following conditions:

- chronic respiratory disease, including asthma;
- chronic heart disease;
- chronic liver disease;
- chronic renal disease;
- diabetes mellitus;
- immunosuppression because of disease (including asplenia or splenic dysfunction) or treatment (including prolonged corticosteroid treatment);
- HIV infection (regardless of immune status).

Influenza immunisation is also recommended for children living in long-stay facilities.

Interactions: Appendix 1 (vaccines).

See section 14.1 for general contra-indications.

Inactivated Influenza Vaccine (Split Virion) (Non-proprietary) PoM

Flu

Injection, suspension of formaldehyde-inactivated influenza virus (split virion), net price 0.25-mL prefilled syringe = £6.29, 0.5-mL prefilled syringe = £6.29

Excipients: may include neomycin and polymixin

Dose

- **By intramuscular injection**
  Child 6–35 months 0.25–0.5 mL; dose repeated after 4-6 weeks if not previously vaccinated
  Child 3–13 years 0.5 mL; dose repeated after 4-6 weeks if not previously vaccinated
  Child 13–18 years 0.5 mL as a single dose
  Note Subcutaneous route used for children with bleeding disorders

Inactivated Influenza Vaccine (Surface Antigen) (Non-proprietary) PoM

Flu or Flu(adj)

Injection, suspension of propiolactone-inactivated influenza virus (surface antigen), net price 0.5-mL prefilled syringe = £3.98

Excipients: may include neomycin, polymyxin B and thiomersal

Dose

- **By intramuscular injection**
  Child 6–35 months 0.25–0.5 mL; dose repeated after 4-6 weeks if not previously vaccinated
  Child 3–13 years 0.5 mL; dose repeated after 4-6 weeks if not previously vaccinated
  Child 13–18 years 0.5 mL as a single dose
  Note Subcutaneous route used for children with bleeding disorders

Agrippal® (Wyeth) PoM

Injection, suspension of formaldehyde-inactivated influenza virus (surface antigen), net price 0.5-mL prefilled syringe = £5.03

Excipients: include kanamycin and neomycin

Dose

- **By intramuscular injection**
  Child 6–35 months 0.25–0.5 mL; dose repeated after 4-6 weeks if not previously vaccinated
  Child 3–13 years 0.5 mL; dose repeated after 4-6 weeks if not previously vaccinated
  Child 13–18 years 0.5 mL as a single dose
  Note Subcutaneous route used for children with bleeding disorders

Begrivac® (Wyeth) PoM

Injection, suspension of formaldehyde-inactivated influenza virus (split virion), net price 0.5-mL prefilled syringe = £5.03

Excipients: include polymyxin B

Dose

- **By intramuscular injection**
  Child 6–35 months 0.25–0.5 mL; dose repeated after 4-6 weeks if not previously vaccinated
  Child 3–13 years 0.5 mL; dose repeated after 4-6 weeks if not previously vaccinated
  Child 13–18 years 0.5 mL as a single dose

Note Subcutaneous route used for children with bleeding disorders

Enzira® (Chiron Vaccines) ▼ PoM

Injection, suspension of inactivated influenza virus (split virion), net price 0.5-mL prefilled syringe = £6.59

Excipients: include neomycin and polymixin B

Dose

- **By intramuscular injection**
  Child 6–35 months 0.25–0.5 mL; dose repeated after 4-6 weeks if not previously vaccinated
  Child 3–13 years 0.5 mL; dose repeated after 4-6 weeks if not previously vaccinated
  Child 13–18 years 0.5 mL as a single dose
  Note Subcutaneous route used for children with bleeding disorders

Fluarix® (GSK) PoM

Injection, suspension of formaldehyde-inactivated influenza virus (split virion), net price 0.5-mL prefilled syringe = £4.49

Excipients: include gentamicin and traces of thiomersal

Dose

- **By intramuscular injection**
  Child 6–35 months 0.25–0.5 mL; dose repeated after 4-6 weeks if not previously vaccinated
  Child 3–13 years 0.5 mL; dose repeated after 4-6 weeks if not previously vaccinated
  Child 13–18 years 0.5 mL as a single dose
  Note Subcutaneous route used for children with bleeding disorders

Influvac Sub-unit® (Solvay) PoM

Injection, suspension of formaldehyde-inactivated influenza virus (surface antigen), net price 0.5-mL prefilled syringe = £5.22

Excipients: include gentamicin

Dose

- **By intramuscular injection**
  Child 6–35 months 0.25–0.5 mL; dose repeated after 4-6 weeks if not previously vaccinated
  Child 3–13 years 0.5 mL; dose repeated after 4-6 weeks if not previously vaccinated
  Child 13–18 years 0.5 mL as a single dose
  Note Subcutaneous route used for children with bleeding disorders

Mastaflu® (MASTA) PoM

Injection, suspension of formaldehyde-inactivated influenza virus (surface antigen), net price 0.5-mL prefilled syringe = £6.50

Excipients: include gentamicin

Dose

- **By intramuscular injection**
  Child 6–35 months 0.25–0.5 mL; dose repeated after 4-6 weeks if not previously vaccinated
  Child 3–13 years 0.5 mL; dose repeated after 4-6 weeks if not previously vaccinated
  Child 13–18 years 0.5 mL as a single dose
  Note Subcutaneous route used for children with bleeding disorders

Measles vaccine

Measles vaccine has been replaced by a combined live measles, mumps and rubella vaccine (MMR vaccine).

Administration of a measles-containing vaccine to children may be associated with a mild measles-like syndrome with a measles-like rash and pyrexia about a week after injection. Much less commonly, convulsions and, very rarely, encephalitis have been reported. Convulsions in infants are much less frequently associated with measles vaccines than with other conditions leading to febrile episodes.

MMR vaccine may be used in the control of outbreaks of measles (see under MMR Vaccine).

Single antigen vaccine
No longer available in the UK

Combined vaccines
See MMR vaccine

Measles, Mumps and Rubella (MMR) vaccine

A combined live **measles, mumps, and rubella vaccine** (MMR vaccine) aims to eliminate measles, mumps and rubella (and congenital rubella syndrome). Every child should receive two doses of MMR vaccine by entry to primary school, unless there is a valid contra-indication (see below) or parental refusal. MMR vaccine should be given irrespective of previous measles, mumps or rubella infection.

The first dose of MMR vaccine is given to infants aged 12–15 months. A second dose is given before starting school at 3–5 years of age (see schedule, section 14.1). Children presenting for pre-school booster who have not received the first dose of MMR vaccine should be given a dose of MMR vaccine followed 3 months later by a second dose. At school-leaving age or at entry into further education, MMR immunisation should be offered to individuals of both sexes who have not received both doses. In a young adult who has received only a single dose of MMR in childhood, a second dose is recommended to achieve full protection.

MMR vaccine should be used to protect against rubella in *seronegative females of child-bearing age* (see schedule, section 14.1). MMR vaccine may also be offered to previously *unimmunised and seronegative post-partum* mothers. Vaccination a few days after delivery is important because about 60% of congenital abnormalities from rubella infection occur in babies of mothers who have borne more than one child. Immigrants arriving after the age of school immunisation are particularly likely to require immunisation.

MMR vaccine may also be used in the control of outbreaks of measles and should be offered to susceptible children including babies aged over 6 months who are contacts of a case, within 3 days of exposure to infection; these children should still receive routine MMR vaccinations at the recommended ages. Household contacts of a case, aged between 6 and 9 months, may receive normal immunoglobulin (section 14.5). MMR vaccine is **not suitable** for prophylaxis following exposure to mumps or rubella since the antibody response to the mumps and rubella components is too slow for effective prophylaxis.

Children with impaired immune response should not receive live vaccines (for advice on HIV see section 14.1). If they have been exposed to measles infection they should be given normal immunoglobulin (section 14.5).

Malaise, fever or a rash may occur after the first dose of MMR vaccine, most commonly about a week after vaccination and lasting about 2 to 3 days (section 14.1). Leaflets are available for parents on advice for reducing fever (including the use of paracetamol). Parotid swelling occurs occasionally, usually in the third week, and rarely, arthropathy 2 to 3 weeks after immunisation. Adverse reactions are considerably less common after the second dose of MMR vaccine than after the first dose.

Idiopathic thrombocytopenic purpura has occurred rarely following MMR vaccination, usually within 6 weeks of the first dose. The risk of developing idiopathic thrombocytopenic purpura after MMR vaccine is much less than the risk of developing it after infection with wild measles, mumps or rubella virus. The CSM has recommended that children who develop idiopathic thrombocytopenic purpura within 6 weeks of the first dose of MMR should undergo serological testing before the second dose is due; if the results suggest incomplete immunity against measles, mumps or rubella then a second dose of MMR is recommended. The Specialist and Reference Microbiology Division, Health Protection Agency offers free serological testing for children who develop idiopathic thrombocytopenic purpura *within 6 weeks* of the first dose of MMR.

Post-vaccination aseptic meningitis was reported (rarely and with complete recovery) following vaccination with MMR vaccine containing Urabe mumps vaccine, which has now been discontinued; no cases have been confirmed in association with the currently used Jeryl Lynn mumps vaccine. Children with post-vaccination symptoms are not infectious.

> Reviews undertaken on behalf of the CSM and the Medical Research Council have not found any evidence of a link between MMR vaccination and bowel disease or autism. The Chief Medical Officers have advised that the MMR vaccine is the safest and best way to protect children against measles, mumps, and rubella. Information (including fact sheets and a list of references) may be obtained from:
> www.immunisation.nhs.uk and www.mmrthefacts.nhs.uk

Contra-indications to MMR include:

- children with severe immunosupression (for advice on vaccines and HIV see section 14.1);
- children who have received another live vaccine by injection within 4 weeks;
- children who have had an anaphylactic reaction to excipients such as gelatin and neomycin;
- if given to girls of child-bearing age, pregnancy should be avoided for 1 month;

MMR vaccine should not be given within 3 months of an immunoglobulin injection because response to the measles component may be reduced.

The Department of Health recommends avoiding rubella vaccination during pregnancy. However, if given inadvertently during pregnancy, then termination is not recommended because extensive studies have failed to link rubella vaccination in early pregnancy with fetal damage.

Note Children with a personal or close family history of convulsions should be given MMR vaccine, provided the parents understand that there may be a febrile response; doctors should seek specialist paediatric advice rather than withhold vaccination; there is increasing evidence that MMR vaccine can be given safely even when the child has had an anaphylactic reaction to food containing egg (dislike of egg or refusal to eat egg is not a contra-indication).

See section 14.1 for general contra-indications.

Measles, Mumps and Rubella Vaccine, Live PoM
MMR(live)

Live measles, mumps, and rubella vaccine

Dose

- **By deep subcutaneous or by intramuscular injection**
  Child 1–18 years 0.5 mL (see schedule, section 14.1)
  Child 6 months–1 year [unlicensed use, for outbreaks of measles, see above], 0.5mL followed by routine doses at usual age (see schedule, section 14.1)

Available from health authorities or direct from Farillon as *MMR II*® (*excipients include* gelatin and neomycin) or *Priorix*® (*excipients include* neomycin)

Meningococcal vaccines

Almost all childhood meningococcal disease in the UK is caused by *Neisseria meningitidis* serogroups B and C. **Meningococcal Group C conjugate vaccine** protects only against infection by serogroup C; it can be given from 2 months of age. After early adulthood the risk of meningococcal disease declines, and immunisation is not generally recommended after the age of 25 years.

Childhood immunisation **Meningococcal Group C conjugate vaccine** provides long-term protection against infection by serogroup C of *Neisseria meningitidis* in children from 2 months of age; it is now a component of the primary course of childhood immunisation. The recommended schedule consists of 3 doses starting at 2 months of age with an interval of 1 month between each dose (see schedule, section 14.1). Infants aged 5–12 months not previously vaccinated should receive 2 doses, with an interval of 1 month between doses. It is recommended that meningococcal group C conjugate vaccine be given to anyone aged under 25 years who has not been vaccinated previously with this vaccine; those over 1 year receive a single dose.

> Important
> See changes to immunisation schedule, p. 677

Meningococcal group C conjugate vaccine is also recommended for individuals with a dysfunctional or absent spleen.

Immunisation for travellers Children travelling to countries of risk (see below) should be immunised with a meningococcal polysaccharide vaccine that covers serotypes **A, C, W135 and Y**. Vaccination is particularly important for those living with local people or visiting an area of risk during outbreaks.

Outbreaks of infection with the W135 strain of meningococcus have occurred in Burkina Faso, West Africa and there have been cases in a number of other African countries. Countries with risk in Africa are listed below but outbreaks may also occur in countries not listed:

> Angola, Benin, Burkina Faso, Burundi, Cameroon, Central African Republic, Chad, Democratic Republic of Congo, Eritrea, Ethiopia, Gambia, Ghana, Guinea, Guinea Bissau, Ivory Coast, Kenya, Mali, Mozambique, Namibia, Niger, Nigeria, Rwanda, Senegal, Sierra Leone, Somalia, Sudan, Tanzania, Togo, Uganda, and Zambia.

Proof of vaccination with the tetravalent (A, C, W135 and Y) meningococcal vaccine is required for those travelling to Saudi Arabia during the Hajj and Umrah pilgrimages (where outbreaks of the W135 strain have occurred).

Travellers should be immunised with the meningococcal polysaccharide vaccine that covers serogroups A, C, W135 and Y, even if they have already received meningococcal group C conjugate vaccine. The response to serotype C in unconjugated meningococcal polysaccharide vaccines given to children aged under 18 months is not as good as in adults.

Contacts of infected individuals and laboratory workers For advice on the immunisation of *close contacts* of cases of meningococcal disease in the UK and on the role of the vaccine in the control of *local outbreaks*, consult Guidelines for Public Health Management of Meningococcal Disease in the UK in *Commun Dis Public Health* 2002; **5**: 187–204. See section 5.1 Table 2 for antibacterial prophylaxis to prevent a secondary case of meningococcal meningitis.

Side-effects Side-effects of meningococcal Group C conjugate vaccine include redness, swelling, and pain at the site of the injection, mild fever, irritability, drowsiness, dizziness, nausea, vomiting, diarrhoea, anorexia, headache, myalgia, rash, urticaria, pruritus, malaise, lymphadenopathy, hypotonia, paraesthesia, hypoaesthesia, and syncope. Hypersensitivity reactions (including anaphylaxis, bronchospasm, and angioedema) and seizures have been reported rarely. Symptoms of meningism have also been reported rarely, but there is no evidence that the vaccine causes meningococcal C meningitis. There have been very rare reports of Stevens-Johnson syndrome. The CSM has advised that vaccination provides benefit in terms of lives saved and disabilities prevented.

Meningococcal polysaccharide A, C, W135 and Y vaccine is associated with injection-site reactions and very rarely headache, fatigue, fever, and drowsiness. Hypersensitivity reactions including anaphylaxis have been reported.

See section 14.1 for general contra-indications.

◢Meningococcal Group C conjugate vaccine

> Important See changes to immunisation schedule, p. 677

Meningitec® (Wyeth) PoM
Injection, suspension of capsular polysaccharide antigen of *Neisseria meningitidis* group C (conjugated to *Corynebacterium diphtheriae* protein), adsorbed onto aluminium phosphate, net price 0.5-mL vial = £17.95

Dose

- **By intramuscular injection**
  Child 2 months–1 year for routine immunisation, 3 doses (each of 0.5 mL) at intervals of 1 month (but see notes above and also schedule, section 14.1)
  Child 1–18 years 0.5 mL as a single dose
  Note Subcutaneous route used for children with bleeding disorders

Available as part of childhood immunisation schedule from Farillon

Menjugate® (Chiron) PoM
Injection, powder for reconstitution, capsular polysaccharide antigen of *Neisseria meningitidis* group C (conjugated to *Corynebacterium diphtheriae* protein), adsorbed onto aluminium hydroxide, single-dose and 10-dose vials

Dose
- **By intramuscular injection**
  Child 2 months–1 year for routine immunisation, 3 doses (each of 0.5 mL) at intervals of 1 month (but see notes above and also schedule, section 14.1)
  Child 1–18 years 0.5 mL as a single dose
  Note Subcutaneous route used for children with bleeding disorders

NeisVac-C® (Baxter) PoM
Injection, suspension of polysaccharide antigen of *Neisseria meningitidis* group C (conjugated to tetanus toxoid protein), adsorbed onto aluminium hydroxide, 0.5-mL prefilled syringe

Dose
- **By intramuscular injection**
  Child 2 months–1 year for routine immunisation, 3 doses (each of 0.5 mL) at intervals of 1 month (but see notes above and also schedule, section 14.1)
  Child 1–18 years 0.5 mL as a single dose
  Note Subcutaneous route used for children with bleeding disorders

Available from Farillon

Meningococcal Group C conjugate vaccine with Haemophilus Influenzae type B vaccine
See *Haemophilus Influenzae* type B vaccine

Meningococcal polysaccharide A, C, W135 and Y vaccine

ACWY Vax® (GSK) PoM
Injection, powder for reconstitution, capsular polysaccharide antigens of *Neisseria meningitidis* groups A, C, W135 and Y, net price single-dose vial (with syringe containing diluent) = £16.73

Dose
- **By deep subcutaneous injection**
  Child 3 months–2 years [unlicensed use] 2 doses of 0.5 mL; antibody response may be suboptimal in this age group
  Child 2–18 years 0.5 mL as a single dose

Mumps vaccine

Single antigen vaccine
No longer available in the UK

Combined vaccine
See MMR Vaccine

Pertussis vaccine

Pertussis vaccine is given as a combination preparation containing other vaccines (see under Diphtheria Vaccines). Acellular vaccines are derived from highly purified components of *Bordetella pertussis.*

For the routine immunisation of infants, primary immunisation with pertussis (whooping cough) vaccine is recommended usually in the form of 3 doses (separated by 1-month intervals) of **diphtheria, tetanus, pertussis (acellular, component), poliomyelitis (inactivated) and haemophilus type b conjugate vaccine (adsorbed)** (see schedule, section 14.1).

A booster dose should be given 3 years after the primary course; children *under 10 years* should receive *either* **adsorbed diphtheria, tetanus, pertussis (acellular, component) and inactivated poliomyelitis vaccine** *or* **adsorbed diphtheria** [low dose], **tetanus, pertussis (acellular, component) and inactivated poliomyelitis vaccine**.

The incidence of local and systemic effects is lower with vaccines containing acellular pertussis components than with the whole-cell pertussis vaccine used previously.

The vaccine should not be withheld from children with a history to a preceding dose of:

- fever, irrespective of severity;
- persistent crying or screaming for more than 3 hours;
- severe local reaction, irrespective of extent.

These side-effects were associated with whole-cell pertussis vaccine.

Predisposition to neurological problems When there is a personal or family history of *febrile* convulsions, there is an increased risk of these occurring during fever from any cause including immunisation. In such children, immunisation is *recommended* but advice on the *prevention of fever* (see Post-immunisation pyrexia, p. 675) should be given before immunisation.

When a child has had a convulsion not associated with fever and the neurological condition is not deteriorating, immunisation is *recommended.*

Where there is a *still evolving neurological problem* including poorly controlled epilepsy, immunisation should be *deferred* and the child referred to a specialist. Immunisation is recommended if a cause for the neurological disorder is found. If a cause is not found, immunisation should be deferred until the condition is stable.

Children with stable neurological disorders (e.g. spina bifida, congenital brain abnormality, and perinatal hypoxic ischaemic encephalopathy) should be immunised according to the recommended schedule.

Older children All children up to the age of 10 years should receive primary immunisation with diphtheria, tetanus, pertussis (acellular, component), poliomyelitis (inactivated) and haemophilus type b conjugate vaccine (adsorbed). Primary immunisation against pertussis is not currently recommended in individuals over 10 years of age.

Combined vaccines

Combined vaccines, see under Diphtheria vaccines

Pneumococcal vaccines

Pneumococcal vaccines protect against infection with *Streptococcus pneumoniae* (pneumococcus); the vaccines contain polysaccharide from capsular pneumococci. Pneumococcal polysaccharide vaccine contains purified polysaccharide from 23 capsular types of pneumococci whereas pneumococcal polysaccharide conjugated vaccine contains polysaccharide from 7 capsular types, the polysaccharide being conjugated to protein.

Pneumococcal vaccination is recommended for individuals at special risk as follows:

- child under 5 years with a history of invasive pneumococcal disease;
- asplenia or splenic dysfunction (including homozygous sickle cell disease and coeliac disease which could lead to splenic dysfunction);
- chronic respiratory disease (includes asthma treated with continuous or frequent use of a systemic corticosteroid);
- chronic heart disease;
- chronic renal disease;
- chronic liver disease;
- diabetes mellitus;
- immune deficiency because of disease (e.g. HIV infection) or treatment (including prolonged systemic corticosteroid treatment);
- presence of cochlear implant;
- presence of CSF shunt or other condition where leakage of cerebrospinal fluid could occur.

> Important
> See changes to immunisation schedule, p. 677

Where possible, the vaccine should be given at least 2 weeks before splenectomy, surgery to insert a CSF shunt, cochlear implant surgery, and chemotherapy; children and carers should be given advice about increased risk of pneumococcal infection. A patient card and information leaflet for patients with asplenia are available from the Department of Health or in Scotland from the Scottish Executive, Public Health Division 1 (Tel (0131) 244 2501). Prophylactic antibacterial therapy against pneumococcal infection should not be stopped after immunisation.

Choice of vaccine A single dose of the 23-valent unconjugated **pneumococcal polysaccharide vaccine** is used to immunise children over 5 years who are at special risk of pneumococcal disease. Children under 5 years who are at special risk should receive the 7-valent **pneumococcal polysaccharide conjugated vaccine** as follows:

- infants from 2 months to 6 months should receive 3 doses (separated by 1-month intervals) of pneumococcal polysaccharide conjugated vaccine, starting at 2 months of age; a further dose is given after the first birthday;
- unimmunised infants 6–11 months should receive 2 doses (separated by 1 month) of pneumococcal polysaccharide conjugated vaccine; a further dose is given after the first birthday and at least 1 month after the previous dose;
- children 1–5 years should receive 2 doses (separated by 2 months) of pneumococcal polysaccharide conjugated vaccine.

All children who have received the pneumococcal polysaccharide conjugated vaccine should receive a single dose of the 23-valent pneumococcal polysaccharide vaccine after their second birthday and at least 2 months after the final dose of the 7-valent pneumococcal polysaccharide conjugated vaccine.

Revaccination In individuals with higher concentrations of antibodies to pneumococcal polysaccharides, revaccination with the 23-valent pneumococcal polysaccharide vaccine more commonly produces adverse reactions. Revaccination is therefore not recommended, except every 5 years in individuals in whom the antibody concentration is likely to decline rapidly (e.g. asplenia, splenic dysfunction and nephrotic syndrome). If there is doubt, the need for revaccination should be discussed with a haematologist, immunologist, or microbiologist.

See section 14.1 for general contra-indications.

Pneumococcal polysaccharide vaccines

Pneumovax® II (Sanofi Pasteur) PoM

Polysaccharide from each of 23 capsular types of pneumococcus, net price 0.5-mL vial = £8.83

Dose

Child under 2 years not recommended (suboptimal response, also safety and efficacy not established)

- **By subcutaneous or intramuscular injection**
  Child 2-18 years 0.5 mL; revaccination, see notes above

Pneumococcal polysaccharide conjugated vaccine

Important See changes to immunisation schedule, p. 677

Prevenar® (Wyeth) ▼ PoM

Polysaccharide from each of 7 capsular types of pneumococcus (conjugated to diphtheria toxoid) adsorbed onto aluminium phosphate, net price 0.5-mL prefilled syringe = £34.50

Dose

- **By intramuscular injection**
  Child 2–6 months 3 doses each of 0.5 mL separated by intervals of 1 month and a further dose in second year of life
  Child 6–11 months 2 doses each of 0.5 mL separated by interval of 1 month and a further dose in second year of life
  Child 1–5 years 2 doses each of 0.5 mL separated by interval of 2 months
  Note Deltoid muscle is preferred site of injection in young children; anterolateral thigh is preferred site in infants
  The dose in BNF for Children may differ from that in product literature

Poliomyelitis vaccines

There are two types of poliomyelitis vaccine, inactivated poliomyelitis vaccine and live (oral) poliomyelitis vaccine. Inactivated poliomyelitis vaccine is now recommended for routine immunisation; it is given by injection and contains inactivated strains of human poliovirus types 1, 2 and 3.

A course of primary immunisation consists of 3 doses of a combined preparation containing inactivated poliomyelitis vaccine (see under Diphtheria Vaccines), starting at 2 months of age with intervals of 1 month between doses (see schedule, section 14.1). A course of 3 doses should also be given to all unimmunised adults; no adult should remain unimmunised against poliomyelitis.

Two booster doses of a preparation containing inactivated poliomyelitis vaccine are recommended, the first before school entry and the second before leaving school (see schedule, section 14.1). Booster doses for adults are not necessary except for those at special risk such as travellers to endemic areas, or laboratory staff likely to be exposed to the viruses, or healthcare workers in possible contact with cases; booster doses should be given to such individuals every 10 years.

Preparations containing inactivated poliomyelitis vaccine may be used to complete an immunisation course initiated with the live (oral) poliomyelitis vaccine. Live (oral) vaccine is available only for use during outbreaks. The live (oral) vaccine poses a very rare risk of vaccine-associated paralytic polio because the attenuated strain of the virus can revert to a virulent form. For this reason the live (oral) vaccine must **not** be used for immunosuppressed individuals or their household contacts. The use of inactivated poliomyelitis vaccine removes the risk of vaccine-associated paralytic polio altogether.

Travellers Unimmunised travellers to areas with a high incidence of poliomyelitis should receive a full course of a preparation containing inactivated poliomyelitis vaccine. Those who have not been vaccinated in the last 10 years should receive a booster dose of adsorbed diphtheria [low dose], tetanus and inactivated poliomyelitis vaccine. A list of countries with a high incidence of poliomyelitis can be obtained from www.travax.scot.nhs.uk or by contacting the National Travel Health Network and Centre.

Inactivated (Salk)

Combined vaccines, see under Diphtheria Vaccines

Inactivated Poliomyelitis Vaccine (Non-proprietary) ▼ PoM

IPV

Injection, inactivated suspension of suitable strains of poliomyelitis virus, types 1, 2, and 3, net price 0.5-mL prefilled syringe = £10.35

Excipients: may include neomycin, polymixin B and streptomycin

Note Not recommended for routine use—combination vaccines are recommended for primary immunisation and for boosters (see schedule, section 14.1)

Live (oral) (Sabin)

Poliomyelitis Vaccine, Live (Oral) (GSK) PoM

OPV

A suspension of suitable live attenuated strains of poliomyelitis virus, types 1, 2, and 3. Available in single-dose and 10-dose containers

Excipients: include neomycin and polymyxin B

Dose

Control of outbreaks

Child 1 month–18 years 3 drops; may be given on a lump of sugar; not to be given with foods which contain preservatives

Note Live poliomyelitis vaccine loses potency once the container has been opened—any vaccine remaining at the end of an immunisation session should be discarded; whenever possible sessions should be arranged to avoid undue wastage.

Rabies vaccine

For advice on prophylaxis against rabies and management following potential exposure to rabies, see Rabies Vaccine, BNF section 14.4.

Rubella vaccine

A combined measles, mumps and rubella vaccine (MMR vaccine) aims to eliminate rubella (German measles) and congenital rubella syndrome. MMR vaccine is used for childhood vaccination as well as for vaccinating adults (including women of child-bearing age) who do not have immunity against rubella.

Single antigen vaccine

No longer available in the UK; the combined live measles, mumps and rubella vaccine is a suitable alternative (see MMR vaccine, p. 689)

Combined vaccines

see MMR vaccine

Smallpox vaccine

Limited supplies of **smallpox vaccine** are held at the Specialist and Reference Microbiology Division, Health Protection Agency (Tel. (020) 8200 4400) for the exclusive use of workers in laboratories where pox viruses (such as vaccinia) are handled.

If a wider use of the vaccine is being considered, *Guidelines for smallpox response and management in the post-eradication era* should be consulted at www.dh.gov.uk

Tetanus vaccines

Tetanus vaccines stimulate production of a protective antitoxin. In general, adsorption on aluminium hydroxide or aluminium phosphate improves antigenicity.

Primary immunisation for children under 10 years consists of 3 doses of a combined preparation containing adsorbed tetanus vaccine, with an interval of 1 month between doses (see schedule, section 14.1).

The recommended schedule of tetanus vaccination not only gives protection against tetanus in childhood but also gives the basic immunity for subsequent booster doses (see schedule, section 14.1).

For primary immunisation of children over 10 years previously unimmunised against tetanus, 3 doses of adsorbed diphtheria [low dose], tetanus and inactivated poliomyelitis vaccine are given with an interval of 1 month between doses (see under Diphtheria Vaccines).

Following routine childhood vaccination, 2 booster doses of a preparation containing adsorbed tetanus vaccine are recommended, the first before school entry and the second before leaving school.

If a child presents for a booster dose but has been vaccinated following a tetanus-prone wound, the vaccine preparation administered at the time of injury should be determined. If this is not possible, the booster should still be given to ensure adequate protection against all antigens in the booster vaccine. An adolescent who has received 5 doses of tetanus vaccine is likely to have life-long immunity.

Active immunisation is important for individuals who may not have completed a course of immunisation. Children over 10 years may be given a course of adsorbed diphtheria [low dose], tetanus and inactivated poliomyelitis vaccine.

Very rarely, tetanus has developed after abdominal surgery; carers of children awaiting elective surgery should be asked about the child's tetanus immunisation status and the child should be immunised if necessary. Parenteral drug abuse is also associated with tetanus; those abusing drugs by injection should be vaccinated if unimmunised. Booster doses should be given if there is any doubt about the immunisation status.

For travel recommendations see section 14.6.

Wounds Wounds are considered to be tetanus-prone if they are sustained more than 6 hours before surgical treatment *or* at any interval after injury and are puncture-type (particularly if contaminated with soil or manure) *or* show much devitalised tissue *or* are septic *or* are compound fractures *or* contain foreign bodies. All wounds should receive thorough cleansing.

- For *clean wounds*, fully immunised individuals (those who have received a total of 5 doses of a tetanus-containing vaccine at appropriate intervals) and those whose primary immunisation is complete (with boosters up to date), do not require tetanus vaccine; individuals whose primary immunisation is incomplete or whose boosters are not up to date require a reinforcing dose of a tetanus-containing vaccine (followed by further doses as required to complete the schedule); non-immunised individuals (or whose immunisation status is not known or who have been fully immunised but are now immunocompromised) should be given a dose of the appropriate tetanus-containing vaccine immediately (followed by completion of the full course of the vaccine if records confirm the need).
- For *tetanus-prone wounds*, management is as for clean wounds with the addition of a dose of tetanus immunoglobulin (section 14.5) given at a different site; in fully immunised individuals and those whose primary immunisation is complete (see above) the immunoglobulin is needed only if the risk of infection is especially high (e.g. contamination with manure). Antibacterial prophylaxis (with benzylpenicillin, co-amoxiclav, or metronidazole) may also be required for tetanus-prone wounds.

See section 14.1 for general contra-indications.

Combined vaccines
See Diphtheria Vaccines

Tick-borne encephalitis vaccine

Tick-borne encephalitis vaccine is licensed for immunisation of those in high-risk areas based on official recommendations (see section 14.6). Children walking or camping in warm forested areas of Central and Eastern Europe and Scandinavia, particularly from April to October when ticks are most prevalent, are at greatest risk of tick-borne encephalitis. Ideally, immunisation should be completed at least one month before travel.

Fever exceeding 40°C may occur, particularly after the first dose of tick-borne encephalitis vaccine. Other side effects include arrhythmias; the vaccine should be used with caution in children with cardiovascular disease. Tick-borne encephalitis vaccine is **contra-indicated** in those with acute febrile infection and severe hypersensitivity to egg protein. See section 14.1 for general contra-indications and side-effects.

FSME-IMMUN® (MASTA) PoM

Injection, suspension, inactivated Neudörfl tick-borne encephalitis virus strain, cultivated in chick embryo cells, net price 0.25-mL prefilled syringe (*FSME-IMMUN Junior®*) = £32.00, 0.5-mL prefilled syringe = £32.00

Excipients: include gentamicin and neomycin

Dose

- **By intramuscular injection into deltoid muscle**
  Child 1–16 years 3 doses of 0.25 mL, second dose after 1–3 months and third dose after a further 5–12 months
  Child 16–18 years 3 doses each of 0.5 mL, second dose after 1–3 months and third dose after further 5–12 months

Immunocompromised (including those receiving immunosuppressants), antibody concentration may be measured 4 weeks after second dose and dose repeated if protective levels not achieved

Note To achieve more rapid protection, second dose may be given 14 days after first dose

First booster dose given within 3 years of third dose, subsequent boosters after 3–5 years

Typhoid vaccines

Typhoid immunisation is advised for children travelling to areas where sanitation standards may be poor, although it is not a substitute for scrupulous personal hygiene (see p. 703).

Capsular **polysaccharide typhoid vaccine** is usually given by *intramuscular* injection. Young children may respond suboptimally to the vaccine, but children aged between 12 and 18 months should be immunised if the risk of typhoid fever is considered high (immunisation is not recommended for infants under 12 months). Booster doses are needed every 3 years on continued exposure. Local reactions, including pain, swelling or erythema, may appear 48–72 hours after administration.

An **oral typhoid vaccine** is also available. It is a **live attenuated** vaccine contained in an enteric-coated capsule. It is taken *by mouth* as 3 doses of one capsule on alternate days, providing protection 7–10 days after the last dose. Protection may persist for up to 3 years in those constantly (or repeatedly) exposed to *Salmonella typhi*, but occasionally travellers require further courses at intervals of 1 year. Oral typhoid vaccine is **contra-indicated** in children who are immunosuppressed (whether due to disease or its treatment) and in acute gastro-intestinal illness; it is inactivated by concomitant administration of anti-bacterials. Administration of a dose of oral typhoid vaccine should be coordinated so that *mefloquine* is not taken for at least 12 hours before or after a dose; vaccination with oral typhoid vaccine should preferably be completed at least 3 days before the first dose of mefloquine or other antimalarials (except proguanil hydrochloride with atovaquone, which may be given concomitantly). Side-effects to oral typhoid vaccine include nausea, vomiting, abdominal pain, diarrhoea, headache, fever and hypersensitivity reactions including, rarely, anaphylaxis.

For general contra-indications to vaccines, see section 14.1.

Polysaccharide vaccine for injection

Typherix® (GSK) PoM

Injection, Vi capsular polysaccharide typhoid vaccine, 50 micrograms/mL virulence poly-saccharide antigen of *Salmonella typhi*, net price 0.5-mL prefilled syringe = £9.93

Dose

- **By intramuscular injection**
  Child under 2 years [unlicensed use], 0.5 mL; response may be suboptimal (see notes above)
  Child 2–18 years 0.5 mL
  Note Subcutaneous route used for children with bleeding disorders

Typhim Vi® (Sanofi Pasteur) PoM

Injection, Vi capsular polysaccharide typhoid vaccine, 50 micrograms/mL virulence poly-saccharide antigen of *Salmonella typhi*, net price 0.5-mL prefilled syringe = £9.49

Dose

- **By intramuscular injection**
  Child under 18 months [unlicensed use], 0.5 mL; response may be suboptimal (see notes above)
  Child 18 months–18 years 0.5 mL
  Note Subcutaneous route used for children with bleeding disorders

Polysaccharide vaccine with hepatitis A vaccine
See Hepatitis A Vaccine

Live oral vaccine

Vivotif® (MASTA) PoM
Capsules, e/c, live attenuated *Salmonella typhi* (Ty21a), net price 3-cap pack = £8.00. Label: 23, 25, counselling, administration

Dose
- **By mouth**
  Child 6–18 years 1 capsule on days 1, 3, and 5
  Counselling. Swallow as soon as possible after placing in mouth with a cold or lukewarm drink; it is important to store capsules in a refrigerator

Varicella–zoster vaccine

Varicella–zoster vaccine (live) is licensed for immunisation against varicella in seronegative individuals. It is not recommended for routine use in children but may be given to seronegative healthy children over 1 year who come into close contact with individuals at high risk of severe varicella infections.

Varicella–zoster vaccine is contra-indicated in pregnancy (avoid pregnancy for 3 months after vaccination). It must not be given to children with primary or acquired immunodeficiency or to children receiving immunosuppressive therapy. For further contra-indications, see section 14.1.

Rarely, the varicella–zoster vaccine virus has been transmitted from the vaccinated individual to close contacts. Therefore, contact with the following should be avoided if a vaccine-related cutaneous rash develops within 4–6 weeks of the first or second dose:

- varicella-susceptible pregnant females;
- individuals at high risk of severe varicella, including those with immunodeficiency or those receiving immunosuppressive therapy.

For reference to specific **varicella–zoster immunoglobulin** see section 14.5.

Varilrix® (GSK) ▼ PoM
Injection, powder for reconstitution, live attenuated varicella–zoster virus (Oka strain) propagated in human diploid cells, net price 0.5-mL vial (with diluent) = £27.31
Excipients: include neomycin

Dose
- **By subcutaneous injection preferably into deltoid region**
  Child 1–12 years (but see notes above), 0.5 mL as a single dose
  Child 13–18 years (see notes above), 2 doses of 0.5 mL separated by an interval of 8 weeks (minimum 6 weeks)

Varivax® (Sanofi Pasteur) ▼ PoM
Injection powder for reconstitution, live attenuated varicella-zoster virus (Oka/Merck strain) propagated in human diploid cells, net price 0.5-mL vial (with diluent) = £32.14
Excipients: include gelatin and neomycin

Dose
- **By subcutaneous injection into deltoid region or higher anterolateral thigh**
  Child 1–12 years (but see notes above) 0.5 mL as a single dose (2 doses separated by 12 weeks in children with asymptomatic HIV infection)
  Child 13–18 years 2 doses of 0.5 mL separated by 4–8 weeks

Yellow fever vaccine

Live yellow fever vaccine is indicated for those travelling or living in areas where infection is endemic (see p. 703) and for laboratory staff who handle the virus or who handle clinical material from suspected cases. Infants under 9 months of age should be vaccinated only if the risk of yellow fever is unavoidable because there is a small risk of encephalitis. The immunity which probably lasts for life is officially accepted for 10 years starting from 10 days after primary immunisation and for a further 10 years immediately after revaccination.

The vaccine should not be given to those with impaired immune responsiveness, or who have had an anaphylactic reaction to egg; it should not be given during pregnancy but if a significant risk of exposure cannot be avoided then vaccination should be delayed to the third trimester if possible (but the need for immunisation usually outweighs risk to the fetus). See section 14.1 for further contra-indications.

Headache, fever, tiredness, and stiffness may occur 4–7 days after vaccination. Other side-effects include myalgia, asthenia, lymphadenopathy, rash, urticaria, and injection-site reactions.

Yellow Fever Vaccine, Live PoM
Yel(live)
Injection, powder for reconstitution, preparation of 17D strain of yellow fever virus grown in fertilized hens eggs

Dose

- **By deep subcutaneous injection**
  Child 9 months–18 years 0.5 mL

Available (only to designated Yellow Fever Vaccination centres) as *Arilvax*® (*excipients: include* gelatin) and *Stamaril*®

14.5 Immunoglobulins

Human immunoglobulins have replaced immunoglobulins of animal origin (antisera) which were frequently associated with hypersensitivity. Injection of immunoglobulins produces immediate protection lasting for several weeks.

Immunoglobulins are produced from pooled human plasma or serum, and are tested and found non-reactive for hepatitis B surface antigen and for antibodies against hepatitis C virus and human immunodeficiency virus (types 1 and 2)

The two types of human immunoglobulin preparation are **normal immunoglobulin** and **specific immunoglobulins.**

Further information about immunoglobulins is included in *Immunisation against Infectious Disease* (see section 14.1) and in the Health Protection Agency's *Immunoglobulin Handbook*: www.hpa.org.uk.

Availability **Normal immunoglobulin** is available from Health Protection and microbiology laboratories only for contacts and the control of outbreaks. It is available commercially for other purposes.

Specific immunoglobulins are available from Health Protection and microbiology laboratories with the exception of **tetanus immunoglobulin** which is distributed through BPL to hospital pharmacies or blood transfusion departments and is also available to general medical practitioners. **Rabies immunoglobulin** is available from the Specialist and Reference Microbiology Division, Health Protection Agency. The large amounts of **hepatitis B immunoglobulin** required by transplant centres should be obtained commercially.

In Scotland all immunoglobulins are available from the *Blood Transfusion Service.* **Tetanus immunoglobulin** is distributed by the *Blood Transfusion Service* to hospitals and general medical practitioners on demand.

Normal immunoglobulin

Human **normal immunoglobulin** ('HNIG') is prepared from pools of at least 1000 donations of human plasma; it contains antibody to measles, mumps, varicella, hepatitis A, and other viruses that are currently prevalent in the general population.

Cautions and side-effects Side-effects of immunoglobulins include malaise, chills, fever, and rarely anaphylaxis. Normal immunoglobulin is **contra-indicated** in patients with known class specific antibody to immunoglobulin A (IgA).

Normal immunoglobulin may **interfere with the immune response to live virus vaccines** which should therefore only be given **at least 3 weeks before or 3 months after** an injection of normal immunoglobulin (this does not apply to yellow fever vaccine since normal immunoglobulin does not contain antibody to this virus).

Uses Normal immunoglobulin is administered by intramuscular injection for the protection of susceptible contacts against **hepatitis A** virus (infectious hepatitis), **measles** and, to a lesser extent, **rubella**.

Special formulations of immunoglobulins for intravenous administration are available for *replacement therapy* for children with congenital agammaglobulinaemia and hypogammaglobulinaemia, for the treatment of idiopathic thrombocytopenic purpura and Kawasaki syndrome (see section 2.9), and for the prophylaxis of infection following bone-marrow transplantation and in children with symptomatic HIV infection who have recurrent bacterial infections. Normal immunoglobulin may also be given intramuscularly or subcutaneously for replacement therapy, but intravenous formulations are normally preferred.

Intravenous immunoglobulin is also used in the treatment of Guillain-Barré syndrome in preference to plasma exchange.

Hepatitis A **Hepatitis A vaccine** is preferred for children at risk of infection (see p. 684) including those visiting areas where the disease is highly endemic (all countries excluding Northern and Western Europe, North America, Japan, Australia, and New Zealand). In unimmunised children, transmission of hepatitis A is reduced by good hygiene. Intramuscular normal immunoglobulin is no longer recommended for routine prophylaxis in travellers but it may be indicated for immunocompromised patients if their antibody response to vaccine is unlikely to be adequate.

Intramuscular normal immunoglobulin is of value in the prevention of infection in close contact of confirmed cases of hepatitis A where there has been a delay in identifying cases or for individuals at high risk of severe disease.

Measles Intramuscular normal immunoglobulin may be given to prevent or attenuate an attack of measles in individuals who do not have adequate immunity. Children with compromised immunity who have come into contact with measles should receive intramuscular normal immunoglobulin as soon as possible after exposure. It is most effective if given within 72 hours but can be effective if given within 6 days. For individuals receiving intravenous immunoglobulin, 100 mg/kg given within 3 weeks before measles exposure should prevent measles. Intramuscular normal immunoglobulin should also be considered for the following individuals if they have been in contact with a confirmed case of measles or with a person associated with a local outbreak:

- non-immune pregnant females
- infants under 9 months

Further advice should be sought from the Communicable Disease Surveillance Centre, Health Protection Agency (tel. (020) 8200 6868).

Individuals with normal immunity who are not in the above categories and who have not been fully immunised against measles, can be given MMR vaccine (section 14.4) for prophylaxis following exposure to measles.

Rubella Intramuscular immunoglobulin after exposure to rubella does **not** prevent infection in non-immune contacts and is **not** recommended for protection of pregnant females exposed to rubella. It may, however, reduce the likelihood of a clinical attack which may possibly reduce the risk to the fetus. It should be used only if termination of pregnancy would be unacceptable to the pregnant individual, when it should be given as soon as possible after exposure. Serological follow-up of recipients is essential. For routine prophylaxis, see MMR vaccine (p. 689).

◢For intramuscular use

Normal Immunoglobulin PoM

Normal immunoglobulin injection. 250-mg vial; 750-mg vial

Dose

To control outbreaks of hepatitis A (see notes above)
- **By deep intramuscular injection**
  Child under 10 years 250 mg
  Child 10–18 years 500 mg

Measles prophylaxis or to attenuate an attack
- **By deep intramuscular injection**
  Child under 1 year 250 mg
  Child 1–3 years 500 mg
  Child 3–18 years 750 mg

Rubella in pregnancy, prevention of clinical attack
- **By deep intramuscular injection**
  750 mg

Available from the Communicable Disease Surveillance Centre and other regional Health Protection Agency offices (for contacts and control of outbreaks only, see above) and from SNBTS (as *Liberim*® *IM*, 250-mg strength only)

◢For subcutaneous use

Subcuvia® (Baxter BioScience) PoM

Normal immunoglobulin injection, net price 5-mL vial = £29.60, 10-mL vial = £59.20

Dose

Antibody deficiency syndromes
- **By subcutaneous injection**
  Consult product literature
  Note May be administered by intramuscular injection (if subcutaneous route not possible) but **not** for patients with bleeding disorders

Subgam® (BPL) PoM

Normal immunoglobulin injection, net price 2-mL vial = £11.20, 5-mL vial = £28.00, 10-mL vial = £56.00

Dose

Antibody deficiency syndromes
- **By subcutaneous injection**
  Consult product literature
  Note May be administered by intramuscular injection (if subcutaneous route not possible) but **not** for patients with bleeding disorders

Vivaglobin® (ZLB Behring) PoM

Normal immunoglobulin injection, net price 10-mL vial = £59.20

Dose

Antibody deficiency syndromes
- **By subcutaneous injection**
  Consult product literature

For intravenous use

Normal Immunoglobulin for Intravenous Use PoM

Brands include *Flebogamma® 5%* (0.5 g, 2.5 g, 5 g, 10 g); *Gammagard® S/D* (0.5 g, 2.5 g, 5 g, 10 g); Human Immunoglobulin (3 g, 5 g, 10 g); *Octagam®* (2.5 g, 5 g, 10 g); *Sandoglobulin®* (1 g, 3 g, 6 g, 12 g); *Sandoglobulin NF®* (6 g, 12 g); *Vigam® S* (2.5 g, 5 g); *Vigam® Liquid* (2.5 g, 5 g, 10 g)

Dose

Kawasaki syndrome
- **By intravenous infusion**
  Child 1 month–12 years 2 g/kg as a single dose within 10 days of onset of symptoms (but children with a delayed diagnosis may also benefit)

Other indications Consult product literature

Specific immunoglobulins

Specific immunoglobulins are prepared by pooling the plasma of selected donors with high levels of the specific antibody required.

Although a hepatitis B vaccine is now available for those at high risk of infection, specific **hepatitis B immunoglobulin** ('HBIG') is available for use in association with hepatitis B vaccine for the prevention of infection in infants born to mothers who have become infected with this virus in pregnancy or who are high-risk carriers (see Hepatitis B Vaccine, p. 686).

Following exposure of an unimmunised individual to an animal in or from a high-risk country, the site of the bite should be washed with soapy water and specific **rabies immunoglobulin** of human origin should be administered; as much of the dose as possible should be injected in and around the cleansed wound. Rabies vaccine should also be given (for details see Rabies Vaccine, BNF section 14.4).

For the management of tetanus-prone wounds, **tetanus immunoglobulin** of human origin ('HTIG') should be used in addition to wound cleansing and, where appropriate, antibacterial prophylaxis and a tetanus-containing vaccine (section 14.4). Tetanus immunoglobulin, together with metronidazole (section 5.1.11) and wound cleansing, should also be used for the treatment of established cases of tetanus.

Varicella–zoster immunoglobulin (VZIG) is recommended for individuals who are at increased risk of severe varicella *and* who have no antibodies to varicella–zoster virus *and* who have significant exposure to chickenpox or herpes zoster. Those at increased risk include neonates of mothers who develop chickenpox in the period 7 days before to 7 days after delivery, those exposed at any stage of pregnancy (but when supplies of VZIG are short, only issued to those exposed in the first 20 weeks' gestation or to those near term), and the immunosuppressed including those who have received corticosteroids in the previous 3 months at the following dose equivalents of prednisolone: *children* 2 mg/kg (or more than 40 mg) daily for at least 1 week or 1 mg/kg daily for 1 month. **Important:** for full details consult *Immunisation against Infectious Disease.* **Varicella–zoster vaccine** is available—see section 14.4

Cytomegalovirus (CMV) immunoglobulin (available on a named-patient basis from SNBTS) is indicated for prophylaxis in patients receiving immunosuppressive treatment.

Hepatitis B

Hepatitis B Immunoglobulin PoM

See notes above

Dose

- **By intramuscular injection**
  (as soon as possible after exposure)

Neonate 200 units as soon as possible after birth; for full details consult *Immunisation against Infectious Disease*

Child 1 month–5 years 200 units

Child 5–10 years 300 units

Child 10–18 years 500 units

Available from selected Health Protection Agency and NHS laboratories (except for Transplant Centres, see p. 699), also available from BPL and SNBTS (as *Liberim HB®*)

Note Hepatitis B immunoglobulin for intravenous use is available from BPL and SNBTS on a named-patient basis.

Rabies

Rabies Immunoglobulin PoM

(Antirabies Immunoglobulin Injection)

See notes above

Dose

20 Units/kg, *by infiltration* in and around the cleansed wound; if the wound not visible or healed or if infiltration of whole volume not possible, give remainder *by intramuscular injection* into anterolateral thigh (remote from vaccination site)

Available from Specialist and Reference Microbiology Division, Health Protection Agency (also from BPL and SNBTS)

Tetanus

Tetanus Immunoglobulin PoM
(Antitetanus Immunoglobulin Injection)
See notes above

Dose

Prophylaxis
- **By intramuscular injection**
250 units, increased to 500 units if more than 24 hours have elapsed or there is risk of heavy contamination or following burns

Therapeutic
- **By intramuscular injection**
150 units/kg (multiple sites)

Available from BPL and from SNBTS (as *Liberim® T*, licensed only for tetanus prophylaxis)

Tetanus Immunoglobulin for Intravenous Use PoM
Used for proven or suspected clinical tetanus

Dose
- **By intravenous infusion**
5000–10 000 Units

Available from BPL and SNBTS on a named-patient basis and from the Northern Ireland Blood Transfusion Service

Varicella–zoster

Varicella–Zoster Immunoglobulin PoM
(Antivaricella–zoster Immunoglobulin)
See notes above

Dose

Prophylaxis (as soon as possible—not later than 10 days after exposure)
- **By deep intramuscular injection**

Neonate 250 mg

Child 1 month–6 years 250 mg

Child 6–11 years 500 mg

Child 11–15 years 750 mg

Child 15–18 years 1 g

Give second dose if further exposure occurs more than 3 weeks after first dose

Note No evidence that effective in treatment of severe disease. Normal immunoglobulin for intravenous use may be used to provide an immediate source of antibody.

Available from selected Health Protection Agency and NHS laboratories (also from BPL, and SNBTS as *Liberim® Z*)

Anti-D (Rh_0) immunoglobulin

Classification not used in BNF for Children

Interferons

Interferon gamma-1b is licensed to reduce the frequency of serious infection in chronic granulomatous disease and in severe malignant osteopetrosis.

INTERFERON GAMMA-1b

(Immune interferon)

Cautions seizure disorders (including seizures associated with fever); cardiac disease (including ischaemia, congestive heart failure, and arrhythmias); monitor before and during treatment: haematological tests (including full blood count, differential white cell count, and platelet count), blood chemistry tests (including renal and liver function tests) and urinalysis; avoid simultaneous administration of foreign proteins including immunological products (risk of exaggerated immune response); **interactions**: Appendix 1 (interferons)

Driving May impair ability to perform skilled tasks; effects may be enhanced by alcohol

Hepatic impairment manufacturer advises caution in severe liver disease

Renal impairment manufacturer advises caution in severe impairment

Pregnancy manufacturer recommends avoid unless compelling reasons; effective contraception should be used by males or females

Breast-feeding manufacturer advises avoid—no information available

Side-effects fever, headache, chills, myalgia, fatigue; nausea, vomiting, arthralgia, rashes and injection-site reactions reported

Indication and dose

See notes above and under Preparations below

Immukin® (Boehringer Ingelheim) PoM
Injection, recombinant human interferon gamma-1b 200 micrograms/mL, net price 0.5-mL vial = £88.00

Dose
- **By subcutaneous injection**

Body surface area 0.5 m² or less 1.5 micrograms/kg 3 times a week

Body surface area greater than 0.5 m² 50 micrograms/m² 3 times a week

Not recommended for infant under 6 months with chronic granulomatous disease

14.6 International travel

Note For advice on **malaria chemoprophylaxis**, see section 5.4.1.

No special immunisation is required for travellers to the United States, Europe, Australia, or New Zealand although all travellers should have immunity to tetanus and poliomyelitis (and childhood immunisations should be up to date). Certain precautions are required in Non-European areas surrounding the Mediterranean, in Africa, the Middle East, Asia, and South America.

Long-term travellers to areas that have a high incidence of **poliomyelitis** or **tuberculosis** should be immunised with the appropriate vaccine; in the case of poliomyelitis previously immunised adults may be given a booster dose of a preparation containing inactivated poliomyelitis vaccine. BCG immunisation is recommended for travellers proposing to stay for longer than one month (or in close contact with the local population) in Asia, Africa, or Central and South America; it should preferably be given three months or more before departure.

Yellow fever immunisation is recommended for travel to the endemic zones of Africa and South America. Many countries require an International Certificate of Vaccination from individuals arriving from, or who have been travelling through, endemic areas, whilst other countries require a certificate from all entering travellers (consult the Department of Health handbook, *Health Information for Overseas Travel*, www.dh.gov.uk).

Immunisation against **meningococcal meningitis** is recommended for a number of areas of the world (for details, see p. 690).

Protection against **hepatitis A** is recommended for travellers to high-risk areas outside Northern and Western Europe, North America, Japan, Australia and New Zealand. Hepatitis A vaccine (see p. 684) is preferred and it is likely to be effective even if given shortly before departure; normal immunoglobulin is no longer given routinely but may be indicated in the immunocompromised (see p. 699). Special care must also be taken with food hygiene (see below).

Hepatitis B vaccine (see p. 686) is recommended for those travelling to areas of high prevalence who plan to remain there for lengthy periods and who may therefore be at increased risk of acquiring infection as the result of medical or dental procedures carried out in those countries. Short-term tourists are not generally at increased risk of infection but may place themselves at risk by their sexual behaviour when abroad.

Prophylactic immunisation against **rabies** (see Rabies Vaccine, BNF section 14.4) is recommended for travellers to enzootic areas on long journeys or to areas out of reach of immediate medical attention.

Travellers who have not had a **tetanus** booster in the last 10 years and are visiting areas where medical attention may not be accessible should receive a booster dose of adsorbed diphtheria [low dose], tetanus and inactivated poliomyelitis vaccine (see p. 681), even if they have received 5 doses of a tetanus-containing vaccine previously.

Typhoid vaccine is indicated for travellers to those countries where typhoid is endemic but the vaccine is no substitute for personal precautions (see below).

There is no requirement for cholera vaccination as a condition for entry into any country, but **oral cholera vaccine** (see p. 681) may be considered for backpackers and those travelling to situations where the risk is greatest (e.g. refugee camps). Regardless of vaccination, travellers to areas where cholera is endemic should take special care with food hygiene (see below).

Advice on **diphtheria**, on **Japanese encephalitis** (NHS vaccine available on named-patient basis from Sanofi Pasteur and MASTA) and on **tick-borne encephalitis** is included in *Health Information for Overseas Travel*, see below.

Food hygiene In areas where sanitation is poor, good food hygiene is important to help prevent hepatitis A, typhoid, cholera, and other diarrhoeal diseases (including travellers' diarrhoea). Food should be freshly prepared and hot, and uncooked vegetables (including green salads) should be avoided; only fruits which can be peeled should be eaten. Only suitable bottled water, or tap water that has been boiled, or treated with sterilising tablets should be used for drinking.

> **Information on health advice for travellers**
> The Department of Health booklet, *Health Advice For Travellers* (code: T6) includes information on immunisation requirements (or recommendations) around the world. The booklet can be obtained from travel agents, post-offices or by telephoning 0800 555 777 (24-hour service); also available on the Internet at:
> www.dh.gov.uk
>
> The Department of Health handbook, *Health Information for Overseas Travel* (2001), which draws together essential information *for healthcare professionals* regarding health advice for travellers, can be obtained from
> The Stationery Office
> PO Box 29, Norwich NR3 1GN
> Telephone orders, 0870 600 5522
> Fax: 0870 600 5533
> www.tso.co.uk

Immunisation requirements change from time to time, and information on the current requirements for any particular country may be obtained from the embassy or legation of the appropriate country or from:

National Travel Health Network and Centre
Hospital for Tropical Diseases
Mortimer Market Centre
Capper Street, off Tottenham Court Road
London, WC1E 6AU.
Tel: (020) 7380 9234
(9 a.m.–noon, 2–4.30 p.m. weekdays for healthcare professionals **only**)
www.nathnac.org

Scottish Centre for Infection and Environmental Health
Clifton House
Clifton Place
Glasgow, G3 7LN.
Tel: (0141) 300 1130
(2 p.m.–4 p.m. weekdays)
www.travax.scot.nhs.uk (registration required. Annual fee may be payable for users outside NHS Scotland)

Welsh Medicines Information Centre
University Hospital of Wales
Cardiff, CF14 4XW.
Tel: (029) 2074 2979 (08.30 a.m.–5 p.m. weekdays for health professionals in Wales **only**)

Department of Health and Social Services
Castle Buildings
Stormont
Belfast, BT4 3PP.
Tel: (028) 9052 0000

15 Anaesthesia

15.1 General anaesthesia

> Note
> The drugs in section 15.1 should be used only by experienced personnel and where adequate resuscitation equipment is available.

It is common practice to administer several drugs with different actions during surgery. An intravenous anaesthetic is usually used for induction, followed by maintenance with an inhalational anaesthetic, often supplemented by other drugs administered intravenously. Specific drugs are often used to produce muscle relaxation; these drugs interfere with spontaneous respiration, and intermittent positive-pressure ventilation is necessary.

Surgery and long-term medication The risk of losing disease control on stopping long-term medication before surgery is often greater than the risk posed by continuing it during surgery. It is vital that the anaesthetist knows about **all** drugs that a child is (or has been) taking.

Children with adrenal atrophy resulting from long-term corticosteroid use (section 6.3.2) may suffer a precipitous fall in blood pressure unless corticosteroid cover is provided during anaesthesia and in the immediate postoperative period. Anaesthetists must therefore know whether a child is, or has been, receiving corticosteroids (including high-dose inhaled corticosteroids).

Other drugs that should normally not be stopped before surgery include drugs for epilepsy, asthma, immunosuppression, and metabolic, endocrine and cardiovascular disorders. Expert advice is required for children receiving antivirals for HIV infection. For general advice on surgery in children with diabetes, see section 6.1.1.

Children taking aspirin or an oral anticoagulant present an increased risk for surgery. In these circumstances, the anaesthetist and surgeon should assess the relative risks and decide jointly whether aspirin or the anticoagulant should be stopped or replaced with heparin therapy.

Drugs that are stopped before surgery include combined oral contraceptives (see Surgery, BNF section 7.3.1 for details). If antidepressants need to be stopped, they should be withdrawn gradually to avoid withdrawal symptoms. Tricyclic antidepressants need not be stopped, but there may be an increased risk of arrhythmias and hypotension (and dangerous interaction with vasopressor drugs); therefore, the anaesthetist should be informed if they are not stopped. Lithium should be stopped 24 hours before major surgery but the normal dose can be continued for minor surgery (with careful monitoring of fluids and electrolytes). Potassium-sparing diuretics may need to be withheld on the morning of surgery because hyperkalaemia may develop if renal perfusion is impaired or if there is tissue damage.

Anaesthesia and skilled tasks Children and their carers should be very carefully warned about the risk of undertaking skilled tasks after the use of sedatives and analgesics during minor outpatient procedures. For intravenous benzodiazepines and for a short general anaesthetic the risk extends to **at least 24 hours** after administration. Responsible persons should be available to take children home. The dangers of taking **alcohol** should also be emphasised.

Prophylaxis of acid aspiration Regurgitation and aspiration of gastric contents (Mendelson's syndrome) is an important complication of general anaesthesia, particularly in obstetrics and emergency surgery and in children with gastro-oesophageal reflux disease.

An **H_2-receptor antagonist** (section 1.3.1) or a **proton pump inhibitor** (section 1.3.5) such as omeprazole may be used before surgery to increase the pH and reduce the volume of gastric fluid. They do not affect the pH of fluid already in the stomach and this limits their value in emergency procedures; oral H_2-receptor antagonists can be given 1–2 hours before the procedure but omeprazole must be given at least 12 hours earlier. Antacids are frequently used to neutralise the acidity of the fluid already in the stomach; 'clear' (non-particulate) antacids such as sodium citrate are preferred. Sodium citrate 300 mmol/litre (88.2 mg/mL) oral solution is licensed for use before general anaesthesia for caesarean section.

Anaesthesia, sedation and resuscitation in dental practice

Anaesthesia, sedation and resuscitation in dental practice

For details see *A Conscious Decision: A review of the use of general anaesthesia and conscious sedation in primary dental care*; report by a group chaired by the Chief Medical Officer and Chief Dental Officer, July 2000 and associated documents.

Further details can also be found in *Conscious Sedation in the Provision of Dental Care*; report of an Expert Group on Sedation for Dentistry (commissioned by the Department of Health), 2003. Both documents are available at www.dh.gov.uk.

Guidance is also included in *Standards for Dental Professionals*, London, General Dental Council, May 2005 (and as amended subsequently).

Gas cylinders

Each gas cylinder bears a label with the name of the gas contained in the cylinder. The name or chemical symbol of the gas appears on the shoulder of the cylinder and is also clearly and indelibly stamped on the cylinder valve.

The colours on the valve end of the cylinder extend down to the shoulder; in the case of mixed gases the colours for the individual gases are applied in four segments, two for each colour.

Gas cylinders should be stored in a cool well-ventilated room, free from flammable materials.

No lubricant of any description should be used on the cylinder valves.

15.1.1 Intravenous anaesthetics

Intravenous anaesthetics may be used either to induce anaesthesia or for maintenance of anaesthesia throughout surgery. Intravenous anaesthetics nearly all produce their effect in one arm-brain circulation time and can cause apnoea and hypotension, and so adequate resuscitative facilities **must** be available. They are **contra-indicated** if the anaesthetist is not confident of being able to maintain the airway. Extreme care is required in surgery of the mouth, pharynx, or larynx and in children with acute circulatory failure (shock) or fixed cardiac output.

Individual requirements vary considerably and the recommended dosage is only a guide. Smaller dosage is indicated in ill, shocked, or debilitated children and in significant hepatic impairment, while robust individuals may require more. To facilitate tracheal intubation, induction is followed by a neuromuscular blocking drug (section 15.1.5).

Total intravenous anaesthesia This is a technique in which major surgery is carried out with all anaesthetic drugs given intravenously. Respiration is controlled, the lungs being inflated with oxygen-enriched air. Muscle relaxants may be used to provide relaxation and prevent reflex muscle movements. The main problem to be overcome is the assessment of depth of anaesthesia.

Anaesthesia and skilled tasks See section 15.1.

Barbiturates

Thiopental sodium (thiopentone sodium) is used widely, but it has no analgesic properties. Induction is generally smooth and rapid, but dose-related cardiorespiratory depression may occur.

Awakening from a moderate dose of thiopental is rapid due to redistribution of the drug into other tissues. However metabolism is slow and some sedative effects may persist for 24 hours. Repeated doses have a cumulative effect particularly in neonates, and recovery is much slower.

THIOPENTAL SODIUM
(Thiopentone sodium)

Cautions see notes above; cardiovascular disease; reconstituted solution is highly alkaline—extravasation causes tissue necrosis and severe pain; avoid intra-arterial injection; **interactions:** Appendix 1 (anaesthetics, general)

Hepatic impairment reduce induction dose in severe liver disease

Pregnancy depresses neonatal respiration in the third trimester—dose should not exceed 250 mg

Contra-indications see notes above; porphyria (section 9.8.2); myotonic dystrophy

Breast-feeding present in milk—manufacturer advises avoid

Side-effects arrhythmias, myocardial depression, laryngeal spasm, cough, sneezing; hypersensitivity reactions; rash, injection-site reactions; excessive doses associated with hypothermia and profound reduction in cerebral function

Licensed use not licensed for use in status epilepticus; not licensed for use by intravenous infusion

Indication and dose

Induction of anaesthesia
- By slow intravenous injection

Neonate 4 mg/kg repeated after 1 minute if necessary

Child 1 month–18 years 4 mg/kg (max. 150 mg) repeated after 1 minute if necessary

Prolonged status epilepticus
- By slow intravenous injection and intravenous infusion

Neonate initially 5 mg/kg followed by continuous intravenous infusion of 2.5 mg/kg/hour, adjusted according to response

Child 1 month–18 years 5 mg/kg followed by continuous intravenous infusion of 2–8 mg/kg/hour, adjusted according to response

Administration For *intravenous injection*, dilute to a concentration of 25 mg/mL with Water for Injections, and give over at least 10–15 seconds; for *intravenous infusion* dilute to a concentration of 2.5 mg/mL with Sodium Chloride 0.9%

Thiopental (Link) PoM
Injection, powder for reconstitution, thiopental sodium, net price 500-mg vial = £3.06

15 Anaesthesia

Other intravenous anaesthetics

Etomidate is an induction agent associated with rapid recovery without a hangover effect. It causes less hypotension than other drugs used for induction. It produces a high incidence of extraneous muscle movement, which can be minimised by an opioid analgesic or a short-acting benzodiazepine given just before induction. Pain on injection can be reduced by injecting into a larger vein or by giving an opioid analgesic just before induction. Etomidate may suppress adrenocortical function, particularly on continuous administration, and it should not be used for maintenance of anaesthesia.

Propofol is associated with rapid recovery without a hangover effect. There is sometimes pain on intravenous injection and significant extraneous muscle movements may occur. Convulsions, anaphylaxis, and delayed recovery from anaesthesia can occur after propofol administration; since the onset of convulsions can be delayed, the CSM has advised special caution after day surgery. Propofol has been associated with bradycardia, occasionally profound; intravenous administration of an antimuscarinic drug may prevent this.

Ketamine is used rarely now. It has good analgesic properties at sub-anaesthetic dosage. It has particular value in children requiring repeated anaesthesia; however, recovery is relatively slow. There is a high incidence of extraneous muscle movements; also cardiovascular stimulation, tachycardia, and raised arterial pressure may occur. The main disadvantage of ketamine is the high incidence of hallucinations, nightmares, and other transient psychotic effects; these can be reduced when drugs such as diazepam are also used. Ketamine is **contra-indicated** in children with hypertension and is best avoided in those prone to hallucinations or nightmares. It also has abuse potential and may lead to dependance.

ETOMIDATE

Cautions see notes above; avoid in porphyria (section 9.8.2); **interactions:** Appendix 1 (anaesthetics, general)

Pregnancy depresses neonatal respiration in third trimester

Breast-feeding avoid for 24 hours after administration

Contra-indications see notes above

Side-effects see notes above

Indication and dose

See under preparations

Etomidate-Lipuro® (Braun) PoM

Injection (emulsion), etomidate 2 mg/mL, net price 10-mL amp = £1.53

Dose

Induction of anaesthesia
- **By slow intravenous injection**
  Child 1 month–18 years 150–300 micrograms/kg; child under 10 years may need up to 400 micrograms/kg

Hypnomidate® (Janssen-Cilag) PoM

Injection, etomidate 2 mg/mL, net price 10-mL amp = £1.50

Excipients: include propylene glycol (see Excipients, p. 3)

Dose

Induction of anaesthesia
- **By slow intravenous injection**
  Child 1 month–18 years 300 micrograms/kg; max. total dose 60 mg

KETAMINE

Cautions see notes above; **interactions:** Appendix 1 (anaesthetics, general)

Pregnancy depresses neonatal respiration in third trimester

Contra-indications see notes above; porphyria (section 9.8.2)

Side-effects see notes above

Indication and dose

Induction and maintenance of anaesthesia (short procedures)
- **By intravenous injection over at least 60 seconds**

  Neonate 1–2 mg/kg produces 5–10 minutes of surgical anaesthesia, adjusted according to response

  Child 1 month–12 years 1–2 mg/kg produces 5–10 minutes of surgical anaesthesia, adjusted according to response

KETAMINE (*continued*)

Child 12–18 years 1–4.5 mg/kg (usually 2 mg/kg) produces 5–10 minutes of surgical anaesthesia, adjusted according to response

- **By intramuscular injection**

Neonate 4 mg/kg usually produces 15 minutes of surgical anaesthesia, adjusted according to response

Child 1 month–18 years 4–13 mg/kg (4 mg/kg sufficient for some diagnostic procedures), adjusted according to response; 10 mg/kg usually produces 12–25 minutes of surgical anaesthesia

Induction and maintenance of anaesthesia (longer procedures)

- **By continuous intravenous infusion**

Neonate initially 0.5–2 mg/kg followed by a continuous intravenous infusion of 500 micrograms/kg/hour adjusted according to response; up to 2 mg/kg/hour may be used to produce deep anaesthesia

Child 1–18 years initially 0.5–2 mg/kg followed by a continuous intravenous infusion of 0.6–2.7 mg/kg/hour adjusted according to response

Administration for *continuous intravenous infusion*, dilute to a concentration of 1 mg/mL with Glucose 5% *or* Sodium Chloride 0.9%

Ketalar® (Pfizer) PoM
Injection, ketamine (as hydrochloride) 10 mg/mL, net price 20-mL vial = £4.22; 50 mg/mL, 10-mL vial = £8.77; 100 mg/mL, 10-mL vial = £16.10

PROPOFOL

Cautions see notes above; monitor blood-lipid concentration if risk of fat overload or if sedation longer than 3 days; **interactions:** Appendix 1 (anaesthetics, general)

Pregnancy depresses neonatal respiration in third trimester

Breast-feeding present in milk but amount probably too small to be harmful

Contra-indications see notes above; not to be used for sedation of ventilated children under 17 years (risk of potentially fatal effects including metabolic acidosis, cardiac failure, rhabdomyolysis, hyperlipidaemia, and hepatomegaly)

Side-effects see notes above; also flushing; transient apnoea during induction; *less commonly* thrombosis, phlebitis; *very rarely* pancreatitis, pulmonary oedema, sexual disinhibition, and discoloration of urine; serious and sometimes fatal side-effects reported with prolonged infusion of doses exceeding 5 mg/kg/hour, including metabolic acidosis, rhabdomyolysis, hyperkalaemia, and cardiac failure

Indication and dose

Induction of anaesthesia

- **By intravenous injection or by intravenous infusion**

Child 1 month–8 years 2.5–4 mg/kg administered slowly until response

Child 8–12 years 2.5 mg/kg administered slowly until response

Child 12–18 years 1.5–2.5 mg/kg at a rate of 20–40 mg every 10 seconds until response

Maintenance of anaesthesia

- **By continuous intravenous infusion**

Child 1 month–3 years 9–15 mg/kg/hour (using *Propofol-Lipuro® 1%* only), adjusted according to response

Child 3–12 years 9–15 mg/kg/hour, adjusted according to response

Child 12–18 years 4–12 mg/kg/hour, adjusted according to response

Sedation in intensive care

- **By continuous intravenous infusion**

Child under 17 years contra-indicated

Child 17–18 years 0.3–4 mg/kg/hour, adjusted according to response

Induction of sedation for surgical and diagnostic procedures (1% emulsion only)

- **By intravenous injection over 1–5 minutes**

Child under 17 years contra-indicated

Child 17–18 years 0.5–1 mg/kg

Maintenance of sedation for surgical and diagnostic procedures (1% emulsion only)

- **By intravenous infusion**

Child under 17 years contra-indicated

Child 17–18 years 1.5–4.5 mg/kg/hour (additionally if rapid increase in sedation required, *by intravenous injection* 10–20 mg)

Administration for *continuous intravenous infusion*; microbiological filter not recommended; **1% emulsion** may be infused undiluted; may also be administered via a Y-piece close to injection site co-administered with Glucose 5% *or* Sodium Chloride 0.9%; *alternatively* dilute to a concentration not less than 2 mg/mL with Glucose 5% (*or* Sodium Chloride 0.9% for *Propofol-Lipuro®*, Braun, Fresenius Kabi, and Zurich brands); use glass or PVC containers (if PVC bag used it should be full—withdraw volume of infusion fluid equal to that of propofol to be added); give within 6 hours of preparation

2% emulsion do not dilute; may be administered via a Y-piece close to injection site co-administered with Glucose 5% *or* Sodium Chloride 0.9%

▢ **PROPOFOL (*continued*)**

Propofol (Non-proprietary) PoM
1% injection (emulsion), propofol 10 mg/mL, net price 20-mL amp = £2.33, 50-mL bottle = £5.82, 100-mL bottle = £11.64

2% injection (emulsion), propofol 20 mg/mL, net price 50-mL vial = £11.64
Brands include *Propofol-Lipuro®*

Diprivan® (AstraZeneca) PoM
1% injection (emulsion), propofol 10 mg/mL, net price 20-mL amp = £3.88, 50-mL vial = £9.70, 50-mL prefilled syringe (for use with *Diprifusor® TCI* system) = £10.67, 100-mL vial = £19.40

2% injection (emulsion), propofol 20 mg/mL, net price 50-mL vial = £19.40, 50-mL prefilled syringe (for use with *Diprifusor® TCI* system) = £20.37

Note *Diprifusor® TCI* ('target controlled infusion') system is for use **only** for induction and maintenance of general anaesthesia in adults

15.1.2 Inhalational anaesthetics

Inhalational anaesthetics may be gases or volatile liquids. They can be used both for induction and maintenance of anaesthesia and may also be used following induction with an intravenous anaesthetic (section 15.1.1).

Gaseous anaesthetics require suitable equipment for storage and administration. They may be supplied via hospital pipelines or from metal cylinders. *Volatile liquid anaesthetics* are administered using calibrated vaporisers, using air, oxygen, or nitrous oxide–oxygen mixtures as the carrier gas. It should be noted that they can all trigger malignant hyperthermia (section 15.1.8).

To prevent hypoxia inhalational anaesthetics must be given with concentrations of oxygen greater than in air.

Anaesthesia and skilled tasks See section 15.1.

Volatile liquid anaesthetics

Halothane is a volatile liquid anaesthetic. Its advantages are that it is potent, induction is smooth, the vapour is non-irritant, and seldom induces coughing or breath-holding. Despite these advantages, however, halothane is much less widely used than previously owing to its association with *severe hepatotoxicity* (**important**: see CSM advice, below).

Halothane causes cardiorespiratory depression. Respiratory depression results in elevation of arterial carbon dioxide tension and perhaps ventricular arrhythmias. Halothane also depresses the cardiac muscle fibres and may cause bradycardia. The result is diminished cardiac output and fall of arterial pressure. Adrenaline (epinephrine) infiltrations should be avoided in children anaesthetised with halothane as ventricular arrhythmias may result.

Halothane produces moderate muscle relaxation, but this may be inadequate for major abdominal surgery and specific muscle relaxants are then used.

> CSM advice (halothane hepatotoxicity)
> In a publication on findings confirming that *severe hepatotoxicity* can follow halothane anaesthesia the CSM has reported that this occurs more frequently after repeated exposures to halothane and has a high mortality. The risk of severe hepatotoxicity appears to be increased by repeated exposures within a short time interval, but even after a long interval (sometimes of several years) susceptible patients have been reported to develop jaundice. Since there is no reliable way of identifying susceptible patients the CSM recommends the following precautions prior to use of halothane:
>
> 1. a careful anaesthetic history should be taken to determine previous exposure and previous reactions to halothane;
> 2. repeated exposure to halothane within a period of **at least** 3 months should be **avoided** unless there are **overriding** clinical circumstances;
> 3. a history of unexplained jaundice or pyrexia in a patient following exposure to halothane is an absolute **contra-indication** to its future use in that patient.

Isoflurane is a less potent volatile liquid anaesthetic than halothane. Heart rhythm is generally stable during isoflurane anaesthesia, but heart-rate may

15 Anaesthesia

rise. Systemic arterial pressure may fall, owing to a decrease in systemic vascular resistance and with less decrease in cardiac output than occurs with halothane. Respiration is depressed. Muscle relaxation is produced and muscle relaxant drugs potentiated. Isoflurane may also cause hepatotoxicity in those sensitised to halogenated anaesthetics but the risk is appreciably smaller than with halothane.

Desflurane is a rapid acting volatile liquid anaesthetic; it is reported to have about one-fifth the potency of isoflurane. Early postoperative pain relief may be required because emergence and recovery are particularly rapid. Owing to limited experience it is not recommended for neurosurgery. It is not recommended for induction in children because cough, breath-holding, apnoea, laryngospasm, and increased secretions can occur. The risk of hepatotoxicity with desflurane in those sensitised to halogenated anaesthetics appears to be remote.

Sevoflurane is a rapid acting volatile liquid anaesthetic. Early postoperative pain relief may be required because emergence and recovery are particularly rapid. Sevoflurane can interact with carbon dioxide absorbents to form compound A, a potentially nephrotoxic vinyl ether. However, in spite of extensive use, no cases of sevoflurane-induced permanent renal injury have been reported and the carbon dioxide absorbents used in the UK produce very low concentrations of compound A.

DESFLURANE

Cautions see notes above; **interactions:** Appendix 1 (anaesthetics, general)

Hepatic impairment reduce dose

Renal impairment reduce dose in moderate impairment

Pregnancy depresses neonatal respiration in third trimester

Contra-indications see notes above; susceptibility to malignant hyperthermia

Side-effects see notes above

Indication and dose

Induction of anaesthesia
- **By inhalation through specifically calibrated vaporiser**

  Child 12–18 years 4–11%, but **not** recommended (see notes above)

Maintenance of anaesthesia
- **By inhalation through specifically calibrated vaporiser**

  Child 1 month–18 years 2–6% in nitrous oxide; 2.5–8.5% in oxygen or oxygen-enriched air; max. 17%

Suprane® (Baxter) PoM

Desflurane, net price 240 mL = £44.41

HALOTHANE

Cautions see notes above (**important:** CSM advice, see notes above); avoid for dental procedures in those under 18 years unless treated in hospital (high risk of arrhythmia); avoid in porphyria (section 9.8.2); **interactions:** Appendix 1 (anaesthetics, general)

Hepatic impairment avoid if history of unexplained pyrexia or jaundice following previous exposure to halothane

Pregnancy depresses neonatal respiration in third trimester

Breast-feeding excreted in milk

Contra-indications see notes above; susceptibility to malignant hyperthermia

Side-effects see notes above

Indication and dose

Induction of anaesthesia
- **By inhalation through specifically calibrated vaporiser**

  Child 12–18 years increased gradually according to response to 2% (up to 4% in child over 16 years) in oxygen or nitrous oxide-oxygen

Maintenance of anaesthesia
- **By inhalation through specifically calibrated vaporiser**

  Child 1 month–18 years 0.5–2%

Halothane (Concord)

Halothane, net price 250 mL = £20.57

ISOFLURANE

Cautions see notes above; **interactions**: Appendix 1 (anaesthetics, general)

Pregnancy depresses neonatal respiration in third trimester

Contra-indications susceptibility to malignant hyperthermia

Side-effects see notes above

Indication and dose

Induction of anaesthesia
- **By inhalation through specifically calibrated vaporiser**

Child 1 month–18 years increased gradually according to response from 0.5% to 3% in oxygen or nitrous oxide-oxygen

Maintenance of anaesthesia
- **By inhalation through specifically calibrated vaporiser**

Child 1 month–18 years 1–2.5% in nitrous oxide-oxygen; additional 0.5–1% may be required if given with oxygen alone; caesarean section, 0.5–0.75% in nitrous oxide-oxygen

Isoflurane (Abbott)
Isoflurane, net price 250 mL = £47.50

AErrane® (Baxter)
Isoflurane, net price 100 mL = £7.98, 250 mL = £30.00

SEVOFLURANE

Cautions see notes above; **interactions**: Appendix 1 (anaesthetics, general)

Renal impairment manufacturer advises use with caution

Pregnancy depresses neonatal respiration in third trimester

Contra-indications see notes above; susceptibility to malignant hyperthermia

Side-effects see notes above; also agitation occurs frequently in children

Indication and dose

Induction of anaesthesia
- **By inhalation through specifically calibrated vaporiser**

Child 1 month–18 years up to 5% (up to 7% in child under 12 years) in oxygen or nitrous oxide-oxygen

Maintenance of anaesthesia
- **By inhalation through specifically calibrated vaporiser**

Child 1 month–18 years 0.5–3%

Sevoflurane (Abbott) PoM
Sevoflurane, net price 250 mL = £123.00

Nitrous oxide

Nitrous oxide is used for maintenance of anaesthesia and, in sub-anaesthetic concentrations, for analgesia. For anaesthesia it is commonly used in a concentration of 50 to 70% in oxygen as part of a balanced technique in association with other inhalational or intravenous agents. Nitrous oxide is unsatisfactory as a sole anaesthetic owing to lack of potency, but is useful as part of a combination of drugs since it allows a significant reduction in dosage.

A mixture of nitrous oxide and oxygen containing 50% of each gas (*Entonox®*, *Equanox®*) is used to produce analgesia without loss of consciousness. Self-administration using a demand valve may be used in children who are able to self-regulate their intake (usually over 5 years of age) for painful dressing changes, as an aid to postoperative physiotherapy, for wound debridement and in emergency ambulances.

Nitrous oxide may have a deleterious effect if used in children with an air-containing closed space since nitrous oxide diffuses into such a space with a resulting increase in pressure. This effect may be dangerous in the presence of a pneumothorax which may enlarge to compromise respiration.

Special care is needed to avoid hypoxia if an anaesthetic machine is being used; machines should incorporate an anti-hypoxia device. Exposure of children to nitrous oxide for prolonged periods, either by continuous or by intermittent administration, may result in megaloblastic anaemia owing to interference with the action of vitamin B_{12}. For the same reason, exposure of theatre staff to nitrous oxide should be minimised. Depression of white cell formation may also occur.

NITROUS OXIDE

Cautions see notes above; **interactions:** Appendix 1 (anaesthetics, general)

Pregnancy depresses neonatal respiration in third trimester

Side-effects see notes above

Licensed use licensed for use in neonates and children

Indication and dose

Maintenance of light anaesthesia
- **By inhalation using suitable anaesthetic apparatus**

Child 1 month–18 years as a mixture with 25–30% oxygen

Analgesia
- **By inhalation using suitable anaesthetic apparatus**

Child up to 18 years (but see notes above) as a mixture with 30–50% oxygen, according to the patient's needs

15.1.3 Antimuscarinic drugs

Antimuscarinic drugs are used (less commonly nowadays) as premedicants to dry bronchial and salivary secretions which are increased by intubation, by surgery to the upper airways, and by some inhalational anaesthetics but they should not be used for this indication in children with cystic fibrosis. Antimuscarinics are also used before or with neostigmine (section 15.1.6) to prevent bradycardia, excessive salivation, and other muscarinic actions of neostigmine. They also prevent bradycardia and hypotension associated with drugs such as halothane, propofol, and suxamethonium.

Atropine is now rarely used for premedication but still has an emergency role in the treatment of vagotonic side-effects. For its role in cardiopulmonary resuscitation, see section 2.7.3.

Hyoscine reduces secretions and also provides a degree of amnesia, sedation and anti-emesis. Unlike atropine it may produce bradycardia rather than tachycardia. In some children hyoscine may cause the central anticholinergic syndrome (excitement, ataxia, hallucinations, behavioural abnormalities, and drowsiness).

Glycopyrronium reduces salivary secretions. When given intravenously it produces less tachycardia than atropine. It is widely used with neostigmine for reversal of non-depolarising muscle relaxants (section 15.1.5).

Glycopyrronium or hyoscine hydrobromide are also used to control excessive secretions in upper airways or hypersalivation in palliative care and in children unable to control posture or with abnormal swallowing reflex; effective dose varies and tolerance may develop. Hyoscine transdermal patches may also be used (section 4.6)

ATROPINE SULPHATE

Cautions use with caution in children especially those with Down's syndrome; gastro-oesophageal reflux disease, diarrhoea, ulcerative colitis, cardiovascular disease, hypertension, conditions characterised by tachycardia (including hyperthyroidism, cardiac insufficiency, cardiac surgery), pyrexia, urinary retention; **interactions:** Appendix 1 (antimuscarinics)

Pregnancy not known to be harmful; manufacturer advises caution

Breast-feeding small amount present in milk—manufacturer advises caution

Duration of action Since atropine has a shorter duration of action than neostigmine, late unopposed bradycardia may result; close monitoring of the patient is necessary

Contra-indications angle-closure glaucoma, myasthenia gravis (but may be used to decrease muscarinic side-effects of anticholinesterases—section 10.2.1), severe ulcerative colitis, paralytic ileus, pyloric stenosis

Side-effects constipation, tachycardia, transient bradycardia (followed by tachycardia, palpitation and arrhythmias), reduced bronchial secretions, urinary urgency and retention, dilatation of the pupils with loss of accommodation, photophobia, dry mouth, flushing, dryness of the skin; *less commonly* nausea, vomiting, giddiness, confusion

Licensed use not licensed for use by oral route; not licensed for use in children under 12 years for intra-operative bradycardia

Indication and dose

Eye (section 11.5)

Premedication
- **By subcutaneous or intramuscular injection 30–60 minutes before induction**

Neonate 10–15 micrograms/kg (subcutaneous route recommended)

15 Anaesthesia

ATROPINE SULPHATE (*continued*)

Child 1 month–12 years 10–30 micrograms/kg (minimum 100 micrograms, max. 600 micrograms)

Child 12–18 years 300–600 micrograms

- **By mouth 1–2 hours before induction**

Neonate 20–40 micrograms/kg

Child 1 month–18 years 20–40 micrograms/kg (max. 900 micrograms)

Intra-operative bradycardia
- **By intravenous injection**

Neonate 20 micrograms/kg

Child 1 month–12 years 10–20 micrograms/kg

Child 12–18 years 300–600 micrograms (larger doses in emergencies)

Control of muscarinic side-effects of neostigmine in reversal of competitive neuromuscular block (but rarely used)
- **By intravenous injection**

Neonate 20 micrograms/kg

Child 1 month–18 years 20 micrograms/kg (max. 1.2 mg)

Administration for administration *by mouth*, injection solution may be given orally

[1]**Atropine** (Non-proprietary) PoM

Injection, atropine sulphate 600 micrograms/mL, net price 1-mL amp = 50p

Note Other strengths also available

Injection, prefilled disposable syringe, atropine sulphate 100 micrograms/mL, net price 5 mL = £4.16, 10 mL = £4.66, 30 mL = £8.52

Brands include *Minijet® Atropine Sulphate*

Injection, prefilled disposable syringe, atropine sulphate 200 micrograms/mL, net price 5 mL = £4.67; 300 micrograms/mL, 10 mL = £4.67; 600 micrograms/mL, 1 mL = £4.67

Oral solution, atropine sulphate 100 micrograms/mL available as a manufactured special from Rosemont

1. PoM restriction does not apply where administration is for saving life in emergency

GLYCOPYRRONIUM BROMIDE

(Glycopyrrolate)

Cautions cardiovascular disease; see also Atropine sulphate; **interactions:** Appendix 1 (antimuscarinics)

Side-effects see under Atropine Sulphate

Licensed use not licensed for use by oral route; not licensed for use in control of upper airways secretion and hypersalivation

Indication and dose

Premedication at induction
- **By intravenous or intramuscular injection**

Neonate 5 micrograms/kg

Child 1 month–18 years 4–8 micrograms/kg (max. 200 micrograms)

Control of muscarinic side-effects of neostigmine in reversal of competitive neuromuscular block
- **By intravenous injection**

Neonate 10 micrograms/kg

Child 1 month–18 years 10 micrograms/kg

Control of upper airways secretion and hypersalivation
- **By mouth**

Child 1 month–18 years 40–100 micrograms/kg 3–4 times daily, adjusted according to response

Administration for administration *by mouth*, injection solution may be given or crushed tablets suspended in water

Glycopyrronium bromide (Non-proprietary)

Tablets, glycopyrronium bromide 1 mg and 2 mg, available from specialist importing company

Robinul® (Anpharm) PoM

Injection, glycopyrronium bromide 200 micrograms/mL, net price 1-mL amp = 60p; 3-mL amp = £1.01

Available as a generic from Antigen

With neostigmine metilsulphate

Section 15.1.6

HYOSCINE HYDROBROMIDE

(Scopolamine hydrobromide)

Cautions see under Hyoscine Hydrobromide (section 4.6); also paralytic ileus, myasthenia gravis, epilepsy

Contra-indications porphyria (section 9.8.2); angle-closure glaucoma

Side-effects see under Atropine Sulphate; bradycardia

Indication and dose

Premedication
- **By subcutaneous or intramuscular injection 30–60 minutes before induction**

Child 1–12 years 15 micrograms/kg (max. 600 micrograms)

Child 12–18 years 200–600 micrograms

Note Same dose may be given by intravenous injection immediately before induction

HYOSCINE HYDROBROMIDE (*continued*)

Motion sickness, Excessive respiratory secretions see p. 234

Hyoscine (Non-proprietary) PoM
Injection, hyoscine hydrobromide 400 micrograms/mL, net price 1-mL amp = £2.71; 600 micrograms/mL, 1-mL amp = £2.81

Preparations
For transdermal and oral preparations see section 4.6

15.1.4 Sedative and analgesic peri-operative drugs

These drugs are given to allay fear and anxiety in the pre-operative period (including the night before operation), to relieve pain and discomfort when present, and to augment the action of subsequent anaesthetic agents. A number of the drugs used also provide some degree of pre-operative amnesia. The choice will vary with the individual child, the nature of the operative procedure, the anaesthetic to be used and other prevailing circumstances such as outpatients, obstetrics, recovery facilities etc. The choice would also vary in elective and emergency operations. Sedative premedication should be avoided in children with a compromised airway, CNS depression or a history of sleep apnoea.

Oral administration is preferred where possible but it is not altogether satisfactory; the rectal route should only be used in exceptional circumstances. Oral alimemazine (trimeprazine, section 3.4.1) is still used but when given alone it may cause postoperative restlessness in the presence of pain.

The use of a suitable local anaesthetic cream (section 15.2) should be considered to avoid pain at injection site.

Anaesthesia and skilled tasks See section 15.1.

Sedation for clinical procedures Anxiety about a clinical procedure can be minimised by using a sedative drug, usually a benzodiazepine, for its anxiolytic and amnesic effect. The child should be **monitored carefully** as soon as the sedative is given until recovery after the procedure; concomitant use of sedatives potentiates the CNS depressant effects of analgesics.

Midazolam is suitable for sedating a child for a procedure lasting no longer than 20 minutes; it is given by mouth 30–60 minutes before the procedure. Alternatively, temazepam may be given by mouth 60–90 minutes before the procedure. If the procedure is likely to last 20–60 minutes, chloral hydrate or triclofos (section 4.1.1) by mouth are effective, especially in children of pre-school age; secobarbital (quinalbarbitone) can be used in older children but the risk of excessive sedation and cardiorespiratory depression is greater.

For a painful procedure, the sedative may be given with a local anaesthetic (administered topically, by infiltration or as a nerve block as appropriate) and an analgesic such as paracetamol or an NSAID. If deep sedation is required and the use of a general anaesthetic (e.g. propofol or ketamine) or a potent opioid (e.g. fentanyl) is needed, they should be used only under the supervision of a specialist experienced in the use of these drugs.

15.1.4.1 Anxiolytics and neuroleptics

Benzodiazepines

Benzodiazepines possess useful properties for premedication including relief of anxiety, sedation, and amnesia; short-acting benzodiazepines taken by mouth are the most common premedicants. They have no analgesic effect so an opioid analgesic may sometimes be required for pain.

Benzodiazepines can alleviate anxiety at doses that do not necessarily cause excessive sedation and they are of particular value during short procedures or during operations under local anaesthesia (including dentistry). Amnesia reduces the likelihood of any unpleasant memories of the procedure (although benzodiazepines, particularly when used for more profound sedation, can sometimes induce sexual fantasies in adolescents). Benzodiazepines are also used in intensive care units for sedation, particularly in those receiving assisted ventilation.

Benzodiazepines may occasionally cause marked respiratory depression and facilities for its treatment are essential; flumazenil (section 15.1.7) is used to antagonise the effects of benzodiazepines. They are best avoided in myasthenia gravis, especially peri-operatively.

Diazepam is used to produce mild sedation with amnesia. It is a long-acting drug with active metabolites and a second period of drowsiness can occur several hours after its administration. Peri-operative use of diazepam is not generally recommended; its effect and timing of response are unreliable and paradoxical effects may occur.

Diazepam is relatively insoluble in water and preparations formulated in organic solvents are painful on intravenous injection and give rise to a high incidence of venous thrombosis (which may not be noticed for several days after the injection). Intramuscular injection of diazepam is painful and absorption is erratic. An emulsion preparation for intravenous injection is less irritant and is followed by a negligible incidence of venous thrombosis; it is not suitable for intramuscular injection. Diazepam is also available as a rectal solution.

Temazepam is given by mouth in older children and has a shorter duration of action and a more rapid onset than diazepam given by mouth. It has been used as a premedicant in inpatient and day-case surgery; anxiolytic and sedative effects last about 90 minutes although there may be residual drowsiness.

Lorazepam produces more prolonged sedation than temazepam and it has marked amnesic effects. It is used as a premedicant the night before major surgery; a further, smaller dose may be required the following morning if any delay in starting surgery is anticipated. Alternatively the first dose may be given early in the morning on the day of operation.

Midazolam is a water-soluble benzodiazepine which is often used by injection in preference to intravenous diazepam; it has a quick onset of action and recovery is faster than from diazepam, making it suitable for day cases. Midazolam can be given by mouth but its bitter acidic taste may need to be disguised. It can also be given intranasally but this route is limited by nasal discomfort. Midazolam is associated with profound sedation when high doses are given or when used with certain other drugs. It can cause severe disinhibition and restlessness in some children. Midazolam is not recommended for prolonged sedation in neonates; drug accumulation is likely to occur.

Dental procedures Anxiolytics diminish tension, anxiety and panic, and may be of benefit in children anxious about the dental procedure. Diazepam is an effective anxiolytic for dental treatment in children but must not be used intravenously; midazolam may also be used by mouth. Diazepam has a longer duration of action than midazolam, and when given at night, diazepam is associated with more residual effects the following day; children and their carers should be carefully warned about the risk of undertaking skilled tasks (**important**: for general advice on anaesthesia and skilled tasks, see p. 706. For futher information on hypnotics and anxiolytics, see p. 202. For further information on hypnotics used for dental procedures, see p. 203.

DIAZEPAM

Cautions see notes above and section 4.1.2 and section 4.8.2

Contra-indications see notes above and section 4.1.2

Side-effects see notes above and section 4.1.2

Licensed use tablets, liquid and injection licensed for use in children for premedication; rectal solution licensed for sedation for procedures

Indication and dose

Premedication and sedation for clinical procedures
- By mouth (before minor or dental surgery, under specialist supervision) 45–60 minutes before procedure

  Child 1 month–12 years 200–300 micrograms/kg (max. 5 mg)

  Child 12–18 years 200–300 micrograms/kg (max. 20 mg)

DIAZEPAM (*continued*)

- **By intravenous injection over 2–4 minutes into large vein (specialist use only); emulsion preparation preferred**
  Child 1 month–12 years 100–200 micrograms/kg (max. 5 mg)
  Child 12–18 years 100–200 micrograms/kg (max. 20 mg)
- **By rectum (as rectal solution)**
  Child 1–3 years 5 mg
  Child 3–12 years 5–10 mg
  Child 12–18 years 10 mg

Preparations
Tablets and oral solution, see Section 4.1.2
Rectal solution and parenteral preparations, see Section 4.8.2

LORAZEPAM

Cautions see notes above and section 4.1.2; **interactions:** Appendix 1 (anxiolytics and hypnotics)

Contra-indications see notes above and under Diazepam (section 4.1.2)

Side-effects see notes above and under Diazepam (section 4.1.2)

Licensed use not licensed for use in children under 5 years by oral route; not licensed for use in children under 12 years by intravenous or intramuscular injection

Indication and dose

See also section 4.8.2

Premedication
- **By mouth**
  Child 1 month–12 years 50–100 micrograms/kg (max. 4 mg) at least 1 hour before surgery
  Child 12–18 years 1–4 mg at least 1 hour before surgery
  Note Same dose may be given the night before surgery in addition to, or to replace, dose before surgery
- **By intravenous or intramuscular injection**
  Child 1 month–18 years 50–100 micrograms/kg (max. 4 mg)
  Note Give intravenous injection 30–45 minutes before surgery; give intramuscular injection 60–90 minutes before surgery

Administration for *intravenous injection*, dilute injection solution with an equal volume of Sodium Chloride 0.9% *or* Water for Injections; give over 3–5 minutes; max. rate 50 micrograms/kg over 3 minutes

Lorazepam (Non-proprietary) PoM
Tablets, lorazepam 1 mg, net price 20 = 89p; 2.5 mg, 20 = £1.24. Label: 2 or 19

Injection, lorazepam 4 mg/mL. Net price 1-mL amp = 37p
Excipients: include benzyl alcohol (avoid in neonates see Excipients, p. 3, propylene glycol
Brands include *Ativan*®
Note For intramuscular injection it should be diluted with an equal volume of water for injections or physiological saline (but only use when oral and intravenous routes not possible)

Extemporaneous formulations available see Extemporaneous Preparations, p. 8

MIDAZOLAM

Cautions cardiac disease; respiratory disease; myasthenia gravis; history of drug or alcohol abuse; reduce dose if debilitated; avoid prolonged use (and abrupt withdrawal thereafter); **interactions:** Appendix 1 (anxiolytics and hypnotics)

Hepatic impairment can precipitate coma

Renal impairment start with small doses in severe renal impairment; increased cerebral sensitivity

Pregnancy use only if clear indication such as seizure control (high doses during late pregnancy or labour may cause neonatal hypothermia, hypotonia, and respiratory depression)

Breast-feeding present in milk—avoid if possible

Contra-indications marked neuromuscular respiratory weakness including unstable myasthenia gravis; severe respiratory depression; acute pulmonary insufficiency

Side-effects gastro-intestinal disturbances, increased appetite, jaundice; hypotension, cardiac arrest, heart rate changes, anaphylaxis, thrombosis; laryngospasm, bronchospasm, respiratory depression and respiratory arrest (particularly with high doses or on rapid injection); drowsiness, confusion, ataxia, amnesia, headache, euphoria, hallucinations, fatigue, dizziness, vertigo, involuntary movements, paradoxical excitement and aggression, dysarthria; urinary retention, incontinence; blood disorders; muscle weakness; visual disturbances; salivation changes; skin reactions; on *intravenous injection*, pain, thrombophlebitis; with *intranasal administration* burning sensation, lacrimation, and severe irritation of nasal mucosa

Licensed use not licensed for use in children under 6 months for premedication, induction of anaesthesia, and conscious sedation; not licensed for use by oral and intranasal routes

Indication and dose

Conscious sedation
- **By mouth**
  Child 1 month–18 years 500 micrograms/kg (max. 20 mg) 30–60 minutes before procedure

MIDAZOLAM (*continued*)

- **Intranasally**

  Child 1 month–18 years 100–150 micrograms/kg in each nostril

- **By rectum**

  Child 6 months–18 years 300–500 micrograms/kg 15–30 minutes before procedure

- **By intravenous injection over 2–3 minutes**

  Child 1 month–6 years initially 50–100 micrograms/kg, increased if necessary in small steps (max. total dose 300 micrograms/kg or 6 mg)

  Child 6–12 years initially 25–50 micrograms/kg, increased in small steps if necessary (max. total dose 10 mg)

  Child 12–18 years initially 2–2.5 mg; increased in steps of 0.5–1 mg if necessary (total dose usually 3.5–7.5 mg)

- **By intramuscular injection**

  Child 1–18 years 50–150 micrograms/kg (max. 300 micrograms/kg)

Premedication

- **By mouth (before minor or dental surgery, under specialist supervision)**

  Child 1 month–18 years 500 micrograms/kg (max. 15 mg) 15–30 minutes before the procedure

- **By deep intramuscular injection**

  Child 6 months–15 years 80–200 micrograms/kg 20–60 minutes before induction (max. 3 mg)

  Child 15–18 years usual dose 2–3 mg 20–60 minutes before induction

- **By rectum**

  Child 6 months–12 years 300–500 micrograms/kg 15–30 minutes before induction

Induction of anaesthesia

- **By slow intravenous injection**

  Child 7–18 years 150 micrograms/kg; increase dose if necessary every 2 minutes (max. 500 micrograms/kg)

Sedation in intensive care

- **By intravenous injection and continuous intravenous infusion**

  Child 1–6 months 60 micrograms/kg/hour *by continuous intravenous infusion* adjusted according to response

  Child 6 months–12 years initially 50–200 micrograms/kg *by slow intravenous injection* over at least 3 minutes followed by 30–120 micrograms/kg/hour *by continuous intravenous infusion* adjusted according to response

  Child 12–18 years initially 30–300 micrograms/kg *by slow intravenous injection* in steps of 1–2.5 mg every 2 minutes followed by 30–200 micrograms/kg/hour *by continuous intravenous infusion* adjusted according to response

  Note Initial dose may not be required and lower maintenance doses needed if opioid analgesics also used; reduce dose (or omit initial dose) in hypovolaemia, vasoconstriction, or hypothermia

Status epilepticus section 4.8.2

Administration for administration *by mouth*, injection solution may be diluted with apple or black currant juice, chocolate sauce, or cola

For *continuous intravenous infusion*, dilute injection solution with Glucose 5% *or* Sodium Chloride 0.9%; for neonates and children under 15 kg body-weight, dilute to a max. concentration of 1 mg/mL

For *intranasal administration*, injection solution may be given

For *rectal administration* of the injection solution, attach a plastic applicator onto the end of a syringe; if the volume to be given rectally is too small, dilute with Water for Injections

Midazolam (Non-proprietary) PoM

Injection, midazolam (as hydrochloride) 1 mg/mL, net price 50-mL vial = £6.30; 5 mg/mL, 2-mL amp = 79p, 5-mL amp = 91p, 10-mL amp = £4.70, 18-mL amp = £6.80

Hypnovel® (Roche) PoM

Injection, midazolam (as hydrochloride) 2 mg/mL, net price 5-mL amp = 75p; 5 mg/mL, 2-mL amp = 90p

Amsed® (Special Products) PoM

Oral liquid, midazolam 2.5 mg/mL, 100 mL

Available as a manufactured special

TEMAZEPAM

Cautions see notes above and under Diazepam (section 4.1.2 and section 4.8.2); **interactions:** Appendix 1 (anxiolytics and hypnotics)

Contra-indications see notes above and under Diazepam (section 4.1.2)

Side-effects see notes above and under Diazepam (section 4.1.2)

Licensed use tablets not licensed for use in children

Indication and dose

Premedication and sedation for clinical procedures

- **By mouth**

  Child 1–12 years 1 mg/kg (max. 30 mg) 1 hour before surgery

  Child 12–18 years 20–30 mg 1 hour before surgery

15 Anaesthesia

TEMAZEPAM (*continued*)

[1]**Temazepam** (Non-proprietary) CD
Tablets, temazepam 10 mg, net price 28-tab pack = 95p; 20 mg, 28-tab pack = £1.65. Label: 19

Oral solution, temazepam 10 mg/5 mL, net price 300 mL = £9.95. Label: 19
Note Sugar-free versions are available and can be ordered by specifying 'sugar-free' on the prescription

Dental prescribing on NHS Temazepam Tablets or Oral Solution may be prescribed

1. See p. 18 for prescribing requirements for temazepam

15.1.4.2 Non-opioid analgesics

Since non-steroidal anti-inflammatory drugs (NSAIDs) do not depress respiration, do not impair gastro-intestinal motility, and do not cause dependence, they may be useful alternatives (or adjuncts) to the use of opioids for the relief of postoperative pain. NSAIDs may be inadequate for the relief of severe pain.

Diclofenac and **ibuprofen** (section 10.1.1) are used to relieve postoperative pain in children; diclofenac can be given parenterally and rectally as well as by mouth. Intramuscular injections of diclofenac are given deep into the gluteal muscle to minimise pain and tissue damage; diclofenac can also be given by intravenous infusion for the treatment or prevention of postoperative pain.

15.1.4.3 Opioid analgesics

Opioid analgesics are now rarely used as premedicants; they are more likely to be administered at induction. Pre-operative use of opioid analgesics is generally limited to children who require control of existing pain. The main side-effects of opioid analgesics are respiratory depression, cardiovascular depression, nausea, and vomiting; for general notes on opioid analgesics and their use in postoperative pain, see section 4.7.2.

For the management of opioid-induced respiratory depression, see section 15.1.7.

Intra-operative analgesia Opioid analgesics such as alfentanil, fentanyl, and remifentanil, given in small doses before or with induction reduce the dose requirement of some drugs used during anaesthesia.

Alfentanil, **fentanyl** and **remifentanil** are particularly useful because they act within 1–2 minutes. The initial doses of alfentanil or fentanyl are followed either by successive intravenous injections or by an intravenous infusion; prolonged infusions increase the duration of effect. Repeated intra-operative doses of alfentanil or fentanyl should be given with care since the respiratory depression can persist into the postoperative period and occasionally it may become apparent for the first time postoperatively when monitoring of the child might be less intensive. Alfentanil, fentanyl, and remifentanil may cause muscle rigidity, particularly of the chest-wall muscle or jaw muscle, which can be managed by the use of muscle relaxants.

In contrast to other opioids which are metabolised in the liver, remifentanil undergoes rapid metabolism by non-specific blood and tissue esterases; its short duration of action allows prolonged administration at high dosage, without accumulation, and with little risk of residual postoperative respiratory depression. Remifentanil should not be given as an intravenous injection intra-operatively, but it is well suited to continuous infusion; a supplementary analgesic will often be required before stopping the infusion.

Neonates The half-life of fentanyl and alfentanil is prolonged in neonates and accumulation is likely with prolonged use.

ALFENTANIL

Cautions see under Morphine Salts (section 4.7.2) and notes above

Contra-indications see section 4.7.2 and notes above

Side-effects see section 4.7.2 and notes above; also hypertension, myoclonic movements; *less commonly* arrhythmias, cough, hiccup, laryngospasm, visual disturbances

Licensed use licensed for use in children (age range not specified by manufacturer)

ALFENTANIL (*continued*)

Indication and dose

To avoid excessive dosage in obese children, dose may need to be calculated on the basis of ideal weight for height

Analgesia especially during short procedures; enhancement of anaesthesia
- By intravenous injection over 30 seconds (with assisted ventilation)

Neonate initially 20–50 micrograms/kg (but lower dose may be effective); supplemental doses up to 15 micrograms/kg

Child 1 month–18 years initially 30–50 micrograms/kg (but lower dose may be effective); supplemental doses up to 15 micrograms/kg

- By intravenous infusion (with assisted ventilation)

Neonate initially 50–100 micrograms/kg over 10 minutes followed by 30–60 micrograms/kg/hour

Child 1 month–18 years initially 50–100 micrograms/kg over 10 minutes followed by 30–60 micrograms/kg/hour

Administration for *continuous or intermittent intravenous infusion* dilute in Glucose 5% *or* Sodium Chloride 0.9% *or* Compound Sodium Lactate

Rapifen® (Janssen-Cilag) CD
Injection, alfentanil (as hydrochloride) 500 micrograms/mL. Net price 2-mL amp = 69p; 10-mL amp = £3.14

Intensive care injection, alfentanil (as hydrochloride) 5 mg/mL. To be diluted before use. Net price 1-mL amp = £2.52

FENTANYL

Cautions see under Morphine Salts (section 4.7.2) and notes above

Contra-indications see section 4.7.2 and notes above

Side-effects see section 4.7.2 and notes above; also myoclonic movements; *less commonly* laryngospasm; *rarely* asystole, insomnia

Licensed use licensed for use in children (age range not specified by manufacturer)

Indication and dose

Analgesia during operation, enhancement of anaesthesia with spontaneous respiration
- By intravenous injection over at least 30 seconds

Neonate initially 1–5 micrograms/kg, then 1 microgram/kg as required

Child 1 month–12 years initially 1–5 micrograms/kg, then 1 microgram/kg as required

Child 12–18 years initially 50–200 micrograms, then 50 micrograms as required

- By intravenous infusion

Child 1 month–18 years 3–5 micrograms/kg/hour adjusted according to response

Analgesia during operation, enhancement of anaesthesia with assisted ventilation
- By intravenous injection over at least 30 seconds

Neonate initially 5–10 micrograms/kg, then 1–3 micrograms/kg as required

Child 1 month–12 years initially 5–10 micrograms/kg, then 1–3 micrograms/kg as required

Child 12–18 years initially 0.3–3.5 mg, then 100–200 micrograms as required

Analgesia and respiratory depressant with assisted ventilation in intensive care
- By intravenous infusion

Neonate initially 10 micrograms/kg over 10 minutes then 1.5 micrograms/kg/hour

Child 1 month–18 years initially 10 micrograms/kg over 10 minutes then 1–6 micrograms/kg/hour adjusted according to response; higher doses may be required in cardiac surgery

Analgesia in other situations section 4.7.2

Administration for *intravenous infusion*, injection solution may be diluted in Glucose 5% *or* Sodium Chloride 0.9%

Fentanyl (Non-proprietary) CD
Injection, fentanyl (as citrate) 50 micrograms/mL, net price 2-mL amp = 54p, 10-mL amp = £1.65

Sublimaze® (Janssen-Cilag) CD
Injection, fentanyl (as citrate) 50 micrograms/mL, net price 2-mL amp = 23p, 10-mL amp = £1.11

REMIFENTANIL

Cautions see under Morphine Salts (section 4.7.2, but no dose adjustment necessary in renal impairment) and notes above

Contra-indications see under Morphine Salts (section 4.7.2) and notes above; left ventricular dysfunction

REMIFENTANIL (*continued*)

Side-effects see under Morphine Salts (section 4.7.2) and notes above; also hypertension, hypoxia; *very rarely* asystole and anaphylaxis

Indication and dose

To avoid excessive dosage in obese children, dose should be calculated on the basis of ideal weight for height

Enhancement and maintenance of anaesthesia
- **By intravenous injection and by continuous intravenous infusion**

  Child 1–12 years initially *intravenous injection* of 0.1–1 micrograms/kg over at least 30 seconds then *intravenous infusion* of 3–80 micrograms/kg/hour according to anaesthetic technique and adjusted according to response; initial dose by intravenous injection omitted if not required

  Child 12–18 years initially *intravenous injection* of 0.1–1 micrograms/kg over at least 30 seconds then *intravenous infusion* of 3–120 micrograms/kg/hour according to anaesthetic technique and adjusted according to response; initial dose by intravenous injection omitted if not required

Administration for *intravenous injection*, reconstitute to a concentration of 1 mg/mL; for *continuous intravenous infusion*, dilute further to a concentration of 20–25 micrograms/mL for **Child 1–12 years**, 20–250 micrograms/mL (usually 50 micrograms/mL) for **Child 12–18 years**, with Glucose 5% *or* Sodium Chloride 0.9% *or* Water for Injections

Ultiva® (GlaxoSmithKline) CD
Injection, powder for reconstitution, remifentanil (as hydrochloride), net price 1-mg vial = £5.12; 2-mg vial = £10.23; 5-mg vial = £25.58

15.1.5 Muscle relaxants

Muscle relaxants used in anaesthesia are also known as **neuromuscular blocking drugs**. By specific blockade of the neuromuscular junction they enable light levels of anaesthesia to be employed with adequate relaxation of the muscles of the abdomen and diaphragm. They also relax the vocal cords and allow the passage of a tracheal tube. Their action differs from the muscle relaxants acting on the spinal cord or brain which are used in musculoskeletal disorders (section 10.2.2).

Children who have received a muscle relaxant should **always** have their respiration assisted or controlled until the drug has been inactivated or antagonised (section 15.1.6).

Non-depolarising muscle relaxants

Non-depolarising muscle relaxants (also known as competitive muscle relaxants) compete with acetylcholine for receptor sites at the neuromuscular junction and their action may be reversed with anticholinesterases such as neostigmine (section 15.1.6). Non-depolarising muscle relaxants may be divided into the **aminosteroid** group comprising pancuronium, rocuronium, and vecuronium, and the **benzylisoquinolinium** group which includes atracurium, cisatracurium, and mivacurium.

Non-depolarising muscle relaxants have a slower onset of action than suxamethonium. These drugs can be classified by their duration of action as short-acting (15–30 minutes), intermediate-acting (30–40 minutes) and long-acting (60–120 minutes), although duration of action is dose-dependent. Drugs with a shorter or intermediate duration of action, such as atracurium and vecuronium, are more widely employed than those with a longer duration of action such as pancuronium.

Non-depolarising muscle relaxants have no sedative or analgesic effects and are not considered to be a triggering factor for malignant hyperthermia.

For children receiving intensive care and who require tracheal intubation and mechanical ventilation, a non-depolarising muscle relaxant is chosen according to its onset of effect, duration of action and side-effects. Rocuronium, with a rapid onset of effect, may facilitate intubation. Atracurium or cisatracurium may be suitable for long-term muscle relaxation since their duration of action is not dependent on elimination by the liver or the kidneys.

Atracurium, a mixture of 10 isomers, is a benzylisoquinolinium muscle relaxant with an intermediate duration of action. It undergoes non-enzymatic metabolism which is independent of liver and kidney function, thus allowing its use in children with hepatic or renal impairment. Cardiovascular effects are associated with significant histamine release. Neonates may be more sensitive to the effects of atracurium and lower doses may be required.

Cisatracurium is a single isomer of atracurium. It is more potent and has a slightly longer duration of action than atracurium and provides greater cardiovascular stability because cisatracurium lacks histamine-releasing effects. In children aged 1 month to 12 years, cisatracurium has a shorter duration of action and produces faster spontaneous recovery.

Mivacurium, a benzylisoquinolinium muscle relaxant, has a short duration of action. It is metabolised by plasma cholinesterase and muscle paralysis is prolonged in individuals deficient in this enzyme. It is not associated with vagolytic activity or ganglionic blockade although histamine release may occur, particularly with rapid injection. In children under 12 years mivacurium has a faster onset, shorter duration of action and produces more rapid spontaneous recovery.

Pancuronium, an aminosteroid muscle relaxant, has a long duration of action and is often used in children receiving long-term mechanical ventilation in intensive care units. It lacks a histamine-releasing effect, but vagolytic and sympathomimetic effects can cause tachycardia and hypertension. The half-life of pancuronium is prolonged in neonates.

Rocuronium exerts an effect within 2 minutes and has the most rapid onset of any of the competitive muscle relaxants. It is an aminosteroid muscle relaxant with an intermediate duration of action. It is reported to have minimal cardiovascular effects; high doses produce mild vagolytic activity. In children under 12 years, rocuronium has a faster onset and shorter duration of action.

Vecuronium, an aminosteroid muscle relaxant, has an intermediate duration of action. It does not generally produce histamine release and lacks cardiovascular effects. In neonates and infants, vecuronium has a faster onset and a longer duration of action; recovery is longer in these children. In neonates and infants under 4 months an initial test dose is recommended, followed by incremental doses until an appropriate response is achieved. Unexpected sustained neuromuscular blockade may occur in neonates.

Cautions Allergic cross-reactivity between neuromuscular blocking agents has been reported; caution is advised in cases of hypersensitivity to these drugs. Their activity is prolonged in children with myasthenia gravis and in hypothermia, therefore lower doses are required. Resistance may develop in children with burns who may require increased doses; low plasma cholinesterase activity in these children requires dose titration for mivacurium. **Interactions:** Appendix 1 (muscle relaxants).

Side-effects Benzylisoquinolinium non-depolarising muscle relaxants (except cisatracurium) are associated with histamine release which can cause skin flushing, hypotension, tachycardia, bronchospasm and rarely, anaphylactoid reactions. Most aminosteroid muscle relaxants produce minimal histamine release. Drugs possessing vagolytic activity can counteract any bradycardia that occurs during surgery.

ATRACURIUM BESILATE

(Atracurium besylate)

Cautions see notes above

Pregnancy does not cross placenta in significant amounts but manufacturer advises use only if potential benefit outweighs risk

Breast-feeding unlikely to be harmful following recovery from neuromuscular block; some manufacturers advise avoiding breast-feeding for 24 hours after administration

Side-effects see notes above

Licensed use not licensed for use in children under 1 month

Indication and dose

To avoid excessive dosage in obese children, dose should be calculated on the basis of ideal weight for height

Muscle relaxation (short to intermediate duration) for surgery or during intensive care

- **By intravenous injection and continuous intravenous infusion**

Neonate initially *by intravenous injection* 300–500 micrograms/kg followed *either by intravenous injection*, 100–200 micrograms/kg repeated as necessary *or by intravenous infusion*, 300–400 micrograms/kg/hour adjusted according to response

ATRACURIUM BESILATE (*continued*)

Child 1 month–18 years initially 300–600 micrograms/kg followed *either by intravenous injection* 100–200 micrograms/kg repeated as necessary *or by intravenous infusion*, 300–600 micrograms/kg/hour adjusted to response; higher doses may be necessary in intensive care

Administration for *continuous intravenous infusion*, dilute to a concentration of 0.5–5 mg/mL with Glucose 5% *or* Sodium Chloride 0.9% *or* Compound Sodium Lactate; stability varies with diluent

Atracurium (Non-proprietary) PoM
Injection, atracurium besilate 10 mg/mL, net price 2.5-mL amp = £1.85; 5-mL amp = £3.37; 25-mL amp = £14.45

Tracrium® (GSK) PoM
Injection, atracurium besilate 10 mg/mL, net price 2.5-mL amp = £1.66; 5-mL amp = £3.00; 25-mL amp = £12.91

CISATRACURIUM

Cautions see notes above

Pregnancy manufacturer advises avoid—no information available

Breast-feeding no information available

Side-effects see notes above

Indication and dose

To avoid excessive dosage in obese children, dose should be calculated on the basis of ideal weight for height

Muscle relaxation for intubation and during surgery

- **By intravenous injection**

Child 1 month–2 years initially 150 micrograms/kg, then 30 micrograms/kg repeated approx. every 20 minutes as necessary

Child 2–12 years initially 150 micrograms/kg (80–100 micrograms/kg if not for intubation), then 20 micrograms/kg repeated approx. every 10 minutes as necessary

Child 12–18 years initially 150 micrograms/kg, then 30 micrograms/kg repeated approx. every 20 minutes as necessary

- **By intravenous infusion**

Child 2–18 years initially 180 micrograms/kg/hour, reduced to 60–120 micrograms/kg/hour when stable; dose reduced by up to 40% if used with isoflurane

Administration for *continuous intravenous infusion*, dilute to a concentration of 0.1–2 mg/mL with Glucose 5% *or* Sodium Chloride 0.9%; solutions of 2 mg/mL and 5 mg/mL may be infused undiluted

Nimbex® (GSK) PoM
Injection, cisatracurium (as besilate) 2 mg/mL, net price 2.5-mL amp = £2.04, 5-mL amp = £3.91, 10-mL amp = £7.55

Forte injection, cisatracurium (as besilate) 5 mg/mL, net price 30-mL vial = £31.09

MIVACURIUM

Cautions see notes above; low plasma cholinesterase activity

Hepatic impairment reduce dose in severe impairment

Renal impairment reduce dose in severe impairment; prolonged paralysis

Pregnancy manufacturer advises avoid—no information available

Side-effects see notes above

Indication and dose

To avoid excessive dosage in obese children, dose should be calculated on the basis of ideal weight for height

Muscle relaxation during surgery

- **By intravenous injection**

Child 2–6 months initially 150 micrograms/kg, then *either by intravenous injection* 100 micrograms/kg repeated every 6–9 minutes as necessary *or by intravenous infusion*, 8–10 micrograms/kg/minute, adjusted if necessary every 3 minutes by 1 microgram/kg/minute to usual dose 11–14 micrograms/kg/minute

Child 6 months–12 years initially 200 micrograms/kg, then *either by intravenous injection* 100 micrograms/kg repeated every 6–9 minutes as necessary *or by intravenous infusion*, 8–10 micrograms/kg/minute, adjusted if necessary every 3 minutes by 1 microgram/kg/minute to usual dose 11–14 micrograms/kg/minute

Child 12–18 years initially 70–250 micrograms/kg, then *either by intravenous injection* 100 micrograms/kg repeated every 15 minutes as necessary *or by intravenous infusion*, 8–10 micrograms/kg/minute, adjusted if necessary every 3 minutes by 1 microgram/kg/minute to usual dose of 6–7 micrograms/kg/minute

Administration for *intravenous injection*, give undiluted or dilute in Glucose 5% *or* Sodium Chloride 0.9%. Doses up to 150 micrograms/kg may be given over 5–15 seconds, higher doses should be given over 30 seconds. In asthma, cardiovascular disease or in those sensitive to reduced arterial blood pressure, give over 60 seconds.

Mivacron® (GSK) PoM
Injection, mivacurium (as chloride) 2 mg/mL, net price 5-mL amp = £2.79; 10-mL amp = £4.51

PANCURONIUM BROMIDE

Cautions see notes above

Hepatic impairment possibly slower onset, higher dose requirement, and prolonged recovery time

Renal impairment prolonged duration of block in severe impairment

Pregnancy crosses placenta in small amounts—manufacturer advises avoid

Breast-feeding no information available—manufacturer advises avoid

Side-effects see notes above

Indication and dose

To avoid excessive dosage in obese children, dose should be calculated on the basis of ideal weight for height

Muscle relaxation during (long duration) surgery

- **By intravenous injection**

Neonate initially 30–100 micrograms/kg, then 10–50 micrograms/kg repeated every 4–6 hours as necessary

Child 1 month–18 years initially 60–100 micrograms/kg, then 10–20 micrograms/kg repeated as required

Administration for *intravenous injection*, give undiluted *or* dilute in Glucose 5% *or* Sodium Chloride 0.9%

Pancuronium (Non-proprietary) PoM
Injection, pancuronium bromide 2 mg/mL, net price 2-mL amp = 65p

ROCURONIUM BROMIDE

Cautions see notes above

Hepatic impairment reduce dose

Renal impairment reduce dose in moderate impairment; prolonged paralysis

Pregnancy manufacturer advises avoid unless potential benefit outweighs risk

Breast-feeding present in milk in *animal* studies—manufacturer advises avoid unless potential benefit outweighs risk

Side-effects see notes above

Indication and dose

To avoid excessive dosage in obese children, dose should be calculated on the basis of ideal weight for height

Muscle relaxation during surgery

- **By intravenous injection**

Child 1 month–18 years initially 600 micrograms/kg, then *either by intravenous injection*, 150 micrograms/kg repeated as required *or by intravenous infusion*, 300–600 micrograms/kg/hour adjusted according to response

Administration for *intravenous administration*, may be diluted with Glucose 5% *or* Sodium Chloride 0.9%

Esmeron® (Organon) PoM
Injection, rocuronium bromide 10 mg/mL, net price 5-mL vial = £3.01, 10-mL vial = £6.01

VECURONIUM BROMIDE

Cautions see notes above

Pregnancy manufacturer advises avoid unless potential benefit outweighs risk—no information available

Side-effects see notes above

Indication and dose

To avoid excessive dosage in obese children, dose should be calculated on the basis of ideal weight for height

Muscle relaxation during surgery

- **By intravenous injection**

Neonate initially 10–20 micrograms/kg, then incremental doses according to response, usually every 2–4 hours

Child 1–4 months initially 10–20 micrograms/kg, then incremental doses according to response, usually every 1–2 hours

Child 5 months–18 years initially 80–100 micrograms/kg, then *either by intravenous injection*, 20–30 micrograms/kg repeated as required *or by intravenous infusion*, 50–80 micrograms/kg/hour, adjusted according to response

Assisted ventilation in intensive care

- **By intravenous injection**

Neonate initially 80–100 micrograms/kg then incremental doses of 30–50 micrograms/kg adjusted according to response usually every 2–4 hours

- **By intravenous infusion**

Child 1 month–18 years initially 80–100 micrograms/kg then 50–80 micrograms/kg/hour, adjusted according to response; up to 200 micrograms/kg/hour may be required

Administration for *continuous intravenous infusion*, dilute to a max. concentration of 40 micrograms/mL with Glucose 5% *or* Sodium Chloride 0.9%, *or* Ringers solution; solution may also be infused undiluted

Norcuron® (Organon) PoM
Injection, powder for reconstitution, vecuronium bromide, net price 10-mg vial = £3.95 (with water for injections)

Depolarising muscle relaxants

Suxamethonium has the most rapid onset of action of any of the muscle relaxants and is ideal if fast onset and brief duration of action are required e.g. with tracheal intubation. Its duration of action is about 2 to 6 minutes following intravenous doses of about 1 mg/kg; repeated doses can be used for longer procedures. Neonates and young children are less sensitive to suxamethonium and a higher dose may be required.

Suxamethonium acts by mimicking acetylcholine at the neuromuscular junction but hydrolysis is much slower than for acetylcholine; depolarisation is therefore prolonged, resulting in neuromuscular blockade. Unlike the non-depolarising muscle relaxants, its action cannot be reversed and recovery is spontaneous; anticholinesterases such as neostigmine potentiate the neuromuscular block.

Suxamethonium should be given after anaesthetic induction because paralysis is usually preceded by painful muscle fasciculations. Bradycardia may occur; pre-medication with atropine (section 15.1.3) reduces bradycardia as well as the excessive salivation associated with suxamethonium use.

Prolonged paralysis may occur in **dual block**, which occurs with high or repeated doses of suxamethonium and is caused by the development of a non-depolarising block following the initial depolarising block; edrophonium (section 15.1.6) may be used to confirm the diagnosis of dual block. Children with myasthenia gravis are resistant to suxamethonium but can develop dual block resulting in delayed recovery. Prolonged paralysis may also occur in those with low or atypical plasma cholinesterase. Assisted ventilation should be continued until muscle function is restored.

SUXAMETHONIUM CHLORIDE

Cautions see notes above; patients with cardiac, respiratory or neuromuscular disease; raised intra-ocular pressure (avoid in penetrating eye injury); severe sepsis (risk of hyperkalaemia); **interactions:** Appendix 1 (muscle relaxants)

Pregnancy mildly prolonged maternal paralysis may occur

Contra-indications family history of malignant hyperthermia, low plasma cholinesterase activity, hyperkalaemia; major trauma, severe burns, neurological disease involving acute wasting of major muscle, prolonged immobilisation—risk of hyperkalaemia, personal or family history of congenital myotonic disease, Duchenne muscular dystrophy

Hepatic impairment prolonged apnoea may occur in severe liver disease because of reduced hepatic synthesis of pseudocholinesterase

Side-effects see notes above; also postoperative muscle pain, myoglobinuria, myoglobinaemia; tachycardia, arrhythmias, cardiac arrest, hypertension, hypotension; bronchospasm, apnoea, prolonged respiratory depression, anaphylactic reactions; hyperkalaemia; hyperthermia; increased gastric pressure; rash, flushing

Indication and dose

Muscle relaxation during surgery

- **By intravenous injection**

Neonate 2 mg/kg produces 5-10 minutes paralysis; 3mg/kg results in full neuromuscular block

Child 1 month–1 year initially 2 mg/kg, maintenance usually 1–2 mg/kg at 5–10 minute intervals as necessary

Child 1–18 years initially 1 mg/kg, then 0.5–1 mg/kg repeated every 5–10 minutes as necessary

- **By intramuscular injection**

Neonate up to 4–5 mg/kg produces 10–30 minutes paralysis (after 2–3 minute delay)

Child 1 month–1 year up to 4–5 mg/kg (paralysis after 2–3 minute delay)

Child 1–12 years up to 4 mg/kg (paralysis after 2–3 minute delay); max. 150 mg

Administration for *intravenous injection*, give undiluted *or* dilute with Glucose 5% *or* Sodium Chloride 0.9%

Suxamethonium Chloride (Non-proprietary) PoM
Injection, suxamethonium chloride 50 mg/mL, net price 2-mL amp = 70p, 2-mL prefilled syringe = £7.35

Anectine® (GSK) PoM
Injection, suxamethonium chloride 50 mg/mL, net price 2-mL amp = 71p

15.1.6 Anticholinesterases used in anaesthesia

Anticholinesterases reverse the effects of the non-depolarising (competitive) muscle relaxant drugs such as pancuronium but they prolong the action of the depolarising muscle relaxant drug suxamethonium.

Edrophonium has a transient action and may be used in the diagnosis of suspected dual block due to suxamethonium. It is also used in the diagnosis of myasthenia gravis (section 10.2.1)

Neostigmine has a longer duration of action than edrophonium. It is the specific drug for reversal of non-depolarising (competitive) blockade. It acts within one minute of intravenous injection and lasts for 20 to 30 minutes; a second dose may then be necessary. Glycopyrronium, or alternatively atropine, (section 15.1.3) should be given before or with neostigmine in order to prevent bradycardia, excessive salivation, and other muscarinic actions of neostigmine.

EDROPHONIUM CHLORIDE

Cautions see section 10.2.1 and notes above; atropine should also be given

Contra-indications see section 10.2.1 and notes above

Side-effects see section 10.2.1 and notes above

Indication and dose

Brief reversal of non-depolarising neuromuscular blockade

- **By intravenous injection over several minutes**
  Child 1 month–18 years 500–700 micrograms/kg (after or with atropine sulphate 7 micrograms/kg, max. 600 micrograms)

Myasthenia gravis (section 10.2.1)

Edrophonium (Cambridge) PoM
Injection, edrophonium chloride 10 mg/mL, net price 1-mL amp = £4.76

NEOSTIGMINE METILSULFATE
(Neostigmine methylsulphate)

Cautions see section 10.2.1 and notes above; atropine should also be given

Contra-indications see section 10.2.1 and notes above

Side-effects see section 10.2.1 and notes above

Indication and dose

Reversal of non-depolarising muscle block

- **By intravenous injection over 1 minute**
  Neonate 50–80 micrograms/kg, with glycopyrronium 10 micrograms/kg or atropine 20 micrograms/kg

  Child 1 month–18 years 50–80 micrograms/kg (under 12 years max. 2.5 mg, 12–18 years max. 5 mg), with glycopyrronium 10 micrograms/kg or atropine 20 micrograms/kg (minimum 100 micrograms, max. 600 micrograms atropine)

Myasthenia gravis section 10.2.1

Administration for *intravenous injection,* give undiluted *or* dilute with Glucose 5% *or* Sodium Chloride 0.9% *or* Water for Injections

Neostigmine (Non-proprietary) PoM
Injection, neostigmine metilsulfate 2.5 mg/mL, net price 1-mL amp = 58p

With glycopyrronium

Robinul-Neostigmine® (Anpharm) PoM
Injection, neostigmine metilsulfate 2.5 mg, glycopyrronium bromide 500 micrograms/mL, net price 1-mL amp = £1.01

Dose

Reversal of non-depolarising neuromuscular blockade

- **By intravenous injection over 10–30 seconds**
  Child 1 month–18 years 0.02 mL/kg (*or* 0.2 mL/kg of a 1 in 10 dilution), dose may be repeated if required (total max. 2 mL)

Administration for *intravenous injection,* may be diluted with Sodium Chloride 0.9% *or* Water for Injections

15.1.7 Antagonists for central and respiratory depression

Respiratory depression is a major concern with opioid analgesics and it may be treated by artificial ventilation or be reversed by an opioid antagonist. **Naloxone** given intravenously immediately reverses opioid-induced respiratory depression but the dose may have to be repeated because of its **short duration of action**; however, naloxone will also antagonise the analgesic effect. Intramuscular injection of naloxone produces a more gradual and prolonged effect but absorption may be erratic. Care is required in children requiring pain relief because naloxone also antagonises the analgesic effect of opioids.

Neonates Naloxone is used in newborn infants to reverse respiratory depression and sedation resulting from the use of opioids by the mother, usually for pain during labour. In neonates the effects of opioids may persist for up to 48 hours and in such cases naloxone is often given by intramuscular injection for its prolonged effect. In severe respiratory depression after birth, breathing should first be established (using artificial means if necessary) and naloxone administered only if use of opioids by the mother is thought to cause the respiratory depression; the infant should be monitored closely and further doses of naloxone administered as necessary.

Flumazenil is a benzodiazepine antagonist for the reversal of the central sedative effects of benzodiazepines after anaesthetic and similar procedures. Flumazenil has a shorter half-life than that of diazepam and midazolam and there is a risk that children may become resedated.

Doxapram (section 3.5.1) is a central and respiratory stimulant but is of limited value.

FLUMAZENIL

Cautions short-acting (repeat doses may be necessary—benzodiazepine effects may persist for at least 24 hours); benzodiazepine dependence (may precipitate withdrawal symptoms); prolonged benzodiazepine therapy for epilepsy (risk of convulsions); history of panic disorders (risk of recurrence); ensure neuromuscular blockade cleared before giving; avoid rapid injection in high-risk or anxious children and following major surgery; head injury (rapid reversal of benzodiazepine sedation may cause convulsions)

Hepatic impairment carefully titrate dose

Pregnancy may cross placenta in small amounts—manufacturer advises avoid unless potential benefit outweighs risk

Contra-indications life-threatening condition (e.g. raised intracranial pressure, status epilepticus) controlled by benzodiazepines

Side-effects nausea, vomiting, and flushing; if wakening too rapid, agitation, anxiety, and fear; transient increase in blood pressure and heart-rate in intensive care patients; very rarely convulsions (particularly in epileptics)

Licensed use not licensed for use in children

Indication and dose

Reversal of sedative effects of benzodiazepines

- **By intravenous injection over 15 seconds (question aetiology if no response to repeated injection)**

Neonate 10 micrograms/kg, repeat at 1-minute intervals if required

Child 1 month–12 years 10 micrograms/kg (max. single dose 200 micrograms), repeated at 1-minute intervals if required; max. total dose of 40 micrograms/kg (1mg) (2mg in intensive care)

Child 12–18 years 200 micrograms, repeated at 1-minute intervals if required; max. total dose 1 mg (2 mg in intensive care)

- **By intravenous infusion, if drowsiness recurs after injection**

Neonate 2–10 micrograms/kg/hour, adjusted according to response

Child 1 month–18 years 2–10 micrograms/kg/hour, adjusted according to response; max. 400 micrograms/hour

Administration for *continuous intravenous infusion*, dilute with Glucose 5% *or* Sodium Chloride 0.9%

Anexate® (Roche) PoM

Injection, flumazenil 100 micrograms/mL, net price 5-mL amp = £14.49

Flumazenil (Non-proprietary) PoM

Injection, flumazenil 100 micrograms/mL, net price 5-mL amp = £14.49

NALOXONE HYDROCHLORIDE

Cautions cardiovascular disease or those receiving cardiotoxic drugs (serious adverse cardiovascular effects reported); maternal physical dependence on opioids (may precipitate withdrawal in newborn); pain (see also under Titration of Dose, below); has short duration of action (see notes above)

Titration of dose In postoperative use, the dose should be titrated for each child in order to obtain sufficient respiratory response; however, naloxone antagonises analgesia

Pregnancy manufacturer advises use only if potential benefit outweighs risk

Side-effects hypotension, hypertension, ventricular tachycardia and fibrilation, cardiac arrest; hyperventilation, dyspnoea, pulmonary oedema; *less commonly* agitation, excitement, paraesthesia

Indication and dose

Reversal of respiratory and CNS depression in infant following maternal opioid use during labour

- **By intramuscular, intravenous or subcutaneous injection**

Neonate 10 micrograms/kg, repeated every 2–3 minutes if required *alternatively by intramuscular injection* (onset of action slower) 200 micrograms (60 micrograms/kg) as a single dose at birth

NALOXONE HYDROCHLORIDE (*continued*)

Reversal of opioid-induced respiratory depression
- **By intravenous injection**

Neonate 10 micrograms/kg, increased and repeated every 2–3 minutes if required

Child 1 month–12 years 10 micrograms/kg; if no response subsequent dose of 100 micrograms/kg

Child 12–18 years 1.5–3 micrograms/kg; if response inadequate, increments of 100 micrograms every 2 minutes

- **By continuous intravenous infusion**

Neonate 5–20 micrograms/kg/hour, adjusted according to response

Child 1 month–18 years 5–20 micrograms/kg/hour, adjusted according to response

See also Emergency treatment of poisoning p. 38

Administration for *continuous intravenous infusion*, dilute to a concentration of 4 micrograms/mL (24 micrograms/mL if fluid restricted) with Glucose 5% *or* Sodium Chloride 0.9%

Naloxone PoM

—see under Emergency Treatment of Poisoning p. 39

15.1.8 Drugs for malignant hyperthermia

Malignant hyperthermia is a rare but potentially lethal complication of anaesthesia. It is characterised by a rapid rise in temperature, increased muscle rigidity, tachycardia, and acidosis. The most common triggers of malignant hyperthermia are the volatile anaesthetics. Suxamethonium has also been implicated, but malignant hyperthermia is more likely if it is given following a volatile anaesthetic. Volatile anaesthetics and suxamethonium should be avoided during anaesthesia in children at high risk of malignant hyperthermia.

Dantrolene is used in the treatment of malignant hyperthermia. It acts on skeletal muscle cells by interfering with calcium efflux, thereby stopping the contractile process.

DANTROLENE SODIUM

Cautions avoid extravasation; **interactions:** Appendix 1 (muscle relaxants)

Pregnancy use only if potential benefit outweighs risk

Breast-feeding present in milk—manufacturer advises avoid

Indication and dose

Malignant hyperthermia
- **By rapid intravenous injection**

Child 1 month–18 years 1 mg/kg, repeated as required to a cumulative max. of 10 mg/kg

Chronic severe muscle spasticity see p. 564

Dantrium Intravenous® (Procter & Gamble Pharm.) PoM

Injection, powder for reconstitution, dantrolene sodium, net price 20-mg vial = £15.08 (hosp. only)

15.2 Local anaesthesia

The use of local anaesthetics by injection or by application to mucous membranes to produce local analgesia is discussed in this section.

See also section 1.7 (anus), section 11.7 (eye), section 12.3 (oropharynx), and section 13.3 (skin).

Use of local anaesthetics Local anaesthetic drugs act by causing a reversible block to conduction along nerve fibres. The drugs used vary widely in their potency, toxicity, duration of action, stability, solubility in water, and ability to penetrate mucous membranes. These variations determine their suitability for use by various routes, e.g. topical (surface), infiltration, intravenous regional anaesthesia (Bier's block), plexus, epidural (extradural) or spinal block. Local anaesthetics may also be used for postoperative pain relief, thereby reducing the need for analgesics such as opioids.

Administration In estimating the safe dosage of these drugs it is important to take account of the rate at which they are absorbed and excreted as well as their potency. The child's age, weight, physique, and clinical condition, the degree of vascularity of the area to which the drug is to be applied, and the duration of administration are other factors which must be taken into account.

Local anaesthetics do not rely on the circulation to transport them to their sites of action, but uptake into the systemic circulation is important in terminating their action and producing toxicity. Following most regional anaesthetic procedures, maximum arterial plasma concentrations of anaesthetic develop within about 10 to 25 minutes, so **careful surveillance** for toxic effects is necessary during the first 30 minutes after injection. Great care must be taken to avoid accidental intravascular injection. Local anaesthesia around the oral cavity may impair swallowing and therefore increase the risk of aspiration.

Epidural anaesthesia is commonly used during surgery, often combined with general anaesthesia, because of its protective effect against the stress response of surgery. It is often used for major surgery in children, including orthopaedic and abdominal surgery.

Toxicity Toxic effects associated with local anaesthetics usually result from excessively high plasma concentrations; single application of topical lidocaine preparations does not generally cause systemic side-effects. Effects initially include a feeling of inebriation and lightheadedness followed by sedation, circumoral paraesthesia and twitching; convulsions can occur in severe reactions. On intravenous injection convulsions and cardiovascular collapse may occur very rapidly. Hypersensitivity reactions occur mainly with the ester-type local anaesthetics such as benzocaine, procaine, and tetracaine (amethocaine); reactions are less frequent with the amide types such as lidocaine (lignocaine), bupivacaine, prilocaine, and ropivacaine.

When prolonged analgesia is required, a long-acting local anaesthetic is preferred to minimise the likelihood of cumulative systemic toxicity. Local anaesthetic injections should be given slowly in order to detect inadvertent intravascular administration. Local anaesthetics should **not** be injected into inflamed or infected tissues nor should they be applied to the traumatised urethra. In such cases absorption into the blood may increase the possibility of systemic side-effects. The local anaesthetic effect may also be reduced by the altered local pH.

Use of vasoconstrictors Most local anaesthetics cause dilation of blood vessels. The addition of a vasoconstrictor such as **adrenaline** (**epinephrine**) diminishes local blood flow, slows the rate of absorption of the local anaesthetic, and prolongs its local effect. Adrenaline must be used in a low concentration (e.g. 1 in 400 000–1 in 200 000) for this purpose and it should **not** be given with a local anaesthetic injection in digits and appendages; it may produce ischaemic necrosis.

When adrenaline is included the final concentration should be no more than 1 in 200 000 (5 micrograms/mL). In dental surgery, up to 1 in 80 000 (12.5 micrograms/mL) of adrenaline is used with local anaesthetics. There is no justification for using higher concentrations.

The total dose of adrenaline should **not** exceed 5 micrograms/kg (1 mL/kg of a 1 in 200 000 solution). For general cautions associated with the use of adrenaline, see section 2.7.3. For drug interactions, see Appendix 1 (sympathomimetics).

Dental anaesthesia **Lidocaine** (lignocaine) is widely used in dental procedures; it is most often used in combination with **adrenaline** (epinephrine). Lidocaine 2% with adrenaline 1 in 80 000 is a safe and effective preparation that has been used for many years.

The local anaesthetics **articaine** (carticaine) and **mepivacaine** are also used in dentistry; they are available in cartridges suitable for dental use. Mepivacaine is available with or without adrenaline (as *Scandonest*®) and articaine is available with adrenaline (as *Septanest*®).

In patients with severe hypertension or unstable cardiac rhythm, the use of adrenaline in a local anaesthetic may be hazardous. For these patients **prilocaine** with or without felypressin can be used but there is no evidence that it is any safer.

Great care should be taken to avoid inadvertent intravenous administration of a preparation containing adrenaline.

There is no clinical evidence of dangerous interactions between adrenaline-containing local anaesthetics and monoamine-oxidase inhibitors (MAOIs) or tricyclic antidepressants.

Lidocaine

Lidocaine (lignocaine) is effectively absorbed from mucous membranes and is a useful surface anaesthetic in concentrations up to 10%. Except for surface anaesthesia and dental anaesthesia, solutions should not usually exceed 1% in strength. The duration of the block (with adrenaline) is about 90 minutes.

Application of a mixture of lidocaine and prilocaine (*EMLA*®) under an occlusive dressing provides surface anaesthesia for 1–2 hours. *EMLA*® does not appear to be effective in providing local anaesthesia for heel lancing in neonates.

LIDOCAINE HYDROCHLORIDE
(Lignocaine hydrochloride)

Cautions epilepsy, respiratory impairment, impaired cardiac conduction, bradycardia, severe shock; porphyria (section 9.8.2); myasthenia gravis; reduce dose in debilitated; resuscitative equipment should be available; see section 2.3.2 for effects on heart; **interactions:** Appendix 1 (lidocaine)

Hepatic impairment manufacturer advises caution—increased risk of side-effects

Renal impairment caution in severe impairment

Pregnancy with large doses, neonatal respiratory depression, hypotonia and bradycardia after paracervical or epidural block

Breast-feeding amount too small to be harmful

Contra-indications hypovolaemia, complete heart block; do not use solutions containing adrenaline for anaesthesia in appendages

Side-effects CNS effects include confusion, respiratory depression and convulsions; hypotension and bradycardia (may lead to cardiac arrest); hypersensitivity reported; see also notes above and section 2.3.2

Licensed use *EMLA*® cream not licensed for use in children under 1 year

Indication and dose

Local anaesthesia
- **By local infiltration (see also Administration p. 728 and *Safe Practice* warning below)**

Neonate according to nature of procedure, up to 3 mg/kg (0.3 mL/kg of 1% solution), repeated not more often than every 4 hours

Child 1 month–12 years according to nature of procedure, up to 3 mg/kg (0.3 mL/kg of 1% solution), repeated not more often than every 4 hours

Child 12–18 years according to nature of procedure, up to 200 mg, repeated not more often than every 4 hours

Ventricular arrhythmias section 2.3.2

Intravenous regional anaesthesia and nerve blocks seek expert advice

Dental anaesthesia seek expert advice

Safe Practice The licensed doses stated above may not be appropriate in some settings and expert advice should be sought

Lidocaine hydrochloride injections

Lidocaine (Non-proprietary) PoM

Injection 0.5%, lidocaine hydrochloride 5 mg/mL, net price 10-mL amp = 35p

Injection 1%, lidocaine hydrochloride 10 mg/mL, net price 2-mL amp = 21p; 5-mL amp = 22p; 10-mL amp = 35p; 10-mL prefilled syringe = £4.53; 20-mL amp = 63p

Injection 2%, lidocaine hydrochloride 20 mg/mL, net price 2-mL amp = 28p; 5-mL amp = 25p

Xylocaine® (AstraZeneca) PoM

Injection 1% with adrenaline 1 in 200 000, anhydrous lidocaine hydrochloride 10 mg/mL, adrenaline 1 in 200 000 (5 micrograms/mL), net price 20-mL vial = 76p

Injection 2% with adrenaline 1 in 200 000, anhydrous lidocaine hydrochloride 20 mg/mL, adrenaline 1 in 200 000 (5 micrograms/mL), net price 20-mL vial = 81p

Lidocaine injections for dental use

Note Consult expert dental sources for specific advice in relation to dose of lidocaine for dental anaesthesia

A variety of lidocaine injections with adrenaline is available in dental cartridges; brand names include *Lignospan Special*®, *Rexocaine*®, *Xylocaine*®, and *Xylotox*®.

Lidocaine for surface anaesthesia

Important. Rapid and extensive absorption may result in systemic side-effects

Lidocaine (Non-proprietary)

Gel, lidocaine hydrochloride 1%, net price 15 mL = £1.30; 2%, 15 mL = £1.30

Dose

Mucocutaneous anaesthesia

Child under 12 years 1–2 mL applied when necessary

Child 12–18 years 2–3 mL applied when necessary

LIDOCAINE HYDROCHLORIDE (*continued*)

Major aphthous ulcers in immunocompromised patients
- **Child under 12 years** 1–2 mL applied when necessary, max. 8 mL in 24 hours
- **Child 12–18 years** 2–3 mL applied when necessary, max. 15 mL in 24 hours;

Ointment, lidocaine hydrochloride 5%, net price 15 g = 88p

Dose

Dental practice
- **Child** rub gently into dry gum

Pain relief (in anal fissures, haemorrhoids, pruritus ani, pruritus vulvae, herpes zoster)
- **Child** 1–2 mL applied when necessary; avoid long-term use

Solution, lidocaine hydrochloride 4%, net price 25 mL = £1.35

Dose

Biopsy in mouth
- **Child** up to 3 mg/kg with suitable spray *or* swab (with adrenaline if necessary); max. 5 mL

Puncture of maxillary sinus or polypectomy
- **Child** up to 3 mg/kg; apply with swab for 2–3 minutes (with adrenaline)

Bronchoscopy and bronchography
- **Child** up to 3 mg/kg; 2–3 mL with suitable spray

Lidocaine and chlorhexidine (Non-proprietary)

Gel, lidocaine hydrochloride 1%, chlorhexidine gluconate solution 0.25%, net price 15 mL = 70p; lidocaine hydrochloride 2%, chlorhexidine gluconate solution 0.25%, 15 mL = 70p

Dose

Urethral catheterisation
- **Child under 12 years** 1–5 mL into urethra at least 5 minutes before catheter insertion

Mucocutaneous anaesthesia
- **Child under 12 years** 1–2 mL applied when necessary
- **Child 12–18 years** 2–3 mL applied when necessary

Major aphthous ulcers in immunocompromised patients
- **Child under 12 years** 1–2 mL, applied when necessary, max. 8 mL in 24 hours
- **Child 12–18 years** 2–3 mL applied when necessary, max. 15 mL in 24 hours

EMLA® (AstraZeneca)

Drug Tariff cream, lidocaine 2.5%, prilocaine 2.5%, net price 5-g tube = £1.73

Surgical pack cream, lidocaine 2.5%, prilocaine 2.5%, net price 30-g tube = £10.25

Premedication pack cream, lidocaine 2.5%, prilocaine 2.5%, net price 5 × 5-g tube with 12 occlusive dressings = £9.75

Cautions not for wounds, mucous membranes, or atopic dermatitis; avoid use near eyes or middle ear; although systemic absorption low, caution in anaemia, in congenital or acquired methaemoglobinaemia or in G6PD deficiency (see also Prilocaine, p. 732)

Side-effects include transient paleness, redness, and oedema

Dose

Anaesthesia before minor skin procedures including venepuncture
- **Child 1–18 years** apply thick layer under occlusive dressing 1–5 hours before procedure (2–5 hours before procedures on large areas e.g. split skin grafting), under 1 month not recommended (risk of methaemoglobinaemia, but unlikely in neonates with mature dermis; see also Cautions above)

Instillagel® (CliniMed)

Gel, lidocaine hydrochloride 2%, chlorhexidine gluconate solution 0.25%, in a sterile lubricant basis in disposable syringe, net price 6-mL syringe = £1.41, 11-mL syringe = £1.58

Excipients: include hydroxybenzoates (parabens)

Laryngojet® (Celltech) PoM

Jet spray 4% (disposable kit for laryngotracheal anaesthesia), lidocaine hydrochloride 40 mg/mL, net price per unit (4-mL vial and disposable sterile cannula with cover and vial injector) = £5.10

Cautions may be rapidly and almost completely absorbed from respiratory tract and systemic side-effects may occur; extreme caution if mucosa has been traumatised or if sepsis present

Xylocaine® (AstraZeneca)

Spray (= pump spray), lidocaine 10% (100 mg/g) supplying 10 mg lidocaine/dose; 500 spray doses per container. Net price 50-mL bottle = £3.13

Note Lidocaine can damage plastic cuffs of endotracheal tubes

Topical 4%, anhydrous lidocaine hydrochloride 40 mg/mL, net price 30-mL bottle = £1.21

Excipients: include hydroxybenzoates (parabens)

Lidocaine for ear, nose, and oropharyngeal use

Lidocaine with Phenylephrine (Non-proprietary)

Topical solution, lidocaine hydrochloride 5%, phenylephrine hydrochloride 0.5%, net price 2.5 mL (with nasal applicator) = £8.73. For cautions, contra-indications and side-effects of phenylephrine, see section 2.7.2

Bupivacaine

The advantage of bupivacaine over other local anaesthetics is its longer duration of action (3–7 hours). It has a slow onset of action, taking up to 30 minutes for full effect. It is often used in lumbar epidural blockade and is particularly suitable for continuous epidural analgesia in labour. It is the principal drug used for spinal anaesthesia.

BUPIVACAINE HYDROCHLORIDE

Cautions see under Lidocaine Hydrochloride and notes above; myocardial depression may be more severe and more resistant to treatment; **interactions:** Appendix 1 (bupivacaine)

Contra-indications see under Lidocaine Hydrochloride and notes above; intravenous regional anaesthesia (Bier's block)

Side-effects see under Lidocaine Hydrochloride and notes above

Indication and dose

Adjusted according to child's physical status and nature of procedure, seek expert advice—**important**: see also under Administration, above

Bupivacaine (Non-proprietary) PoM
Injection, anhydrous bupivacaine hydrochloride 2.5 mg/mL (0.25%), net price 10 mL = 82p; 5 mg/mL (0.5%), 10 mL = 94p
Note Bupivacaine hydrochloride injection 0.25% and 0.5% are available in glass or plastic ampoules, and sterile-wrapped glass ampoules

Infusion, anhydrous bupivacaine hydrochloride 1 mg/mL (0.1%), net price 100 mL = £8.41, 250 mL = £10.59; 1.25 mg/mL (0.125%), 250 mL = £10.80

Marcain® (AstraZeneca) PoM
Injection, anhydrous bupivacaine hydrochloride 2.5 mg/mL (*Marcain® 0.25%*), net price 10-mL *Polyamp®* = £1.06; 5 mg/mL (*Marcain® 0.5%*), 10-mL *Polyamp®* = £1.21

Marcain Heavy® (AstraZeneca) PoM
Injection, anhydrous bupivacaine hydrochloride 5 mg, glucose 80 mg/mL, net price 4-mL amp = 93p

With adrenaline

Bupivacaine and Adrenaline (Non-proprietary) PoM
Injection, anhydrous bupivacaine hydrochloride 2.5 mg/mL (0.25%), adrenaline 1 in 200 000 (5 micrograms/mL), net price 10-mL amp = £1.23

Injection, anhydrous bupivacaine hydrochloride 5 mg/mL (0.5%), adrenaline 1 in 200 000 (5 micrograms/mL), net price 10-mL amp = £1.40

Levobupivacaine

Levobupivacaine, an isomer of bupivacaine, has anaesthetic and analgesic properties similar to bupivacaine but is thought to have fewer adverse effects.

LEVOBUPIVACAINE

Note Levobupivacaine is an isomer of bupivacaine

Cautions see under Lidocaine Hydrochloride and notes above; **interactions:** Appendix 1 (levobupivacaine)

Contra-indications see under Lidocaine Hydrochloride and notes above; intravenous regional anaesthesia (Bier's block); paracervical block in obstetrics

Side-effects see under Lidocaine Hydrochloride and notes above

Licensed use not licensed for use in children by epidural infusion

Indication and dose

Adjusted according to child's physical status and nature of procedure, seek expert advice—**important**: see also under Administration, above

Chirocaine® (Abbott) ▼ PoM
Injection, levobupivacaine (as hydrochloride) 2.5 mg/mL, net price 10-mL amp = £1.66; 5 mg/mL, 10-mL amp = £1.90; 7.5 mg/mL, 10-mL amp = £2.85

Infusion, levobupivacaine (as hydrochloride) 625 micrograms/mL, net price 100 mL = £7.80, 200 mL = £10.40; 1.25 mg/mL, net price 100 mL = £8.54, 200 mL = £12.20

Prilocaine

Prilocaine is a local anaesthetic of low toxicity which is similar to lidocaine (lignocaine). If used in high doses, methaemoglobinaemia may occur which can be treated with intravenous injection of methylthioninium chloride (methylene blue) 1% using a dose of 1 mg/kg. Neonates and infants under 6 months are particularly susceptible to methaemoglobinaemia.

PRILOCAINE HYDROCHLORIDE

Cautions see under Lidocaine Hydrochloride and notes above; severe or untreated hypertension, severe heart disease; concomitant drugs which cause methaemoglobinaemia; hepatic impairment; renal impairment; **interactions:** Appendix 1 (prilocaine)

Contra-indications see under Lidocaine Hydrochloride and notes above; anaemia or congenital or acquired methaemoglobinaemia

Side-effects see under Lidocaine Hydrochloride and notes above; ocular toxicity (including blindness) reported with excessively high strengths used for ophthalmic procedures

PRILOCAINE HYDROCHLORIDE (*continued*)

Indication and dose

Infiltration anaesthesia (higher strengths for dental use only), Nerve block
adjusted according to site of operation and response of patient, to max. 400 mg used alone, or 300 mg if used with felypressin

Citanest® (AstraZeneca) PoM
Injection 1%, prilocaine hydrochloride 10 mg/mL, net price 50-mL multidose vial = £2.01

Dose

Child 6 months–12 years up to 5 mg/kg adjusted according to site of administration and response; max. 400 mg

Child 12–18 years 100–200 mg/minute, or in incremental doses, to max. total dose 400 mg (adjusted according to site of administration and response)

For dental use

Citanest® (Dentsply) PoM
Injection 4%, prilocaine hydrochloride 40 mg/mL, net price 2-mL cartridge = 16p

Dose

Dental infiltration and dental nerve block
Child under 10 years 1 mL, adjusted according to response
Child 10–18 years 1–2 mL (max. 10 mL), adjusted according to response

Citanest with Octapressin® (Dentsply) PoM
Injection 3%, prilocaine hydrochloride 30 mg/mL, felypressin 0.03 unit/mL, net price 2-mL cartridge and self-aspirating cartridge (both) = 16p

Dose

Dental infiltration and dental nerve block
Child under 10 years 1–2 mL, adjusted according to response
Child 10–18 years 1–5 mL (max. 10 mL), adjusted according to response

Ropivacaine

Ropivacaine is an amide-type local anaesthetic agent similar to bupivacaine. It is less cardiotoxic than bupivacaine, but also less potent.

ROPIVACAINE HYDROCHLORIDE

Cautions see Lidocaine Hydrochloride and notes above; **interactions**: Appendix 1 (ropivacaine)

Contra-indications see Lidocaine Hydrochloride and notes above; intravenous regional anaesthesia (Bier's block); paracervical block in obstetrics

Side-effects see Lidocaine Hydrochloride and notes above

Licensed use not licensed for use in children by epidural infusion

Indication and dose

Adjust according to child's physical status and nature of procedure, **important**—seek expert advice, see also under Administration on p. 729

Naropin® (AstraZeneca) PoM
Injection, ropivacaine hydrochloride 2 mg/mL, net price 10-mL *Polyamp®* = £1.37; 7.5 mg/mL, 10-mL *Polyamp®* = £2.65; 10 mg/mL, 10-mL *Polyamp®* = £3.20

Epidural infusion, ropivacaine hydrochloride 2 mg/mL, net price 200-mL *Polybag®* = £14.45

Tetracaine

Tetracaine (amethocaine) is an effective local anaesthetic for topical application; a 4% gel is indicated for anaesthesia prior to venepuncture or venous cannulation. Tetracaine remains effective for 4–6 hours after a single application in most children. It does not appear to be effective prior to neonatal heal lancing.

Tetracaine is rapidly absorbed from mucous membranes and should **never** be applied to inflamed, traumatised, or highly vascular surfaces. It should **never** be used to provide anaesthesia for bronchoscopy or cystoscopy, as lidocaine (lignocaine) is a safer alternative. It is used in ophthalmology (section 11.7) and in skin preparations (section 13.3). Hypersensitivity to tetracaine has been reported.

TETRACAINE
(Amethocaine)

Cautions see notes above

Contra-indications see notes above

Side-effects see notes above; also erythema, oedema and pruritus; very rarely blistering
Important. Rapid and extensive absorption may result in systemic side-effects (see also notes above)

Dose

Neonate apply contents of tube (or appropriate proportion) to site of venepuncture or venous cannulation and cover with occlusive dressing; remove gel and dressing after 30 minutes for venepuncture and after 45 minutes for venous cannulation

Child 1 month–18 years apply contents of tube to site of venepuncture or venous cannulation and cover with occlusive dressing; remove gel and dressing after 30 minutes for venepuncture and after 45 minutes for venous cannulation

Ametop® (S&N Hlth.)
Gel, tetracaine 4%, net price 1.5-g tube = £1.08

A1 Interactions

Two or more drugs given at the same time may exert their effects independently or may interact. The interaction may be potentiation or antagonism of one drug by another, or occasionally some other effect. Adverse drug interactions should be reported to the CSM as for other adverse drug reactions.

Drug interactions may be **pharmacodynamic** or **pharmacokinetic**.

Pharmacodynamic interactions

These are interactions between drugs which have similar or antagonistic pharmacological effects or side-effects. They may be due to competition at receptor sites, or occur between drugs acting on the same physiological system. They are usually predictable from a knowledge of the pharmacology of the interacting drugs; in general, those demonstrated with one drug are likely to occur with related drugs. They occur to a greater or lesser extent in most patients who receive the interacting drugs.

Pharmacokinetic interactions

These occur when one drug alters the absorption, distribution, metabolism, or excretion of another, thus increasing or reducing the amount of drug available to produce its pharmacological effects. They are not easily predicted and many of them affect only a small proportion of patients taking the combination of drugs. Pharmacokinetic interactions occurring with one drug cannot be assumed to occur with related drugs unless their pharmacokinetic properties are known to be similar.

Pharmacokinetic interactions are of several types:

Affecting absorption The rate of absorption or the total amount absorbed can both be altered by drug interactions. Delayed absorption is rarely of clinical importance unless high peak plasma concentrations are required (e.g. when giving an analgesic). Reduction in the total amount absorbed, however, may result in ineffective therapy.

Due to changes in protein binding To a variable extent most drugs are loosely bound to plasma proteins. Protein-binding sites are non-specific and one drug can displace another thereby increasing its proportion free to diffuse from plasma to its site of action. This only produces a detectable increase in effect if it is an extensively bound drug (more than 90%) that is not widely distributed throughout the body. Even so displacement rarely produces more than transient potentiation because this increased concentration of free drug results in an increased rate of elimination.

Displacement from protein binding plays a part in the potentiation of warfarin by sulphonamides, and tolbutamide but the importance of these interactions is due mainly to the fact that warfarin metabolism is also inhibited.

Affecting metabolism Many drugs are metabolised in the liver. Induction of the hepatic microsomal enzyme system by one drug can gradually increase the rate of metabolism of another, resulting in lower plasma concentrations and a reduced effect. On withdrawal of the inducer plasma concentrations increase and toxicity may occur. Barbiturates, griseofulvin, many antiepileptics, and rifampicin are the most important enzyme inducers. Drugs affected include warfarin and the oral contraceptives.

Conversely when one drug inhibits the metabolism of another higher plasma concentrations are produced, rapidly resulting in an increased effect with risk of toxicity. Some drugs which potentiate warfarin and phenytoin do so by this mechanism.

Isoenzymes of the hepatic cytochrome P450 system interact with a wide range of drugs. Drugs may be substrates, inducers or inhibitors of the different isoenzymes. A great deal of *in-vitro* information is available on the effect of drugs on the isoenzymes; however, since drugs are eliminated by a number of different metabolic routes as well as renal excretion, the clinical effects of interactions cannot be predicted accurately from laboratory data on the cytochrome P450 isoenzymes. Except where a combination of drugs is specifically contra-indicated, the BNF presents only interactions that have been reported in clinical practice. In all cases the possibility of an interaction must be considered if toxic effects occur or if the activity of a drug diminishes.

Affecting renal excretion Drugs are eliminated through the kidney both by glomerular filtration and by active tubular secretion. Competition occurs between those which share active transport mechanisms in the proximal tubule. For example, salicylates and some other NSAIDs delay the excretion of methotrexate; serious methotrexate toxicity is possible.

Relative importance of interactions

Many drug interactions are harmless and many of those which are potentially harmful only occur in a small proportion of patients; moreover, the severity of an interaction varies from one patient to another. Drugs with a small therapeutic ratio (e.g. phenytoin) and those which require careful control of dosage (e.g. anticoagulants, antihypertensives, and antidiabetics) are most often involved.

Patients at increased risk from drug interactions include those with impaired renal or liver function.

Hazardous interactions The symbol • has been placed against interactions that are **potentially hazardous** and where combined administration of the drugs involved should be **avoided** (or only undertaken with caution and appropriate monitoring).

Interactions that have no symbol do not usually have serious consequences.

List of drug interactions

The following is an alphabetical list of drugs and their interactions; to avoid excessive cross-referencing each drug or group is listed twice: in the alphabetical list and also against the drug or group with which it interacts.

For explanation of symbol • see above

Abacavir
- Analgesics: abacavir possibly reduces plasma concentration of methadone
- Antibacterials: plasma concentration of abacavir possibly reduced by rifampicin
- Antiepileptics: plasma concentration of abacavir possibly reduced by phenytoin
- • Antivirals: plasma concentration of abacavir reduced by •tipranavir
- Barbiturates: plasma concentration of abacavir possibly reduced by phenobarbital

Acarbose *see* Antidiabetics

ACE Inhibitors
- Alcohol: enhanced hypotensive effect when ACE inhibitors given with alcohol
- Aldesleukin: enhanced hypotensive effect when ACE inhibitors given with aldesleukin
- Allopurinol: increased risk of toxicity when captopril given with allopurinol especially in renal impairment
- Alpha-blockers: enhanced hypotensive effect when ACE inhibitors given with alpha-blockers
- Anaesthetics, General: enhanced hypotensive effect when ACE inhibitors given with general anaesthetics
- Analgesics: increased risk of renal impairment when ACE inhibitors given with NSAIDs, also hypotensive effect antagonised; increased risk of hyperkalaemia when ACE inhibitors given with ketorolac; risk of renal impairment when ACE inhibitors given with aspirin (in doses over 300 mg daily), also hypotensive effect antagonised
- Angiotensin-II Receptor Antagonists: enhanced hypotensive effect when ACE inhibitors given with angiotensin-II receptor antagonists
- Antacids: absorption of ACE inhibitors possibly reduced by antacids; absorption of captopril, enalapril and fosinopril reduced by antacids
- Anti-arrhythmics: increased risk of toxicity when captopril given with procainamide especially in renal impairment
- Antibacterials: plasma concentration of active metabolite of imidapril reduced by rifampicin (reduced antihypertensive effect); quinapril tablets reduce absorption of tetracyclines (quinapril tablets contain magnesium carbonate)
- Anticoagulants: increased risk of hyperkalaemia when ACE inhibitors given with heparins
- Antidepressants: hypotensive effect of ACE inhibitors possibly enhanced by MAOIs
- Antidiabetics: ACE inhibitors possibly enhance hypoglycaemic effect of insulin, metformin and sulphonylureas
- Antipsychotics: enhanced hypotensive effect when ACE inhibitors given with antipsychotics

ACE Inhibitors *(continued)*
- Anxiolytics and Hypnotics: enhanced hypotensive effect when ACE inhibitors given with anxiolytics and hypnotics
- Beta-blockers: enhanced hypotensive effect when ACE inhibitors given with beta-blockers
- Calcium-channel Blockers: enhanced hypotensive effect when ACE inhibitors given with calcium-channel blockers
- Cardiac Glycosides: captopril possibly increases plasma concentration of digoxin
- • Ciclosporin: increased risk of hyperkalaemia when ACE inhibitors given with •ciclosporin
- Clonidine: enhanced hypotensive effect when ACE inhibitors given with clonidine; antihypertensive effect of captopril possibly delayed by previous treatment with clonidine
- Corticosteroids: hypotensive effect of ACE inhibitors antagonised by corticosteroids
- Cytotoxics: increased risk of leucopenia when captopril given with azathioprine
- Diazoxide: enhanced hypotensive effect when ACE inhibitors given with diazoxide
- • Diuretics: enhanced hypotensive effect when ACE inhibitors given with •diuretics; increased risk of severe hyperkalaemia when ACE inhibitors given with •potassium-sparing diuretics and aldosterone antagonists (monitor potassium concentration with low-dose spironolactone in heart failure)
- Dopaminergics: enhanced hypotensive effect when ACE inhibitors given with levodopa
- Epoetin: antagonism of hypotensive effect and increased risk of hyperkalaemia when ACE inhibitors given with epoetin
- • Lithium: ACE inhibitors reduce excretion of •lithium (increased plasma concentration)
- Methyldopa: enhanced hypotensive effect when ACE inhibitors given with methyldopa
- Moxisylyte (thymoxamine): enhanced hypotensive effect when ACE inhibitors given with moxisylyte
- Moxonidine: enhanced hypotensive effect when ACE inhibitors given with moxonidine
- Muscle Relaxants: enhanced hypotensive effect when ACE inhibitors given with baclofen or tizanidine
- Nitrates: enhanced hypotensive effect when ACE inhibitors given with nitrates
- Oestrogens: hypotensive effect of ACE inhibitors antagonised by oestrogens
- • Potassium Salts: increased risk of severe hyperkalaemia when ACE inhibitors given with •potassium salts
- Probenecid: excretion of captopril reduced by probenecid
- Progestogens: risk of hyperkalaemia when ACE inhibitors given with drospirenone (monitor serum potassium during first cycle)
- Prostaglandins: enhanced hypotensive effect when ACE inhibitors given with alprostadil
- Vasodilator Antihypertensives: enhanced hypotensive effect when ACE inhibitors given with hydralazine, minoxidil or nitroprusside

Acebutolol *see* Beta-blockers

Aceclofenac *see* NSAIDs

Acemetacin *see* NSAIDs

Acenocoumarol (nicoumalone) *see* Coumarins

Acetazolamide *see* Diuretics

Aciclovir

Note. Interactions do not apply to topical aciclovir preparations

Note. Valaciclovir interactions as for aciclovir

Aciclovir *(continued)*
- Ciclosporin: increased risk of nephrotoxicity when aciclovir given with ciclosporin
- Cytotoxics: plasma concentration of aciclovir increased by mycophenolate mofetil, also plasma concentration of inactive metabolite of mycophenolate mofetil increased
- Probenecid: excretion of aciclovir reduced by probenecid (increased plasma concentration)

Acitretin *see* Retinoids

Acrivastine *see* Antihistamines

Adalimumab
- • Anakinra: avoid concomitant use of adalimumab with •anakinra
- • Vaccines: avoid concomitant use of adalimumab with live •vaccines (see p. 675)

Adenosine

Note. Possibility of interaction with drugs tending to impair myocardial conduction
- Anaesthetics, Local: increased myocardial depression when anti-arrhythmics given with bupivacaine, levobupivacaine or prilocaine
- • Anti-arrhythmics: increased myocardial depression when anti-arrhythmics given with other •anti-arrhythmics
- • Antipsychotics: increased risk of ventricular arrhythmias when anti-arrhythmics that prolong the QT interval given with •antipsychotics that prolong the QT interval
- • Beta-blockers: increased myocardial depression when anti-arrhythmics given with •beta-blockers
- • Dipyridamole: effect of adenosine enhanced and extended by •dipyridamole (important risk of toxicity)
- $5HT_3$ Antagonists: caution with anti-arrhythmics advised by manufacturer of tropisetron (risk of ventricular arrhythmias)
- Theophylline: anti-arrhythmic effect of adenosine antagonised by theophylline

Adrenaline (epinephrine) *see* Sympathomimetics

Adrenergic Neurone Blockers
- Alcohol: enhanced hypotensive effect when adrenergic neurone blockers given with alcohol
- Alpha-blockers: enhanced hypotensive effect when adrenergic neurone blockers given with alpha-blockers
- • Anaesthetics, General: enhanced hypotensive effect when adrenergic neurone blockers given with •general anaesthetics
- Analgesics: hypotensive effect of adrenergic neurone blockers antagonised by NSAIDs
- Angiotensin-II Receptor Antagonists: enhanced hypotensive effect when adrenergic neurone blockers given with angiotensin-II receptor antagonists
- Antidepressants: enhanced hypotensive effect when adrenergic neurone blockers given with MAOIs; hypotensive effect of adrenergic neurone blockers antagonised by tricyclics
- Antipsychotics: hypotensive effect of adrenergic neurone blockers antagonised by haloperidol; hypotensive effect of adrenergic neurone blockers antagonised by higher doses of chlorpromazine; enhanced hypotensive effect when adrenergic neurone blockers given with phenothiazines
- Anxiolytics and Hypnotics: enhanced hypotensive effect when adrenergic neurone blockers given with anxiolytics and hypnotics
- Beta-blockers: enhanced hypotensive effect when adrenergic neurone blockers given with beta-blockers

Adrenergic Neurone Blockers *(continued)*
- Calcium-channel Blockers: enhanced hypotensive effect when adrenergic neurone blockers given with calcium-channel blockers
- Clonidine: enhanced hypotensive effect when adrenergic neurone blockers given with clonidine
- Corticosteroids: hypotensive effect of adrenergic neurone blockers antagonised by corticosteroids
- Diazoxide: enhanced hypotensive effect when adrenergic neurone blockers given with diazoxide
- Diuretics: enhanced hypotensive effect when adrenergic neurone blockers given with diuretics
- Dopaminergics: enhanced hypotensive effect when adrenergic neurone blockers given with levodopa
- Methyldopa: enhanced hypotensive effect when adrenergic neurone blockers given with methyldopa
- Moxisylyte (thymoxamine): enhanced hypotensive effect when adrenergic neurone blockers given with moxisylyte
- Moxonidine: enhanced hypotensive effect when adrenergic neurone blockers given with moxonidine
- Muscle Relaxants: enhanced hypotensive effect when adrenergic neurone blockers given with baclofen or tizanidine
- Nitrates: enhanced hypotensive effect when adrenergic neurone blockers given with nitrates
- Oestrogens: hypotensive effect of adrenergic neurone blockers antagonised by oestrogens
- Pizotifen: hypotensive effect of adrenergic neurone blockers antagonised by pizotifen
- Prostaglandins: enhanced hypotensive effect when adrenergic neurone blockers given with alprostadil
- • Sympathomimetics: hypotensive effect of adrenergic neurone blockers antagonised by •ephedrine, •isometheptene, •metaraminol, •methylphenidate, •noradrenaline (norepinephrine), •oxymetazoline, •phenylephrine, •phenylpropanolamine, •pseudoephedrine and •xylometazoline
- Vasodilator Antihypertensives: enhanced hypotensive effect when adrenergic neurone blockers given with hydralazine, minoxidil or nitroprusside

Adsorbents *see* Kaolin

Agalsidase Beta
- Anti-arrhythmics: effects of agalsidase beta possibly inhibited by amiodarone (manufacturer of agalsidase beta advises avoid concomitant use)
- Antibacterials: effects of agalsidase beta possibly inhibited by gentamicin (manufacturer of agalsidase beta advises avoid concomitant use)
- Antimalarials: effects of agalsidase beta possibly inhibited by chloroquine and hydroxychloroquine (manufacturer of agalsidase beta advises avoid concomitant use)

Alcohol
- ACE Inhibitors: enhanced hypotensive effect when alcohol given with ACE inhibitors
- Adrenergic Neurone Blockers: enhanced hypotensive effect when alcohol given with adrenergic neurone blockers
- Alpha-blockers: increased sedative effect when alcohol given with indoramin; enhanced hypotensive effect when alcohol given with alpha-blockers
- Analgesics: enhanced hypotensive and sedative effects when alcohol given with opioid analgesics
- Angiotensin-II Receptor Antagonists: enhanced hypotensive effect when alcohol given with angiotensin-II receptor antagonists
- • Antibacterials: disulfiram-like reaction when alcohol given with metronidazole; possibility of disulfiram-like reaction when alcohol given with tinidazole; increased risk of convulsions when alcohol given with •cycloserine
- • Anticoagulants: major changes in consumption of alcohol may affect anticoagulant control with •coumarins or •phenindione
- • Antidepressants: some beverages containing alcohol and some dealcoholised beverages contain tyramine which interacts with •MAOIs (hypertensive crisis)—if no tyramine, enhanced hypotensive effect; sedative effects possibly increased when alcohol given with SSRIs; increased sedative effect when alcohol given with •mirtazapine, •tricyclic-related antidepressants or •tricyclics
- Antidiabetics: alcohol enhances hypoglycaemic effect of antidiabetics; increased risk of lactic acidosis when alcohol given with metformin; flushing, in susceptible subjects, when alcohol given with chlorpropamide
- Antiepileptics: alcohol possibly increases CNS side-effects of carbamazepine; increased sedative effect when alcohol given with primidone
- Antifungals: effects of alcohol possibly enhanced by griseofulvin
- Antihistamines: increased sedative effect when alcohol given with antihistamines (possibly less effect with non-sedating antihistamines)
- Antimuscarinics: increased sedative effect when alcohol given with hyoscine
- Antipsychotics: increased sedative effect when alcohol given with antipsychotics
- Anxiolytics and Hypnotics: increased sedative effect when alcohol given with anxiolytics and hypnotics
- Barbiturates: increased sedative effect when alcohol given with barbiturates
- Beta-blockers: enhanced hypotensive effect when alcohol given with beta-blockers
- Calcium-channel Blockers: enhanced hypotensive effect when alcohol given with calcium-channel blockers; plasma concentration of alcohol possibly increased by verapamil
- Clonidine: enhanced hypotensive effect when alcohol given with clonidine
- Cytotoxics: disulfiram-like reaction when alcohol given with procarbazine
- Diazoxide: enhanced hypotensive effect when alcohol given with diazoxide
- Disulfiram: disulfiram reaction when alcohol given with disulfiram (see BNF section 4.10)
- Diuretics: enhanced hypotensive effect when alcohol given with diuretics
- Dopaminergics: alcohol reduces tolerance to bromocriptine
- Levamisole: possibility of disulfiram-like reaction when alcohol given with levamisole
- Lofexidine: increased sedative effect when alcohol given with lofexidine
- Methyldopa: enhanced hypotensive effect when alcohol given with methyldopa

Alcohol *(continued)*
- Moxonidine: enhanced hypotensive effect when alcohol given with moxonidine
- Muscle Relaxants: increased sedative effect when alcohol given with baclofen, methocarbamol or tizanidine
- Nabilone: increased sedative effect when alcohol given with nabilone
- Nicorandil: alcohol possibly enhances hypotensive effect of nicorandil
- Nitrates: enhanced hypotensive effect when alcohol given with nitrates
- • Paraldehyde: increased sedative effect when alcohol given with •paraldehyde
- Retinoids: presence of alcohol causes etretinate to be formed from acitretin
- Vasodilator Antihypertensives: enhanced hypotensive effect when alcohol given with hydralazine, minoxidil or nitroprusside

Aldesleukin
- ACE Inhibitors: enhanced hypotensive effect when aldesleukin given with ACE inhibitors
- Alpha-blockers: enhanced hypotensive effect when aldesleukin given with alpha-blockers
- Angiotensin-II Receptor Antagonists: enhanced hypotensive effect when aldesleukin given with angiotensin-II receptor antagonists
- Beta-blockers: enhanced hypotensive effect when aldesleukin given with beta-blockers
- Calcium-channel Blockers: enhanced hypotensive effect when aldesleukin given with calcium-channel blockers
- Clonidine: enhanced hypotensive effect when aldesleukin given with clonidine
- Diazoxide: enhanced hypotensive effect when aldesleukin given with diazoxide
- Diuretics: enhanced hypotensive effect when aldesleukin given with diuretics
- Methyldopa: enhanced hypotensive effect when aldesleukin given with methyldopa
- Moxonidine: enhanced hypotensive effect when aldesleukin given with moxonidine
- Nitrates: enhanced hypotensive effect when aldesleukin given with nitrates
- Vasodilator Antihypertensives: enhanced hypotensive effect when aldesleukin given with hydralazine, minoxidil or nitroprusside

Alendronic Acid *see* Bisphosphonates

Alfentanil *see* Opioid Analgesics

Alfuzosin *see* Alpha-blockers

Alimemazine (trimeprazine) *see* Antihistamines

Alkylating Drugs *see* Busulfan, Cyclophosphamide, Ifosfamide, Melphalan, and Thiotepa

Allopurinol
- ACE Inhibitors: increased risk of toxicity when allopurinol given with captopril especially in renal impairment
- Antibacterials: increased risk of rash when allopurinol given with amoxicillin or ampicillin
- Anticoagulants: allopurinol possibly enhances anticoagulant effect of coumarins
- Antivirals: allopurinol possibly increases plasma concentration of didanosine
- Ciclosporin: allopurinol possibly increases plasma concentration of ciclosporin (risk of nephrotoxicity)
- • Cytotoxics: allopurinol enhances effects and increases toxicity of •azathioprine and •mercaptopurine (reduce dose of azathioprine and mercaptopurine); avoidance of allopurinol advised by manufacturer of •capecitabine

Allopurinol *(continued)*
- Diuretics: increased risk of hypersensitivity when allopurinol given with thiazides and related diuretics especially in renal impairment
- Theophylline: allopurinol possibly increases plasma concentration of theophylline

Almotriptan *see* $5HT_1$ Agonists

Alpha$_2$-adrenoceptor Stimulants
- Antidepressants: manufacturer of apraclonidine and brimonidine advises avoid concomitant use with MAOIs; manufacturer of apraclonidine and brimonidine advises avoid concomitant use with tricyclic-related antidepressants; manufacturer of apraclonidine and brimonidine advises avoid concomitant use with tricyclics

Alpha-blockers
- ACE Inhibitors: enhanced hypotensive effect when alpha-blockers given with ACE inhibitors
- Adrenergic Neurone Blockers: enhanced hypotensive effect when alpha-blockers given with adrenergic neurone blockers
- Alcohol: enhanced hypotensive effect when alpha-blockers given with alcohol; increased sedative effect when indoramin given with alcohol
- Aldesleukin: enhanced hypotensive effect when alpha-blockers given with aldesleukin
- • Anaesthetics, General: enhanced hypotensive effect when alpha-blockers given with •general anaesthetics
- Analgesics: hypotensive effect of alpha-blockers antagonised by NSAIDs
- Angiotensin-II Receptor Antagonists: enhanced hypotensive effect when alpha-blockers given with angiotensin-II receptor antagonists
- • Antidepressants: enhanced hypotensive effect when alpha-blockers given with MAOIs; manufacturer of indoramin advises avoid concomitant use with •MAOIs
- Antipsychotics: enhanced hypotensive effect when alpha-blockers given with antipsychotics
- Anxiolytics and Hypnotics: enhanced hypotensive and sedative effects when alpha-blockers given with anxiolytics and hypnotics
- • Beta-blockers: enhanced hypotensive effect when alpha-blockers given with •beta-blockers, also increased risk of first-dose hypotension with post-synaptic alpha-blockers such as prazosin
- • Calcium-channel Blockers: enhanced hypotensive effect when alpha-blockers given with •calcium-channel blockers, also increased risk of first-dose hypotension with post-synaptic alpha-blockers such as prazosin
- Cardiac Glycosides: prazosin increases plasma concentration of digoxin
- Clonidine: enhanced hypotensive effect when alpha-blockers given with clonidine
- Corticosteroids: hypotensive effect of alpha-blockers antagonised by corticosteroids
- Diazoxide: enhanced hypotensive effect when alpha-blockers given with diazoxide
- • Diuretics: enhanced hypotensive effect when alpha-blockers given with •diuretics, also increased risk of first-dose hypotension with post-synaptic alpha-blockers such as prazosin
- Dopaminergics: enhanced hypotensive effect when alpha-blockers given with levodopa
- Methyldopa: enhanced hypotensive effect when alpha-blockers given with methyldopa
- • Moxisylyte (thymoxamine): possible severe postural hypotension when alpha-blockers given with •moxisylyte

Alpha-blockers *(continued)*
- Moxonidine: enhanced hypotensive effect when alpha-blockers given with moxonidine
- Muscle Relaxants: enhanced hypotensive effect when alpha-blockers given with baclofen or tizanidine
- Nitrates: enhanced hypotensive effect when alpha-blockers given with nitrates
- Oestrogens: hypotensive effect of alpha-blockers antagonised by oestrogens
- Prostaglandins: enhanced hypotensive effect when alpha-blockers given with alprostadil
- • Sildenafil: enhanced hypotensive effect when alpha-blockers given with •sildenafil (avoid alpha-blockers for 4 hours after sildenafil)
- • Sympathomimetics: avoid concomitant use of tolazoline with •adrenaline (epinephrine) or •dopamine
- • Tadalafil: enhanced hypotensive effect when alpha-blockers given with •tadalafil—avoid concomitant use
- • Ulcer-healing Drugs: effects of tolazoline antagonised by •cimetidine and •ranitidine
- • Vardenafil: enhanced hypotensive effect when alpha-blockers (excludes tamsulosin) given with •vardenafil—avoid vardenafil for 6 hours after alpha-blockers
- Vasodilator Antihypertensives: enhanced hypotensive effect when alpha-blockers given with hydralazine, minoxidil or nitroprusside

Alpha-blockers (post-synaptic) *see* Alpha-blockers
Alprazolam *see* Anxiolytics and Hypnotics
Alprostadil *see* Prostaglandins
Aluminium Hydroxide *see* Antacids
Amantadine
- Antimuscarinics: increased risk of antimuscarinic side-effects when amantadine given with antimuscarinics
- Antipsychotics: increased risk of extrapyramidal side-effects when amantadine given with antipsychotics
- Bupropion: increased risk of side-effects when amantadine given with bupropion
- Domperidone: increased risk of extrapyramidal side-effects when amantadine given with domperidone
- • Memantine: increased risk of CNS toxicity when amantadine given with •memantine (manufacturer of memantine advises avoid concomitant use); effects of dopaminergics possibly enhanced by memantine
- Methyldopa: increased risk of extrapyramidal side-effects when amantadine given with methyldopa; antiparkinsonian effect of dopaminergics antagonised by methyldopa
- Metoclopramide: increased risk of extrapyramidal side-effects when amantadine given with metoclopramide
- Tetrabenazine: increased risk of extrapyramidal side-effects when amantadine given with tetrabenazine

Amikacin *see* Aminoglycosides
Amiloride *see* Diuretics
Aminoglycosides
- Agalsidase Beta: gentamicin possibly inhibits effects of agalsidase beta (manufacturer of agalsidase beta advises avoid concomitant use)
- Analgesics: plasma concentration of amikacin and gentamicin in neonates possibly increased by indometacin
- Antibacterials: neomycin reduces absorption of phenoxymethylpenicillin; increased risk of nephrotoxicity when aminoglycosides given with colistin or polymyxins; increased risk of nephrotoxicity and ototoxicity when aminoglycosides given with capreomycin, teicoplanin or vancomycin
- • Anticoagulants: experience in anticoagulant clinics suggests that INR possibly altered when neomycin (given for local action on gut) is given with •coumarins or •phenindione
- Antidiabetics: neomycin possibly enhances hypoglycaemic effect of acarbose, also severity of gastro-intestinal effects increased
- Antifungals: increased risk of nephrotoxicity when aminoglycosides given with amphotericin
- Bisphosphonates: increased risk of hypocalcaemia when aminoglycosides given with bisphosphonates
- Cardiac Glycosides: gentamicin possibly increases plasma concentration of digoxin; neomycin reduces absorption of digoxin
- • Ciclosporin: increased risk of nephrotoxicity when aminoglycosides given with •ciclosporin
- • Cytotoxics: neomycin possibly reduces absorption of methotrexate; increased risk of nephrotoxicity and possibly of ototoxicity when aminoglycosides given with •platinum compounds
- • Diuretics: increased risk of otoxicity when aminoglycosides given with •loop diuretics
- • Muscle Relaxants: aminoglycosides enhance effects of •non-depolarising muscle relaxants and •suxamethonium
- Oestrogens: antibacterials that do not induce liver enzymes possibly reduce contraceptive effect of oestrogens (risk probably small, see BNF section 7.3.1)
- • Parasympathomimetics: aminoglycosides antagonise effects of •neostigmine and •pyridostigmine
- • Tacrolimus: increased risk of nephrotoxicity when aminoglycosides given with •tacrolimus
- Vitamins: neomycin possibly reduces absorption of vitamin A

Aminophylline *see* Theophylline
Aminosalicylates
- Cardiac Glycosides: sulfasalazine possibly reduces absorption of digoxin
- Cytotoxics: possible increased risk of leucopenia when aminosalicylates given with azathioprine or mercaptopurine
- Folates: sulfasalazine possibly reduces absorption of folic acid

Amiodarone

Note. Amiodarone has a long half-life; there is a potential for drug interactions to occur for several weeks (or even months) after treatment with it has been stopped

- Agalsidase Beta: amiodarone possibly inhibits effects of agalsidase beta (manufacturer of agalsidase beta advises avoid concomitant use)
- Anaesthetics, Local: increased myocardial depression when anti-arrhythmics given with bupivacaine, levobupivacaine or prilocaine
- • Anti-arrhythmics: increased myocardial depression when anti-arrhythmics given with other •anti-arrhythmics; increased risk of ventricular arrhythmias when amiodarone given with •disopyramide—avoid concomitant use; amiodarone increases plasma concentration of •flecainide (halve dose of flecainide); amiodarone increases plasma concentration of •procainamide and •quinidine (increased risk of ventricular arrhythmias—avoid concomitant use)

Amiodarone *(continued)*
- • Antibacterials: increased risk of ventricular arrhythmias when amiodarone given with parenteral •erythromycin—avoid concomitant use; increased risk of ventricular arrhythmias when amiodarone given with •moxifloxacin—avoid concomitant use; increased risk of ventricular arrhythmias when amiodarone given with •sulfamethoxazole and •trimethoprim (as co-trimoxazole)—avoid concomitant use of co-trimoxazole
- • Anticoagulants: amiodarone inhibits metabolism of •coumarins and •phenindione (enhanced anticoagulant effect)
- • Antidepressants: increased risk of ventricular arrhythmias when amiodarone given with •tricyclics—avoid concomitant use
- • Antiepileptics: amiodarone inhibits metabolism of •phenytoin (increased plasma concentration)
- • Antihistamines: increased risk of ventricular arrhythmias when amiodarone given with •mizolastine—avoid concomitant use
- • Antimalarials: avoidance of amiodarone advised by manufacturer of •artemether/lumefantrine (risk of ventricular arrhythmias); increased risk of ventricular arrhythmias when amiodarone given with •chloroquine and hydroxychloroquine, •mefloquine or •quinine—avoid concomitant use
- • Antipsychotics: increased risk of ventricular arrhythmias when anti-arrhythmics that prolong the QT interval given with •antipsychotics that prolong the QT interval; increased risk of ventricular arrhythmias when amiodarone given with •amisulpride, •haloperidol, •phenothiazines, •pimozide or •sertindole—avoid concomitant use
- • Antivirals: plasma concentration of amiodarone possibly increased by •amprenavir (increased risk of ventricular arrhythmias—avoid concomitant use); plasma concentration of amiodarone possibly increased by •atazanavir; increased risk of ventricular arrhythmias when amiodarone given with •nelfinavir—avoid concomitant use; plasma concentration of amiodarone increased by •ritonavir (increased risk of ventricular arrhythmias—avoid concomitant use)
- • Beta-blockers: increased risk of bradycardia, AV block and myocardial depression when amiodarone given with •beta-blockers; increased myocardial depression when anti-arrhythmics given with •beta-blockers; increased risk of ventricular arrhythmias when amiodarone given with •sotalol—avoid concomitant use
- • Calcium-channel Blockers: increased risk of bradycardia, AV block and myocardial depression when amiodarone given with •diltiazem or •verapamil
- • Cardiac Glycosides: amiodarone increases plasma concentration of •digoxin (halve dose of digoxin)
- Ciclosporin: amiodarone possibly increases plasma concentration of ciclosporin
- Diuretics: increased cardiac toxicity with amiodarone if hypokalaemia occurs with acetazolamide, loop diuretics or thiazides and related diuretics; amiodarone increases plasma concentration of eplerenone (reduce dose of eplerenone)
- • Dolasetron: increased risk of ventricular arrhythmias when amiodarone given with •dolasetron—avoid concomitant use

Amiodarone *(continued)*
- $5HT_3$ Antagonists: caution with anti-arrhythmics advised by manufacturer of tropisetron (risk of ventricular arrhythmias)
- • Ivabradine: increased risk of ventricular arrhythmias when amiodarone given with •ivabradine
- • Lipid-regulating Drugs: increased risk of myopathy when amiodarone given with •simvastatin
- • Lithium: manufacturer of amiodarone advises avoid concomitant use with •lithium (risk of ventricular arrhythmias)
- Orlistat: plasma concentration of amiodarone possibly reduced by orlistat
- • Pentamidine Isetionate: increased risk of ventricular arrhythmias when amiodarone given with •pentamidine isetionate—avoid concomitant use
- Thyroid Hormones: for concomitant use of amiodarone and thyroid hormones see p. 106
- Ulcer-healing Drugs: plasma concentration of amiodarone increased by cimetidine

Amisulpride *see* Antipsychotics
Amitriptyline *see* Antidepressants, Tricyclic
Amlodipine *see* Calcium-channel Blockers
Amobarbital *see* Barbiturates
Amoxapine *see* Antidepressants, Tricyclic
Amoxicillin *see* Penicillins
Amphotericin

Note. Close monitoring required with concomitant administration of nephrotoxic drugs or cytotoxics

- Antibacterials: increased risk of nephrotoxicity when amphotericin given with aminoglycosides or polymyxins; possible increased risk of nephrotoxicity when amphotericin given with vancomycin
- Antifungals: amphotericin reduces renal excretion and increases cellular uptake of flucytosine (toxicity possibly increased); effects of amphotericin possibly antagonised by imidazoles and triazoles
- • Cardiac Glycosides: hypokalaemia caused by amphotericin increases cardiac toxicity with •cardiac glycosides
- • Ciclosporin: increased risk of nephrotoxicity when amphotericin given with •ciclosporin
- • Corticosteroids: increased risk of hypokalaemia when amphotericin given with •corticosteroids—avoid concomitant use unless corticosteroids needed to control reactions
- Diuretics: increased risk of hypokalaemia when amphotericin given with loop diuretics or thiazides and related diuretics
- Pentamidine Isetionate: possible increased risk of nephrotoxicity when amphotericin given with pentamidine isetionate
- • Tacrolimus: increased risk of nephrotoxicity when amphotericin given with •tacrolimus

Ampicillin *see* Penicillins
Amprenavir

Note. Fosamprenavir is a prodrug of amprenavir

- Analgesics: amprenavir reduces plasma concentration of methadone
- Antacids: absorption of amprenavir possibly reduced by antacids
- • Anti-arrhythmics: amprenavir possibly increases plasma concentration of •amiodarone, •flecainide, •propafenone and •quinidine (increased risk of ventricular arrhythmias—avoid concomitant use); amprenavir possibly increases plasma concentration of •lidocaine (lignocaine)—avoid concomitant use

Appendix 1

Amprenavir *(continued)*

- • Antibacterials: plasma concentration of both drugs increased when amprenavir given with erythromycin; amprenavir increases plasma concentration of •rifabutin (reduce dose of rifabutin); plasma concentration of amprenavir significantly reduced by •rifampicin—avoid concomitant use; amprenavir possibly increases plasma concentration of dapsone
- Anticoagulants: amprenavir may enhance or reduce anticoagulant effect of coumarins
- • Antidepressants: plasma concentration of amprenavir reduced by •St John's wort—avoid concomitant use; amprenavir possibly increases side-effects of tricyclics
- Antiepileptics: plasma concentration of amprenavir possibly reduced by carbamazepine and phenytoin
- Antifungals: amprenavir increases plasma concentration of ketoconazole; amprenavir possibly increases plasma concentration of itraconazole
- Antihistamines: amprenavir possibly increases plasma concentration of loratadine
- • Antimalarials: avoidance of amprenavir advised by manufacturer of •artemether/lumefantrine
- Antimuscarinics: avoidance of amprenavir advised by manufacturer of tolterodine
- • Antipsychotics: amprenavir possibly inhibits metabolism of •aripiprazole (reduce dose of aripiprazole); amprenavir possibly increases plasma concentration of clozapine; amprenavir increases plasma concentration of •pimozide and •sertindole (increased risk of ventricular arrhythmias—avoid concomitant use)
- • Antivirals: plasma concentration of amprenavir reduced by efavirenz and •tipranavir; plasma concentration of amprenavir reduced by lopinavir, effect on lopinavir plasma concentration not predictable; plasma concentration of amprenavir possibly reduced by nevirapine; plasma concentration of amprenavir increased by ritonavir
- • Anxiolytics and Hypnotics: increased risk of prolonged sedation and respiratory depression when amprenavir given with •alprazolam, clonazepam, •diazepam, •flurazepam or •midazolam
- Barbiturates: plasma concentration of amprenavir possibly reduced by phenobarbital
- Calcium-channel Blockers: amprenavir possibly increases plasma concentration of diltiazem, nicardipine, nifedipine and nimodipine
- • Cilostazol: amprenavir possibly increases plasma concentration of •cilostazol—avoid concomitant use
- • Ergot Alkaloids: increased risk of ergotism when amprenavir given with •ergotamine and methysergide—avoid concomitant use
- • Lipid-regulating Drugs: possible increased risk of myopathy when amprenavir given with atorvastatin; possible increased risk of myopathy when amprenavir given with •simvastatin—avoid concomitant use
- Oestrogens: amprenavir possibly reduces contraceptive effect of oestrogens
- Progestogens: amprenavir possibly reduces contraceptive effect of progestogens
- Sildenafil: amprenavir possibly increases plasma concentration of sildenafil— reduce initial dose of sildenafil
- Tadalafil: amprenavir possibly increases plasma concentration of tadalafil

Amprenavir *(continued)*

- Ulcer-healing Drugs: amprenavir possibly increases plasma concentration of cimetidine
- Vardenafil: amprenavir possibly increases plasma concentration of vardenafil

Anabolic Steroids

- • Anticoagulants: anabolic steroids enhance anticoagulant effect of •coumarins and •phenindione
- Antidiabetics: anabolic steroids possibly enhance hypoglycaemic effect of antidiabetics

Anaesthetics, General

Note. See also Surgery and Long-term Medication, p. 705

- ACE Inhibitors: enhanced hypotensive effect when general anaesthetics given with ACE inhibitors
- • Adrenergic Neurone Blockers: enhanced hypotensive effect when general anaesthetics given with •adrenergic neurone blockers
- • Alpha-blockers: enhanced hypotensive effect when general anaesthetics given with •alpha-blockers
- Angiotensin-II Receptor Antagonists: enhanced hypotensive effect when general anaesthetics given with angiotensin-II receptor antagonists
- Antibacterials: general anaesthetics possibly potentiate hepatotoxicity of isoniazid; effects of thiopental enhanced by sulphonamides; hypersensitivity-like reactions can occur when general anaesthetics given with intravenous vancomycin
- • Antidepressants: Because of hazardous interactions between general anaesthetics and •MAOIs, MAOIs should normally be stopped 2 weeks before surgery; increased risk of arrhythmias and hypotension when general anaesthetics given with tricyclics
- • Antipsychotics: enhanced hypotensive effect when general anaesthetics given with •antipsychotics
- Anxiolytics and Hypnotics: increased sedative effect when general anaesthetics given with anxiolytics and hypnotics
- Beta-blockers: enhanced hypotensive effect when general anaesthetics given with beta-blockers
- • Calcium-channel Blockers: enhanced hypotensive effect when general anaesthetics or isoflurane given with calcium-channel blockers; general anaesthetics enhance hypotensive effect of •verapamil (also AV delay)
- Clonidine: enhanced hypotensive effect when general anaesthetics given with clonidine
- • Cytotoxics: nitrous oxide increases antifolate effect of •methotrexate—avoid concomitant use
- Diazoxide: enhanced hypotensive effect when general anaesthetics given with diazoxide
- Diuretics: enhanced hypotensive effect when general anaesthetics given with diuretics
- • Dopaminergics: increased risk of arrhythmias when volatile liquid general anaesthetics given with •levodopa
- Ergot Alkaloids: halothane reduces effects of ergometrine on the parturient uterus
- • Memantine: increased risk of CNS toxicity when ketamine given with •memantine (manufacturer of memantine advises avoid concomitant use)
- Methyldopa: enhanced hypotensive effect when general anaesthetics given with methyldopa
- Moxonidine: enhanced hypotensive effect when general anaesthetics given with moxonidine

Anaesthetics, General *(continued)*
Muscle Relaxants: volatile liquid general anaesthetics enhance effects of non-depolarising muscle relaxants and suxamethonium
Nitrates: enhanced hypotensive effect when general anaesthetics given with nitrates
Oxytocin: oxytocic effect possibly reduced, also enhanced hypotensive effect and risk of arrhythmias when volatile liquid general anaesthetics given with oxytocin
• Sympathomimetics: increased risk of arrhythmias when volatile liquid general anaesthetics given with •adrenaline (epinephrine); increased risk of hypertension when volatile liquid general anaesthetics given with •methylphenidate
Theophylline: increased risk of convulsions when ketamine given with theophylline; increased risk of arrhythmias when halothane given with theophylline
Vasodilator Antihypertensives: enhanced hypotensive effect when general anaesthetics given with hydralazine, minoxidil or nitroprusside

Anaesthetics, General (intravenous) *see* Anaesthetics, General

Anaesthetics, General (volatile liquids) *see* Anaesthetics, General

Anaesthetics, Local *see* Bupivacaine, Levobupivacaine, Lidocaine (lignocaine), Prilocaine, and Ropivacaine

Anagrelide
• Cilostazol: manufacturer of anagrelide advises avoid concomitant use with •cilostazol
• Phosphodiesterase Inhibitors: manufacturer of anagrelide advises avoid concomitant use with •enoximone and •milrinone

Anakinra
• Adalimumab: avoid concomitant use of anakinra with •adalimumab
• Etanercept: increased risk of side-effects when anakinra given with •etanercept—avoid concomitant use
• Infliximab: avoid concomitant use of anakinra with •infliximab
• Vaccines: avoid concomitant use of anakinra with live •vaccines (see p. 675)

Analgesics *see* Aspirin, Nefopam, NSAIDs, Opioid Analgesics, and Paracetamol

Angiotensin-II Receptor Antagonists
ACE Inhibitors: enhanced hypotensive effect when angiotensin-II receptor antagonists given with ACE inhibitors
Adrenergic Neurone Blockers: enhanced hypotensive effect when angiotensin-II receptor antagonists given with adrenergic neurone blockers
Alcohol: enhanced hypotensive effect when angiotensin-II receptor antagonists given with alcohol
Aldesleukin: enhanced hypotensive effect when angiotensin-II receptor antagonists given with aldesleukin
Alpha-blockers: enhanced hypotensive effect when angiotensin-II receptor antagonists given with alpha-blockers
Anaesthetics, General: enhanced hypotensive effect when angiotensin-II receptor antagonists given with general anaesthetics
Analgesics: increased risk of renal impairment when angiotensin-II receptor antagonists given with NSAIDs, also hypotensive effect antagonised; increased risk of hyperkalaemia when angiotensin-II receptor antagonists given with ketorolac; risk of renal impairment when

Angiotensin-II Receptor Antagonists
Analgesics *(continued)*
angiotensin-II receptor antagonists given with aspirin (in doses over 300 mg daily), also hypotensive effect antagonised
Anticoagulants: increased risk of hyperkalaemia when angiotensin-II receptor antagonists given with heparin
Antidepressants: hypotensive effect of angiotensin-II receptor antagonists possibly enhanced by MAOIs
Antipsychotics: enhanced hypotensive effect when angiotensin-II receptor antagonists given with antipsychotics
Anxiolytics and Hypnotics: enhanced hypotensive effect when angiotensin-II receptor antagonists given with anxiolytics and hypnotics
Beta-blockers: enhanced hypotensive effect when angiotensin-II receptor antagonists given with beta-blockers
Calcium-channel Blockers: enhanced hypotensive effect when angiotensin-II receptor antagonists given with calcium-channel blockers
• Cardiac Glycosides: telmisartan increases plasma concentration of •digoxin
• Ciclosporin: increased risk of hyperkalaemia when angiotensin-II receptor antagonists given with •ciclosporin
Clonidine: enhanced hypotensive effect when angiotensin-II receptor antagonists given with clonidine
Corticosteroids: hypotensive effect of angiotensin-II receptor antagonists antagonised by corticosteroids
Diazoxide: enhanced hypotensive effect when angiotensin-II receptor antagonists given with diazoxide
• Diuretics: enhanced hypotensive effect when angiotensin-II receptor antagonists given with •diuretics; increased risk of hyperkalaemia when angiotensin-II receptor antagonists given with •potassium-sparing diuretics and aldosterone antagonists
Dopaminergics: enhanced hypotensive effect when angiotensin-II receptor antagonists given with levodopa
Epoetin: antagonism of hypotensive effect and increased risk of hyperkalaemia when angiotensin-II receptor antagonists given with epoetin
• Lithium: angiotensin-II receptor antagonists reduce excretion of •lithium (increased plasma concentration)
Methyldopa: enhanced hypotensive effect when angiotensin-II receptor antagonists given with methyldopa
Moxisylyte (thymoxamine): enhanced hypotensive effect when angiotensin-II receptor antagonists given with moxisylyte
Moxonidine: enhanced hypotensive effect when angiotensin-II receptor antagonists given with moxonidine
Muscle Relaxants: enhanced hypotensive effect when angiotensin-II receptor antagonists given with baclofen or tizanidine
Nitrates: enhanced hypotensive effect when angiotensin-II receptor antagonists given with nitrates
Oestrogens: hypotensive effect of angiotensin-II receptor antagonists antagonised by oestrogens

Angiotensin-II Receptor Antagonists *(continued)*
- • Potassium Salts: increased risk of hyperkalaemia when angiotensin-II receptor antagonists given with •potassium salts
- Progestogens: risk of hyperkalaemia when angiotensin-II receptor antagonists given with drospirenone (monitor serum potassium during first cycle)
- Prostaglandins: enhanced hypotensive effect when angiotensin-II receptor antagonists given with alprostadil
- Vasodilator Antihypertensives: enhanced hypotensive effect when angiotensin-II receptor antagonists given with hydralazine, minoxidil or nitroprusside

Anion-exchange Resins *see* Colestipol and Colestyramine

Antacids

Note. Antacids should preferably not be taken at the same time as other drugs since they may impair absorption

- ACE Inhibitors: antacids possibly reduce absorption of ACE inhibitors; antacids reduce absorption of captopril, enalapril and fosinopril
- Analgesics: antacids reduce absorption of diflunisal; alkaline urine due to some antacids increases excretion of aspirin
- Anti-arrhythmics: alkaline urine due to some antacids reduces excretion of quinidine (plasma concentration of quinidine occasionally increased)
- Antibacterials: antacids reduce absorption of azithromycin, cefaclor, cefpodoxime, ciprofloxacin, isoniazid, levofloxacin, moxifloxacin, norfloxacin, ofloxacin, rifampicin and tetracyclines; oral magnesium salts (as magnesium trisilicate) reduce absorption of nitrofurantoin
- Antiepileptics: antacids reduce absorption of gabapentin and phenytoin
- Antifungals: antacids reduce absorption of itraconazole and ketoconazole
- Antihistamines: antacids reduce absorption of fexofenadine
- Antimalarials: antacids reduce absorption of chloroquine and hydroxychloroquine; oral magnesium salts (as magnesium trisilicate) reduce absorption of proguanil
- Antipsychotics: antacids reduce absorption of phenothiazines and sulpiride
- Antivirals: antacids possibly reduce absorption of amprenavir; antacids possibly reduce plasma concentration of atazanavir; antacids reduce absorption of tipranavir
- Bile Acids: antacids possibly reduce absorption of bile acids
- Bisphosphonates: antacids reduce absorption of bisphosphonates
- Cardiac Glycosides: antacids possibly reduce absorption of digoxin
- Corticosteroids: antacids reduce absorption of deflazacort
- Cytotoxics: antacids reduce absorption of mycophenolate mofetil
- Dipyridamole: antacids possibly reduce absorption of dipyridamole
- Iron: oral magnesium salts (as magnesium trisilicate) reduce absorption of *oral* iron
- Lipid-regulating Drugs: antacids reduce absorption of rosuvastatin
- Lithium: sodium bicarbonate increases excretion of lithium (reduced plasma concentration)
- Penicillamine: antacids reduce absorption of penicillamine

Antacids *(continued)*
- Ulcer-healing Drugs: antacids possibly reduce absorption of lansoprazole

Antazoline *see* Antihistamines

Anti-arrhythmics *see* Adenosine, Amiodarone, Bretylium, Disopyramide, Flecainide, Lidocaine (lignocaine), Mexiletine, Procainamide, Propafenone, and Quinidine

Antibacterials *see* individual drugs

Antibiotics (cytotoxic) *see* Bleomycin, Doxorubicin, Epirubicin

Anticoagulants *see* Coumarins, Heparins, and Phenindione

Antidepressants *see* Antidepressants, SSRI; Antidepressants, Tricyclic; Antidepressants, Tricyclic (related); MAOIs; Mirtazapine; Moclobemide; Reboxetine; St John's Wort; Tryptophan; Venlafaxine

Antidepressants, Noradrenaline Re-uptake Inhibitors *see* Reboxetine

Antidepressants, SSRI
- Alcohol: sedative effects possibly increased when SSRIs given with alcohol
- Anaesthetics, Local: fluvoxamine inhibits metabolism of ropivacaine—avoid prolonged administration of ropivacaine
- • Analgesics: increased risk of bleeding when SSRIs given with •NSAIDs or •aspirin; fluvoxamine possibly increases plasma concentration of methadone; increased risk of CNS toxicity when SSRIs given with •tramadol
- • Anti-arrhythmics: fluoxetine increases plasma concentration of flecainide; fluvoxamine inhibits metabolism of •mexiletine (increased risk of toxicity); paroxetine possibly inhibits metabolism of propafenone (increased risk of toxicity)
- • Anticoagulants: SSRIs possibly enhance anticoagulant effect of •coumarins
- • Antidepressants: avoidance of fluvoxamine advised by manufacturer of •reboxetine; possible increased serotonergic effects when SSRIs given with duloxetine; fluvoxamine inhibits metabolism of •duloxetine—avoid concomitant use; sertraline should not be started until 2 weeks after stopping •MAOIs, also MAOIs should not be started until at least 2 weeks after stopping sertraline; citalopram, escitalopram, fluvoxamine or paroxetine should not be started until 2 weeks after stopping •MAOIs, also MAOIs should not be started until at least 1 week after stopping citalopram, escitalopram, fluvoxamine or paroxetine; fluoxetine should not be started until 2 weeks after stopping •MAOIs, also MAOIs should not be started until at least 5 weeks after stopping fluoxetine; CNS effects of SSRIs increased by •MAOIs (risk of serious toxicity); increased risk of CNS toxicity when escitalopram given with •moclobemide, preferably avoid concomitant use; after stopping citalopram, fluvoxamine or paroxetine do not start •moclobemide for at least 1 week; after stopping fluoxetine do not start •moclobemide for 5 weeks; after stopping sertraline do not start •moclobemide for 2 weeks; increased serotonergic effects when SSRIs given with •St John's wort—avoid concomitant use; SSRIs increase plasma concentration of some •tricyclics; agitation and nausea may occur when SSRIs given with •tryptophan
- • Antiepileptics: SSRIs antagonise anticonvulsant effect of •antiepileptics (convulsive threshold lowered); fluoxetine and fluvoxamine increase

Antidepressants, SSRI
- Antiepileptics *(continued)* plasma concentration of •carbamazepine; plasma concentration of paroxetine reduced by carbamazepine, phenytoin and primidone; fluoxetine and fluvoxamine increase plasma concentration of •phenytoin

Antihistamines: antidepressant effect of SSRIs possibly antagonised by cyproheptadine
- Antimalarials: avoidance of antidepressants advised by manufacturer of •artemether/lumefantrine

Antimuscarinics: paroxetine increases plasma concentration of procyclidine
- Antipsychotics: fluoxetine increases plasma concentration of •clozapine, •haloperidol, risperidone, •sertindole and •zotepine; paroxetine inhibits metabolism of perphenazine (reduce dose of perphenazine); fluoxetine and paroxetine possibly inhibit metabolism of •aripiprazole (reduce dose of aripiprazole); fluvoxamine, paroxetine and sertraline increase plasma concentration of •clozapine; citalopram possibly increases plasma concentration of clozapine (increased risk of toxicity); fluvoxamine increases plasma concentration of olanzapine; sertraline increases plasma concentration of •pimozide (increased risk of ventricular arrhythmias—avoid concomitant use); paroxetine possibly increases plasma concentration of risperidone (increased risk of toxicity); paroxetine increases plasma concentration of •sertindole
- Antivirals: plasma concentration of sertraline reduced by efavirenz; plasma concentration of SSRIs possibly increased by •ritonavir

Anxiolytics and Hypnotics: fluvoxamine increases plasma concentration of some benzodiazepines; sedative effects possibly increased when sertraline given with zolpidem

Barbiturates: SSRIs antagonise anticonvulsant effect of barbiturates (convulsive threshold lowered); plasma concentration of paroxetine reduced by phenobarbital

Beta-blockers: paroxetine possibly increases plasma concentration of metoprolol (enhanced effect); citalopram and escitalopram increase plasma concentration of metoprolol; fluvoxamine increases plasma concentration of propranolol
- Dopaminergics: caution with paroxetine advised by manufacturer of entacapone; increased risk of CNS toxicity when SSRIs given with •rasagiline; fluvoxamine should not be started until 2 weeks after stopping •rasagiline; fluoxetine should not be started until 2 weeks after stopping •rasagiline, also rasagiline should not be started until at least 5 weeks after stopping fluoxetine; increased risk of hypertension and CNS excitation when fluoxetine given with •selegiline (selegiline should not be started until 5 weeks after stopping fluoxetine, avoid fluoxetine for 2 weeks after stopping selegiline); theoretical risk of serotonin syndrome if citalopram given with selegiline (especially if dose of selegiline exceeds 10 mg daily); manufacturer of escitalopram advises caution with selegiline; increased risk of hypertension and CNS excitation when paroxetine or sertraline given with •selegiline (selegiline should not be started until 2 weeks after stopping paroxetine or sertraline, avoid paroxetine or sertraline for 2 weeks after

Antidepressants, SSRI
- Dopaminergics *(continued)* stopping selegiline); increased risk of hypertension and CNS excitation when fluvoxamine given with •selegiline (selegiline should not be started until 1 week after stopping fluvoxamine, avoid fluvoxamine for 2 weeks after stopping selegiline)
- $5HT_1$ Agonists: fluvoxamine inhibits the metabolism of frovatriptan; possible increased serotonergic effects when SSRIs given with frovatriptan; increased risk of CNS toxicity when citalopram, escitalopram, fluoxetine, fluvoxamine or paroxetine given with •sumatriptan; increased risk of CNS toxicity when sertraline given with •sumatriptan (manufacturer of sertraline advises avoid concomitant use); fluvoxamine possibly inhibits metabolism of zolmitriptan (reduce dose of zolmitriptan)
- Lithium: Increased risk of CNS effects when SSRIs given with •lithium (lithium toxicity reported)

Parasympathomimetics: paroxetine increases plasma concentration of galantamine
- Sibutramine: increased risk of CNS toxicity when SSRIs given with •sibutramine (manufacturer of sibutramine advises avoid concomitant use)

Sympathomimetics: metabolism of SSRIs possibly inhibited by methylphenidate
- Theophylline: fluvoxamine increases plasma concentration of •theophylline (concomitant use should usually be avoided, but where not possible halve theophylline dose and monitor plasma-theophylline concentration)

Ulcer-healing Drugs: plasma concentration of citalopram, escitalopram and sertraline increased by cimetidine; plasma concentration of escitalopram increased by omeprazole

Antidepressants, SSRI (related) *see* Duloxetine and Venlafaxine

Antidepressants, Tricyclic

Adrenergic Neurone Blockers: tricyclics antagonise hypotensive effect of adrenergic neurone blockers
- Alcohol: increased sedative effect when tricyclics given with •alcohol

$Alpha_2$-adrenoceptor Stimulants: avoidance of tricyclics advised by manufacturer of apraclonidine and brimonidine

Anaesthetics, General: increased risk of arrhythmias and hypotension when tricyclics given with general anaesthetics
- Analgesics: increased risk of CNS toxicity when tricyclics given with •tramadol; side-effects possibly increased when tricyclics given with nefopam; sedative effects possibly increased when tricyclics given with opioid analgesics
- Anti-arrhythmics: increased risk of ventricular arrhythmias when tricyclics given with •amiodarone—avoid concomitant use; increased risk of ventricular arrhythmias when tricyclics given with •disopyramide, •flecainide, •procainamide or •quinidine; increased risk of arrhythmias when tricyclics given with •propafenone
- Antibacterials: increased risk of ventricular arrhythmias when tricyclics given with •moxifloxacin—avoid concomitant use; plasma concentration of tricyclics possibly reduced by rifampicin
- Anticoagulants: tricyclics may enhance or reduce anticoagulant effect of •coumarins

Antidepressants, Tricyclic *(continued)*

- Antidepressants: possible increased serotonergic effects when amitriptyline or clomipramine given with duloxetine; increased risk of hypertension and CNS excitation when tricyclics given with •MAOIs, tricyclics should not be started until 2 weeks after stopping MAOIs (3 weeks if starting clomipramine or imipramine), also MAOIs should not be started for at least 1–2 weeks after stopping tricyclics (3 weeks in the case of clomipramine or imipramine); after stopping tricyclics do not start •moclobemide for at least 1 week; plasma concentration of some tricyclics increased by •SSRIs; plasma concentration of amitriptyline reduced by St John's wort
- Antiepileptics: tricyclics antagonise anticonvulsant effect of •antiepileptics (convulsive threshold lowered); metabolism of tricyclics accelerated by •carbamazepine (reduced plasma concentration and reduced effect); plasma concentration of tricyclics possibly reduced by •phenytoin; tricyclics antagonises anticonvulsant effect of •primidone (convulsive threshold lowered), also metabolism of tricyclics possibly accelerated (reduced plasma concentration)

Antifungals: plasma concentration of imipramine and nortriptyline possibly increased by terbinafine

Antihistamines: increased antimuscarinic and sedative effects when tricyclics given with antihistamines

- Antimalarials: avoidance of antidepressants advised by manufacturer of •artemether/lumefantrine

Antimuscarinics: increased risk of antimuscarinic side-effects when tricyclics given with antimuscarinics

- Antipsychotics: plasma concentration of tricyclics increased by •antipsychotics—possibly increased risk of ventricular arrhythmias; possibly increased antimuscarinic side-effects when tricyclics given with clozapine; increased risk of antimuscarinic side-effects when tricyclics given with phenothiazines; increased risk of ventricular arrhythmias when tricyclics given with •pimozide—avoid concomitant use
- Antivirals: side-effects of tricyclics possibly increased by amprenavir; plasma concentration of tricyclics possibly increased by •ritonavir

Anxiolytics and Hypnotics: increased sedative effect when tricyclics given with anxiolytics and hypnotics

- Barbiturates: tricyclics antagonises anticonvulsant effect of •barbiturates (convulsive threshold lowered), also metabolism of tricyclics possibly accelerated (reduced plasma concentration)
- Beta-blockers: increased risk of ventricular arrhythmias when tricyclics given with •sotalol

Calcium-channel Blockers: plasma concentration of tricyclics possibly increased by diltiazem and verapamil; plasma concentration of imipramine increased by diltiazem and verapamil

- Clonidine: tricyclics antagonise hypotensive effect of •clonidine, also increased risk of hypertension on clonidine withdrawal

Disulfiram: metabolism of tricyclics inhibited by disulfiram (increased plasma concentration); concomitant amitriptyline reported to increase disulfiram reaction with alcohol

Antidepressants, Tricyclic *(continued)*

Diuretics: increased risk of postural hypotension when tricyclics given with diuretics

- Dopaminergics: caution with tricyclics advised by manufacturer of entacapone; increased risk of CNS toxicity when tricyclics given with •rasagiline; CNS toxicity reported when tricyclics given with •selegiline

Lithium: risk of toxicity when tricyclics given with lithium

Muscle Relaxants: tricyclics enhance muscle relaxant effect of baclofen

Nicorandil: tricyclics possibly enhance hypotensive effect of nicorandil

Nitrates: tricyclics reduce effects of sublingual tablets of nitrates (failure to dissolve under tongue owing to dry mouth)

Oestrogens: antidepressant effect of tricyclics antagonised by oestrogens (but side-effects of tricyclics possibly increased due to increased plasma concentration)

- Sibutramine: increased risk of CNS toxicity when tricyclics given with •sibutramine (manufacturer of sibutramine advises avoid concomitant use)
- Sympathomimetics: increased risk of hypertension and arrhythmias when tricyclics given with •adrenaline (epinephrine) (but local anaesthetics with adrenaline appear to be safe); metabolism of tricyclics possibly inhibited by methylphenidate; increased risk of hypertension and arrhythmias when tricyclics given with •noradrenaline (norepinephrine)

Thyroid Hormones: effects of tricyclics possibly enhanced by thyroid hormones; effects of amitriptyline and imipramine enhanced by thyroid hormones

Ulcer-healing Drugs: plasma concentration of tricyclics possibly increased by cimetidine; metabolism of amitriptyline, doxepin, imipramine and nortriptyline inhibited by cimetidine (increased plasma concentration)

Antidepressants, Tricyclic (related)

- Alcohol: increased sedative effect when tricyclic-related antidepressants given with •alcohol

Alpha$_2$-adrenoceptor Stimulants: avoidance of tricyclic-related antidepressants advised by manufacturer of apraclonidine and brimonidine

- Antidepressants: tricyclic-related antidepressants should not be started until 2 weeks after stopping •MAOIs, also MAOIs should not be started until at least 1–2 weeks after stopping tricyclic-related antidepressants; after stopping tricyclic-related antidepressants do not start •moclobemide for at least 1 week
- Antiepileptics: tricyclic-related antidepressants possibly antagonise anticonvulsant effect of •antiepileptics (convulsive threshold lowered); plasma concentration of mianserin reduced by •carbamazepine and •phenytoin; metabolism of mianserin accelerated by •primidone (reduced plasma concentration)

Antihistamines: possible increased antimuscarinic and sedative effects when tricyclic-related antidepressants given with antihistamines

- Antimalarials: avoidance of antidepressants advised by manufacturer of •artemether/lumefantrine

Antimuscarinics: possibly increased antimuscarinic side-effects when tricyclic-related antidepressants given with antimuscarinics

Antidepressants, Tricyclic (related) *(continued)*
- Antipsychotics: increased risk of ventricular arrhythmias when maprotiline given with •pimozide—avoid concomitant use
  Anxiolytics and Hypnotics: increased sedative effect when tricyclic-related antidepressants given with anxiolytics and hypnotics
- Barbiturates: tricyclic-related antidepressants possibly antagonise anticonvulsant effect of •barbiturates (convulsive threshold lowered); metabolism of mianserin accelerated by •phenobarbital (reduced plasma concentration)
  Diazoxide: enhanced hypotensive effect when tricyclic-related antidepressants given with diazoxide
  Dopaminergics: caution with maprotiline advised by manufacturer of entacapone
  Nitrates: tricyclic-related antidepressants possibly reduce effects of sublingual tablets of nitrates (failure to dissolve under tongue owing to dry mouth)
- Sibutramine: increased risk of CNS toxicity when tricyclic-related antidepressants given with •sibutramine (manufacturer of sibutramine advises avoid concomitant use)
  Vasodilator Antihypertensives: enhanced hypotensive effect when tricyclic-related antidepressants given with hydralazine or nitroprusside

Antidiabetics
  ACE Inhibitors: hypoglycaemic effect of insulin, metformin and sulphonylureas possibly enhanced by ACE inhibitors
  Alcohol: hypoglycaemic effect of antidiabetics enhanced by alcohol; increased risk of lactic acidosis when metformin given with alcohol; flushing, in susceptible subjects, when chlorpropamide given with alcohol
  Anabolic Steroids: hypoglycaemic effect of antidiabetics possibly enhanced by anabolic steroids
- Analgesics: effects of sulphonylureas possibly enhanced by •NSAIDs
  Anti-arrhythmics: hypoglycaemic effect of gliclazide, insulin and metformin possibly enhanced by disopyramide
- Antibacterials: hypoglycaemic effect of acarbose possibly enhanced by neomycin, also severity of gastro-intestinal effects increased; effects of repaglinide enhanced by clarithromycin; effects of glibenclamide possibly enhanced by ciprofloxacin and norfloxacin; plasma concentration of nateglinide and repaglinide reduced by rifampicin; plasma concentration of rosiglitazone reduced by •rifampicin—consider increasing dose of rosiglitazone; effects of sulphonylureas enhanced by •chloramphenicol; metabolism of sulphonylureas possibly accelerated by •rifamycins (reduced effect); metabolism of chlorpropamide and tolbutamide accelerated by •rifamycins (reduced effect); effects of sulphonylureas rarely enhanced by sulphonamides and trimethoprim
- Anticoagulants: hypoglycaemic effect of sulphonylureas possibly enhanced by •coumarins, also possible changes to anticoagulant effect
  Antidepressants: hypoglycaemic effect of insulin, metformin and sulphonylureas enhanced by MAOIs; hypoglycaemic effect of antidiabetics possibly enhanced by MAOIs
  Antiepileptics: tolbutamide transiently increases plasma concentration of phenytoin (possibility of toxicity)

Antidiabetics *(continued)*
- Antifungals: plasma concentration of sulphonylureas increased by •fluconazole and •miconazole; hypoglycaemic effect of gliclazide and glipizide enhanced by •miconazole— avoid concomitant use; hypoglycaemic effect of nateglinide possibly enhanced by fluconazole; plasma concentration of sulphonylureas possibly increased by voriconazole
  Antihistamines: thrombocyte count depressed when metformin given with ketotifen
  Antipsychotics: hypoglycaemic effect of sulphonylureas possibly antagonised by phenothiazines
  Antivirals: plasma concentration of tolbutamide possibly increased by ritonavir
  Aprepitant: plasma concentration of tolbutamide reduced by aprepitant
  Beta-blockers: warning signs of hypoglycaemia (such as tremor) with antidiabetics may be masked when given with beta-blockers; hypoglycaemic effect of insulin enhanced by beta-blockers
- Bosentan: plasma concentration of both drugs reduced when glibenclamide given with •bosentan (avoid concomitant use)
  Calcium-channel Blockers: glucose tolerance occasionally impaired when insulin given with nifedipine
  Cardiac Glycosides: acarbose possibly reduces plasma concentration of digoxin
  Corticosteroids: hypoglycaemic effect of antidiabetics antagonised by corticosteroids
  Cytotoxics: metabolism of rosiglitazone possibly inhibited by paclitaxel
  Diazoxide: hypoglycaemic effect of antidiabetics antagonised by diazoxide
  Diuretics: hypoglycaemic effect of antidiabetics antagonised by loop diuretics and thiazides and related diuretics; increased risk of hyponatraemia when chlorpropamide given with potassium-sparing diuretics and aldosterone antagonists plus thiazide; increased risk of hyponatraemia when chlorpropamide given with thiazides and related diuretics plus potassium-sparing diuretic
  Hormone Antagonists: requirements for insulin, metformin, repaglinide and sulphonylureas possibly reduced by lanreotide; requirements for insulin, metformin, repaglinide and sulphonylureas possibly reduced by octreotide
  Leflunomide: hypoglycaemic effect of tolbutamide possibly enhanced by leflunomide
- Lipid-regulating Drugs: hypoglycaemic effect of acarbose possibly enhanced by colestyramine; hypoglycaemic effect of nateglinide possibly enhanced by gemfibrozil; increased risk of severe hypoglycaemia when repaglinide given with •gemfibrozil—avoid concomitant use; plasma concentration of rosiglitazone increased by •gemfibrozil (consider reducing dose of rosiglitazone); may be improved glucose tolerance and an additive effect when insulin or sulphonylureas given with fibrates
  Oestrogens: hypoglycaemic effect of antidiabetics antagonised by oestrogens
  Orlistat: avoidance of acarbose advised by manufacturer of orlistat
  Pancreatin: hypoglycaemic effect of acarbose antagonised by pancreatin
  Probenecid: hypoglycaemic effect of chlorpropamide possibly enhanced by probenecid
  Progestogens: hypoglycaemic effect of antidiabetics antagonised by progestogens

Antidiabetics *(continued)*
- • Sulfinpyrazone: effects of sulphonylureas enhanced by •sulfinpyrazone
- Testosterone: hypoglycaemic effect of antidiabetics possibly enhanced by testosterone
- Ulcer-healing Drugs: excretion of metformin reduced by cimetidine (increased plasma concentration); hypoglycaemic effect of sulphonylureas enhanced by cimetidine

Antiepileptics *see* Carbamazepine, Ethosuximide, Gabapentin, Lamotrigine, Levetiracetam, Oxcarbazepine, Phenytoin, Primidone, Tiagabine, Topiramate, Valproate, Vigabatrin, and Zonisamide

Antifungals *see* Amphotericin; Antifungals, Imidazole; Antifungals, Triazole; Caspofungin; Flucytosine; Griseofulvin; Terbinafine

Antifungals, Imidazole
- • Analgesics: ketoconazole inhibits metabolism of alfentanil (risk of prolonged or delayed respiratory depression); ketoconazole inhibits metabolism of •buprenorphine (reduce dose of buprenorphine)
- Antacids: absorption of ketoconazole reduced by antacids
- • Anti-arrhythmics: miconazole increases plasma concentration of •quinidine (increased risk of ventricular arrhythmias—avoid concomitant use)
- • Antibacterials: metabolism of ketoconazole accelerated by •rifampicin (reduced plasma concentration), also plasma concentration of rifampicin may be reduced by ketoconazole; plasma concentration of ketoconazole possibly reduced by isoniazid
- • Anticoagulants: ketoconazole enhances anticoagulant effect of •coumarins; miconazole enhances anticoagulant effect of •coumarins (miconazole oral gel and possibly vaginal formulations absorbed)
- • Antidepressants: avoidance of imidazoles advised by manufacturer of •reboxetine; ketoconazole increases plasma concentration of mirtazapine
- • Antidiabetics: miconazole enhances hypoglycaemic effect of •gliclazide and •glipizide—avoid concomitant use; miconazole increases plasma concentration of •sulphonylureas
- • Antiepileptics: miconazole possibly increases plasma concentration of carbamazepine; miconazole enhances anticonvulsant effect of •phenytoin (plasma concentration of phenytoin increased); plasma concentration of ketoconazole reduced by •phenytoin
- Antifungals: imidazoles possibly antagonise effects of amphotericin
- • Antihistamines: manufacturer of loratadine advises ketoconazole possibly increases plasma concentration of loratadine; imidazoles possibly inhibit metabolism of •mizolastine (avoid concomitant use); ketoconazole inhibits metabolism of •mizolastine—avoid concomitant use
- • Antimalarials: avoidance of imidazoles advised by manufacturer of •artemether/lumefantrine
- Antimuscarinics: absorption of ketoconazole reduced by antimuscarinics; ketoconazole increases plasma concentration of solifenacin; avoidance of ketoconazole advised by manufacturer of tolterodine
- • Antipsychotics: ketoconazole inhibits metabolism of •aripiprazole (reduce dose of aripiprazole); increased risk of ventricular arrhythmias when imidazoles given with

Antifungals, Imidazole
- • Antipsychotics *(continued)* •pimozide—avoid concomitant use; imidazoles possibly increase plasma concentration of quetiapine (reduce dose of quetiapine); possible increased risk of ventricular arrhythmias when imidazoles given with •sertindole—avoid concomitant use; increased risk of ventricular arrhythmias when ketoconazole given with •sertindole—avoid concomitant use
- • Antivirals: plasma concentration of ketoconazole increased by amprenavir; ketoconazole inhibits the metabolism of indinavir; plasma concentration of ketoconazole reduced by •nevirapine—avoid concomitant use; combination of ketoconazole with •ritonavir may increase plasma concentration of either drug (or both); imidazoles possibly increase plasma concentration of saquinavir; ketoconazole increases plasma concentration of saquinavir
- • Anxiolytics and Hypnotics: ketoconazole increases plasma concentration of •midazolam (risk of prolonged sedation)
- Aprepitant: ketoconazole increases plasma concentration of aprepitant
- Bosentan: ketoconazole possibly increases plasma concentration of bosentan
- • Calcium-channel Blockers: ketoconazole inhibits metabolism of •felodipine (increased plasma concentration); avoidance of ketoconazole advised by manufacturer of lercanidipine; ketoconazole possibly inhibits metabolism of dihydropyridines (increased plasma concentration)
- • Ciclosporin: ketoconazole inhibits metabolism of •ciclosporin (increased plasma concentration); miconazole possibly inhibits metabolism of •ciclosporin (increased plasma concentration)
- • Cilostazol: ketoconazole possibly increases plasma concentration of •cilostazol—avoid concomitant use
- Cinacalcet: ketoconazole inhibits metabolism of cinacalcet (increased plasma concentration)
- Corticosteroids: ketoconazole possibly inhibits metabolism of corticosteroids; ketoconazole increases plasma concentration of inhaled budesonide and mometasone; ketoconazole inhibits the metabolism of methylprednisolone
- Cytotoxics: *in vitro* studies suggest a possible interaction between ketoconazole and docetaxel (consult docetaxel product literature); ketoconazole inhibits metabolism of erlotinib (increased plasma concentration); ketoconazole increases plasma concentration of imatinib
- • Diuretics: ketoconazole increases plasma concentration of •eplerenone—avoid concomitant use
- • Ergot Alkaloids: increased risk of ergotism when imidazoles given with •ergotamine and methysergide—avoid concomitant use
- • $5HT_1$ Agonists: ketoconazole increases plasma concentration of almotriptan (increased risk of toxicity); ketoconazole increases plasma concentration of •eletriptan (risk of toxicity)—avoid concomitant use
- • Ivabradine: ketoconazole increases plasma concentration of •ivabradine—avoid concomitant use
- • Lipid-regulating Drugs: possible increased risk of myopathy when imidazoles given with atorvastatin or simvastatin; increased risk of myopathy when ketoconazole given with

Antifungals, Imidazole

- Lipid-regulating Drugs *(continued)* •simvastatin (avoid concomitant use); possible increased risk of myopathy when miconazole given with •simvastatin—avoid concomitant use
- Oestrogens: anecdotal reports of contraceptive failure when imidazoles or ketoconazole given with oestrogens
- Parasympathomimetics: ketoconazole increases plasma concentration of galantamine
- Sildenafil: ketoconazole increases plasma concentration of sildenafil—reduce initial dose of sildenafil
- • Sirolimus: ketoconazole increases plasma concentration of •sirolimus—avoid concomitant use; miconazole increases plasma concentration of •sirolimus
- • Tacrolimus: imidazoles possibly increase plasma concentration of •tacrolimus; ketoconazole increases plasma concentration of •tacrolimus
- Tadalafil: ketoconazole increases plasma concentration of tadalafil
- • Theophylline: ketoconazole possibly increases plasma concentration of •theophylline
- Ulcer-healing Drugs: absorption of ketoconazole reduced by histamine H_2-antagonists, proton pump inhibitors and sucralfate
- • Vardenafil: ketoconazole increases plasma concentration of •vardenafil—avoid concomitant use

Antifungals, Polyene *see* Amphotericin

Antifungals, Triazole

Note. In general, fluconazole interactions relate to multiple-dose treatment

- • Analgesics: fluconazole increases plasma concentration of celecoxib (halve dose of celecoxib); fluconazole increases plasma concentration of parecoxib (reduce dose of parecoxib); fluconazole inhibits metabolism of alfentanil (risk of prolonged or delayed respiratory depression); itraconazole possibly inhibits metabolism of alfentanil; voriconazole increases plasma concentration of •methadone (consider reducing dose of methadone)
- Antacids: absorption of itraconazole reduced by antacids
- • Anti-arrhythmics: itraconazole and voriconazole increase plasma concentration of •quinidine (increased risk of ventricular arrhythmias—avoid concomitant use)
- • Antibacterials: plasma concentration of itraconazole increased by clarithromycin; triazoles possibly increase plasma concentration of •rifabutin (increased risk of uveitis—reduce rifabutin dose); voriconazole increases plasma concentration of •rifabutin, also rifabutin reduces plasma concentration of voriconazole (increase dose of voriconazole and also monitor for rifabutin toxicity); fluconazole increases plasma concentration of •rifabutin (increased risk of uveitis—reduce rifabutin dose); plasma concentration of itraconazole reduced by •rifabutin—avoid concomitant use; plasma concentration of voriconazole reduced by •rifampicin—avoid concomitant use; metabolism of fluconazole and itraconazole accelerated by •rifampicin (reduced plasma concentration)
- • Anticoagulants: fluconazole, itraconazole and voriconazole enhance anticoagulant effect of •coumarins
- • Antidepressants: avoidance of triazoles advised by manufacturer of •reboxetine

Antifungals, Triazole *(continued)*

- • Antidiabetics: fluconazole possibly enhances hypoglycaemic effect of nateglinide; fluconazole increases plasma concentration of •sulphonylureas; voriconazole possibly increases plasma concentration of sulphonylureas
- • Antiepileptics: plasma concentration of voriconazole possibly reduced by •carbamazepine and •primidone—avoid concomitant use; plasma concentration of itraconazole possibly reduced by carbamazepine; voriconazole increases plasma concentration of •phenytoin, also phenytoin reduces plasma concentration of voriconazole (increase dose of voriconazole and also monitor for phenytoin toxicity); plasma concentration of itraconazole reduced by •phenytoin—avoid concomitant use; fluconazole increases plasma concentration of •phenytoin (consider reducing dose of phenytoin)
- Antifungals: triazoles possibly antagonise effects of amphotericin
- • Antihistamines: itraconazole inhibits metabolism of •mizolastine—avoid concomitant use
- • Antimalarials: avoidance of triazoles advised by manufacturer of •artemether/lumefantrine
- Antimuscarinics: itraconazole increases plasma concentration of solifenacin; avoidance of itraconazole advised by manufacturer of tolterodine
- • Antipsychotics: itraconazole possibly inhibits metabolism of •aripiprazole (reduce dose of aripiprazole); increased risk of ventricular arrhythmias when triazoles given with •pimozide—avoid concomitant use; triazoles possibly increase plasma concentration of quetiapine (reduce dose of quetiapine); possible increased risk of ventricular arrhythmias when triazoles given with •sertindole—avoid concomitant use; increased risk of ventricular arrhythmias when itraconazole given with •sertindole—avoid concomitant use
- • Antivirals: plasma concentration of itraconazole possibly increased by amprenavir; plasma concentration of voriconazole reduced by •efavirenz, also plasma concentration of efavirenz increased (avoid concomitant use); itraconazole increases plasma concentration of •indinavir (consider reducing dose of indinavir); fluconazole increases plasma concentration of •nevirapine, ritonavir and tipranavir; plasma concentration of voriconazole reduced by •ritonavir—avoid concomitant use; combination of itraconazole with •ritonavir may increase plasma concentration of either drug (or both); triazoles possibly increase plasma concentration of saquinavir; fluconazole increases plasma concentration of •zidovudine (increased risk of toxicity)
- • Anxiolytics and Hypnotics: itraconazole increases plasma concentration of alprazolam; fluconazole and itraconazole increase plasma concentration of •midazolam (risk of prolonged sedation); itraconazole increases plasma concentration of buspirone (reduce dose of buspirone)
- • Barbiturates: plasma concentration of itraconazole possibly reduced by phenobarbital; plasma concentration of voriconazole possibly reduced by •phenobarbital—avoid concomitant use
- • Bosentan: fluconazole increases plasma concentration of •bosentan—avoid concomitant

Antifungals, Triazole
- Bosentan *(continued)* use; itraconazole possibly increases plasma concentration of bosentan
- Calcium-channel Blockers: negative inotropic effect possibly increased when itraconazole given with calcium-channel blockers; itraconazole inhibits metabolism of •felodipine (increased plasma concentration); avoidance of itraconazole advised by manufacturer of lercanidipine; itraconazole possibly inhibits metabolism of dihydropyridines (increased plasma concentration)
- Cardiac Glycosides: itraconazole increases plasma concentration of •digoxin
- Ciclosporin: fluconazole, itraconazole and voriconazole inhibit metabolism of •ciclosporin (increased plasma concentration)

Corticosteroids: itraconazole possibly inhibits metabolism of corticosteroids and methylprednisolone; itraconazole increases plasma concentration of inhaled budesonide
- Cytotoxics: itraconazole inhibits metabolism of busulfan (increased risk of toxicity); itraconazole possibly increases side-effects of cyclophosphamide; itraconazole possibly inhibits metabolism of •vincristine (increased risk of neurotoxicity)
- Diuretics: fluconazole increases plasma concentration of eplerenone (reduce dose of eplerenone); itraconazole increases plasma concentration of •eplerenone—avoid concomitant use; plasma concentration of fluconazole increased by hydrochlorothiazide
- Ergot Alkaloids: increased risk of ergotism when triazoles given with •ergotamine and methysergide—avoid concomitant use
- $5HT_1$ Agonists: itraconazole increases plasma concentration of •eletriptan (risk of toxicity)—avoid concomitant use
- Ivabradine: fluconazole increases plasma concentration of ivabradine—reduce initial dose of ivabradine; itraconazole possibly increases plasma concentration of •ivabradine—avoid concomitant use
- Lipid-regulating Drugs: possible increased risk of myopathy when triazoles given with atorvastatin or simvastatin; increased risk of myopathy when itraconazole given with •atorvastatin or •simvastatin (avoid concomitant use)

Oestrogens: anecdotal reports of contraceptive failure when fluconazole or itraconazole given with oestrogens

Sildenafil: itraconazole increases plasma concentration of sildenafil—reduce initial dose of sildenafil
- Sirolimus: itraconazole and voriconazole increase plasma concentration of •sirolimus—avoid concomitant use
- Tacrolimus: triazoles possibly increase plasma concentration of •tacrolimus; fluconazole and voriconazole increase plasma concentration of •tacrolimus

Tadalafil: itraconazole possibly increases plasma concentration of tadalafil
- Theophylline: fluconazole possibly increases plasma concentration of •theophylline

Ulcer-healing Drugs: voriconazole increases plasma concentration of omeprazole (reduce dose of omeprazole); absorption of itraconazole reduced by histamine H_2-antagonists and proton pump inhibitors

Antifungals, Triazole *(continued)*
- Vardenafil: itraconazole possibly increases plasma concentration of •vardenafil—avoid concomitant use

Antihistamines

Note. Sedative interactions apply to a lesser extent to the non-sedating antihistamines. Interactions do not generally apply to antihistamines used for topical action (including inhalation)

Alcohol: increased sedative effect when antihistamines given with alcohol (possibly less effect with non-sedating antihistamines)

Antacids: absorption of fexofenadine reduced by antacids
- Anti-arrhythmics: increased risk of ventricular arrhythmias when mizolastine given with •amiodarone, •disopyramide, •flecainide, •mexiletine, •procainamide, •propafenone or •quinidine—avoid concomitant use
- Antibacterials: manufacturer of loratadine advises plasma concentration possibly increased by erythromycin; metabolism of mizolastine inhibited by •erythromycin—avoid concomitant use; increased risk of ventricular arrhythmias when mizolastine given with •moxifloxacin—avoid concomitant use; metabolism of mizolastine possibly inhibited by •macrolides (avoid concomitant use)

Antidepressants: increased antimuscarinic and sedative effects when antihistamines given with MAOIs or tricyclics; cyproheptadine possibly antagonises antidepressant effect of SSRIs; possible increased antimuscarinic and sedative effects when antihistamines given with tricyclic-related antidepressants

Antidiabetics: thrombocyte count depressed when ketotifen given with metformin
- Antifungals: manufacturer of loratadine advises plasma concentration possibly increased by ketoconazole; metabolism of mizolastine inhibited by •itraconazole or •ketoconazole—avoid concomitant use; metabolism of mizolastine possibly inhibited by •imidazoles (avoid concomitant use)

Antimuscarinics: increased risk of antimuscarinic side-effects when antihistamines given with antimuscarinics

Antivirals: plasma concentration of loratadine possibly increased by amprenavir; plasma concentration of chlorphenamine (chlorpheniramine) possibly increased by lopinavir; plasma concentration of non-sedating antihistamines possibly increased by ritonavir

Anxiolytics and Hypnotics: increased sedative effect when antihistamines given with anxiolytics and hypnotics
- Beta-blockers: increased risk of ventricular arrhythmias when mizolastine given with •sotalol—avoid concomitant use

Betahistine: antihistamines theoretically antagonise effect of betahistine

Ulcer-healing Drugs: manufacturer of loratadine advises plasma concentration possibly increased by cimetidine

Antihistamines, Non-sedating *see* Antihistamines

Antihistamines, Sedating *see* Antihistamines

Antimalarials *see* Artemether with Lumefantrine, Chloroquine and Hydroxychloroquine, Mefloquine, Primaquine, Proguanil, and Quinine

Adsorbents: absorption of chloroquine and hydroxychloroquine reduced by kaolin

Agalsidase Beta: chloroquine and hydroxychloroquine possibly inhibit effects of

Antihistamines

Agalsidase Beta *(continued)*
agalsidase beta (manufacturer of agalsidase beta advises avoid concomitant use)

Antacids: absorption of chloroquine and hydroxychloroquine reduced by antacids; absorption of proguanil reduced by oral magnesium salts (as magnesium trisilicate)

• Anti-arrhythmics: increased risk of ventricular arrhythmias when chloroquine and hydroxychloroquine, mefloquine or quinine given with •amiodarone—avoid concomitant use; manufacturer of artemether/lumefantrine advises avoid concomitant use with •amiodarone, •disopyramide, •flecainide, •procainamide or •quinidine (risk of ventricular arrhythmias); quinine increases plasma concentration of •flecainide; increased risk of ventricular arrhythmias when mefloquine given with •quinidine

• Antibacterials: increased risk of ventricular arrhythmias when chloroquine and hydroxychloroquine, mefloquine or quinine given with •moxifloxacin—avoid concomitant use; manufacturer of artemether/lumefantrine advises avoid concomitant use with •macrolides and •quinolones; increased antifolate effect when pyrimethamine (includes Fansidar®) given with •sulphonamides; increased antifolate effect when pyrimethamine given with •trimethoprim

Anticoagulants: isolated reports that proguanil may enhance anticoagulant effect of warfarin

• Antidepressants: manufacturer of artemether/lumefantrine advises avoid concomitant use with •antidepressants

• Antiepileptics: possible increased risk of convulsions when chloroquine and hydroxychloroquine given with antiepileptics; mefloquine antagonises anticonvulsant effect of •antiepileptics, •carbamazepine and •valproate; pyrimethamine antagonises anticonvulsant effect of •phenytoin, also increased antifolate effect

• Antifungals: manufacturer of artemether/lumefantrine advises avoid concomitant use with •imidazoles and •triazoles

• Antimalarials: avoidance of antimalarials advised by manufacturer of •artemether/lumefantrine; increased risk of convulsions when chloroquine and hydroxychloroquine given with •mefloquine; increased antifolate effect when proguanil given with pyrimethamine; increased risk of convulsions when mefloquine given with •quinine (but should not prevent the use of intravenous quinine in severe cases)

• Antipsychotics: manufacturer of artemether/lumefantrine advises avoid concomitant use with •antipsychotics; increased risk of ventricular arrhythmias when mefloquine or quinine given with •pimozide—avoid concomitant use

• Antivirals: manufacturer of artemether/lumefantrine advises avoid concomitant use with •amprenavir, •atazanavir, •indinavir, •lopinavir, •nelfinavir, •ritonavir and •saquinavir; possible increased risk of ventricular arrhythmias when artemether/lumefantrine given with •tipranavir—avoid concomitant use; increased antifolate effect when pyrimethamine given with zidovudine

• Beta-blockers: increased risk of bradycardia when mefloquine given with beta-blockers; manufacturer of artemether/lumefantrine advises avoid concomitant use with •metoprolol and •sotalol

Calcium-channel Blockers: possible increased risk of bradycardia when mefloquine given with calcium-channel blockers

• Cardiac Glycosides: quinine increases plasma concentration of •digoxin; possible increased risk of bradycardia when mefloquine given with digoxin; chloroquine and hydroxychloroquine possibly increase plasma concentration of •digoxin

• Ciclosporin: chloroquine and hydroxychloroquine increase plasma concentration of •ciclosporin (increased risk of toxicity)

• Cytotoxics: pyrimethamine increases antifolate effect of •methotrexate

• Grapefruit Juice: metabolism of artemether/lumefantrine possibly inhibited by •grapefruit juice (avoid concomitant use)

• Ivabradine: increased risk of ventricular arrhythmias when mefloquine given with •ivabradine

Laronidase: chloroquine and hydroxychloroquine possibly inhibit effects of laronidase (manufacturer of laronidase advises avoid concomitant use)

Mepacrine: plasma concentration of primaquine increased by mepacrine (increased risk of toxicity)

Muscle Relaxants: quinine possibly enhances effects of suxamethonium

Parasympathomimetics: chloroquine and hydroxychloroquine have potential to increase symptoms of myasthenia gravis and thus diminish effect of neostigmine and pyridostigmine

• Ulcer-healing Drugs: manufacturer of artemether/lumefantrine advises avoid concomitant use with •cimetidine; metabolism of chloroquine and hydroxychloroquine and quinine inhibited by cimetidine (increased plasma concentration)

Antimetabolites *see* Cytarabine, Fludarabine, Fluorouracil, Mercaptopurine, Methotrexate, and Tioguanine

Antimuscarinics

Note. Many drugs have antimuscarinic effects; concomitant use of two or more such drugs can increase side-effects such as dry mouth, urine retention, and constipation; concomitant use can also lead to confusion in the elderly. Interactions do not generally apply to antimuscarinics used by inhalation

Alcohol: increased sedative effect when hyoscine given with alcohol

Analgesics: increased risk of antimuscarinic side-effects when antimuscarinics given with nefopam

Anti-arrhythmics: increased risk of antimuscarinic side-effects when antimuscarinics given with disopyramide; atropine delays absorption of mexiletine

Antibacterials: manufacturer of tolterodine advises avoid concomitant use with clarithromycin and erythromycin

Antidepressants: plasma concentration of procyclidine increased by paroxetine; increased risk of antimuscarinic side-effects when antimuscarinics given with MAOIs or tricyclics; possibly increased antimuscarinic side-effects when antimuscarinics given with tricyclic-related antidepressants

Antimuscarinics *(continued)*

Antifungals: antimuscarinics reduce absorption of ketoconazole; plasma concentration of solifenacin increased by itraconazole and ketoconazole; manufacturer of tolterodine advises avoid concomitant use with itraconazole and ketoconazole

Antihistamines: increased risk of antimuscarinic side-effects when antimuscarinics given with antihistamines

Antipsychotics: antimuscarinics possibly reduce effects of haloperidol; increased risk of antimuscarinic side-effects when antimuscarinics given with clozapine; antimuscarinics reduce plasma concentration of phenothiazines, but risk of antimuscarinic side-effects increased

Antivirals: manufacturer of tolterodine advises avoid concomitant use with amprenavir, indinavir, lopinavir, nelfinavir, ritonavir and saquinavir; plasma concentration of solifenacin increased by nelfinavir and ritonavir

Domperidone: antimuscarinics antagonise effects of domperidone on gastro-intestinal activity

Dopaminergics: increased risk of antimuscarinic side-effects when antimuscarinics given with amantadine; antimuscarinics possibly reduce absorption of levodopa

Memantine: effects of antimuscarinics possibly enhanced by memantine

Metoclopramide: antimuscarinics antagonise effects of metoclopramide on gastro-intestinal activity

Nitrates: antimuscarinics possibly reduce effects of sublingual tablets of nitrates (failure to dissolve under tongue owing to dry mouth)

Parasympathomimetics: antimuscarinics antagonise effects of parasympathomimetics

Antipsychotics

Note. Increased risk of toxicity with myelosuppressive drugs

Note. Avoid concomitant use of clozapine with drugs that have a substantial potential for causing agranulocytosis

ACE Inhibitors: enhanced hypotensive effect when antipsychotics given with ACE inhibitors

Adrenergic Neurone Blockers: enhanced hypotensive effect when phenothiazines given with adrenergic neurone blockers; higher doses of chlorpromazine antagonise hypotensive effect of adrenergic neurone blockers; haloperidol antagonises hypotensive effect of adrenergic neurone blockers

Adsorbents: absorption of phenothiazines possibly reduced by kaolin

Alcohol: increased sedative effect when antipsychotics given with alcohol

Alpha-blockers: enhanced hypotensive effect when antipsychotics given with alpha-blockers

• Anaesthetics, General: enhanced hypotensive effect when antipsychotics given with •general anaesthetics

Analgesics: possible severe drowsiness when haloperidol given with indometacin; increased risk of convulsions when antipsychotics given with tramadol; enhanced hypotensive and sedative effects when antipsychotics given with opioid analgesics

Angiotensin-II Receptor Antagonists: enhanced hypotensive effect when antipsychotics given with angiotensin-II receptor antagonists

Antacids: absorption of phenothiazines and sulpiride reduced by antacids

• Anti-arrhythmics: increased risk of ventricular arrhythmias when antipsychotics that prolong the QT interval given with •anti-arrhythmics that prolong the QT interval; increased risk of ventricular arrhythmias when amisulpride, haloperidol, phenothiazines, pimozide or sertindole given with •amiodarone—avoid concomitant use; increased risk of ventricular arrhythmias when phenothiazines given with •disopyramide, •procainamide or •quinidine; increased risk of ventricular arrhythmias when amisulpride, pimozide or sertindole given with •disopyramide—avoid concomitant use; increased risk of arrhythmias when clozapine given with •flecainide; increased risk of ventricular arrhythmias when amisulpride, pimozide or sertindole given with •procainamide—avoid concomitant use; increased risk of ventricular arrhythmias when amisulpride, pimozide or sertindole given with •quinidine—avoid concomitant use; metabolism of aripiprazole inhibited by •quinidine (reduce dose of aripiprazole)

• Antibacterials: increased risk of ventricular arrhythmias when pimozide given with •clarithromycin, •moxifloxacin or •telithromycin—avoid concomitant use; increased risk of ventricular arrhythmias when sertindole given with •erythromycin or •moxifloxacin—avoid concomitant use; increased risk of ventricular arrhythmias when amisulpride given with parenteral •erythromycin—avoid concomitant use; plasma concentration of clozapine possibly increased by •erythromycin (possible increased risk of convulsions); possible increased risk of ventricular arrhythmias when pimozide given with •erythromycin—avoid concomitant use; plasma concentration of olanzapine possibly increased by ciprofloxacin; increased risk of ventricular arrhythmias when haloperidol or phenothiazines given with •moxifloxacin—avoid concomitant use; plasma concentration of aripiprazole possibly reduced by •rifabutin and •rifampicin—increase dose of aripiprazole; plasma concentration of clozapine possibly reduced by rifampicin; metabolism of haloperidol accelerated by •rifampicin (reduced plasma concentration); avoid concomitant use of clozapine with •chloramphenicol or •sulphonamides (increased risk of agranulocytosis); possible increased risk of ventricular arrhythmias when sertindole given with •macrolides—avoid concomitant use; plasma concentration of quetiapine possibly increased by macrolides (reduce dose of quetiapine)

• Antidepressants: plasma concentration of clozapine possibly increased by citalopram (increased risk of toxicity); metabolism of aripiprazole possibly inhibited by •fluoxetine and •paroxetine (reduce dose of aripiprazole); plasma concentration of clozapine, haloperidol, risperidone, sertindole and zotepine increased by •fluoxetine; plasma concentration of clozapine and olanzapine increased by •fluvoxamine; plasma concentration of clozapine and sertindole increased by •paroxetine; plasma concentration of risperidone possibly increased by paroxetine (increased risk of toxicity); metabolism of perphenazine inhibited by paroxetine (reduce dose of perphenazine); plasma concentration of clozapine increased by •sertraline and

Antipsychotics

- Antidepressants *(continued)*
  •venlafaxine; plasma concentration of pimozide increased by •sertraline (increased risk of ventricular arrhythmias—avoid concomitant use); plasma concentration of haloperidol increased by venlafaxine; increased risk of ventricular arrhythmias when pimozide given with •maprotiline or •tricyclics—avoid concomitant use; clozapine possibly increases CNS effects of •MAOIs; plasma concentration of aripiprazole possibly reduced by •St John's wort—increase dose of aripiprazole; possibly increased antimuscarinic side-effects when clozapine given with tricyclics; antipsychotics increase plasma concentration of •tricyclics—possibly increased risk of ventricular arrhythmias; increased risk of antimuscarinic side-effects when phenothiazines given with tricyclics

Antidiabetics: phenothiazines possibly antagonise hypoglycaemic effect of sulphonylureas

- Antiepileptics: antipsychotics antagonise anticonvulsant effect of •carbamazepine, •ethosuximide, •oxcarbazepine, •phenytoin, •primidone and •valproate (convulsive threshold lowered); metabolism of haloperidol, olanzapine, quetiapine, risperidone and sertindole accelerated by carbamazepine (reduced plasma concentration); metabolism of clozapine accelerated by •carbamazepine (reduced plasma concentration), also avoid concomitant use of drugs with substantial potential for causing agranulocytosis; plasma concentration of aripiprazole reduced by •carbamazepine—increase dose of aripiprazole; metabolism of clozapine, quetiapine and sertindole accelerated by phenytoin (reduced plasma concentration); plasma concentration of aripiprazole possibly reduced by •phenytoin and •primidone—increase dose of aripiprazole; metabolism of haloperidol accelerated by primidone (reduced plasma concentration); increased risk of neutropenia when olanzapine given with •valproate
- Antifungals: metabolism of aripiprazole inhibited by •ketoconazole (reduce dose of aripiprazole); increased risk of ventricular arrhythmias when sertindole given with •itraconazole or •ketoconazole—avoid concomitant use; metabolism of aripiprazole possibly inhibited by •itraconazole (reduce dose of aripiprazole); possible increased risk of ventricular arrhythmias when sertindole given with •imidazoles or •triazoles—avoid concomitant use; plasma concentration of quetiapine possibly increased by imidazoles and triazoles (reduce dose of quetiapine); increased risk of ventricular arrhythmias when pimozide given with •imidazoles or •triazoles—avoid concomitant use
- Antimalarials: avoidance of antipsychotics advised by manufacturer of •artemether/lumefantrine; increased risk of ventricular arrhythmias when pimozide given with •mefloquine or •quinine—avoid concomitant use

Antimuscarinics: increased risk of antimuscarinic side-effects when clozapine given with antimuscarinics; plasma concentration of phenothiazines reduced by antimuscarinics, but risk of antimuscarinic side-effects increased; effects of haloperidol possibly reduced by antimuscarinics

- Antipsychotics: avoid concomitant use of clozapine with depot formulation of •flupentixol, •fluphenazine, •haloperidol, •pipotiazine, •risperidone or •zuclopenthixol as cannot be withdrawn quickly if neutropenia occurs; increased risk of ventricular arrhythmias when sertindole given with •amisulpride—avoid concomitant use; increased risk of ventricular arrhythmias when pimozide given with •phenothiazines—avoid concomitant use
- Antivirals: metabolism of aripiprazole possibly inhibited by •amprenavir, •atazanavir, •indinavir, •lopinavir, •nelfinavir, •ritonavir and •saquinavir (reduce dose of aripiprazole); plasma concentration of pimozide and sertindole increased by •amprenavir (increased risk of ventricular arrhythmias—avoid concomitant use); plasma concentration of clozapine possibly increased by amprenavir; plasma concentration of pimozide possibly increased by •atazanavir—avoid concomitant use; plasma concentration of pimozide possibly increased by •efavirenz, •indinavir, •nelfinavir and •saquinavir (increased risk of ventricular arrhythmias—avoid concomitant use); plasma concentration of aripiprazole possibly reduced by •efavirenz and •nevirapine—increase dose of aripiprazole; plasma concentration of sertindole increased by •indinavir, •lopinavir, •nelfinavir, •ritonavir and •saquinavir (increased risk of ventricular arrhythmias—avoid concomitant use); plasma concentration of pimozide increased by •ritonavir (increased risk of ventricular arrhythmias—avoid concomitant use); plasma concentration of clozapine increased by •ritonavir (increased risk of toxicity)—avoid concomitant use; plasma concentration of antipsychotics possibly increased by •ritonavir
- Anxiolytics and Hypnotics: increased sedative effect when antipsychotics given with anxiolytics and hypnotics; plasma concentration of zotepine increased by diazepam; increased risk of hypotension, bradycardia and respiratory depression when intramuscular olanzapine given with parenteral •benzodiazepines; plasma concentration of haloperidol increased by buspirone
- Aprepitant: avoidance of pimozide advised by manufacturer of •aprepitant
- Barbiturates: antipsychotics antagonise anticonvulsant effect of •barbiturates (convulsive threshold lowered); plasma concentration of aripiprazole possibly reduced by •phenobarbital—increase dose of aripiprazole; metabolism of haloperidol accelerated by phenobarbital (reduced plasma concentration)
- Beta-blockers: enhanced hypotensive effect when phenothiazines given with beta-blockers; plasma concentration of both drugs may increase when chlorpromazine given with •propranolol; increased risk of ventricular arrhythmias when amisulpride, phenothiazines, pimozide or sertindole given with •sotalol

Calcium-channel Blockers: enhanced hypotensive effect when antipsychotics given with calcium-channel blockers

Clonidine: enhanced hypotensive effect when phenothiazines given with clonidine

Antipsychotics *(continued)*

- Cytotoxics: avoid concomitant use of clozapine with •cytotoxics (increased risk of agranulocytosis)

Desferrioxamine: manufacturer of levomepromazine (methotrimeprazine) advises avoid concomitant use with desferrioxamine; avoidance of prochlorperazine advised by manufacturer of desferrioxamine

Diazoxide: enhanced hypotensive effect when phenothiazines given with diazoxide

- Diuretics: risk of ventricular arrhythmias with amisulpride or sertindole increased by hypokalaemia caused by •diuretics; risk of ventricular arrhythmias with pimozide increased by hypokalaemia caused by •diuretics (avoid concomitant use); enhanced hypotensive effect when phenothiazines given with diuretics

Dopaminergics: increased risk of extrapyramidal side-effects when antipsychotics given with amantadine; antipsychotics antagonise effects of apomorphine, levodopa, lisuride and pergolide; antipsychotics antagonise hypoprolactinaemic and antiparkinsonian effects of bromocriptine and cabergoline; manufacturer of amisulpride advises avoid concomitant use of levodopa (antagonism of effect); avoidance of antipsychotics advised by manufacturer of pramipexole and ropinirole (antagonism of effect)

- Ivabradine: increased risk of ventricular arrhythmias when pimozide or sertindole given with •ivabradine
- Lithium: increased risk of ventricular arrhythmias when sertindole given with •lithium—avoid concomitant use; increased risk of extrapyramidal side-effects and possibly neurotoxicity when clozapine, haloperidol or phenothiazines given with lithium; increased risk of extrapyramidal side-effects when sulpiride given with lithium

Memantine: effects of antipsychotics possibly reduced by memantine

Methyldopa: enhanced hypotensive effect when antipsychotics given with methyldopa (also increased risk of extrapyramidal effects)

Metoclopramide: increased risk of extrapyramidal side-effects when antipsychotics given with metoclopramide

Moxonidine: enhanced hypotensive effect when phenothiazines given with moxonidine

Muscle Relaxants: promazine possibly enhances effects of suxamethonium

Nitrates: enhanced hypotensive effect when phenothiazines given with nitrates

- Penicillamine: avoid concomitant use of clozapine with •penicillamine (increased risk of agranulocytosis)
- Pentamidine Isetionate: increased risk of ventricular arrhythmias when amisulpride given with •pentamidine isetionate—avoid concomitant use
- Sibutramine: increased risk of CNS toxicity when antipsychotics given with •sibutramine (manufacturer of sibutramine advises avoid concomitant use)

Sodium Benzoate: haloperidol possibly reduces effects of sodium benzoate

Sodium Phenylbutyrate: haloperidol possibly reduces effects of sodium phenylbutyrate

Sympathomimetics: antipsychotics antagonise hypertensive effect of sympathomimetics

Antipsychotics *(continued)*

Tetrabenazine: increased risk of extrapyramidal side-effects when antipsychotics given with tetrabenazine

- Ulcer-healing Drugs: effects of antipsychotics, chlorpromazine and clozapine possibly enhanced by cimetidine; increased risk of ventricular arrhythmias when sertindole given with •cimetidine—avoid concomitant use; plasma concentration of clozapine possibly reduced by omeprazole; absorption of sulpiride reduced by sucralfate

Vasodilator Antihypertensives: enhanced hypotensive effect when phenothiazines given with hydralazine, minoxidil or nitroprusside

Antivirals *see* Abacavir, Aciclovir, Amprenavir, Atazanavir, Cidofovir, Didanosine, Efavirenz, Emtricitabine, Famciclovir, Foscarnet, Ganciclovir, Indinavir, Lamivudine, Lopinavir, Nelfinavir, Nevirapine, Ribavirin, Ritonavir, Saquinavir, Stavudine, Tenofovir, Tipranavir, Valaciclovir, and Zidovudine

Anxiolytics and Hypnotics

ACE Inhibitors: enhanced hypotensive effect when anxiolytics and hypnotics given with ACE inhibitors

Adrenergic Neurone Blockers: enhanced hypotensive effect when anxiolytics and hypnotics given with adrenergic neurone blockers

Alcohol: increased sedative effect when anxiolytics and hypnotics given with alcohol

Alpha-blockers: enhanced hypotensive and sedative effects when anxiolytics and hypnotics given with alpha-blockers

Anaesthetics, General: increased sedative effect when anxiolytics and hypnotics given with general anaesthetics

Analgesics: increased sedative effect when anxiolytics and hypnotics given with opioid analgesics

Angiotensin-II Receptor Antagonists: enhanced hypotensive effect when anxiolytics and hypnotics given with angiotensin-II receptor antagonists

- Antibacterials: metabolism of midazolam inhibited by •clarithromycin, •erythromycin, •quinupristin/dalfopristin and •telithromycin (increased plasma concentration with increased sedation); plasma concentration of buspirone increased by erythromycin (reduce dose of buspirone); metabolism of zopiclone inhibited by erythromycin and quinupristin/dalfopristin; metabolism of benzodiazepines possibly accelerated by rifampicin (reduced plasma concentration); metabolism of diazepam accelerated by rifampicin (reduced plasma concentration); metabolism of buspirone and zaleplon possibly accelerated by rifampicin; metabolism of zolpidem accelerated by rifampicin (reduced plasma concentration and reduced effect); metabolism of diazepam inhibited by isoniazid

Anticoagulants: chloral and triclofos may transiently enhance anticoagulant effect of coumarins

Antidepressants: plasma concentration of some benzodiazepines increased by fluvoxamine; sedative effects possibly increased when zolpidem given with sertraline; manufacturer of buspirone advises avoid concomitant use with MAOIs; increased sedative effect when anxiolytics and hypnotics given with mirtazapine, tricyclic-related antidepressants or tricyclics

Anxiolytics and Hypnotics *(continued)*
Antiepileptics: plasma concentration of clonazepam often reduced by carbamazepine, phenytoin and primidone; benzodiazepines possibly increase or decrease plasma concentration of phenytoin; diazepam increases or decreases plasma concentration of phenytoin
• Antifungals: plasma concentration of midazolam increased by •fluconazole, •itraconazole and •ketoconazole (risk of prolonged sedation); plasma concentration of alprazolam increased by itraconazole; plasma concentration of buspirone increased by itraconazole (reduce dose of buspirone)
Antihistamines: increased sedative effect when anxiolytics and hypnotics given with antihistamines
• Antipsychotics: increased sedative effect when anxiolytics and hypnotics given with antipsychotics; buspirone increases plasma concentration of haloperidol; increased risk of hypotension, bradycardia and respiratory depression when parenteral benzodiazepines given with intramuscular •olanzapine; diazepam increases plasma concentration of zotepine
• Antivirals: increased risk of prolonged sedation and respiratory depression when alprazolam, clonazepam, diazepam, flurazepam or midazolam given with •amprenavir; increased risk of prolonged sedation when midazolam given with •efavirenz, •indinavir or •nelfinavir—avoid concomitant use; increased risk of prolonged sedation when alprazolam given with •indinavir—avoid concomitant use; plasma concentration of alprazolam, diazepam, flurazepam, midazolam and zolpidem possibly increased by •ritonavir (risk of extreme sedation and respiratory depression —avoid concomitant use); plasma concentration of anxiolytics and hypnotics possibly increased by •ritonavir; plasma concentration of buspirone increased by ritonavir (increased risk of toxicity); plasma concentration of midazolam increased by •saquinavir (risk of prolonged sedation)
Barbiturates: plasma concentration of clonazepam often reduced by phenobarbital
Beta-blockers: enhanced hypotensive effect when anxiolytics and hypnotics given with beta-blockers
Calcium-channel Blockers: enhanced hypotensive effect when anxiolytics and hypnotics given with calcium-channel blockers; midazolam increases absorption of lercanidipine; metabolism of midazolam inhibited by diltiazem and verapamil (increased plasma concentration with increased sedation); plasma concentration of buspirone increased by diltiazem and verapamil (reduce dose of buspirone)
Cardiac Glycosides: alprazolam increases plasma concentration of digoxin (increased risk of toxicity)
Clonidine: enhanced hypotensive effect when anxiolytics and hypnotics given with clonidine
Diazoxide: enhanced hypotensive effect when anxiolytics and hypnotics given with diazoxide
Disulfiram: metabolism of benzodiazepines inhibited by disulfiram (increased sedative effects); increased risk of temazepam toxicity when given with disulfiram
Diuretics: enhanced hypotensive effect when anxiolytics and hypnotics given with diuretics; administration of chloral or triclofos with parenteral furosemide (frusemide) may displace thyroid hormone from binding sites
Dopaminergics: benzodiazepines possibly antagonise effects of levodopa
Grapefruit Juice: plasma concentration of buspirone increased by grapefruit juice
Lofexidine: increased sedative effect when anxiolytics and hypnotics given with lofexidine
Methyldopa: enhanced hypotensive effect when anxiolytics and hypnotics given with methyldopa
Moxonidine: enhanced hypotensive effect when anxiolytics and hypnotics given with moxonidine; sedative effects possibly increased when benzodiazepines given with moxonidine
Muscle Relaxants: increased sedative effect when anxiolytics and hypnotics given with baclofen or tizanidine
Nabilone: increased sedative effect when anxiolytics and hypnotics given with nabilone
Nitrates: enhanced hypotensive effect when anxiolytics and hypnotics given with nitrates
Theophylline: effects of benzodiazepines possibly reduced by theophylline
Ulcer-healing Drugs: metabolism of benzodiazepines, clomethiazole and zaleplon inhibited by cimetidine (increased plasma concentration); metabolism of diazepam possibly inhibited by esomeprazole and omeprazole (increased plasma concentration)
Vasodilator Antihypertensives: enhanced hypotensive effect when anxiolytics and hypnotics given with hydralazine, minoxidil or nitroprusside

Apomorphine
Antipsychotics: effects of apomorphine antagonised by antipsychotics
Dopaminergics: effects of apomorphine possibly enhanced by entacapone
Memantine: effects of dopaminergics possibly enhanced by memantine
Methyldopa: antiparkinsonian effect of dopaminergics antagonised by methyldopa
Nitrates: sublingual apomorphine enhances hypotensive effect of nitrates

Apraclonidine *see* Alpha$_2$-adrenoceptor Stimulants

Aprepitant
Antibacterials: plasma concentration of aprepitant possibly increased by clarithromycin and telithromycin; plasma concentration of aprepitant reduced by rifampicin
Anticoagulants: aprepitant possibly reduces anticoagulant effect of warfarin
• Antidepressants: manufacturer of aprepitant advises avoid concomitant use with •St John's wort
Antidiabetics: aprepitant reduces plasma concentration of tolbutamide
Antiepileptics: plasma concentration of aprepitant possibly reduced by carbamazepine and phenytoin
Antifungals: plasma concentration of aprepitant increased by ketoconazole
• Antipsychotics: manufacturer of aprepitant advises avoid concomitant use with •pimozide
Antivirals: plasma concentration of aprepitant possibly increased by ritonavir
Barbiturates: plasma concentration of aprepitant possibly reduced by phenobarbital

Aprepitant *(continued)*
Corticosteroids: aprepitant inhibits metabolism of dexamethasone and methylprednisolone (reduce dose of dexamethasone and methylprednisolone)
• Oestrogens: aprepitant possibly causes contraceptive failure of hormonal contraceptives containing •oestrogens (alternative contraception recommended)
• Progestogens: aprepitant possibly causes contraceptive failure of hormonal contraceptives containing •progestogens (alternative contraception recommended)

Aripiprazole *see* Antipsychotics

Artemether with Lumefantrine
• Anti-arrhythmics: manufacturer of artemether/lumefantrine advises avoid concomitant use with •amiodarone, •disopyramide, •flecainide, •procainamide or •quinidine (risk of ventricular arrhythmias)
• Antibacterials: manufacturer of artemether/lumefantrine advises avoid concomitant use with •macrolides and •quinolones
• Antidepressants: manufacturer of artemether/lumefantrine advises avoid concomitant use with •antidepressants
• Antifungals: manufacturer of artemether/lumefantrine advises avoid concomitant use with •imidazoles and •triazoles
• Antimalarials: manufacturer of artemether/lumefantrine advises avoid concomitant use with •antimalarials
• Antipsychotics: manufacturer of artemether/lumefantrine advises avoid concomitant use with •antipsychotics
• Antivirals: manufacturer of artemether/lumefantrine advises avoid concomitant use with •amprenavir, •atazanavir, •indinavir, •lopinavir, •nelfinavir, •ritonavir and •saquinavir; possible increased risk of ventricular arrhythmias when artemether/lumefantrine given with •tipranavir—avoid concomitant use
• Beta-blockers: manufacturer of artemether/lumefantrine advises avoid concomitant use with •metoprolol and •sotalol
• Grapefruit Juice: metabolism of artemether/lumefantrine possibly inhibited by •grapefruit juice (avoid concomitant use)
• Ulcer-healing Drugs: manufacturer of artemether/lumefantrine advises avoid concomitant use with •cimetidine

Aspirin
ACE Inhibitors: risk of renal impairment when aspirin (in doses over 300 mg daily) given with ACE inhibitors, also hypotensive effect antagonised
Adsorbents: absorption of aspirin possibly reduced by kaolin
• Analgesics: avoid concomitant use of aspirin with •NSAIDs (increased side-effects); antiplatelet effect of aspirin possibly reduced by ibuprofen
Angiotensin-II Receptor Antagonists: risk of renal impairment when aspirin (in doses over 300 mg daily) given with angiotensin-II receptor antagonists, also hypotensive effect antagonised
Antacids: excretion of aspirin increased by alkaline urine due to some antacids
• Anticoagulants: increased risk of bleeding when aspirin given with •coumarins or •phenindione (due to antiplatelet effect); aspirin enhances anticoagulant effect of •heparins

Aspirin *(continued)*
• Antidepressants: increased risk of bleeding when aspirin given with •SSRIs or •venlafaxine
Antiepileptics: aspirin enhances effects of phenytoin and valproate
Cilostazol: manufacturer of cilostazol recommends dose of aspirin should not exceed 80 mg daily when given with cilostazol
Clopidogrel: increased risk of bleeding when aspirin given with clopidogrel
Corticosteroids: increased risk of gastro-intestinal bleeding and ulceration when aspirin given with corticosteroids, also corticosteroids reduce plasma concentration of salicylate
• Cytotoxics: aspirin reduces excretion of •methotrexate (increased risk of toxicity)
Diuretics: aspirin antagonises diuretic effect of spironolactone; increased risk of toxicity when high-dose aspirin given with carbonic anhydrase inhibitors
Iloprost: increased risk of bleeding when aspirin given with iloprost
Leukotriene Antagonists: aspirin increases plasma concentration of zafirlukast
Metoclopramide: rate of absorption of aspirin increased by metoclopramide (enhanced effect)
Mifepristone: avoidance of aspirin advised by manufacturer of mifepristone
Probenecid: aspirin antagonises effects of probenecid
Sibutramine: increased risk of bleeding when aspirin given with sibutramine
Sulfinpyrazone: aspirin antagonises effects of sulfinpyrazone

Atazanavir
Antacids: plasma concentration of atazanavir possibly reduced by antacids
• Anti-arrhythmics: atazanavir possibly increases plasma concentration of •amiodarone and •lidocaine (lignocaine); atazanavir possibly increases plasma concentration of •quinidine—avoid concomitant use
• Antibacterials: plasma concentration of both drugs increased when atazanavir given with clarithromycin; atazanavir increases plasma concentration of •rifabutin (reduce dose of rifabutin); plasma concentration of atazanavir reduced by •rifampicin—avoid concomitant use
Anticoagulants: atazanavir may enhance or reduce anticoagulant effect of warfarin
• Antidepressants: plasma concentration of atazanavir reduced by •St John's wort—avoid concomitant use
• Antimalarials: avoidance of atazanavir advised by manufacturer of •artemether/lumefantrine
• Antipsychotics: atazanavir possibly inhibits metabolism of •aripiprazole (reduce dose of aripiprazole); atazanavir possibly increases plasma concentration of •pimozide—avoid concomitant use
• Antivirals: plasma concentration of atazanavir reduced by efavirenz—increase dose of atazanavir; avoid concomitant use of atazanavir with •indinavir; plasma concentration of atazanavir possibly reduced by •nevirapine—avoid concomitant use; atazanavir increases plasma concentration of saquinavir; plasma concentration of atazanavir reduced by tenofovir
• Calcium-channel Blockers: atazanavir increases plasma concentration of •diltiazem (reduce dose of diltiazem); atazanavir possibly increases plasma concentration of verapamil

Atazanavir *(continued)*
- • Ciclosporin: atazanavir possibly increases plasma concentration of •ciclosporin
- • Cytotoxics: atazanavir possibly inhibits metabolism of •irinotecan (increased risk of toxicity)
- • Ergot Alkaloids: atazanavir possibly increases plasma concentration of •ergot alkaloids—avoid concomitant use
- • Lipid-regulating Drugs: possible increased risk of myopathy when atazanavir given with atorvastatin; increased risk of myopathy when atazanavir given with •simvastatin (avoid concomitant use)
- • Oestrogens: atazanavir increases plasma concentration of •ethinylestradiol—avoid concomitant use
- • Sildenafil: atazanavir possibly increases side-effects of •sildenafil
- • Sirolimus: atazanavir possibly increases plasma concentration of •sirolimus
- • Tacrolimus: atazanavir possibly increases plasma concentration of •tacrolimus
- • Ulcer-healing Drugs: plasma concentration of atazanavir significantly reduced by •omeprazole—avoid concomitant use; plasma concentration of atazanavir possibly reduced by histamine H_2-antagonists; plasma concentration of atazanavir possibly reduced by •proton pump inhibitors—avoid concomitant use

Atenolol *see* Beta-blockers

Atomoxetine
- • Antidepressants: atomoxetine should not be started until 2 weeks after stopping •MAOIs, also MAOIs should not be started until at least 2 weeks after stopping atomoxetine
- Sympathomimetics, $Beta_2$: Increased risk of cardiovascular side-effects when atomoxetine given with parenteral salbutamol

Atorvastatin *see* Statins

Atovaquone
- • Antibacterials: plasma concentration of atovaquone reduced by •rifabutin and •rifampicin (possible therapeutic failure of atovaquone); plasma concentration of atovaquone reduced by tetracycline
- Antivirals: atovaquone possibly reduces plasma concentration of indinavir; atovaquone possibly inhibits metabolism of zidovudine (increased plasma concentration)
- Metoclopramide: plasma concentration of atovaquone reduced by metoclopramide

Atracurium *see* Muscle Relaxants

Atropine *see* Antimuscarinics

Azathioprine
- ACE Inhibitors: increased risk of leucopenia when azathioprine given with captopril
- • Allopurinol: enhanced effects and increased toxicity of azathioprine when given with •allopurinol (reduce dose of azathioprine)
- Aminosalicylates: possible increased risk of leucopenia when azathioprine given with aminosalicylates
- • Antibacterials: increased risk of haematological toxicity when azathioprine given with •sulfamethoxazole (as co-trimoxazole); increased risk of haematological toxicity when azathioprine given with •trimethoprim (also with co-trimoxazole)
- • Anticoagulants: azathioprine possibly reduces anticoagulant effect of •coumarins
- Antiepileptics: cytotoxics possibly reduce absorption of phenytoin

Azathioprine *(continued)*
- • Antipsychotics: avoid concomitant use of cytotoxics with •clozapine (increased risk of agranulocytosis)
- Cardiac Glycosides: cytotoxics reduce absorption of digoxin tablets

Azelastine *see* Antihistamines

Azithromycin *see* Macrolides

Aztreonam
- • Anticoagulants: aztreonam possibly enhances anticoagulant effect of •coumarins
- Oestrogens: antibacterials that do not induce liver enzymes possibly reduce contraceptive effect of oestrogens (risk probably small, see BNF section 7.3.1)

Baclofen *see* Muscle Relaxants

Balsalazide *see* Aminosalicylates

Bambuterol *see* Sympathomimetics, $Beta_2$

Barbiturates
- Alcohol: increased sedative effect when barbiturates given with alcohol
- Anti-arrhythmics: barbiturates accelerate metabolism of disopyramide and quinidine (reduced plasma concentration)
- • Antibacterials: barbiturates accelerate metabolism of •chloramphenicol, doxycycline and metronidazole (reduced plasma concentration); phenobarbital reduces plasma concentration of •telithromycin (avoid during and for 2 weeks after phenobarbital)
- • Anticoagulants: barbiturates accelerate metabolism of •coumarins (reduced anticoagulant effect)
- • Antidepressants: phenobarbital reduces plasma concentration of paroxetine; phenobarbital accelerates metabolism of •mianserin (reduced plasma concentration); anticonvulsant effect of barbiturates possibly antagonised by MAOIs and •tricyclic-related antidepressants (convulsive threshold lowered); anticonvulsant effect of barbiturates antagonised by SSRIs (convulsive threshold lowered); plasma concentration of phenobarbital reduced by •St John's wort—avoid concomitant use; anticonvulsant effect of barbiturates antagonised by •tricyclics (convulsive threshold lowered), also metabolism of tricyclics possibly accelerated (reduced plasma concentration)
- Antiepileptics: phenobarbital reduces plasma concentration of carbamazepine, lamotrigine, tiagabine and zonisamide; phenobarbital possibly reduces plasma concentration of ethosuximide; plasma concentration of phenobarbital increased by oxcarbazepine, also plasma concentration of an active metabolite of oxcarbazepine reduced; plasma concentration of phenobarbital often increased by phenytoin, plasma concentration of phenytoin often reduced but may be increased; increased sedative effect when barbiturates given with primidone; plasma concentration of phenobarbital increased by valproate (also plasma concentration of valproate reduced); plasma concentration of phenobarbital possibly reduced by vigabatrin
- • Antifungals: phenobarbital possibly reduces plasma concentration of itraconazole; phenobarbital possibly reduces plasma concentration of •voriconazole—avoid concomitant use; phenobarbital reduces absorption of griseofulvin (reduced effect)
- • Antipsychotics: anticonvulsant effect of barbiturates antagonised by •antipsychotics (convulsive threshold lowered); phenobarbital

Barbiturates
- • Antipsychotics *(continued)* accelerates metabolism of haloperidol (reduced plasma concentration); phenobarbital possibly reduces plasma concentration of •aripiprazole—increase dose of aripiprazole
- • Antivirals: phenobarbital possibly reduces plasma concentration of abacavir, amprenavir and •lopinavir; barbiturates possibly reduce plasma concentration of •indinavir, •nelfinavir and •saquinavir
- Anxiolytics and Hypnotics: phenobarbital often reduces plasma concentration of clonazepam
- Aprepitant: phenobarbital possibly reduces plasma concentration of aprepitant
- • Calcium-channel Blockers: barbiturates reduce effects of •felodipine and •isradipine; barbiturates probably reduce effects of •dihydropyridines, •diltiazem and •verapamil
- Cardiac Glycosides: barbiturates accelerate metabolism of digitoxin (reduced effect)
- • Ciclosporin: barbiturates accelerate metabolism of •ciclosporin (reduced effect)
- • Corticosteroids: barbiturates accelerate metabolism of •corticosteroids (reduced effect)
- Cytotoxics: phenobarbital possibly reduces plasma concentration of etoposide
- • Diuretics: phenobarbital reduces plasma concentration of •eplerenone—avoid concomitant use; increased risk of osteomalacia when phenobarbital given with carbonic anhydrase inhibitors
- Folates: plasma concentration of phenobarbital possibly reduced by folates
- Hormone Antagonists: barbiturates accelerate metabolism of gestrinone (reduced plasma concentration); barbiturates possibly accelerate metabolism of toremifene (reduced plasma concentration)
- $5HT_3$ Antagonists: phenobarbital reduces plasma concentration of tropisetron
- Leukotriene Antagonists: phenobarbital reduces plasma concentration of montelukast
- Memantine: effects of barbiturates possibly reduced by memantine
- • Oestrogens: barbiturates accelerate metabolism of •oestrogens (reduced contraceptive effect—see BNF section 7.3.1)
- • Progestogens: barbiturates accelerate metabolism of •progestogens (reduced contraceptive effect—see BNF section 7.3.1)
- Sympathomimetics: plasma concentration of phenobarbital possibly increased by methylphenidate
- Theophylline: barbiturates accelerate metabolism of theophylline (reduced effect)
- Thyroid Hormones: barbiturates accelerate metabolism of thyroid hormones (may increase requirements for thyroid hormones in hypothyroidism)
- Tibolone: barbiturates accelerate metabolism of tibolone (reduced plasma concentration)
- Vitamins: barbiturates possibly increase requirements for vitamin D

Beclometasone *see* Corticosteroids
Belladonna Alkaloids *see* Antimuscarinics
Bendroflumethiazide (bendrofluazide) *see* Diuretics
Benperidol *see* Antipsychotics
Benzatropine (benztropine) *see* Antimuscarinics
Benzodiazepines *see* Anxiolytics and Hypnotics
Benzthiazide *see* Diuretics
Benzylpenicillin *see* Penicillins

Beta-blockers

Note. Since systemic absorption may follow topical application of beta-blockers to the eye the possibility of interactions, in particular, with drugs such as verapamil should be borne in mind

- ACE Inhibitors: enhanced hypotensive effect when beta-blockers given with ACE inhibitors
- Adrenergic Neurone Blockers: enhanced hypotensive effect when beta-blockers given with adrenergic neurone blockers
- Alcohol: enhanced hypotensive effect when beta-blockers given with alcohol
- Aldesleukin: enhanced hypotensive effect when beta-blockers given with aldesleukin
- • Alpha-blockers: enhanced hypotensive effect when beta-blockers given with •alpha-blockers, also increased risk of first-dose hypotension with post-synaptic alpha-blockers such as prazosin
- Anaesthetics, General: enhanced hypotensive effect when beta-blockers given with general anaesthetics
- • Anaesthetics, Local: propranolol increases risk of •bupivacaine toxicity
- Analgesics: hypotensive effect of beta-blockers antagonised by NSAIDs; plasma concentration of esmolol possibly increased by morphine
- Angiotensin-II Receptor Antagonists: enhanced hypotensive effect when beta-blockers given with angiotensin-II receptor antagonists
- • Anti-arrhythmics: increased myocardial depression when beta-blockers given with •anti-arrhythmics; increased risk of ventricular arrhythmias when sotalol given with •amiodarone, •disopyramide, •procainamide or •quinidine—avoid concomitant use; increased risk of bradycardia, AV block and myocardial depression when beta-blockers given with •amiodarone; increased risk of myocardial depression and bradycardia when beta-blockers given with •flecainide; propranolol increases risk of •lidocaine (lignocaine) toxicity; plasma concentration of metoprolol and propranolol increased by propafenone
- • Antibacterials: increased risk of ventricular arrhythmias when sotalol given with •moxifloxacin—avoid concomitant use; metabolism of bisoprolol and propranolol accelerated by rifampicin (plasma concentration significantly reduced)
- • Antidepressants: plasma concentration of metoprolol increased by citalopram and escitalopram; plasma concentration of propranolol increased by fluvoxamine; plasma concentration of metoprolol possibly increased by paroxetine (enhanced effect); enhanced hypotensive effect when beta-blockers given with MAOIs; increased risk of ventricular arrhythmias when sotalol given with •tricyclics
- Antidiabetics: beta-blockers may mask warning signs of hypoglycaemia (such as tremor) with antidiabetics; beta-blockers enhance hypoglycaemic effect of insulin
- • Antihistamines: increased risk of ventricular arrhythmias when sotalol given with •mizolastine—avoid concomitant use
- • Antimalarials: avoidance of metoprolol and sotalol advised by manufacturer of •artemether/lumefantrine; increased risk of bradycardia when beta-blockers given with mefloquine
- • Antipsychotics: plasma concentration of both drugs may increase when propranolol given with •chlorpromazine; increased risk of

Beta-blockers
- • Antipsychotics *(continued)* ventricular arrhythmias when sotalol given with •amisulpride, •phenothiazines, •pimozide or •sertindole; enhanced hypotensive effect when beta-blockers given with phenothiazines
- Anxiolytics and Hypnotics: enhanced hypotensive effect when beta-blockers given with anxiolytics and hypnotics
- • Calcium-channel Blockers: enhanced hypotensive effect when beta-blockers given with calcium-channel blockers; possible severe hypotension and heart failure when beta-blockers given with •nifedipine or •nisoldipine; increased risk of AV block and bradycardia when beta-blockers given with •diltiazem; asystole, severe hypotension and heart failure when beta-blockers given with •verapamil (see p. 136)
- Cardiac Glycosides: increased risk of AV block and bradycardia when beta-blockers given with cardiac glycosides
- • Ciclosporin: carvedilol increases plasma concentration of •ciclosporin
- • Clonidine: increased risk of withdrawal hypertension when beta-blockers given with •clonidine (withdraw beta-blockers several days before slowly withdrawing clonidine)
- Corticosteroids: hypotensive effect of beta-blockers antagonised by corticosteroids
- Diazoxide: enhanced hypotensive effect when beta-blockers given with diazoxide
- • Diuretics: enhanced hypotensive effect when beta-blockers given with diuretics; risk of ventricular arrhythmias with sotalol increased by hypokalaemia caused by •loop diuretics or •thiazides and related diuretics
- • Dolasetron: increased risk of ventricular arrhythmias when sotalol given with •dolasetron—avoid concomitant use
- Dopaminergics: enhanced hypotensive effect when beta-blockers given with levodopa
- Ergot Alkaloids: increased peripheral vasoconstriction when beta-blockers given with ergotamine and methysergide
- $5HT_1$ Agonists: propranolol possibly increases plasma concentration of rizatriptan (reduce dose of rizatriptan)
- $5HT_3$ Antagonists: caution with beta-blockers advised by manufacturer of tropisetron (risk of ventricular arrhythmias)
- • Ivabradine: increased risk of ventricular arrhythmias when sotalol given with •ivabradine
- Methyldopa: enhanced hypotensive effect when beta-blockers given with methyldopa
- • Moxisylyte (thymoxamine): possible severe postural hypotension when beta-blockers given with •moxisylyte
- Moxonidine: enhanced hypotensive effect when beta-blockers given with moxonidine
- Muscle Relaxants: propranolol enhances effects of muscle relaxants; enhanced hypotensive effect when beta-blockers given with baclofen; possible enhanced hypotensive effect and bradycardia when beta-blockers given with tizanidine
- Nitrates: enhanced hypotensive effect when beta-blockers given with nitrates
- Oestrogens: hypotensive effect of beta-blockers antagonised by oestrogens
- Parasympathomimetics: propranolol antagonises effects of neostigmine and pyridostigmine; increased risk of arrhythmias when beta-blockers given with pilocarpine
- Prostaglandins: enhanced hypotensive effect when beta-blockers given with alprostadil
- • Sympathomimetics: severe hypertension when beta-blockers given with •adrenaline (epinephrine) or •noradrenaline (norepinephrine) especially with non-selective beta-blockers; possible severe hypertension when beta-blockers given with •dobutamine especially with non-selective beta-blockers
- Ulcer-healing Drugs: plasma concentration of labetalol, metoprolol and propranolol increased by cimetidine
- Vasodilator Antihypertensives: enhanced hypotensive effect when beta-blockers given with hydralazine, minoxidil or nitroprusside

Betahistine
- Antihistamines: effect of betahistine theoretically antagonised by antihistamines

Betamethasone *see* Corticosteroids

Betaxolol *see* Beta-blockers

Bethanechol *see* Parasympathomimetics

Bexarotene
- Antiepileptics: cytotoxics possibly reduce absorption of phenytoin
- • Antipsychotics: avoid concomitant use of cytotoxics with •clozapine (increased risk of agranulocytosis)
- Cardiac Glycosides: cytotoxics reduce absorption of digoxin tablets
- • Lipid-regulating Drugs: plasma concentration of bexarotene increased by •gemfibrozil—avoid concomitant use

Bezafibrate *see* Fibrates

Bicalutamide
- Anticoagulants: bicalutamide possibly enhances anticoagulant effect of coumarins

Biguanides *see* Antidiabetics

Bile Acids *see* Ursodeoxycholic Acid

Bisoprolol *see* Beta-blockers

Bisphosphonates
- Analgesics: bioavailability of tiludronic acid increased by indometacin
- Antacids: absorption of bisphosphonates reduced by antacids
- Antibacterials: increased risk of hypocalcaemia when bisphosphonates given with aminoglycosides
- Calcium Salts: absorption of bisphosphonates reduced by calcium salts
- Iron: absorption of bisphosphonates reduced by *oral* iron

Bleomycin
- Antiepileptics: cytotoxics possibly reduce absorption of phenytoin
- • Antipsychotics: avoid concomitant use of cytotoxics with •clozapine (increased risk of agranulocytosis)
- Cardiac Glycosides: cytotoxics reduce absorption of digoxin tablets
- • Cytotoxics: increased pulmonary toxicity when bleomycin given with •cisplatin

Bosentan
- Anticoagulants: manufacturer of bosentan recommends monitoring anticoagulant effect of coumarins
- • Antidiabetics: plasma concentration of both drugs reduced when bosentan given with •glibenclamide (avoid concomitant use)

Bosentan *(continued)*
- • Antifungals: plasma concentration of bosentan possibly increased by itraconazole and ketoconazole; plasma concentration of bosentan increased by •fluconazole—avoid concomitant use
- Antivirals: plasma concentration of bosentan possibly increased by ritonavir
- • Ciclosporin: plasma concentration of bosentan increased by •ciclosporin (also plasma concentration of ciclosporin reduced—avoid concomitant use)
- Lipid-regulating Drugs: bosentan reduces plasma concentration of simvastatin
- • Oestrogens: bosentan possibly causes contraceptive failure of hormonal contraceptives containing •oestrogens (alternative contraception recommended)
- • Progestogens: bosentan possibly causes contraceptive failure of hormonal contraceptives containing •progestogens (alternative contraception recommended)

Brimonidine *see* Alpha$_2$-adrenoceptor Stimulants

Brinzolamide *see* Diuretics

Bromocriptine
- Alcohol: tolerance of bromocriptine reduced by alcohol
- Antibacterials: plasma concentration of bromocriptine increased by erythromycin (increased risk of toxicity); plasma concentration of bromocriptine possibly increased by macrolides (increased risk of toxicity)
- Antipsychotics: hypoprolactinaemic and antiparkinsonian effects of bromocriptine antagonised by antipsychotics
- Domperidone: hypoprolactinaemic effect of bromocriptine possibly antagonised by domperidone
- Hormone Antagonists: plasma concentration of bromocriptine increased by octreotide
- Memantine: effects of dopaminergics possibly enhanced by memantine
- Methyldopa: antiparkinsonian effect of dopaminergics antagonised by methyldopa
- Metoclopramide: hypoprolactinaemic effect of bromocriptine antagonised by metoclopramide
- • Sympathomimetics: risk of toxicity when bromocriptine given with •isometheptene or •phenylpropanolamine

Buclizine *see* Antihistamines

Budesonide *see* Corticosteroids

Bumetanide *see* Diuretics

Bupivacaine
- Anti-arrhythmics: increased myocardial depression when bupivacaine given with anti-arrhythmics
- • Beta-blockers: increased risk of bupivacaine toxicity when given with •propranolol

Buprenorphine *see* Opioid Analgesics

Bupropion

Note. Bupropion should be administered with extreme caution to patients receiving other medication known to lower the seizure threshold—see CSM advice BNF section 4.10 and Cautions, Contra-indications and Side-effects of individual drugs

- • Antidepressants: manufacturer of bupropion advises avoid for 2 weeks after stopping •MAOIs; manufacturer of bupropion advises avoid concomitant use with •moclobemide
- Antiepileptics: plasma concentration of bupropion reduced by carbamazepine and phenytoin; metabolism of bupropion inhibited by valproate

Bupropion *(continued)*
- • Antivirals: plasma concentration of bupropion increased by •ritonavir (risk of toxicity)—avoid concomitant use
- Dopaminergics: increased risk of side-effects when bupropion given with amantadine or levodopa

Buspirone *see* Anxiolytics and Hypnotics

Busulfan
- Analgesics: metabolism of *intravenous* busulfan possibly inhibited by paracetamol (manufacturer of *intravenous* busulfan advises caution within 72 hours of paracetamol)
- Antiepileptics: plasma concentration of busulfan possibly reduced by phenytoin; cytotoxics possibly reduce absorption of phenytoin
- Antifungals: metabolism of busulfan inhibited by itraconazole (increased risk of toxicity)
- • Antipsychotics: avoid concomitant use of cytotoxics with •clozapine (increased risk of agranulocytosis)
- Cardiac Glycosides: cytotoxics reduce absorption of digoxin tablets
- Cytotoxics: increased risk of hepatotoxicity when busulfan given with tioguanine

Butobarbital *see* Barbiturates

Butyrophenones *see* Antipsychotics

Cabergoline
- Antibacterials: plasma concentration of cabergoline increased by erythromycin (increased risk of toxicity); plasma concentration of cabergoline possibly increased by macrolides (increased risk of toxicity)
- Antipsychotics: hypoprolactinaemic and antiparkinsonian effects of cabergoline antagonised by antipsychotics
- Domperidone: hypoprolactinaemic effect of cabergoline possibly antagonised by domperidone
- Memantine: effects of dopaminergics possibly enhanced by memantine
- Methyldopa: antiparkinsonian effect of dopaminergics antagonised by methyldopa
- Metoclopramide: hypoprolactinaemic effect of cabergoline antagonised by metoclopramide

Calcium Salts

Note. see also Antacids

- Antibacterials: calcium salts reduce absorption of ciprofloxacin and tetracycline
- Bisphosphonates: calcium salts reduce absorption of bisphosphonates
- Cardiac Glycosides: large intravenous doses of calcium salts can precipitate arrhythmias when given with cardiac glycosides
- Corticosteroids: absorption of calcium salts reduced by corticosteroids
- Diuretics: increased risk of hypercalcaemia when calcium salts given with thiazides and related diuretics
- Fluorides: calcium salts reduce absorption of fluorides
- Iron: calcium salts reduce absorption of *oral* iron
- Thyroid Hormones: calcium salts reduce absorption of levothyroxine (thyroxine)
- Zinc: calcium salts reduce absorption of zinc

Calcium-channel Blockers

Note. Dihydropyridine calcium-channel blockers include amlodipine, felodipine, isradipine, lacidipine, lercanidipine, nicardipine, nifedipine, nimodipine, and nisoldipine

- ACE Inhibitors: enhanced hypotensive effect when calcium-channel blockers given with ACE inhibitors

Calcium-channel Blockers *(continued)*

Adrenergic Neurone Blockers: enhanced hypotensive effect when calcium-channel blockers given with adrenergic neurone blockers

Alcohol: enhanced hypotensive effect when calcium-channel blockers given with alcohol; verapamil possibly increases plasma concentration of alcohol

Aldesleukin: enhanced hypotensive effect when calcium-channel blockers given with aldesleukin

• Alpha-blockers: enhanced hypotensive effect when calcium-channel blockers given with •alpha-blockers, also increased risk of first-dose hypotension with post-synaptic alpha-blockers such as prazosin

• Anaesthetics, General: enhanced hypotensive effect when calcium-channel blockers given with general anaesthetics or isoflurane; hypotensive effect of verapamil enhanced by •general anaesthetics (also AV delay)

Analgesics: hypotensive effect of calcium-channel blockers antagonised by NSAIDs; diltiazem inhibits metabolism of alfentanil (risk of prolonged or delayed respiratory depression)

Angiotensin-II Receptor Antagonists: enhanced hypotensive effect when calcium-channel blockers given with angiotensin-II receptor antagonists

• Anti-arrhythmics: increased risk of bradycardia, AV block and myocardial depression when diltiazem or verapamil given with •amiodarone; increased risk of myocardial depression and asystole when verapamil given with •disopyramide or •flecainide; verapamil increases plasma concentration of •quinidine (extreme hypotension may occur); nifedipine reduces plasma concentration of quinidine

• Antibacterials: metabolism of verapamil possibly inhibited by •clarithromycin and •erythromycin (increased risk of toxicity); metabolism of felodipine possibly inhibited by erythromycin (increased plasma concentration); manufacturer of lercanidipine advises avoid concomitant use with erythromycin; metabolism of diltiazem, nifedipine, nimodipine and verapamil accelerated by •rifampicin (plasma concentration significantly reduced); metabolism of isradipine, nicardipine and nisoldipine possibly accelerated by •rifampicin (possible significantly reduced plasma concentration); plasma concentration of nifedipine increased by •quinupristin/dalfopristin

Antidepressants: diltiazem and verapamil increase plasma concentration of imipramine; enhanced hypotensive effect when calcium-channel blockers given with MAOIs; diltiazem and verapamil possibly increase plasma concentration of tricyclics

Antidiabetics: glucose tolerance occasionally impaired when nifedipine given with insulin

• Antiepileptics: effects of dihydropyridines, nicardipine and nifedipine probably reduced by carbamazepine; effects of felodipine and isradipine reduced by carbamazepine; diltiazem and verapamil enhance effects of •carbamazepine; effects of felodipine, isradipine and verapamil reduced by phenytoin; effects of dihydropyridines, nicardipine and nifedipine probably reduced by •phenytoin; diltiazem increases plasma concentration of •phenytoin but also effect of diltiazem reduced; plasma concentration of nisoldipine reduced by phenytoin; effects of felodipine and isradipine reduced by •primidone; effects of dihydropyridines, diltiazem and verapamil probably reduced by •primidone

• Antifungals: metabolism of dihydropyridines possibly inhibited by itraconazole and ketoconazole (increased plasma concentration); metabolism of felodipine inhibited by •itraconazole and •ketoconazole (increased plasma concentration); manufacturer of lercanidipine advises avoid concomitant use with itraconazole and ketoconazole; negative inotropic effect possibly increased when calcium-channel blockers given with itraconazole

Antimalarials: possible increased risk of bradycardia when calcium-channel blockers given with mefloquine

Antipsychotics: enhanced hypotensive effect when calcium-channel blockers given with antipsychotics

• Antivirals: plasma concentration of diltiazem, nicardipine, nifedipine and nimodipine possibly increased by amprenavir; plasma concentration of diltiazem increased by •atazanavir (reduce dose of diltiazem); plasma concentration of verapamil possibly increased by atazanavir; manufacturer of lercanidipine advises avoid concomitant use with ritonavir; plasma concentration of calcium-channel blockers possibly increased by •ritonavir

Anxiolytics and Hypnotics: enhanced hypotensive effect when calcium-channel blockers given with anxiolytics and hypnotics; diltiazem and verapamil inhibit metabolism of midazolam (increased plasma concentration with increased sedation); absorption of lercanidipine increased by midazolam; diltiazem and verapamil increase plasma concentration of buspirone (reduce dose of buspirone)

• Barbiturates: effects of dihydropyridines, diltiazem and verapamil probably reduced by •barbiturates; effects of felodipine and isradipine reduced by •barbiturates

• Beta-blockers: enhanced hypotensive effect when calcium-channel blockers given with beta-blockers; increased risk of AV block and bradycardia when diltiazem given with •beta-blockers; asystole, severe hypotension and heart failure when verapamil given with •beta-blockers (see p. 136); possible severe hypotension and heart failure when nifedipine or nisoldipine given with •beta-blockers

Calcium-channel Blockers: plasma concentration of both drugs may increase when diltiazem given with nifedipine

• Cardiac Glycosides: nifedipine possibly increases plasma concentration of •digoxin; diltiazem, lercanidipine and nicardipine increase plasma concentration of •digoxin; verapamil increases plasma concentration of •digoxin, also increased risk of AV block and bradycardia

• Ciclosporin: diltiazem, nicardipine and verapamil increase plasma concentration of •ciclosporin; combination of lercanidipine with •ciclosporin may increase plasma concentration of either drug (or both)—avoid concomitant use; plasma concentration of nifedipine possibly increased by ciclosporin (increased risk of toxicity including gingival hyperplasia)

Calcium-channel Blockers *(continued)*
- • Cilostazol: diltiazem increases plasma concentration of •cilostazol—avoid concomitant use
- Clonidine: enhanced hypotensive effect when calcium-channel blockers given with clonidine
- Corticosteroids: hypotensive effect of calcium-channel blockers antagonised by corticosteroids
- Cytotoxics: nifedipine possibly inhibits metabolism of vincristine
- Diazoxide: enhanced hypotensive effect when calcium-channel blockers given with diazoxide
- Diuretics: enhanced hypotensive effect when calcium-channel blockers given with diuretics; diltiazem and verapamil increase plasma concentration of eplerenone (reduce dose of eplerenone)
- Dopaminergics: enhanced hypotensive effect when calcium-channel blockers given with levodopa
- Grapefruit Juice: plasma concentration of felodipine, isradipine, lacidipine, lercanidipine, nicardipine, nifedipine, nimodipine, nisoldipine and verapamil increased by grapefruit juice
- Hormone Antagonists: diltiazem and verapamil increase plasma concentration of dutasteride
- • Ivabradine: diltiazem and verapamil increase plasma concentration of •ivabradine—avoid concomitant use
- • Lipid-regulating Drugs: possible increased risk of myopathy when diltiazem given with simvastatin; increased risk of myopathy when verapamil given with •simvastatin
- Lithium: neurotoxicity may occur when diltiazem or verapamil given with lithium without increased plasma concentration of lithium
- • Magnesium (parenteral): profound hypotension reported with concomitant use of nifedipine and •parenteral magnesium in pre-eclampsia
- Methyldopa: enhanced hypotensive effect when calcium-channel blockers given with methyldopa
- Moxisylyte (thymoxamine): enhanced hypotensive effect when calcium-channel blockers given with moxisylyte
- Moxonidine: enhanced hypotensive effect when calcium-channel blockers given with moxonidine
- Muscle Relaxants: verapamil enhances effects of non-depolarising muscle relaxants and suxamethonium; enhanced hypotensive effect when calcium-channel blockers given with baclofen or tizanidine; risk of arrhythmias when diltiazem given with intravenous dantrolene; hypotension, myocardial depression, and hyperkalaemia when verapamil given with intravenous dantrolene; nifedipine enhances effects of non-depolarising muscle relaxants
- Nitrates: enhanced hypotensive effect when calcium-channel blockers given with nitrates
- Oestrogens: hypotensive effect of calcium-channel blockers antagonised by oestrogens
- Prostaglandins: enhanced hypotensive effect when calcium-channel blockers given with alprostadil
- Sildenafil: enhanced hypotensive effect when amlodipine given with sildenafil
- • Sirolimus: diltiazem increases plasma concentration of •sirolimus; plasma concentration of both drugs increased when verapamil given with •sirolimus

Calcium-channel Blockers *(continued)*
- • Tacrolimus: diltiazem and nifedipine increase plasma concentration of •tacrolimus; felodipine possibly increases plasma concentration of tacrolimus
- • Theophylline: calcium-channel blockers possibly increase plasma concentration of •theophylline (enhanced effect); diltiazem increases plasma concentration of theophylline; verapamil increases plasma concentration of •theophylline (enhanced effect)
- Ulcer-healing Drugs: metabolism of calcium-channel blockers possibly inhibited by cimetidine (increased plasma concentration)
- Vardenafil: enhanced hypotensive effect when nifedipine given with vardenafil
- Vasodilator Antihypertensives: enhanced hypotensive effect when calcium-channel blockers given with hydralazine, minoxidil or nitroprusside

Calcium-channel Blockers (dihydropyridines) *see* Calcium-channel Blockers

Candesartan *see* Angiotensin-II Receptor Antagonists

Capecitabine *see* Fluorouracil

Capreomycin
- Antibacterials: increased risk of nephrotoxicity when capreomycin given with colistin or polymyxins; increased risk of nephrotoxicity and ototoxicity when capreomycin given with aminoglycosides or vancomycin
- Cytotoxics: increased risk of nephrotoxicity and ototoxicity when capreomycin given with platinum compounds
- Oestrogens: antibacterials that do not induce liver enzymes possibly reduce contraceptive effect of oestrogens (risk probably small, see BNF section 7.3.1)

Captopril *see* ACE Inhibitors

Carbamazepine
- Alcohol: CNS side-effects of carbamazepine possibly increased by alcohol
- • Analgesics: effects of carbamazepine enhanced by •dextropropoxyphene; carbamazepine reduces plasma concentration of methadone; carbamazepine reduces effects of tramadol
- • Antibacterials: plasma concentration of carbamazepine increased by •clarithromycin and •erythromycin; plasma concentration of carbamazepine reduced by •rifabutin; carbamazepine accelerates metabolism of doxycycline (reduced effect); plasma concentration of carbamazepine increased by •isoniazid (also possibly increased isoniazid hepatotoxicity); carbamazepine reduces plasma concentration of •telithromycin (avoid during and for 2 weeks after carbamazepine)
- • Anticoagulants: carbamazepine accelerates metabolism of •coumarins (reduced anticoagulant effect)
- • Antidepressants: plasma concentration of carbamazepine increased by •fluoxetine and •fluvoxamine; carbamazepine reduces plasma concentration of •mianserin, mirtazapine and paroxetine; manufacturer of carbamazepine advises avoid for 2 weeks after stopping •MAOIs, also antagonism of anticonvulsant effect; anticonvulsant effect of antiepileptics possibly antagonised by MAOIs and •tricyclic-related antidepressants (convulsive threshold lowered); anticonvulsant effect of antiepileptics antagonised by •SSRIs and •tricyclics (convulsive threshold lowered); plasma concentration of carbamazepine reduced by •St John's

Carbamazepine
- Antidepressants *(continued)* wort—avoid concomitant use; carbamazepine accelerates metabolism of •tricyclics (reduced plasma concentration and reduced effect)

Antiepileptics: carbamazepine possibly reduces plasma concentration of ethosuximide; carbamazepine often reduces plasma concentration of lamotrigine, also plasma concentration of an active metabolite of carbamazepine sometimes raised (but evidence is conflicting); plasma concentration of carbamazepine sometimes reduced by oxcarbazepine (but concentration of an active metabolite of carbamazepine may be increased), also plasma concentration of an active metabolite of oxcarbazepine often reduced; plasma concentration of both drugs often reduced when carbamazepine given with phenytoin, also plasma concentration of phenytoin may be increased; plasma concentration of carbamazepine often reduced by primidone, also plasma concentration of primidone sometimes reduced (but concentration of an active metabolite of primidone often increased); carbamazepine reduces plasma concentration of tiagabine; carbamazepine often reduces plasma concentration of topiramate; carbamazepine reduces plasma concentration of valproate, also plasma concentration of active metabolite of carbamazepine increased; carbamazepine reduces plasma concentration of zonisamide, effect on carbamazepine plasma concentration not predictable

- Antifungals: plasma concentration of carbamazepine possibly increased by miconazole; carbamazepine possibly reduces plasma concentration of itraconazole; carbamazepine possibly reduces plasma concentration of •voriconazole—avoid concomitant use; carbamazepine possibly reduces plasma concentration of caspofungin—consider increasing dose of caspofungin
- Antimalarials: possible increased risk of convulsions when antiepileptics given with chloroquine and hydroxychloroquine; anticonvulsant effect of antiepileptics and carbamazepine antagonised by •mefloquine
- Antipsychotics: anticonvulsant effect of carbamazepine antagonised by •antipsychotics (convulsive threshold lowered); carbamazepine accelerates metabolism of haloperidol, olanzapine, quetiapine, risperidone and sertindole (reduced plasma concentration); carbamazepine reduces plasma concentration of •aripiprazole—increase dose of aripiprazole; carbamazepine accelerates metabolism of •clozapine (reduced plasma concentration), also avoid concomitant use of drugs with substantial potential for causing agranulocytosis
- Antivirals: carbamazepine possibly reduces plasma concentration of amprenavir, indinavir, lopinavir, nelfinavir and saquinavir; plasma concentration of both drugs reduced when carbamazepine given with efavirenz; plasma concentration of carbamazepine possibly increased by •ritonavir

Anxiolytics and Hypnotics: carbamazepine often reduces plasma concentration of clonazepam

Aprepitant: carbamazepine possibly reduces plasma concentration of aprepitant

Carbamazepine *(continued)*

Barbiturates: plasma concentration of carbamazepine reduced by phenobarbital

Bupropion: carbamazepine reduces plasma concentration of bupropion

- Calcium-channel Blockers: carbamazepine reduces effects of felodipine and isradipine; carbamazepine probably reduces effects of dihydropyridines, nicardipine and nifedipine; effects of carbamazepine enhanced by •diltiazem and •verapamil

Cardiac Glycosides: carbamazepine accelerates metabolism of digitoxin (reduced effect)

- Ciclosporin: carbamazepine accelerates metabolism of •ciclosporin (reduced plasma concentration)
- Corticosteroids: carbamazepine accelerates metabolism of •corticosteroids (reduced effect)
- Diuretics: increased risk of hyponatraemia when carbamazepine given with diuretics; plasma concentration of carbamazepine increased by •acetazolamide; carbamazepine reduces plasma concentration of •eplerenone—avoid concomitant use
- Hormone Antagonists: metabolism of carbamazepine inhibited by •danazol (increased risk of toxicity); carbamazepine accelerates metabolism of gestrinone (reduced plasma concentration); carbamazepine possibly accelerates metabolism of toremifene (reduced plasma concentration)

$5HT_3$ Antagonists: carbamazepine accelerates metabolism of ondansetron (reduced effect)

Lithium: neurotoxicity may occur when carbamazepine given with lithium without increased plasma concentration of lithium

Muscle Relaxants: carbamazepine antagonises muscle relaxant effect of non-depolarising muscle relaxants (accelerated recovery from neuromuscular blockade)

- Oestrogens: carbamazepine accelerates metabolism of •oestrogens (reduced contraceptive effect—see BNF section 7.3.1)
- Progestogens: carbamazepine accelerates metabolism of •progestogens (reduced contraceptive effect—see BNF section 7.3.1)

Retinoids: plasma concentration of carbamazepine possibly reduced by isotretinoin

Theophylline: carbamazepine accelerates metabolism of theophylline (reduced effect)

Thyroid Hormones: carbamazepine accelerates metabolism of thyroid hormones (may increase requirements for thyroid hormones in hypothyroidism)

Tibolone: carbamazepine accelerates metabolism of tibolone (reduced plasma concentration)

- Ulcer-healing Drugs: metabolism of carbamazepine inhibited by •cimetidine (increased plasma concentration)

Vitamins: carbamazepine possibly increases requirements for vitamin D

Carbapenems *see* Ertapenem, Imipenem with Cilastatin, and Meropenem

Carbonic Anhydrase Inhibitors *see* Diuretics

Carboplatin *see* Platinum Compounds

Carboprost *see* Prostaglandins

Cardiac Glycosides

ACE Inhibitors: plasma concentration of digoxin possibly increased by captopril

Alpha-blockers: plasma concentration of digoxin increased by prazosin

Aminosalicylates: absorption of digoxin possibly reduced by sulfasalazine

Cardiac Glycosides *(continued)*
Analgesics: plasma concentration of cardiac glycosides possibly increased by NSAIDs, also possible exacerbation of heart failure and reduction of renal function
• Angiotensin-II Receptor Antagonists: plasma concentration of digoxin increased by •telmisartan
Antacids: absorption of digoxin possibly reduced by antacids
• Anti-arrhythmics: plasma concentration of digoxin increased by •amiodarone, •propafenone and •quinidine (halve dose of digoxin)
Antibacterials: plasma concentration of digoxin possibly increased by gentamicin, telithromycin and trimethoprim; absorption of digoxin reduced by neomycin; plasma concentration of digoxin possibly reduced by rifampicin; plasma concentration of digoxin increased by macrolides (increased risk of toxicity); metabolism of digitoxin accelerated by rifamycins (reduced effect)
• Antidepressants: plasma concentration of digoxin reduced by •St John's wort—avoid concomitant use
Antidiabetics: plasma concentration of digoxin possibly reduced by acarbose
Antiepileptics: metabolism of digitoxin accelerated by carbamazepine, phenytoin and primidone (reduced effect); plasma concentration of digoxin possibly reduced by phenytoin
• Antifungals: increased cardiac toxicity with cardiac glycosides if hypokalaemia occurs with •amphotericin; plasma concentration of digoxin increased by •itraconazole
• Antimalarials: plasma concentration of digoxin possibly increased by •chloroquine and hydroxychloroquine; possible increased risk of bradycardia when digoxin given with mefloquine; plasma concentration of digoxin increased by •quinine
Anxiolytics and Hypnotics: plasma concentration of digoxin increased by alprazolam (increased risk of toxicity)
Barbiturates: metabolism of digitoxin accelerated by barbiturates (reduced effect)
Beta-blockers: increased risk of AV block and bradycardia when cardiac glycosides given with beta-blockers
Calcium Salts: arrhythmias can be precipitated when cardiac glycosides given with large intravenous doses of calcium salts
• Calcium-channel Blockers: plasma concentration of digoxin increased by •diltiazem, •lercanidipine and •nicardipine; plasma concentration of digoxin possibly increased by •nifedipine; plasma concentration of digoxin increased by •verapamil, also increased risk of AV block and bradycardia
• Ciclosporin: plasma concentration of digoxin increased by •ciclosporin (increased risk of toxicity)
Corticosteroids: increased risk of hypokalaemia when cardiac glycosides given with corticosteroids
Cytotoxics: absorption of digoxin tablets reduced by cytotoxics
• Diuretics: increased cardiac toxicity with cardiac glycosides if hypokalaemia occurs with •acetazolamide, •loop diuretics or •thiazides and related diuretics; plasma concentration of digitoxin possibly affected by spironolactone; plasma concentration of digoxin increased by •spironolactone
Lipid-regulating Drugs: absorption of cardiac glycosides possibly reduced by colestipol and colestyramine; plasma concentration of digoxin possibly increased by atorvastatin
Muscle Relaxants: risk of ventricular arrhythmias when cardiac glycosides given with suxamethonium; possible increased risk of bradycardia when cardiac glycosides given with tizanidine
Penicillamine: plasma concentration of digoxin possibly reduced by penicillamine
Sympathomimetics, Beta$_2$: plasma concentration of digoxin possibly reduced by salbutamol
Ulcer-healing Drugs: plasma concentration of digoxin possibly slightly increased by proton pump inhibitors; absorption of cardiac glycosides possibly reduced by sucralfate

Carisoprodol *see* Muscle Relaxants
Carteolol *see* Beta-blockers
Carvedilol *see* Beta-blockers
Caspofungin
Antibacterials: plasma concentration of caspofungin initially increased and then reduced by rifampicin (consider increasing dose of caspofungin)
Antiepileptics: plasma concentration of caspofungin possibly reduced by carbamazepine and phenytoin—consider increasing dose of caspofungin
Antivirals: plasma concentration of caspofungin possibly reduced by efavirenz and nevirapine—consider increasing dose of caspofungin
• Ciclosporin: plasma concentration of caspofungin increased by •ciclosporin (manufacturer of caspofungin recommends monitoring liver enzymes)
Corticosteroids: plasma concentration of caspofungin possibly reduced by dexamethasone—consider increasing dose of caspofungin
• Tacrolimus: caspofungin reduces plasma concentration of •tacrolimus

Cefaclor *see* Cephalosporins
Cefadroxil *see* Cephalosporins
Cefalexin *see* Cephalosporins
Cefixime *see* Cephalosporins
Cefotaxime *see* Cephalosporins
Cefpodoxime *see* Cephalosporins
Cefprozil *see* Cephalosporins
Cefradine *see* Cephalosporins
Ceftazidime *see* Cephalosporins
Ceftriaxone *see* Cephalosporins
Cefuroxime *see* Cephalosporins
Celecoxib *see* NSAIDs
Celiprolol *see* Beta-blockers
Cephalosporins
Antacids: absorption of cefaclor and cefpodoxime reduced by antacids
• Anticoagulants: cephalosporins possibly enhance anticoagulant effect of •coumarins
Oestrogens: antibacterials that do not induce liver enzymes possibly reduce contraceptive effect of oestrogens (risk probably small, see BNF section 7.3.1)
Probenecid: excretion of cephalosporins reduced by probenecid (increased plasma concentration)
Ulcer-healing Drugs: absorption of cefpodoxime reduced by histamine H_2-antagonists

Cetirizine *see* Antihistamines

Chloral *see* Anxiolytics and Hypnotics

Chloramphenicol

Antibacterials: metabolism of chloramphenicol accelerated by rifampicin (reduced plasma concentration)

• Anticoagulants: chloramphenicol enhances anticoagulant effect of •coumarins

• Antidiabetics: chloramphenicol enhances effects of •sulphonylureas

• Antiepileptics: chloramphenicol increases plasma concentration of •phenytoin (increased risk of toxicity); metabolism of chloramphenicol accelerated by •primidone (reduced plasma concentration)

• Antipsychotics: avoid concomitant use of chloramphenicol with •clozapine (increased risk of agranulocytosis)

• Barbiturates: metabolism of chloramphenicol accelerated by •barbiturates (reduced plasma concentration)

• Ciclosporin: chloramphenicol possibly increases plasma concentration of •ciclosporin

Hydroxocobalamin: chloramphenicol reduces response to hydroxocobalamin

Oestrogens: antibacterials that do not induce liver enzymes possibly reduce contraceptive effect of oestrogens (risk probably small, see BNF section 7.3.1)

• Tacrolimus: chloramphenicol possibly increases plasma concentration of •tacrolimus

Chlordiazepoxide *see* Anxiolytics and Hypnotics

Chloroquine and Hydroxychloroquine

Adsorbents: absorption of chloroquine and hydroxychloroquine reduced by kaolin

Agalsidase Beta: chloroquine and hydroxychloroquine possibly inhibit effects of agalsidase beta (manufacturer of agalsidase beta advises avoid concomitant use)

Antacids: absorption of chloroquine and hydroxychloroquine reduced by antacids

• Anti-arrhythmics: increased risk of ventricular arrhythmias when chloroquine and hydroxychloroquine given with •amiodarone—avoid concomitant use

• Antibacterials: increased risk of ventricular arrhythmias when chloroquine and hydroxychloroquine given with •moxifloxacin—avoid concomitant use

Antiepileptics: possible increased risk of convulsions when chloroquine and hydroxychloroquine given with antiepileptics

• Antimalarials: avoidance of antimalarials advised by manufacturer of •artemether/lumefantrine; increased risk of convulsions when chloroquine and hydroxychloroquine given with •mefloquine

• Cardiac Glycosides: chloroquine and hydroxychloroquine possibly increase plasma concentration of •digoxin

• Ciclosporin: chloroquine and hydroxychloroquine increase plasma concentration of •ciclosporin (increased risk of toxicity)

Laronidase: chloroquine and hydroxychloroquine possibly inhibit effects of laronidase (manufacturer of laronidase advises avoid concomitant use)

Parasympathomimetics: chloroquine and hydroxychloroquine have potential to increase symptoms of myasthenia gravis and thus diminish effect of neostigmine and pyridostigmine

Chloroquine and Hydroxychloroquine *(continued)*

Ulcer-healing Drugs: metabolism of chloroquine and hydroxychloroquine inhibited by cimetidine (increased plasma concentration)

Chlorothiazide *see* Diuretics

Chlorphenamine (chlorpheniramine) *see* Antihistamines

Chlorpromazine *see* Antipsychotics

Chlorpropamide *see* Antidiabetics

Chlortalidone *see* Diuretics

Chlortetracycline *see* Tetracyclines

Ciclesonide *see* Corticosteroids

Ciclosporin

• ACE Inhibitors: increased risk of hyperkalaemia when ciclosporin given with •ACE inhibitors

Allopurinol: plasma concentration of ciclosporin possibly increased by allopurinol (risk of nephrotoxicity)

• Analgesics: increased risk of nephrotoxicity when ciclosporin given with •NSAIDs; ciclosporin increases plasma concentration of •diclofenac (halve dose of diclofenac)

• Angiotensin-II Receptor Antagonists: increased risk of hyperkalaemia when ciclosporin given with •angiotensin-II receptor antagonists

Anti-arrhythmics: plasma concentration of ciclosporin possibly increased by amiodarone and propafenone

• Antibacterials: metabolism of ciclosporin inhibited by •clarithromycin and •erythromycin (increased plasma concentration); metabolism of ciclosporin accelerated by •rifampicin (reduced plasma concentration); plasma concentration of ciclosporin possibly reduced by •sulfadiazine; plasma concentration of ciclosporin possibly increased by •chloramphenicol, •doxycycline and •telithromycin; increased risk of nephrotoxicity when ciclosporin given with •aminoglycosides, •polymyxins, •quinolones, •sulphonamides or •vancomycin; metabolism of ciclosporin possibly inhibited by •macrolides (increased plasma concentration); plasma concentration of ciclosporin increased by •quinupristin/dalfopristin; increased risk of nephrotoxicity when ciclosporin given with •trimethoprim, also plasma concentration of ciclosporin reduced by intravenous trimethoprim

• Antidepressants: plasma concentration of ciclosporin reduced by •St John's wort—avoid concomitant use

• Antiepileptics: metabolism of ciclosporin accelerated by •carbamazepine and •phenytoin (reduced plasma concentration); plasma concentration of ciclosporin possibly reduced by oxcarbazepine; metabolism of ciclosporin accelerated by •primidone (reduced effect)

• Antifungals: metabolism of ciclosporin inhibited by •fluconazole, •itraconazole, •ketoconazole and •voriconazole (increased plasma concentration); metabolism of ciclosporin possibly inhibited by •miconazole (increased plasma concentration); increased risk of nephrotoxicity when ciclosporin given with •amphotericin; ciclosporin increases plasma concentration of •caspofungin (manufacturer of caspofungin recommends monitoring liver enzymes); plasma concentration of ciclosporin possibly reduced by griseofulvin

• Antimalarials: plasma concentration of ciclosporin increased by •chloroquine and hydroxychloroquine (increased risk of toxicity)

• Antivirals: increased risk of nephrotoxicity when ciclosporin given with aciclovir; plasma con-

Ciclosporin
• Antivirals *(continued)*
centration of ciclosporin possibly increased by •atazanavir, •nelfinavir and •ritonavir; plasma concentration of both drugs increased when ciclosporin given with •saquinavir
• Barbiturates: metabolism of ciclosporin accelerated by •barbiturates (reduced effect)
• Beta-blockers: plasma concentration of ciclosporin increased by •carvedilol
• Bile Acids: absorption of ciclosporin increased by •ursodeoxycholic acid
• Bosentan: ciclosporin increases plasma concentration of •bosentan (also plasma concentration of ciclosporin reduced—avoid concomitant use)
• Calcium-channel Blockers: combination of ciclosporin with •lercanidipine may increase plasma concentration of either drug (or both)—avoid concomitant use; plasma concentration of ciclosporin increased by •diltiazem, •nicardipine and •verapamil; ciclosporin possibly increases plasma concentration of nifedipine (increased risk of toxicity including gingival hyperplasia)
• Cardiac Glycosides: ciclosporin increases plasma concentration of •digoxin (increased risk of toxicity)
• Colchicine: possible increased risk of nephrotoxicity and myotoxicity when ciclosporin given with •colchicine (increased plasma concentration of ciclosporin)
• Corticosteroids: plasma concentration of ciclosporin increased by high-dose •methylprednisolone (risk of convulsions); ciclosporin increases plasma concentration of prednisolone
• Cytotoxics: increased risk of nephrotoxicity when ciclosporin given with •melphalan; increased risk of neurotoxicity when ciclosporin given with •doxorubicin; risk of toxicity when ciclosporin given with •methotrexate; *in vitro* studies suggest a possible interaction between ciclosporin and docetaxel (consult docetaxel product literature); ciclosporin possibly increases plasma concentration of etoposide (increased risk of toxicity)
• Diuretics: increased risk of hyperkalaemia when ciclosporin given with •potassium-sparing diuretics and aldosterone antagonists; increased risk of nephrotoxicity and possibly hypermagnesaemia when ciclosporin given with thiazides and related diuretics
• Grapefruit Juice: plasma concentration of ciclosporin increased by •grapefruit juice (increased risk of toxicity)
• Hormone Antagonists: metabolism of ciclosporin inhibited by •danazol (increased plasma concentration); plasma concentration of ciclosporin reduced by lanreotide and •octreotide
• Lipid-regulating Drugs: increased risk of renal impairment when ciclosporin given with fenofibrate; increased risk of myopathy when ciclosporin given with •rosuvastatin (avoid concomitant use); plasma concentration of both drugs may increase when ciclosporin given with •ezetimibe; increased risk of myopathy when ciclosporin given with •statins
• Metoclopramide: plasma concentration of ciclosporin increased by •metoclopramide
• Modafinil: plasma concentration of ciclosporin reduced by •modafinil

Ciclosporin *(continued)*
Oestrogens: plasma concentration of ciclosporin possibly increased by oestrogens
• Orlistat: absorption of ciclosporin possibly reduced by •orlistat
• Potassium Salts: increased risk of hyperkalaemia when ciclosporin given with •potassium salts
• Progestogens: metabolism of ciclosporin inhibited by •progestogens (increased plasma concentration)
Sirolimus: ciclosporin increases plasma concentration of sirolimus
• Tacrolimus: plasma concentration of ciclosporin increased by •tacrolimus (increased risk of toxicity)—avoid concomitant use
• Ulcer-healing Drugs: plasma concentration of ciclosporin possibly increased by •cimetidine; plasma concentration of ciclosporin possibly affected by omeprazole

Cidofovir
Antivirals: combination of cidofovir with tenofovir may increase plasma concentration of either drug (or both)

Cilazapril *see* ACE Inhibitors

Cilostazol
• Anagrelide: avoidance of cilostazol advised by manufacturer of •anagrelide
Analgesics: manufacturer of cilostazol recommends dose of concomitant aspirin should not exceed 80 mg daily
• Antibacterials: plasma concentration of cilostazol increased by •erythromycin (also plasma concentration of erythromycin reduced)—avoid concomitant use
• Antifungals: plasma concentration of cilostazol possibly increased by •ketoconazole—avoid concomitant use
• Antivirals: plasma concentration of cilostazol possibly increased by •amprenavir, •indinavir, •lopinavir, •nelfinavir, •ritonavir and •saquinavir—avoid concomitant use
• Calcium-channel Blockers: plasma concentration of cilostazol increased by •diltiazem—avoid concomitant use
• Ulcer-healing Drugs: plasma concentration of cilostazol possibly increased by •cimetidine and •lansoprazole—avoid concomitant use; plasma concentration of cilostazol increased by •omeprazole (risk of toxicity)—avoid concomitant use

Cimetidine *see* Histamine H_2-antagonists

Cinacalcet
Antifungals: metabolism of cinacalcet inhibited by ketoconazole (increased plasma concentration)
Tobacco: metabolism of cinacalcet increased by tobacco smoking (reduced plasma concentration)

Cinnarizine *see* Antihistamines
Ciprofibrate *see* Fibrates
Ciprofloxacin *see* Quinolones
Cisatracurium *see* Muscle Relaxants
Cisplatin *see* Platinum Compounds
Citalopram *see* Antidepressants, SSRI
Clarithromycin *see* Macrolides
Clemastine *see* Antihistamines

Clindamycin
• Muscle Relaxants: clindamycin enhances effects of •non-depolarising muscle relaxants and •suxamethonium
Oestrogens: antibacterials that do not induce liver enzymes possibly reduce contraceptive effect of oestrogens (risk probably small, see BNF section 7.3.1)

Clindamycin *(continued)*
Parasympathomimetics: clindamycin antagonises effects of neostigmine and pyridostigmine
Clobazam *see* Anxiolytics and Hypnotics
Clomethiazole *see* Anxiolytics and Hypnotics
Clomipramine *see* Antidepressants, Tricyclic
Clonazepam *see* Anxiolytics and Hypnotics
Clonidine
ACE Inhibitors: enhanced hypotensive effect when clonidine given with ACE inhibitors; previous treatment with clonidine possibly delays antihypertensive effect of captopril
Adrenergic Neurone Blockers: enhanced hypotensive effect when clonidine given with adrenergic neurone blockers
Alcohol: enhanced hypotensive effect when clonidine given with alcohol
Aldesleukin: enhanced hypotensive effect when clonidine given with aldesleukin
Alpha-blockers: enhanced hypotensive effect when clonidine given with alpha-blockers
Anaesthetics, General: enhanced hypotensive effect when clonidine given with general anaesthetics
Analgesics: hypotensive effect of clonidine antagonised by NSAIDs
Angiotensin-II Receptor Antagonists: enhanced hypotensive effect when clonidine given with angiotensin-II receptor antagonists
• Antidepressants: enhanced hypotensive effect when clonidine given with MAOIs; hypotensive effect of clonidine antagonised by •tricyclics, also increased risk of hypertension on clonidine withdrawal
Antipsychotics: enhanced hypotensive effect when clonidine given with phenothiazines
Anxiolytics and Hypnotics: enhanced hypotensive effect when clonidine given with anxiolytics and hypnotics
• Beta-blockers: increased risk of withdrawal hypertension when clonidine given with •beta-blockers (withdraw beta-blockers several days before slowly withdrawing clonidine)
Calcium-channel Blockers: enhanced hypotensive effect when clonidine given with calcium-channel blockers
Corticosteroids: hypotensive effect of clonidine antagonised by corticosteroids
Diazoxide: enhanced hypotensive effect when clonidine given with diazoxide
Diuretics: enhanced hypotensive effect when clonidine given with diuretics
Dopaminergics: enhanced hypotensive effect when clonidine given with levodopa
Methyldopa: enhanced hypotensive effect when clonidine given with methyldopa
Moxisylyte (thymoxamine): enhanced hypotensive effect when clonidine given with moxisylyte
Moxonidine: enhanced hypotensive effect when clonidine given with moxonidine
Muscle Relaxants: enhanced hypotensive effect when clonidine given with baclofen or tizanidine
Nitrates: enhanced hypotensive effect when clonidine given with nitrates
Oestrogens: hypotensive effect of clonidine antagonised by oestrogens
Prostaglandins: enhanced hypotensive effect when clonidine given with alprostadil
• Sympathomimetics: possible risk of hypertension when clonidine given with adrenaline (epinephrine) or noradrenaline (norepinephrine); serious adverse events reported with concomitant use of clonidine and •methylphenidate (causality not established)

Clonidine
• Sympathomimetics *(continued)*
Vasodilator Antihypertensives: enhanced hypotensive effect when clonidine given with hydralazine, minoxidil or nitroprusside
Clopamide *see* Diuretics
Clopidogrel
Analgesics: increased risk of bleeding when clopidogrel given with NSAIDs or aspirin
• Anticoagulants: manufacturer of clopidogrel advises avoid concomitant use with •warfarin; antiplatelet action of clopidogrel enhances anticoagulant effect of •coumarins and •phenindione; increased risk of bleeding when clopidogrel given with heparins
Dipyridamole: increased risk of bleeding when clopidogrel given with dipyridamole
Iloprost: increased risk of bleeding when clopidogrel given with iloprost
Clotrimazole *see* Antifungals, Imidazole
Clozapine *see* Antipsychotics
Co-amoxiclav *see* Penicillins
Co-beneldopa *see* Levodopa
Co-careldopa *see* Levodopa
Codeine *see* Opioid Analgesics
Co-fluampicil *see* Penicillins
Colchicine
• Antibacterials: increased risk of colchicine toxicity when given with •clarithromycin or •erythromycin
• Ciclosporin: possible increased risk of nephrotoxicity and myotoxicity when colchicine given with •ciclosporin (increased plasma concentration of ciclosporin)
Colestipol
Note. Other drugs should be taken at least 1 hour before or 4-6 hours after colestipol to reduce possible interference with absorption
Bile Acids: colestipol possibly reduces absorption of bile acids
Cardiac Glycosides: colestipol possibly reduces absorption of cardiac glycosides
Diuretics: colestipol reduces absorption of thiazides and related diuretics (give at least 2 hours apart)
Thyroid Hormones: colestipol reduces absorption of thyroid hormones
Colestyramine
Note. Other drugs should be taken at least 1 hour before or 4-6 hours after colestyramine to reduce possible interference with absorption
Analgesics: colestyramine increases the excretion of meloxicam; colestyramine reduces absorption of paracetamol
Antibacterials: colestyramine antagonises effects of oral vancomycin
• Anticoagulants: colestyramine may enhance or reduce anticoagulant effect of •coumarins and •phenindione
Antidiabetics: colestyramine possibly enhances hypoglycaemic effect of acarbose
Antiepileptics: colestyramine possibly reduces absorption of valproate
Bile Acids: colestyramine possibly reduces absorption of bile acids
Cardiac Glycosides: colestyramine possibly reduces absorption of cardiac glycosides
Cytotoxics: colestyramine reduces absorption of mycophenolate mofetil

Colestyramine *(continued)*

Diuretics: colestyramine reduces absorption of thiazides and related diuretics (give at least 2 hours apart)

Leflunomide: colestyramine significantly decreases effect of leflunomide (enhanced elimination)—avoid unless drug elimination desired

Raloxifene: colestyramine reduces absorption of raloxifene (manufacturer of raloxifene advises avoid concomitant administration)

Thyroid Hormones: colestyramine reduces absorption of thyroid hormones

Colistin *see* Polymyxins

Contraceptives, oral *see* Oestrogens and Progestogens

Corticosteroids

Note. Interactions do not generally apply to corticosteroids used for topical action (including inhalation) unless specified

ACE Inhibitors: corticosteroids antagonise hypotensive effect of ACE inhibitors

Adrenergic Neurone Blockers: corticosteroids antagonise hypotensive effect of adrenergic neurone blockers

Alpha-blockers: corticosteroids antagonise hypotensive effect of alpha-blockers

Analgesics: increased risk of gastro-intestinal bleeding and ulceration when corticosteroids given with NSAIDs; increased risk of gastro-intestinal bleeding and ulceration when corticosteroids given with aspirin, also corticosteroids reduce plasma concentration of salicylate

Angiotensin-II Receptor Antagonists: corticosteroids antagonise hypotensive effect of angiotensin-II receptor antagonists

Antacids: absorption of deflazacort reduced by antacids

• Antibacterials: plasma concentration of methylprednisolone possibly increased by clarithromycin; metabolism of corticosteroids possibly inhibited by erythromycin; metabolism of methylprednisolone inhibited by erythromycin; metabolism of corticosteroids accelerated by •rifamycins (reduced effect)

• Anticoagulants: corticosteroids may enhance or reduce anticoagulant effect of •coumarins (high-dose corticosteroids enhance anticoagulant effect)

Antidiabetics: corticosteroids antagonise hypoglycaemic effect of antidiabetics

• Antiepileptics: metabolism of corticosteroids accelerated by •carbamazepine, •phenytoin and •primidone (reduced effect)

• Antifungals: metabolism of corticosteroids possibly inhibited by itraconazole and ketoconazole; plasma concentration of inhaled budesonide and mometasone increased by ketoconazole; metabolism of methylprednisolone inhibited by ketoconazole; increased risk of hypokalaemia when corticosteroids given with •amphotericin—avoid concomitant use unless amphotericin needed to control reactions; plasma concentration of inhaled budesonide increased by itraconazole; metabolism of methylprednisolone possibly inhibited by itraconazole; dexamethasone possibly reduces plasma concentration of caspofungin—consider increasing dose of caspofungin

• Antivirals: dexamethasone possibly reduces plasma concentration of indinavir, lopinavir and saquinavir; plasma concentration of corticosteroids, dexamethasone and prednisolone possibly increased by ritonavir; plasma concentration of inhaled and intranasal budesonide and fluticasone increased by •ritonavir

Aprepitant: metabolism of dexamethasone and methylprednisolone inhibited by aprepitant (reduce dose of dexamethasone and methylprednisolone)

• Barbiturates: metabolism of corticosteroids accelerated by •barbiturates (reduced effect)

Beta-blockers: corticosteroids antagonise hypotensive effect of beta-blockers

Calcium Salts: corticosteroids reduce absorption of calcium salts

Calcium-channel Blockers: corticosteroids antagonise hypotensive effect of calcium-channel blockers

Cardiac Glycosides: increased risk of hypokalaemia when corticosteroids given with cardiac glycosides

• Ciclosporin: high-dose methylprednisolone increases plasma concentration of •ciclosporin (risk of convulsions); plasma concentration of prednisolone increased by ciclosporin

Clonidine: corticosteroids antagonise hypotensive effect of clonidine

• Cytotoxics: increased risk of haematological toxicity when corticosteroids given with •methotrexate

Diazoxide: corticosteroids antagonise hypotensive effect of diazoxide

Diuretics: corticosteroids antagonise diuretic effect of diuretics; increased risk of hypokalaemia when corticosteroids given with acetazolamide, loop diuretics or thiazides and related diuretics

Methyldopa: corticosteroids antagonise hypotensive effect of methyldopa

Mifepristone: effect of corticosteroids (including inhaled corticosteroids) may be reduced for 3–4 days after mifepristone

Moxonidine: corticosteroids antagonise hypotensive effect of moxonidine

Nitrates: corticosteroids antagonise hypotensive effect of nitrates

Oestrogens: plasma concentration of corticosteroids increased by oral contraceptives containing oestrogens

Sodium Benzoate: corticosteroids possibly reduce effects of sodium benzoate

Sodium Phenylbutyrate: corticosteroids possibly reduce effects of sodium phenylbutyrate

Somatropin: corticosteroids may inhibit growth-promoting effect of somatropin

Sympathomimetics: metabolism of dexamethasone accelerated by ephedrine

Sympathomimetics, Beta$_2$: increased risk of hypokalaemia when corticosteroids given with high doses of beta$_2$ sympathomimetics—for CSM advice (hypokalaemia) see p. 167

Theophylline: increased risk of hypokalaemia when corticosteroids given with theophylline

• Vaccines: high doses of corticosteroids impair immune response to •vaccines, avoid concomitant use with live vaccines (see p. 675)

Vasodilator Antihypertensives: corticosteroids antagonise hypotensive effect of hydralazine, minoxidil and nitroprusside

Cortisone *see* Corticosteroids

Co-trimoxazole *see* Trimethoprim and Sulfamethoxazole

Coumarins

Note. Change in patient's clinical condition, particularly associated with liver disease, intercurrent illness, or drug administration, necessitates more frequent testing. Major changes in diet (especially involving salads and vegetables) and in alcohol consumption may also affect anticoagulant control

- • Alcohol: anticoagulant control with coumarins may be affected by major changes in consumption of •alcohol
- Allopurinol: anticoagulant effect of coumarins possibly enhanced by allopurinol
- • Anabolic Steroids: anticoagulant effect of coumarins enhanced by •anabolic steroids
- • Analgesics: anticoagulant effect of coumarins possibly enhanced by •NSAIDs, •celecoxib, •dextropropoxyphene, •diflunisal, •etodolac, •etoricoxib, •flurbiprofen, •ibuprofen, •lumiracoxib, •mefenamic acid, •meloxicam, •parecoxib, •piroxicam and •sulindac; anticoagulant effect of coumarins possibly enhanced by •diclofenac, also increased risk of haemorrhage with intravenous diclofenac (avoid concomitant use); increased risk of bleeding when coumarins given with •ketorolac (avoid concomitant use); anticoagulant effect of coumarins enhanced by •tramadol; increased risk of bleeding when coumarins given with •aspirin (due to antiplatelet effect); anticoagulant effect of coumarins possibly enhanced by prolonged regular use of paracetamol
- • Anti-arrhythmics: metabolism of coumarins inhibited by •amiodarone (enhanced anticoagulant effect); anticoagulant effect of coumarins enhanced by •propafenone; anticoagulant effect of coumarins possibly enhanced by •quinidine
- • Antibacterials: experience in anticoagulant clinics suggests that INR possibly altered when coumarins are given with •neomycin (given for local action on gut); anticoagulant effect of coumarins enhanced by •chloramphenicol, •ciprofloxacin, •clarithromycin, •erythromycin, •metronidazole, •nalidixic acid, •norfloxacin, •ofloxacin and •sulphonamides; anticoagulant effect of coumarins possibly enhanced by •aztreonam, •cephalosporins, levofloxacin, •macrolides, •tetracyclines and trimethoprim; studies have failed to demonstrate an interaction with coumarins, but common experience in anticoagulant clinics is that INR can be altered by a course of broad-spectrum penicillins such as ampicillin; metabolism of coumarins accelerated by •rifamycins (reduced anticoagulant effect)
- • Antidepressants: anticoagulant effect of warfarin possibly enhanced by •venlafaxine; anticoagulant effect of coumarins possibly enhanced by •SSRIs; anticoagulant effect of coumarins reduced by •St John's wort (avoid concomitant use); anticoagulant effect of warfarin enhanced by mirtazapine; anticoagulant effect of coumarins may be enhanced or reduced by •tricyclics
- • Antidiabetics: coumarins possibly enhance hypoglycaemic effect of •sulphonylureas, also possible changes to anticoagulant effect
- • Antiepileptics: metabolism of coumarins accelerated by •carbamazepine and •primidone (reduced anticoagulant effect); metabolism of coumarins accelerated by •phenytoin (possibility of reduced anticoagulant effect, but enhancement also reported); anticoagulant effect of coumarins possibly enhanced by valproate

Coumarins

- • Antifungals: anticoagulant effect of coumarins enhanced by •fluconazole, •itraconazole, •ketoconazole and •voriconazole; anticoagulant effect of coumarins enhanced by •miconazole (miconazole oral gel and possibly vaginal formulations absorbed); anticoagulant effect of coumarins reduced by •griseofulvin
- Antimalarials: isolated reports that anticoagulant effect of warfarin may be enhanced by proguanil
- • Antivirals: anticoagulant effect of coumarins may be enhanced or reduced by amprenavir; anticoagulant effect of warfarin may be enhanced or reduced by atazanavir, •nevirapine and •ritonavir; anticoagulant effect of coumarins possibly enhanced by •ritonavir; anticoagulant effect of warfarin possibly enhanced by saquinavir
- Anxiolytics and Hypnotics: anticoagulant effect of coumarins may transiently be enhanced by chloral and triclofos
- Aprepitant: anticoagulant effect of warfarin possibly reduced by aprepitant
- • Barbiturates: metabolism of coumarins accelerated by •barbiturates (reduced anticoagulant effect)
- Bosentan: monitoring anticoagulant effect of coumarins recommended by manufacturer of bosentan
- • Clopidogrel: anticoagulant effect of coumarins enhanced due to antiplatelet action of •clopidogrel; avoidance of warfarin advised by manufacturer of •clopidogrel
- • Corticosteroids: anticoagulant effect of coumarins may be enhanced or reduced by •corticosteroids (high-dose corticosteroids enhance anticoagulant effect)
- • Cranberry Juice: anticoagulant effect of coumarins possibly enhanced by •cranberry juice—avoid concomitant use
- • Cytotoxics: anticoagulant effect of coumarins possibly enhanced by •etoposide, •fluorouracil and •ifosfamide; anticoagulant effect of coumarins possibly reduced by •azathioprine, •mercaptopurine and •mitotane; increased risk of bleeding when coumarins given with •erlotinib; replacement of warfarin with a heparin advised by manufacturer of imatinib (possibility of enhanced warfarin effect)
- • Dipyridamole: anticoagulant effect of coumarins enhanced due to antiplatelet action of •dipyridamole
- • Disulfiram: anticoagulant effect of coumarins enhanced by •disulfiram
- • Dopaminergics: anticoagulant effect of warfarin enhanced by •entacapone
- • Enteral Foods: anticoagulant effect of coumarins antagonised by vitamin K (present in some •enteral feeds)
- • Hormone Antagonists: anticoagulant effect of coumarins possibly enhanced by bicalutamide and •toremifene; metabolism of coumarins inhibited by •danazol (enhanced anticoagulant effect); anticoagulant effect of coumarins enhanced by •flutamide and •tamoxifen
- Iloprost: anticoagulant effect of coumarins possibly enhanced by iloprost

Appendix 1

Coumarins *(continued)*
Leflunomide: anticoagulant effect of warfarin possibly enhanced by leflunomide
Leukotriene Antagonists: anticoagulant effect of warfarin enhanced by zafirlukast
• Levamisole: anticoagulant effect of warfarin possibly enhanced by •levamisole
• Lipid-regulating Drugs: anticoagulant effect of coumarins may be enhanced or reduced by •colestyramine; anticoagulant effect of warfarin may be transiently reduced by atorvastatin; anticoagulant effect of coumarins enhanced by •fibrates, •fluvastatin and simvastatin; anticoagulant effect of coumarins possibly enhanced by •rosuvastatin; anticoagulant effect of warfarin possibly enhanced by ezetimibe
• Oestrogens: anticoagulant effect of coumarins antagonised by •oestrogens
Orlistat: monitoring anticoagulant effect of coumarins recommended by manufacturer of orlistat
• Progestogens: anticoagulant effect of coumarins antagonised by •progestogens
Raloxifene: anticoagulant effect of coumarins antagonised by raloxifene
• Retinoids: anticoagulant effect of coumarins possibly reduced by •acitretin
Sibutramine: increased risk of bleeding when anticoagulants given with sibutramine
• Sulfinpyrazone: anticoagulant effect of coumarins enhanced by •sulfinpyrazone
• Sympathomimetics: anticoagulant effect of coumarins possibly enhanced by •methylphenidate
Terpene Mixture: anticoagulant effect of coumarins possibly reduced by Rowachol®
• Testolactone: anticoagulant effect of coumarins enhanced by •testolactone
• Testosterone: anticoagulant effect of coumarins enhanced by •testosterone
• Thyroid Hormones: anticoagulant effect of coumarins enhanced by •thyroid hormones
Ubidecarenone: anticoagulant effect of warfarin may be enhanced or reduced by ubidecarenone
• Ulcer-healing Drugs: metabolism of coumarins inhibited by •cimetidine (enhanced anticoagulant effect); anticoagulant effect of coumarins possibly enhanced by •esomeprazole and •omeprazole; absorption of coumarins possibly reduced by •sucralfate (reduced anticoagulant effect)
Vaccines: anticoagulant effect of warfarin possibly enhanced by influenza vaccine
• Vitamins: anticoagulant effect of coumarins antagonised by •vitamin K

Cranberry Juice
• Anticoagulants: cranberry juice possibly enhances anticoagulant effect of •coumarins—avoid concomitant use

Cyclizine *see* Antihistamines
Cyclopenthiazide *see* Diuretics
Cyclopentolate *see* Antimuscarinics

Cyclophosphamide
Antiepileptics: cytotoxics possibly reduce absorption of phenytoin
Antifungals: side-effects of cyclophosphamide possibly increased by itraconazole
• Antipsychotics: avoid concomitant use of cytotoxics with •clozapine (increased risk of agranulocytosis)
Cardiac Glycosides: cytotoxics reduce absorption of digoxin tablets

Cyclophosphamide *(continued)*
• Cytotoxics: increased toxicity when high-dose cyclophosphamide given with •pentostatin—avoid concomitant use
Muscle Relaxants: cyclophosphamide enhances effects of suxamethonium

Cycloserine
• Alcohol: increased risk of convulsions when cycloserine given with •alcohol
Antibacterials: increased risk of CNS toxicity when cycloserine given with isoniazid
Oestrogens: antibacterials that do not induce liver enzymes possibly reduce contraceptive effect of oestrogens (risk probably small, see BNF section 7.3.1)

Cyproheptadine *see* Antihistamines

Cytarabine
Antiepileptics: cytotoxics possibly reduce absorption of phenytoin
Antifungals: cytarabine possibly reduces plasma concentration of flucytosine
• Antipsychotics: avoid concomitant use of cytotoxics with •clozapine (increased risk of agranulocytosis)
Cardiac Glycosides: cytotoxics reduce absorption of digoxin tablets
Cytotoxics: intracellular concentration of cytarabine increased by fludarabine

Cytotoxics *see* individual drugs

Dairy Products
Antibacterials: dairy products reduces absorption of ciprofloxacin and norfloxacin; dairy products reduces absorption of tetracyclines (except doxycycline and minocycline)

Dalteparin *see* Heparins

Danazol
• Anticoagulants: danazol inhibits metabolism of •coumarins (enhanced anticoagulant effect)
• Antiepileptics: danazol inhibits metabolism of •carbamazepine (increased risk of toxicity)
• Ciclosporin: danazol inhibits metabolism of •ciclosporin (increased plasma concentration)
• Lipid-regulating Drugs: possible increased risk of myopathy when danazol given with •simvastatin
Tacrolimus: danazol possibly increases plasma concentration of tacrolimus

Dantrolene *see* Muscle Relaxants

Dapsone
Antibacterials: plasma concentration of dapsone reduced by rifamycins; plasma concentration of both drugs may increase when dapsone given with trimethoprim
Antivirals: plasma concentration of dapsone possibly increased by amprenavir
Oestrogens: antibacterials that do not induce liver enzymes possibly reduce contraceptive effect of oestrogens (risk probably small, see BNF section 7.3.1)
Probenecid: excretion of dapsone reduced by probenecid (increased risk of side-effects)

Darbepoetin *see* Epoetin
Deflazacort *see* Corticosteroids
Demeclocycline *see* Tetracyclines

Desferrioxamine
Antipsychotics: avoidance of desferrioxamine advised by manufacturer of levomepromazine (methotrimeprazine); manufacturer of desferrioxamine advises avoid concomitant use with prochlorperazine

Desflurane *see* Anaesthetics, General
Desloratadine *see* Antihistamines

Desmopressin
- Analgesics: effects of desmopressin enhanced by indometacin
- Loperamide: plasma concentration of *oral* desmopressin increased by loperamide

Desogestrel *see* Progestogens
Dexamethasone *see* Corticosteroids
Dexamfetamine *see* Sympathomimetics
Dexibuprofen *see* NSAIDs
Dexketoprofen *see* NSAIDs
Dextromethorphan *see* Opioid Analgesics
Dextropropoxyphene *see* Opioid Analgesics
Diamorphine *see* Opioid Analgesics
Diazepam *see* Anxiolytics and Hypnotics

Diazoxide
- ACE Inhibitors: enhanced hypotensive effect when diazoxide given with ACE inhibitors
- Adrenergic Neurone Blockers: enhanced hypotensive effect when diazoxide given with adrenergic neurone blockers
- Alcohol: enhanced hypotensive effect when diazoxide given with alcohol
- Aldesleukin: enhanced hypotensive effect when diazoxide given with aldesleukin
- Alpha-blockers: enhanced hypotensive effect when diazoxide given with alpha-blockers
- Anaesthetics, General: enhanced hypotensive effect when diazoxide given with general anaesthetics
- Analgesics: hypotensive effect of diazoxide antagonised by NSAIDs
- Angiotensin-II Receptor Antagonists: enhanced hypotensive effect when diazoxide given with angiotensin-II receptor antagonists
- Antidepressants: enhanced hypotensive effect when diazoxide given with MAOIs or tricyclic-related antidepressants
- Antidiabetics: diazoxide antagonises hypoglycaemic effect of antidiabetics
- Antiepileptics: diazoxide reduces plasma concentration of phenytoin, also effect of diazoxide may be reduced
- Antipsychotics: enhanced hypotensive effect when diazoxide given with phenothiazines
- Anxiolytics and Hypnotics: enhanced hypotensive effect when diazoxide given with anxiolytics and hypnotics
- Beta-blockers: enhanced hypotensive effect when diazoxide given with beta-blockers
- Calcium-channel Blockers: enhanced hypotensive effect when diazoxide given with calcium-channel blockers
- Clonidine: enhanced hypotensive effect when diazoxide given with clonidine
- Corticosteroids: hypotensive effect of diazoxide antagonised by corticosteroids
- Diuretics: enhanced hypotensive effect when diazoxide given with diuretics
- Dopaminergics: enhanced hypotensive effect when diazoxide given with levodopa
- Methyldopa: enhanced hypotensive effect when diazoxide given with methyldopa
- Moxisylyte (thymoxamine): enhanced hypotensive effect when diazoxide given with moxisylyte
- Moxonidine: enhanced hypotensive effect when diazoxide given with moxonidine
- Muscle Relaxants: enhanced hypotensive effect when diazoxide given with baclofen or tizanidine
- Nitrates: enhanced hypotensive effect when diazoxide given with nitrates

Diazoxide *(continued)*
- Oestrogens: hypotensive effect of diazoxide antagonised by oestrogens
- Prostaglandins: enhanced hypotensive effect when diazoxide given with alprostadil
- Vasodilator Antihypertensives: enhanced hypotensive effect when diazoxide given with hydralazine, minoxidil or nitroprusside

Diclofenac *see* NSAIDs
Dicycloverine (dicyclomine) *see* Antimuscarinics

Didanosine
Note. Antacids in tablet formulation may affect absorption of other drugs
- Allopurinol: plasma concentration of didanosine possibly increased by allopurinol
- • Antivirals: plasma concentration of didanosine possibly increased by ganciclovir; increased risk of side-effects when didanosine given with •stavudine; plasma concentration of didanosine increased by •tenofovir (increased risk of toxicity)—avoid concomitant use; plasma concentration of didanosine reduced by •tipranavir
- • Cytotoxics: increased risk of toxicity when didanosine given with •hydroxycarbamide—avoid concomitant use

Diflunisal *see* NSAIDs
Digitoxin *see* Cardiac Glycosides
Digoxin *see* Cardiac Glycosides
Dihydrocodeine *see* Opioid Analgesics
Diltiazem *see* Calcium-channel Blockers

Dimercaprol
- • Iron: avoid concomitant use of dimercaprol with •iron

Dinoprostone *see* Prostaglandins
Diphenoxylate *see* Opioid Analgesics
Diphenylpyraline *see* Antihistamines
Dipipanone *see* Opioid Analgesics
Dipivefrine *see* Sympathomimetics

Dipyridamole
- Antacids: absorption of dipyridamole possibly reduced by antacids
- • Anti-arrhythmics: dipyridamole enhances and extends the effects of •adenosine (important risk of toxicity)
- • Anticoagulants: antiplatelet action of dipyridamole enhances anticoagulant effect of •coumarins and •phenindione; dipyridamole enhances anticoagulant effect of heparins
- Clopidogrel: increased risk of bleeding when dipyridamole given with clopidogrel
- Cytotoxics: dipyridamole possibly reduces effects of fludarabine

Disodium Etidronate *see* Bisphosphonates
Disodium Pamidronate *see* Bisphosphonates

Disopyramide
- Anaesthetics, Local: increased myocardial depression when anti-arrhythmics given with bupivacaine, levobupivacaine or prilocaine
- • Anti-arrhythmics: increased myocardial depression when anti-arrhythmics given with other •anti-arrhythmics; increased risk of ventricular arrhythmias when disopyramide given with •amiodarone—avoid concomitant use
- • Antibacterials: plasma concentration of disopyramide possibly increased by •clarithromycin (increased risk of toxicity); plasma concentration of disopyramide increased by •erythromycin (increased risk of toxicity); increased risk of ventricular arrhythmias when disopyramide given with •moxifloxacin or •quinupristin/dalfopristin—avoid concomitant use; metabolism of disopyramide accelerated by •rifamycins (reduced plasma concentration)

Disopyramide *(continued)*
- • Antidepressants: increased risk of ventricular arrhythmias when disopyramide given with •tricyclics
- Antidiabetics: disopyramide possibly enhances hypoglycaemic effect of gliclazide, insulin and metformin
- Antiepileptics: plasma concentration of disopyramide reduced by phenytoin; metabolism of disopyramide accelerated by primidone (reduced plasma concentration)
- • Antihistamines: increased risk of ventricular arrhythmias when disopyramide given with •mizolastine—avoid concomitant use
- • Antimalarials: avoidance of disopyramide advised by manufacturer of •artemether/lumefantrine (risk of ventricular arrhythmias)
- Antimuscarinics: increased risk of antimuscarinic side-effects when disopyramide given with antimuscarinics
- • Antipsychotics: increased risk of ventricular arrhythmias when anti-arrhythmics that prolong the QT interval given with •antipsychotics that prolong the QT interval; increased risk of ventricular arrhythmias when disopyramide given with •amisulpride, •pimozide or •sertindole—avoid concomitant use; increased risk of ventricular arrhythmias when disopyramide given with •phenothiazines
- • Antivirals: plasma concentration of disopyramide possibly increased by •ritonavir (increased risk of toxicity)
- Barbiturates: metabolism of disopyramide accelerated by barbiturates (reduced plasma concentration)
- • Beta-blockers: increased myocardial depression when anti-arrhythmics given with •beta-blockers; increased risk of ventricular arrhythmias when disopyramide given with •sotalol—avoid concomitant use
- • Calcium-channel Blockers: increased risk of myocardial depression and asystole when disopyramide given with •verapamil
- • Diuretics: increased cardiac toxicity with disopyramide if hypokalaemia occurs with •acetazolamide, •loop diuretics or •thiazides and related diuretics
- • Dolasetron: increased risk of ventricular arrhythmias when disopyramide given with •dolasetron—avoid concomitant use
- $5HT_3$ Antagonists: caution with anti-arrhythmics advised by manufacturer of tropisetron (risk of ventricular arrhythmias)
- • Ivabradine: increased risk of ventricular arrhythmias when disopyramide given with •ivabradine
- Nitrates: disopyramide reduces effects of sublingual tablets of nitrates (failure to dissolve under tongue owing to dry mouth)

Distigmine *see* Parasympathomimetics

Disulfiram
- Alcohol: disulfiram reaction when disulfiram given with alcohol (see BNF section 4.10)
- Antibacterials: psychotic reaction reported when disulfiram given with metronidazole
- • Anticoagulants: disulfiram enhances anticoagulant effect of •coumarins
- Antidepressants: increased disulfiram reaction with alcohol reported with concomitant amitriptyline; disulfiram inhibits metabolism of tricyclics (increased plasma concentration)
- • Antiepileptics: disulfiram inhibits metabolism of •phenytoin (increased risk of toxicity)

Disulfiram *(continued)*
- Anxiolytics and Hypnotics: disulfiram increases risk of temazepam toxicity; disulfiram inhibits metabolism of benzodiazepines (increased sedative effects)
- • Paraldehyde: risk of toxicity when disulfiram given with •paraldehyde
- Theophylline: disulfiram inhibits metabolism of theophylline (increased risk of toxicity)

Diuretics

Note. Since systemic absorption may follow topical application of brinzolamide to the eye, the possibility of interactions should be borne in mind

Note. Since systemic absorption may follow topical application of dorzolamide to the eye, the possibility of interactions should be borne in mind
- • ACE Inhibitors: enhanced hypotensive effect when diuretics given with •ACE inhibitors; increased risk of severe hyperkalaemia when potassium-sparing diuretics and aldosterone antagonists given with •ACE inhibitors (monitor potassium concentration with low-dose spironolactone in heart failure)
- Adrenergic Neurone Blockers: enhanced hypotensive effect when diuretics given with adrenergic neurone blockers
- Alcohol: enhanced hypotensive effect when diuretics given with alcohol
- Aldesleukin: enhanced hypotensive effect when diuretics given with aldesleukin
- Allopurinol: increased risk of hypersensitivity when thiazides and related diuretics given with allopurinol especially in renal impairment
- • Alpha-blockers: enhanced hypotensive effect when diuretics given with •alpha-blockers, also increased risk of first-dose hypotension with post-synaptic alpha-blockers such as prazosin
- Anaesthetics, General: enhanced hypotensive effect when diuretics given with general anaesthetics
- • Analgesics: possibly increased risk of hyperkalaemia when potassium-sparing diuretics and aldosterone antagonists given with NSAIDs; diuretics increase risk of nephrotoxicity of NSAIDs, also antagonism of diuretic effect; effects of diuretics antagonised by indometacin and ketorolac; increased risk of hyperkalaemia when potassium-sparing diuretics and aldosterone antagonists given with indometacin; occasional reports of reduced renal function when triamterene given with •indometacin—avoid concomitant use; increased risk of toxicity when carbonic anhydrase inhibitors given with high-dose aspirin; diuretic effect of spironolactone antagonised by aspirin
- • Angiotensin-II Receptor Antagonists: enhanced hypotensive effect when diuretics given with •angiotensin-II receptor antagonists; increased risk of hyperkalaemia when potassium-sparing diuretics and aldosterone antagonists given with •angiotensin-II receptor antagonists
- • Anti-arrhythmics: plasma concentration of eplerenone increased by amiodarone (reduce dose of eplerenone); hypokalaemia caused by acetazolamide, loop diuretics or thiazides and related diuretics increases cardiac toxicity with amiodarone; hypokalaemia caused by acetazolamide, loop diuretics or thiazides and related diuretics increases cardiac toxicity with •disopyramide; hypokalaemia caused by acetazolamide, loop diuretics or thiazides and related diuretics increases cardiac toxicity with •flecainide; hypokalaemia caused by acetazol-

Diuretics

- Anti-arrhythmics *(continued)* amide, loop diuretics or thiazides and related diuretics antagonises action of •lidocaine (lignocaine); hypokalaemia caused by acetazolamide, loop diuretics or thiazides and related diuretics antagonises action of •mexiletine; hypokalaemia caused by loop diuretics or thiazides and related diuretics increases cardiac toxicity with •quinidine; acetazolamide possibly reduces excretion of •quinidine (increased plasma concentration), also cardiotoxicity of quinidine increased in hypokalaemia
- Antibacterials: plasma concentration of eplerenone increased by •clarithromycin and •telithromycin—avoid concomitant use; plasma concentration of eplerenone increased by erythromycin (reduce dose of eplerenone); plasma concentration of eplerenone reduced by •rifampicin—avoid concomitant use; avoidance of diuretics advised by manufacturer of lymecycline; increased risk of otoxicity when loop diuretics given with •aminoglycosides, •polymyxins or •vancomycin; acetazolamide antagonises effects of •methenamine; increased risk of hyperkalaemia when eplerenone given with trimethoprim
- Antidepressants: possible increased risk of hypokalaemia when loop diuretics or thiazides and related diuretics given with reboxetine; enhanced hypotensive effect when diuretics given with MAOIs; plasma concentration of eplerenone reduced by •St John's wort—avoid concomitant use; increased risk of postural hypotension when diuretics given with tricyclics

Antidiabetics: loop diuretics and thiazides and related diuretics antagonise hypoglycaemic effect of antidiabetics; increased risk of hyponatraemia when thiazides and related diuretics plus potassium-sparing diuretic given with chlorpropamide; increased risk of hyponatraemia when potassium-sparing diuretics and aldosterone antagonists plus thiazide given with chlorpropamide

- Antiepileptics: acetazolamide increases plasma concentration of •carbamazepine; plasma concentration of eplerenone reduced by •carbamazepine and •phenytoin—avoid concomitant use; increased risk of hyponatraemia when diuretics given with carbamazepine; increased risk of osteomalacia when carbonic anhydrase inhibitors given with phenytoin or primidone; acetazolamide possibly reduces plasma concentration of primidone
- Antifungals: plasma concentration of eplerenone increased by •itraconazole and •ketoconazole—avoid concomitant use; increased risk of hypokalaemia when loop diuretics or thiazides and related diuretics given with amphotericin; hydrochlorothiazide increases plasma concentration of fluconazole; plasma concentration of eplerenone increased by fluconazole (reduce dose of eplerenone)
- Antipsychotics: hypokalaemia caused by diuretics increases risk of ventricular arrhythmias with •amisulpride or •sertindole; enhanced hypotensive effect when diuretics given with phenothiazines; hypokalaemia caused by diuretics increases risk of ventricular arrhythmias with •pimozide (avoid concomitant use)

Diuretics *(continued)*

- Antivirals: plasma concentration of eplerenone increased by •nelfinavir and •ritonavir—avoid concomitant use; plasma concentration of eplerenone increased by saquinavir (reduce dose of eplerenone)

Anxiolytics and Hypnotics: enhanced hypotensive effect when diuretics given with anxiolytics and hypnotics; administration of parenteral furosemide (frusemide) with chloral or triclofos may displace thyroid hormone from binding sites

- Barbiturates: plasma concentration of eplerenone reduced by •phenobarbital—avoid concomitant use; increased risk of osteomalacia when carbonic anhydrase inhibitors given with phenobarbital
- Beta-blockers: enhanced hypotensive effect when diuretics given with beta-blockers; hypokalaemia caused by loop diuretics or thiazides and related diuretics increases risk of ventricular arrhythmias with •sotalol

Calcium Salts: increased risk of hypercalcaemia when thiazides and related diuretics given with calcium salts

Calcium-channel Blockers: enhanced hypotensive effect when diuretics given with calcium-channel blockers; plasma concentration of eplerenone increased by diltiazem and verapamil (reduce dose of eplerenone)

- Cardiac Glycosides: hypokalaemia caused by acetazolamide, loop diuretics or thiazides and related diuretics increases cardiac toxicity with •cardiac glycosides; spironolactone possibly affects plasma concentration of digitoxin; spironolactone increases plasma concentration of •digoxin
- Ciclosporin: increased risk of nephrotoxicity and possibly hypermagnesaemia when thiazides and related diuretics given with ciclosporin; increased risk of hyperkalaemia when potassium-sparing diuretics and aldosterone antagonists given with •ciclosporin

Clonidine: enhanced hypotensive effect when diuretics given with clonidine

Corticosteroids: diuretic effect of diuretics antagonised by corticosteroids; increased risk of hypokalaemia when acetazolamide, loop diuretics or thiazides and related diuretics given with corticosteroids

Cytotoxics: avoidance of spironolactone advised by manufacturer of mitotane (antagonism of effect); increased risk of nephrotoxicity and ototoxicity when diuretics given with platinum compounds

Diazoxide: enhanced hypotensive effect when diuretics given with diazoxide

Diuretics: increased risk of hypokalaemia when loop diuretics or thiazides and related diuretics given with acetazolamide; profound diuresis possible when metolazone given with furosemide (frusemide); increased risk of hypokalaemia when thiazides and related diuretics given with loop diuretics

Dopaminergics: enhanced hypotensive effect when diuretics given with levodopa

Hormone Antagonists: increased risk of hypercalcaemia when thiazides and related diuretics given with toremifene; increased risk of hyperkalaemia when potassium-sparing diuretics and aldosterone antagonists given with trilostane

Diuretics *(continued)*

Lipid-regulating Drugs: absorption of thiazides and related diuretics reduced by colestipol and colestyramine (give at least 2 hours apart)

• Lithium: loop diuretics and thiazides and related diuretics reduce excretion of •lithium (increased plasma concentration and risk of toxicity)—loop diuretics safer than thiazides; potassium-sparing diuretics and aldosterone antagonists reduce excretion of •lithium (increased plasma concentration and risk of toxicity); acetazolamide increases the excretion of •lithium

Methyldopa: enhanced hypotensive effect when diuretics given with methyldopa

Moxisylyte (thymoxamine): enhanced hypotensive effect when diuretics given with moxisylyte

Moxonidine: enhanced hypotensive effect when diuretics given with moxonidine

Muscle Relaxants: enhanced hypotensive effect when diuretics given with baclofen or tizanidine

Nitrates: enhanced hypotensive effect when diuretics given with nitrates

Oestrogens: diuretic effect of diuretics antagonised by oestrogens

• Potassium Salts: increased risk of hyperkalaemia when potassium-sparing diuretics and aldosterone antagonists given with •potassium salts

Progestogens: risk of hyperkalaemia when potassium-sparing diuretics and aldosterone antagonists given with drospirenone (monitor serum potassium during first cycle)

Prostaglandins: enhanced hypotensive effect when diuretics given with alprostadil

Sympathomimetics, Beta$_2$: increased risk of hypokalaemia when acetazolamide, loop diuretics or thiazides and related diuretics given with high doses of beta$_2$ sympathomimetics—for CSM advice (hypokalaemia) see p. 167

• Tacrolimus: increased risk of hyperkalaemia when potassium-sparing diuretics and aldosterone antagonists given with •tacrolimus

Theophylline: increased risk of hypokalaemia when acetazolamide, loop diuretics or thiazides and related diuretics given with theophylline

Vasodilator Antihypertensives: enhanced hypotensive effect when diuretics given with hydralazine, minoxidil or nitroprusside

Vitamins: increased risk of hypercalcaemia when thiazides and related diuretics given with vitamin D

Diuretics, Loop *see* Diuretics

Diuretics, Potassium-sparing and Aldosterone Antagonists *see* Diuretics

Diuretics, Thiazide and related *see* Diuretics

Dobutamine *see* Sympathomimetics

Docetaxel

Antibacterials: *in vitro* studies suggest a possible interaction between docetaxel and erythromycin (consult docetaxel product literature)

Antiepileptics: cytotoxics possibly reduce absorption of phenytoin

Antifungals: *in vitro* studies suggest a possible interaction between docetaxel and ketoconazole (consult docetaxel product literature)

• Antipsychotics: avoid concomitant use of cytotoxics with •clozapine (increased risk of agranulocytosis)

Docetaxel *(continued)*

Cardiac Glycosides: cytotoxics reduce absorption of digoxin tablets

Ciclosporin: *in vitro* studies suggest a possible interaction between docetaxel and ciclosporin (consult docetaxel product literature)

Dolasetron

• Anti-arrhythmics: increased risk of ventricular arrhythmias when dolasetron given with •amiodarone, •disopyramide, •flecainide, •lidocaine (lignocaine), •mexiletine, •procainamide or •propafenone—avoid concomitant use

• Beta-blockers: increased risk of ventricular arrhythmias when dolasetron given with •sotalol—avoid concomitant use

Domperidone

Analgesics: effects of domperidone on gastro-intestinal activity antagonised by opioid analgesics

Antimuscarinics: effects of domperidone on gastro-intestinal activity antagonised by antimuscarinics

Dopaminergics: increased risk of extrapyramidal side-effects when domperidone given with amantadine; domperidone possibly antagonises hypoprolactinaemic effects of bromocriptine and cabergoline

Donepezil *see* Parasympathomimetics

Dopamine *see* Sympathomimetics

Dopaminergics *see* Amantadine, Apomorphine, Bromocriptine, Cabergoline, Entacapone, Levodopa, Lisuride, Pergolide, Pramipexole, Quinagolide, Ropinirole, Rasagiline, Selegiline, and Tolcapone e

Dopexamine *see* Sympathomimetics

Dorzolamide *see* Diuretics

Dosulepin (dothiepin) *see* Antidepressants, Tricyclic

Doxapram

Antidepressants: effects of doxapram enhanced by MAOIs

Sympathomimetics: increased risk of hypertension when doxapram given with sympathomimetics

Theophylline: increased CNS stimulation when doxapram given with theophylline

Doxazosin *see* Alpha-blockers

Doxepin *see* Antidepressants, Tricyclic

Doxorubicin

Antiepileptics: cytotoxics possibly reduce absorption of phenytoin

• Antipsychotics: avoid concomitant use of cytotoxics with •clozapine (increased risk of agranulocytosis)

Antivirals: doxorubicin possibly inhibits effects of stavudine

Cardiac Glycosides: cytotoxics reduce absorption of digoxin tablets

• Ciclosporin: increased risk of neurotoxicity when doxorubicin given with •ciclosporin

Doxycycline *see* Tetracyclines

Drospirenone *see* Progestogens

Drotrecogin Alfa

• Anticoagulants: manufacturer of drotrecogin alfa advises avoid concomitant use with high doses of •heparin—consult product literature

Duloxetine

Analgesics: possible increased serotonergic effects when duloxetine given with pethidine or tramadol

• Antibacterials: metabolism of duloxetine inhibited by •ciprofloxacin—avoid concomitant use

Duloxetine *(continued)*
- • Antidepressants: metabolism of duloxetine inhibited by •fluvoxamine—avoid concomitant use; possible increased serotonergic effects when duloxetine given with SSRIs, St John's wort, amitriptyline, clomipramine, •moclobemide, tryptophan or venlafaxine; duloxetine should not be started until 2 weeks after stopping •MAOIs, also MAOIs should not be started until at least 5 days after stopping duloxetine; after stopping SSRI-related antidepressants do not start •moclobemide for at least 1 week
- • Antimalarials: avoidance of antidepressants advised by manufacturer of •artemether/lumefantrine
- $5HT_1$ Agonists: possible increased serotonergic effects when duloxetine given with $5HT_1$ agonists
- • Sibutramine: increased risk of CNS toxicity when SSRI-related antidepressants given with •sibutramine (manufacturer of sibutramine advises avoid concomitant use)

Dutasteride
- Calcium-channel Blockers: plasma concentration of dutasteride increased by diltiazem and verapamil

Dydrogesterone *see* Progestogens

Edrophonium *see* Parasympathomimetics

Efalizumab
- • Vaccines: discontinue efalizumab 8 weeks before and until 2 weeks after vaccination with live or live-attenuated •vaccines

Efavirenz
- Analgesics: efavirenz reduces plasma concentration of methadone
- Antibacterials: increased risk of rash when efavirenz given with clarithromycin; efavirenz reduces plasma concentration of rifabutin—increase dose of rifabutin; plasma concentration of efavirenz reduced by rifampicin—increase dose of efavirenz
- • Antidepressants: efavirenz reduces plasma concentration of sertraline; plasma concentration of efavirenz reduced by •St John's wort—avoid concomitant use
- Antiepileptics: plasma concentration of both drugs reduced when efavirenz given with carbamazepine
- • Antifungals: efavirenz reduces plasma concentration of •voriconazole, also plasma concentration of efavirenz increased (avoid concomitant use); efavirenz possibly reduces plasma concentration of caspofungin—consider increasing dose of caspofungin
- • Antipsychotics: efavirenz possibly reduces plasma concentration of •aripiprazole—increase dose of aripiprazole; efavirenz possibly increases plasma concentration of •pimozide (increased risk of ventricular arrhythmias—avoid concomitant use)
- Antivirals: efavirenz reduces plasma concentration of amprenavir, indinavir and lopinavir; efavirenz reduces plasma concentration of atazanavir—increase dose of atazanavir; plasma concentration of efavirenz reduced by nevirapine; toxicity of efavirenz increased by ritonavir, monitor liver function tests; efavirenz significantly reduces plasma concentration of saquinavir
- • Anxiolytics and Hypnotics: increased risk of prolonged sedation when efavirenz given with •midazolam—avoid concomitant use

Efavirenz *(continued)*
- • Ergot Alkaloids: increased risk of ergotism when efavirenz given with •ergot alkaloids—avoid concomitant use
- Grapefruit Juice: plasma concentration of efavirenz possibly increased by grapefruit juice
- Lipid-regulating Drugs: efavirenz reduces plasma concentration of atorvastatin, pravastatin and simvastatin
- Oestrogens: efavirenz possibly reduces contraceptive effect of oestrogens

Eletriptan *see* $5HT_1$ Agonists

Emtricitabine
- Antivirals: manufacturer of emtricitabine advises avoid concomitant use with lamivudine

Enalapril *see* ACE Inhibitors

Enoxaparin *see* Heparins

Enoximone *see* Phosphodiesterase Inhibitors

Entacapone
- • Anticoagulants: entacapone enhances anticoagulant effect of •warfarin
- • Antidepressants: manufacturer of entacapone advises caution with maprotiline, moclobemide, paroxetine, tricyclics and venlafaxine; avoid concomitant use of entacapone with non-selective •MAOIs
- Dopaminergics: entacapone possibly enhances effects of apomorphine; entacapone possibly reduces plasma concentration of rasagiline; manufacturer of entacapone advises max. dose of 10 mg selegiline if used concomitantly
- Iron: absorption of entacapone reduced by *oral* iron
- Memantine: effects of dopaminergics possibly enhanced by memantine
- Methyldopa: entacapone possibly enhances effects of methyldopa; antiparkinsonian effect of dopaminergics antagonised by methyldopa
- Sympathomimetics: entacapone possibly enhances effects of adrenaline (epinephrine), dobutamine, dopamine and noradrenaline (norepinephrine)

Enteral Foods
- • Anticoagulants: the presence of vitamin K in some enteral feeds can antagonise the anticoagulant effect of •coumarins and •phenindione
- Antiepileptics: enteral feeds possibly reduce absorption of phenytoin

Ephedrine *see* Sympathomimetics

Epinephrine (adrenaline) *see* Sympathomimetics

Epirubicin
- Antiepileptics: cytotoxics possibly reduce absorption of phenytoin
- • Antipsychotics: avoid concomitant use of cytotoxics with •clozapine (increased risk of agranulocytosis)
- Cardiac Glycosides: cytotoxics reduce absorption of digoxin tablets
- • Ulcer-healing Drugs: plasma concentration of epirubicin increased by •cimetidine

Eplerenone *see* Diuretics

Epoetin
- ACE Inhibitors: antagonism of hypotensive effect and increased risk of hyperkalaemia when epoetin given with ACE inhibitors
- Angiotensin-II Receptor Antagonists: antagonism of hypotensive effect and increased risk of hyperkalaemia when epoetin given with angiotensin-II receptor antagonists

Eprosartan *see* Angiotensin-II Receptor Antagonists

Eptifibatide
- Iloprost: increased risk of bleeding when eptifibatide given with iloprost

Appendix 1

Ergometrine *see* Ergot Alkaloids
Ergot Alkaloids
Anaesthetics, General: effects of ergometrine on the parturient uterus reduced by halothane
• Antibacterials: increased risk of ergotism when ergotamine and methysergide given with •macrolides or •telithromycin—avoid concomitant use; avoidance of ergotamine and methysergide advised by manufacturer of •quinupristin/dalfopristin; increased risk of ergotism when ergotamine and methysergide given with tetracyclines
Antidepressants: possible risk of hypertension when ergotamine and methysergide given with reboxetine
• Antifungals: increased risk of ergotism when ergotamine and methysergide given with •imidazoles or •triazoles—avoid concomitant use
• Antivirals: increased risk of ergotism when ergotamine and methysergide given with •amprenavir, •indinavir, •nelfinavir, •ritonavir or •saquinavir—avoid concomitant use; plasma concentration of ergot alkaloids possibly increased by •atazanavir—avoid concomitant use; increased risk of ergotism when ergot alkaloids given with •efavirenz—avoid concomitant use
Beta-blockers: increased peripheral vasoconstriction when ergotamine and methysergide given with beta-blockers
• $5HT_1$ Agonists: increased risk of vasospasm when ergotamine and methysergide given with •almotriptan, •rizatriptan, •sumatriptan or •zolmitriptan (avoid ergotamine and methysergide for 6 hours after almotriptan, rizatriptan, sumatriptan or zolmitriptan, avoid almotriptan, rizatriptan, sumatriptan or zolmitriptan for 24 hours after ergotamine and methysergide); increased risk of vasospasm when ergotamine and methysergide given with •eletriptan or •frovatriptan (avoid ergotamine and methysergide for 24 hours after eletriptan or frovatriptan, avoid eletriptan or frovatriptan for 24 hours after ergotamine and methysergide)
Sympathomimetics: increased risk of ergotism when ergotamine and methysergide given with sympathomimetics
• Ulcer-healing Drugs: increased risk of ergotism when ergotamine and methysergide given with •cimetidine—avoid concomitant use

Ergotamine and Methysergide *see* Ergot Alkaloids
Erlotinib
• Analgesics: increased risk of bleeding when erlotinib given with •NSAIDs
Antibacterials: metabolism of erlotinib accelerated by rifampicin (reduced plasma concentration)
• Anticoagulants: increased risk of bleeding when erlotinib given with •coumarins
Antiepileptics: cytotoxics possibly reduce absorption of phenytoin
Antifungals: metabolism of erlotinib inhibited by ketoconazole (increased plasma concentration)
• Antipsychotics: avoid concomitant use of cytotoxics with •clozapine (increased risk of agranulocytosis)
Cardiac Glycosides: cytotoxics reduce absorption of digoxin tablets

Ertapenem
Antiepileptics: ertapenem possibly reduces plasma concentration of valproate

Ertapenem *(continued)*
Oestrogens: antibacterials that do not induce liver enzymes possibly reduce contraceptive effect of oestrogens (risk probably small, see BNF section 7.3.1)

Erythromycin *see* Macrolides
Erythropoietin *see* Epoetin
Escitalopram *see* Antidepressants, SSRI
Esmolol *see* Beta-blockers
Esomeprazole *see* Proton Pump Inhibitors
Estradiol *see* Oestrogens
Estriol *see* Oestrogens
Estrone *see* Oestrogens
Estropipate *see* Oestrogens
Etanercept
• Anakinra: increased risk of side-effects when etanercept given with •anakinra—avoid concomitant use
• Vaccines: avoid concomitant use of etanercept with live •vaccines (see p. 675)

Ethinylestradiol *see* Oestrogens
Ethosuximide
• Antibacterials: metabolism of ethosuximide inhibited by •isoniazid (increased plasma concentration and risk of toxicity)
• Antidepressants: anticonvulsant effect of antiepileptics possibly antagonised by MAOIs and •tricyclic-related antidepressants (convulsive threshold lowered); anticonvulsant effect of antiepileptics antagonised by •SSRIs and •tricyclics (convulsive threshold lowered)
• Antiepileptics: plasma concentration of ethosuximide possibly reduced by carbamazepine and primidone; plasma concentration of ethosuximide possibly reduced by •phenytoin, also plasma concentration of phenytoin possibly increased; plasma concentration of ethosuximide possibly increased by valproate
• Antimalarials: possible increased risk of convulsions when antiepileptics given with chloroquine and hydroxychloroquine; anticonvulsant effect of antiepileptics antagonised by •mefloquine
• Antipsychotics: anticonvulsant effect of ethosuximide antagonised by •antipsychotics (convulsive threshold lowered)
Barbiturates: plasma concentration of ethosuximide possibly reduced by phenobarbital

Etodolac *see* NSAIDs
Etomidate *see* Anaesthetics, General
Etonogestrel *see* Progestogens
Etoposide
• Anticoagulants: etoposide possibly enhances anticoagulant effect of •coumarins
Antiepileptics: plasma concentration of etoposide possibly reduced by phenytoin; cytotoxics possibly reduce absorption of phenytoin
• Antipsychotics: avoid concomitant use of cytotoxics with •clozapine (increased risk of agranulocytosis)
Barbiturates: plasma concentration of etoposide possibly reduced by phenobarbital
Cardiac Glycosides: cytotoxics reduce absorption of digoxin tablets
Ciclosporin: plasma concentration of etoposide possibly increased by ciclosporin (increased risk of toxicity)

Etoricoxib *see* NSAIDs
Etynodiol *see* Progestogens
Exemestane
Antibacterials: plasma concentration of exemestane possibly reduced by rifampicin

Ezetimibe
Anticoagulants: ezetimibe possibly enhances anticoagulant effect of warfarin
• Ciclosporin: plasma concentration of both drugs may increase when ezetimibe given with •ciclosporin
• Lipid-regulating Drugs: manufacturer of ezetimibe advises avoid concomitant use with •fibrates

Famciclovir
Probenecid: excretion of famciclovir possibly reduced by probenecid (increased plasma concentration)

Famotidine *see* Histamine H_2-antagonists
Felodipine *see* Calcium-channel Blockers
Fenbufen *see* NSAIDs
Fenofibrate *see* Fibrates
Fenoprofen *see* NSAIDs
Fenoterol *see* Sympathomimetics, $Beta_2$
Fentanyl *see* Opioid Analgesics
Ferrous Salts *see* Iron
Fexofenadine *see* Antihistamines

Fibrates
• Anticoagulants: fibrates enhance anticoagulant effect of •coumarins and •phenindione
• Antidiabetics: gemfibrozil increases plasma concentration of •rosiglitazone (consider reducing dose of rosiglitazone); fibrates may improve glucose tolerance and have an additive effect with insulin or sulphonylureas; gemfibrozil possibly enhances hypoglycaemic effect of nateglinide; increased risk of severe hypoglycaemia when gemfibrozil given with •repaglinide—avoid concomitant use
Ciclosporin: increased risk of renal impairment when fenofibrate given with ciclosporin
• Cytotoxics: gemfibrozil increases plasma concentration of •bexarotene—avoid concomitant use
• Lipid-regulating Drugs: avoidance of fibrates advised by manufacturer of •ezetimibe; increased risk of myopathy when fibrates given with •statins; increased risk of myopathy when gemfibrozil given with •statins (preferably avoid concomitant use)

Filgrastim
Note. Pegfilgrastim interactions as for filgrastim
Cytotoxics: neutropenia possibly exacerbated when filgrastim given with fluorouracil

Flavoxate *see* Antimuscarinics

Flecainide
Anaesthetics, Local: increased myocardial depression when anti-arrhythmics given with bupivacaine, levobupivacaine or prilocaine
• Anti-arrhythmics: increased myocardial depression when anti-arrhythmics given with other •anti-arrhythmics; plasma concentration of flecainide increased by •amiodarone (halve dose of flecainide)
• Antidepressants: plasma concentration of flecainide increased by fluoxetine; increased risk of ventricular arrhythmias when flecainide given with •tricyclics
• Antihistamines: increased risk of ventricular arrhythmias when flecainide given with •mizolastine—avoid concomitant use
• Antimalarials: avoidance of flecainide advised by manufacturer of •artemether/lumefantrine (risk of ventricular arrhythmias); plasma concentration of flecainide increased by •quinine
• Antipsychotics: increased risk of ventricular arrhythmias when anti-arrhythmics that prolong the QT interval given with •antipsychotics that prolong the QT interval; increased risk of arrhythmias when flecainide given with •clozapine
• Antivirals: plasma concentration of flecainide possibly increased by •amprenavir (increased risk of ventricular arrhythmias—avoid concomitant use); plasma concentration of flecainide increased by •ritonavir (increased risk of ventricular arrhythmias—avoid concomitant use)
• Beta-blockers: increased risk of myocardial depression and bradycardia when flecainide given with •beta-blockers; increased myocardial depression when anti-arrhythmics given with •beta-blockers
• Calcium-channel Blockers: increased risk of myocardial depression and asystole when flecainide given with •verapamil
• Diuretics: increased cardiac toxicity with flecainide if hypokalaemia occurs with •acetazolamide, •loop diuretics or •thiazides and related diuretics
• Dolasetron: increased risk of ventricular arrhythmias when flecainide given with •dolasetron—avoid concomitant use
$5HT_3$ Antagonists: caution with anti-arrhythmics advised by manufacturer of tropisetron (risk of ventricular arrhythmias)
Ulcer-healing Drugs: metabolism of flecainide inhibited by cimetidine (increased plasma concentration)

Flucloxacillin *see* Penicillins
Fluconazole *see* Antifungals, Triazole

Flucytosine
Antifungals: renal excretion of flucytosine decreased and cellular uptake increased by amphotericin (toxicity possibly increased)
Cytotoxics: plasma concentration of flucytosine possibly reduced by cytarabine

Fludarabine
Antiepileptics: cytotoxics possibly reduce absorption of phenytoin
• Antipsychotics: avoid concomitant use of cytotoxics with •clozapine (increased risk of agranulocytosis)
Cardiac Glycosides: cytotoxics reduce absorption of digoxin tablets
• Cytotoxics: fludarabine increases intracellular concentration of cytarabine; increased pulmonary toxicity when fludarabine given with •pentostatin (unacceptably high incidence of fatalities)
Dipyridamole: effects of fludarabine possibly reduced by dipyridamole

Fludrocortisone *see* Corticosteroids
Flunisolide *see* Corticosteroids

Fluorides
Calcium Salts: absorption of fluorides reduced by calcium salts

Fluorouracil
Note. Capecitabine is a prodrug of fluorouracil
Note. Tegafur is a prodrug of fluorouracil
• Allopurinol: manufacturer of capecitabine advises avoid concomitant use with •allopurinol
Antibacterials: metabolism of fluorouracil inhibited by metronidazole (increased toxicity)
• Anticoagulants: fluorouracil possibly enhances anticoagulant effect of •coumarins
Antiepileptics: cytotoxics possibly reduce absorption of phenytoin; fluorouracil possibly inhibits metabolism of phenytoin (increased risk of toxicity)

Fluorouracil *(continued)*
- • Antipsychotics: avoid concomitant use of cytotoxics with •clozapine (increased risk of agranulocytosis)
- Cardiac Glycosides: cytotoxics reduce absorption of digoxin tablets
- Filgrastim: neutropenia possibly exacerbated when fluorouracil given with filgrastim
- • Temoporfin: increased skin photosensitivity when topical fluorouracil used with •temoporfin
- Ulcer-healing Drugs: metabolism of fluorouracil inhibited by cimetidine (increased plasma concentration)

Fluoxetine *see* Antidepressants, SSRI
Flupentixol *see* Antipsychotics
Fluphenazine *see* Antipsychotics
Flurazepam *see* Anxiolytics and Hypnotics
Flurbiprofen *see* NSAIDs
Flutamide
- • Anticoagulants: flutamide enhances anticoagulant effect of •coumarins

Fluticasone *see* Corticosteroids
Fluvastatin *see* Statins
Fluvoxamine *see* Antidepressants, SSRI
Folates
- Aminosalicylates: absorption of folic acid possibly reduced by sulfasalazine
- Antiepileptics: folates possibly reduce plasma concentration of phenytoin and primidone
- Barbiturates: folates possibly reduce plasma concentration of phenobarbital

Folic Acid *see* Folates
Folinic Acid *see* Folates
Formoterol (eformoterol) *see* Sympathomimetics, Beta$_2$
Fosamprenavir *see* Amprenavir
Foscarnet
- Antivirals: avoidance of foscarnet advised by manufacturer of lamivudine

Fosinopril *see* ACE Inhibitors
Fosphenytoin *see* Phenytoin
Framycetin *see* Aminoglycosides
Frovatriptan *see* 5HT$_1$ Agonists
Furosemide (frusemide) *see* Diuretics
Fusidic Acid
- Antivirals: plasma concentration of both drugs may increase when fusidic acid given with ritonavir
- Lipid-regulating Drugs: possible increased risk of myopathy when fusidic acid given with atorvastatin or simvastatin
- Oestrogens: antibacterials that do not induce liver enzymes possibly reduce contraceptive effect of oestrogens (risk probably small, see BNF section 7.3.1)

Gabapentin
- Antacids: absorption of gabapentin reduced by antacids
- • Antidepressants: anticonvulsant effect of antiepileptics possibly antagonised by MAOIs and •tricyclic-related antidepressants (convulsive threshold lowered); anticonvulsant effect of antiepileptics antagonised by •SSRIs and •tricyclics (convulsive threshold lowered)
- • Antimalarials: possible increased risk of convulsions when antiepileptics given with chloroquine and hydroxychloroquine; anticonvulsant effect of antiepileptics antagonised by •mefloquine

Galantamine *see* Parasympathomimetics
Ganciclovir

Note. Increased risk of myelosuppression with other myelosuppressive drugs—consult product literature
Note. Valganciclovir interactions as for ganciclovir

- • Antibacterials: increased risk of convulsions when ganciclovir given with •imipenem with cilastatin
- • Antivirals: ganciclovir possibly increases plasma concentration of didanosine; avoidance of intravenous ganciclovir advised by manufacturer of lamivudine; profound myelosuppression when ganciclovir given with •zidovudine (if possible avoid concomitant administration, particularly during initial ganciclovir therapy)
- Cytotoxics: plasma concentration of ganciclovir possibly increased by mycophenolate mofetil, also plasma concentration of inactive metabolite of mycophenolate mofetil possibly increased
- Probenecid: excretion of ganciclovir reduced by probenecid (increased plasma concentration and risk of toxicity)

Gemeprost *see* Prostaglandins
Gemfibrozil *see* Fibrates
Gentamicin *see* Aminoglycosides
Gestodene *see* Progestogens
Gestrinone
- Antibacterials: metabolism of gestrinone accelerated by rifampicin (reduced plasma concentration)
- Antiepileptics: metabolism of gestrinone accelerated by carbamazepine, phenytoin and primidone (reduced plasma concentration)
- Barbiturates: metabolism of gestrinone accelerated by barbiturates (reduced plasma concentration)

Glibenclamide *see* Antidiabetics
Gliclazide *see* Antidiabetics
Glimepiride *see* Antidiabetics
Glipizide *see* Antidiabetics
Gliquidone *see* Antidiabetics
Glyceryl Trinitrate *see* Nitrates
Glycopyrronium *see* Antimuscarinics
Grapefruit Juice
- • Antimalarials: grapefruit juice possibly inhibits metabolism of •artemether/lumefantrine (avoid concomitant use)
- Antivirals: grapefruit juice possibly increases plasma concentration of efavirenz
- Anxiolytics and Hypnotics: grapefruit juice increases plasma concentration of buspirone
- Calcium-channel Blockers: grapefruit juice increases plasma concentration of felodipine, isradipine, lacidipine, lercanidipine, nicardipine, nifedipine, nimodipine, nisoldipine and verapamil
- • Ciclosporin: grapefruit juice increases plasma concentration of •ciclosporin (increased risk of toxicity)
- Ivabradine: grapefruit juice increases plasma concentration of ivabradine
- • Lipid-regulating Drugs: grapefruit juice increases plasma concentration of •simvastatin—avoid concomitant use
- Sildenafil: grapefruit juice possibly increases plasma concentration of sildenafil
- • Sirolimus: grapefruit juice increases plasma concentration of •sirolimus—avoid concomitant use
- • Tacrolimus: grapefruit juice increases plasma concentration of •tacrolimus
- Tadalafil: grapefruit juice possibly increases plasma concentration of tadalafil

Grapefruit Juice *(continued)*
- • Vardenafil: grapefruit juice possibly increases plasma concentration of •vardenafil—avoid concomitant use

Griseofulvin
- Alcohol: griseofulvin possibly enhances effects of alcohol
- • Anticoagulants: griseofulvin reduces anticoagulant effect of •coumarins
- Antiepileptics: absorption of griseofulvin reduced by primidone (reduced effect)
- Barbiturates: absorption of griseofulvin reduced by phenobarbital (reduced effect)
- Ciclosporin: griseofulvin possibly reduces plasma concentration of ciclosporin
- • Oestrogens: griseofulvin accelerates metabolism of •oestrogens (reduced contraceptive effect—see BNF section 7.3.1)
- • Progestogens: griseofulvin accelerates metabolism of •progestogens (reduced contraceptive effect—see BNF section 7.3.1)

Guanethidine *see* Adrenergic Neurone Blockers
Haloperidol *see* Antipsychotics
Halothane *see* Anaesthetics, General
Heparin *see* Heparins

Heparins
- ACE Inhibitors: increased risk of hyperkalaemia when heparins given with ACE inhibitors
- • Analgesics: possible increased risk of bleeding when heparins given with NSAIDs; increased risk of haemorrhage when heparins given with intravenous •diclofenac (avoid concomitant use, including low-dose heparin); increased risk of haemorrhage when heparins given with •ketorolac (avoid concomitant use, including low-dose heparin); anticoagulant effect of heparins enhanced by •aspirin
- Angiotensin-II Receptor Antagonists: increased risk of hyperkalaemia when heparin given with angiotensin-II receptor antagonists
- Clopidogrel: increased risk of bleeding when heparins given with clopidogrel
- Dipyridamole: anticoagulant effect of heparins enhanced by dipyridamole
- • Drotrecogin Alfa: avoidance of concomitant use of high doses of heparin with drotrecogin alfa advised by manufacturer of •drotrecogin alfa—consult product literature
- Iloprost: anticoagulant effect of heparins possibly enhanced by iloprost
- • Nitrates: anticoagulant effect of heparins reduced by infusion of •glyceryl trinitrate
- Sibutramine: increased risk of bleeding when anticoagulants given with sibutramine

Histamine H_2-antagonists
- • Alpha-blockers: cimetidine and ranitidine antagonise effects of •tolazoline
- Analgesics: cimetidine inhibits metabolism of opioid analgesics (increased plasma concentration)
- • Anti-arrhythmics: cimetidine increases plasma concentration of amiodarone, •procainamide, •propafenone and •quinidine; cimetidine inhibits metabolism of flecainide (increased plasma concentration); cimetidine increases plasma concentration of •lidocaine (lignocaine) (increased risk of toxicity)
- Antibacterials: histamine H_2-antagonists reduce absorption of cefpodoxime; cimetidine increases plasma concentration of erythromycin (increased risk of toxicity, including deafness); cimetidine inhibits metabolism of metronidazole (increased plasma concentration); metabolism of cimetidine accelerated by

Histamine H_2-antagonists
- Antibacterials *(continued)* rifampicin (reduced plasma concentration); ranitidine bismuth citrate reduces absorption of tetracyclines
- • Anticoagulants: cimetidine inhibits metabolism of •coumarins (enhanced anticoagulant effect)
- Antidepressants: cimetidine increases plasma concentration of citalopram, escitalopram, mirtazapine and sertraline; cimetidine inhibits metabolism of amitriptyline, doxepin, imipramine and nortriptyline (increased plasma concentration); cimetidine increases plasma concentration of moclobemide (halve dose of moclobemide); cimetidine possibly increases plasma concentration of tricyclics
- Antidiabetics: cimetidine reduces excretion of metformin (increased plasma concentration); cimetidine enhances hypoglycaemic effect of sulphonylureas
- • Antiepileptics: cimetidine inhibits metabolism of •carbamazepine, •phenytoin and •valproate (increased plasma concentration)
- Antifungals: histamine H_2-antagonists reduce absorption of itraconazole and ketoconazole; cimetidine increases plasma concentration of terbinafine
- Antihistamines: manufacturer of loratadine advises cimetidine possibly increases plasma concentration of loratadine
- • Antimalarials: avoidance of cimetidine advised by manufacturer of •artemether/lumefantrine; cimetidine inhibits metabolism of chloroquine and hydroxychloroquine and quinine (increased plasma concentration)
- • Antipsychotics: cimetidine possibly enhances effects of antipsychotics, chlorpromazine and clozapine; increased risk of ventricular arrhythmias when cimetidine given with •sertindole—avoid concomitant use
- Antivirals: plasma concentration of cimetidine possibly increased by amprenavir; histamine H_2-antagonists possibly reduce plasma concentration of atazanavir
- Anxiolytics and Hypnotics: cimetidine inhibits metabolism of benzodiazepines, clomethiazole and zaleplon (increased plasma concentration)
- Beta-blockers: cimetidine increases plasma concentration of labetalol, metoprolol and propranolol
- Calcium-channel Blockers: cimetidine possibly inhibits metabolism of calcium-channel blockers (increased plasma concentration)
- • Ciclosporin: cimetidine possibly increases plasma concentration of •ciclosporin
- • Cilostazol: cimetidine possibly increases plasma concentration of •cilostazol—avoid concomitant use
- • Cytotoxics: cimetidine increases plasma concentration of •epirubicin; cimetidine inhibits metabolism of fluorouracil (increased plasma concentration)
- Dopaminergics: cimetidine reduces excretion of pramipexole (increased plasma concentration)
- • Ergot Alkaloids: increased risk of ergotism when cimetidine given with •ergotamine and methysergide—avoid concomitant use
- Hormone Antagonists: absorption of cimetidine possibly delayed by octreotide
- $5HT_1$ Agonists: cimetidine inhibits metabolism of zolmitriptan (reduce dose of zolmitriptan)

Histamine H_2-antagonists *(continued)*
Mebendazole: cimetidine possibly inhibits metabolism of mebendazole (increased plasma concentration)
Sildenafil: cimetidine increases plasma concentration of sildenafil (reduce initial dose of sildenafil)
• Theophylline: cimetidine inhibits metabolism of •theophylline (increased plasma concentration)
Thyroid Hormones: cimetidine reduces absorption of levothyroxine (thyroxine)

Homatropine *see* Antimuscarinics

Hormone Antagonists *see* Bicalutamide, Danazol, Dutasteride, Exemestane, Flutamide, Gestrinone, Lanreotide, Octreotide, Tamoxifen, Toremifene, and Trilostane

$5HT_1$ Agonists
• Antibacterials: plasma concentration of eletriptan increased by •clarithromycin and •erythromycin (risk of toxicity)—avoid concomitant use; metabolism of zolmitriptan possibly inhibited by quinolones (reduce dose of zolmitriptan)
• Antidepressants: increased risk of CNS toxicity when sumatriptan given with •citalopram, •escitalopram, •fluoxetine, •fluvoxamine or •paroxetine; metabolism of frovatriptan inhibited by fluvoxamine; metabolism of zolmitriptan possibly inhibited by fluvoxamine (reduce dose of zolmitriptan); increased risk of CNS toxicity when sumatriptan given with •sertraline (manufacturer of sertraline advises avoid concomitant use); possible increased serotonergic effects when $5HT_1$ agonists given with duloxetine; risk of CNS toxicity when rizatriptan or sumatriptan given with •MAOIs (avoid rizatriptan or sumatriptan for 2 weeks after MAOIs); increased risk of CNS toxicity when zolmitriptan given with •MAOIs; risk of CNS toxicity when rizatriptan or sumatriptan given with •moclobemide (avoid rizatriptan or sumatriptan for 2 weeks after moclobemide); risk of CNS toxicity when zolmitriptan given with •moclobemide (reduce dose of zolmitriptan); possible increased serotonergic effects when frovatriptan given with SSRIs; increased serotonergic effects when $5HT_1$ agonists given with •St John's wort—avoid concomitant use
• Antifungals: plasma concentration of eletriptan increased by •itraconazole and •ketoconazole (risk of toxicity)—avoid concomitant use; plasma concentration of almotriptan increased by ketoconazole (increased risk of toxicity)
• Antivirals: plasma concentration of eletriptan increased by •indinavir, •nelfinavir and •ritonavir (risk of toxicity)—avoid concomitant use
Beta-blockers: plasma concentration of rizatriptan possibly increased by propranolol (reduce dose of rizatriptan)
• Ergot Alkaloids: increased risk of vasospasm when eletriptan or frovatriptan given with •ergotamine and methysergide (avoid ergotamine and methysergide for 24 hours after eletriptan or frovatriptan, avoid eletriptan or frovatriptan for 24 hours after ergotamine and methysergide); increased risk of vasospasm when almotriptan, rizatriptan, sumatriptan or zolmitriptan given with •ergotamine and methysergide (avoid ergotamine and methysergide for 6 hours after almotriptan, rizatriptan, sumatriptan or zolmitriptan, avoid almotriptan, rizatriptan, sumatriptan or zolmitriptan for 24 hours after ergotamine and methysergide)
Ulcer-healing Drugs: metabolism of zolmitriptan inhibited by cimetidine (reduce dose of zolmitriptan)

$5HT_3$ Antagonists *see* Ondansetron and Tropisetron

Hydralazine *see* Vasodilator Antihypertensives

Hydrochlorothiazide *see* Diuretics

Hydrocortisone *see* Corticosteroids

Hydroflumethiazide *see* Diuretics

Hydromorphone *see* Opioid Analgesics

Hydrotalcite *see* Antacids

Hydroxocobalamin
Antibacterials: response to hydroxocobalamin reduced by chloramphenicol

Hydroxycarbamide
Antiepileptics: cytotoxics possibly reduce absorption of phenytoin
• Antipsychotics: avoid concomitant use of cytotoxics with •clozapine (increased risk of agranulocytosis)
• Antivirals: increased risk of toxicity when hydroxycarbamide given with •didanosine and •stavudine—avoid concomitant use
Cardiac Glycosides: cytotoxics reduce absorption of digoxin tablets

Hydroxychloroquine *see* Chloroquine and Hydroxychloroquine

Hydroxyzine *see* Antihistamines

Hyoscine *see* Antimuscarinics

Ibandronic Acid *see* Bisphosphonates

Ibuprofen *see* NSAIDs

Ifosfamide
• Anticoagulants: ifosfamide possibly enhances anticoagulant effect of •coumarins
Antiepileptics: cytotoxics possibly reduce absorption of phenytoin
• Antipsychotics: avoid concomitant use of cytotoxics with •clozapine (increased risk of agranulocytosis)
Cardiac Glycosides: cytotoxics reduce absorption of digoxin tablets

Iloprost
Analgesics: increased risk of bleeding when iloprost given with NSAIDs or aspirin
Anticoagulants: iloprost possibly enhances anticoagulant effect of coumarins and heparins; increased risk of bleeding when iloprost given with phenindione
Clopidogrel: increased risk of bleeding when iloprost given with clopidogrel
Eptifibatide: increased risk of bleeding when iloprost given with eptifibatide
Tirofiban: increased risk of bleeding when iloprost given with tirofiban

Imatinib
• Antibacterials: plasma concentration of imatinib reduced by •rifampicin—avoid concomitant use
Anticoagulants: manufacturer of imatinib advises replacement of warfarin with a heparin (possibility of enhanced warfarin effect)
• Antiepileptics: cytotoxics possibly reduce absorption of phenytoin; plasma concentration of imatinib reduced by •phenytoin—avoid concomitant use
Antifungals: plasma concentration of imatinib increased by ketoconazole
• Antipsychotics: avoid concomitant use of cytotoxics with •clozapine (increased risk of agranulocytosis)

Imatinib *(continued)*
Cardiac Glycosides: cytotoxics reduce absorption of digoxin tablets
Lipid-regulating Drugs: imatinib increases plasma concentration of simvastatin
Imidapril *see* ACE Inhibitors
Imipenem with Cilastatin
• Antivirals: increased risk of convulsions when imipenem with cilastatin given with •ganciclovir
Oestrogens: antibacterials that do not induce liver enzymes possibly reduce contraceptive effect of oestrogens (risk probably small, see BNF section 7.3.1)
Imipramine *see* Antidepressants, Tricyclic
Immunoglobulins
Note. For advice on immunoglobulins and live virus vaccines, see under Normal Immunoglobulin, p. 699
Immunosuppressants (antiproliferative) *see* Azathioprine and Mycophenolate Mofetil
Indapamide *see* Diuretics
Indinavir
• Antibacterials: indinavir increases plasma concentration of •rifabutin, also plasma concentration of indinavir decreased (reduce dose of rifabutin and increase dose of indinavir); metabolism of indinavir accelerated by •rifampicin (reduced plasma concentration—avoid concomitant use)
• Antidepressants: plasma concentration of indinavir reduced by •St John's wort—avoid concomitant use
• Antiepileptics: plasma concentration of indinavir possibly reduced by carbamazepine, phenytoin and •primidone
• Antifungals: metabolism of indinavir inhibited by ketoconazole; plasma concentration of indinavir increased by •itraconazole (consider reducing dose of indinavir)
• Antimalarials: avoidance of indinavir advised by manufacturer of •artemether/lumefantrine
Antimuscarinics: avoidance of indinavir advised by manufacturer of tolterodine
• Antipsychotics: indinavir possibly inhibits metabolism of •aripiprazole (reduce dose of aripiprazole); indinavir possibly increases plasma concentration of •pimozide (increased risk of ventricular arrhythmias—avoid concomitant use); indinavir increases plasma concentration of •sertindole (increased risk of ventricular arrhythmias—avoid concomitant use)
• Antivirals: avoid concomitant use of indinavir with •atazanavir; plasma concentration of indinavir reduced by efavirenz and nevirapine; combination of indinavir with nelfinavir may increase plasma concentration of either drug (or both); plasma concentration of indinavir increased by ritonavir; indinavir increases plasma concentration of saquinavir
• Anxiolytics and Hypnotics: increased risk of prolonged sedation when indinavir given with •alprazolam or •midazolam—avoid concomitant use
Atovaquone: plasma concentration of indinavir possibly reduced by atovaquone
• Barbiturates: plasma concentration of indinavir possibly reduced by •barbiturates
• Cilostazol: indinavir possibly increases plasma concentration of •cilostazol—avoid concomitant use
Corticosteroids: plasma concentration of indinavir possibly reduced by dexamethasone

Indinavir *(continued)*
• Ergot Alkaloids: increased risk of ergotism when indinavir given with •ergotamine and methysergide—avoid concomitant use
• $5HT_1$ Agonists: indinavir increases plasma concentration of •eletriptan (risk of toxicity)—avoid concomitant use
• Lipid-regulating Drugs: possible increased risk of myopathy when indinavir given with atorvastatin; increased risk of myopathy when indinavir given with •simvastatin (avoid concomitant use)
Sildenafil: indinavir increases plasma concentration of sildenafil—reduce initial dose of sildenafil
• Vardenafil: indinavir increases plasma concentration of •vardenafil—avoid concomitant use
Indometacin *see* NSAIDs
Indoramin *see* Alpha-blockers
Infliximab
• Anakinra: avoid concomitant use of infliximab with •anakinra
• Vaccines: avoid concomitant use of infliximab with live •vaccines (see p. 675)
Influenza Vaccine *see* Vaccines
Insulin *see* Antidiabetics
Interferon Alfa *see* Interferons
Interferon Gamma *see* Interferons
Interferons
Note. Peginterferon alfa interactions as for interferon alfa
Theophylline: interferon alfa inhibits metabolism of theophylline (increased plasma concentration)
Vaccines: manufacturer of interferon gamma advises avoid concomitant use with vaccines
Ipratropium *see* Antimuscarinics
Irbesartan *see* Angiotensin-II Receptor Antagonists
Irinotecan
Antiepileptics: cytotoxics possibly reduce absorption of phenytoin
• Antipsychotics: avoid concomitant use of cytotoxics with •clozapine (increased risk of agranulocytosis)
• Antivirals: metabolism of irinotecan possibly inhibited by •atazanavir (increased risk of toxicity)
Cardiac Glycosides: cytotoxics reduce absorption of digoxin tablets
Iron
Antacids: absorption of *oral* iron reduced by oral magnesium salts (as magnesium trisilicate)
Antibacterials: *oral* iron reduces absorption of ciprofloxacin, levofloxacin, moxifloxacin, norfloxacin and ofloxacin; *oral* iron reduces absorption of tetracyclines, also absorption of *oral* iron reduced by tetracyclines
Bisphosphonates: *oral* iron reduces absorption of bisphosphonates
Calcium Salts: absorption of *oral* iron reduced by calcium salts
• Dimercaprol: avoid concomitant use of iron with •dimercaprol
Dopaminergics: *oral* iron reduces absorption of entacapone; *oral* iron possibly reduces absorption of levodopa
Methyldopa: *oral* iron antagonises hypotensive effect of methyldopa
Penicillamine: *oral* iron reduces absorption of penicillamine
Thyroid Hormones: *oral* iron reduces absorption of levothyroxine (thyroxine) (give at least 2 hours apart)
Trientine: absorption of *oral* iron reduced by trientine

Iron *(continued)*
Zinc: *oral* iron reduces absorption of zinc, also absorption of *oral* iron reduced by zinc
Isocarboxazid *see* MAOIs
Isoflurane *see* Anaesthetics, General
Isometheptene *see* Sympathomimetics
Isoniazid
Anaesthetics, General: hepatotoxicity of isoniazid possibly potentiated by general anaesthetics
Antacids: absorption of isoniazid reduced by antacids
Antibacterials: increased risk of CNS toxicity when isoniazid given with cycloserine
• Antiepileptics: isoniazid increases plasma concentration of •carbamazepine (also possibly increased isoniazid hepatotoxicity); isoniazid inhibits metabolism of •ethosuximide (increased plasma concentration and risk of toxicity); isoniazid inhibits metabolism of •phenytoin (increased plasma concentration)
Antifungals: isoniazid possibly reduces plasma concentration of ketoconazole
Anxiolytics and Hypnotics: isoniazid inhibits the metabolism of diazepam
Oestrogens: antibacterials that do not induce liver enzymes possibly reduce contraceptive effect of oestrogens (risk probably small, see BNF section 7.3.1)
Theophylline: isoniazid possibly increases plasma concentration of theophylline
Isosorbide Dinitrate *see* Nitrates
Isosorbide Mononitrate *see* Nitrates
Isotretinoin *see* Retinoids
Isradipine *see* Calcium-channel Blockers
Itraconazole *see* Antifungals, Triazole
Ivabradine
• Anti-arrhythmics: increased risk of ventricular arrhythmias when ivabradine given with •amiodarone, •disopyramide or •quinidine
• Antibacterials: plasma concentration of ivabradine possibly increased by •clarithromycin and •telithromycin—avoid concomitant use; increased risk of ventricular arrhythmias when ivabradine given with •erythromycin—avoid concomitant use
Antidepressants: plasma concentration of ivabradine reduced by St John's wort—avoid concomitant use
• Antifungals: plasma concentration of ivabradine increased by •ketoconazole—avoid concomitant use; plasma concentration of ivabradine increased by fluconazole—reduce initial dose of ivabradine; plasma concentration of ivabradine possibly increased by •itraconazole—avoid concomitant use
• Antimalarials: increased risk of ventricular arrhythmias when ivabradine given with •mefloquine
• Antipsychotics: increased risk of ventricular arrhythmias when ivabradine given with •pimozide or •sertindole
• Antivirals: plasma concentration of ivabradine possibly increased by •nelfinavir and •ritonavir—avoid concomitant use
• Beta-blockers: increased risk of ventricular arrhythmias when ivabradine given with •sotalol
• Calcium-channel Blockers: plasma concentration of ivabradine increased by •diltiazem and •verapamil—avoid concomitant use
Grapefruit Juice: plasma concentration of ivabradine increased by grapefruit juice

Ivabradine *(continued)*
• Pentamidine Isetionate: increased risk of ventricular arrhythmias when ivabradine given with •pentamidine isetionate
Kaolin
Analgesics: kaolin possibly reduces absorption of aspirin
Anti-arrhythmics: kaolin possibly reduces absorption of quinidine
Antibacterials: kaolin possibly reduces absorption of tetracyclines
Antimalarials: kaolin reduces absorption of chloroquine and hydroxychloroquine
Antipsychotics: kaolin possibly reduces absorption of phenothiazines
Ketamine *see* Anaesthetics, General
Ketoconazole *see* Antifungals, Imidazole
Ketoprofen *see* NSAIDs
Ketorolac *see* NSAIDs
Ketotifen *see* Antihistamines
Labetalol *see* Beta-blockers
Lacidipine *see* Calcium-channel Blockers
Lamivudine
Antibacterials: plasma concentration of lamivudine increased by trimethoprim (as co-trimoxazole)—avoid concomitant use of high-dose co-trimoxazole
Antivirals: avoidance of lamivudine advised by manufacturer of emtricitabine; manufacturer of lamivudine advises avoid concomitant use with foscarnet; manufacturer of lamivudine advises avoid concomitant use of intravenous ganciclovir
Lamotrigine
• Antibacterials: plasma concentration of lamotrigine reduced by •rifampicin
• Antidepressants: anticonvulsant effect of antiepileptics possibly antagonised by MAOIs and •tricyclic-related antidepressants (convulsive threshold lowered); anticonvulsant effect of antiepileptics antagonised by •SSRIs and •tricyclics (convulsive threshold lowered)
Antiepileptics: plasma concentration of lamotrigine often reduced by carbamazepine and oxcarbazepine, also plasma concentration of an active metabolite of carbamazepine and oxcarbazepine sometimes raised (but evidence is conflicting); plasma concentration of lamotrigine reduced by phenytoin and primidone; plasma concentration of lamotrigine increased by valproate
• Antimalarials: possible increased risk of convulsions when antiepileptics given with chloroquine and hydroxychloroquine; anticonvulsant effect of antiepileptics antagonised by •mefloquine
Barbiturates: plasma concentration of lamotrigine reduced by phenobarbital
• Oestrogens: plasma concentration of lamotrigine reduced by •oestrogens
• Progestogens: plasma concentration of lamotrigine reduced by •progestogens
Lanreotide
Antidiabetics: lanreotide possibly reduces requirements for insulin, metformin, repaglinide and sulphonylureas
Ciclosporin: lanreotide reduces plasma concentration of ciclosporin
Lansoprazole *see* Proton Pump Inhibitors
Laronidase
Anaesthetics, Local: effects of laronidase possibly inhibited by procaine (manufacturer of laronidase advises avoid concomitant use)

Laronidase *(continued)*
Antimalarials: effects of laronidase possibly inhibited by chloroquine and hydroxychloroquine (manufacturer of laronidase advises avoid concomitant use)

Leflunomide
Note. Increased risk of toxicity with other haematotoxic and hepatotoxic drugs
Anticoagulants: leflunomide possibly enhances anticoagulant effect of warfarin
Antidiabetics: leflunomide possibly enhances hypoglycaemic effect of tolbutamide
Antiepileptics: leflunomide possibly increases plasma concentration of phenytoin
Lipid-regulating Drugs: the effect of leflunomide is significantly decreased by colestyramine (enhanced elimination)—avoid unless drug elimination desired
• Vaccines: avoid concomitant use of leflunomide with live •vaccines (see p. 675)

Lercanidipine *see* Calcium-channel Blockers

Leukotriene Antagonists
Analgesics: plasma concentration of zafirlukast increased by aspirin
Antibacterials: plasma concentration of zafirlukast reduced by erythromycin
Anticoagulants: zafirlukast enhances anticoagulant effect of warfarin
Antiepileptics: plasma concentration of montelukast reduced by primidone
Barbiturates: plasma concentration of montelukast reduced by phenobarbital
Theophylline: zafirlukast possibly increases plasma concentration of theophylline, also plasma concentration of zafirlukast reduced

Levamisole
Alcohol: possibility of disulfiram-like reaction when levamisole given with alcohol
• Anticoagulants: levamisole possibly enhances anticoagulant effect of •warfarin
Antiepileptics: levamisole possibly increases plasma concentration of phenytoin

Levetiracetam
• Antidepressants: anticonvulsant effect of antiepileptics possibly antagonised by MAOIs and •tricyclic-related antidepressants (convulsive threshold lowered); anticonvulsant effect of antiepileptics antagonised by •SSRIs and •tricyclics (convulsive threshold lowered)
• Antimalarials: possible increased risk of convulsions when antiepileptics given with chloroquine and hydroxychloroquine; anticonvulsant effect of antiepileptics antagonised by •mefloquine

Levobunolol *see* Beta-blockers

Levobupivacaine
Anti-arrhythmics: increased myocardial depression when levobupivacaine given with anti-arrhythmics

Levocetirizine *see* Antihistamines

Levodopa
ACE Inhibitors: enhanced hypotensive effect when levodopa given with ACE inhibitors
Adrenergic Neurone Blockers: enhanced hypotensive effect when levodopa given with adrenergic neurone blockers
Alpha-blockers: enhanced hypotensive effect when levodopa given with alpha-blockers
• Anaesthetics, General: increased risk of arrhythmias when levodopa given with •volatile liquid general anaesthetics
Angiotensin-II Receptor Antagonists: enhanced hypotensive effect when levodopa given with angiotensin-II receptor antagonists

Levodopa *(continued)*
• Antidepressants: risk of hypertensive crisis when levodopa given with •MAOIs, avoid levodopa for at least 2 weeks after stopping MAOIs; increased risk of side-effects when levodopa given with moclobemide
Antiepileptics: effects of levodopa possibly reduced by phenytoin
Antimuscarinics: absorption of levodopa possibly reduced by antimuscarinics
Antipsychotics: effects of levodopa antagonised by antipsychotics; avoidance of levodopa advised by manufacturer of amisulpride (antagonism of effect)
Anxiolytics and Hypnotics: effects of levodopa possibly antagonised by benzodiazepines
Beta-blockers: enhanced hypotensive effect when levodopa given with beta-blockers
Bupropion: increased risk of side-effects when levodopa given with bupropion
Calcium-channel Blockers: enhanced hypotensive effect when levodopa given with calcium-channel blockers
Clonidine: enhanced hypotensive effect when levodopa given with clonidine
Diazoxide: enhanced hypotensive effect when levodopa given with diazoxide
Diuretics: enhanced hypotensive effect when levodopa given with diuretics
Dopaminergics: enhanced effects and increased toxicity of levodopa when given with selegiline (reduce dose of levodopa)
Iron: absorption of levodopa possibly reduced by *oral* iron
Memantine: effects of dopaminergics possibly enhanced by memantine
Methyldopa: enhanced hypotensive effect when levodopa given with methyldopa; antiparkinsonian effect of dopaminergics antagonised by methyldopa
Moxonidine: enhanced hypotensive effect when levodopa given with moxonidine
Muscle Relaxants: possible agitation, confusion and hallucinations when levodopa given with baclofen
Nitrates: enhanced hypotensive effect when levodopa given with nitrates
Vasodilator Antihypertensives: enhanced hypotensive effect when levodopa given with hydralazine, minoxidil or nitroprusside
Vitamins: effects of levodopa reduced by pyridoxine when given without dopa-decarboxylase inhibitor

Levofloxacin *see* Quinolones

Levomepromazine (methotrimeprazine) *see* Antipsychotics

Levonorgestrel *see* Progestogens

Levothyroxine (thyroxine) *see* Thyroid Hormones

Lidocaine (lignocaine)
Note. Interactions less likely when lidocaine used topically
Anaesthetics, Local: increased myocardial depression when anti-arrhythmics given with bupivacaine, levobupivacaine or prilocaine
• Anti-arrhythmics: increased myocardial depression when anti-arrhythmics given with other •anti-arrhythmics
• Antibacterials: increased risk of ventricular arrhythmias when lidocaine (lignocaine) given with •quinupristin/dalfopristin—avoid concomitant use
• Antipsychotics: increased risk of ventricular arrhythmias when anti-arrhythmics that

Lidocaine (lignocaine)
- Antipsychotics *(continued)*
  prolong the QT interval given with •antipsychotics that prolong the QT interval
- Antivirals: plasma concentration of lidocaine (lignocaine) possibly increased by •amprenavir—avoid concomitant use; plasma concentration of lidocaine (lignocaine) possibly increased by •atazanavir and lopinavir
- Beta-blockers: increased myocardial depression when anti-arrhythmics given with •beta-blockers; increased risk of lidocaine (lignocaine) toxicity when given with •propranolol
- Diuretics: action of lidocaine (lignocaine) antagonised by hypokalaemia caused by •acetazolamide, •loop diuretics or •thiazides and related diuretics
- Dolasetron: increased risk of ventricular arrhythmias when lidocaine (lignocaine) given with •dolasetron—avoid concomitant use

$5HT_3$ Antagonists: caution with anti-arrhythmics advised by manufacturer of tropisetron (risk of ventricular arrhythmias)

Muscle Relaxants: neuromuscular blockade enhanced and prolonged when lidocaine (lignocaine) given with suxamethonium

- Ulcer-healing Drugs: plasma concentration of lidocaine (lignocaine) increased by •cimetidine (increased risk of toxicity)

Linezolid

Note. Linezolid is a reversible, non-selective MAO inhibitor—see interactions of MAOIs

Oestrogens: antibacterials that do not induce liver enzymes possibly reduce contraceptive effect of oestrogens (risk probably small, see BNF section 7.3.1)

Liothyronine *see* Thyroid Hormones

Lipid-regulating Drugs *see* Colestipol, Colestyramine, Ezetimibe, Fibrates, Nicotinic Acid, and Statins

Lisinopril *see* ACE Inhibitors

Lisuride

Antipsychotics: effects of lisuride antagonised by antipsychotics

Memantine: effects of dopaminergics possibly enhanced by memantine

Methyldopa: antiparkinsonian effect of dopaminergics antagonised by methyldopa

Lithium
- ACE Inhibitors: excretion of lithium reduced by •ACE inhibitors (increased plasma concentration)
- Analgesics: excretion of lithium probably reduced by •NSAIDs (increased risk of toxicity); excretion of lithium reduced by •diclofenac, •ibuprofen, •indometacin, •mefenamic acid, •naproxen, •parecoxib and •piroxicam (increased risk of toxicity); excretion of lithium reduced by •ketorolac (increased risk of toxicity)—avoid concomitant use
- Angiotensin-II Receptor Antagonists: excretion of lithium reduced by •angiotensin-II receptor antagonists (increased plasma concentration)

Antacids: excretion of lithium increased by sodium bicarbonate (reduced plasma concentration)

- Anti-arrhythmics: avoidance of lithium advised by manufacturer of •amiodarone (risk of ventricular arrhythmias)

Antibacterials: increased risk of lithium toxicity when given with metronidazole

- Antidepressants: increased risk of CNS effects when lithium given with •SSRIs (lithium toxicity reported); risk of toxicity when lithium given with tricyclics

Antiepileptics: neurotoxicity may occur when lithium given with carbamazepine or phenytoin without increased plasma concentration of lithium

- Antipsychotics: increased risk of extrapyramidal side-effects and possibly neurotoxicity when lithium given with clozapine, haloperidol or phenothiazines; increased risk of ventricular arrhythmias when lithium given with •sertindole—avoid concomitant use; increased risk of extrapyramidal side-effects when lithium given with sulpiride

Calcium-channel Blockers: neurotoxicity may occur when lithium given with diltiazem or verapamil without increased plasma concentration of lithium

- Diuretics: excretion of lithium increased by •acetazolamide; excretion of lithium reduced by •loop diuretics and •thiazides and related diuretics (increased plasma concentration and risk of toxicity)—loop diuretics safer than thiazides; excretion of lithium reduced by •potassium-sparing diuretics and aldosterone antagonists (increased plasma concentration and risk of toxicity)
- Methyldopa: neurotoxicity may occur when lithium given with •methyldopa without increased plasma concentration of lithium

Muscle Relaxants: lithium enhances effects of muscle relaxants; hyperkinesis caused by lithium possibly aggravated by baclofen

Parasympathomimetics: lithium antagonises effects of neostigmine and pyridostigmine

Theophylline: excretion of lithium increased by theophylline (reduced plasma concentration)

Lofepramine *see* Antidepressants, Tricyclic

Lofexidine

Alcohol: increased sedative effect when lofexidine given with alcohol

Anxiolytics and Hypnotics: increased sedative effect when lofexidine given with anxiolytics and hypnotics

Loperamide

Desmopressin: loperamide increases plasma concentration of *oral* desmopressin

Lopinavir

Note. In combination with ritonavir as Kaletra® (ritonavir is present to inhibit lopinavir metabolism and increase plasma-lopinavir concentration)—see also Ritonavir

Anti-arrhythmics: lopinavir possibly increases plasma concentration of lidocaine (lignocaine)

- Antibacterials: plasma concentration of lopinavir reduced by •rifampicin—avoid concomitant use
- Antidepressants: plasma concentration of lopinavir reduced by •St John's wort—avoid concomitant use
- Antiepileptics: plasma concentration of lopinavir possibly reduced by carbamazepine, phenytoin and •primidone

Antihistamines: lopinavir possibly increases plasma concentration of chlorphenamine (chlorpheniramine)

- Antimalarials: avoidance of lopinavir advised by manufacturer of •artemether/lumefantrine

Antimuscarinics: avoidance of lopinavir advised by manufacturer of tolterodine

- Antipsychotics: lopinavir possibly inhibits metabolism of •aripiprazole (reduce dose of aripiprazole); lopinavir increases plasma con-

Lopinavir
- • Antipsychotics *(continued)* centration of •sertindole (increased risk of ventricular arrhythmias—avoid concomitant use)
- • Antivirals: lopinavir reduces plasma concentration of amprenavir, effect on lopinavir plasma concentration not predictable; plasma concentration of lopinavir reduced by efavirenz, nevirapine and •tipranavir; plasma concentration of lopinavir reduced by nelfinavir, also plasma concentration of active metabolite of nelfinavir increased; lopinavir increases plasma concentration of saquinavir and tenofovir
- • Barbiturates: plasma concentration of lopinavir possibly reduced by •phenobarbital
- • Cilostazol: lopinavir possibly increases plasma concentration of •cilostazol—avoid concomitant use
- Corticosteroids: plasma concentration of lopinavir possibly reduced by dexamethasone
- • Lipid-regulating Drugs: possible increased risk of myopathy when lopinavir given with atorvastatin; possible increased risk of myopathy when lopinavir given with •simvastatin—avoid concomitant use
- Sirolimus: lopinavir possibly increases plasma concentration of sirolimus

Loprazolam *see* Anxiolytics and Hypnotics
Loratadine *see* Antihistamines
Lorazepam *see* Anxiolytics and Hypnotics
Lormetazepam *see* Anxiolytics and Hypnotics
Losartan *see* Angiotensin-II Receptor Antagonists
Lumefantrine *see* Artemether with Lumefantrine
Lumiracoxib *see* NSAIDs
Lymecycline *see* Tetracyclines

Macrolides

Note. See also Telithromycin

Note. Interactions do not apply to small amounts of erythromycin used topically

- Analgesics: erythromycin increases plasma concentration of alfentanil
- Antacids: absorption of azithromycin reduced by antacids
- • Anti-arrhythmics: increased risk of ventricular arrhythmias when parenteral erythromycin given with •amiodarone—avoid concomitant use; clarithromycin possibly increases plasma concentration of •disopyramide (increased risk of toxicity); erythromycin increases plasma concentration of •disopyramide (increased risk of toxicity); increased risk of ventricular arrhythmias when parenteral erythromycin given with •quinidine; increased risk of ventricular arrhythmias when clarithromycin given with •quinidine
- • Antibacterials: increased risk of ventricular arrhythmias when parenteral erythromycin given with •moxifloxacin—avoid concomitant use; macrolides possibly increase plasma concentration of •rifabutin (increased risk of uveitis—reduce rifabutin dose); clarithromycin increases plasma concentration of •rifabutin (increased risk of uveitis—reduce rifabutin dose); plasma concentration of clarithromycin reduced by rifamycins
- • Anticoagulants: macrolides possibly enhance anticoagulant effect of •coumarins; clarithromycin and erythromycin enhance anticoagulant effect of •coumarins
- • Antidepressants: avoidance of macrolides advised by manufacturer of •reboxetine

Macrolides *(continued)*
- Antidiabetics: clarithromycin enhances effects of repaglinide
- • Antiepileptics: clarithromycin and erythromycin increase plasma concentration of •carbamazepine; clarithromycin inhibits metabolism of phenytoin (increased plasma concentration); erythromycin possibly inhibits metabolism of valproate (increased plasma concentration)
- Antifungals: clarithromycin increases plasma concentration of itraconazole
- • Antihistamines: manufacturer of loratadine advises erythromycin possibly increases plasma concentration of loratadine; macrolides possibly inhibit metabolism of •mizolastine (avoid concomitant use); erythromycin inhibits metabolism of •mizolastine—avoid concomitant use
- • Antimalarials: avoidance of macrolides advised by manufacturer of •artemether/lumefantrine
- Antimuscarinics: avoidance of clarithromycin and erythromycin advised by manufacturer of tolterodine
- • Antipsychotics: increased risk of ventricular arrhythmias when parenteral erythromycin given with •amisulpride—avoid concomitant use; erythromycin possibly increases plasma concentration of •clozapine (possible increased risk of convulsions); increased risk of ventricular arrhythmias when clarithromycin given with •pimozide—avoid concomitant use; possible increased risk of ventricular arrhythmias when erythromycin given with •pimozide—avoid concomitant use; macrolides possibly increase plasma concentration of quetiapine (reduce dose of quetiapine); possible increased risk of ventricular arrhythmias when macrolides given with •sertindole—avoid concomitant use; increased risk of ventricular arrhythmias when erythromycin given with •sertindole—avoid concomitant use
- • Antivirals: plasma concentration of both drugs increased when erythromycin given with amprenavir; plasma concentration of both drugs increased when clarithromycin given with atazanavir; increased risk of rash when clarithromycin given with efavirenz; plasma concentration of azithromycin and erythromycin possibly increased by ritonavir; plasma concentration of clarithromycin increased by •ritonavir (reduce dose of clarithromycin in renal impairment); plasma concentration of clarithromycin increased by •tipranavir (reduce dose of clarithromycin in renal impairment), also clarithromycin increases plasma concentration of tipranavir; clarithromycin tablets reduce absorption of zidovudine
- • Anxiolytics and Hypnotics: clarithromycin and erythromycin inhibit metabolism of •midazolam (increased plasma concentration with increased sedation); erythromycin increases plasma concentration of buspirone (reduce dose of buspirone); erythromycin inhibits the metabolism of zopiclone
- Aprepitant: clarithromycin possibly increases plasma concentration of aprepitant
- • Calcium-channel Blockers: erythromycin possibly inhibits metabolism of felodipine (increased plasma concentration); avoidance of erythromycin advised by manufacturer of lercanidipine; clarithromycin and erythromycin possibly inhibit metabolism of •verapamil (increased risk of toxicity)

Macrolides *(continued)*

Cardiac Glycosides: macrolides increase plasma concentration of digoxin (increased risk of toxicity)
- Ciclosporin: macrolides possibly inhibit metabolism of •ciclosporin (increased plasma concentration); clarithromycin and erythromycin inhibit metabolism of •ciclosporin (increased plasma concentration)
- Cilostazol: erythromycin increases plasma concentration of •cilostazol (also plasma concentration of erythromycin reduced)—avoid concomitant use
- Colchicine: clarithromycin or erythromycin increase risk of •colchicine toxicity

Corticosteroids: erythromycin possibly inhibits metabolism of corticosteroids; erythromycin inhibits the metabolism of methylprednisolone; clarithromycin possibly increases plasma concentration of methylprednisolone
- Cytotoxics: *in vitro* studies suggest a possible interaction between erythromycin and docetaxel (consult docetaxel product literature); erythromycin increases toxicity of •vinblastine—avoid concomitant use
- Diuretics: clarithromycin increases plasma concentration of •eplerenone—avoid concomitant use; erythromycin increases plasma concentration of eplerenone (reduce dose of eplerenone)

Dopaminergics: macrolides possibly increase plasma concentration of bromocriptine and cabergoline (increased risk of toxicity); erythromycin increases plasma concentration of bromocriptine and cabergoline (increased risk of toxicity)
- Ergot Alkaloids: increased risk of ergotism when macrolides given with •ergotamine and methysergide—avoid concomitant use
- $5HT_1$ Agonists: clarithromycin and erythromycin increase plasma concentration of •eletriptan (risk of toxicity)—avoid concomitant use
- Ivabradine: clarithromycin possibly increases plasma concentration of •ivabradine—avoid concomitant use; increased risk of ventricular arrhythmias when erythromycin given with •ivabradine—avoid concomitant use

Leukotriene Antagonists: erythromycin reduces plasma concentration of zafirlukast
- Lipid-regulating Drugs: clarithromycin increases plasma concentration of atorvastatin; possible increased risk of myopathy when erythromycin given with atorvastatin; erythromycin reduces plasma concentration of rosuvastatin; increased risk of myopathy when clarithromycin or erythromycin given with •simvastatin (avoid concomitant use)

Oestrogens: antibacterials that do not induce liver enzymes possibly reduce contraceptive effect of oestrogens (risk probably small, see BNF section 7.3.1)

Parasympathomimetics: erythromycin increases plasma concentration of galantamine

Sildenafil: erythromycin increases plasma concentration of sildenafil—reduce initial dose of sildenafil
- Sirolimus: clarithromycin increases plasma concentration of •sirolimus—avoid concomitant use; plasma concentration of both drugs increased when erythromycin given with •sirolimus
- Tacrolimus: clarithromycin and erythromycin increase plasma concentration of •tacrolimus

Macrolides *(continued)*

Tadalafil: clarithromycin and erythromycin possibly increase plasma concentration of tadalafil
- Theophylline: azithromycin possibly increases plasma concentration of theophylline; clarithromycin inhibits metabolism of •theophylline (increased plasma concentration); erythromycin inhibits metabolism of •theophylline (increased plasma concentration), if erythromycin given by mouth, also decreased plasma-erythromycin concentration

Ulcer-healing Drugs: plasma concentration of erythromycin increased by cimetidine (increased risk of toxicity, including deafness); plasma concentration of both drugs increased when clarithromycin given with omeprazole

Vardenafil: erythromycin increases plasma concentration of vardenafil (reduce dose of vardenafil)

Magnesium (parenteral)
- Calcium-channel Blockers: profound hypotension reported with concomitant use of parenteral magnesium and •nifedipine in pre-eclampsia

Muscle Relaxants: parenteral magnesium enhances effects of non-depolarising muscle relaxants and suxamethonium

Magnesium Salts (oral) *see* Antacids

MAOIs

Note. For interactions of reversible MAO-A inhibitors (RIMAs) see Moclobemide, and for interactions of MAO-B inhibitors see Rasagiline and Selegiline; the antibacterial Linezolid is a reversible, non-selective MAO inhibitor

ACE Inhibitors: MAOIs possibly enhance hypotensive effect of ACE inhibitors

Adrenergic Neurone Blockers: enhanced hypotensive effect when MAOIs given with adrenergic neurone blockers
- Alcohol: MAOIs interact with tyramine found in some beverages containing •alcohol and some dealcoholised beverages (hypertensive crisis)—if no tyramine, enhanced hypotensive effect

$Alpha_2$-adrenoceptor Stimulants: avoidance of MAOIs advised by manufacturer of apraclonidine and brimonidine
- Alpha-blockers: avoidance of MAOIs advised by manufacturer of •indoramin; enhanced hypotensive effect when MAOIs given with alpha-blockers
- Anaesthetics, General: Because of hazardous interactions between MAOIs and •general anaesthetics, MAOIs should normally be stopped 2 weeks before surgery
- Analgesics: CNS excitation or depression (hypertension or hypotension) when MAOIs given with •pethidine—avoid concomitant use and for 2 weeks after stopping MAOIs; avoidance of MAOIs advised by manufacturer of •nefopam; possible CNS excitation or depression (hypertension or hypotension) when MAOIs given with •opioid analgesics—avoid concomitant use and for 2 weeks after stopping MAOIs

Angiotensin-II Receptor Antagonists: MAOIs possibly enhance hypotensive effect of angiotensin-II receptor antagonists
- Antidepressants: increased risk of hypertension and CNS excitation when MAOIs given with •reboxetine (MAOIs should not be started until 1 week after stopping reboxetine, avoid reboxetine for 2 weeks after stopping MAOIs); after stopping MAOIs do not start •cital-

MAOIs

- Antidepressants *(continued)* opram, •escitalopram, •fluvoxamine or •paroxetine for 2 weeks, also MAOIs should not be started until at least 1 week after stopping citalopram, escitalopram, fluvoxamine or paroxetine; after stopping MAOIs do not start •fluoxetine for 2 weeks, also MAOIs should not be started until at least 5 weeks after stopping fluoxetine; after stopping MAOIs do not start •mirtazapine or •sertraline for 2 weeks, also MAOIs should not be started until at least 2 weeks after stopping mirtazapine or sertraline; after stopping MAOIs do not start •duloxetine for 2 weeks, also MAOIs should not be started until at least 5 days after stopping duloxetine; enhanced CNS effects and toxicity when MAOIs given with •venlafaxine (venlafaxine should not be started until 2 weeks after stopping MAOIs, avoid MAOIs for 1 week after stopping venlafaxine); MAOIs can cause increased risk of hypertension and CNS excitation when given with other •MAOIs (avoid for at least 2 weeks after stopping previous MAOIs and then start at a reduced dose); after stopping MAOIs do not start •moclobemide for at least 1 week; MAOIs increase CNS effects of •SSRIs (risk of serious toxicity); after stopping MAOIs do not start •tricyclic-related antidepressants for 2 weeks, also MAOIs should not be started until at least 1–2 weeks after stopping tricyclic-related antidepressants; increased risk of hypertension and CNS excitation when MAOIs given with •tricyclics, tricyclics should not be started until 2 weeks after stopping MAOIs (3 weeks if starting clomipramine or imipramine), also MAOIs should not be started for at least 1–2 weeks after stopping tricyclics (3 weeks in the case of clomipramine or imipramine); CNS excitation and confusion when MAOIs given with •tryptophan (reduce dose of tryptophan)

Antidiabetics: MAOIs possibly enhance hypoglycaemic effect of antidiabetics; MAOIs enhance hypoglycaemic effect of insulin, metformin and sulphonylureas

- Antiepileptics: MAOIs possibly antagonise anticonvulsant effect of antiepileptics (convulsive threshold lowered); avoidance for 2 weeks after stopping MAOIs advised by manufacturer of •carbamazepine, also antagonism of anticonvulsant effect; avoidance of MAOIs advised by manufacturer of •oxcarbazepine

Antihistamines: increased antimuscarinic and sedative effects when MAOIs given with antihistamines

- Antimalarials: avoidance of antidepressants advised by manufacturer of •artemether/lumefantrine

Antimuscarinics: increased risk of antimuscarinic side-effects when MAOIs given with antimuscarinics

- Antipsychotics: CNS effects of MAOIs possibly increased by •clozapine

Anxiolytics and Hypnotics: avoidance of MAOIs advised by manufacturer of buspirone

- Atomoxetine: after stopping MAOIs do not start •atomoxetine for 2 weeks, also MAOIs should not be started until at least 2 weeks after stopping atomoxetine

Barbiturates: MAOIs possibly antagonise anticonvulsant effect of barbiturates (convulsive threshold lowered)

MAOIs *(continued)*

Beta-blockers: enhanced hypotensive effect when MAOIs given with beta-blockers

- Bupropion: avoidance of bupropion for 2 weeks after stopping MAOIs advised by manufacturer of •bupropion

Calcium-channel Blockers: enhanced hypotensive effect when MAOIs given with calcium-channel blockers

Clonidine: enhanced hypotensive effect when MAOIs given with clonidine

Diazoxide: enhanced hypotensive effect when MAOIs given with diazoxide

Diuretics: enhanced hypotensive effect when MAOIs given with diuretics

- Dopaminergics: avoid concomitant use of non-selective MAOIs with •entacapone; risk of hypertensive crisis when MAOIs given with •levodopa, avoid levodopa for at least 2 weeks after stopping MAOIs; risk of hypertensive crisis when MAOIs given with •rasagiline, avoid MAOIs for at least 2 weeks after stopping rasagiline; enhanced hypotensive effect when MAOIs given with selegiline; avoid concomitant use of MAOIs with tolcapone

Doxapram: MAOIs enhance effects of doxapram

- $5HT_1$ Agonists: risk of CNS toxicity when MAOIs given with •rizatriptan or •sumatriptan (avoid rizatriptan or sumatriptan for 2 weeks after MAOIs); increased risk of CNS toxicity when MAOIs given with •zolmitriptan
- Methyldopa: avoidance of MAOIs advised by manufacturer of •methyldopa

Moxonidine: enhanced hypotensive effect when MAOIs given with moxonidine

Muscle Relaxants: phenelzine enhances effects of suxamethonium

Nicorandil: enhanced hypotensive effect when MAOIs given with nicorandil

Nitrates: enhanced hypotensive effect when MAOIs given with nitrates

- Sibutramine: increased CNS toxicity when MAOIs given with •sibutramine (manufacturer of sibutramine advises avoid concomitant use), also avoid sibutramine for 2 weeks after stopping MAOIs
- Sympathomimetics: risk of hypertensive crisis when MAOIs given with •dexamfetamine, •dopamine, •dopexamine, •ephedrine, •isometheptene, •methylphenidate, •phenylephrine, •phenylpropanolamine, •pseudoephedrine or •sympathomimetics
- Tetrabenazine: risk of CNS excitation and hypertension when MAOIs given with •tetrabenazine

Vasodilator Antihypertensives: enhanced hypotensive effect when MAOIs given with hydralazine, minoxidil or nitroprusside

MAOIs, reversible *see* Moclobemide

Maprotiline *see* Antidepressants, Tricyclic (related)

Mebendazole

Ulcer-healing Drugs: metabolism of mebendazole possibly inhibited by cimetidine (increased plasma concentration)

Meclozine *see* Antihistamines

Medroxyprogesterone *see* Progestogens

Mefenamic Acid *see* NSAIDs

Mefloquine

- Anti-arrhythmics: increased risk of ventricular arrhythmias when mefloquine given with •amiodarone—avoid concomitant use; increased risk of ventricular arrhythmias when mefloquine given with •quinidine

Mefloquine *(continued)*
- • Antibacterials: increased risk of ventricular arrhythmias when mefloquine given with •moxifloxacin—avoid concomitant use
- • Antiepileptics: mefloquine antagonises anticonvulsant effect of •antiepileptics, •carbamazepine and •valproate
- • Antimalarials: avoidance of antimalarials advised by manufacturer of •artemether/lumefantrine; increased risk of convulsions when mefloquine given with •chloroquine and hydroxychloroquine; increased risk of convulsions when mefloquine given with •quinine (but should not prevent the use of intravenous quinine in severe cases)
- • Antipsychotics: increased risk of ventricular arrhythmias when mefloquine given with •pimozide—avoid concomitant use
- Beta-blockers: increased risk of bradycardia when mefloquine given with beta-blockers
- Calcium-channel Blockers: possible increased risk of bradycardia when mefloquine given with calcium-channel blockers
- Cardiac Glycosides: possible increased risk of bradycardia when mefloquine given with digoxin
- • Ivabradine: increased risk of ventricular arrhythmias when mefloquine given with •ivabradine

Megestrol *see* Progestogens

Meloxicam *see* NSAIDs

Melphalan
- Antibacterials: increased risk of melphalan toxicity when given with nalidixic acid
- Antiepileptics: cytotoxics possibly reduce absorption of phenytoin
- • Antipsychotics: avoid concomitant use of cytotoxics with •clozapine (increased risk of agranulocytosis)
- Cardiac Glycosides: cytotoxics reduce absorption of digoxin tablets
- • Ciclosporin: increased risk of nephrotoxicity when melphalan given with •ciclosporin

Memantine
- • Anaesthetics, General: increased risk of CNS toxicity when memantine given with •ketamine (manufacturer of memantine advises avoid concomitant use)
- • Analgesics: increased risk of CNS toxicity when memantine given with •dextromethorphan (manufacturer of memantine advises avoid concomitant use)
- Antiepileptics: memantine possibly reduces effects of primidone
- Antimuscarinics: memantine possibly enhances effects of antimuscarinics
- Antipsychotics: memantine possibly reduces effects of antipsychotics
- Barbiturates: memantine possibly reduces effects of barbiturates
- • Dopaminergics: memantine possibly enhances effects of dopaminergics and selegiline; increased risk of CNS toxicity when memantine given with •amantadine (manufacturer of memantine advises avoid concomitant use)
- Muscle Relaxants: memantine possibly modifies effects of baclofen and dantrolene

Mepacrine
- Antimalarials: mepacrine increases plasma concentration of primaquine (increased risk of toxicity)

Meprobamate *see* Anxiolytics and Hypnotics

Meptazinol *see* Opioid Analgesics

Mercaptopurine
- • Allopurinol: enhanced effects and increased toxicity of mercaptopurine when given with •allopurinol (reduce dose of mercaptopurine)
- Aminosalicylates: possible increased risk of leucopenia when mercaptopurine given with aminosalicylates
- • Antibacterials: increased risk of haematological toxicity when mercaptopurine given with •sulfamethoxazole (as co-trimoxazole); increased risk of haematological toxicity when mercaptopurine given with •trimethoprim (also with co-trimoxazole)
- • Anticoagulants: mercaptopurine possibly reduces anticoagulant effect of •coumarins
- Antiepileptics: cytotoxics possibly reduce absorption of phenytoin
- • Antipsychotics: avoid concomitant use of cytotoxics with •clozapine (increased risk of agranulocytosis)
- Cardiac Glycosides: cytotoxics reduce absorption of digoxin tablets

Meropenem
- Antiepileptics: meropenem reduces plasma concentration of valproate
- Oestrogens: antibacterials that do not induce liver enzymes possibly reduce contraceptive effect of oestrogens (risk probably small, see BNF section 7.3.1)
- Probenecid: excretion of meropenem reduced by probenecid (manufacturers of meropenem advise avoid concomitant use)

Mesalazine *see* Aminosalicylates

Mestranol *see* Oestrogens

Metaraminol *see* Sympathomimetics

Metformin *see* Antidiabetics

Methadone *see* Opioid Analgesics

Methenamine
- • Antibacterials: increased risk of crystalluria when methenamine given with •sulphonamides
- • Diuretics: effects of methenamine antagonised by •acetazolamide
- Oestrogens: antibacterials that do not induce liver enzymes possibly reduce contraceptive effect of oestrogens (risk probably small, see BNF section 7.3.1)
- Potassium Salts: avoid concomitant use of methenamine with potassium citrate

Methocarbamol *see* Muscle Relaxants

Methotrexate
- • Anaesthetics, General: antifolate effect of methotrexate increased by •nitrous oxide—avoid concomitant use
- • Analgesics: excretion of methotrexate probably reduced by •NSAIDs (increased risk of toxicity); excretion of methotrexate reduced by •aspirin, •diclofenac, •ibuprofen, •indometacin, •ketoprofen, •meloxicam and •naproxen (increased risk of toxicity)
- • Antibacterials: absorption of methotrexate possibly reduced by neomycin; excretion of methotrexate possibly reduced by ciprofloxacin (increased risk of toxicity); increased risk of haematological toxicity when methotrexate given with •sulfamethoxazole (as co-trimoxazole); increased risk of methotrexate toxicity when given with doxycycline, sulphonamides or tetracycline; excretion of methotrexate reduced by penicillins (increased risk of toxicity); increased risk of haematological toxicity when methotrexate given with •trimethoprim (also with co-trimoxazole)

Methotrexate *(continued)*
- Antiepileptics: cytotoxics possibly reduce absorption of phenytoin; antifolate effect of methotrexate increased by phenytoin
- • Antimalarials: antifolate effect of methotrexate increased by •pyrimethamine
- • Antipsychotics: avoid concomitant use of cytotoxics with •clozapine (increased risk of agranulocytosis)
- Cardiac Glycosides: cytotoxics reduce absorption of digoxin tablets
- • Ciclosporin: risk of toxicity when methotrexate given with •ciclosporin
- • Corticosteroids: increased risk of haematological toxicity when methotrexate given with •corticosteroids
- • Cytotoxics: increased pulmonary toxicity when methotrexate given with •cisplatin
- • Probenecid: excretion of methotrexate reduced by •probenecid (increased risk of toxicity)
- • Retinoids: plasma concentration of methotrexate increased by •acitretin (also increased risk of hepatotoxicity)—avoid concomitant use
- Theophylline: methotrexate possibly increases plasma concentration of theophylline
- Ulcer-healing Drugs: excretion of methotrexate possibly reduced by omeprazole (increased risk of toxicity)

Methoxamine *see* Sympathomimetics

Methyldopa
- ACE Inhibitors: enhanced hypotensive effect when methyldopa given with ACE inhibitors
- Adrenergic Neurone Blockers: enhanced hypotensive effect when methyldopa given with adrenergic neurone blockers
- Alcohol: enhanced hypotensive effect when methyldopa given with alcohol
- Aldesleukin: enhanced hypotensive effect when methyldopa given with aldesleukin
- Alpha-blockers: enhanced hypotensive effect when methyldopa given with alpha-blockers
- Anaesthetics, General: enhanced hypotensive effect when methyldopa given with general anaesthetics
- Analgesics: hypotensive effect of methyldopa antagonised by NSAIDs
- Angiotensin-II Receptor Antagonists: enhanced hypotensive effect when methyldopa given with angiotensin-II receptor antagonists
- • Antidepressants: manufacturer of methyldopa advises avoid concomitant use with •MAOIs
- Antipsychotics: enhanced hypotensive effect when methyldopa given with antipsychotics (also increased risk of extrapyramidal effects)
- Anxiolytics and Hypnotics: enhanced hypotensive effect when methyldopa given with anxiolytics and hypnotics
- Beta-blockers: enhanced hypotensive effect when methyldopa given with beta-blockers
- Calcium-channel Blockers: enhanced hypotensive effect when methyldopa given with calcium-channel blockers
- Clonidine: enhanced hypotensive effect when methyldopa given with clonidine
- Corticosteroids: hypotensive effect of methyldopa antagonised by corticosteroids
- Diazoxide: enhanced hypotensive effect when methyldopa given with diazoxide
- Diuretics: enhanced hypotensive effect when methyldopa given with diuretics
- Dopaminergics: methyldopa antagonises antiparkinsonian effect of dopaminergics; increased risk of extrapyramidal side-effects when methyldopa given with amantadine;

Methyldopa
- Dopaminergics *(continued)* effects of methyldopa possibly enhanced by entacapone; enhanced hypotensive effect when methyldopa given with levodopa
- Iron: hypotensive effect of methyldopa antagonised by *oral* iron
- • Lithium: neurotoxicity may occur when methyldopa given with •lithium without increased plasma concentration of lithium
- Moxisylyte (thymoxamine): enhanced hypotensive effect when methyldopa given with moxisylyte
- Moxonidine: enhanced hypotensive effect when methyldopa given with moxonidine
- Muscle Relaxants: enhanced hypotensive effect when methyldopa given with baclofen or tizanidine
- Nitrates: enhanced hypotensive effect when methyldopa given with nitrates
- Oestrogens: hypotensive effect of methyldopa antagonised by oestrogens
- Prostaglandins: enhanced hypotensive effect when methyldopa given with alprostadil
- • Sympathomimetics, Beta$_2$: acute hypotension reported when methyldopa given with infusion of •salbutamol
- Vasodilator Antihypertensives: enhanced hypotensive effect when methyldopa given with hydralazine, minoxidil or nitroprusside

Methylphenidate *see* Sympathomimetics

Methylprednisolone *see* Corticosteroids

Methysergide *see* Ergot Alkaloids

Metipranolol *see* Beta-blockers

Metoclopramide
- Analgesics: metoclopramide increases rate of absorption of aspirin (enhanced effect); effects of metoclopramide on gastro-intestinal activity antagonised by opioid analgesics; metoclopramide increases rate of absorption of paracetamol
- Antimuscarinics: effects of metoclopramide on gastro-intestinal activity antagonised by antimuscarinics
- Antipsychotics: increased risk of extrapyramidal side-effects when metoclopramide given with antipsychotics
- Atovaquone: metoclopramide reduces plasma concentration of atovaquone
- • Ciclosporin: metoclopramide increases plasma concentration of •ciclosporin
- Dopaminergics: increased risk of extrapyramidal side-effects when metoclopramide given with amantadine; metoclopramide antagonises hypoprolactinaemic effects of bromocriptine and cabergoline; metoclopramide antagonises antiparkinsonian effect of pergolide; metoclopramide antagonises antiparkinsonian effect of ropinirole (manufacturers of ropinirole advise avoid concomitant use)
- Muscle Relaxants: metoclopramide enhances effects of suxamethonium
- Tetrabenazine: increased risk of extrapyramidal side-effects when metoclopramide given with tetrabenazine

Metolazone *see* Diuretics

Metoprolol *see* Beta-blockers

Metronidazole
- Alcohol: disulfiram-like reaction when metronidazole given with alcohol
- • Anticoagulants: metronidazole enhances anticoagulant effect of •coumarins

Metronidazole *(continued)*
• Antiepileptics: metronidazole inhibits metabolism of •phenytoin (increased plasma concentration); metabolism of metronidazole accelerated by primidone (reduced plasma concentration)
Barbiturates: metabolism of metronidazole accelerated by barbiturates (reduced plasma concentration)
Cytotoxics: metronidazole inhibits metabolism of fluorouracil (increased toxicity)
Disulfiram: psychotic reaction reported when metronidazole given with disulfiram
Lithium: metronidazole increases risk of lithium toxicity
Oestrogens: antibacterials that do not induce liver enzymes possibly reduce contraceptive effect of oestrogens (risk probably small, see BNF section 7.3.1)
Ulcer-healing Drugs: metabolism of metronidazole inhibited by cimetidine (increased plasma concentration)

Mexiletine
Anaesthetics, Local: increased myocardial depression when anti-arrhythmics given with bupivacaine, levobupivacaine or prilocaine
Analgesics: absorption of mexiletine delayed by opioid analgesics
• Anti-arrhythmics: increased myocardial depression when anti-arrhythmics given with other •anti-arrhythmics
Antibacterials: metabolism of mexiletine accelerated by rifampicin (reduced plasma concentration)
• Antidepressants: metabolism of mexiletine inhibited by •fluvoxamine (increased risk of toxicity)
Antiepileptics: metabolism of mexiletine accelerated by phenytoin (reduced plasma concentration)
• Antihistamines: increased risk of ventricular arrhythmias when mexiletine given with •mizolastine—avoid concomitant use
Antimuscarinics: absorption of mexiletine delayed by atropine
• Antipsychotics: increased risk of ventricular arrhythmias when anti-arrhythmics that prolong the QT interval given with •antipsychotics that prolong the QT interval
• Antivirals: plasma concentration of mexiletine possibly increased by •ritonavir (increased risk of toxicity)
• Beta-blockers: increased myocardial depression when anti-arrhythmics given with •beta-blockers
• Diuretics: action of mexiletine antagonised by hypokalaemia caused by •acetazolamide, •loop diuretics or •thiazides and related diuretics
• Dolasetron: increased risk of ventricular arrhythmias when mexiletine given with •dolasetron—avoid concomitant use
$5HT_3$ Antagonists: caution with anti-arrhythmics advised by manufacturer of tropisetron (risk of ventricular arrhythmias)
Theophylline: mexiletine increases plasma concentration of theophylline

Mianserin *see* Antidepressants, Tricyclic (related)
Miconazole *see* Antifungals, Imidazole
Midazolam *see* Anxiolytics and Hypnotics
Mifepristone
Analgesics: manufacturer of mifepristone advises avoid concomitant use with NSAIDs and aspirin

Mifepristone *(continued)*
Corticosteroids: mifepristone may reduce effect of corticosteroids (including inhaled corticosteroids) for 3–4 days

Milrinone *see* Phosphodiesterase Inhibitors
Minocycline *see* Tetracyclines
Minoxidil *see* Vasodilator Antihypertensives
Mirtazapine
• Alcohol: increased sedative effect when mirtazapine given with •alcohol
Anticoagulants: mirtazapine enhances anticoagulant effect of warfarin
• Antidepressants: mirtazapine should not be started until 2 weeks after stopping •MAOIs, also MAOIs should not be started until at least 2 weeks after stopping mirtazapine; after stopping mirtazapine do not start •moclobemide for at least 1 week
Antiepileptics: plasma concentration of mirtazapine reduced by carbamazepine and phenytoin
Antifungals: plasma concentration of mirtazapine increased by ketoconazole
• Antimalarials: avoidance of antidepressants advised by manufacturer of •artemether/lumefantrine
Anxiolytics and Hypnotics: increased sedative effect when mirtazapine given with anxiolytics and hypnotics
• Sibutramine: increased risk of CNS toxicity when mirtazapine given with •sibutramine (manufacturer of sibutramine advises avoid concomitant use)
Ulcer-healing Drugs: plasma concentration of mirtazapine increased by cimetidine

Mitotane
• Anticoagulants: mitotane possibly reduces anticoagulant effect of •coumarins
Antiepileptics: cytotoxics possibly reduce absorption of phenytoin
• Antipsychotics: avoid concomitant use of cytotoxics with •clozapine (increased risk of agranulocytosis)
Cardiac Glycosides: cytotoxics reduce absorption of digoxin tablets
Diuretics: manufacturer of mitotane advises avoid concomitant use of spironolactone (antagonism of effect)

Mivacurium *see* Muscle Relaxants
Mizolastine *see* Antihistamines
Moclobemide
• Analgesics: possible CNS excitation or depression (hypertension or hypotension) when moclobemide given with •dextromethorphan or •pethidine—avoid concomitant use; possible CNS excitation or depression (hypertension or hypotension) when moclobemide given with •opioid analgesics
• Antidepressants: moclobemide should not be started for at least 1 week after stopping •MAOIs, •SSRI-related antidepressants, •citalopram, •fluvoxamine, •mirtazapine, •paroxetine, •tricyclic-related antidepressants or •tricyclics; increased risk of CNS toxicity when moclobemide given with •escitalopram, preferably avoid concomitant use; moclobemide should not be started until 5 weeks after stopping •fluoxetine; moclobemide should not be started until 2 weeks after stopping •sertraline; possible increased serotonergic effects when moclobemide given with •duloxetine
• Antimalarials: avoidance of antidepressants advised by manufacturer of •artemether/lumefantrine

Moclobemide *(continued)*
- • Bupropion: avoidance of moclobemide advised by manufacturer of •bupropion
- • Dopaminergics: caution with moclobemide advised by manufacturer of entacapone; increased risk of side-effects when moclobemide given with levodopa; avoid concomitant use of moclobemide with •selegiline
- • $5HT_1$ Agonists: risk of CNS toxicity when moclobemide given with •rizatriptan or •sumatriptan (avoid rizatriptan or sumatriptan for 2 weeks after moclobemide); risk of CNS toxicity when moclobemide given with •zolmitriptan (reduce dose of zolmitriptan)
- • Sibutramine: increased CNS toxicity when moclobemide given with •sibutramine (manufacturer of sibutramine advises avoid concomitant use), also avoid sibutramine for 2 weeks after stopping moclobemide
- • Sympathomimetics: risk of hypertensive crisis when moclobemide given with •dexamfetamine, •dopamine, •dopexamine, •ephedrine, •isometheptene, •methylphenidate, •phenylephrine, •phenylpropanolamine, •pseudoephedrine or •sympathomimetics

Ulcer-healing Drugs: plasma concentration of moclobemide increased by cimetidine (halve dose of moclobemide)

Modafinil

Antiepileptics: modafinil possibly increases plasma concentration of phenytoin
- • Ciclosporin: modafinil reduces plasma concentration of •ciclosporin
- • Oestrogens: modafinil accelerates metabolism of •oestrogens (reduced contraceptive effect—see BNF section 7.3.1)

Moexipril *see* ACE Inhibitors
Mometasone *see* Corticosteroids
Monobactams *see* Aztreonam
Montelukast *see* Leukotriene Antagonists
Morphine *see* Opioid Analgesics
Moxifloxacin *see* Quinolones

Moxisylyte (thymoxamine)

ACE Inhibitors: enhanced hypotensive effect when moxisylyte given with ACE inhibitors

Adrenergic Neurone Blockers: enhanced hypotensive effect when moxisylyte given with adrenergic neurone blockers
- • Alpha-blockers: possible severe postural hypotension when moxisylyte given with •alpha-blockers

Angiotensin-II Receptor Antagonists: enhanced hypotensive effect when moxisylyte given with angiotensin-II receptor antagonists
- • Beta-blockers: possible severe postural hypotension when moxisylyte given with •beta-blockers

Calcium-channel Blockers: enhanced hypotensive effect when moxisylyte given with calcium-channel blockers

Clonidine: enhanced hypotensive effect when moxisylyte given with clonidine

Diazoxide: enhanced hypotensive effect when moxisylyte given with diazoxide

Diuretics: enhanced hypotensive effect when moxisylyte given with diuretics

Methyldopa: enhanced hypotensive effect when moxisylyte given with methyldopa

Moxonidine: enhanced hypotensive effect when moxisylyte given with moxonidine

Nitrates: enhanced hypotensive effect when moxisylyte given with nitrates

Moxisylyte (thymoxamine) *(continued)*

Vasodilator Antihypertensives: enhanced hypotensive effect when moxisylyte given with hydralazine, minoxidil or nitroprusside

Moxonidine

ACE Inhibitors: enhanced hypotensive effect when moxonidine given with ACE inhibitors

Adrenergic Neurone Blockers: enhanced hypotensive effect when moxonidine given with adrenergic neurone blockers

Alcohol: enhanced hypotensive effect when moxonidine given with alcohol

Aldesleukin: enhanced hypotensive effect when moxonidine given with aldesleukin

Alpha-blockers: enhanced hypotensive effect when moxonidine given with alpha-blockers

Anaesthetics, General: enhanced hypotensive effect when moxonidine given with general anaesthetics

Analgesics: hypotensive effect of moxonidine antagonised by NSAIDs

Angiotensin-II Receptor Antagonists: enhanced hypotensive effect when moxonidine given with angiotensin-II receptor antagonists

Antidepressants: enhanced hypotensive effect when moxonidine given with MAOIs

Antipsychotics: enhanced hypotensive effect when moxonidine given with phenothiazines

Anxiolytics and Hypnotics: enhanced hypotensive effect when moxonidine given with anxiolytics and hypnotics; sedative effects possibly increased when moxonidine given with benzodiazepines

Beta-blockers: enhanced hypotensive effect when moxonidine given with beta-blockers

Calcium-channel Blockers: enhanced hypotensive effect when moxonidine given with calcium-channel blockers

Clonidine: enhanced hypotensive effect when moxonidine given with clonidine

Corticosteroids: hypotensive effect of moxonidine antagonised by corticosteroids

Diazoxide: enhanced hypotensive effect when moxonidine given with diazoxide

Diuretics: enhanced hypotensive effect when moxonidine given with diuretics

Dopaminergics: enhanced hypotensive effect when moxonidine given with levodopa

Methyldopa: enhanced hypotensive effect when moxonidine given with methyldopa

Moxisylyte (thymoxamine): enhanced hypotensive effect when moxonidine given with moxisylyte

Muscle Relaxants: enhanced hypotensive effect when moxonidine given with baclofen or tizanidine

Nitrates: enhanced hypotensive effect when moxonidine given with nitrates

Oestrogens: hypotensive effect of moxonidine antagonised by oestrogens

Prostaglandins: enhanced hypotensive effect when moxonidine given with alprostadil

Vasodilator Antihypertensives: enhanced hypotensive effect when moxonidine given with hydralazine, minoxidil or nitroprusside

Muscle Relaxants

ACE Inhibitors: enhanced hypotensive effect when baclofen or tizanidine given with ACE inhibitors

Adrenergic Neurone Blockers: enhanced hypotensive effect when baclofen or tizanidine given with adrenergic neurone blockers

Muscle Relaxants *(continued)*

Alcohol: increased sedative effect when baclofen, methocarbamol or tizanidine given with alcohol

Alpha-blockers: enhanced hypotensive effect when baclofen or tizanidine given with alpha-blockers

Anaesthetics, General: effects of non-depolarising muscle relaxants and suxamethonium enhanced by volatile liquid general anaesthetics

Analgesics: excretion of baclofen possibly reduced by NSAIDs (increased risk of toxicity); excretion of baclofen reduced by ibuprofen (increased risk of toxicity)

Angiotensin-II Receptor Antagonists: enhanced hypotensive effect when baclofen or tizanidine given with angiotensin-II receptor antagonists

• Anti-arrhythmics: neuromuscular blockade enhanced and prolonged when suxamethonium given with lidocaine (lignocaine); effects of muscle relaxants enhanced by •procainamide and •quinidine

• Antibacterials: effects of non-depolarising muscle relaxants and suxamethonium enhanced by piperacillin; effects of non-depolarising muscle relaxants and suxamethonium enhanced by •aminoglycosides; effects of non-depolarising muscle relaxants and suxamethonium enhanced by •clindamycin; effects of non-depolarising muscle relaxants and suxamethonium enhanced by •polymyxins; effects of suxamethonium enhanced by •vancomycin

Antidepressants: effects of suxamethonium enhanced by phenelzine; muscle relaxant effect of baclofen enhanced by tricyclics

Antiepileptics: muscle relaxant effect of non-depolarising muscle relaxants antagonised by carbamazepine and phenytoin (accelerated recovery from neuromuscular blockade)

Antimalarials: effects of suxamethonium possibly enhanced by quinine

Antipsychotics: effects of suxamethonium possibly enhanced by promazine

Anxiolytics and Hypnotics: increased sedative effect when baclofen or tizanidine given with anxiolytics and hypnotics

Beta-blockers: enhanced hypotensive effect when baclofen given with beta-blockers; possible enhanced hypotensive effect and bradycardia when tizanidine given with beta-blockers; effects of muscle relaxants enhanced by propranolol

Calcium-channel Blockers: enhanced hypotensive effect when baclofen or tizanidine given with calcium-channel blockers; effects of non-depolarising muscle relaxants enhanced by nifedipine and verapamil; risk of arrhythmias when intravenous dantrolene given with diltiazem; hypotension, myocardial depression, and hyperkalaemia when intravenous dantrolene given with verapamil; effects of suxamethonium enhanced by verapamil

Cardiac Glycosides: possible increased risk of bradycardia when tizanidine given with cardiac glycosides; risk of ventricular arrhythmias when suxamethonium given with cardiac glycosides

Clonidine: enhanced hypotensive effect when baclofen or tizanidine given with clonidine

Cytotoxics: effects of suxamethonium enhanced by cyclophosphamide and thiotepa

Muscle Relaxants *(continued)*

Diazoxide: enhanced hypotensive effect when baclofen or tizanidine given with diazoxide

Diuretics: enhanced hypotensive effect when baclofen or tizanidine given with diuretics

Dopaminergics: possible agitation, confusion and hallucinations when baclofen given with levodopa

Lithium: effects of muscle relaxants enhanced by lithium; baclofen possibly aggravates hyperkinesis caused by lithium

Magnesium (parenteral): effects of non-depolarising muscle relaxants and suxamethonium enhanced by parenteral magnesium

Memantine: effects of baclofen and dantrolene possibly modified by memantine

Methyldopa: enhanced hypotensive effect when baclofen or tizanidine given with methyldopa

Metoclopramide: effects of suxamethonium enhanced by metoclopramide

Moxonidine: enhanced hypotensive effect when baclofen or tizanidine given with moxonidine

Nitrates: enhanced hypotensive effect when baclofen or tizanidine given with nitrates

Parasympathomimetics: effects of suxamethonium possibly enhanced by donepezil; effects of non-depolarising muscle relaxants possibly antagonised by donepezil; effects of suxamethonium enhanced by edrophonium, galantamine, neostigmine, pyridostigmine and rivastigmine; effects of non-depolarising muscle relaxants antagonised by edrophonium, neostigmine, pyridostigmine and rivastigmine

Sympathomimetics, Beta$_2$: effects of suxamethonium enhanced by bambuterol

Vasodilator Antihypertensives: enhanced hypotensive effect when baclofen or tizanidine given with hydralazine; enhanced hypotensive effect when baclofen or tizanidine given with minoxidil; enhanced hypotensive effect when baclofen or tizanidine given with nitroprusside

Muscle Relaxants, depolarising *see* Muscle Relaxants

Muscle Relaxants, non-depolarising *see* Muscle Relaxants

Mycophenolate Mofetil

Antacids: absorption of mycophenolate mofetil reduced by antacids

Antiepileptics: cytotoxics possibly reduce absorption of phenytoin

• Antipsychotics: avoid concomitant use of cytotoxics with •clozapine (increased risk of agranulocytosis)

Antivirals: mycophenolate mofetil increases plasma concentration of aciclovir, also plasma concentration of inactive metabolite of mycophenolate mofetil increased; mycophenolate mofetil possibly increases plasma concentration of ganciclovir, also plasma concentration of inactive metabolite of mycophenolate mofetil possibly increased

Cardiac Glycosides: cytotoxics reduce absorption of digoxin tablets

Lipid-regulating Drugs: absorption of mycophenolate mofetil reduced by colestyramine

Nabilone

Alcohol: increased sedative effect when nabilone given with alcohol

Anxiolytics and Hypnotics: increased sedative effect when nabilone given with anxiolytics and hypnotics

Nabumetone *see* NSAIDs

Nadolol *see* Beta-blockers

Nalidixic Acid *see* Quinolones
Nandrolone *see* Anabolic Steroids
Naproxen *see* NSAIDs
Naratriptan *see* $5HT_1$ Agonists
Nateglinide *see* Antidiabetics
Nebivolol *see* Beta-blockers
Nefopam
- Antidepressants: manufacturer of nefopam advises avoid concomitant use with •MAOIs; side-effects possibly increased when nefopam given with tricyclics

Antimuscarinics: increased risk of antimuscarinic side-effects when nefopam given with antimuscarinics

Nelfinavir

Analgesics: nelfinavir reduces plasma concentration of methadone
- Anti-arrhythmics: increased risk of ventricular arrhythmias when nelfinavir given with •amiodarone or •quinidine—avoid concomitant use
- Antibacterials: nelfinavir increases plasma concentration of •rifabutin (halve dose of rifabutin); plasma concentration of nelfinavir significantly reduced by •rifampicin—avoid concomitant use
- Antidepressants: plasma concentration of nelfinavir reduced by •St John's wort—avoid concomitant use
- Antiepileptics: plasma concentration of nelfinavir possibly reduced by carbamazepine and •primidone; nelfinavir reduces plasma concentration of phenytoin
- Antimalarials: avoidance of nelfinavir advised by manufacturer of •artemether/lumefantrine

Antimuscarinics: nelfinavir increases plasma concentration of solifenacin; avoidance of nelfinavir advised by manufacturer of tolterodine
- Antipsychotics: nelfinavir possibly inhibits metabolism of •aripiprazole (reduce dose of aripiprazole); nelfinavir possibly increases plasma concentration of •pimozide (increased risk of ventricular arrhythmias—avoid concomitant use); nelfinavir increases plasma concentration of •sertindole (increased risk of ventricular arrhythmias—avoid concomitant use)

Antivirals: combination of nelfinavir with indinavir, ritonavir or saquinavir may increase plasma concentration of either drug (or both); nelfinavir reduces plasma concentration of lopinavir, also plasma concentration of active metabolite of nelfinavir increased
- Anxiolytics and Hypnotics: increased risk of prolonged sedation when nelfinavir given with •midazolam—avoid concomitant use
- Barbiturates: plasma concentration of nelfinavir possibly reduced by •barbiturates
- Ciclosporin: nelfinavir possibly increases plasma concentration of •ciclosporin
- Cilostazol: nelfinavir possibly increases plasma concentration of •cilostazol—avoid concomitant use

Cytotoxics: nelfinavir increases plasma concentration of paclitaxel
- Diuretics: nelfinavir increases plasma concentration of •eplerenone—avoid concomitant use
- Ergot Alkaloids: increased risk of ergotism when nelfinavir given with •ergotamine and methysergide—avoid concomitant use

Nelfinavir *(continued)*
- $5HT_1$ Agonists: nelfinavir increases plasma concentration of •eletriptan (risk of toxicity)—avoid concomitant use
- Ivabradine: nelfinavir possibly increases plasma concentration of •ivabradine—avoid concomitant use
- Lipid-regulating Drugs: possible increased risk of myopathy when nelfinavir given with atorvastatin; increased risk of myopathy when nelfinavir given with •simvastatin (avoid concomitant use)
- Oestrogens: nelfinavir accelerates metabolism of •oestrogens (reduced contraceptive effect—see BNF section 7.3.1)

Progestogens: nelfinavir possibly reduces contraceptive effect of progestogens

Sildenafil: nelfinavir possibly increases plasma concentration of sildenafil— reduce initial dose of sildenafil
- Tacrolimus: nelfinavir possibly increases plasma concentration of •tacrolimus

Neomycin *see* Aminoglycosides
Neostigmine *see* Parasympathomimetics
Netilmicin *see* Aminoglycosides
Nevirapine

Analgesics: nevirapine possibly reduces plasma concentration of methadone
- Antibacterials: plasma concentration of nevirapine reduced by •rifampicin—avoid concomitant use
- Anticoagulants: nevirapine may enhance or reduce anticoagulant effect of •warfarin
- Antidepressants: plasma concentration of nevirapine reduced by •St John's wort—avoid concomitant use
- Antifungals: nevirapine reduces plasma concentration of •ketoconazole—avoid concomitant use; plasma concentration of nevirapine increased by •fluconazole; nevirapine possibly reduces plasma concentration of caspofungin—consider increasing dose of caspofungin
- Antipsychotics: nevirapine possibly reduces plasma concentration of •aripiprazole—increase dose of aripiprazole
- Antivirals: nevirapine possibly reduces plasma concentration of amprenavir; nevirapine possibly reduces plasma concentration of •atazanavir—avoid concomitant use; nevirapine reduces plasma concentration of efavirenz, indinavir, lopinavir and saquinavir
- Oestrogens: nevirapine accelerates metabolism of •oestrogens (reduced contraceptive effect—see BNF section 7.3.1)
- Progestogens: nevirapine accelerates metabolism of •progestogens (reduced contraceptive effect—see BNF section 7.3.1)

Nicardipine *see* Calcium-channel Blockers
Nicorandil

Alcohol: hypotensive effect of nicorandil possibly enhanced by alcohol

Antidepressants: enhanced hypotensive effect when nicorandil given with MAOIs; hypotensive effect of nicorandil possibly enhanced by tricyclics
- Sildenafil: hypotensive effect of nicorandil significantly enhanced by •sildenafil (avoid concomitant use)
- Tadalafil: hypotensive effect of nicorandil significantly enhanced by •tadalafil (avoid concomitant use)
- Vardenafil: possible increased hypotensive effect when nicorandil given with •vardenafil—avoid concomitant use

Nicorandil *(continued)*
Vasodilator Antihypertensives: possible enhanced hypotensive effect when nicorandil given with hydralazine, minoxidil or nitroprusside

Nicotinic Acid
Note. Interactions apply to lipid-regulating doses of nicotinic acid

• Lipid-regulating Drugs: increased risk of myopathy when nicotinic acid given with •statins (applies to lipid regulating doses of nicotinic acid)

Nifedipine *see* Calcium-channel Blockers
Nimodipine *see* Calcium-channel Blockers
Nisoldipine *see* Calcium-channel Blockers

Nitrates
ACE Inhibitors: enhanced hypotensive effect when nitrates given with ACE inhibitors
Adrenergic Neurone Blockers: enhanced hypotensive effect when nitrates given with adrenergic neurone blockers
Alcohol: enhanced hypotensive effect when nitrates given with alcohol
Aldesleukin: enhanced hypotensive effect when nitrates given with aldesleukin
Alpha-blockers: enhanced hypotensive effect when nitrates given with alpha-blockers
Anaesthetics, General: enhanced hypotensive effect when nitrates given with general anaesthetics
Analgesics: hypotensive effect of nitrates antagonised by NSAIDs
Angiotensin-II Receptor Antagonists: enhanced hypotensive effect when nitrates given with angiotensin-II receptor antagonists
Anti-arrhythmics: effects of sublingual tablets of nitrates reduced by disopyramide (failure to dissolve under tongue owing to dry mouth)
• Anticoagulants: infusion of glyceryl trinitrate reduces anticoagulant effect of •heparins
Antidepressants: enhanced hypotensive effect when nitrates given with MAOIs; effects of sublingual tablets of nitrates possibly reduced by tricyclic-related antidepressants (failure to dissolve under tongue owing to dry mouth); effects of sublingual tablets of nitrates reduced by tricyclics (failure to dissolve under tongue owing to dry mouth)
Antimuscarinics: effects of sublingual tablets of nitrates possibly reduced by antimuscarinics (failure to dissolve under tongue owing to dry mouth)
Antipsychotics: enhanced hypotensive effect when nitrates given with phenothiazines
Anxiolytics and Hypnotics: enhanced hypotensive effect when nitrates given with anxiolytics and hypnotics
Beta-blockers: enhanced hypotensive effect when nitrates given with beta-blockers
Calcium-channel Blockers: enhanced hypotensive effect when nitrates given with calcium-channel blockers
Clonidine: enhanced hypotensive effect when nitrates given with clonidine
Corticosteroids: hypotensive effect of nitrates antagonised by corticosteroids
Diazoxide: enhanced hypotensive effect when nitrates given with diazoxide
Diuretics: enhanced hypotensive effect when nitrates given with diuretics
Dopaminergics: hypotensive effect of nitrates enhanced by sublingual apomorphine; enhanced hypotensive effect when nitrates given with levodopa

Nitrates *(continued)*
Methyldopa: enhanced hypotensive effect when nitrates given with methyldopa
Moxisylyte (thymoxamine): enhanced hypotensive effect when nitrates given with moxisylyte
Moxonidine: enhanced hypotensive effect when nitrates given with moxonidine
Muscle Relaxants: enhanced hypotensive effect when nitrates given with baclofen or tizanidine
Oestrogens: hypotensive effect of nitrates antagonised by oestrogens
Prostaglandins: enhanced hypotensive effect when nitrates given with alprostadil
• Sildenafil: hypotensive effect of nitrates significantly enhanced by •sildenafil (avoid concomitant use)
• Tadalafil: hypotensive effect of nitrates significantly enhanced by •tadalafil (avoid concomitant use)
• Vardenafil: possible increased hypotensive effect when nitrates given with •vardenafil—avoid concomitant use
Vasodilator Antihypertensives: enhanced hypotensive effect when nitrates given with hydralazine, minoxidil or nitroprusside

Nitrazepam *see* Anxiolytics and Hypnotics

Nitrofurantoin
Antacids: absorption of nitrofurantoin reduced by oral magnesium salts (as magnesium trisilicate)
Oestrogens: antibacterials that do not induce liver enzymes possibly reduce contraceptive effect of oestrogens (risk probably small, see BNF section 7.3.1)
Probenecid: excretion of nitrofurantoin reduced by probenecid (increased risk of side-effects)
Sulfinpyrazone: excretion of nitrofurantoin reduced by sulfinpyrazone (increased risk of toxicity)

Nitroimidazoles *see* Metronidazole and Tinidazole
Nitroprusside *see* Vasodilator Antihypertensives
Nitrous Oxide *see* Anaesthetics, General
Nizatidine *see* Histamine H_2-antagonists
Noradrenaline (norepinephrine) *see* Sympathomimetics
Norelgestromin *see* Progestogens
Norepinephrine (noradrenaline) *see* Sympathomimetics
Norethisterone *see* Progestogens
Norfloxacin *see* Quinolones
Norgestimate *see* Progestogens
Norgestrel *see* Progestogens
Nortriptyline *see* Antidepressants, Tricyclic

NSAIDs
Note. See also Aspirin. Interactions do not generally apply to topical NSAIDs
ACE Inhibitors: increased risk of renal impairment when NSAIDs given with ACE inhibitors, also hypotensive effect antagonised; increased risk of hyperkalaemia when ketorolac given with ACE inhibitors
Adrenergic Neurone Blockers: NSAIDs antagonise hypotensive effect of adrenergic neurone blockers
Alpha-blockers: NSAIDs antagonise hypotensive effect of alpha-blockers
• Analgesics: avoid concomitant use of NSAIDs with •NSAIDs or •aspirin (increased side-effects); avoid concomitant use of NSAIDs with •ketorolac (increased side-effects and haemorrhage); ibuprofen possibly reduces antiplatelet effect of aspirin
Angiotensin-II Receptor Antagonists: increased risk of renal impairment when NSAIDs given

NSAIDs

Angiotensin-II Receptor Antagonists *(continued)* with angiotensin-II receptor antagonists, also hypotensive effect antagonised; increased risk of hyperkalaemia when ketorolac given with angiotensin-II receptor antagonists

Antacids: absorption of diflunisal reduced by antacids

• Antibacterials: indometacin possibly increases plasma concentration of amikacin and gentamicin in neonates; plasma concentration of etoricoxib reduced by rifampicin; possible increased risk of convulsions when NSAIDs given with •quinolones

• Anticoagulants: celecoxib, diflunisal, etodolac, etoricoxib, flurbiprofen, ibuprofen, lumiracoxib, mefenamic acid, meloxicam, parecoxib, piroxicam and sulindac possibly enhance anticoagulant effect of •coumarins; diclofenac possibly enhances anticoagulant effect of •coumarins, also increased risk of haemorrhage with intravenous diclofenac (avoid concomitant use); NSAIDs possibly enhance anticoagulant effect of •coumarins and •phenindione; increased risk of bleeding when ketorolac given with •coumarins (avoid concomitant use); increased risk of haemorrhage when intravenous diclofenac given with •heparins (avoid concomitant use, including low-dose heparin); possible increased risk of bleeding when NSAIDs given with heparins; increased risk of haemorrhage when ketorolac given with •heparins (avoid concomitant use, including low-dose heparin); diclofenac enhances anticoagulant effect of •phenindione, also increased risk of haemorrhage with intravenous diclofenac (avoid concomitant use); ketorolac enhances anticoagulant effect of •phenindione (increased risk of haemorrhage—avoid concomitant use)

• Antidepressants: increased risk of bleeding when NSAIDs given with •SSRIs or •venlafaxine

• Antidiabetics: NSAIDs possibly enhance effects of •sulphonylureas

• Antiepileptics: NSAIDs possibly enhance effects of •phenytoin

Antifungals: plasma concentration of parecoxib increased by fluconazole (reduce dose of parecoxib); plasma concentration of celecoxib increased by fluconazole (halve dose of celecoxib)

Antipsychotics: possible severe drowsiness when indometacin given with haloperidol

• Antivirals: plasma concentration of piroxicam increased by •ritonavir (risk of toxicity)—avoid concomitant use; plasma concentration of NSAIDs possibly increased by ritonavir; increased risk of haematological toxicity when NSAIDs given with zidovudine

Beta-blockers: NSAIDs antagonise hypotensive effect of beta-blockers

Bisphosphonates: indometacin increases bioavailability of tiludronic acid

Calcium-channel Blockers: NSAIDs antagonise hypotensive effect of calcium-channel blockers

Cardiac Glycosides: NSAIDs possibly increase plasma concentration of cardiac glycosides, also possible exacerbation of heart failure and reduction of renal function

• Ciclosporin: increased risk of nephrotoxicity when NSAIDs given with •ciclosporin; plasma concentration of diclofenac increased by •ciclosporin (halve dose of diclofenac)

NSAIDs *(continued)*

Clonidine: NSAIDs antagonise hypotensive effect of clonidine

Clopidogrel: increased risk of bleeding when NSAIDs given with clopidogrel

Corticosteroids: increased risk of gastro-intestinal bleeding and ulceration when NSAIDs given with corticosteroids

• Cytotoxics: NSAIDs probably reduce excretion of •methotrexate (increased risk of toxicity); diclofenac, ibuprofen, indometacin, ketoprofen, meloxicam and naproxen reduce excretion of •methotrexate (increased risk of toxicity); increased risk of bleeding when NSAIDs given with •erlotinib

Desmopressin: indometacin enhances effects of desmopressin

Diazoxide: NSAIDs antagonise hypotensive effect of diazoxide

• Diuretics: risk of nephrotoxicity of NSAIDs increased by diuretics, also antagonism of diuretic effect; indometacin and ketorolac antagonise effects of diuretics; occasional reports of reduced renal function when indometacin given with •triamterene—avoid concomitant use; possibly increased risk of hyperkalaemia when NSAIDs given with potassium-sparing diuretics and aldosterone antagonists; increased risk of hyperkalaemia when indometacin given with potassium-sparing diuretics and aldosterone antagonists

Iloprost: increased risk of bleeding when NSAIDs given with iloprost

Lipid-regulating Drugs: excretion of meloxicam increased by colestyramine

• Lithium: NSAIDs probably reduce excretion of •lithium (increased risk of toxicity); diclofenac, ibuprofen, indometacin, mefenamic acid, naproxen, parecoxib and piroxicam reduce excretion of •lithium (increased risk of toxicity); ketorolac reduces excretion of •lithium (increased risk of toxicity)—avoid concomitant use

Methyldopa: NSAIDs antagonise hypotensive effect of methyldopa

Mifepristone: avoidance of NSAIDs advised by manufacturer of mifepristone

Moxonidine: NSAIDs antagonise hypotensive effect of moxonidine

Muscle Relaxants: NSAIDs possibly reduce excretion of baclofen (increased risk of toxicity); ibuprofen reduces excretion of baclofen (increased risk of toxicity)

Nitrates: NSAIDs antagonise hypotensive effect of nitrates

Oestrogens: etoricoxib increases plasma concentration of ethinylestradiol

Penicillamine: possible increased risk of nephrotoxicity when NSAIDs given with penicillamine

• Pentoxifylline (oxpentifylline): possible increased risk of bleeding when NSAIDs given with pentoxifylline (oxpentifylline); increased risk of bleeding when ketorolac given with •pentoxifylline (oxpentifylline) (avoid concomitant use)

• Probenecid: excretion of indometacin, ketoprofen and naproxen reduced by •probenecid (increased plasma concentration); excretion of ketorolac reduced by •probenecid (increased plasma concentration)—avoid concomitant use

Progestogens: risk of hyperkalaemia when NSAIDs given with drospirenone (monitor serum potassium during first cycle)

NSAIDs *(continued)*

Sibutramine: increased risk of bleeding when NSAIDs given with sibutramine

• Tacrolimus: possible increased risk of nephrotoxicity when NSAIDs given with tacrolimus; increased risk of nephrotoxicity when ibuprofen given with •tacrolimus

Vasodilator Antihypertensives: NSAIDs antagonise hypotensive effect of hydralazine, minoxidil and nitroprusside

Octreotide

Antidiabetics: octreotide possibly reduces requirements for insulin, metformin, repaglinide and sulphonylureas

• Ciclosporin: octreotide reduces plasma concentration of •ciclosporin

Dopaminergics: octreotide increases plasma concentration of bromocriptine

Ulcer-healing Drugs: octreotide possibly delays absorption of cimetidine

Oestrogens

Note. Interactions of combined oral contraceptives may also apply to combined contraceptive patches; in case of hormone replacement therapy low dose unlikely to induce interactions

ACE Inhibitors: oestrogens antagonise hypotensive effect of ACE inhibitors

Adrenergic Neurone Blockers: oestrogens antagonise hypotensive effect of adrenergic neurone blockers

Alpha-blockers: oestrogens antagonise hypotensive effect of alpha-blockers

Analgesics: plasma concentration of ethinylestradiol increased by etoricoxib

Angiotensin-II Receptor Antagonists: oestrogens antagonise hypotensive effect of angiotensin-II receptor antagonists

• Antibacterials: contraceptive effect of oestrogens possibly reduced by antibacterials that do not induce liver enzymes (risk probably small, see BNF section 7.3.1); metabolism of oestrogens accelerated by •rifamycins (reduced contraceptive effect—see BNF section 7.3.1)

• Anticoagulants: oestrogens antagonise anticoagulant effect of •coumarins and •phenindione

• Antidepressants: contraceptive effect of oestrogens reduced by •St John's wort (avoid concomitant use); oestrogens antagonise antidepressant effect of tricyclics (but side-effects of tricyclics possibly increased due to increased plasma concentration)

Antidiabetics: oestrogens antagonise hypoglycaemic effect of antidiabetics

• Antiepileptics: metabolism of oestrogens accelerated by •carbamazepine, •oxcarbazepine, •phenytoin, •primidone and •topiramate (reduced contraceptive effect—see BNF section 7.3.1); oestrogens reduce plasma concentration of •lamotrigine

• Antifungals: anecdotal reports of contraceptive failure when oestrogens given with fluconazole, imidazoles, itraconazole or ketoconazole; metabolism of oestrogens accelerated by •griseofulvin (reduced contraceptive effect—see BNF section 7.3.1); occasional reports of breakthrough bleeding when oestrogens (used for contraception) given with terbinafine

• Antivirals: contraceptive effect of oestrogens possibly reduced by amprenavir and efavirenz; plasma concentration of ethinylestradiol increased by •atazanavir—avoid concomitant use; metabolism of oestrogens accelerated by •nelfinavir, •nevirapine and •ritonavir

Oestrogens

• Antivirals *(continued)*
(reduced contraceptive effect—see BNF section 7.3.1)

• Aprepitant: possible contraceptive failure of hormonal contraceptives containing oestrogens when given with •aprepitant (alternative contraception recommended)

• Barbiturates: metabolism of oestrogens accelerated by •barbiturates (reduced contraceptive effect—see BNF section 7.3.1)

Beta-blockers: oestrogens antagonise hypotensive effect of beta-blockers

Bile Acids: elimination of cholesterol in bile increased when oestrogens given with bile acids

• Bosentan: possible contraceptive failure of hormonal contraceptives containing oestrogens when given with •bosentan (alternative contraception recommended)

Calcium-channel Blockers: oestrogens antagonise hypotensive effect of calcium-channel blockers

Ciclosporin: oestrogens possibly increase plasma concentration of ciclosporin

Clonidine: oestrogens antagonise hypotensive effect of clonidine

Corticosteroids: oral contraceptives containing oestrogens increase plasma concentration of corticosteroids

Diazoxide: oestrogens antagonise hypotensive effect of diazoxide

Diuretics: oestrogens antagonise diuretic effect of diuretics

Dopaminergics: oestrogens increase plasma concentration of ropinirole; oestrogens increase plasma concentration of selegiline (increased risk of toxicity)

Lipid-regulating Drugs: plasma concentration of ethinylestradiol increased by rosuvastatin

Methyldopa: oestrogens antagonise hypotensive effect of methyldopa

• Modafinil: metabolism of oestrogens accelerated by •modafinil (reduced contraceptive effect—see BNF section 7.3.1)

Moxonidine: oestrogens antagonise hypotensive effect of moxonidine

Nitrates: oestrogens antagonise hypotensive effect of nitrates

Somatropin: oestrogens (when used as oral replacement therapy) may increase dose requirements of somatropin

Tacrolimus: contraceptive effect of oestrogens possibly reduced by tacrolimus

Theophylline: oestrogens reduce excretion of theophylline (increased plasma concentration)

Vasodilator Antihypertensives: oestrogens antagonise hypotensive effect of hydralazine, minoxidil and nitroprusside

Oestrogens, conjugated *see* Oestrogens

Ofloxacin *see* Quinolones

Olanzapine *see* Antipsychotics

Olmesartan *see* Angiotensin-II Receptor Antagonists

Olsalazine *see* Aminosalicylates

Omeprazole *see* Proton Pump Inhibitors

Ondansetron

Analgesics: ondansetron possibly antagonises effects of tramadol

Antibacterials: metabolism of ondansetron accelerated by rifampicin (reduced effect)

Ondansetron *(continued)*
Antiepileptics: metabolism of ondansetron accelerated by carbamazepine and phenytoin (reduced effect)

Opioid Analgesics
Alcohol: enhanced hypotensive and sedative effects when opioid analgesics given with alcohol
Anti-arrhythmics: opioid analgesics delay absorption of mexiletine
Antibacterials: plasma concentration of alfentanil increased by erythromycin; avoidance of premedication with opioid analgesics advised by manufacturer of ciprofloxacin (reduced plasma concentration of ciprofloxacin) when ciprofloxacin used for surgical prophylaxis; metabolism of methadone accelerated by rifampicin (reduced effect)
• Anticoagulants: tramadol enhances anticoagulant effect of •coumarins; dextropropoxyphene possibly enhances anticoagulant effect of •coumarins
• Antidepressants: plasma concentration of methadone possibly increased by fluvoxamine; possible increased serotonergic effects when pethidine or tramadol given with duloxetine; CNS excitation or depression (hypertension or hypotension) when pethidine given with •MAOIs—avoid concomitant use and for 2 weeks after stopping MAOIs; possible CNS excitation or depression (hypertension or hypotension) when opioid analgesics given with •MAOIs—avoid concomitant use and for 2 weeks after stopping MAOIs; possible CNS excitation or depression (hypertension or hypotension) when opioid analgesics given with •moclobemide; possible CNS excitation or depression (hypertension or hypotension) when dextromethorphan or pethidine given with •moclobemide—avoid concomitant use; increased risk of CNS toxicity when tramadol given with •SSRIs or •tricyclics; sedative effects possibly increased when opioid analgesics given with tricyclics
• Antiepileptics: effects of tramadol reduced by carbamazepine; plasma concentration of methadone reduced by carbamazepine; dextropropoxyphene enhances effects of •carbamazepine; metabolism of methadone accelerated by phenytoin (reduced effect and risk of withdrawal effects)
• Antifungals: metabolism of alfentanil inhibited by fluconazole and ketoconazole (risk of prolonged or delayed respiratory depression); metabolism of buprenorphine inhibited by •ketoconazole (reduce dose of buprenorphine); metabolism of alfentanil possibly inhibited by itraconazole; plasma concentration of methadone increased by •voriconazole (consider reducing dose of methadone)
Antipsychotics: enhanced hypotensive and sedative effects when opioid analgesics given with antipsychotics; increased risk of convulsions when tramadol given with antipsychotics
• Antivirals: plasma concentration of methadone possibly reduced by abacavir and nevirapine; plasma concentration of methadone reduced by amprenavir, efavirenz, nelfinavir and ritonavir; plasma concentration of fentanyl increased by •ritonavir; plasma concentration of dextropropoxyphene increased by •ritonavir (risk of toxicity)—avoid concomitant use; plasma concentration of opioid analgesics (except methadone) possibly increased by •ritonavir; plasma concentration of pethidine reduced by •ritonavir, but plasma concentration of toxic pethidine metabolite increased (avoid concomitant use); methadone possibly increases plasma concentration of zidovudine
Anxiolytics and Hypnotics: increased sedative effect when opioid analgesics given with anxiolytics and hypnotics
Beta-blockers: morphine possibly increases plasma concentration of esmolol
Calcium-channel Blockers: metabolism of alfentanil inhibited by diltiazem (risk of prolonged or delayed respiratory depression)
Domperidone: opioid analgesics antagonise effects of domperidone on gastro-intestinal activity
• Dopaminergics: risk of CNS toxicity when pethidine given with •rasagiline (avoid pethidine for 2 weeks after rasagiline); avoid concomitant use of dextromethorphan with •rasagiline; hyperpyrexia and CNS toxicity reported when pethidine given with •selegiline (avoid concomitant use); caution with tramadol advised by manufacturer of selegiline
$5HT_3$ Antagonists: effects of tramadol possibly antagonised by ondansetron
• Memantine: increased risk of CNS toxicity when dextromethorphan given with •memantine (manufacturer of memantine advises avoid concomitant use)
Metoclopramide: opioid analgesics antagonise effects of metoclopramide on gastro-intestinal activity
Ulcer-healing Drugs: metabolism of opioid analgesics inhibited by cimetidine (increased plasma concentration)

Orciprenaline *see* Sympathomimetics

Orlistat
Anti-arrhythmics: orlistat possibly reduces plasma concentration of amiodarone
Anticoagulants: manufacturer of orlistat recommends monitoring anticoagulant effect of coumarins
Antidiabetics: manufacturer of orlistat advises avoid concomitant use with acarbose
• Ciclosporin: orlistat possibly reduces absorption of •ciclosporin

Orphenadrine *see* Antimuscarinics

Oxaliplatin *see* Platinum Compounds

Oxandrolone *see* Anabolic Steroids

Oxazepam *see* Anxiolytics and Hypnotics

Oxcarbazepine
• Antidepressants: anticonvulsant effect of antiepileptics possibly antagonised by MAOIs and •tricyclic-related antidepressants (convulsive threshold lowered); manufacturer of oxcarbazepine advises avoid concomitant use with •MAOIs; anticonvulsant effect of antiepileptics antagonised by •SSRIs and •tricyclics (convulsive threshold lowered)
Antiepileptics: oxcarbazepine sometimes reduces plasma concentration of carbamazepine (but concentration of an active metabolite of carbamazepine may be increased), also plasma concentration of an active metabolite of oxcarbazepine often reduced; oxcarbazepine often reduces plasma concentration of lamotrigine, also plasma concentration of an active metabolite of oxcarbazepine sometimes raised (but evidence is conflicting); oxcarba-

Oxcarbazepine
Antiepileptics *(continued)*
zepine increases plasma concentration of phenytoin, also plasma concentration of an active metabolite of oxcarbazepine reduced; oxcarbazepine increases plasma concentration of an active metabolite of primidone, also plasma concentration of an active metabolite of oxcarbazepine reduced; plasma concentration of an active metabolite of oxcarbazepine sometimes reduced by valproate
• Antimalarials: possible increased risk of convulsions when antiepileptics given with chloroquine and hydroxychloroquine; anticonvulsant effect of antiepileptics antagonised by •mefloquine
• Antipsychotics: anticonvulsant effect of oxcarbazepine antagonised by •antipsychotics (convulsive threshold lowered)
Barbiturates: oxcarbazepine increases plasma concentration of phenobarbital, also plasma concentration of an active metabolite of oxcarbazepine reduced
Ciclosporin: oxcarbazepine possibly reduces plasma concentration of ciclosporin
• Oestrogens: oxcarbazepine accelerates metabolism of •oestrogens (reduced contraceptive effect—see BNF section 7.3.1)
• Progestogens: oxcarbazepine accelerates metabolism of •progestogens (reduced contraceptive effect—see BNF section 7.3.1)

Oxprenolol *see* Beta-blockers
Oxybutynin *see* Antimuscarinics
Oxycodone *see* Opioid Analgesics
Oxymetazoline *see* Sympathomimetics
Oxytetracycline *see* Tetracyclines

Oxytocin
Anaesthetics, General: oxytocic effect possibly reduced, also enhanced hypotensive effect and risk of arrhythmias when oxytocin given with volatile liquid general anaesthetics
Prostaglandins: uterotonic effect of oxytocin potentiated by prostaglandins
Sympathomimetics: risk of hypertension when oxytocin given with vasoconstrictor sympathomimetics (due to enhanced vasopressor effect)

Paclitaxel
Antidiabetics: paclitaxel possibly inhibits metabolism of rosiglitazone
Antiepileptics: cytotoxics possibly reduce absorption of phenytoin
• Antipsychotics: avoid concomitant use of cytotoxics with •clozapine (increased risk of agranulocytosis)
Antivirals: plasma concentration of paclitaxel increased by nelfinavir and ritonavir
Cardiac Glycosides: cytotoxics reduce absorption of digoxin tablets

Pancreatin
Antidiabetics: pancreatin antagonises hypoglycaemic effect of acarbose

Pancuronium *see* Muscle Relaxants
Pantoprazole *see* Proton Pump Inhibitors
Papaveretum *see* Opioid Analgesics

Paracetamol
Anticoagulants: prolonged regular use of paracetamol possibly enhances anticoagulant effect of coumarins
Cytotoxics: paracetamol possibly inhibits metabolism of *intravenous* busulfan (manufacturer of *intravenous* busulfan advises caution within 72 hours of paracetamol)

Paracetamol *(continued)*
Lipid-regulating Drugs: absorption of paracetamol reduced by colestyramine
Metoclopramide: rate of absorption of paracetamol increased by metoclopramide

Paraldehyde
• Alcohol: increased sedative effect when paraldehyde given with •alcohol
• Disulfiram: risk of toxicity when paraldehyde given with •disulfiram

Parasympathomimetics
Anti-arrhythmics: effects of neostigmine and pyridostigmine antagonised by procainamide; effects of neostigmine and pyridostigmine possibly antagonised by propafenone; effects of neostigmine and pyridostigmine antagonised by quinidine
• Antibacterials: plasma concentration of galantamine increased by erythromycin; effects of neostigmine and pyridostigmine antagonised by •aminoglycosides; effects of neostigmine and pyridostigmine antagonised by clindamycin; effects of neostigmine and pyridostigmine antagonised by •polymyxins
Antidepressants: plasma concentration of galantamine increased by paroxetine
Antifungals: plasma concentration of galantamine increased by ketoconazole
Antimalarials: effects of neostigmine and pyridostigmine may be diminished because of potential for chloroquine and hydroxychloroquine to increase symptoms of myasthenia gravis
Antimuscarinics: effects of parasympathomimetics antagonised by antimuscarinics
Beta-blockers: increased risk of arrhythmias when pilocarpine given with beta-blockers; effects of neostigmine and pyridostigmine antagonised by propranolol
Lithium: effects of neostigmine and pyridostigmine antagonised by lithium
Muscle Relaxants: donepezil possibly enhances effects of suxamethonium; edrophonium, galantamine, neostigmine, pyridostigmine and rivastigmine enhance effects of suxamethonium; donepezil possibly antagonises effects of non-depolarising muscle relaxants ; edrophonium, neostigmine, pyridostigmine and rivastigmine antagonise effects of non-depolarising muscle relaxants

Parecoxib *see* NSAIDs
Paroxetine *see* Antidepressants, SSRI
Pegfilgrastim *see* Filgrastim
Peginterferon Alfa *see* Interferons

Penicillamine
Analgesics: possible increased risk of nephrotoxicity when penicillamine given with NSAIDs
Antacids: absorption of penicillamine reduced by antacids
• Antipsychotics: avoid concomitant use of penicillamine with •clozapine (increased risk of agranulocytosis)
Cardiac Glycosides: penicillamine possibly reduces plasma concentration of digoxin
Iron: absorption of penicillamine reduced by *oral* iron
Zinc: penicillamine reduces absorption of zinc, also absorption of penicillamine reduced by zinc

Penicillins
Allopurinol: increased risk of rash when amoxicillin or ampicillin given with allopurinol
Antibacterials: absorption of phenoxymethylpenicillin reduced by neomycin

Penicillins *(continued)*
Anticoagulants: common experience in anticoagulant clinics is that INR can be altered by a course of broad-spectrum penicillins such as ampicillin, although studies have failed to demonstrate an interaction with coumarins or phenindione
Cytotoxics: penicillins reduce excretion of methotrexate (increased risk of toxicity)
Muscle Relaxants: piperacillin enhances effects of non-depolarising muscle relaxants and suxamethonium
Oestrogens: antibacterials that do not induce liver enzymes possibly reduce contraceptive effect of oestrogens (risk probably small, see BNF section 7.3.1)
Probenecid: excretion of penicillins reduced by probenecid (increased plasma concentration)
Sulfinpyrazone: excretion of penicillins reduced by sulfinpyrazone

Pentamidine Isetionate
• Anti-arrhythmics: increased risk of ventricular arrhythmias when pentamidine isetionate given with •amiodarone—avoid concomitant use
• Antibacterials: increased risk of ventricular arrhythmias when pentamidine isetionate given with •moxifloxacin—avoid concomitant use
Antifungals: possible increased risk of nephrotoxicity when pentamidine isetionate given with amphotericin
• Antipsychotics: increased risk of ventricular arrhythmias when pentamidine isetionate given with •amisulpride—avoid concomitant use
• Ivabradine: increased risk of ventricular arrhythmias when pentamidine isetionate given with •ivabradine

Pentazocine *see* Opioid Analgesics

Pentostatin
Antiepileptics: cytotoxics possibly reduce absorption of phenytoin
• Antipsychotics: avoid concomitant use of cytotoxics with •clozapine (increased risk of agranulocytosis)
Cardiac Glycosides: cytotoxics reduce absorption of digoxin tablets
• Cytotoxics: increased toxicity when pentostatin given with high-dose •cyclophosphamide—avoid concomitant use; increased pulmonary toxicity when pentostatin given with •fludarabine (unacceptably high incidence of fatalities)

Pentoxifylline (oxpentifylline)
• Analgesics: possible increased risk of bleeding when pentoxifylline (oxpentifylline) given with NSAIDs; increased risk of bleeding when pentoxifylline (oxpentifylline) given with •ketorolac (avoid concomitant use)
Theophylline: pentoxifylline (oxpentifylline) increases plasma concentration of theophylline

Pergolide
Antipsychotics: effects of pergolide antagonised by antipsychotics
Memantine: effects of dopaminergics possibly enhanced by memantine
Methyldopa: antiparkinsonian effect of dopaminergics antagonised by methyldopa
Metoclopramide: antiparkinsonian effect of pergolide antagonised by metoclopramide

Pericyazine *see* Antipsychotics
Perindopril *see* ACE Inhibitors
Perphenazine *see* Antipsychotics
Pethidine *see* Opioid Analgesics
Phenazocine *see* Opioid Analgesics
Phenelzine *see* MAOIs

Phenindione
Note. Change in patient's clinical condition particularly associated with liver disease, intercurrent illness, or drug administration, necessitates more frequent testing. Major changes in diet (especially involving salads and vegetables) and in alcohol consumption may also affect anticoagulant control
• Alcohol: anticoagulant control with phenindione may be affected by major changes in consumption of •alcohol
• Anabolic Steroids: anticoagulant effect of phenindione enhanced by •anabolic steroids
• Analgesics: anticoagulant effect of phenindione possibly enhanced by •NSAIDs; anticoagulant effect of phenindione enhanced by •diclofenac, also increased risk of haemorrhage with intravenous diclofenac (avoid concomitant use); anticoagulant effect of phenindione enhanced by •ketorolac (increased risk of haemorrhage—avoid concomitant use); increased risk of bleeding when phenindione given with •aspirin (due to antiplatelet effect)
• Anti-arrhythmics: metabolism of phenindione inhibited by •amiodarone (enhanced anticoagulant effect)
• Antibacterials: experience in anticoagulant clinics suggests that INR possibly altered when phenindione is given with •neomycin (given for local action on gut); anticoagulant effect of phenindione possibly enhanced by levofloxacin and •tetracyclines; studies have failed to demonstrate an interaction with phenindione, but common experience in anticoagulant clinics is that INR can be altered by a course of broad-spectrum penicillins such as ampicillin
• Antivirals: anticoagulant effect of phenindione possibly enhanced by •ritonavir
• Clopidogrel: anticoagulant effect of phenindione enhanced due to antiplatelet action of •clopidogrel
• Dipyridamole: anticoagulant effect of phenindione enhanced due to antiplatelet action of •dipyridamole
• Enteral Foods: anticoagulant effect of phenindione antagonised by vitamin K (present in some •enteral feeds)
Iloprost: increased risk of bleeding when phenindione given with iloprost
• Lipid-regulating Drugs: anticoagulant effect of phenindione may be enhanced or reduced by •colestyramine; anticoagulant effect of phenindione possibly enhanced by •rosuvastatin; anticoagulant effect of phenindione enhanced by •fibrates
• Oestrogens: anticoagulant effect of phenindione antagonised by •oestrogens
• Progestogens: anticoagulant effect of phenindione antagonised by •progestogens
Sibutramine: increased risk of bleeding when anticoagulants given with sibutramine
• Testolactone: anticoagulant effect of phenindione enhanced by •testolactone
• Testosterone: anticoagulant effect of phenindione enhanced by •testosterone
• Thyroid Hormones: anticoagulant effect of phenindione enhanced by •thyroid hormones
• Vitamins: anticoagulant effect of phenindione antagonised by •vitamin K

Phenobarbital *see* Barbiturates
Phenoperidine *see* Opioid Analgesics

Phenothiazines *see* Antipsychotics
Phenoxybenzamine *see* Alpha-blockers
Phenoxymethylpenicillin *see* Penicillins
Phentolamine *see* Alpha-blockers
Phenylephrine *see* Sympathomimetics
Phenylpropanolamine *see* Sympathomimetics
Phenytoin

- • Analgesics: effects of phenytoin possibly enhanced by •NSAIDs; phenytoin accelerates metabolism of methadone (reduced effect and risk of withdrawal effects); effects of phenytoin enhanced by aspirin
- Antacids: absorption of phenytoin reduced by antacids
- • Anti-arrhythmics: metabolism of phenytoin inhibited by •amiodarone (increased plasma concentration); phenytoin reduces plasma concentration of disopyramide; phenytoin accelerates metabolism of mexiletine and •quinidine (reduced plasma concentration)
- • Antibacterials: metabolism of phenytoin inhibited by clarithromycin, •isoniazid and •metronidazole (increased plasma concentration); plasma concentration of phenytoin increased or decreased by ciprofloxacin; phenytoin accelerates metabolism of doxycycline (reduced plasma concentration); plasma concentration of phenytoin increased by •chloramphenicol (increased risk of toxicity); metabolism of phenytoin accelerated by •rifamycins (reduced plasma concentration); plasma concentration of phenytoin possibly increased by sulphonamides; phenytoin reduces plasma concentration of •telithromycin (avoid during and for 2 weeks after phenytoin); plasma concentration of phenytoin increased by •trimethoprim (also increased antifolate effect)
- • Anticoagulants: phenytoin accelerates metabolism of •coumarins (possibility of reduced anticoagulant effect, but enhancement also reported)
- • Antidepressants: plasma concentration of phenytoin increased by •fluoxetine and •fluvoxamine; phenytoin reduces plasma concentration of •mianserin, mirtazapine and paroxetine; anticonvulsant effect of antiepileptics possibly antagonised by MAOIs and •tricyclic-related antidepressants (convulsive threshold lowered); anticonvulsant effect of antiepileptics antagonised by •SSRIs and •tricyclics (convulsive threshold lowered); plasma concentration of phenytoin reduced by •St John's wort—avoid concomitant use; phenytoin possibly reduces plasma concentration of •tricyclics
- Antidiabetics: plasma concentration of phenytoin transiently increased by tolbutamide (possibility of toxicity)
- • Antiepileptics: plasma concentration of both drugs often reduced when phenytoin given with carbamazepine, also plasma concentration of phenytoin may be increased; plasma concentration of phenytoin possibly increased by •ethosuximide, also plasma concentration of ethosuximide possibly reduced; phenytoin reduces plasma concentration of lamotrigine, tiagabine and zonisamide; plasma concentration of phenytoin increased by oxcarbazepine, also plasma concentration of an active metabolite of oxcarbazepine reduced; phenytoin possibly reduces plasma concentration of primidone (but concentration of an active

Phenytoin

- • Antiepileptics *(continued)* metabolite increased), plasma concentration of phenytoin often reduced but may be increased; plasma concentration of phenytoin increased by •topiramate (also plasma concentration of topiramate reduced); plasma concentration of phenytoin increased or possibly reduced when given with valproate, also plasma concentration of valproate reduced; plasma concentration of phenytoin reduced by vigabatrin
- • Antifungals: phenytoin reduces plasma concentration of •ketoconazole; anticonvulsant effect of phenytoin enhanced by •miconazole (plasma concentration of phenytoin increased); plasma concentration of phenytoin increased by •fluconazole (consider reducing dose of phenytoin); phenytoin reduces plasma concentration of •itraconazole—avoid concomitant use; plasma concentration of phenytoin increased by •voriconazole, also phenytoin reduces plasma concentration of voriconazole (increase dose of voriconazole and also monitor for phenytoin toxicity); phenytoin possibly reduces plasma concentration of caspofungin—consider increasing dose of caspofungin
- • Antimalarials: possible increased risk of convulsions when antiepileptics given with chloroquine and hydroxychloroquine; anticonvulsant effect of antiepileptics antagonised by •mefloquine; anticonvulsant effect of phenytoin antagonised by •pyrimethamine, also increased antifolate effect
- • Antipsychotics: anticonvulsant effect of phenytoin antagonised by •antipsychotics (convulsive threshold lowered); phenytoin possibly reduces plasma concentration of •aripiprazole—increase dose of aripiprazole; phenytoin accelerates metabolism of clozapine, quetiapine and sertindole (reduced plasma concentration)
- Antivirals: phenytoin possibly reduces plasma concentration of abacavir, amprenavir, indinavir, lopinavir and saquinavir; plasma concentration of phenytoin reduced by nelfinavir; plasma concentration of phenytoin increased or decreased by zidovudine
- Anxiolytics and Hypnotics: phenytoin often reduces plasma concentration of clonazepam; plasma concentration of phenytoin increased or decreased by diazepam; plasma concentration of phenytoin possibly increased or decreased by benzodiazepines
- Aprepitant: phenytoin possibly reduces plasma concentration of aprepitant
- Barbiturates: phenytoin often increases plasma concentration of phenobarbital, plasma concentration of phenytoin often reduced but may be increased
- Bupropion: phenytoin reduces plasma concentration of bupropion
- • Calcium-channel Blockers: phenytoin reduces effects of felodipine, isradipine and verapamil; phenytoin probably reduces effects of dihydropyridines, nicardipine and •nifedipine; phenytoin reduces plasma concentration of nisoldipine; plasma concentration of phenytoin increased by •diltiazem but also effect of diltiazem reduced
- Cardiac Glycosides: phenytoin accelerates metabolism of digitoxin (reduced

Phenytoin
Cardiac Glycosides *(continued)* effect); phenytoin possibly reduces plasma concentration of digoxin
• Ciclosporin: phenytoin accelerates metabolism of •ciclosporin (reduced plasma concentration)
• Corticosteroids: phenytoin accelerates metabolism of •corticosteroids (reduced effect)
• Cytotoxics: phenytoin possibly reduces plasma concentration of busulfan and etoposide; metabolism of phenytoin possibly inhibited by fluorouracil (increased risk of toxicity); phenytoin increases antifolate effect of methotrexate; absorption of phenytoin possibly reduced by cytotoxics; phenytoin reduces plasma concentration of •imatinib—avoid concomitant use
Diazoxide: plasma concentration of phenytoin reduced by diazoxide, also effect of diazoxide may be reduced
• Disulfiram: metabolism of phenytoin inhibited by •disulfiram (increased risk of toxicity)
• Diuretics: phenytoin reduces plasma concentration of •eplerenone—avoid concomitant use; increased risk of osteomalacia when phenytoin given with carbonic anhydrase inhibitors
Dopaminergics: phenytoin possibly reduces effects of levodopa
Enteral Foods: absorption of phenytoin possibly reduced by enteral feeds
Folates: plasma concentration of phenytoin possibly reduced by folates
Hormone Antagonists: phenytoin accelerates metabolism of gestrinone (reduced plasma concentration); phenytoin possibly accelerates metabolism of toremifene
$5HT_3$ Antagonists: phenytoin accelerates metabolism of ondansetron (reduced effect)
Leflunomide: plasma concentration of phenytoin possibly increased by leflunomide
Levamisole: plasma concentration of phenytoin possibly increased by levamisole
Lipid-regulating Drugs: combination of phenytoin with fluvastatin may increase plasma concentration of either drug (or both)
Lithium: neurotoxicity may occur when phenytoin given with lithium without increased plasma concentration of lithium
Modafinil: plasma concentration of phenytoin possibly increased by modafinil
Muscle Relaxants: phenytoin antagonises muscle relaxant effect of non-depolarising muscle relaxants (accelerated recovery from neuromuscular blockade)
• Oestrogens: phenytoin accelerates metabolism of •oestrogens (reduced contraceptive effect—see BNF section 7.3.1)
• Progestogens: phenytoin accelerates metabolism of •progestogens (reduced contraceptive effect—see BNF section 7.3.1)
• Sulfinpyrazone: plasma concentration of phenytoin increased by •sulfinpyrazone
Sympathomimetics: plasma concentration of phenytoin increased by methylphenidate
• Theophylline: plasma concentration of both drugs reduced when phenytoin given with •theophylline
Thyroid Hormones: phenytoin accelerates metabolism of thyroid hormones (may increase requirements in hypothyroidism), also plasma concentration of phenytoin possibly increased

Phenytoin *(continued)*
Tibolone: phenytoin accelerates metabolism of tibolone
• Ulcer-healing Drugs: metabolism of phenytoin inhibited by •cimetidine (increased plasma concentration); effects of phenytoin enhanced by •esomeprazole; effects of phenytoin possibly enhanced by omeprazole; absorption of phenytoin reduced by •sucralfate
Vaccines: effects of phenytoin enhanced by influenza vaccine
Vitamins: phenytoin possibly increases requirements for vitamin D

Phosphodiesterase Inhibitors
• Anagrelide: avoidance of enoximone and milrinone advised by manufacturer of •anagrelide

Physostigmine *see* Parasympathomimetics
Pilocarpine *see* Parasympathomimetics
Pimozide *see* Antipsychotics
Pindolol *see* Beta-blockers
Pioglitazone *see* Antidiabetics
Piperacillin *see* Penicillins
Pipotiazine *see* Antipsychotics
Piroxicam *see* NSAIDs
Pivmecillinam *see* Penicillins

Pizotifen
Adrenergic Neurone Blockers: pizotifen antagonises hypotensive effect of adrenergic neurone blockers

Platinum Compounds
• Antibacterials: increased risk of nephrotoxicity and possibly of ototoxicity when platinum compounds given with •aminoglycosides or •polymyxins; increased risk of nephrotoxicity and ototoxicity when platinum compounds given with capreomycin; increased risk of nephrotoxicity and possibly of ototoxicity when cisplatin given with vancomycin
Antiepileptics: cytotoxics possibly reduce absorption of phenytoin
• Antipsychotics: avoid concomitant use of cytotoxics with •clozapine (increased risk of agranulocytosis)
Cardiac Glycosides: cytotoxics reduce absorption of digoxin tablets
• Cytotoxics: increased pulmonary toxicity when cisplatin given with •bleomycin and •methotrexate
Diuretics: increased risk of nephrotoxicity and ototoxicity when platinum compounds given with diuretics

Polymyxin B *see* Polymyxins

Polymyxins
Antibacterials: increased risk of nephrotoxicity when colistin or polymyxins given with aminoglycosides; increased risk of nephrotoxicity when colistin or polymyxins given with capreomycin; increased risk of nephrotoxicity and ototoxicity when colistin given with teicoplanin or vancomycin; increased risk of nephrotoxicity when polymyxins given with vancomycin
Antifungals: increased risk of nephrotoxicity when polymyxins given with amphotericin
• Ciclosporin: increased risk of nephrotoxicity when polymyxins given with •ciclosporin
• Cytotoxics: increased risk of nephrotoxicity and possibly of ototoxicity when polymyxins given with •platinum compounds
• Diuretics: increased risk of otoxicity when polymyxins given with •loop diuretics
• Muscle Relaxants: polymyxins enhance effects of •non-depolarising muscle relaxants and •suxamethonium

Polymyxins *(continued)*
Oestrogens: antibacterials that do not induce liver enzymes possibly reduce contraceptive effect of oestrogens (risk probably small, see BNF section 7.3.1)
• Parasympathomimetics: polymyxins antagonise effects of •neostigmine and •pyridostigmine

Potassium Aminobenzoate
Antibacterials: potassium aminobenzoate inhibits effects of sulphonamides

Potassium Bicarbonate *see* Potassium Salts
Potassium Chloride *see* Potassium Salts
Potassium Citrate *see* Potassium Salts

Potassium Salts
Note. Includes salt substitutes
• ACE Inhibitors: increased risk of severe hyperkalaemia when potassium salts given with •ACE inhibitors
• Angiotensin-II Receptor Antagonists: increased risk of hyperkalaemia when potassium salts given with •angiotensin-II receptor antagonists
Antibacterials: avoid concomitant use of potassium citrate with methenamine
• Ciclosporin: increased risk of hyperkalaemia when potassium salts given with •ciclosporin
• Diuretics: increased risk of hyperkalaemia when potassium salts given with •potassium-sparing diuretics and aldosterone antagonists
• Tacrolimus: increased risk of hyperkalaemia when potassium salts given with •tacrolimus

Pramipexole
Antipsychotics: manufacturer of pramipexole advises avoid concomitant use of antipsychotics (antagonism of effect)
Memantine: effects of dopaminergics possibly enhanced by memantine
Methyldopa: antiparkinsonian effect of dopaminergics antagonised by methyldopa
Ulcer-healing Drugs: excretion of pramipexole reduced by cimetidine (increased plasma concentration)

Pravastatin *see* Statins
Prazosin *see* Alpha-blockers
Prednisolone *see* Corticosteroids

Prilocaine
Anti-arrhythmics: increased myocardial depression when prilocaine given with anti-arrhythmics
Antibacterials: increased risk of methaemoglobinaemia when prilocaine given with sulphonamides

Primaquine
• Antimalarials: avoidance of antimalarials advised by manufacturer of •artemether/lumefantrine
Mepacrine: plasma concentration of primaquine increased by mepacrine (increased risk of toxicity)

Primidone
Alcohol: increased sedative effect when primidone given with alcohol
Anti-arrhythmics: primidone accelerates metabolism of disopyramide and quinidine (reduced plasma concentration)
• Antibacterials: primidone accelerates metabolism of •chloramphenicol, doxycycline and metronidazole (reduced plasma concentration); primidone reduces plasma concentration of •telithromycin (avoid during and for 2 weeks after primidone)
• Anticoagulants: primidone accelerates metabolism of •coumarins (reduced anticoagulant effect)
• Antidepressants: primidone reduces plasma concentration of paroxetine; primidone accelerates metabolism of •mianserin (reduced plasma concentration); anticonvulsant effect of antiepileptics possibly antagonised by MAOIs and •tricyclic-related antidepressants (convulsive threshold lowered); anticonvulsant effect of antiepileptics antagonised by •SSRIs and •tricyclics (convulsive threshold lowered); plasma concentration of active metabolite of primidone reduced by •St John's wort—avoid concomitant use; anticonvulsant effect of primidone antagonised by •tricyclics (convulsive threshold lowered), also metabolism of tricyclics possibly accelerated (reduced plasma concentration)
• Antiepileptics: primidone often reduces plasma concentration of carbamazepine, also plasma concentration of primidone sometimes reduced (but concentration of an active metabolite of primidone often increased); primidone possibly reduces plasma concentration of ethosuximide; primidone reduces plasma concentration of lamotrigine and tiagabine; plasma concentration of an active metabolite of primidone increased by oxcarbazepine, also plasma concentration of an active metabolite of oxcarbazepine reduced; plasma concentration of primidone possibly reduced by phenytoin (but concentration of an active metabolite increased), plasma concentration of phenytoin often reduced but may be increased; plasma concentration of primidone possibly increased by •valproate (plasma concentration of active metabolite of primidone increased), also plasma concentration of valproate reduced; plasma concentration of primidone possibly reduced by vigabatrin
• Antifungals: primidone possibly reduces plasma concentration of •voriconazole—avoid concomitant use; primidone reduces absorption of griseofulvin (reduced effect)
• Antimalarials: possible increased risk of convulsions when antiepileptics given with chloroquine and hydroxychloroquine; anticonvulsant effect of antiepileptics antagonised by •mefloquine
• Antipsychotics: anticonvulsant effect of primidone antagonised by •antipsychotics (convulsive threshold lowered); primidone accelerates metabolism of haloperidol (reduced plasma concentration); primidone possibly reduces plasma concentration of •aripiprazole—increase dose of aripiprazole
• Antivirals: primidone possibly reduces plasma concentration of •indinavir, •lopinavir, •nelfinavir and •saquinavir
Anxiolytics and Hypnotics: primidone often reduces plasma concentration of clonazepam
Barbiturates: increased sedative effect when primidone given with barbiturates
• Calcium-channel Blockers: primidone reduces effects of •felodipine and •isradipine; primidone probably reduces effects of •dihydropyridines, •diltiazem and •verapamil
Cardiac Glycosides: primidone accelerates metabolism of digitoxin (reduced effect)
• Ciclosporin: primidone accelerates metabolism of •ciclosporin (reduced effect)
• Corticosteroids: primidone accelerates metabolism of •corticosteroids (reduced effect)
Diuretics: plasma concentration of primidone possibly reduced by acetazolamide; increased

Primidone
Diuretics *(continued)*
risk of osteomalacia when primidone given with carbonic anhydrase inhibitors
Folates: plasma concentration of primidone possibly reduced by folates
Hormone Antagonists: primidone accelerates metabolism of gestrinone and toremifene (reduced plasma concentration)
$5HT_3$ Antagonists: primidone reduces plasma concentration of tropisetron
Leukotriene Antagonists: primidone reduces plasma concentration of montelukast
Memantine: effects of primidone possibly reduced by memantine
• Oestrogens: primidone accelerates metabolism of •oestrogens (reduced contraceptive effect—see BNF section 7.3.1)
• Progestogens: primidone accelerates metabolism of •progestogens (reduced contraceptive effect—see BNF section 7.3.1)
Sympathomimetics: plasma concentration of primidone possibly increased by methylphenidate
Theophylline: primidone accelerates metabolism of theophylline (reduced effect)
Thyroid Hormones: primidone accelerates metabolism of thyroid hormones (may increase requirements for thyroid hormones in hypothyroidism)
Tibolone: primidone accelerates metabolism of tibolone (reduced plasma concentration)
Vitamins: primidone possibly increases requirements for vitamin D

Probenecid
ACE Inhibitors: probenecid reduces excretion of captopril
• Analgesics: probenecid reduces excretion of •indometacin, •ketoprofen and •naproxen (increased plasma concentration); probenecid reduces excretion of •ketorolac (increased plasma concentration)—avoid concomitant use; effects of probenecid antagonised by aspirin
Antibacterials: probenecid reduces excretion of meropenem (manufacturers of meropenem advise avoid concomitant use); probenecid reduces excretion of cephalosporins, ciprofloxacin, nalidixic acid, norfloxacin and penicillins (increased plasma concentration); probenecid reduces excretion of dapsone and nitrofurantoin (increased risk of side-effects); effects of probenecid antagonised by pyrazinamide
Antidiabetics: probenecid possibly enhances hypoglycaemic effect of chlorpropamide
Antivirals: probenecid reduces excretion of aciclovir (increased plasma concentration); probenecid possibly reduces excretion of famciclovir (increased plasma concentration); probenecid reduces excretion of ganciclovir and zidovudine (increased plasma concentration and risk of toxicity)
• Cytotoxics: probenecid reduces excretion of •methotrexate (increased risk of toxicity)
Sodium Benzoate: probenecid possibly reduces excretion of conjugate formed by sodium benzoate
Sodium Phenylbutyrate: probenecid possibly reduces excretion of conjugate formed by sodium phenylbutyrate

Procainamide
ACE Inhibitors: increased risk of toxicity when procainamide given with captopril especially in renal impairment
Anaesthetics, Local: increased myocardial depression when anti-arrhythmics given with bupivacaine, levobupivacaine or prilocaine
• Anti-arrhythmics: increased myocardial depression when anti-arrhythmics given with other •anti-arrhythmics; plasma concentration of procainamide increased by •amiodarone (increased risk of ventricular arrhythmias—avoid concomitant use)
• Antibacterials: increased risk of ventricular arrhythmias when procainamide given with •moxifloxacin—avoid concomitant use; plasma concentration of procainamide increased by trimethoprim
• Antidepressants: increased risk of ventricular arrhythmias when procainamide given with •tricyclics
• Antihistamines: increased risk of ventricular arrhythmias when procainamide given with •mizolastine—avoid concomitant use
• Antimalarials: avoidance of procainamide advised by manufacturer of •artemether/lumefantrine (risk of ventricular arrhythmias)
• Antipsychotics: increased risk of ventricular arrhythmias when anti-arrhythmics that prolong the QT interval given with •antipsychotics that prolong the QT interval; increased risk of ventricular arrhythmias when procainamide given with •amisulpride, •pimozide or •sertindole—avoid concomitant use; increased risk of ventricular arrhythmias when procainamide given with •phenothiazines
• Beta-blockers: increased myocardial depression when anti-arrhythmics given with •beta-blockers; increased risk of ventricular arrhythmias when procainamide given with •sotalol—avoid concomitant use
• Dolasetron: increased risk of ventricular arrhythmias when procainamide given with •dolasetron—avoid concomitant use
$5HT_3$ Antagonists: caution with anti-arrhythmics advised by manufacturer of tropisetron (risk of ventricular arrhythmias)
• Muscle Relaxants: procainamide enhances effects of •muscle relaxants
Parasympathomimetics: procainamide antagonises effects of neostigmine and pyridostigmine
• Ulcer-healing Drugs: plasma concentration of procainamide increased by •cimetidine

Procaine
Laronidase: procaine possibly inhibits effects of laronidase (manufacturer of laronidase advises avoid concomitant use)

Procarbazine
Alcohol: disulfiram-like reaction when procarbazine given with alcohol
Antiepileptics: cytotoxics possibly reduce absorption of phenytoin
• Antipsychotics: avoid concomitant use of cytotoxics with •clozapine (increased risk of agranulocytosis)
Cardiac Glycosides: cytotoxics reduce absorption of digoxin tablets

Prochlorperazine *see* Antipsychotics
Procyclidine *see* Antimuscarinics
Progesterone *see* Progestogens
Progestogens
Note. Interactions of combined oral contraceptives may also apply to combined contraceptive patches

Progestogens *(continued)*
ACE Inhibitors: risk of hyperkalaemia when drospirenone given with ACE inhibitors (monitor serum potassium during first cycle)
Analgesics: risk of hyperkalaemia when drospirenone given with NSAIDs (monitor serum potassium during first cycle)
Angiotensin-II Receptor Antagonists: risk of hyperkalaemia when drospirenone given with angiotensin-II receptor antagonists (monitor serum potassium during first cycle)
• Antibacterials: metabolism of progestogens accelerated by •rifamycins (reduced contraceptive effect—see BNF section 7.3.1)
• Anticoagulants: progestogens antagonise anticoagulant effect of •coumarins and •phenindione
• Antidepressants: contraceptive effect of progestogens reduced by •St John's wort (avoid concomitant use)
Antidiabetics: progestogens antagonise hypoglycaemic effect of antidiabetics
• Antiepileptics: metabolism of progestogens accelerated by •carbamazepine, •oxcarbazepine, •phenytoin, •primidone and •topiramate (reduced contraceptive effect—see BNF section 7.3.1); progestogens reduce plasma concentration of •lamotrigine
• Antifungals: metabolism of progestogens accelerated by •griseofulvin (reduced contraceptive effect—see BNF section 7.3.1); occasional reports of breakthrough bleeding when progestogens (used for contraception) given with terbinafine
• Antivirals: contraceptive effect of progestogens possibly reduced by amprenavir and nelfinavir; metabolism of progestogens accelerated by •nevirapine (reduced contraceptive effect—see BNF section 7.3.1)
• Aprepitant: possible contraceptive failure of hormonal contraceptives containing progestogens when given with •aprepitant (alternative contraception recommended)
• Barbiturates: metabolism of progestogens accelerated by •barbiturates (reduced contraceptive effect—see BNF section 7.3.1)
• Bosentan: possible contraceptive failure of hormonal contraceptives containing progestogens when given with •bosentan (alternative contraception recommended)
• Ciclosporin: progestogens inhibit metabolism of •ciclosporin (increased plasma concentration)
Diuretics: risk of hyperkalaemia when drospirenone given with potassium-sparing diuretics and aldosterone antagonists (monitor serum potassium during first cycle)
Dopaminergics: progestogens increase plasma concentration of selegiline (increased risk of toxicity)
Lipid-regulating Drugs: plasma concentration of norgestrel increased by rosuvastatin
• Retinoids: efficacy of low dose progestogens may be reduced by •tretinoin but need not affect prescribing of combined oral contraceptives, there is no compelling evidence of interaction between isotretinoin and combined oral contraceptives
Tacrolimus: contraceptive effect of progestogens possibly reduced by tacrolimus

Proguanil
Antacids: absorption of proguanil reduced by oral magnesium salts (as magnesium trisilicate)
Anticoagulants: isolated reports that proguanil may enhance anticoagulant effect of warfarin

Proguanil *(continued)*
• Antimalarials: avoidance of antimalarials advised by manufacturer of •artemether/lumefantrine; increased antifolate effect when proguanil given with pyrimethamine

Promazine *see* Antipsychotics
Promethazine *see* Antihistamines
Propafenone
Anaesthetics, Local: increased myocardial depression when anti-arrhythmics given with bupivacaine, levobupivacaine or prilocaine
• Anti-arrhythmics: increased myocardial depression when anti-arrhythmics given with other •anti-arrhythmics; plasma concentration of propafenone increased by quinidine
• Antibacterials: metabolism of propafenone accelerated by •rifampicin (reduced effect)
• Anticoagulants: propafenone enhances anticoagulant effect of •coumarins
• Antidepressants: metabolism of propafenone possibly inhibited by paroxetine (increased risk of toxicity); increased risk of arrhythmias when propafenone given with •tricyclics
• Antihistamines: increased risk of ventricular arrhythmias when propafenone given with •mizolastine—avoid concomitant use
• Antipsychotics: increased risk of ventricular arrhythmias when anti-arrhythmics that prolong the QT interval given with •antipsychotics that prolong the QT interval
• Antivirals: plasma concentration of propafenone possibly increased by •amprenavir (increased risk of ventricular arrhythmias—avoid concomitant use); plasma concentration of propafenone increased by •ritonavir (increased risk of ventricular arrhythmias—avoid concomitant use)
• Beta-blockers: increased myocardial depression when anti-arrhythmics given with •beta-blockers; propafenone increases plasma concentration of metoprolol and propranolol
• Cardiac Glycosides: propafenone increases plasma concentration of •digoxin (halve dose of digoxin)
Ciclosporin: propafenone possibly increases plasma concentration of ciclosporin
• Dolasetron: increased risk of ventricular arrhythmias when propafenone given with •dolasetron—avoid concomitant use
$5HT_3$ Antagonists: caution with anti-arrhythmics advised by manufacturer of tropisetron (risk of ventricular arrhythmias)
Parasympathomimetics: propafenone possibly antagonises effects of neostigmine and pyridostigmine
Theophylline: propafenone increases plasma concentration of theophylline
• Ulcer-healing Drugs: plasma concentration of propafenone increased by •cimetidine

Propantheline *see* Antimuscarinics
Propiverine *see* Antimuscarinics
Propofol *see* Anaesthetics, General
Propranolol *see* Beta-blockers
Prostaglandins
ACE Inhibitors: enhanced hypotensive effect when alprostadil given with ACE inhibitors
Adrenergic Neurone Blockers: enhanced hypotensive effect when alprostadil given with adrenergic neurone blockers
Alpha-blockers: enhanced hypotensive effect when alprostadil given with alpha-blockers
Angiotensin-II Receptor Antagonists: enhanced hypotensive effect when alprostadil given with angiotensin-II receptor antagonists

Prostaglandins *(continued)*
Beta-blockers: enhanced hypotensive effect when alprostadil given with beta-blockers
Calcium-channel Blockers: enhanced hypotensive effect when alprostadil given with calcium-channel blockers
Clonidine: enhanced hypotensive effect when alprostadil given with clonidine
Diazoxide: enhanced hypotensive effect when alprostadil given with diazoxide
Diuretics: enhanced hypotensive effect when alprostadil given with diuretics
Methyldopa: enhanced hypotensive effect when alprostadil given with methyldopa
Moxonidine: enhanced hypotensive effect when alprostadil given with moxonidine
Nitrates: enhanced hypotensive effect when alprostadil given with nitrates
Oxytocin: prostaglandins potentiate uterotonic effect of oxytocin
Vasodilator Antihypertensives: enhanced hypotensive effect when alprostadil given with hydralazine, minoxidil or nitroprusside

Proton Pump Inhibitors
Antacids: absorption of lansoprazole possibly reduced by antacids
Antibacterials: plasma concentration of both drugs increased when omeprazole given with clarithromycin
• Anticoagulants: esomeprazole and omeprazole possibly enhance anticoagulant effect of •coumarins
Antidepressants: omeprazole increases plasma concentration of escitalopram
• Antiepileptics: esomeprazole enhances effects of •phenytoin; omeprazole possibly enhances effects of phenytoin
Antifungals: proton pump inhibitors reduce absorption of itraconazole and ketoconazole; plasma concentration of omeprazole increased by voriconazole (reduce dose of omeprazole)
Antipsychotics: omeprazole possibly reduces plasma concentration of clozapine
• Antivirals: proton pump inhibitors possibly reduce plasma concentration of •atazanavir—avoid concomitant use; omeprazole significantly reduces plasma concentration of •atazanavir—avoid concomitant use
Anxiolytics and Hypnotics: esomeprazole and omeprazole possibly inhibit metabolism of diazepam (increased plasma concentration)
Cardiac Glycosides: proton pump inhibitors possibly slightly increase plasma concentration of digoxin
Ciclosporin: omeprazole possibly affects plasma concentration of ciclosporin
• Cilostazol: omeprazole increases plasma concentration of •cilostazol (risk of toxicity)—avoid concomitant use; lansoprazole possibly increases plasma concentration of •cilostazol—avoid concomitant use
Cytotoxics: omeprazole possibly reduces excretion of methotrexate (increased risk of toxicity)
Tacrolimus: omeprazole possibly increases plasma concentration of tacrolimus
Ulcer-healing Drugs: absorption of lansoprazole possibly reduced by sucralfate

Pseudoephedrine *see* Sympathomimetics

Pyrazinamide
Oestrogens: antibacterials that do not induce liver enzymes possibly reduce contraceptive effect of oestrogens (risk probably small, see BNF section 7.3.1)

Pyrazinamide *(continued)*
Probenecid: pyrazinamide antagonises effects of probenecid
Sulfinpyrazone: pyrazinamide antagonises effects of sulfinpyrazone

Pyridostigmine *see* Parasympathomimetics

Pyridoxine *see* Vitamins

Pyrimethamine
• Antibacterials: increased antifolate effect when pyrimethamine (includes Fansidar®) given with •sulphonamides; increased antifolate effect when pyrimethamine given with •trimethoprim
• Antiepileptics: pyrimethamine antagonises anticonvulsant effect of •phenytoin, also increased antifolate effect
• Antimalarials: avoidance of antimalarials advised by manufacturer of •artemether/lumefantrine; increased antifolate effect when pyrimethamine given with proguanil
Antivirals: increased antifolate effect when pyrimethamine given with zidovudine
• Cytotoxics: pyrimethamine increases antifolate effect of •methotrexate

Quetiapine *see* Antipsychotics

Quinagolide
Memantine: effects of dopaminergics possibly enhanced by memantine
Methyldopa: antiparkinsonian effect of dopaminergics antagonised by methyldopa

Quinapril *see* ACE Inhibitors

Quinidine
Adsorbents: absorption of quinidine possibly reduced by kaolin
Anaesthetics, Local: increased myocardial depression when anti-arrhythmics given with bupivacaine, levobupivacaine or prilocaine
Antacids: excretion of quinidine reduced by alkaline urine due to some antacids (plasma concentration of quinidine occasionally increased)
• Anti-arrhythmics: increased myocardial depression when anti-arrhythmics given with other •anti-arrhythmics; plasma concentration of quinidine increased by •amiodarone (increased risk of ventricular arrhythmias—avoid concomitant use); quinidine increases plasma concentration of propafenone
• Antibacterials: increased risk of ventricular arrhythmias when quinidine given with •clarithromycin; increased risk of ventricular arrhythmias when quinidine given with parenteral •erythromycin; increased risk of ventricular arrhythmias when quinidine given with •moxifloxacin or •quinupristin/dalfopristin—avoid concomitant use; metabolism of quinidine accelerated by •rifamycins (reduced plasma concentration)
• Anticoagulants: quinidine possibly enhances anticoagulant effect of •coumarins
• Antidepressants: increased risk of ventricular arrhythmias when quinidine given with •tricyclics
• Antiepileptics: metabolism of quinidine accelerated by •phenytoin and primidone (reduced plasma concentration)
• Antifungals: plasma concentration of quinidine increased by •itraconazole, •miconazole and •voriconazole (increased risk of ventricular arrhythmias—avoid concomitant use)
• Antihistamines: increased risk of ventricular arrhythmias when quinidine given with •mizolastine—avoid concomitant use
• Antimalarials: avoidance of quinidine advised by manufacturer of •artemether/lumefantrine

Quinidine

- Antimalarials *(continued)*
  (risk of ventricular arrhythmias); increased risk of ventricular arrhythmias when quinidine given with •mefloquine
- Antipsychotics: increased risk of ventricular arrhythmias when anti-arrhythmics that prolong the QT interval given with •antipsychotics that prolong the QT interval; increased risk of ventricular arrhythmias when quinidine given with •amisulpride, •pimozide or •sertindole—avoid concomitant use; quinidine inhibits metabolism of •aripiprazole (reduce dose of aripiprazole); increased risk of ventricular arrhythmias when quinidine given with •phenothiazines
- Antivirals: plasma concentration of quinidine possibly increased by •amprenavir (increased risk of ventricular arrhythmias—avoid concomitant use); plasma concentration of quinidine possibly increased by •atazanavir—avoid concomitant use; increased risk of ventricular arrhythmias when quinidine given with •nelfinavir—avoid concomitant use; plasma concentration of quinidine increased by •ritonavir (increased risk of ventricular arrhythmias—avoid concomitant use)

Barbiturates: metabolism of quinidine accelerated by barbiturates (reduced plasma concentration)

- Beta-blockers: increased myocardial depression when anti-arrhythmics given with •beta-blockers; increased risk of ventricular arrhythmias when quinidine given with •sotalol—avoid concomitant use
- Calcium-channel Blockers: plasma concentration of quinidine reduced by nifedipine; plasma concentration of quinidine increased by •verapamil (extreme hypotension may occur)
- Cardiac Glycosides: quinidine increases plasma concentration of •digoxin (halve dose of digoxin)
- Diuretics: excretion of quinidine possibly reduced by •acetazolamide (increased plasma concentration), also cardiotoxicity of quinidine increased in hypokalaemia; increased cardiac toxicity with quinidine if hypokalaemia occurs with •loop diuretics or •thiazides and related diuretics

$5HT_3$ Antagonists: caution with anti-arrhythmics advised by manufacturer of tropisetron (risk of ventricular arrhythmias)

- Ivabradine: increased risk of ventricular arrhythmias when quinidine given with •ivabradine
- Muscle Relaxants: quinidine enhances effects of •muscle relaxants

Parasympathomimetics: quinidine antagonises effects of neostigmine and pyridostigmine

- Ulcer-healing Drugs: plasma concentration of quinidine increased by •cimetidine

Quinine

- Anti-arrhythmics: increased risk of ventricular arrhythmias when quinine given with •amiodarone—avoid concomitant use; quinine increases plasma concentration of •flecainide
- Antibacterials: increased risk of ventricular arrhythmias when quinine given with •moxifloxacin—avoid concomitant use
- Antimalarials: avoidance of antimalarials advised by manufacturer of •artemether/lumefantrine; increased risk of convulsions when quinine given with •mefloquine (but should not prevent the use of intravenous quinine in severe cases)
- Antipsychotics: increased risk of ventricular arrhythmias when quinine given with •pimozide—avoid concomitant use
- Cardiac Glycosides: quinine increases plasma concentration of •digoxin

Muscle Relaxants: quinine possibly enhances effects of suxamethonium

Ulcer-healing Drugs: metabolism of quinine inhibited by cimetidine (increased plasma concentration)

Quinolones

- Analgesics: possible increased risk of convulsions when quinolones given with •NSAIDs; manufacturer of ciprofloxacin advises avoid premedication with opioid analgesics (reduced plasma concentration of ciprofloxacin) when ciprofloxacin used for surgical prophylaxis

Antacids: absorption of ciprofloxacin, levofloxacin, moxifloxacin, norfloxacin and ofloxacin reduced by antacids

- Anti-arrhythmics: increased risk of ventricular arrhythmias when moxifloxacin given with •amiodarone, •disopyramide, •procainamide or •quinidine—avoid concomitant use
- Antibacterials: increased risk of ventricular arrhythmias when moxifloxacin given with parenteral •erythromycin—avoid concomitant use
- Anticoagulants: ciprofloxacin, nalidixic acid, norfloxacin and ofloxacin enhance anticoagulant effect of •coumarins; levofloxacin possibly enhances anticoagulant effect of coumarins and phenindione
- Antidepressants: ciprofloxacin inhibits metabolism of •duloxetine—avoid concomitant use; increased risk of ventricular arrhythmias when moxifloxacin given with •tricyclics—avoid concomitant use

Antidiabetics: ciprofloxacin and norfloxacin possibly enhance effects of glibenclamide

Antiepileptics: ciprofloxacin increases or decreases plasma concentration of phenytoin

- Antihistamines: increased risk of ventricular arrhythmias when moxifloxacin given with •mizolastine—avoid concomitant use
- Antimalarials: avoidance of quinolones advised by manufacturer of •artemether/lumefantrine; increased risk of ventricular arrhythmias when moxifloxacin given with •chloroquine and hydroxychloroquine, •mefloquine or •quinine—avoid concomitant use
- Antipsychotics: increased risk of ventricular arrhythmias when moxifloxacin given with •haloperidol, •phenothiazines, •pimozide or •sertindole—avoid concomitant use; ciprofloxacin possibly increases plasma concentration of olanzapine
- Beta-blockers: increased risk of ventricular arrhythmias when moxifloxacin given with •sotalol—avoid concomitant use

Calcium Salts: absorption of ciprofloxacin reduced by calcium salts

- Ciclosporin: increased risk of nephrotoxicity when quinolones given with •ciclosporin

Cytotoxics: nalidixic acid increases risk of melphalan toxicity; ciprofloxacin possibly reduces excretion of methotrexate (increased risk of toxicity)

Quinolones *(continued)*

Dairy Products: absorption of ciprofloxacin and norfloxacin reduced by dairy products

$5HT_1$ Agonists: quinolones possibly inhibit metabolism of zolmitriptan (reduce dose of zolmitriptan)

Iron: absorption of ciprofloxacin, levofloxacin, moxifloxacin, norfloxacin and ofloxacin reduced by *oral* iron

Oestrogens: antibacterials that do not induce liver enzymes possibly reduce contraceptive effect of oestrogens (risk probably small, see BNF section 7.3.1)

• Pentamidine Isetionate: increased risk of ventricular arrhythmias when moxifloxacin given with •pentamidine isetionate—avoid concomitant use

Probenecid: excretion of ciprofloxacin, nalidixic acid and norfloxacin reduced by probenecid (increased plasma concentration)

Strontium Ranelate: absorption of quinolones reduced by strontium ranelate (manufacturer of strontium ranelate advises avoid concomitant use)

• Theophylline: possible increased risk of convulsions when quinolones given with •theophylline; ciprofloxacin and norfloxacin increase plasma concentration of •theophylline

Ulcer-healing Drugs: absorption of ciprofloxacin, levofloxacin, moxifloxacin, norfloxacin and ofloxacin reduced by sucralfate

Zinc: absorption of ciprofloxacin, levofloxacin, moxifloxacin, norfloxacin and ofloxacin reduced by zinc

Quinupristin with Dalfopristin

• Anti-arrhythmics: increased risk of ventricular arrhythmias when quinupristin/dalfopristin given with •disopyramide, •lidocaine (lignocaine) or •quinidine—avoid concomitant use

Antibacterials: manufacturer of quinupristin/dalfopristin recommends monitoring liver function when given with rifampicin

Antivirals: quinupristin/dalfopristin possibly increases plasma concentration of saquinavir

• Anxiolytics and Hypnotics: quinupristin/dalfopristin inhibits metabolism of •midazolam (increased plasma concentration with increased sedation); quinupristin/dalfopristin inhibits the metabolism of zopiclone

• Calcium-channel Blockers: quinupristin/dalfopristin increases plasma concentration of •nifedipine

• Ciclosporin: quinupristin/dalfopristin increases plasma concentration of •ciclosporin

• Ergot Alkaloids: manufacturer of quinupristin/dalfopristin advises avoid concomitant use with •ergotamine and methysergide

Oestrogens: antibacterials that do not induce liver enzymes possibly reduce contraceptive effect of oestrogens (risk probably small, see BNF section 7.3.1)

• Tacrolimus: quinupristin/dalfopristin increases plasma concentration of •tacrolimus

Rabeprazole *see* Proton Pump Inhibitors

Raloxifene

Anticoagulants: raloxifene antagonises anticoagulant effect of coumarins

Lipid-regulating Drugs: absorption of raloxifene reduced by colestyramine (manufacturer of raloxifene advises avoid concomitant administration)

Ramipril *see* ACE Inhibitors

Ranitidine *see* Histamine H_2-antagonists

Ranitidine Bismuth Citrate *see* Histamine H_2-antagonists

Rasagiline

Note. Rasagiline is a MAO-B inhibitor

• Analgesics: avoid concomitant use of rasagiline with •dextromethorphan; risk of CNS toxicity when rasagiline given with •pethidine (avoid pethidine for 2 weeks after rasagiline)

• Antidepressants: after stopping rasagiline do not start •fluoxetine for 2 weeks, also rasagiline should not be started until at least 5 weeks after stopping fluoxetine; after stopping rasagiline do not start •fluvoxamine for 2 weeks; risk of hypertensive crisis when rasagiline given with •MAOIs, avoid MAOIs for at least 2 weeks after stopping rasagiline; increased risk of CNS toxicity when rasagiline given with •SSRIs or •tricyclics

Dopaminergics: plasma concentration of rasagiline possibly reduced by entacapone

Memantine: effects of dopaminergics possibly enhanced by memantine

Methyldopa: antiparkinsonian effect of dopaminergics antagonised by methyldopa

• Sympathomimetics: avoid concomitant use of rasagiline with •sympathomimetics

Reboxetine

• Antibacterials: manufacturer of reboxetine advises avoid concomitant use with •macrolides

• Antidepressants: manufacturer of reboxetine advises avoid concomitant use with •fluvoxamine; increased risk of hypertension and CNS excitation when reboxetine given with •MAOIs (MAOIs should not be started until 1 week after stopping reboxetine, avoid reboxetine for 2 weeks after stopping MAOIs)

• Antifungals: manufacturer of reboxetine advises avoid concomitant use with •imidazoles and •triazoles

• Antimalarials: avoidance of antidepressants advised by manufacturer of •artemether/lumefantrine

Diuretics: possible increased risk of hypokalaemia when reboxetine given with loop diuretics or thiazides and related diuretics

Ergot Alkaloids: possible risk of hypertension when reboxetine given with ergotamine and methysergide

• Sibutramine: increased risk of CNS toxicity when noradrenaline re-uptake inhibitors given with •sibutramine (manufacturer of sibutramine advises avoid concomitant use)

Remifentanil *see* Opioid Analgesics

Repaglinide *see* Antidiabetics

Retinoids

Alcohol: etretinate formed from acitretin in presence of alcohol

• Antibacterials: possible increased risk of benign intracranial hypertension when retinoids given with •tetracyclines (avoid concomitant use)

• Anticoagulants: acitretin possibly reduces anticoagulant effect of •coumarins

Antiepileptics: isotretinoin possibly reduces plasma concentration of carbamazepine

• Cytotoxics: acitretin increases plasma concentration of •methotrexate (also increased risk of hepatotoxicity)—avoid concomitant use

• Progestogens: oral tretinoin may reduce contraceptive efficacy of low dose •progestogens but need not affect prescribing of combined oral contraceptives, there is no compelling evi-

Retinoids
• Progestogens *(continued)*
dence of interaction between isotretinoin and combined oral contraceptives
Vitamins: risk of hypervitaminosis A when retinoids given with vitamin A

Reviparin *see* Heparins

Ribavirin
• Antivirals: ribavirin possibly inhibits effects of •stavudine; ribavirin possibly inhibits effects of •zidovudine (manufacturer of zidovudine advises avoid concomitant use)

Rifabutin *see* Rifamycins

Rifampicin *see* Rifamycins

Rifamycins
ACE Inhibitors: rifampicin reduces plasma concentration of active metabolite of imidapril (reduced antihypertensive effect)
Analgesics: rifampicin reduces plasma concentration of etoricoxib; rifampicin accelerates metabolism of methadone (reduced effect)
Antacids: absorption of rifampicin reduced by antacids
• Anti-arrhythmics: rifamycins accelerate metabolism of •disopyramide and •quinidine (reduced plasma concentration); rifampicin accelerates metabolism of mexiletine (reduced plasma concentration); rifampicin accelerates metabolism of •propafenone (reduced effect)
• Antibacterials: rifamycins reduce plasma concentration of clarithromycin and dapsone; plasma concentration of rifabutin increased by •clarithromycin (increased risk of uveitis—reduce rifabutin dose); rifampicin accelerates metabolism of chloramphenicol (reduced plasma concentration); plasma concentration of rifabutin possibly increased by •macrolides (increased risk of uveitis—reduce rifabutin dose); monitoring of liver function with rifampicin recommended by manufacturer of quinupristin/dalfopristin; rifampicin reduces plasma concentration of •telithromycin (avoid during and for 2 weeks after rifampicin)
• Anticoagulants: rifamycins accelerate metabolism of •coumarins (reduced anticoagulant effect)
Antidepressants: rifampicin possibly reduces plasma concentration of tricyclics
• Antidiabetics: rifamycins accelerate metabolism of •chlorpropamide and •tolbutamide (reduced effect);
rifampicin reduces plasma concentration of •rosiglitazone—consider increasing dose of rosiglitazone; rifampicin reduces plasma concentration of nateglinide and repaglinide; rifamycins possibly accelerate metabolism of •sulphonylureas (reduced effect)
• Antiepileptics: rifabutin reduces plasma concentration of •carbamazepine; rifampicin reduces plasma concentration of •lamotrigine; rifamycins accelerate metabolism of •phenytoin (reduced plasma concentration)
• Antifungals: rifampicin accelerates metabolism of •ketoconazole (reduced plasma concentration), also plasma concentration of rifampicin may be reduced by ketoconazole; plasma concentration of rifabutin increased by •fluconazole (increased risk of uveitis—reduce rifabutin dose); rifampicin accelerates metabolism of •fluconazole and •itraconazole (reduced plasma concentration); rifabutin reduces plasma concentration of •itraconazole—avoid concomitant use; plasma concentration of rifabutin increased by •voriconazole, also rifabutin reduces plasma concentration of voriconazole (increase dose of voriconazole and also monitor for rifabutin toxicity); rifampicin reduces plasma concentration of •voriconazole—avoid concomitant use; rifampicin initially increases and then reduces plasma concentration of caspofungin (consider increasing dose of caspofungin); rifampicin reduces plasma concentration of terbinafine; plasma concentration of rifabutin possibly increased by •triazoles (increased risk of uveitis—reduce rifabutin dose)
• Antipsychotics: rifampicin accelerates metabolism of •haloperidol (reduced plasma concentration); rifabutin and rifampicin possibly reduce plasma concentration of •aripiprazole—increase dose of aripiprazole; rifampicin possibly reduces plasma concentration of clozapine
• Antivirals: rifampicin possibly reduces plasma concentration of abacavir; rifampicin significantly reduces plasma concentration of •amprenavir, •nelfinavir and •saquinavir—avoid concomitant use; plasma concentration of rifabutin increased by •amprenavir, •atazanavir and •tipranavir (reduce dose of rifabutin); rifampicin reduces plasma concentration of •atazanavir, •lopinavir and •nevirapine—avoid concomitant use; plasma concentration of rifabutin reduced by efavirenz—increase dose of rifabutin; rifampicin reduces plasma concentration of efavirenz—increase dose of efavirenz; rifampicin accelerates metabolism of •indinavir (reduced plasma concentration—avoid concomitant use); plasma concentration of rifabutin increased by •indinavir, also plasma concentration of indinavir decreased (reduce dose of rifabutin and increase dose of indinavir); plasma concentration of rifabutin increased by •nelfinavir (halve dose of rifabutin); plasma concentration of rifabutin increased by •ritonavir (risk of uveitis—avoid concomitant use); rifabutin significantly reduces plasma concentration of •saquinavir—avoid concomitant use unless another protease inhibitor also given e.g. ritonavir; rifampicin possibly reduces plasma concentration of •tipranavir—avoid concomitant use; avoidance of rifampicin advised by manufacturer of zidovudine
Anxiolytics and Hypnotics: rifampicin accelerates metabolism of diazepam (reduced plasma concentration); rifampicin possibly accelerates metabolism of benzodiazepines (reduced plasma concentration); rifampicin possibly accelerates metabolism of buspirone and zaleplon; rifampicin accelerates metabolism of zolpidem (reduced plasma concentration and reduced effect)
Aprepitant: rifampicin reduces plasma concentration of aprepitant
• Atovaquone: rifabutin and rifampicin reduce plasma concentration of •atovaquone (possible therapeutic failure of atovaquone)
Beta-blockers: rifampicin accelerates metabolism of bisoprolol and propranolol (plasma concentration significantly reduced)
• Calcium-channel Blockers: rifampicin possibly accelerates metabolism of •isradipine, •nicardipine and •nisoldipine (possible signifi-

Rifamycins

- Calcium-channel Blockers *(continued)* cantly reduced plasma concentration); rifampicin accelerates metabolism of •diltiazem, •nifedipine, •nimodipine and •verapamil (plasma concentration significantly reduced)
  Cardiac Glycosides: rifamycins accelerate metabolism of digitoxin (reduced effect); rifampicin possibly reduces plasma concentration of digoxin
- Ciclosporin: rifampicin accelerates metabolism of •ciclosporin (reduced plasma concentration)
- Corticosteroids: rifamycins accelerate metabolism of •corticosteroids (reduced effect)
- Cytotoxics: rifampicin accelerates metabolism of erlotinib (reduced plasma concentration); rifampicin reduces plasma concentration of •imatinib—avoid concomitant use
- Diuretics: rifampicin reduces plasma concentration of •eplerenone—avoid concomitant use
  Hormone Antagonists: rifampicin possibly reduces plasma concentration of exemestane; rifampicin accelerates metabolism of gestrinone (reduced plasma concentration)
  $5HT_3$ Antagonists: rifampicin accelerates metabolism of ondansetron (reduced effect); rifampicin reduces plasma concentration of tropisetron
  Lipid-regulating Drugs: rifampicin accelerates metabolism of fluvastatin (reduced effect)
- Oestrogens: rifamycins accelerate metabolism of •oestrogens (reduced contraceptive effect—see BNF section 7.3.1); antibacterials that do not induce liver enzymes possibly reduce contraceptive effect of oestrogens (risk probably small, see BNF section 7.3.1)
- Progestogens: rifamycins accelerate metabolism of •progestogens (reduced contraceptive effect—see BNF section 7.3.1)
- Sirolimus: rifabutin and rifampicin reduce plasma concentration of •sirolimus—avoid concomitant use
- Tacrolimus: rifampicin reduces plasma concentration of •tacrolimus
  Tadalafil: rifampicin reduces plasma concentration of tadalafil
  Theophylline: rifampicin accelerates metabolism of theophylline (reduced plasma concentration)
  Thyroid Hormones: rifampicin accelerates metabolism of levothyroxine (thyroxine) (may increase requirements for levothyroxine (thyroxine) in hypothyroidism)
  Tibolone: rifampicin accelerates metabolism of tibolone (reduced plasma concentration)
  Ulcer-healing Drugs: rifampicin accelerates metabolism of cimetidine (reduced plasma concentration)

Risedronate Sodium *see* Bisphosphonates
Risperidone *see* Antipsychotics
Ritodrine *see* Sympathomimetics, $Beta_2$
Ritonavir

- Analgesics: ritonavir possibly increases plasma concentration of NSAIDs; ritonavir increases plasma concentration of •dextropropoxyphene and •piroxicam (risk of toxicity)—avoid concomitant use; ritonavir increases plasma concentration of •fentanyl; ritonavir reduces plasma concentration of methadone; ritonavir reduces plasma concentration of •pethidine, but increases plasma concentration of toxic metabolite of pethidine (avoid concomitant use); ritonavir possibly increases plasma concentration of •opioid analgesics (except methadone)
- Anti-arrhythmics: ritonavir increases plasma concentration of •amiodarone, •flecainide, •propafenone and •quinidine (increased risk of ventricular arrhythmias—avoid concomitant use); ritonavir possibly increases plasma concentration of •disopyramide and •mexiletine (increased risk of toxicity)
- Antibacterials: ritonavir possibly increases plasma concentration of azithromycin and erythromycin; ritonavir increases plasma concentration of •clarithromycin (reduce dose of clarithromycin in renal impairment); ritonavir increases plasma concentration of •rifabutin (risk of uveitis—avoid concomitant use); plasma concentration of both drugs may increase when ritonavir given with fusidic acid
- Anticoagulants: ritonavir may enhance or reduce anticoagulant effect of •warfarin; ritonavir possibly enhances anticoagulant effect of •coumarins and •phenindione
- Antidepressants: ritonavir possibly increases plasma concentration of •SSRIs and •tricyclics; plasma concentration of ritonavir reduced by •St John's wort—avoid concomitant use
  Antidiabetics: ritonavir possibly increases plasma concentration of tolbutamide
- Antiepileptics: ritonavir possibly increases plasma concentration of •carbamazepine
- Antifungals: combination of ritonavir with •itraconazole or •ketoconazole may increase plasma concentration of either drug (or both); plasma concentration of ritonavir increased by fluconazole; ritonavir reduces plasma concentration of •voriconazole—avoid concomitant use
  Antihistamines: ritonavir possibly increases plasma concentration of non-sedating antihistamines
- Antimalarials: avoidance of ritonavir advised by manufacturer of •artemether/lumefantrine
  Antimuscarinics: ritonavir increases plasma concentration of solifenacin; avoidance of ritonavir advised by manufacturer of tolterodine
- Antipsychotics: ritonavir possibly increases plasma concentration of •antipsychotics; ritonavir possibly inhibits metabolism of •aripiprazole (reduce dose of aripiprazole); ritonavir increases plasma concentration of •clozapine (increased risk of toxicity)—avoid concomitant use; ritonavir increases plasma concentration of •pimozide and •sertindole (increased risk of ventricular arrhythmias—avoid concomitant use)
- Antivirals: ritonavir increases plasma concentration of amprenavir, indinavir and •saquinavir; ritonavir increases toxicity of efavirenz, monitor liver function tests; combination of ritonavir with nelfinavir may increase plasma concentration of either drug (or both)
- Anxiolytics and Hypnotics: ritonavir possibly increases plasma concentration of •anxiolytics and hypnotics; ritonavir possibly increases plasma concentration of •alprazolam, •diazepam, •flurazepam, •midazolam and •zolpidem (risk of extreme sedation and respiratory depression —avoid concomitant use); ritonavir increases plasma concentration of buspirone (increased risk of toxicity)

Ritonavir *(continued)*

Aprepitant: ritonavir possibly increases plasma concentration of aprepitant

Bosentan: ritonavir possibly increases plasma concentration of bosentan

• Bupropion: ritonavir increases plasma concentration of •bupropion (risk of toxicity)—avoid concomitant use

• Calcium-channel Blockers: ritonavir possibly increases plasma concentration of •calcium-channel blockers; avoidance of ritonavir advised by manufacturer of lercanidipine

• Ciclosporin: ritonavir possibly increases plasma concentration of •ciclosporin

• Cilostazol: ritonavir possibly increases plasma concentration of •cilostazol—avoid concomitant use

• Corticosteroids: ritonavir possibly increases plasma concentration of corticosteroids, dexamethasone and prednisolone; ritonavir increases plasma concentration of inhaled and intranasal budesonide and •fluticasone

Cytotoxics: ritonavir increases plasma concentration of paclitaxel

• Diuretics: ritonavir increases plasma concentration of •eplerenone—avoid concomitant use

• Ergot Alkaloids: increased risk of ergotism when ritonavir given with •ergotamine and methysergide—avoid concomitant use

• $5HT_1$ Agonists: ritonavir increases plasma concentration of •eletriptan (risk of toxicity)—avoid concomitant use

• Ivabradine: ritonavir possibly increases plasma concentration of •ivabradine—avoid concomitant use

• Lipid-regulating Drugs: possible increased risk of myopathy when ritonavir given with atorvastatin; increased risk of myopathy when ritonavir given with •simvastatin (avoid concomitant use)

• Oestrogens: ritonavir accelerates metabolism of •oestrogens (reduced contraceptive effect—see BNF section 7.3.1)

• Sildenafil: ritonavir significantly increases plasma concentration of •sildenafil—avoid concomitant use

Sympathomimetics: ritonavir possibly increases plasma concentration of dexamfetamine

• Tacrolimus: ritonavir possibly increases plasma concentration of •tacrolimus

Tadalafil: ritonavir increases plasma concentration of tadalafil

• Theophylline: ritonavir accelerates metabolism of •theophylline (reduced plasma concentration)

• Vardenafil: ritonavir possibly increases plasma concentration of •vardenafil—avoid concomitant use

Rivastigmine *see* Parasympathomimetics

Rizatriptan *see* $5HT_1$ Agonists

Rocuronium *see* Muscle Relaxants

Ropinirole

Antipsychotics: manufacturer of ropinirole advises avoid concomitant use of antipsychotics (antagonism of effect)

Memantine: effects of dopaminergics possibly enhanced by memantine

Methyldopa: antiparkinsonian effect of dopaminergics antagonised by methyldopa

Metoclopramide: antiparkinsonian effect of ropinirole antagonised by metoclopramide (manufacturers of ropinirole advise avoid concomitant use)

Ropinirole *(continued)*

Oestrogens: plasma concentration of ropinirole increased by oestrogens

Ropivacaine

Antidepressants: metabolism of ropivacaine inhibited by fluvoxamine—avoid prolonged administration of ropivacaine

Rosiglitazone *see* Antidiabetics

Rosuvastatin *see* Statins

Rowachol®

Anticoagulants: Rowachol® possibly reduces anticoagulant effect of coumarins

St John's Wort

• Antibacterials: St John's wort reduces plasma concentration of •telithromycin (avoid during and for 2 weeks after St John's wort)

• Anticoagulants: St John's wort reduces anticoagulant effect of •coumarins (avoid concomitant use)

• Antidepressants: possible increased serotonergic effects when St John's wort given with duloxetine; St John's wort reduces plasma concentration of amitriptyline; increased serotonergic effects when St John's wort given with •SSRIs—avoid concomitant use

• Antiepileptics: St John's wort reduces plasma concentration of •carbamazepine and •phenytoin—avoid concomitant use; St John's wort reduces plasma concentration of active metabolite of •primidone—avoid concomitant use

• Antimalarials: avoidance of antidepressants advised by manufacturer of •artemether/lumefantrine

• Antipsychotics: St John's wort possibly reduces plasma concentration of •aripiprazole—increase dose of aripiprazole

• Antivirals: St John's wort reduces plasma concentration of •amprenavir, •atazanavir, •efavirenz, •indinavir, •lopinavir, •nelfinavir, •nevirapine, •ritonavir and •saquinavir—avoid concomitant use; St John's wort possibly reduces plasma concentration of •tipranavir—avoid concomitant use

• Aprepitant: avoidance of St John's wort advised by manufacturer of •aprepitant

• Barbiturates: St John's wort reduces plasma concentration of •phenobarbital—avoid concomitant use

• Cardiac Glycosides: St John's wort reduces plasma concentration of •digoxin—avoid concomitant use

• Ciclosporin: St John's wort reduces plasma concentration of •ciclosporin—avoid concomitant use

• Diuretics: St John's wort reduces plasma concentration of •eplerenone—avoid concomitant use

• $5HT_1$ Agonists: increased serotonergic effects when St John's wort given with •$5HT_1$ agonists—avoid concomitant use

Ivabradine: St John's wort reduces plasma concentration of ivabradine—avoid concomitant use

Lipid-regulating Drugs: St John's wort reduces plasma concentration of simvastatin

• Oestrogens: St John's wort reduces contraceptive effect of •oestrogens (avoid concomitant use)

• Progestogens: St John's wort reduces contraceptive effect of •progestogens (avoid concomitant use)

St John's Wort *(continued)*
- • Tacrolimus: St John's wort reduces plasma concentration of •tacrolimus—avoid concomitant use
- • Theophylline: St John's wort reduces plasma concentration of •theophylline—avoid concomitant use

Salbutamol *see* Sympathomimetics, $Beta_2$

Salmeterol *see* Sympathomimetics, $Beta_2$

Saquinavir
- • Antibacterials: plasma concentration of saquinavir significantly reduced by •rifabutin—avoid concomitant use unless another protease inhibitor also given e.g. ritonavir; plasma concentration of saquinavir significantly reduced by •rifampicin—avoid concomitant use; plasma concentration of saquinavir possibly increased by quinupristin/dalfopristin
- Anticoagulants: saquinavir possibly enhances anticoagulant effect of warfarin
- • Antidepressants: plasma concentration of saquinavir reduced by •St John's wort—avoid concomitant use
- • Antiepileptics: plasma concentration of saquinavir possibly reduced by carbamazepine, phenytoin and •primidone
- Antifungals: plasma concentration of saquinavir increased by ketoconazole; plasma concentration of saquinavir possibly increased by imidazoles and triazoles
- • Antimalarials: avoidance of saquinavir advised by manufacturer of •artemether/lumefantrine
- Antimuscarinics: avoidance of saquinavir advised by manufacturer of tolterodine
- • Antipsychotics: saquinavir possibly inhibits metabolism of •aripiprazole (reduce dose of aripiprazole); saquinavir possibly increases plasma concentration of •pimozide (increased risk of ventricular arrhythmias—avoid concomitant use); saquinavir increases plasma concentration of •sertindole (increased risk of ventricular arrhythmias—avoid concomitant use)
- • Antivirals: plasma concentration of saquinavir increased by atazanavir, indinavir, lopinavir and •ritonavir; plasma concentration of saquinavir significantly reduced by efavirenz; combination of saquinavir with nelfinavir may increase plasma concentration of either drug (or both); plasma concentration of saquinavir reduced by nevirapine and •tipranavir
- • Anxiolytics and Hypnotics: saquinavir increases plasma concentration of •midazolam (risk of prolonged sedation)
- • Barbiturates: plasma concentration of saquinavir possibly reduced by •barbiturates
- • Ciclosporin: plasma concentration of both drugs increased when saquinavir given with •ciclosporin
- • Cilostazol: saquinavir possibly increases plasma concentration of •cilostazol—avoid concomitant use
- Corticosteroids: plasma concentration of saquinavir possibly reduced by dexamethasone
- Diuretics: saquinavir increases plasma concentration of eplerenone (reduce dose of eplerenone)
- • Ergot Alkaloids: increased risk of ergotism when saquinavir given with •ergotamine and methysergide—avoid concomitant use
- • Lipid-regulating Drugs: possible increased risk of myopathy when saquinavir given with atorvastatin; increased risk of myopathy when saquinavir given with •simvastatin (avoid concomitant use)
- Sildenafil: saquinavir possibly increases plasma concentration of sildenafil— reduce initial dose of sildenafil
- • Tacrolimus: saquinavir increases plasma concentration of •tacrolimus (consider reducing dose of tacrolimus)
- Tadalafil: saquinavir possibly increases plasma concentration of tadalafil— reduce initial dose of tadalafil
- Vardenafil: saquinavir possibly increases plasma concentration of vardenafil— reduce initial dose of vardenafil

Secobarbital *see* Barbiturates

Selegiline

Note. Selegiline is a MAO-B inhibitor
- • Analgesics: hyperpyrexia and CNS toxicity reported when selegiline given with •pethidine (avoid concomitant use); manufacturer of selegiline advises caution with tramadol
- • Antidepressants: theoretical risk of serotonin syndrome if selegiline given with citalopram (especially if dose of selegiline exceeds 10 mg daily); caution with selegiline advised by manufacturer of escitalopram; increased risk of hypertension and CNS excitation when selegiline given with •fluoxetine (selegiline should not be started until 5 weeks after stopping fluoxetine, avoid fluoxetine for 2 weeks after stopping selegiline); increased risk of hypertension and CNS excitation when selegiline given with •fluvoxamine or •venlafaxine (selegiline should not be started until 1 week after stopping fluvoxamine or venlafaxine, avoid fluvoxamine or venlafaxine for 2 weeks after stopping selegiline); increased risk of hypertension and CNS excitation when selegiline given with •paroxetine or •sertraline (selegiline should not be started until 2 weeks after stopping paroxetine or sertraline, avoid paroxetine or sertraline for 2 weeks after stopping selegiline); enhanced hypotensive effect when selegiline given with MAOIs; avoid concomitant use of selegiline with •moclobemide; CNS toxicity reported when selegiline given with •tricyclics
- Dopaminergics: max. dose of 10 mg selegiline advised by manufacturer of entacapone if used concomitantly; selegiline enhances effects and increases toxicity of levodopa (reduce dose of levodopa)
- Memantine: effects of dopaminergics and selegiline possibly enhanced by memantine
- Methyldopa: antiparkinsonian effect of dopaminergics antagonised by methyldopa
- Oestrogens: plasma concentration of selegiline increased by oestrogens (increased risk of toxicity)
- Progestogens: plasma concentration of selegiline increased by progestogens (increased risk of toxicity)
- • Sympathomimetics: risk of hypertensive crisis when selegiline given with •dopamine

Sertindole *see* Antipsychotics

Sertraline *see* Antidepressants, SSRI

Sevoflurane *see* Anaesthetics, General

Sibutramine
- Analgesics: increased risk of bleeding when sibutramine given with NSAIDs or aspirin
- Anticoagulants: increased risk of bleeding when sibutramine given with anticoagulants

Sibutramine *(continued)*
- • Antidepressants: increased CNS toxicity when sibutramine given with •MAOIs or •moclobemide (manufacturer of sibutramine advises avoid concomitant use), also avoid sibutramine for 2 weeks after stopping MAOIs or moclobemide; increased risk of CNS toxicity when sibutramine given with •SSRI-related antidepressants, •SSRIs, •mirtazapine, •noradrenaline re-uptake inhibitors, •tricyclic-related antidepressants, •tricyclics or •tryptophan (manufacturer of sibutramine advises avoid concomitant use)
- • Antipsychotics: increased risk of CNS toxicity when sibutramine given with •antipsychotics (manufacturer of sibutramine advises avoid concomitant use)

Sildenafil
- • Alpha-blockers: enhanced hypotensive effect when sildenafil given with •alpha-blockers (avoid alpha-blockers for 4 hours after sildenafil)
- Antibacterials: plasma concentration of sildenafil increased by erythromycin—reduce initial dose of sildenafil
- Antifungals: plasma concentration of sildenafil increased by itraconazole and ketoconazole—reduce initial dose of sildenafil
- • Antivirals: plasma concentration of sildenafil possibly increased by amprenavir, nelfinavir and saquinavir— reduce initial dose of sildenafil; side-effects of sildenafil possibly increased by •atazanavir; plasma concentration of sildenafil increased by indinavir—reduce initial dose of sildenafil; plasma concentration of sildenafil significantly increased by •ritonavir—avoid concomitant use
- Calcium-channel Blockers: enhanced hypotensive effect when sildenafil given with amlodipine
- Grapefruit Juice: plasma concentration of sildenafil possibly increased by grapefruit juice
- • Nicorandil: sildenafil significantly enhances hypotensive effect of •nicorandil (avoid concomitant use)
- • Nitrates: sildenafil significantly enhances hypotensive effect of •nitrates (avoid concomitant use)
- Ulcer-healing Drugs: plasma concentration of sildenafil increased by cimetidine (reduce initial dose of sildenafil)

Simvastatin *see* Statins

Sirolimus
- • Antibacterials: plasma concentration of sirolimus increased by •clarithromycin and •telithromycin—avoid concomitant use; plasma concentration of both drugs increased when sirolimus given with •erythromycin; plasma concentration of sirolimus reduced by •rifabutin and •rifampicin—avoid concomitant use
- • Antifungals: plasma concentration of sirolimus increased by •itraconazole, •ketoconazole and •voriconazole—avoid concomitant use; plasma concentration of sirolimus increased by •miconazole
- • Antivirals: plasma concentration of sirolimus possibly increased by •atazanavir and lopinavir
- • Calcium-channel Blockers: plasma concentration of sirolimus increased by •diltiazem; plasma concentration of both drugs increased when sirolimus given with •verapamil
- Ciclosporin: plasma concentration of sirolimus increased by ciclosporin

Sirolimus *(continued)*
- • Grapefruit Juice: plasma concentration of sirolimus increased by •grapefruit juice—avoid concomitant use

Sodium Benzoate
- Antiepileptics: effects of sodium benzoate possibly reduced by valproate
- Antipsychotics: effects of sodium benzoate possibly reduced by haloperidol
- Corticosteroids: effects of sodium benzoate possibly reduced by corticosteroids
- Probenecid: excretion of conjugate formed by sodium benzoate possibly reduced by probenecid

Sodium Bicarbonate *see* Antacids

Sodium Clodronate *see* Bisphosphonates

Sodium Phenylbutyrate
- Antiepileptics: effects of sodium phenylbutyrate possibly reduced by valproate
- Antipsychotics: effects of sodium phenylbutyrate possibly reduced by haloperidol
- Corticosteroids: effects of sodium phenylbutyrate possibly reduced by corticosteroids
- Probenecid: excretion of conjugate formed by sodium phenylbutyrate possibly reduced by probenecid

Sodium Polystyrene Sulphonate
- Thyroid Hormones: sodium polystyrene sulphonate reduces absorption of levothyroxine (thyroxine)

Sodium Valproate *see* Valproate

Solifenacin *see* Antimuscarinics

Somatropin
- Corticosteroids: growth-promoting effect of somatropin may be inhibited by corticosteroids
- Oestrogens: increased doses of somatropin may be needed when given with oestrogens (when used as oral replacement therapy)

Sotalol *see* Beta-blockers

Spironolactone *see* Diuretics

Statins
- Antacids: absorption of rosuvastatin reduced by antacids
- • Anti-arrhythmics: increased risk of myopathy when simvastatin given with •amiodarone
- • Antibacterials: plasma concentration of atorvastatin increased by clarithromycin; increased risk of myopathy when simvastatin given with •clarithromycin, •erythromycin or •telithromycin (avoid concomitant use); plasma concentration of rosuvastatin reduced by erythromycin; possible increased risk of myopathy when atorvastatin given with erythromycin or fusidic acid; metabolism of fluvastatin accelerated by rifampicin (reduced effect); possible increased risk of myopathy when simvastatin given with fusidic acid; increased risk of myopathy when atorvastatin given with •telithromycin (avoid concomitant use)
- • Anticoagulants: atorvastatin may transiently reduce anticoagulant effect of warfarin; rosuvastatin possibly enhances anticoagulant effect of •coumarins and •phenindione; fluvastatin and simvastatin enhance anticoagulant effect of •coumarins
- Antidepressants: plasma concentration of simvastatin reduced by St John's wort
- Antiepileptics: combination of fluvastatin with phenytoin may increase plasma concentration of either drug (or both)
- • Antifungals: increased risk of myopathy when simvastatin given with •itraconazole or •ketoconazole (avoid concomitant use); possible

Appendix 1

Statins

• Antifungals *(continued)*
increased risk of myopathy when simvastatin given with •miconazole—avoid concomitant use; increased risk of myopathy when atorvastatin given with •itraconazole (avoid concomitant use); possible increased risk of myopathy when atorvastatin or simvastatin given with imidazoles; possible increased risk of myopathy when atorvastatin or simvastatin given with triazoles

• Antivirals: possible increased risk of myopathy when atorvastatin given with amprenavir, atazanavir, indinavir, lopinavir, nelfinavir, ritonavir or saquinavir; possible increased risk of myopathy when simvastatin given with •amprenavir or •lopinavir—avoid concomitant use; increased risk of myopathy when simvastatin given with •atazanavir, •indinavir, •nelfinavir, •ritonavir or •saquinavir (avoid concomitant use); plasma concentration of atorvastatin, pravastatin and simvastatin reduced by efavirenz

Bosentan: plasma concentration of simvastatin reduced by bosentan

• Calcium-channel Blockers: possible increased risk of myopathy when simvastatin given with diltiazem; increased risk of myopathy when simvastatin given with •verapamil

Cardiac Glycosides: atorvastatin possibly increases plasma concentration of digoxin

• Ciclosporin: increased risk of myopathy when statins given with •ciclosporin; increased risk of myopathy when rosuvastatin given with •ciclosporin (avoid concomitant use)

Cytotoxics: plasma concentration of simvastatin increased by imatinib

• Grapefruit Juice: plasma concentration of simvastatin increased by •grapefruit juice—avoid concomitant use

• Hormone Antagonists: possible increased risk of myopathy when simvastatin given with •danazol

• Lipid-regulating Drugs: increased risk of myopathy when statins given with •gemfibrozil (preferably avoid concomitant use); increased risk of myopathy when statins given with •fibrates; increased risk of myopathy when statins given with •nicotinic acid (applies to lipid regulating doses of nicotinic acid)

Oestrogens: rosuvastatin increases plasma concentration of ethinylestradiol

Progestogens: rosuvastatin increases plasma concentration of norgestrel

Stavudine

• Antivirals: increased risk of side-effects when stavudine given with •didanosine; effects of stavudine possibly inhibited by •ribavirin; effects of stavudine possibly inhibited by •zidovudine (manufacturers advise avoid concomitant use)

• Cytotoxics: effects of stavudine possibly inhibited by doxorubicin; increased risk of toxicity when stavudine given with •hydroxycarbamide—avoid concomitant use

Streptomycin *see* Aminoglycosides

Strontium Ranelate

Antibacterials: strontium ranelate reduces absorption of quinolones and tetracyclines (manufacturer of strontium ranelate advises avoid concomitant use)

Sucralfate

Antibacterials: sucralfate reduces absorption of ciprofloxacin, levofloxacin, moxifloxacin, norfloxacin, ofloxacin and tetracyclines

• Anticoagulants: sucralfate possibly reduces absorption of •coumarins (reduced anticoagulant effect)

• Antiepileptics: sucralfate reduces absorption of •phenytoin

Antifungals: sucralfate reduces absorption of ketoconazole

Antipsychotics: sucralfate reduces absorption of sulpiride

Cardiac Glycosides: sucralfate possibly reduces absorption of cardiac glycosides

Thyroid Hormones: sucralfate reduces absorption of levothyroxine (thyroxine)

Ulcer-healing Drugs: sucralfate possibly reduces absorption of lansoprazole

Sulfadiazine *see* Sulphonamides

Sulfadoxine *see* Sulphonamides

Sulfamethoxazole *see* Sulphonamides

Sulfasalazine *see* Aminosalicylates

Sulfinpyrazone

Analgesics: effects of sulfinpyrazone antagonised by aspirin

Antibacterials: sulfinpyrazone reduces excretion of nitrofurantoin (increased risk of toxicity); sulfinpyrazone reduces excretion of penicillins; effects of sulfinpyrazone antagonised by pyrazinamide

• Anticoagulants: sulfinpyrazone enhances anticoagulant effect of •coumarins

• Antidiabetics: sulfinpyrazone enhances effects of •sulphonylureas

• Antiepileptics: sulfinpyrazone increases plasma concentration of •phenytoin

Theophylline: sulfinpyrazone reduces plasma concentration of theophylline

Sulindac *see* NSAIDs

Sulphonamides

Anaesthetics, General: sulphonamides enhance effects of thiopental

Anaesthetics, Local: increased risk of methaemoglobinaemia when sulphonamides given with prilocaine

• Anti-arrhythmics: increased risk of ventricular arrhythmias when sulfamethoxazole (as co-trimoxazole) given with •amiodarone—avoid concomitant use of co-trimoxazole

• Antibacterials: increased risk of crystalluria when sulphonamides given with •methenamine

• Anticoagulants: sulphonamides enhance anticoagulant effect of •coumarins

Antidiabetics: sulphonamides rarely enhance the effects of sulphonylureas

Antiepileptics: sulphonamides possibly increase plasma concentration of phenytoin

• Antimalarials: increased antifolate effect when sulphonamides given with •pyrimethamine (includes Fansidar®)

• Antipsychotics: avoid concomitant use of sulphonamides with •clozapine (increased risk of agranulocytosis)

• Ciclosporin: increased risk of nephrotoxicity when sulphonamides given with •ciclosporin; sulfadiazine possibly reduces plasma concentration of •ciclosporin

• Cytotoxics: increased risk of haematological toxicity when sulfamethoxazole (as co-trimoxazole) given with •azathioprine, •mercaptopurine or •methotrexate; sulphonamides increase risk of methotrexate toxicity

Sulphonamides *(continued)*
Oestrogens: antibacterials that do not induce liver enzymes possibly reduce contraceptive effect of oestrogens (risk probably small, see BNF section 7.3.1)
Potassium Aminobenzoate: effects of sulphonamides inhibited by potassium aminobenzoate

Sulphonylureas *see* Antidiabetics
Sulpiride *see* Antipsychotics
Sumatriptan *see* $5HT_1$ Agonists
Suxamethonium *see* Muscle Relaxants

Sympathomimetics
• Adrenergic Neurone Blockers: ephedrine, isometheptene, metaraminol, methylphenidate, noradrenaline (norepinephrine), oxymetazoline, phenylephrine, phenylpropanolamine, pseudoephedrine and xylometazoline antagonise hypotensive effect of •adrenergic neurone blockers
• Alpha-blockers: avoid concomitant use of adrenaline (epinephrine) or dopamine with •tolazoline
• Anaesthetics, General: increased risk of arrhythmias when adrenaline (epinephrine) given with •volatile liquid general anaesthetics; increased risk of hypertension when methylphenidate given with •volatile liquid general anaesthetics
• Anticoagulants: methylphenidate possibly enhances anticoagulant effect of •coumarins
• Antidepressants: risk of hypertensive crisis when dexamfetamine, dopamine, dopexamine, ephedrine, isometheptene, methylphenidate, phenylephrine, phenylpropanolamine, pseudoephedrine or sympathomimetics given with •MAOIs; risk of hypertensive crisis when dexamfetamine, dopamine, dopexamine, ephedrine, isometheptene, methylphenidate, phenylephrine, phenylpropanolamine, pseudoephedrine or sympathomimetics given with •moclobemide; methylphenidate possibly inhibits metabolism of SSRIs and tricyclics; increased risk of hypertension and arrhythmias when noradrenaline (norepinephrine) given with •tricyclics; increased risk of hypertension and arrhythmias when adrenaline (epinephrine) given with •tricyclics (but local anaesthetics with adrenaline appear to be safe)
Antiepileptics: methylphenidate increases plasma concentration of phenytoin; methylphenidate possibly increases plasma concentration of primidone
Antipsychotics: hypertensive effect of sympathomimetics antagonised by antipsychotics
Antivirals: plasma concentration of dexamfetamine possibly increased by ritonavir
Barbiturates: methylphenidate possibly increases plasma concentration of phenobarbital
• Beta-blockers: severe hypertension when adrenaline (epinephrine) or noradrenaline (norepinephrine) given with •beta-blockers especially with non-selective beta-blockers; possible severe hypertension when dobutamine given with •beta-blockers especially with non-selective beta-blockers
• Clonidine: possible risk of hypertension when adrenaline (epinephrine) or noradrenaline (norepinephrine) given with clonidine; serious adverse events reported with concomitant use of methylphenidate and •clonidine (causality not established)
Corticosteroids: ephedrine accelerates metabolism of dexamethasone

Sympathomimetics *(continued)*
• Dopaminergics: risk of toxicity when isometheptene or phenylpropanolamine given with •bromocriptine; effects of adrenaline (epinephrine), dobutamine, dopamine and noradrenaline (norepinephrine) possibly enhanced by entacapone; avoid concomitant use of sympathomimetics with •rasagiline; risk of hypertensive crisis when dopamine given with •selegiline
Doxapram: increased risk of hypertension when sympathomimetics given with doxapram
Ergot Alkaloids: increased risk of ergotism when sympathomimetics given with ergotamine and methysergide
Oxytocin: risk of hypertension when vasoconstrictor sympathomimetics given with oxytocin (due to enhanced vasopressor effect)
• Sympathomimetics: effects of adrenaline (epinephrine) possibly enhanced by •dopexamine; dopexamine possibly enhances effects of •noradrenaline (norepinephrine)
Theophylline: avoidance of ephedrine in children advised by manufacturer of theophylline

Sympathomimetics, Beta$_2$
Atomoxetine: Increased risk of cardiovascular side-effects when parenteral salbutamol given with atomoxetine
Cardiac Glycosides: salbutamol possibly reduces plasma concentration of digoxin
Corticosteroids: increased risk of hypokalaemia when high doses of beta$_2$ sympathomimetics given with corticosteroids—for CSM advice (hypokalaemia) see p. 167
Diuretics: increased risk of hypokalaemia when high doses of beta$_2$ sympathomimetics given with acetazolamide, loop diuretics or thiazides and related diuretics—for CSM advice (hypokalaemia) see p. 167
• Methyldopa: acute hypotension reported when infusion of salbutamol given with •methyldopa
Muscle Relaxants: bambuterol enhances effects of suxamethonium
Theophylline: increased risk of hypokalaemia when high doses of beta$_2$ sympathomimetics given with theophylline—for CSM advice (hypokalaemia) see p. 167

Tacrolimus
Note. Interactions do not generally apply to tacrolimus used topically; risk of facial flushing and skin irritation with alcohol consumption (p. 640) does not apply to tacrolimus taken systemically
• Analgesics: possible increased risk of nephrotoxicity when tacrolimus given with NSAIDs; increased risk of nephrotoxicity when tacrolimus given with •ibuprofen
• Antibacterials: plasma concentration of tacrolimus increased by •clarithromycin, •erythromycin and •quinupristin/dalfopristin; plasma concentration of tacrolimus reduced by •rifampicin; increased risk of nephrotoxicity when tacrolimus given with •aminoglycosides; plasma concentration of tacrolimus possibly increased by •chloramphenicol and •telithromycin
• Antidepressants: plasma concentration of tacrolimus reduced by •St John's wort—avoid concomitant use
• Antifungals: plasma concentration of tacrolimus increased by •fluconazole, •ketoconazole and •voriconazole; increased risk of nephrotoxicity when tacrolimus given with •amphotericin; plasma concentration of tacrolimus reduced by •caspofungin; plasma concentration of tacro-

Tacrolimus
- Antifungals *(continued)* limus possibly increased by •imidazoles and •triazoles
- Antivirals: plasma concentration of tacrolimus possibly increased by •atazanavir, •nelfinavir and •ritonavir; plasma concentration of tacrolimus increased by •saquinavir (consider reducing dose of tacrolimus)
- Calcium-channel Blockers: plasma concentration of tacrolimus possibly increased by felodipine; plasma concentration of tacrolimus increased by •diltiazem and •nifedipine
- Ciclosporin: tacrolimus increases plasma concentration of •ciclosporin (increased risk of toxicity)—avoid concomitant use
- Diuretics: increased risk of hyperkalaemia when tacrolimus given with •potassium-sparing diuretics and aldosterone antagonists
- Grapefruit Juice: plasma concentration of tacrolimus increased by •grapefruit juice

Hormone Antagonists: plasma concentration of tacrolimus possibly increased by danazol

Oestrogens: tacrolimus possibly reduces contraceptive effect of oestrogens
- Potassium Salts: increased risk of hyperkalaemia when tacrolimus given with •potassium salts

Progestogens: tacrolimus possibly reduces contraceptive effect of progestogens

Ulcer-healing Drugs: plasma concentration of tacrolimus possibly increased by omeprazole

Tadalafil
- Alpha-blockers: enhanced hypotensive effect when tadalafil given with •alpha-blockers—avoid concomitant use

Antibacterials: plasma concentration of tadalafil possibly increased by clarithromycin and erythromycin; plasma concentration of tadalafil reduced by rifampicin

Antifungals: plasma concentration of tadalafil increased by ketoconazole; plasma concentration of tadalafil possibly increased by itraconazole

Antivirals: plasma concentration of tadalafil possibly increased by amprenavir; plasma concentration of tadalafil increased by ritonavir; plasma concentration of tadalafil possibly increased by saquinavir— reduce initial dose of tadalafil

Grapefruit Juice: plasma concentration of tadalafil possibly increased by grapefruit juice
- Nicorandil: tadalafil significantly enhances hypotensive effect of •nicorandil (avoid concomitant use)
- Nitrates: tadalafil significantly enhances hypotensive effect of •nitrates (avoid concomitant use)

Tamoxifen
- Anticoagulants: tamoxifen enhances anticoagulant effect of •coumarins

Tamsulosin *see* Alpha-blockers

Taxanes *see* Docetaxel and Paclitaxel

Tegafur with uracil *see* Fluorouracil

Teicoplanin

Antibacterials: increased risk of nephrotoxicity and ototoxicity when teicoplanin given with aminoglycosides or colistin

Oestrogens: antibacterials that do not induce liver enzymes possibly reduce contraceptive effect of oestrogens (risk probably small, see BNF section 7.3.1)

Telithromycin
- Antibacterials: plasma concentration of telithromycin reduced by •rifampicin (avoid during and for 2 weeks after rifampicin)
- Antidepressants: plasma concentration of telithromycin reduced by •St John's wort (avoid during and for 2 weeks after St John's wort)
- Antiepileptics: plasma concentration of telithromycin reduced by •carbamazepine, •phenytoin and •primidone (avoid during and for 2 weeks after carbamazepine, phenytoin and primidone)
- Antipsychotics: increased risk of ventricular arrhythmias when telithromycin given with •pimozide—avoid concomitant use
- Anxiolytics and Hypnotics: telithromycin inhibits metabolism of •midazolam (increased plasma concentration with increased sedation)

Aprepitant: telithromycin possibly increases plasma concentration of aprepitant
- Barbiturates: plasma concentration of telithromycin reduced by •phenobarbital (avoid during and for 2 weeks after phenobarbital)

Cardiac Glycosides: telithromycin possibly increases plasma concentration of digoxin
- Ciclosporin: telithromycin possibly increases plasma concentration of •ciclosporin
- Diuretics: telithromycin increases plasma concentration of •eplerenone—avoid concomitant use
- Ergot Alkaloids: increased risk of ergotism when telithromycin given with •ergotamine and methysergide—avoid concomitant use
- Ivabradine: telithromycin possibly increases plasma concentration of •ivabradine—avoid concomitant use
- Lipid-regulating Drugs: increased risk of myopathy when telithromycin given with •atorvastatin or •simvastatin (avoid concomitant use)

Oestrogens: antibacterials that do not induce liver enzymes possibly reduce contraceptive effect of oestrogens (risk probably small, see BNF section 7.3.1)
- Sirolimus: telithromycin increases plasma concentration of •sirolimus—avoid concomitant use
- Tacrolimus: telithromycin possibly increases plasma concentration of •tacrolimus

Telmisartan *see* Angiotensin-II Receptor Antagonists

Temazepam *see* Anxiolytics and Hypnotics

Temoporfin
- Cytotoxics: increased skin photosensitivity when temoporfin given with topical •fluorouracil

Temozolomide

Antiepileptics: cytotoxics possibly reduce absorption of phenytoin; plasma concentration of temozolomide increased by valproate
- Antipsychotics: avoid concomitant use of cytotoxics with •clozapine (increased risk of agranulocytosis)

Cardiac Glycosides: cytotoxics reduce absorption of digoxin tablets

Tenofovir
- Antivirals: tenofovir reduces plasma concentration of atazanavir; combination of tenofovir with cidofovir may increase plasma concentration of either drug (or both); tenofovir increases plasma concentration of •didanosine (increased risk of toxicity)—avoid concomitant use; plasma concentration of tenofovir increased by lopinavir

Appendix 1

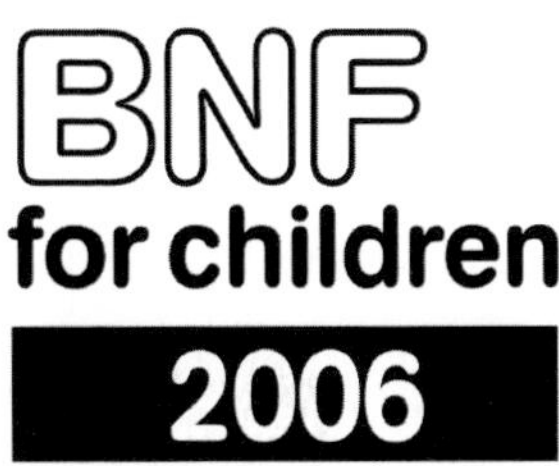

The layout of this second edition of *BNF for Children* (BNFC) has undergone numerous changes to improve the speed and accuracy of information retrieval. A great many of these changes have resulted from comments by users of the first edition. We canvassed feedback by means of a questionnaire in every copy of BNFC. Independent market research provided us with further valuable insight from key users in the community and in secondary-care facilities. Finally, we carefully processed formal and informal, spontaneous and prompted comments from a wide range of readers.

In the first edition, the flow of text, particularly on pages with a mixture of single-column and two-column layout was confusing. Although we have retained the mix of single- and double-columns, careful use of rules across the page now makes it much easier to follow the text from one column to the next.

Our market research revealed that in most instances readers want to simply look up the dose. Changes to the layout of the doses should now make it much easier to pick out a specific condition and the dose relevant to a child of a given age. Better use is made of tinted panels and colour to improve navigation. Nevertheless, it remains as important as ever to read the dosage information with great care and to heed the listed warnings and side-effects: mistakes from cursory or inattentive reading can seriously compromise clinical care.

More space has been devoted in this edition to the administration of medicines to children. In addition to information on the intravenous infusion of drugs, advice is also given on uncommon (but, in children, necessary) ways of giving a medicine by mouth.

Readers will notice that BNFC includes a number of 'Safe Practice' boxes which highlight particular, unusual hazards associated with medicines.

The layout of BNFC will continue to evolve in the light of users' needs. Do please write to us with suggestions (see below for address).

New in this edition

For a list of significant changes for this edition, turn to page ix.

Emergency care in the community

In the glossy reference pages at the back of the book, there is now guidance on the community management of paediatric emergencies such as anaphylaxis and meningitis. This new section provides doses of drugs used in such emergencies.

Immunisation schedule

The Department of Health has announced plans to introduce routine childhood immunisation against pneumococcal disease and to change the immunisation schedule for Haemophilus influenzae type b vaccine and for meningococcal group C vaccine (letter from the Chief Medical Officer 8 February 2006; Gateway reference 6126). The date for the introduction of these changes has yet to be decided.

In the circumstances it has not been possible to include details of the new immunisation schedule—readers should check the Department of Health website for up-to-date information.

Croup

It is now considered that the use of dexamethasone is beneficial even in mild croup (Bjornson CL, Klassen TP, *et al*. A randomized trial of a single dose of oral dexamethasone for mild croup. *N Engl J Med* 2004; **351**: 1306–13). Although soluble prednisolone tablets are easier to give, a recent study suggests that a single dose of dexamethasone might be of greater benefit than a single dose of prednisolone (Sparrow A, Geelhoed GC. Prednisolone versus dexamethasone in croup: a randomised equivalence trial. *Arch Dis Child* published online on 19 April 2006). Advice in BNFC reflects the results of these studies.

Cystic fibrosis

Advice on the management of children with cystic fibrosis has been introduced in a number of places in BNFC. In particular, Table 1, section 5.1 now includes recommendations for the initial treatment of respiratory-tract infections in cystic fibrosis and Table 2 suggests which antibacterials can be used to prevent *Staphylococcus aureus* lung infections.

Severe hyperkalaemia

Severe hyperkalaemia requires urgent and effective management. BNFC gives advice on intravenous infusion of soluble insulin together with glucose to reduce the potassium concentration (p. 501). Calcium gluconate is infused to manage arrhythmias resulting from hyperkalaemia. BNFC also mentions salbutamol as an alternative when insulin cannot be used.

Marketing authorisations

Considerable confusion exists about the use of medicines outside the scope of their marketing authorisation (or product licence). BNFC provides guidance on this (pp. 2–3). Where a medicine is not licensed for use in particular circumstances, this is shown under the 'Licensed use' heading.

The terms of the marketing authorisation apply principally to the supplier of the medicine (marketing authorisation holder) and should not restrict appropriate clinical use of a medicine outside the licence; however, in these circumstances, the clinician's responsibility increases.

Cardiopulmonary resuscitation

European guidelines on cardiopulmonary resuscitation, published last year, have been adopted by the Resuscitation Council (UK). Revised algorithms based on the new guidelines (*Resuscitation* 2005; **67**(suppl.1): S97–133) and covering newborn life support, paediatric basic life support, and paediatric advanced life support are shown in the glossy reference pages at the back of the book.

Atomoxetine

In September 2005, the Committee on Safety of Medicines (whose function has now passed to the Commission on Human Medicines) wrote to health professionals about the risk of suicidal thoughts and behaviour in children taking atomoxetine for attention deficit hyperactivity disorder. BNFC (p. 225) includes advice that patients and their carers should look out for and report adverse changes of mood or behaviour. In February 2006 the Commission on Human Medicine pointed out (CEM/CMO/2006/) that atomoxetine is associated with a small risk of seizures and of prolonging the QT interval. BNFC reflects these warnings.

Feedback

We welcome constructive comments from readers. If you have suggestions on how the content of the BNFC might be improved, please write to:

The Executive Editor
BNF Publications
Royal Pharmaceutical Society of Great Britain
1 Lambeth High Street
LONDON SE1 7JN
Email: bnfc@bnf.org

To report a fault with your printed copy of the BNFC please contact John Wilson on 020 7572 2354 or email john.wilson@rpsgb.org

Distribution of BNFCs

The UK health departments distribute BNFCs to NHS hospitals, doctors, surgeons, and community pharmacies. In England, BNFCs are mailed individually to NHS general practitioners and community pharmacies; contact the DH Publication Orderline on 08701 555 455 for extra copies or changes relating to mailed BNFCs. In Wales, telephone the Business Services Centre on 01495 332 000.

Pharmaid

Numerous requests have been received from developing countries for BNFCs. The Pharmaid scheme of the Commonwealth Pharmaceutical Association will dispatch old BNFCs to Commonwealth countries. BNFCs will be collected from certain community pharmacies in November. For further details check the health press or contact:

Betty Falconbridge
Tel: 020 7572 2364
Email: admin@commonwealthpharmacy.org

Tenoxicam *see* NSAIDs
Terazosin *see* Alpha-blockers
Terbinafine
Antibacterials: plasma concentration of terbinafine reduced by rifampicin
Antidepressants: terbinafine possibly increases plasma concentration of imipramine and nortriptyline
Oestrogens: occasional reports of breakthrough bleeding when terbinafine given with oestrogens (when used for contraception)
Progestogens: occasional reports of breakthrough bleeding when terbinafine given with progestogens (when used for contraception)
Ulcer-healing Drugs: plasma concentration of terbinafine increased by cimetidine
Terbutaline *see* Sympathomimetics, $Beta_2$
Terpene Mixture *see* Rowachol®
Testolactone
• Anticoagulants: testolactone enhances anticoagulant effect of •coumarins and •phenindione
Testosterone
• Anticoagulants: testosterone enhances anticoagulant effect of •coumarins and •phenindione
Antidiabetics: testosterone possibly enhances hypoglycaemic effect of antidiabetics
Tetrabenazine
• Antidepressants: risk of CNS excitation and hypertension when tetrabenazine given with •MAOIs
Antipsychotics: increased risk of extrapyramidal side-effects when tetrabenazine given with antipsychotics
Dopaminergics: increased risk of extrapyramidal side-effects when tetrabenazine given with amantadine
Metoclopramide: increased risk of extrapyramidal side-effects when tetrabenazine given with metoclopramide
Tetracosactide *see* Corticosteroids
Tetracycline *see* Tetracyclines
Tetracyclines
ACE Inhibitors: absorption of tetracyclines reduced by quinapril tablets (quinapril tablets contain magnesium carbonate)
Adsorbents: absorption of tetracyclines possibly reduced by kaolin
Antacids: absorption of tetracyclines reduced by antacids
• Anticoagulants: tetracyclines possibly enhance anticoagulant effect of •coumarins and •phenindione
Antiepileptics: metabolism of doxycycline accelerated by carbamazepine (reduced effect); metabolism of doxycycline accelerated by phenytoin and primidone (reduced plasma concentration)
Atovaquone: tetracycline reduces plasma concentration of atovaquone
Barbiturates: metabolism of doxycycline accelerated by barbiturates (reduced plasma concentration)
Calcium Salts: absorption of tetracycline reduced by calcium salts
• Ciclosporin: doxycycline possibly increases plasma concentration of •ciclosporin
Cytotoxics: doxycycline or tetracycline increase risk of methotrexate toxicity
Dairy Products: absorption of tetracyclines (except doxycycline and minocycline) reduced by dairy products

Tetracyclines *(continued)*
Diuretics: manufacturer of lymecycline advises avoid concomitant use with diuretics
Ergot Alkaloids: increased risk of ergotism when tetracyclines given with ergotamine and methysergide
Iron: absorption of tetracyclines reduced by *oral* iron, also absorption of *oral* iron reduced by tetracyclines
Oestrogens: antibacterials that do not induce liver enzymes possibly reduce contraceptive effect of oestrogens (risk probably small, see BNF section 7.3.1)
• Retinoids: possible increased risk of benign intracranial hypertension when tetracyclines given with •retinoids (avoid concomitant use)
Strontium Ranelate: absorption of tetracyclines reduced by strontium ranelate (manufacturer of strontium ranelate advises avoid concomitant use)
Ulcer-healing Drugs: absorption of tetracyclines reduced by ranitidine bismuth citrate, sucralfate and tripotassium dicitratobismuthate
Zinc: absorption of tetracyclines reduced by zinc, also absorption of zinc reduced by tetracyclines
Theophylline
Allopurinol: plasma concentration of theophylline possibly increased by allopurinol
Anaesthetics, General: increased risk of convulsions when theophylline given with ketamine; increased risk of arrhythmias when theophylline given with halothane
Anti-arrhythmics: theophylline antagonises anti-arrhythmic effect of adenosine; plasma concentration of theophylline increased by mexiletine and propafenone
• Antibacterials: plasma concentration of theophylline possibly increased by azithromycin and isoniazid; metabolism of theophylline inhibited by •clarithromycin (increased plasma concentration); metabolism of theophylline inhibited by •erythromycin (increased plasma concentration), if erythromycin given by mouth, also decreased plasma-erythromycin concentration; plasma concentration of theophylline increased by •ciprofloxacin and •norfloxacin; metabolism of theophylline accelerated by rifampicin (reduced plasma concentration); possible increased risk of convulsions when theophylline given with •quinolones
• Antidepressants: plasma concentration of theophylline increased by •fluvoxamine (concomitant use should usually be avoided, but where not possible halve theophylline dose and monitor plasma-theophylline concentration); plasma concentration of theophylline reduced by •St John's wort—avoid concomitant use
• Antiepileptics: metabolism of theophylline accelerated by carbamazepine and primidone (reduced effect); plasma concentration of both drugs reduced when theophylline given with •phenytoin
• Antifungals: plasma concentration of theophylline possibly increased by •fluconazole and •ketoconazole
• Antivirals: metabolism of theophylline accelerated by •ritonavir (reduced plasma concentration)
Anxiolytics and Hypnotics: theophylline possibly reduces effects of benzodiazepines
Barbiturates: metabolism of theophylline accelerated by barbiturates (reduced effect)

Theophylline *(continued)*
- • Calcium-channel Blockers: plasma concentration of theophylline possibly increased by •calcium-channel blockers (enhanced effect); plasma concentration of theophylline increased by diltiazem; plasma concentration of theophylline increased by •verapamil (enhanced effect)
- Corticosteroids: increased risk of hypokalaemia when theophylline given with corticosteroids
- Cytotoxics: plasma concentration of theophylline possibly increased by methotrexate
- Disulfiram: metabolism of theophylline inhibited by disulfiram (increased risk of toxicity)
- Diuretics: increased risk of hypokalaemia when theophylline given with acetazolamide, loop diuretics or thiazides and related diuretics
- Doxapram: increased CNS stimulation when theophylline given with doxapram
- Interferons: metabolism of theophylline inhibited by interferon alfa (increased plasma concentration)
- Leukotriene Antagonists: plasma concentration of theophylline possibly increased by zafirlukast, also plasma concentration of zafirlukast reduced
- Lithium: theophylline increases excretion of lithium (reduced plasma concentration)
- Oestrogens: excretion of theophylline reduced by oestrogens (increased plasma concentration)
- Pentoxifylline (oxpentifylline): plasma concentration of theophylline increased by pentoxifylline (oxpentifylline)
- Sulfinpyrazone: plasma concentration of theophylline reduced by sulfinpyrazone
- Sympathomimetics: manufacturer of theophylline advises avoid concomitant use with ephedrine in children
- Sympathomimetics, Beta$_2$: increased risk of hypokalaemia when theophylline given with high doses of beta$_2$ sympathomimetics—for CSM advice (hypokalaemia) see p. 167
- Tobacco: metabolism of theophylline increased by tobacco smoking (reduced plasma concentration)
- • Ulcer-healing Drugs: metabolism of theophylline inhibited by •cimetidine (increased plasma concentration)
- Vaccines: plasma concentration of theophylline possibly increased by influenza vaccine

Thiazolidinediones *see* Antidiabetics

Thiopental *see* Anaesthetics, General

Thiotepa
- Antiepileptics: cytotoxics possibly reduce absorption of phenytoin
- • Antipsychotics: avoid concomitant use of cytotoxics with •clozapine (increased risk of agranulocytosis)
- Cardiac Glycosides: cytotoxics reduce absorption of digoxin tablets
- Muscle Relaxants: thiotepa enhances effects of suxamethonium

Thioxanthenes *see* Antipsychotics

Thyroid Hormones
- Anti-arrhythmics: for concomitant use of thyroid hormones and amiodarone see p. 106
- Antibacterials: metabolism of levothyroxine (thyroxine) accelerated by rifampicin (may increase requirements for levothyroxine (thyroxine) in hypothyroidism)
- • Anticoagulants: thyroid hormones enhance anticoagulant effect of •coumarins and •phenindione
- Antidepressants: thyroid hormones enhance effects of amitriptyline and imipramine; thyroid hormones possibly enhance effects of tricyclics
- Antiepileptics: metabolism of thyroid hormones accelerated by carbamazepine and primidone (may increase requirements for thyroid hormones in hypothyroidism); metabolism of thyroid hormones accelerated by phenytoin (may increase requirements in hypothyroidism), also plasma concentration of phenytoin possibly increased
- Barbiturates: metabolism of thyroid hormones accelerated by barbiturates (may increase requirements for thyroid hormones in hypothyroidism)
- Calcium Salts: absorption of levothyroxine (thyroxine) reduced by calcium salts
- Iron: absorption of levothyroxine (thyroxine) reduced by *oral* iron (give at least 2 hours apart)
- Lipid-regulating Drugs: absorption of thyroid hormones reduced by colestipol and colestyramine
- Sodium Polystyrene Sulphonate: absorption of levothyroxine (thyroxine) reduced by sodium polystyrene sulphonate
- Ulcer-healing Drugs: absorption of levothyroxine (thyroxine) reduced by cimetidine and sucralfate

Tiagabine
- • Antidepressants: anticonvulsant effect of antiepileptics possibly antagonised by MAOIs and •tricyclic-related antidepressants (convulsive threshold lowered); anticonvulsant effect of antiepileptics antagonised by •SSRIs and •tricyclics (convulsive threshold lowered)
- Antiepileptics: plasma concentration of tiagabine reduced by carbamazepine, phenytoin and primidone
- • Antimalarials: possible increased risk of convulsions when antiepileptics given with chloroquine and hydroxychloroquine; anticonvulsant effect of antiepileptics antagonised by •mefloquine
- Barbiturates: plasma concentration of tiagabine reduced by phenobarbital

Tiaprofenic Acid *see* NSAIDs

Tibolone
- Antibacterials: metabolism of tibolone accelerated by rifampicin (reduced plasma concentration)
- Antiepileptics: metabolism of tibolone accelerated by carbamazepine and primidone (reduced plasma concentration); metabolism of tibolone accelerated by phenytoin
- Barbiturates: metabolism of tibolone accelerated by barbiturates (reduced plasma concentration)

Ticarcillin *see* Penicillins

Tiludronic Acid *see* Bisphosphonates

Timolol *see* Beta-blockers

Tinidazole
- Alcohol: possibility of disulfiram-like reaction when tinidazole given with alcohol
- Oestrogens: antibacterials that do not induce liver enzymes possibly reduce contraceptive effect of oestrogens (risk probably small, see BNF section 7.3.1)

Tinzaparin *see* Heparins

Tioguanine
- Antiepileptics: cytotoxics possibly reduce absorption of phenytoin

Tioguanine *(continued)*
• Antipsychotics: avoid concomitant use of cytotoxics with •clozapine (increased risk of agranulocytosis)
Cardiac Glycosides: cytotoxics reduce absorption of digoxin tablets
Cytotoxics: increased risk of hepatotoxicity when tioguanine given with busulfan

Tiotropium *see* Antimuscarinics

Tipranavir
Antacids: absorption of tipranavir reduced by antacids
• Antibacterials: tipranavir increases plasma concentration of •clarithromycin (reduce dose of clarithromycin in renal impairment), also plasma concentration of tipranavir increased by clarithromycin; tipranavir increases plasma concentration of •rifabutin (reduce dose of rifabutin); plasma concentration of tipranavir possibly reduced by •rifampicin—avoid concomitant use
• Antidepressants: plasma concentration of tipranavir possibly reduced by •St John's wort—avoid concomitant use
Antifungals: plasma concentration of tipranavir increased by fluconazole
• Antimalarials: possible increased risk of ventricular arrhythmias when tipranavir given with •artemether/lumefantrine—avoid concomitant use
• Antivirals: tipranavir reduces plasma concentration of •abacavir, •amprenavir, •didanosine, •lopinavir, •saquinavir and •zidovudine

Tirofiban
Iloprost: increased risk of bleeding when tirofiban given with iloprost

Tizanidine *see* Muscle Relaxants

Tobacco
Cinacalcet: tobacco smoking increases cinacalcet metabolism (reduced plasma concentration)
Theophylline: tobacco smoking increases theophylline metabolism (reduced plasma concentration)

Tobramycin *see* Aminoglycosides

Tolazoline *see* Alpha-blockers

Tolbutamide *see* Antidiabetics

Tolcapone
Antidepressants: avoid concomitant use of tolcapone with MAOIs
Memantine: effects of dopaminergics possibly enhanced by memantine
Methyldopa: antiparkinsonian effect of dopaminergics antagonised by methyldopa

Tolfenamic Acid *see* NSAIDs

Tolterodine *see* Antimuscarinics

Topiramate
• Antidepressants: anticonvulsant effect of antiepileptics possibly antagonised by MAOIs and •tricyclic-related antidepressants (convulsive threshold lowered); anticonvulsant effect of antiepileptics antagonised by •SSRIs and •tricyclics (convulsive threshold lowered)
• Antiepileptics: plasma concentration of topiramate often reduced by carbamazepine; topiramate increases plasma concentration of •phenytoin (also plasma concentration of topiramate reduced)
• Antimalarials: possible increased risk of convulsions when antiepileptics given with chloroquine and hydroxychloroquine; anticonvulsant effect of antiepileptics antagonised by •mefloquine

Topiramate *(continued)*
• Oestrogens: topiramate accelerates metabolism of •oestrogens (reduced contraceptive effect—see BNF section 7.3.1)
• Progestogens: topiramate accelerates metabolism of •progestogens (reduced contraceptive effect—see BNF section 7.3.1)

Torasemide *see* Diuretics

Toremifene
• Anticoagulants: toremifene possibly enhances anticoagulant effect of •coumarins
Antiepileptics: metabolism of toremifene possibly accelerated by carbamazepine (reduced plasma concentration); metabolism of toremifene possibly accelerated by phenytoin; metabolism of toremifene accelerated by primidone (reduced plasma concentration)
Barbiturates: metabolism of toremifene possibly accelerated by barbiturates (reduced plasma concentration)
Diuretics: increased risk of hypercalcaemia when toremifene given with thiazides and related diuretics

Tramadol *see* Opioid Analgesics

Trandolapril *see* ACE Inhibitors

Tranylcypromine *see* MAOIs

Trazodone *see* Antidepressants, Tricyclic (related)

Tretinoin *see* Retinoids

Triamcinolone *see* Corticosteroids

Triamterene *see* Diuretics

Triclofos *see* Anxiolytics and Hypnotics

Trientine
Iron: trientine reduces absorption of *oral* iron
Zinc: trientine reduces absorption of zinc, also absorption of trientine reduced by zinc

Trifluoperazine *see* Antipsychotics

Trihexyphenidyl (benzhexol) *see* Antimuscarinics

Trilostane
Diuretics: increased risk of hyperkalaemia when trilostane given with potassium-sparing diuretics and aldosterone antagonists

Trimethoprim
• Anti-arrhythmics: increased risk of ventricular arrhythmias when trimethoprim (as co-trimoxazole) given with •amiodarone—avoid concomitant use of co-trimoxazole; trimethoprim increases plasma concentration of procainamide
Antibacterials: plasma concentration of both drugs may increase when trimethoprim given with dapsone
Anticoagulants: trimethoprim possibly enhances anticoagulant effect of coumarins
Antidiabetics: trimethoprim rarely enhances the effects of sulphonylureas
• Antiepileptics: trimethoprim increases plasma concentration of •phenytoin (also increased antifolate effect)
• Antimalarials: increased antifolate effect when trimethoprim given with •pyrimethamine
Antivirals: trimethoprim (as co-trimoxazole) increases plasma concentration of lamivudine—avoid concomitant use of high-dose co-trimoxazole
Cardiac Glycosides: trimethoprim possibly increases plasma concentration of digoxin
• Ciclosporin: increased risk of nephrotoxicity when trimethoprim given with •ciclosporin, also plasma concentration of ciclosporin reduced by intravenous trimethoprim
• Cytotoxics: increased risk of haematological toxicity when trimethoprim (also with co-trimoxazole) given with •azathioprine, •mercaptopurine or •methotrexate

Trimethoprim *(continued)*
Diuretics: increased risk of hyperkalaemia when trimethoprim given with eplerenone
Oestrogens: antibacterials that do not induce liver enzymes possibly reduce contraceptive effect of oestrogens (risk probably small, see BNF section 7.3.1)

Trimipramine *see* Antidepressants, Tricyclic

Tripotassium Dicitratobismuthate
Antibacterials: tripotassium dicitratobismuthate reduces absorption of tetracyclines

Tropicamide *see* Antimuscarinics

Tropisetron
Anti-arrhythmics: manufacturer of tropisetron advises caution with anti-arrhythmics (risk of ventricular arrhythmias)
Antibacterials: plasma concentration of tropisetron reduced by rifampicin
Antiepileptics: plasma concentration of tropisetron reduced by primidone
Barbiturates: plasma concentration of tropisetron reduced by phenobarbital
Beta-blockers: manufacturer of tropisetron advises caution with beta-blockers (risk of ventricular arrhythmias)

Trospium *see* Antimuscarinics

Tryptophan
• Antidepressants: possible increased serotonergic effects when tryptophan given with duloxetine; CNS excitation and confusion when tryptophan given with •MAOIs (reduce dose of tryptophan); agitation and nausea may occur when tryptophan given with •SSRIs
• Antimalarials: avoidance of antidepressants advised by manufacturer of •artemether/lumefantrine
• Sibutramine: increased risk of CNS toxicity when tryptophan given with •sibutramine (manufacturer of sibutramine advises avoid concomitant use)

Typhoid Vaccine *see* Vaccines

Ubidecarenone
Anticoagulants: ubidecarenone may enhance or reduce anticoagulant effect of warfarin

Ulcer-healing Drugs *see* Carbenoxolone, Histamine H_2-antagonists, Proton Pump Inhibitors, Sucralfate, and Tripotassium Dicitratobismuthate

Ursodeoxycholic Acid
Antacids: absorption of bile acids possibly reduced by antacids
• Ciclosporin: ursodeoxycholic acid increases absorption of •ciclosporin
Lipid-regulating Drugs: absorption of bile acids possibly reduced by colestipol and colestyramine
Oestrogens: elimination of cholesterol in bile increased when bile acids given with oestrogens

Vaccines
Note. For a general warning on live vaccines and high doses of corticosteroids or other immunosuppressive drugs, see p. 675 ; for advice on live vaccines and immunoglobulins, see under Normal Immunoglobulin, p. 699
Note. For interactions of oral typhoid vaccine see p. 697
• Adalimumab: avoid concomitant use of live vaccines with •adalimumab (see p. 675)
• Anakinra: avoid concomitant use of live vaccines with •anakinra (see p. 675)
Anticoagulants: influenza vaccine possibly enhances anticoagulant effect of warfarin
Antiepileptics: influenza vaccine enhances effects of phenytoin

Vaccines *(continued)*
• Corticosteroids: immune response to vaccines impaired by high doses of •corticosteroids, avoid concomitant use with live vaccines (see p. 675)
• Efalizumab: live or live-attenuated vaccines should be given 2 weeks before •efalizumab or withheld until 8 weeks after discontinuation
• Etanercept: avoid concomitant use of live vaccines with •etanercept (see p. 675)
• Infliximab: avoid concomitant use of live vaccines with •infliximab (see p. 675)
Interferons: avoidance of vaccines advised by manufacturer of interferon gamma
• Leflunomide: avoid concomitant use of live vaccines with •leflunomide (see p. 675)
Theophylline: influenza vaccine possibly increases plasma concentration of theophylline

Valaciclovir *see* Aciclovir

Valganciclovir *see* Ganciclovir

Valproate
Analgesics: effects of valproate enhanced by aspirin
Antibacterials: plasma concentration of valproate possibly reduced by ertapenem; plasma concentration of valproate reduced by meropenem; metabolism of valproate possibly inhibited by erythromycin (increased plasma concentration)
Anticoagulants: valproate possibly enhances anticoagulant effect of coumarins
• Antidepressants: anticonvulsant effect of antiepileptics possibly antagonised by MAOIs and •tricyclic-related antidepressants (convulsive threshold lowered); anticonvulsant effect of antiepileptics antagonised by •SSRIs and •tricyclics (convulsive threshold lowered)
• Antiepileptics: plasma concentration of valproate reduced by carbamazepine, also plasma concentration of active metabolite of carbamazepine increased; valproate possibly increases plasma concentration of ethosuximide; valproate increases plasma concentration of lamotrigine; valproate sometimes reduces plasma concentration of an active metabolite of oxcarbazepine; valproate increases or possibly decreases plasma concentration of phenytoin, also plasma concentration of valproate reduced; valproate possibly increases plasma concentration of •primidone (plasma concentration of active metabolite of primidone increased), also plasma concentration of valproate reduced
• Antimalarials: possible increased risk of convulsions when antiepileptics given with chloroquine and hydroxychloroquine; anticonvulsant effect of antiepileptics and valproate antagonised by •mefloquine
• Antipsychotics: anticonvulsant effect of valproate antagonised by •antipsychotics (convulsive threshold lowered); increased risk of neutropenia when valproate given with •olanzapine
Antivirals: valproate possibly increases plasma concentration of zidovudine (increased risk of toxicity)
Barbiturates: valproate increases plasma concentration of phenobarbital (also plasma concentration of valproate reduced)
Bupropion: valproate inhibits the metabolism of bupropion
Cytotoxics: valproate increases plasma concentration of temozolomide

Valproate *(continued)*
Lipid-regulating Drugs: absorption of valproate possibly reduced by colestyramine
Sodium Benzoate: valproate possibly reduces effects of sodium benzoate
Sodium Phenylbutyrate: valproate possibly reduces effects of sodium phenylbutyrate
• Ulcer-healing Drugs: metabolism of valproate inhibited by •cimetidine (increased plasma concentration)

Valsartan *see* Angiotensin-II Receptor Antagonists

Vancomycin
Anaesthetics, General: hypersensitivity-like reactions can occur when intravenous vancomycin given with general anaesthetics
Antibacterials: increased risk of nephrotoxicity and ototoxicity when vancomycin given with aminoglycosides, capreomycin or colistin; increased risk of nephrotoxicity when vancomycin given with polymyxins
Antifungals: possible increased risk of nephrotoxicity when vancomycin given with amphotericin
• Ciclosporin: increased risk of nephrotoxicity when vancomycin given with •ciclosporin
Cytotoxics: increased risk of nephrotoxicity and possibly of ototoxicity when vancomycin given with cisplatin
• Diuretics: increased risk of otoxicity when vancomycin given with •loop diuretics
Lipid-regulating Drugs: effects of oral vancomycin antagonised by colestyramine
• Muscle Relaxants: vancomycin enhances effects of •suxamethonium
Oestrogens: antibacterials that do not induce liver enzymes possibly reduce contraceptive effect of oestrogens (risk probably small, see BNF section 7.3.1)

Vardenafil
• Alpha-blockers: enhanced hypotensive effect when vardenafil given with •alpha-blockers (exludes tamsulosin)—avoid vardenafil for 6 hours after alpha-blockers
Antibacterials: plasma concentration of vardenafil increased by erythromycin (reduce dose of vardenafil)
• Antifungals: plasma concentration of vardenafil increased by •ketoconazole—avoid concomitant use; plasma concentration of vardenafil possibly increased by •itraconazole—avoid concomitant use
• Antivirals: plasma concentration of vardenafil possibly increased by amprenavir; plasma concentration of vardenafil increased by •indinavir—avoid concomitant use; plasma concentration of vardenafil possibly increased by •ritonavir—avoid concomitant use; plasma concentration of vardenafil possibly increased by saquinavir— reduce initial dose of vardenafil
Calcium-channel Blockers: enhanced hypotensive effect when vardenafil given with nifedipine
• Grapefruit Juice: plasma concentration of vardenafil possibly increased by •grapefruit juice—avoid concomitant use
• Nicorandil: possible increased hypotensive effect when vardenafil given with •nicorandil—avoid concomitant use
• Nitrates: possible increased hypotensive effect when vardenafil given with •nitrates—avoid concomitant use

Vasodilator Antihypertensives
ACE Inhibitors: enhanced hypotensive effect when hydralazine, minoxidil or nitroprusside given with ACE inhibitors
Adrenergic Neurone Blockers: enhanced hypotensive effect when hydralazine, minoxidil or nitroprusside given with adrenergic neurone blockers
Alcohol: enhanced hypotensive effect when hydralazine, minoxidil or nitroprusside given with alcohol
Aldesleukin: enhanced hypotensive effect when hydralazine, minoxidil or nitroprusside given with aldesleukin
Alpha-blockers: enhanced hypotensive effect when hydralazine, minoxidil or nitroprusside given with alpha-blockers
Anaesthetics, General: enhanced hypotensive effect when hydralazine, minoxidil or nitroprusside given with general anaesthetics
Analgesics: hypotensive effect of hydralazine, minoxidil and nitroprusside antagonised by NSAIDs
Angiotensin-II Receptor Antagonists: enhanced hypotensive effect when hydralazine, minoxidil or nitroprusside given with angiotensin-II receptor antagonists
Antidepressants: enhanced hypotensive effect when hydralazine, minoxidil or nitroprusside given with MAOIs; enhanced hypotensive effect when hydralazine or nitroprusside given with tricyclic-related antidepressants
Antipsychotics: enhanced hypotensive effect when hydralazine, minoxidil or nitroprusside given with phenothiazines
Anxiolytics and Hypnotics: enhanced hypotensive effect when hydralazine, minoxidil or nitroprusside given with anxiolytics and hypnotics
Beta-blockers: enhanced hypotensive effect when hydralazine, minoxidil or nitroprusside given with beta-blockers
Calcium-channel Blockers: enhanced hypotensive effect when hydralazine, minoxidil or nitroprusside given with calcium-channel blockers
Clonidine: enhanced hypotensive effect when hydralazine, minoxidil or nitroprusside given with clonidine
Corticosteroids: hypotensive effect of hydralazine, minoxidil and nitroprusside antagonised by corticosteroids
Diazoxide: enhanced hypotensive effect when hydralazine, minoxidil or nitroprusside given with diazoxide
Diuretics: enhanced hypotensive effect when hydralazine, minoxidil or nitroprusside given with diuretics
Dopaminergics: enhanced hypotensive effect when hydralazine, minoxidil or nitroprusside given with levodopa
Methyldopa: enhanced hypotensive effect when hydralazine, minoxidil or nitroprusside given with methyldopa
Moxisylyte (thymoxamine): enhanced hypotensive effect when hydralazine, minoxidil or nitroprusside given with moxisylyte
Moxonidine: enhanced hypotensive effect when hydralazine, minoxidil or nitroprusside given with moxonidine
Muscle Relaxants: enhanced hypotensive effect when hydralazine, minoxidil or nitroprusside given with baclofen; enhanced hypotensive

Vasodilator Antihypertensives
Muscle Relaxants *(continued)*
effect when hydralazine, minoxidil or nitroprusside given with tizanidine
Nicorandil: possible enhanced hypotensive effect when hydralazine, minoxidil or nitroprusside given with nicorandil
Nitrates: enhanced hypotensive effect when hydralazine, minoxidil or nitroprusside given with nitrates
Oestrogens: hypotensive effect of hydralazine, minoxidil and nitroprusside antagonised by oestrogens
Prostaglandins: enhanced hypotensive effect when hydralazine, minoxidil or nitroprusside given with alprostadil
Vasodilator Antihypertensives: enhanced hypotensive effect when hydralazine given with minoxidil or nitroprusside; enhanced hypotensive effect when minoxidil given with nitroprusside

Vecuronium *see* Muscle Relaxants

Venlafaxine
• Analgesics: increased risk of bleeding when venlafaxine given with •NSAIDs or •aspirin
• Anticoagulants: venlafaxine possibly enhances anticoagulant effect of •warfarin
• Antidepressants: possible increased serotonergic effects when venlafaxine given with duloxetine; enhanced CNS effects and toxicity when venlafaxine given with •MAOIs (venlafaxine should not be started until 2 weeks after stopping MAOIs, avoid MAOIs for 1 week after stopping venlafaxine); after stopping SSRI-related antidepressants do not start •moclobemide for at least 1 week
• Antimalarials: avoidance of antidepressants advised by manufacturer of •artemether/lumefantrine
• Antipsychotics: venlafaxine increases plasma concentration of •clozapine and haloperidol
• Dopaminergics: caution with venlafaxine advised by manufacturer of entacapone; increased risk of hypertension and CNS excitation when venlafaxine given with •selegiline (selegiline should not be started until 1 week after stopping venlafaxine, avoid venlafaxine for 2 weeks after stopping selegiline)
• Sibutramine: increased risk of CNS toxicity when SSRI-related antidepressants given with •sibutramine (manufacturer of sibutramine advises avoid concomitant use)

Verapamil *see* Calcium-channel Blockers

Vigabatrin
• Antidepressants: anticonvulsant effect of antiepileptics possibly antagonised by MAOIs and •tricyclic-related antidepressants (convulsive threshold lowered); anticonvulsant effect of antiepileptics antagonised by •SSRIs and •tricyclics (convulsive threshold lowered)
Antiepileptics: vigabatrin reduces plasma concentration of phenytoin; vigabatrin possibly reduces plasma concentration of primidone
• Antimalarials: possible increased risk of convulsions when antiepileptics given with chloroquine and hydroxychloroquine; anticonvulsant effect of antiepileptics antagonised by •mefloquine
Barbiturates: vigabatrin possibly reduces plasma concentration of phenobarbital

Vinblastine
• Antibacterials: toxicity of vinblastine increased by •erythromycin—avoid concomitant use

Vinblastine *(continued)*
Antiepileptics: cytotoxics possibly reduce absorption of phenytoin
• Antipsychotics: avoid concomitant use of cytotoxics with •clozapine (increased risk of agranulocytosis)
Cardiac Glycosides: cytotoxics reduce absorption of digoxin tablets

Vincristine
Antiepileptics: cytotoxics possibly reduce absorption of phenytoin
• Antifungals: metabolism of vincristine possibly inhibited by •itraconazole (increased risk of neurotoxicity)
• Antipsychotics: avoid concomitant use of cytotoxics with •clozapine (increased risk of agranulocytosis)
Calcium-channel Blockers: metabolism of vincristine possibly inhibited by nifedipine
Cardiac Glycosides: cytotoxics reduce absorption of digoxin tablets

Vitamin A *see* Vitamins

Vitamin D *see* Vitamins

Vitamin K (Phytomenadione) *see* Vitamins

Vitamins
Antibacterials: absorption of vitamin A possibly reduced by neomycin
• Anticoagulants: vitamin K antagonises anticoagulant effect of •coumarins and •phenindione
Antiepileptics: vitamin D requirements possibly increased when given with carbamazepine, phenytoin or primidone
Barbiturates: vitamin D requirements possibly increased when given with barbiturates
Diuretics: increased risk of hypercalcaemia when vitamin D given with thiazides and related diuretics
Dopaminergics: pyridoxine reduces effects of levodopa when given without dopa-decarboxylase inhibitor
Retinoids: risk of hypervitaminosis A when vitamin A given with retinoids

Voriconazole *see* Antifungals, Triazole

Warfarin *see* Coumarins

Xipamide *see* Diuretics

Xylometazoline *see* Sympathomimetics

Zafirlukast *see* Leukotriene Antagonists

Zaleplon *see* Anxiolytics and Hypnotics

Zidovudine
Note. Increased risk of toxicity with nephrotoxic and myelosuppressive drugs - for further details consult product literature
Analgesics: increased risk of haematological toxicity when zidovudine given with NSAIDs; plasma concentration of zidovudine possibly increased by methadone
Antibacterials: absorption of zidovudine reduced by clarithromycin tablets; manufacturer of zidovudine advises avoid concomitant use with rifampicin
Antiepileptics: zidovudine increases or decreases plasma concentration of phenytoin; plasma concentration of zidovudine possibly increased by valproate (increased risk of toxicity)
• Antifungals: plasma concentration of zidovudine increased by •fluconazole (increased risk of toxicity)
Antimalarials: increased antifolate effect when zidovudine given with pyrimethamine
• Antivirals: profound myelosuppression when zidovudine given with •ganciclovir (if possible avoid concomitant administration, particularly

Zidovudine
- Antivirals *(continued)*
  during initial ganciclovir therapy); effects of zidovudine possibly inhibited by •ribavirin (manufacturer of zidovudine advises avoid concomitant use); zidovudine possibly inhibits effects of •stavudine (manufacturers advise avoid concomitant use); plasma concentration of zidovudine reduced by •tipranavir

Atovaquone: metabolism of zidovudine possibly inhibited by atovaquone (increased plasma concentration)

Probenecid: excretion of zidovudine reduced by probenecid (increased plasma concentration and risk of toxicity)

Zinc

Antibacterials: zinc reduces absorption of ciprofloxacin, levofloxacin, moxifloxacin, norfloxacin and ofloxacin; zinc reduces absorption of tetracyclines, also absorption of zinc reduced by tetracyclines

Calcium Salts: absorption of zinc reduced by calcium salts

Iron: absorption of zinc reduced by *oral* iron, also absorption of *oral* iron reduced by zinc

Penicillamine: absorption of zinc reduced by penicillamine, also absorption of penicillamine reduced by zinc

Zinc *(continued)*

Trientine: absorption of zinc reduced by trientine, also absorption of trientine reduced by zinc

Zoledronic Acid *see* Bisphosphonates

Zolmitriptan *see* $5HT_1$ Agonists

Zolpidem *see* Anxiolytics and Hypnotics

Zonisamide
- Antidepressants: anticonvulsant effect of antiepileptics possibly antagonised by MAOIs and •tricyclic-related antidepressants (convulsive threshold lowered); anticonvulsant effect of antiepileptics antagonised by •SSRIs and •tricyclics (convulsive threshold lowered)

Antiepileptics: plasma concentration of zonisamide reduced by carbamazepine, effect on carbamazepine plasma concentration not predictable; plasma concentration of zonisamide reduced by phenytoin

- Antimalarials: possible increased risk of convulsions when antiepileptics given with chloroquine and hydroxychloroquine; anticonvulsant effect of antiepileptics antagonised by •mefloquine

Barbiturates: plasma concentration of zonisamide reduced by phenobarbital

Zopiclone *see* Anxiolytics and Hypnotics

Zotepine *see* Antipsychotics

Zuclopenthixol *see* Antipsychotics

A2 Borderline substances

In certain conditions some foods (and toilet preparations) have characteristics of drugs and the Advisory Committee on Borderline Substances advises as to the circumstances in which such substances may be regarded as drugs. Prescriptions issued in accordance with the Committee's advice and endorsed 'ACBS' will normally not be investigated.

General Practitioners are reminded that the ACBS recommends products on the basis that they may be regarded as drugs for the management of specified conditions. Doctors should satisfy themselves that the products can safely be prescribed, that patients are adequately monitored and that, where necessary, expert hospital supervision is available.

Foods which may be prescribed on FP10, GP10 (Scotland), or when available WP10 (Wales)

Note These are food products which the ACBS has approved. The clinical condition for which the product has approval follows each entry.

Foods included in this Appendix may contain cariogenic sugars and appropriate oral hygiene measures should be taken.

Note Feeds containing more than 6 g/100 mL protein or 2 g/100 mL fibre should be avoided in children unless recommended by an appropriate specialist or dietician.

Enteral foods and supplements

Calogen® (Nutricia Clinical)

Emulsion, arachis oil (peanut oil) 50% in water, net price, 250 mL = £4.45; 500 mL = £8.73 (natural, banana, strawberry or butterscotch flavour).

For disease-related malnutrition, malabsorption states or other conditions requiring fortification with a high-fat supplement with or without fluid and electrolyte restrictions

Caloreen® (Nestlé Clinical)

Powder, water-soluble dextrins, 390 kcal/100 g, with less than 1.8 mmol of Na^+ and 0.3 mmol of K^+/100 g. Gluten-, lactose-, and fructose-free. Net price 500 g = £3.02.

For disease-related malnutrition, malabsorption states or other conditions requiring fortification with a high or readily available carbohydrate supplement

Calshake® (Fresenius Kabi)

Powder, protein 4 g, carbohydrate 58 g, fat 20.4 g, energy 1809 kJ (432 kcal)/87 g. Gluten-free. Strawberry, vanilla, neutral, and banana flavours, net price 87-g sachet = £1.82; also available chocolate flavour (protein 4 g, carbohydrate 58 g, fat 20.4 g, fibre 1.6 g, energy 1809 kJ (432 kcal)/90 g = £1.82.

For disease-related malnutrition, malabsorption states or other conditions requiring fortification with a fat/carbohydrate supplement

Clinutren® 1.5 (Nestlé Clinical)

Liquid, protein 5.5 g, carbohydrate 21 g, fat 5 g, energy 630 kJ (150 kcal)/100 mL with vitamins and minerals. Gluten-free; clinically lactose-free. Flavours: apricot, banana, chocolate, coffee, strawberry-raspberry or vanilla, net price 4 × 200-mL pot = £5.60.

For indications see *Clinutren Fruit*

Clinutren® Dessert (Nestlé Clinical)

Semi-solid, protein 12 g, carbohydrate 19 g, fat 3.3 g, energy 650 kJ (160 kcal)/ 125 g with vitamins and minerals. Gluten-free. Flavours: caramel, chocolate, peach or vanilla, net price 4 × 125-g pot = £4.20.

For use as a nutritional supplement prescribed on medical grounds for: short-bowel syndrome, intractable malabsorption, pre-operative preparation of undernourished patients, proven inflammatory bowel disease, following total gastrectomy, dysphagia, bowel fistulas, disease-related malnutrition, continuous ambulatory peritoneal dialysis (CAPD), haemodialysis. Not suitable for any child under 3 years; maximum of 3 units daily for children aged 3 to 6 years

Clinutren® 1.5 Fibre (Nestlé Clinical)

Liquid, protein 5.7 g, carbohydrate 19 g, fat 5.9 g, fibre 2.6 g, energy 630 kJ (150 kcal)/100 mL with vitamins, minerals and trace elements. Gluten-free; clinically lactose-free. Flavours: vanilla or plum, net price 4 × 200-mL pot = £5.60.

For use as the sole source of nutrition or as a necessary nutritional supplement prescribed on medical grounds for: short-bowel syndrome, intractable malabsorption, pre-operative preparation of undernourished patients, proven inflammatory bowel disease, following total gastrectomy, dysphagia, bowel fistulas, disease-related malnutrition. Not suitable for any child under 3 years; not suitable as a sole source of nutrition for patients under 6 years

Clinutren® Fruit (Nestlé Clinical)

Liquid, protein 4 g, carbohydrate 27 g, fat less than 0.2 g, energy 520 kJ (125 kcal)/100 mL with vitamins and minerals. Gluten-free. Low-lactose. Flavours: grapefruit, orange, pear-cherry, or raspberry-blackcurrant, net price 4 × 200-mL cup = £6.00.

For use as a nutritional supplement prescribed on medical grounds for: short-bowel syndrome, intractable malabsorption, pre-operative preparation of undernourished patients, proven inflammatory bowel disease, following total gastrectomy, dysphagia, bowel fistulas, disease-related malnutrition. Not suitable for any child under 3 years; maximum of 3 units daily for children aged 3 to 6 years

Clinutren® ISO (Nestlé Clinical)

Liquid, protein 3.8 g, carbohydrate 14 g, fat 3.3 g, energy 420 kJ (100 kcal)/100 mL with vitamins and minerals. Gluten-free. Flavours: chocolate or vanilla, net price 4 × 200-mL pot = £4.72.

For use as a sole source of nutrition or as a necessary nutritional supplement prescribed on medical grounds for: short-bowel syndrome, intractable malabsorption, pre-operative preparation of undernourished patients, proven inflammatory bowel disease, following total gastrectomy, dysphagia, bowel fistulas, disease-related malnutrition. Not suitable for any child under 3 years; not suitable as a sole source of nutrition for patients under 6 years; maximum of 3 units daily for children aged 3 to 6 years

Clinutren Junior® (Nestlé Clinical)

Powder, protein 13.9 g, carbohydrate 62.2 g, fat 18.3 g, energy 1950 kJ (467 kcal)/100 g with vitamins, minerals and trace elements. Gluten-free; clinically lactose-free. Flavour: vanilla, net price 400 g = £9.72.

For use as a sole source of nutrition or as a nutritional supplement prescribed on medical grounds for: short bowel syndrome, intractable malabsorption, pre-operative preparation of undernourished patients, proven inflammatory bowel disease, following total gastrectomy, dysphagia, bowel fistulas, disease-related malnutrition, and growth failure in children aged 1 to 10 years.

Duobar® (SHS)

Bar, protein-free (phenylalanine nil added), carbohydrate 49.9 g, fat 49.9 g, energy 2692 kJ (648 kcal)/100 g. Low sodium and potassium. Strawberry, toffee, or neutral flavours. Net price 45-g bar = £1.34.

For disease-related malnutrition, malabsorption states or other conditions requiring fortification with fat/carbohydrate supplement

Duocal® (SHS)

Liquid, emulsion providing carbohydrate 23.4 g, fat 7.1 g, energy 661 kJ (158 kcal)/100 mL. Low-electrolyte, gluten-, lactose-, and protein-free. Net price 250 mL = £2.74; 1 litre = £9.77

MCT Powder, carbohydrate 74 g, fat 23.2 g (of which MCT 83%), energy 2042 kJ (486 kcal)/100 g. Low electrolyte, gluten-, protein- and lactose-free. Net price 400 g = £14.69

Super Soluble Powder, carbohydrate 72.7 g, fat 22.3 g, energy 2061 kJ (492 kcal)/100 g. Low electrolyte, gluten-, protein-, and lactose-free. Net price 400 g = £12.36

All for disease-related malnutrition, malabsorption states or other conditions requiring fortification with fat/carbohydrate supplement

Elemental 028® (SHS)

028 Powder, amino acids 12%, carbohydrate 70.5–72%, fat 6.64%, energy 1544–1568 kJ (364–370 kcal)/100 g with vitamins and minerals. For preparation with water before use. Net price 100-g box (orange flavoured or plain) = £4.03

For use as the sole source of nutrition or as a nutritional supplement prescribed on medical grounds for: short-bowel syndrome, intractable malabsorption, proven inflammatory bowel disease, bowel fistulas. Not to be prescribed for any child under 1 year; use with caution for children up to 5 years

Note See also Flavour Sachets, for use with unflavoured amino acid and peptide products from SHS

Elemental 028® Extra (SHS)

Liquid, amino acids 3 g, carbohydrate 11 g, fat 3.48 g, energy 358 kJ (86 kcal)/100 mL, with vitamins, minerals, and trace elements. Flavours: grapefruit, orange and pineapple, summer fruits. Net price 250-mL carton = £2.51

Powder, amino acids 15%, carbohydrate 59%, fat 17.45%, energy 1860 kJ (443 kcal)/100 g, with vitamins, minerals, and trace elements. For preparation with water before use. Net price 100 g (plain) = £4.76; also available in banana, citrus, or orange flavours (carbohydrate 55%, energy 1793 kJ (427 kcal)/100 g), 100 g = £4.88

All for use as the sole source of nutrition or as a nutritional supplement prescribed on medical grounds for: short-bowel syndrome, intractable malabsorption, proven inflammatory bowel disease, bowel fistulas. Not to be prescribed for any child under 1 year; use with caution for children up to 5 years

Note see also Flavour Sachets, for use with unflavoured amino acid and peptide products from SHS

Emsogen® (SHS)

Powder, amino acids 15%, carbohydrate 60%, fat 16.4%, energy 1839 kJ (438 kcal)/100 g, with vitamins, minerals, and trace elements. For preparation with water before use. Net price 100 g = £5.03; also available orange-flavoured (carbohydrate 55%, energy 1754 kJ (418 kcal)/100 g), 100 g = £5.03.

For use as the sole source of nutrition or as a nutritional supplement prescribed on medical grounds for short-bowel syndrome, intractable malabsorption, proven inflammatory bowel disease, bowel fistulas. Not to be prescribed for any child under 1 year; use with caution for children up to 5 years

Enlive Plus® (Abbott)

Liquid, protein 4.8 g, carbohydrate 32.7 g, energy 638 kJ (150 kcal)/100 mL, with vitamins, minerals and trace elements. Fat- and gluten-free; clinically lactose-free. Flavours: apple, fruit punch, grapefruit, lemon and lime, orange, peach, pineapple, strawberry, net price 220-mL Tetrapak® = £1.66.

For use as a nutritional supplement prescribed on medical grounds for: short-bowel syndrome, intractable malabsorption, pre-operative preparation of undernourished patients, proven inflammatory bowel disease, following total gastrectomy, dysphagia, bowel fistulas, disease-related malnutrition. Not for use in galactosaemia. Not to be prescribed for any child under 1 year; use with caution for children up to 5 years

Enmix Plus Commence® (Abbott)

Starter pack, contains: *Ensure Plus* milkshake-style (4 flavours), yoghurt-style (2 flavours); *Enlive Plus* (4 flavours) – see *Ensure Plus®* and *Enlive Plus®* for product information, net price 1 pack (10 × 220 mL) = £16.18.

Intended as an initial 5- to 10-day supply to establish patient preferences. For use as a nutritional supplement prescribed on medical grounds for: short-bowel syndrome, intractable malabsorption, pre-operative preparation of undernourished patients, proven inflammatory bowel disease, following total gastrectomy, dysphagia, bowel fistulas, disease-related malnutrition. Not to be prescribed for any child under 1 year; use with caution for children up to 5 years

Enrich® (Abbott)

Liquid with dietary fibre, providing protein 3.8 g, carbohydrate 14 g, fat 3.5 g, fibre 1.4 g, energy 432 kJ (102 kcal)/100 mL with vitamins and minerals. Lactose- and gluten-free. Vanilla flavour. Net price 250-mL can = £2.24.

For use as the sole source of nutrition or as a nutritional supplement prescribed on medical grounds for: short-bowel syndrome, intractable malabsorption, pre-operative preparation of patients who are undernourished, proven inflammatory bowel disease, following total gastrectomy, dysphagia, disease-related malnutrition. Not to be prescribed for any child under 1 year; use with caution for children up to 5 years

Enrich Plus® (Abbott)

Liquid with dietary fibre, providing protein 6.25 g, carbohydrate 20.2 g, fat 4.92 g, fibre 1.25 g, energy 642 kJ (153 kcal)/100 mL with vitamins and minerals. Lactose- and gluten-free. Vanilla, chocolate, fruits of the forest, raspberry, strawberry, and banana flavours. Net price 200-mL Tetrapak® = £1.71.

For use as a nutritional supplement for patients with disease-related malnutrition, continuous ambulatory peritoneal dialysis (CAPD), short-bowel syndrome, intractable malabsorption, dysphagia, proven inflammatory bowel disease, bowel fistulas, gastrectomy, and pre-operative preparation of undernourished patients. Not to be prescribed for any child under 1 year; use with caution for children up to 5 years

Enshake® (Abbott)

Powder, protein 16 g, carbohydrate 78.4 g, fat 24.7 g, energy 2519 kJ (600 kcal)/310 mL serving (serving = 1 sachet reconstituted with 240mL whole milk), with vitamins, minerals and trace elements. Gluten-free. Flavours:

banana, chocolate, strawberry, vanilla, net price 96.5-g sachet = £1.82.

For use as a nutritional supplement prescribed on medical grounds for: disease-related malnutrition, malabsorption states or other conditions requiring fortification with a fat/carbohydrate supplement. Not suitable for children under 1 year

Ensure® (Abbott)

Liquid, protein 4 g, fat 3.4 g, carbohydrate 13.6 g, energy 423 kJ (100 kcal)/100 mL with minerals and vitamins, lactose- and gluten-free. Vanilla, coffee, eggnog, nut, chicken, mushroom, and asparagus flavours. Net price 250-mL can = £1.92; 500-mL ready-to-hang (vanilla) = £3.74

For use as the sole source of nutrition or as a nutritional supplement prescribed on medical grounds for: short-bowel syndrome, intractable malabsorption, pre-operative preparation of patients who are undernourished, proven inflammatory bowel disease, following total gastrectomy, dysphagia, bowel fistulas, disease-related malnutrition. Not to be prescribed for any child under 1 year; use with caution for children up to 5 years

Ensure Plus® (Abbott)

Liquid, protein 6.3 g, fat 4.9 g, carbohydrate 20.2 g, with vitamins and minerals, lactose- and gluten-free, energy 632 kJ (150 kcal)/100 mL. Vanilla flavour, (formulations may vary slightly). Net price 220-mL Tetrapak® = £1.59; 250-mL can = £2.10; 500-mL ready-to-hang (unflavoured) = £3.91; 1-litre ready-to-hang (unflavoured) = £7.63; 1.5-litre ready-to-hang (unflavoured) = £11.44. Caramel, chocolate, strawberry, banana, fruit of the forest, raspberry, orange, coffee, blackcurrant, peach, vanilla or neutral flavours. Net price 220-mL Tetrapak® = £1.59.

Yoghurt Style, protein 6.3 g, fat 4.9 g, carbohydrate 20.2 g, with vitamins, minerals and trace elements, gluten-free, clinically lactose-free, energy 632 kJ (150 kcal)/100 mL. Orange, peach, pineapple, or strawberry flavour, net price 220-mL Tetrapak® = £1.59.

Both as nutritional supplements prescribed on medical grounds for: short-bowel syndrome, intractable malabsorption, pre-operative preparation of patients who are undernourished, proven inflammatory bowel disease, following total gastrectomy, dysphagia, bowel fistulas, disease-related malnutrition, continuous ambulatory peritoneal dialysis (CAPD), and haemodialysis. Not to be prescribed for any child under 1 year; use with caution for children up to 5 years

Foodlink Complete (Foodlink)

Powder, protein 21.9 g, carbohydrate 57.3 g, fat 13.3 g, energy 1838 kJ (436.5 kcal)/100 g with vitamins and minerals, Flavours: banana, chocolate, natural, or strawberry, net price 450-g carton = £3.19; also available, vanilla with fibre, protein 19.5 g, carbohydrate 60.2 g, fat 12.3 g, fibre 8 g, energy 1804 kJ (428 kcal)/100 g = £3.75.

As a nutritional supplement prescribed on medical grounds for: short-bowel syndrome, intractable malabsorption, pre-operative preparation of undernourished patients, proven inflammatory bowel disease, following total gastrectomy, dysphagia, bowel fistulas, disease-related malnutrition. Not to be prescribed for any child under 1 year; use with caution for children up to 5 years

Formance® (Abbott)

Semi-solid, protein 4 g, carbohydrate 27 g, fat 5 g, energy 703 kJ (167 kcal)/113 g with vitamins and minerals. Gluten-free. Vanilla and butterscotch flavours. Net price 113-g pot = £1.40.

As a nutritional supplement prescribed on medical grounds for: short-bowel syndrome, intractable malabsorption, pre-operative preparation of patients who are undernourished, proven inflammatory bowel disease, following total gastrectomy, dysphagia, bowel fistulas, disease-related malnutrition, continuous ambulatory peritoneal dialysis (CAPD), and haemodialysis. Not to be prescribed for any child under 1 year; use with caution for children up to 5 years

Forticreme® (Nutricia Clinical)

Semi-solid, protein 10 g, carbohydrate 19 g, fat 5 g, energy 680 kJ (160 kcal)/100 g with vitamins and minerals. Gluten-free. Vanilla, chocolate, coffee, banana, and forest fruit flavours, net price 4 × 125-g pot = £6.37.

As a nutritional supplement prescribed on medical grounds for: short-bowel syndrome, intractable malabsorption, pre-operative preparation of patients who are undernourished, proven inflammatory bowel disease, following total gastrectomy, dysphagia, bowel fistulas, disease-related malnutrition, continuous ambulatory peritoneal dialysis (CAPD) and haemodialysis. Not to be prescribed for any child under 3 years; use with caution for children aged 3 to 5 years

Fortifresh® (Nutricia Clinical)

Liquid, protein 12 g, carbohydrate 37.4 g, fat 11.6 g, energy 1260 kJ (300 kcal)/200 mL with vitamins, minerals and trace elements. Gluten-free. Flavours: blackcurrant, peach and orange, pineapple, raspberry, and vanilla and lemon, net price 200 mL carton = £1.64.

For use as a sole source of nutrition or as a nutritional supplement prescribed on medical grounds for: short-bowel syndrome, intractable malabsorption, pre-operative preparation of patients who are undernourished, inflammatory bowel disease, following total gastrectomy, dysphagia, bowel fistulas, disease-related malnutrition. Not to be prescribed for any child under 3 years; use with caution for children aged 3 to 5 years; not suitable as a sole source of nutrition in children under 6 years

Fortijuce® (Nutricia Clinical)

Liquid, protein 4 g, carbohydrate 33.5 g, energy 630 kJ (150 kcal)/100 mL, with vitamins, minerals and trace elements. Fat-free. Flavours: apricot, blackcurrant, lemon and lime, peach and orange, pineapple, apple and pear, and forest fruits. Net price 200-mL carton = £1.64.

As a nutritional supplement prescribed on medical grounds for: short-bowel syndrome, intractable malabsorption, pre-operative preparation of patients who are undernourished, proven inflammatory bowel disease, following total gastrectomy, dysphagia, bowel fistulas, disease-related malnutrition. Not to be prescribed for any child under 3 years; use with caution for children up to 5 years

Fortimel® (Nutricia Clinical)

Liquid, protein 20 g, carbohydrate 20.6 g (chocolate flavour has 20.8 g), fat 4.2 g, energy 840 kJ (200 kcal)/200 mL with vitamins and minerals. Gluten-free. Vanilla, strawberry, coffee, chocolate, and forest fruits flavours. Net price 200-mL carton = £1.39.

As a nutritional supplement prescribed on medical grounds for: short-bowel syndrome, intractable malabsorption, pre-operative preparation of patients who are undernourished, proven inflammatory bowel disease, following total gastrectomy, dysphagia, bowel fistulas, disease-related malnutrition. Not to be prescribed for any child under 3 years; use with caution for children up to 5 years

Fortini® (Nutricia Clinical)

Liquid, protein 3.4 g, carbohydrate 18.8 g, fat 6.8 g, energy 630 kJ (150 kcal)/100 mL with vitamins, minerals, and trace elements. Gluten- and lactose-free. Flavours: strawberry or vanilla, net price 200 mL = £2.38.

For use as a sole source of nutrition or as a nutritional supplement prescribed on medical grounds for: disease-related malnutrition, and growth failure. For children aged 1–6 years (8–20 kg body-weight)

Fortini Multifibre® (Nutricia Clinical)

Liquid, protein 3.4 g, carbohydrate 18.8 g, fat 6.8 g, fibre 1.5 g, energy 630 kJ (150 kcal)/ 100 mL with vitamins, minerals, and trace elements. Gluten- and lactose-free. Flavours: banana, chocolate, strawberry, and vanilla, net price 200-mL = £2.50.

For indications see Fortini liquid

Fortisip® Bottle (Nutricia Clinical)

Liquid, protein 12 g, carbohydrate 36.8 g, fat 11.6 g, energy 1260 kJ (300 kcal)/200 mL, with vitamins, minerals and trace elements. Gluten-free; clinically lactose-free. Vanilla, banana, chocolate, orange, strawberry, tropical fruits, toffee, and neutral flavours, net price 200 mL = £1.63.

As a nutritional supplement prescribed on medical grounds for: short-bowel syndrome, intractable malabsorption, pre-operative preparation of patients who are undernourished, proven inflammatory bowel disease, following total gastrectomy, dysphagia, bowel fistulas, disease-related malnutrition. Not to be prescribed for any child under 3 years; use with caution for children aged 3 to 5 years

Fortisip® Multi Fibre (Nutricia Clinical)
Liquid, protein 12 g, carbohydrate 36.8 g, fat 11.6 g, fibre 4.6 g, energy 1260 kJ (300 kcal)/200 mL, with vitamins, minerals and trace elements. Gluten-free, clinically lactose-free. Banana, chicken, orange, strawberry, tomato, vanilla flavours; also available chocolate flavour (protein 10 g, carbohydrate 36 g, fat 13 g, fibre 4.5 g, energy 1260 kJ (300 kcal)/200 mL, net price 200 mL = £1.69.

As a sole source of nutrition or as a nutritional supplement prescribed on medical grounds for: short-bowel syndrome, intractable malabsorption, pre-operative preparation of undernourished patients, proven inflammatory bowel disease, following total gastrectomy, dysphagia, disease-related malnutrition. Not to be prescribed for any child under 3 years; use with caution for children aged 3 to 5 years

Fortisip® Protein (Nutricia Clinical)
Liquid, protein 10 g, carbohydrate 14.7 g, fat 3.5 g, energy 550 kJ (130 kcal)/100 mL, with vitamins, minerals and trace elements. Gluten-free. Chocolate, forest fruits, strawberry, and vanilla flavour, net price 200 mL = £1.54.

As a nutritional supplement prescribed on medical grounds for: short-bowel syndrome, intractable malabsorption, pre-operative preparation of undernourished patients, proven inflammatory bowel disease, following total gastrectomy, dysphagia, bowel fistulas, disease-related malnutrition. Not to be prescribed for any child under 3 years

Frebini® Energy (Fresenius Kabi)
Sip feed, protein 3.75 g, carbohydrate 18.8 g, fat 6.65 g, energy 630 kJ (150 kcal)/100 mL, with vitamins, minerals and trace elements. Gluten-free; clinically lactose-free. Flavours: banana or strawberry. Net price 200-mL carton = £2.16.

Tube feed, protein 3.75 g, carbohydrate 18.75 g, fat 6.7 g, energy 630 kJ (150 kcal)/100 mL, with vitamins, minerals and trace elements. Gluten-free; clinically lactose-free. Flavour: neutral, net price 500-mL EasyBag® = £5.70.

For use as a sole source of nutrition or as a nutritional supplement for children aged 1 to 10 years or 8–30kg with disease-related malnutrition and/or growth failure, proven inflammatory bowel disease, following total gastrectomy, short-bowel syndrome, intractable malabsorption, dysphagia, bowel fistulas, and for pre-operative preparation of malnourished patients. Not to be prescribed for any child under 1 year

Frebini® Energy Fibre (Fresenius Kabi)
Sip feed, protein 3.75 g, carbohydrate 18.8 g, fat 6.65 g, fibre 1.1 g, energy 630 kJ (150 kcal)/100 mL, with vitamins, minerals and trace elements. Gluten-free; clinically lactose-free. Chocolate flavour, net price 200-mL carton = £2.21.

Tube feed, protein 3.75 g, carbohydrate 18.75 g, fat 6.7 g, fibre 1.13 g, energy 630 kJ (150 kcal)/100 mL, with vitamins, minerals and trace elements. Gluten-free, clinically lactose-free. Flavour: neutral, net price 500-mL EasyBag® = £6.10.

For indications see *Frebini Energy®*

Frebini® Original (Fresenius Kabi)
Liquid, tube feed, protein 2.5 g, carbohydrate 13.5 g, fat 4 g, energy 420 kJ (100 kcal)/100 mL, with vitamins, minerals and trace elements. Flavour: neutral, net price 500-mL EasyBag® = £4.55

For use as the sole source of nutrition or as a nutritional supplement for children aged 1–10 years or 8–30kg with short-bowel syndrome, intractable malabsorption, pre-operative preparation of patients who are undernourished, proven inflammatory bowel disease, following total gastrectomy, dysphagia, bowel fistulas, disease-related malnutrition and/or growth failure. Not to be prescribed for any child under 1 year

Frebini® Original Fibre (Fresenius Kabi)
Tube feed, protein 2.5 g, carbohydrate 12.5 g, fat 4.4 g, fibre 750 mg, energy 420 kJ (100 kcal)/100 mL, with vitamins, minerals and trace elements. Gluten-free, clinically lactose-free. Neutral flavour, net price 500-mL EasyBag® = £5.05

For use as a sole source of nutrition or as a nutritional supplement for children aged 1–10 years or 8–30kg with disease-related malnutrition and/or growth failure, proven inflammatory bowel disease, following total gastrectomy, short-bowel syndrome, intractable malabsorption, dysphagia, bowel fistulas, and pre-operative preparation of malnourished patients. Not to be prescribed for any child under 1 year

Fresubin® Energy (Fresenius Kabi)
Liquid, protein 5.65 g, carbohydrate 18.8 g, fat 5.83 g, energy 630 kJ (150 kcal)/100 mL, with vitamins and minerals. Net price 200-mL carton = £1.55 (flavours: vanilla, strawberry, butterscotch, blackcurrant, banana, orange, pineapple, chocolate-mint, vegetable cream, and neutral): 500-mL bottle = £3.80 (flavour: neutral); 500-mL EasyBag® = £3.88; 1-litre EasyBag® = £7.70; 1.5-litre EasyBag® = £9.60.

For use as sole source of nutrition or as a nutritional supplement prescribed on medical grounds for: short-bowel syndrome, intractable malabsorption, pre-operative preparation of undernourished patients, proven inflammatory bowel disease, following total gastrectomy, dysphagia, bowel fistulas, disease-related malnutrition. Not to be prescribed for any child under 1 year; use with caution for children under 5 years

Fresubin® Energy Fibre (Fresenius Kabi)
Sip feed, protein 5.65 g, carbohydrate 18.8 g, fat 5.83 g, fibre 2.5 g, energy 630 kJ (150 kcal)/100 mL, with vitamins, minerals and trace elements. Gluten-free; clinically lactose-free. Flavours: banana, cappucino, chocolate, lemon, strawberry, vanilla. Net price 200-mL carton = £1.70.

For indications see *Fresubin® Energy*

Tube feed, protein 5.6 g, carbohydrate 18.8 g, fat 5.8 g, fibre 2 g, energy 630 kJ (150 kcal)/100 mL, with vitamins, minerals and trace elements. Gluten-free; clinically lactose-free. Unflavoured, net price 500-mL EasyBag® = £4.00; 1-litre EasyBag® = £7.99; 1.5-litre EasyBag® = £10.60.

For indications see *Fresubin® Energy*

Fresubin HP Energy® (Fresenius Kabi)
Liquid, protein 7.5 g, carbohydrate 17 g, fat 6 g, energy 630 kJ (150 kcal)/100 mL with vitamins, minerals, and trace elements. Gluten-free and low lactose. Vanilla flavour. Net price 500-mL bottle = £3.67; 500-mL EasyBag® = £3.72; 1-litre EasyBag® = £7.44.

As a nutritional supplement prescribed on medical grounds for: short-bowel syndrome, intractable malabsorption, pre-operative preparation of patients who are undernourished, proven inflammatory bowel disease, following total gastrectomy, dysphagia, bowel fistulas, disease-related malnutrition, continuous ambulatory peritoneal dialysis (CAPD), and haemodialysis. Not to be prescribed for any child under 1 year; use with caution for children up to 5 years

Fresubin® 1000 Complete (Fresenius Kabi)
Liquid, tube feed, protein 5.5 g, carbohydrate 12.5 g, fat 3.1 g, fibre 2 g, energy 420 kJ (100 kcal)/100mL with vitamins, minerals and trace elements. Gluten-free, clinically lactose-free, net price 1-litre EasyBag® = £8.20.

For use as the sole source of nutrition or as a nutritional supplement prescribed on medical grounds for: short-bowel syndrome, intractable malabsorption, pre-operative preparation of undernourished patients, proven inflammatory bowel disease, following total gastrectomy, dysphagia, bowel fistulas, disease-related malnutrition. Not to be prescribed for any child under 1 year; use with caution for children up to 5 years

Fresubin® 1200 Complete (Fresenius Kabi)
Liquid, tube feed, protein 4 g, carbohydrate 10 g, fat 2.7 g, fibre 2 g, energy 336 kJ (80 kcal)/100 mL with vitamins, minerals and trace elements. Gluten-free, clinically lactose-free, net price 1.5-litre EasyBag® = £10.20.

For use as the sole source of nutrition or as a nutritional supplement prescribed on medical grounds for: short-bowel syndrome, intractable malabsorption, pre-operative preparation of undernourished patients, proven inflammatory bowel disease, following total gastrectomy, bowel fistulas, disease-related malnutrition. Not to be prescribed for any child under 5 years

Fresubin® Original (Fresenius Kabi)
Liquid, protein 3.8 g, carbohydrate 13.8 g, fat 3.4 g, energy 420 kJ (100 kcal)/100 mL with vitamins and minerals. Gluten-free, low lactose and cholesterol. Net price 200-mL carton (nut, peach, blackcurrant, chocolate, mocha, and vanilla flavours) = £1.55; 500-mL bottle (neutral flavour) = £3.08; 500-mL EasyBag® = £2.99; 1-litre EasyBag® = £5.97; 1.5-litre EasyBag® = £8.96

For use as the sole source of nutrition or as a nutritional supplement prescribed on medical grounds for: short-bowel syndrome, intractable malabsorption, pre-operative preparation of patients who are undernourished, proven inflammatory bowel disease, following total gastrectomy, dysphagia, bowel fistulas, and disease-related malnutrition. Not to be prescribed for any child under 1 year; use with caution for children up to 5 years

Fresubin® Original Fibre (Fresenius Kabi)
Liquid with dietary fibre, protein 3.8 g, carbohydrate 13.8 g, fat 3.4 g, energy 420 kJ (100 kcal)/100 mL, with vitamins and minerals. Flavour: neutral. Net price 500-mL bottle = £3.48; 500-mL EasyBag® = £3.62; 1-litre EasyBag® = £7.24; 1.5-litre EasyBag® = £10.20.

For use as sole source of nutrition or as a nutritional supplement prescribed on medical grounds for: short-bowel syndrome, intractable malabsorption, pre-operative preparation of patients who are undernourished, proven inflammatory bowel disease, following total gastrectomy, dysphagia, disease-related malnutrition. Not to be prescribed for any child under 2 years; use with caution for children up to 5 years

Fresubin Protein Energy Drink (Fresenius Kabi)
Liquid, protein 10 g, carbohydrate 12.4 g, fat 6.7 g, energy 630 kJ (150 kcal)/100 mL, with vitamins, minerals and trace elements. Gluten- and lactose-free. Chocolate, strawberry, and vanilla flavours, net price 200-mL = £1.58.

As a necessary nutritional supplement prescribed on medical grounds for: short-bowel syndrome, intractable malabsorption, pre-operative preparation of undernourished patients, proven inflammatory bowel disease, following total gastrectomy, dysphagia, bowel fistulas, disease-related malnutrition, continuous ambulatory peritoneal dialysis (CAPD), haemodialysis. Not to be prescribed for any child under 1 year; use with caution for children up to 5 years of age

Infatrini® (Nutricia Clinical)
Liquid, protein 2.6 g, carbohydrate 10.3 g, fat 5.4 g, energy 420 kJ (100 kcal)/100 mL with vitamins, minerals and trace elements. Gluten-free. Net price 100 mL bottle = 88p, 200-mL Tetrapak® = £1.75

For use as a sole source of nutrition or as a nutritional supplement prescribed on medical grounds for: failure to thrive, disease-related malnutrition and malabsorption. Manufacturer advises suitable for infants up to 8 kg body weight (0–12 months of age)

Isosource® Energy (Novartis Consumer Health)
Liquid, protein 5.7 g, carbohydrate 20 g, fat 6.2 g, energy 660 kJ (160 kcal)/100 mL with vitamins, minerals and trace elements. Gluten-free; clinically lactose-free. Net price 500-mL flexible pouch = £3.72, 1-litre flexible pouch = £7.44.

For indications see *Isosource Standard*

Isosource® Energy Fibre (Novartis Consumer Health)
Liquid, tube feed, protein 4.9 g, carbohydrate 20.2 g, fat 5.5 g, fibre, 1.5 g, energy 630 kJ (150 kcal)/100 mL with vitamins, minerals and trace elements. Gluten-free; clinically lactose-free. Net price 500-mL flexible pouch = £4.04, 1-litre flexible pouch = £8.08.

For use as the sole source of nutrition or as a nutritional supplement prescribed on medical grounds for: short-bowel syndrome, intractable malabsorption, pre-operative preparation of undernourished patients, proven inflammatory bowel disease, following total gastrectomy, dysphagia, disease-related malnutrition. Not to be prescribed for any child under 1 year; use with caution for children up to 5 years

Isosource® Fibre (Novartis Consumer Health)
Liquid , protein 3.8 g, carbohydrate 13.6 g, fat 3.4 g, fibre 1.4 g, energy 422 kJ (100 kcal)/100 mL with vitamins, minerals and trace elements. Gluten-free; clinically lactose-free. Net price 500-mL flexible pouch = £3.45, 1-litre flexible pouch = £6.90.

For indications see *Isosource Standard*

Isosource® Junior (Novartis Consumer Health)
Liquid, protein 2.7 g, carbohydrate 17 g, fat 4.7 g, energy 512 kJ (122 kcal)/100 mL with vitamins, minerals and trace elements. Gluten-free; clinically lactose-free. Net price 500-mL flexible pouch = £5.17.

Nutritionally complete feed for disease-related malnutrition, short-bowel syndrome, intractable malabsorption, pre-operative preparation of undernourished patients, proven inflammatory bowel disease, following total gastrectomy, dysphagia, bowel fistulas, growth failure, for children aged 1 to 6 years or 8 to 20 kg

Isosource® Standard (Novartis Consumer Health)
Liquid, protein 4.1 g, carbohydrate 14.2 g, fat 3.5 g, energy 441 kJ (105 kcal)/100 mL with vitamins, minerals and trace elements. Gluten-free; clinically lactose-free. Net price 500-mL flexible pouch = £3.03, 1-litre flexible pouch = £6.06.

For use as a sole source of nutrition or as a nutritional supplement prescribed on medical grounds for: short-bowel syndrome, intractable malabsorption, pre-operative preparation of undernourished patients, proven inflammatory bowel disease, following total gastrectomy, dysphagia, bowel fistulas, disease-related malnutrition. Not to be prescribed for any child under 1 year; use with caution for children up to 5 years

Jevity® (Abbott)
Liquid, protein 4 g, fat 3.5 g, carbohydrate 14.8 g, dietary fibre 1.1 g, energy 441 kJ (106 kcal)/100 mL, with vitamins and minerals. Gluten-, lactose-, and sucrose-free. Net price 500-mL ready-to-hang = £3.53, 1-litre ready-to-hang = £6.82, 1.5-litre ready-to-hang = £10.23.

For use as the sole source of nutrition or as a nutritional supplement prescribed on medical grounds for: short-bowel syndrome, intractable malabsorption, pre-operative preparation of patients who are undernourished, proven inflammatory bowel disease, bowel fistulas, following total gastrectomy, dysphagia, disease-related malnutrition. Not to be prescribed for any child under 2 years; use with caution for children up to 5 years

Jevity 1.5 kcal® (Abbott)
Liquid, tube feed, protein 6.38 g, carbohydrate 21.1 g, fat 4.9 g, fibre 1.2 g, energy 640 kJ (152 kcal)/100 mL, with vitamins, minerals and trace elements. Gluten- and lactose-free. Net price 500-mL ready-to-hang = £4.42, 1-litre ready-to-hang = £8.20, 1.5-litre ready-to-hang = £12.80.

For use as the sole source of nutrition or as a nutritional supplement prescribed on medical grounds for: short-bowel syndrome, intractable malabsorption, pre-operative preparation of undernourished patients, proven inflammatory bowel disease, bowel fistulas, following total gastrectomy, dysphagia, disease-related malnutrition. Not to be prescribed for any child under 2 years; use with caution for children up to 10 years

Jevity Plus® (Abbott)
Liquid, protein 5.6 g, carbohydrate 16.1 g, fat 3.9 g, dietary fibre 1.2 g, energy 504 kJ (120 kcal)/100 mL, with vitamins and minerals. Gluten- and lactose-free. Net price 500-mL ready-to-hang = £4.00, 1-litre ready-to-hang = £8.18, 1.5-litre ready-to-hang = £12.28.

For indications see under *Jevity®*.

Jevity Promote® (Abbott)
Liquid, protein 5.55 g, carbohydrate 11.98 g, fat 3.32 g, dietary fibre 1.7 g, energy 427 kJ (101 kcal)/100 mL, with vitamins and minerals. Gluten-free, clinically lactose-free. Net price 1-litre ready-to-hang = £8.00.
For use as the sole source of nutrition or as a nutritional supplement prescribed on medical grounds for: short-bowel syndrome, intractable malabsorption, pre-operative preparation of undernourished patients, proven inflammatory bowel disease, following total gastrectomy, dysphagia, disease-related malnutrition, bowel fistulas. Not to be prescribed for any child under 2 years; use with caution for children up to 10 years

Kindergen® (SHS)
Powder, protein 7.5 g, carbohydrate 60.5 g, fat 26.1 g, energy 2060 kJ (492 kcal)/100 g with vitamins and minerals. Net price 400 g = £19.86.
For complete nutritional support or supplementary feeding for infants and children with chronic renal failure who are receiving peritoneal rapid overnight dialysis

Maxijul® (SHS)
Liquid, carbohydrate 50%, with potassium 0.004%, sodium 0.023%. Gluten-, lactose-, and fructose-free. Flavours: blackcurrant, lemon and lime, orange, and natural. Net price 200 mL = £1.12
LE Powder, modification of *Maxijul®* with lower concentrations of sodium and potassium. Net price 200 g = £3.82, 2 kg = £26.62
Super Soluble Powder, glucose polymer, potassium 0.004%, sodium 0.046%. Gluten-, lactose-, and fructose-free. Net price 4 × 132-g sachet pack = £4.41, 200 g = £1.78, 2.5 kg = £15.66, 25 kg = £106.35
All for disease-related malnutrition; malabsorption states or other conditions requiring fortification with high or readily available carbohydrate supplement

Modulen IBD® (Nestlé)
Powder, protein 18 g, carbohydrate 54 g, fat 23 g, energy 2040 kJ (500 kcal)/100 g with vitamins, minerals and trace elements. Net price 400 g = £9.72.
For use as the sole source of nutrition during the active phase of Crohn's disease and for nutritional support during the remission phase in patients who are malnourished. Not to be prescribed for any child under one year; use with caution for children up to 5 years
May be flavoured with Nestlé Nutrition Flavour Mix (see under *Peptamen*)

Novasource® Forte (Novartis Consumer Health)
Liquid, protein 6 g, carbohydrate 18.3 g, fat 5.9 g, fibre 2.2 g, energy 631 kJ (150 kcal)/100 mL with vitamins, minerals and trace elements. Gluten-free; low-lactose, net price 500-mL flexible pouch = £4.36.
For use as a sole source of nutrition or as a nutritional supplement prescribed on medical grounds for: short-bowel syndrome, intractable malabsorption, pre-operative preparation of undernourished patients, proven inflammatory bowel disease, following total gastrectomy, dysphagia, bowel fistulas, disease-related malnutrition, neoplasia-related cachexia. Not to be prescribed for any child under 1 year; use with caution for children up to 5 years

Novasource GI Control® (Novartis Consumer Health)
Liquid, protein 4.1 g, carbohydrate 14.2 g, fat 3.5 g, fibre 2.2 g, energy 440 kJ (100 kcal)/100 mL with vitamins minerals and trace elements. Gluten-free; clinically lactose-free, net price 500-mL bottle = £4.39, 500-mL flexible pouch = £4.70.
For use as a sole source of nutrition or as a nutritional supplement prescribed on medical grounds for: short-bowel syndrome, intractable malabsorption, pre-operative preparation of undernourished patients, proven inflammatory bowel disease, following total gastrectomy, dysphagia, bowel fistulas, disease-related malnutrition. Not to be prescribed for any child under 1 year; use with caution for children up to 5 years

Nutrini® (Nutricia Clinical)
Liquid, protein 2.75 g, carbohydrate 12.3 g, fat 4.4 g, energy 420 kJ (100 kcal)/100 mL. Gluten- and sucrose-free; clinically lactose-free. Net price 200-mL bottle = £1.93, 500-mL pack = £4.83.
For use as the sole source of nutrition or as a nutritional supplement prescribed on medical grounds for: short-bowel syndrome, intractable malabsorption, pre-operative preparation of undernourished patients, proven inflammatory bowel disease, following total gastrectomy, dysphagia, bowel fistulas, disease-related malnutrition and/or growth failure. For children aged between 1 to 6 years or 8–20 kg body-weight

Nutrini® Energy (Nutricia Clinical)
Liquid, protein 4.1 g, carbohydrate 18.5 g, fat 6.7 g, energy 630 kJ (150 kcal)/100 mL. Gluten- and sucrose-free; clinically lactose-free. Net price 200-mL bottle = £2.38, 500-mL pack = £5.95.
For use as the sole source of nutrition or as a nutritional supplement prescribed on medical grounds for: short-bowel syndrome, intractable malabsorption, pre-operative preparation of undernourished patients, following total gastrectomy, dysphagia, bowel fistulas, disease-related malnutrition and growth failure. For children aged 1 to 6 years or between 8–20 kg body-weight

Nutrini® Energy Multi Fibre (Nutricia Clinical)
Liquid, tube feed, protein 4.1 g, carbohydrate 18.5 g, fat 6.7 g, fibre 0.75 g, energy 630 kJ (150 kcal)/100 mL with vitamins, minerals and trace elements. Gluten- and lactose-free, net price 200-mL bottle = £2.58, 500-mL pack = £6.44.
For short-bowel syndrome, intractable malabsorption, pre-operative preparation of undernourished patients, total gastrectomy, dysphagia, disease-related malnutrition, and growth failure. For children aged 1 to 6 years or between 8–20 kg body-weight

Nutrini® Low Energy Multi Fibre (Nutricia Clinical)
Liquid, tube feed, protein 2.06 g, carbohydrate 9.3 g, fat 3.3 g, fibre 0.75 g, energy 315 kJ (75 kcal)/100 mL with vitamins, minerals and trace elements. Gluten- and lactose-free, net price 200-mL bottle = £1.87, 500-mL pack = £4.71
For indications see *Nutrini Multi Fibre*

Nutrini® Multi Fibre (Nutricia Clinical)
Liquid, protein 2.75 g, carbohydrate 12.3 g, fat 4.4 g, fibre 750 mg, energy 420 kJ (100 kcal)/100 mL. Gluten- and sucrose-free; clinically lactose-free. Net price 200-mL bottle = £2.14, 500-mL pack = £5.35.
For use as a sole source of nutrition or as a nutritional supplement prescribed on medical grounds for: short-bowel syndrome, intractable malabsorption, pre-operative preparation of undernourished patients, total gastrectomy, dysphagia, disease-related malnutrition and growth failure. For children aged 1 to 6 years or 8–20 kg body-weight

Nutriprem 2® (Cow & Gate)
Liquid, protein 2 g, carbohydrate 7.5 g, fat 4.1 g, energy 310 kJ (75 kcal)/100 mL, with vitamins, minerals, and trace elements, net price 200-mL Tetrapak® = £1.32. Also available to hospitals-only as a sterilised prepared feed in 100-mL bottles
Powder, protein 2 g, carbohydrate 7.4 g, fat 4.1 g, energy 310 kJ (75 kcal) per 100 mL when reconstituted, with vitamins and minerals. Net price 900 g = £8.80.
For catch-up growth in pre-term infants (less than 35 weeks at birth), and small-for-gestational-age infants, until 6 months corrected age

Nutrison® Energy (Nutricia Clinical)
Liquid, protein 6 g, carbohydrate 18.5 g, fat 5.8 g, energy 630 kJ (150 kcal)/100 mL with vitamins, minerals and trace elements. Gluten- and sucrose-free; clinically lactose-free. Net price 500-mL bottle = £3.77; 500-mL pack = £4.04; 1-litre pack = £7.55; 1.5-litre pack = £11.32.
As a nutritional supplement prescribed on medical grounds for: short-bowel syndrome, intractable malabsorption, pre-operative preparation of undernourished

patients, proven inflammatory bowel disease, following total gastrectomy, dysphagia, bowel fistulas, disease-related malnutrition. Not to be prescribed for any child under 1 year; use with caution for children aged 1 to 6 years

Nutrison® Energy Multi Fibre (Nutricia Clinical)
Liquid, protein 6 g, carbohydrate 18.5 g, fat 5.8 g, fibre 1.5 g, energy 630 kJ (150 kcal)/100 mL with vitamins, minerals, and trace elements. Gluten-free and clinically lactose-free. Net price 500-mL bottle = £4.20; 500-mL pack = £4.48; 1-litre pack = £8.39; 1.5-litre pack = £13.45.
For use as the sole source of nutrition or as a nutritional supplement prescribed on medical grounds for: short-bowel syndrome, intractable malabsorption, pre-operative preparation of undernourished patients, proven inflammatory bowel disease, following total gastrectomy, dysphagia, disease-related malnutrition. Not to be prescribed for any child under 1 year; use with caution for children aged 1 to 6 years

Nutrison MCT® (Nutricia Clinical)
Liquid, protein 5 g, carbohydrate 12.6 g, fat 3.3 g, energy 420 kJ (100 kcal)/100 mL with vitamins, minerals and trace elements. Gluten- and fructose-free, clinically lactose-free. Net price 1-litre pack = £7.05.
For indications see *Nutrison Energy*. Not to be prescribed for any child under 1 year; use with caution for children aged 1 to 6 years

Nutrison® Multi Fibre (Nutricia Clinical)
Liquid, protein 4 g, carbohydrate 12.3 g, fat 3.9 g, fibre 1.5 g, energy 420 kJ (100 kcal)/100 mL with vitamins, minerals and trace elements. Gluten- and sucrose-free; clinically lactose-free. Net price 500-mL bottle = £3.40; 500-mL pack = £3.63; 1-litre pack = £6.79; 1.5-litre pack = £10.19.
For indications see *Nutrison Standard* excluding bowel fistulas. Not to be prescribed for any child under 1 year; use with caution for children aged 1 to 6 years

Nutrison® Protein Plus (Nutricia Clinical)
Liquid, protein 6.3 g, carbohydrate 14.2 g, fat 4.9 g, energy 525 kJ (125 kcal)/100 mL, with vitamins, minerals and trace elements. Gluten- and lactose-free. Net price l-litre pack = £7.45.
For use in the dietary management of disease-related malnutrition. Not suitable for infants under 1 year; use with caution in children aged 1 to 6 years

Nutrison® Protein Plus Multi Fibre (Nutricia Clinical)
Liquid, protein 6.3 g, carbohydrate 14.2 g, fat 4.9 g, fibre 1.5 g, energy 525 kJ (125 kcal)/100 mL, with vitamins, minerals and trace elements. Gluten- and clinically lactose-free. Net price l-litre pack = £8.29.
For use in the dietary management of disease-related malnutrition. Not suitable for infants under 1 year; use with caution in children aged 1 to 6 years

Nutrison® Soya (Nutricia Clinical)
Liquid, protein 4 g, carbohydrate 12.3 g, fat 3.9 g, energy 420 kJ (100 kcal)/100 mL, with vitamins, minerals and trace elements. Gluten- and sucrose-free; clinically lactose-free. Net price 500-mL bottle = £3.75; 1-litre pack = £7.50.
For use as the sole source of nutrition or as a nutritional supplement prescribed on medical grounds for: cow's milk protein and lactose intolerance, short-bowel syndrome, intractable malabsorption, pre-operative preparation of undernourished patients, proven inflammatory bowel disease, following total gastrectomy, dysphagia, bowel fistulas, disease-related malnutrition. Not to be prescribed for any child under 1 year; use with caution for children aged 1 to 6 years

Nutrison® Standard (Nutricia Clinical)
Liquid, protein 4 g, carbohydrate 12.3 g, fat 3.9 g, energy 425 kJ (100 kcal)/100 mL, with vitamins, minerals and trace elements. Gluten- and sucrose-free; clinically lactose-free. Net price 500-mL bottle = £3.12; 500-mL pack = £3.36; 1-litre pack = £6.09; 1.5-litre pack = £9.14.
For use as the sole source of nutrition or as a nutritional supplement prescribed on medical grounds for: short-bowel syndrome, intractable malabsorption, pre-operative preparation of undernourished patients, proven inflammatory bowel disease, following total gastrectomy, dysphagia, bowel fistulas, disease-related malnutrition. Not to be prescribed for any child under 1 year; use with caution for children aged 1 to 6 years

Nutrison® 1000 Complete Multi Fibre (Nutricia Clinical)
Liquid, protein 5.5 g, carbohydrate 11.3 g, fat 3.7 g, fibre 2 g, energy 420 kJ (100 kcal)/100 mL, with vitamins, minerals and trace elements. Gluten- and clinically lactose-free, net price l-litre pack = £8.05.
For use as the sole source of nutrition or as a nutritional supplement prescribed on medical grounds for: short-bowel syndrome, intractable malabsorption, pre-operative preparation of undernourished patients, proven inflammatory bowel disease, following total gastrectomy, dysphagia, disease-related malnutrition. Not to be prescribed for any child under 1 year; use with caution for children aged 1 to 6 years

Nutrison® 1200 Complete Multi Fibre (Nutricia Clinical)
Liquid, protein 5.5 g, carbohydrate 15 g, fat 4.3 g, fibre 2 g, energy 505 kJ (120 kcal)/100 mL, with vitamins, minerals and trace elements. Gluten- and clinically lactose-free, net price 500-mL bottle = £4.03; l-litre pack = £8.05; 1.5-litre pack = £12.08.
As a sole source of nutrition or as a nutritional supplement prescribed on medical grounds for: short-bowel syndrome, intractable malabsorption, pre-operative preparation of undernourished patients, proven inflammatory bowel disease, following total gastrectomy, dysphagia, disease-related malnutrition. Not to be prescribed for any child under 1 year; use with caution for children aged 1 to 6 years

Osmolite® (Abbott)
Liquid, protein 4 g, carbohydrate 13.56 g, fat 3.4 g, energy 424 kJ (100 kcal)/100 mL with vitamins and minerals. Gluten- and lactose-free. Net price 250-mL can = £1.69; 500-mL bottle = £3.10, 1-litre bottle = £5.99, 1.5-litre bottle = £8.99.
For use as the sole source of nutrition or as a nutritional supplement prescribed on medical grounds for: short-bowel syndrome, intractable malabsorption, pre-operative preparation of undernourished patients, proven inflammatory bowel disease, following total gastrectomy, bowel fistulas, disease-related malnutrition, dysphagia. Not to be prescribed for any child under 1 year; use with caution for children up to 5 years

Osmolite Plus® (Abbott)
Liquid, protein 5.6 g, carbohydrate 15.8 g, fat 3.9 g, energy 508 kJ (121 kcal)/100 mL with vitamins, minerals and trace elements. Gluten-free and clinically lactose-free. Net price 500-mL ready-to-hang = £3.73, 1-litre ready-to-hang = £7.20, 1.5-litre ready-to-hang = £10.79.
For indications see *Osmolite*

Paediasure® (Abbott)
Liquid, protein 2.8 g, carbohydrate 11 g, fat 5 g, energy 422 kJ (101 kcal)/100 mL with vitamins and minerals. Gluten-free, clinically lactose-free. Flavours: vanilla (can, ready-to-hang and Tetrapaks®), strawberry, chocolate and banana (Tetrapaks®). Net price 250-mL can = £2.34, 500-mL ready-to-hang = £4.69, 200-mL Tetrapaks® = £1.88.
For use as the sole source of nutrition or as a nutritional supplement prescribed on medical grounds for children aged 1 to 10 years for short-bowel syndrome, intractable malabsorption, pre-operative preparation of undernourished patients, dysphagia, bowel fistulas, and disease-related malnutrition and/or growth failure. Not to be prescribed for any child under 1 year

Paediasure® Fibre (Abbott)
Liquid, protein 2.8 g, carbohydrate 11.16 g, fat 5 g, fibre 520 mg, energy 422 kJ (101 kcal)/100 mL with vitamins and minerals. Gluten-free, clinically lactose-free. Flavours: vanilla (ready-to-hang and Tetrapak®), banana (Tetrapak®) strawberry (Tetrapak®). Net price 500-mL ready-to-hang = £5.20, 200-mL Tetrapak® = £2.08.
For indications see *Paediasure*

Paediasure® Plus (Abbott)
Liquid, protein 4.2 g, carbohydrate 16.7 g, fat 7.5 g, energy 632 kJ (151 kcal)/100 mL with vitamins and minerals. Gluten-free, clinically lactose-free. Flavours: vanilla (ready-to-hang and Tetrapak®), strawberry (Tetrapak®). Net price 200-mL Tetrapak® = £2.30, 500-mL ready-to-hang = £5.87.

For indications see *Paediasure liquid*

Paediasure® Plus Fibre (Abbott)
Sip feed, protein 4.2 g, carbohydrate 16.4 g, fat 7.47 g, fibre 1.1g, energy 626 kJ (150 kcal)/100 mL with vitamins and minerals. Gluten-free, clinically lactose-free, net price 200-mL Tetrapak® = £2.50.

Tube feed, protein 4.2 g, carbohydrate 16.7 g, fat 7.5 g, fibre 1.1 g, energy 629 kJ (150 kcal)/100 mL with vitamins and minerals. Gluten-free, clinically lactose-free, net price 500-mL ready-to-hang = £6.25.

As a sole source of nutrition, or as a nutritional supplement for children aged 1 to 10 years, or 8–30 kg body-weight, with disease-related malnutrition and/or growth failure, short-bowel syndrome, intractable malabsorption, dysphagia, bowel fistulas, pre-operative preparation of undernourished patients. Not to be prescribed for any child under 1 year.

Peptamen® (Nestlé Clinical)
Liquid, protein 4 g, carbohydrate 12.7 g, fat 3.7 g, energy 420 kJ (100 kcal)/100 mL, with vitamins, minerals and trace elements. Lactose- and gluten-free. Flavours: unflavoured (can), vanilla (cup, see also *Flavour Sachets*). Net price 375-mL can = £3.88, 200-mL cup = £2.25; 500-mL (Dripac-Flex) = £4.57, 1-litre = £8.23.

For use as the sole source of nutrition or as a nutritional supplement prescribed on medical grounds for: short-bowel syndrome, intractable malabsorption, proven inflammatory bowel disease, bowel fistulas. Not to be prescribed for any child under 1 year; use with caution for children up to 5 years

Nestlé Nutrition Flavour Mix for use with *Peptamen Liquid* 200-mL cup and *Modulen IBD*. Flavours: banana, chocolate, coffee, lemon and lime, strawberry. Net price 60 g = £5.62

Peptisorb® (Nutricia Clinical)
Liquid, protein 4 g, carbohydrate 17.6 g, fat 1.7 g, energy 425 kJ (100 kcal)/100 mL with vitamins, minerals and trace elements. Gluten-free. Net price 500-mL bottle = £4.86; 500-mL pack = £5.34; 1-litre pack = £9.65.

For use as the sole source of nutrition or as a nutritional supplement prescribed on medical grounds for: short-bowel syndrome, intractable malabsorption, proven inflammatory bowel disease, bowel fistulas. Not to be prescribed for any child under 1 year; use with caution for children up to 5 years

Perative® (Abbott)
Liquid, providing protein 6.67 g, carbohydrate 17.7 g, fat 3.7 g, energy 552 kJ (131 kcal)/100 mL, with vitamins and minerals. Gluten-free, unflavoured. Net price 500-mL ready-to-hang = £5.36, 1-litre ready-to-hang = £10.72.

For use as a nutritional supplement prescribed on medical grounds for: short-bowel syndrome, intractable malabsorption, pre-operative preparation of patients who are undernourished, proven inflammatory bowel disease, following total gastrectomy, bowel fistulas, disease-related malnutrition. Not to be prescribed for any child under 5 years

Polycal® (Nutricia Clinical)
Powder, glucose, maltose, and polysaccharides, providing 1630 kJ (384 kcal)/100 g. Net price 400 g = £3.24

Liquid, glucose polymers providing carbohydrate 61.9 g/100 mL. Low-electrolyte, protein-free. Flavours: orange and neutral. Net price 200 mL = £1.29

Both for disease-related malnutrition; malabsorption states or other conditions requiring fortification with a high or readily available carbohydrate supplement

Polycose® (Abbott)
Powder, glucose polymers, providing carbohydrate 94 g, energy 1598 kJ (376 kcal)/100 g. Net price 350-g can = £3.30.

For disease-related malnutrition; malabsorption states or other conditions requiring fortification with a high or readily available carbohydrate supplement

PremCare® (Heinz)
Powder, protein 1.85 g, carbohydrate 7.24 g, fat 3.96 g, energy 301 kJ (72 kcal) per 100 mL when reconstituted, with vitamins and minerals. Gluten-, sucrose-, and lactose-free. Net price 450 g = £3.29.

For catch-up growth in pre-term infants (less than 35 weeks at birth), and small-for-gestational-age infants, until 6 months post-natal age

Pro-Cal® (Vitaflo)
Powder, protein 13.5 g, carbohydrate 26.8 g, fat 56.2 g, energy 2788 kJ (667 kcal)/100 g, net price 25 x 15 g sachets = £11.73, 510 g = £10.86, 1.5 kg = £21.15, 12.5 kg = £140, 25 kg = £250.

For disease-related malnutrition, malabsorption states or other conditions requiring fortification with a fat/carbohydrate supplement. Not to be prescribed for any child under 1 year; use with caution for young children up to 5 years

ProSure® (Abbott)
Liquid, protein 6.65 g, carbohydrate 19.4 g, fat 2.56 g, fibre 0.97 g, energy 528 kJ (125 kcal)/100 mL with vitamins, minerals, and trace elements. Gluten-free, clinically lactose-free. Vanilla, orange, or banana flavour, net price, 240-mL Tetrapak® = £2.70; 500-mL ready-to-hang = £5.63 (vanilla only).

As a nutritional supplement for patients with cancer cachexia. Not to be prescribed for children under 1 year; use with caution in children under 4 years

Provide® Xtra (Fresenius Kabi)
Liquid, protein 3.75 g, carbohydrate 27.5 g, energy 525 kJ (125 kcal)/100 mL with vitamins, minerals and trace elements. Gluten-free. Apple, blackcurrant, carrot-apple, cherry, citrus cola, lemon & lime, melon, orange & pineapple, or tomato flavour. Net price 200-mL carton = £1.58.

As a nutritional supplement prescribed on medical grounds for: short-bowel syndrome, intractable malabsorption, pre-operative preparation of patients who are undernourished, proven inflammatory bowel disease, following total gastrectomy, dysphagia, bowel fistulas, disease-related malnutrition. Not to be prescribed for any child under 1 year; use with caution for children up to 5 years

QuickCal® (Vitaflo)
Powder, protein 4.6 g, carbohydrate 17 g, fat 77 g, energy 3260 kJ (780 kcal)/100 g, net price 25 × 13-g sachets = £10.55.

For disease-related malnutrition, malabsorption states or other conditions requiring fortification with a fat/carbohydrate supplement. Not to be prescribed for any child under 1 year; use with caution for young children up to 5 years

Resource® Benefiber® (Novartis Consumer Health)
Powder, soluble dietary fibre, carbohydrate 19 g, fibre 78 g, energy 323 kJ (76 kcal)/100 g with minerals. Gluten-free; low lactose, net price 250 g pack = £8.76, 16 x 8-g sachets = £5.72.

As a nutritional supplement prescribed on medical grounds for: short-bowel syndrome, intractable malabsorption, pre-operative preparation of undernourished patients, proven inflammatory bowel disease, following total gastrectomy, bowel fistulas, disease-related malnutrition. Not to be prescribed for children under 5 years

Resource® Energy Dessert (Novartis Consumer Health)
Semi-solid, protein 4.8 g, carbohydrate 21.2 g, fat 6.24 g, energy 671 kJ (160 kcal)/100 g with vitamins, minerals, and trace elements. Gluten-free; low lactose. Flavours:

caramel, chocolate, or vanilla, net price 125-g cup = £1.35.

For use as a nutritional supplement prescribed on medical grounds for: disease-related malnutrition, short-bowel syndrome, intractable malabsorption, proven inflammatory bowel disease, bowel fistulas, dysphagia, pre-operative preparation of undernourished patients, after total gastrectomy, continuous ambulatory peritoneal dialysis (CAPD), haemodialysis. Not to be prescribed for any child under 1 year; use with caution for children up to 5 years

Resource® Fruit Flavour Drink (Novartis Consumer Health)

Liquid, protein 4 g, carbohydrate 33.5 g, energy 638 kJ (150 kcal)/100 mL with vitamins, minerals, and trace elements. Fat- and gluten-free; low lactose. Flavours: apple, orange, or pineapple, net price 125-g carton = £1.49.

For use as a nutritional supplement prescribed on medical grounds for: disease-related malnutrition, short-bowel syndrome, intractable malabsorption, proven inflammatory bowel disease, bowel fistulas, dysphagia, pre-operative preparation of undernourished patients, after total gastrectomy. Not to be prescribed for any child under 3 years; use with caution for children up to 5 years

Resource® Junior (Novartis Consumer Health)

Liquid, protein 3 g, carbohydrate 20.6 g, fat 6.2 g, energy 631 kJ (150 kcal)/100 mL with vitamins, minerals, and trace elements. Gluten-free; clinically lactose-free. Flavours: chocolate, strawberry, or vanilla, net price 200-mL carton = £1.69.

For use as a sole source of nutrition or as a nutritional supplement prescribed on medical grounds for: disease-related malnutrition, short-bowel syndrome, intractable malabsorption, pre-operative preparation of undernourished patients, proven inflammatory bowel disease, following total gastrectomy, bowel fistulas, and dysphagia. Not to be prescribed for any child under 1 year

Resource® Protein Extra (Novartis Consumer Health)

Liquid, protein 9.4 g, carbohydrate 14 g, fat 3.5 g, energy 530 kJ (125 kcal)/100 mL with vitamins, minerals and trace elements. Gluten-free; low lactose. Flavours: apricot, chocolate, summer fruits, or vanilla. Net price 200-mL carton = £1.29.

For use as a nutritional supplement prescribed on medical grounds for: disease-related malnutrition, short-bowel syndrome, intractable malabsorption, proven inflammatory bowel disease, bowel fistulas, dysphagia, pre-operative preparation of undernourished patients, after total gastrectomy. Not to be prescribed for any child under 1 year; use with caution for children up to 5 years

Appendix 2

Resource® Shake (Novartis Consumer Health)

Liquid, protein 5.1 g, carbohydrate 22.6 g, fat 7 g, energy 731 kJ (174 kcal)/100 mL with vitamins, minerals and trace elements. Gluten-free; low lactose. Flavours: banana, chocolate, lemon, strawberry, summer fruits, toffee, or vanilla. Net price 175-mL carton = £1.46.

For use as a nutritional supplement prescribed on medical grounds for: disease-related malnutrition, short-bowel syndrome, intractable malabsorption, proven inflammatory bowel disease, bowel fistulas, dysphagia, pre-operative preparation of undernourished patients, after total gastrectomy. Not to be prescribed for any child under 1 year; use with caution for children up to 5 years

Scandishake® Mix (Nutricia Clinical)

Powder, protein 11.7 g, carbohydrate 66.8 g, fat 30.4 g, energy 2457 kJ (588 kcal)/unflavoured serving (serving = 1 sachet reconstituted with 240 mL whole milk; protein, carbohydrate, and energy values vary with flavour). Flavours: banana, caramel, chocolate, strawberry, vanilla, and unflavoured. Net price 85-g sachet = £1.90.

For disease-related malnutrition; malabsorption states or other conditions requiring fortification with a fat/carbohydrate supplement

SMA High Energy® (SMA Nutrition)

Liquid, protein 2 g, carbohydrate 9.8 g, fat 4.9 g, energy 382 kJ (91 kcal)/100mL, with vitamins and minerals. Net price 250 mL = £1.80.

For disease-related malnutrition, malabsorption, and growth failure

Survimed OPD® (Fresenius Kabi)

Liquid, protein 4.5 g, carbohydrate 15 g, fat 2.6 g, energy 420 kJ (100 kcal)/100 mL, with vitamins, minerals, and trace elements. Gluten-free, and low lactose. Net price 500-mL EasyBag® = £5.00.

As a nutritional supplement prescribed on medical grounds for: short-bowel syndrome, intractable malabsorption, pre-operative preparation of patients who are undernourished, proven inflammatory bowel disease, following total gastrectomy, dysphagia, bowel fistulas, disease-related malnutrition. Not to be prescribed for any child under 1 year; use with caution for children up to 5 years

Tentrini® (Nutricia Clinical)

Liquid, tube feed, protein 3.3 g, carbohydrate 12.3 g, fat 4.2 g, energy 420 kJ (100 kcal)/100 mL, with vitamins, minerals and trace elements. Gluten- and lactose-free. Unflavoured, net price 500-mL bottle or pack = £4.24

For short-bowel syndrome, intractable malabsorption, pre-operative preparation of undernourished patients, inflammatory bowel disease, total gastrectomy, dysphagia, bowel fistulas, disease-related malnutrition, and growth failure. For children between 21–45 kg body-weight

Tentrini® Energy (Nutricia Clinical)

Liquid, tube feed, protein 4.9 g, carbohydrate 18.5 g, fat 6.3 g, energy 630 kJ (150 kcal)/100 mL, with vitamins, minerals and trace elements. Gluten- and lactose-free. Unflavoured, net price 500-mL bottle or pack = £5.25

For indications see *Tentrini*

Tentrini® Energy Multi Fibre (Nutricia Clinical)

Liquid, tube feed, protein 4.9 g, carbohydrate 18.5 g, fat 6.3 g, fibre 1.12 g, energy 630 kJ (150 kcal)/100 mL, with vitamins, minerals and trace elements. Gluten- and lactose-free. Unflavoured, net price 500-mL bottle or pack = £5.79

For indications see *Tentrini Multi Fibre*

Tentrini® Multi Fibre (Nutricia Clinical)

Liquid, tube feed, protein 3.3 g, carbohydrate 12.3 g, fat 4.2 g, fibre 1.12 g, energy 420 kJ (100 kcal)/100 mL, with vitamins, minerals and trace elements. Gluten- and lactose-free. Unflavoured, net price 500-mL bottle or pack = £4.66

For short-bowel syndrome, intractable malabsorption, pre-operative preparation of undernourished patients, inflammatory bowel disease, total gastrectomy, dysphagia, disease-related malnutrition, and growth failure. Not to be prescribed for any child under 1 year; use with caution for children under 7 years or 21 kg

Vitajoule® (Vitaflo)

Powder, glucose polymers, providing carbohydrate 96 g, energy 1610 kJ (380 kcal)/100 g. Net price 500 g = £3.24, 2.5 kg = £16.15, 25 kg = £99.00.

For disease-related malnutrition; malabsorption states or other conditions requiring fortification with a high or readily available carbohydrate supplement

Vitasavoury® (Vitaflo)

Powder, protein 12 g, carbohydrate 24 g, fat 54 g, energy 2610 kJ (630 kcal)/100 g, net price 10 x 50-g sachets = £14.63, 24 x 33-g ready cups = £24.28. Flavours: chicken, leek and potato, mushroom, vegetable.

As a nutritional supplement for disease-related malnutrition, malabsorption states or other conditions requiring fortification with a fat/carbohydrate supplement. Not to be prescribed for any child under 1 year; use with caution for young children up to 5 years

Feed thickeners and pre-thickened foods

Carobel, Instant® (Cow & Gate)
Powder, carob seed flour. Net price 135 g = £2.63.
For thickening feeds in the treatment of vomiting

Clinutren® Thickened Drinks (Nestlé Clinical)
Liquid, modified maize starch, gluten-free. Flavours: orange, peppermint, and tea, net price 4 × 125 g = £1.96.
Thickening of foods and fluids in dysphagia. Not to be used for children under 3 years

Clinutren® Thickener (Nestlé Clinical)
Powder, modified maize starch, gluten-free, net price 300 g = £4.53.
Thickening of foods and fluids in dysphagia. Not to be used for children under 3 years

Enfamil AR® (Mead Johnson)
AR (Anti-Reflux), powder, protein 1.7 g, fat 3.5 g, carbohydrate 7.6 g, energy 285 kJ (68 kcal)/100 mL with vitamins, minerals and trace elements, net price 400 g = £2.76.
For significant reflux disease. For use not in excess of a 6-month period. Not to be used in conjunction with any other thickener or antacid product.

Nestargel® (Nestlé)
Powder, carob seed flour 96.5%, calcium lactate 3.5%. Net price 125 g = £2.99.
For thickening feeds in the treatment of vomiting

Nutilis® (Nutricia Clinical)
Powder, modified maize starch, gluten- and lactose-free, net price 20 × 9-g sachets = £5.00.
For thickening of foods in dysphagia. Not to be prescribed for children under 3 years

Resource® Thickened Drink (Novartis Consumer Health)
Liquid, carbohydrate 22 g, energy: orange 383 kJ (89 kcal); apple 375 kJ (89 kcal)/100 mL. Syrup and custard consistencies. Gluten-free; clinically lactose free, net price 12 × 114-mL cups = £7.08.
For dysphagia. Not suitable for children under 1 year

Resource® Thickened Squash (Novartis Consumer Health)
Liquid, syrup consistency: carbohydrate 16.9 g, energy 287 kJ (68 kcal)/100 mL; custard consistency: carbohydrate 17.8 g, energy 303 kJ (71 kcal)/100 mL. Gluten-free; clinically lactose-free. Orange and lemon flavour, net price 1.89-litre bottle = £3.99.
For dysphagia. Not suitable for children under 1 year

Resource® ThickenUp® (Novartis Consumer Health)
Powder, modified maize starch. Gluten- and lactose-free, net price 227 g = £3.90; 75 × 6.4-g sachet = £15.75.
For thickening of foods in dysphagia. Not to be prescribed for children under 1 year

SMA Staydown® (SMA Nutrition)
Powder, protein 12.4 g, fat 27.9 g, carbohydrate 54.3 g, energy 2166 kJ (518 kcal)/100g, with vitamins, minerals, and trace elements. Net price 900 g = £5.74.
For significant reflux disease. Not to be used for more than 6 months or in conjunction with any other thickener or antacid product

Thick and Easy® (Fresenius Kabi)
Powder. Modified maize starch, net price 225-g can = £3.99; 100 × 9-g sachets = £26.35; 4.54 kg = £70.53.
Dairy. Pre-thickened milk, net price 250 mL = £1.38
Thickened Juices, liquid, modified food starch. Flavours: apple, blackcurrant, cranberry, kiwi-strawberry, and orange, net price 118-mL pot = 52p; 1.42-litre bottle = £3.61.
For thickening of foods in dysphagia. Not to be prescribed for children under 1 year except in cases of failure to thrive

Thixo-D® (Sutherland)
Powder, modified maize starch, gluten-free. Net price 375-g tub = £5.79.
For thickening of foods in dysphagia. Not to be prescribed for children under 1 year except in cases of failure to thrive

Vitaquick® (Vitaflo)
Powder. Modified maize starch. Net price 300 g = £5.85; 2 kg = £30.72; 6 kg = £78.60.
For thickening of foods in dysphagia. Not to be prescribed for children under 1 year except in cases of failure to thrive

Hypoproteinaemia (biochemically proven)

Casilan 90® (Heinz)
Powder, whole protein, containing all essential amino acids, 90% with less than 0.1% Na^+. Net price 250 g = £4.69.
For biochemically proven hypoproteinaemia

Dialamine® (SHS)
Powder, essential amino acids 30%, with carbohydrate 62%, energy 1500 kJ (360 kcal)/100 g, with ascorbic acid, minerals, and trace elements. Flavour: orange. Net price 200 g = £25.11.
For oral feeding where essential amino acid supplements are required; e.g. chronic renal failure, hypoproteinaemia, wound fistula leakage with excessive protein loss, conditions requiring a controlled nitrogen intake, and haemodialysis

Maxipro Super Soluble® (SHS)
Powder, whey protein and additional amino acids (protein equivalent 80%). Net price 200 g = £8.64; 1 kg = £34.66.
For biochemically proven hypoproteinaemia. Not to be prescribed for any child under 1 year; unsuitable as a sole source of nutrition

Maxisorb® (SHS)
Powder, protein 12 g, carbohydrate 9 g, fat 6 g, energy 579 kJ (138 kcal)/30 g with minerals. Vanilla, strawberry and chocolate flavours. Net price 5 × 30-g sachets = £3.63.
For biochemically proven hypoproteinaemia. Not to be prescribed for any child under 1 year; use with caution for children up to 5 years

ProMod® (Abbott, SHS)
Powder, protein 75 g, carbohydrate 7.5 g, fat 6.9 g/100 g. Gluten-free. Net price 275-g can = £8.82.
For biochemically proven hypoproteinaemia

Protifar® (Nutricia Clinical)
Powder, protein 88.5%. Low lactose, gluten- and sucrose-free. Net price 225 g = £6.58.
For biochemically proven hypoproteinaemia

Renapro® (KoRa)
Powder, whey protein providing protein 92 g, carbohydrate less than 300 mg, fat 500 mg, 1562 kJ (367 kcal)/100 g. Net price 20-g sachet = £2.32.
For dialysis and hypoproteinaemia. Not suitable for infants and children under 1 year

Vitapro® (Vitaflo)
Powder, whole milk proteins, containing all essential amino acids, 75%. Net price 250 g = £6.49, 2 kg = £50.90.
For biochemically proven hypoproteinaemia

Foods and supplements for special diets

Alembicol D® (Alembic Products)
Fractionated coconut oil. Net price 5 kg = £125.55.
For steatorrhoea associated with cystic fibrosis of the pancreas, intestinal lymphangiectasia, surgery of the intestine, chronic liver disease, liver cirrhosis, other proven malabsorption syndromes; in a ketogenic diet in the management of epilepsy; type 1 hyperlipoproteinaemia

Caprilon® (SHS)
Powder, protein 11.8%, carbohydrate 55.1%, fat 28.3% (medium chain triglycerides 21.3%). Low in lactose, gluten- and sucrose-free. Used as a 12.7% solution. Net price 420 g = £12.46.
For disorders in which a high intake of MCT is beneficial

Corn flour and corn starch
For hypoglycaemia associated with glycogen-storage disease

Energivit® (SHS)
Powder, protein-free, carbohydrate 66.7 g, fat 25 g, energy 2059 kJ, (492 kcal)/100 g with vitamins, minerals and trace elements, net price 400 g = £15.04.
For infants requiring additional enegy, vitamins, minerals and trace elements following a protein restricted diet

Generaid® (SHS)
Powder, whey protein and additional branched-chain amino acids (protein equivalent 81%). Net price 200 g (unflavoured) = £20.92. See also Flavour Sachets.
For patients with chronic liver disease and/or porto-hepatic encephalopathy

Generaid Plus® (SHS)
Powder, whey protein and additional branched-chain amino acids (protein equivalent 11%) carbohydrate 62%, fat 19% with vitamins, minerals and trace elements. Net price 400 g = £14.96.
For children over 1 year with hepatic disorders

Liquigen® (SHS)
Emulsion, medium chain triglycerides 52%. Net price 250 mL = £6.34; 1 litre = £26.60.
For steatorrhoea associated with cystic fibrosis of the pancreas; intestinal lymphangiectasia, surgery of the intestine; chronic liver disease and liver cirrhosis; other proven malabsorption syndromes; ketogenic diet in the management of epilepsy; type I hyperlipoproteinaemia

MCT Oil
Triglycerides from medium chain fatty acids. For steatorrhoea associated with cystic fibrosis of the pancreas; intestinal lymphangiectasia; surgery of the intestine; chronic liver disease and liver cirrhosis; other proven malabsorption syndromes; in a ketogenic diet in the management of epilepsy; in type I hyperlipoproteinaemia
Available from SHS (net price 500 mL = £9.79)

MCT Pepdite® (SHS)
Powder, essential and non-essential amino acids, peptides, medium chain triglycerides, monoglyceride of sunflower oil, with carbohydrate, fat, vitamins, minerals, and trace elements. Flavour Sachets available.
MCT Pepdite 0–2. Net price 400 g = £13.96
MCT Pepdite 1+. Net price 400 g = £13.96
Both for disorders in which a high intake of medium chain triglyceride is beneficial

Metabolic Mineral Mixture® (SHS)
Powder, essential mineral salts. Net price 100 g = £8.67.
For mineral supplementation in synthetic diets

Monogen® (SHS)
Powder, protein 11.4 g, carbohydrate 68 g, fat 11.4 g (of which MCT 93%), energy 1772 kJ (420 kcal)/100 g, with vitamins, minerals and trace elements. Net price 400 g = £13.89.
For long-chain acyl-CoA dehydrogenase deficiency (LCAD), carnitine palmitoyl transferase deficiency (CPTD), primary and secondary lipoprotin lipase deficiency

Nepro® (Abbott)
Liquid, protein 7 g, carbohydrate 20.6 g, fat 9.6 g, energy 840 kJ (200 kcal)/100 mL with vitamins and minerals. Net price 237-mL can = £2.28; 500–mL ready-to-hang = £4.81.
For patients with chronic renal failure who are on haemodialysis or continuous ambulatory peritoneal dialysis (CAPD), or patients with cirrhosis or other conditions requiring a high energy, low fluid, low electrolyte diet

Paediatric Seravit® (SHS)
Powder, vitamins, minerals, low sodium and potassium, and trace elements. Net price 200 g (unflavoured) = £12.24; pineapple flavour, 200 g = £13.04.
For vitamin and mineral supplementation in restrictive therapeutic diets in infants and children

Phlexyvits® (SHS)
Powder, vitamins, minerals and trace elements, net price 30 × 7-g sachets = £48.94.
For use as a vitamin and mineral component of restricted therapeutic diets in older children from the age of around 11 years and over and adults with phenylketonuria and similar amino acid abnormalities

Renamil® (KoRa)
Powder, protein 4.7 g, carbohydrate 70.2 g, fat 18.7 g, 1984 kJ (468 kcal)/100 g, with vitamins and minerals. Net price 1 kg = £25.40.
For chronic renal failure. Not suitable for infants and children under 1 year

Suplena® (Abbott)
Liquid, protein 3 g, carbohydrate 25.5 g, fat 9.6 g, energy 841 kJ (201 kcal)/100 mL. Flavour: vanilla. Net price 237-mL can = £2.28.
For patients with chronic or acute renal failure who are not undergoing dialysis; chronic or acute liver disease with fluid restriction; other conditions requiring a high-energy, low-protein, low-electrolyte, low-volume enteral feed

Special foods for conditions of intolerance

Colief® (Britannia)
Liquid, lactase 50 000 units/g, net price 7-mL dropper bottle = £7.00
For the relief of symptoms associated with lactose intolerance in infants, provided that lactose intolerance is confirmed by the presence of reducing substances and/or excessive acid in stools, a low concentration of the corresponding disaccharide enzyme on intestinal biopsy or by breath hydrogen test or lactose intolerance test. For dosage and administration details, consult product literature

Comminuted Chicken Meat (SHS)
Suspension (aqueous). Net price 150 g = £2.56.
For carbohydrate intolerance in association with possible or proven intolerance of milk; glucose and galactose intolerance

Enfamil Lactofree® (Mead Johnson)
Powder, protein 1.42 g, fat 3.7 g, carbohydrate 7.2 g, energy 280 kJ (68 kcal)/100 mL with vitamins, minerals and trace elements. Lactose- and sucrose-free, net price 400 g = £2.76.
For proven lactose intolerance

Farley's Soya Formula (Heinz)
Powder, providing protein 2%, carbohydrate 7%, fat 3.8% with vitamins and minerals when reconstituted. Gluten-, sucrose-, and lactose-free. Net price 450 g = £3.38.
For proven lactose and associated sucrose intolerance in pre-school children, galactokinase deficiency, galactosaemia, and cow's milk protein intolerance

Fructose
(Laevulose)
For proven glucose/galactose intolerance

Galactomin 17® (SHS)
Powder, protein 14.5 g, fat 25.9 g, carbohydrate 56.9 g, mineral salts 3.4 g/100 g. Used as a 13.1% solution with additional vitamins in place of milk. Net price 400 g = £11.48.
For proven lactose intolerance in preschool children, galactosaemia and galactokinase deficiency

Galactomin 19® (SHS)
Powder, protein 14.6 g, fat 30.8 g, carbohydrate 49.7 g (fructose as carbohydrate source), mineral salts 2.1 g/100 g, with vitamins. Used as a 12.9% solution in place of milk. Net price 400 g = £30.24.
For glucose plus galactose intolerance

Glucose
(Dextrose monohydrate)
Net price 100 g = 39p.
For glycogen storage disease and sucrose/isomaltose intolerance

InfaSoy® (Cow & Gate)
Powder, carbohydrate 7.1%, fat 3.6%, and protein 1.8% with vitamins and minerals when used as a 12.7% solution. Net price 450 g = £3.77; 900 g = £7.23.
For proven lactose and associated sucrose intolerance in preschool children, galactokinase deficiency, galactosaemia, and proven whole cow's milk sensitivity

Isomil® (Abbott)
Powder, protein 1.8%, carbohydrate 6.9%, fat 3.7% with vitamins and minerals when reconstituted. Lactose-free. Net price 400 g = £3.38.
For proven lactose intolerance in preschool children, galactokinase deficiency, galactosaemia, and proven whole cow's milk sensitivity

Locasol® (SHS)
Powder, protein 14.6 g, carbohydrate 56.5 g, fat 26.1 g, mineral salts 1.9 g, not more than 55 mg of Ca^{2+}/100 g and vitamins. Used as a 13.1% solution in place of milk. Net price 400 g = £15.96.
For calcium intolerance

Neocate® (SHS)
Powder, essential and non-essential amino acids, maltodextrin, fat, vitamins, minerals, and trace elements. Net price 400 g = £19.98.
For proven whole protein intolerance, short-bowel syndrome, intractable malabsorption, and other gastro-intestinal disorders where an elemental diet is specifically indicated; for use in children under 1 year

Neocate® Advance (SHS)
Powder, essential and non-essential amino acids, carbohydrate, fat, vitamins, minerals and trace elements. Milk protein-, soy- and lactose-free. Net price 100 g = £4.10; banana-vanilla flavour 15 x 50 g = £33.24.
For proven whole protein intolerance, short-bowel syndrome, intractable malabsorption, and other gastro-intestinal disorders where an elemental diet is specifically indicated; for use in children under 1 year

Nutramigen® 1 (Mead Johnson)
Powder, protein 1.9 g, carbohydrate 7.5 g, fat 3.4 g, energy 280 kJ (68 kcal)/100 mL with vitamins and minerals. Gluten-, sucrose-, and lactose-free. Net price 400 g = £7.81.
For disaccharide and/or whole protein intolerance where additional medium chain triglyceride is not indicated

Nutramigen® 2 (Mead Johnson)
Powder, protein 2.3 g, carbohydrate 7.8 g, fat 3.5 g energy 301 kJ (72 kcal) per 100 mL when normal dilution used, with vitamins, minerals and trace elements. Gluten-, sucrose-, and lactose-free, net price 400 g = £7.81.
For disaccharide and/or whole protein intolerance where additional medium chain triglyceride is not indicated. Not suitable for infants under 6 months

Pepdite® (SHS)
Powder, peptides, essential and non-essential amino acids, with carbohydrate, fat, vitamins, minerals, and trace elements. Flavour Sachets available.
Pepdite (birth to 1 year). Providing 1925 kJ (472 kcal)/100 g. Net price 400 g = £12.83
Pepdite 1+. Providing 1787 kJ (439 kcal)/100 g. Net price 400 g = £13.48; 15 x 57 g (banana flavour) = £32.70
Both for disaccharide and/or whole protein intolerance, or where amino acids or peptides are indicated in conjunction with medium chain triglycerides

Pepti® (Cow & Gate)
Powder, protein equivalent 12.4 g, fat 28.5 g, carbohydrate 54.2 g, energy 2185 kJ (522 kcal)/100 g, with vitamins, minerals, and trace elements. Used as a solution in place of milk, net price 900 g = £15.98.
For the dietary management of established cows' milk protein intolerance with or without proven secondary lactose intolerance

Pepti-Junior® (Cow & Gate)
Powder, protein 15.3 g, fat 28.3 g, carbohydrate 55.1 g, energy 2140 kJ (507 kcal)/100 g with vitamins and minerals. Used as a 13.1% solution in place of milk. Net price 450 g = £8.80.
For disaccharide and/or whole protein intolerance or where amino acids and peptides are indicated in conjunction with medium chain triglycerides

Pregestimil® (Mead Johnson)
Powder, protein 12.8%, carbohydrate 61.6%, fat 18.3% with vitamins and minerals. Gluten-, sucrose-, and lactose-free. Net price 400 g = £8.91.
For disaccharide and/or whole protein intolerance or where amino acids or peptides are indicated in conjunction with medium chain triglycerides

Prejomin® (Milupa)
Granules, protein 13.5 g, carbohydrate 57 g, fat 24 g, energy 2085 kJ (497 kcal)/100 g, with vitamins and minerals. Gluten-free. For preparation with water before use. Net price 400 g = £9.44.
For disaccharide and/or whole protein intolerance where additional medium chain triglyceride is not indicated

Prosobee® (Mead Johnson)
Powder, protein 1.76 g, carbohydrate 6.8 g, fat 3.7 g, energy 285 kJ (68 kcal)/100 mL with vitamins and minerals. Gluten-, sucrose-, and lactose-free. Net price 400 g = £3.51.
For proven lactose and associated sucrose intolerance in pre-school children, galactokinase deficiency, galactosaemia, and proven whole cow's milk sensitivity

SMA LF® (SMA Nutrition)
Powder, protein 1.5 g, carbohydrate 7.2 g, fat 3.6 g, energy 282 kJ (67 kcal)/100 mL, with vitamins and minerals. Net price 430 g = £3.99.
For proven lactose intolerance

Wysoy® (Wyeth)
Powder, carbohydrate 6.9%, fat 3.6%, and protein 2.1% with vitamins and minerals when reconstituted. Net price 430 g = £3.98; 860 g = £7.58.
For proven lactose and associated sucrose intolerance in preschool children, galactokinase deficiency, galactosaemia and proven whole cow's milk sensitivity

Gluten-sensitive enteropathies

Aproten® (Ultrapharm)
Gluten-free. Flour. Net price 500 g = £4.99.
For gluten-sensitive enteropathies including steatorrhoea due to gluten sensitivity, coeliac disease, and dermatitis herpetiformis

Arnott® (Ultrapharm)
Rice Cookies, gluten-free. Net price 200 g = £2.06.
For gluten-sensitive enteropathies including steatorrhoea due to gluten sensitivity, coeliac disease, and dermatitis herpetiformis

Baker's Delight®
Gluten-free. Bread, net price 100 g = 80p.
For established gluten enteropathy

Barkat® (Gluten Free Foods Ltd)
Gluten-free. Bread mix, net price 500 g = £4.12. Multi Grain Bread, 450 g = £2.99. Rice bread (sliced), brown or white, 450 g = £2.99. Rice pizza crust, brown or white, 150 g = £2.21.
For gluten-sensitive enteropathies including steatorrhoea due to gluten sensitivity, coeliac disease, and dermatitis herpetiformis

Bercoeli® (Bercoeli)
Gluten- and wheat-free. White sliced loaf = £1.89. Brown rice bread loaf = £1.96. Pizza bases, 3 = £2.07.
For established gluten enteropathy with coexisting established wheat sensitivity only

Bi-Aglut® (Novartis Consumer Health)
Gluten-free. Biscuits, net price 180 g = £2.89. Crackers, 150 g = £2.36. Cracker toast, 240 g = £4.18. Pasta (fusilli, macaroni, penne, spaghetti), 500 g = £5.23.
For gluten-sensitive enteropathies including steatorrhoea due to gluten sensitivity, coeliac disease, and dermatitis herpetiformis

Dietary Specials (Nutrition Point)
Gluten-free. Bread. Loaf, sliced (brown, white or multigrain) 400 g = £2.50; bread rolls, long (white) 3 = £1.55. Bread mix, net price 500 g = £4.75; cracker bread, 150 g = £1.80; cake mix (white), 750 g = £4.75; white mix, 500 g = £4.75; digestive biscuits, 150 g = £1.70. Tea biscuits, 220 g = £2.00. Pasta (spaghetti, penne, fusilli), 500 g = £3.20
For gluten-sensitive enteropathies including steatorrhoea due to gluten sensitivity, coeliac disease, and dermatitis herpetiformis

Ener-G® (General Dietary)
Gluten-free. Cookies (vanilla flavour), net price 435 g = £4.88. Dinner Rolls (× 6), 280 g = £2.90; Rice bread (sliced), brown, 474 g = £4.28; white, 456 g = £4.28. Rice loaf (sliced), 612 g = £4.28. Seattle brown loaf, 600 g = £4.93. Tapioca bread (sliced), 480 g = £4.28. Rice pasta (macaroni, shells, small shells, and lasagne), 454 g = £3.98; spaghetti, 447 g = £3.98; tagliatelle, 400 g = £3.98; vermicelli, 300 g = £3.98; cannelloni, 335 g = £3.98. Brown rice pasta: lasagne, 454 g = £3.98; macaroni, 454 g = £3.98; spaghetti, 447 g = £3.98. Xanthan gum, 170 g = £6.76.
For gluten-sensitive enteropathies including steatorrhoea due to gluten sensitivity, coeliac disease, and dermatitis herpetiformis

Gluten-free. Pizza bases, 372 g = £3.75. Six flour bread loaf, 576 g = £3.60. Seattle brown rolls (round or long), 4 x 119 g = £3.00
For established gluten enteropathy with coexisting established wheat sensitivity only

Gadsby's
Gluten-free. White bread flour, net price 1 kg = £4.99. White sliced bread, 400 g = £2.50. White bread rolls, 4 × 75 g = £2.00
For established gluten enteropathy

Glutafin® (Nutricia Dietary)
Gluten-free. Biscuits, savoury, 125 g = £1.70; 150 g = £2.32. Biscuits, digestive, sweet or tea, 150 g = £1.70. Biscuits, 200 g = £3.31. Biscuits, shortbread, 125 g = £1.47. Cake mix, 500 g = £5.31. Crackers, 200 g = £2.76. High fibre crackers, 200 g = £2.31. Pasta (penne, shells, spirals, spaghetti), 500 g = £5.36; (lasagne, tagliatelle), 250 g = £2.81. Pizza bases, 2 × 110 g = £3.83.

Select Gluten-free. Fibre loaf (sliced or unsliced), 400 g = £2.73; part-baked, 400 g = £3.06. Fresh Bread, white loaf, (sliced), 400 g = £2.94. Seeded loaf, 400 g = £2.97. White loaf (sliced or unsliced), 400 g = £2.73; part-baked, 400 g = £3.06. Fibre rolls, 4 = £3.06; (part-baked), 4 = £3.06; long, 2 = £3.06. White rolls, 4 = £3.06; (part-baked), 4 = £3.06; long, 2 = £3.06. Mixes (bread, cake, fibre, fibre bread, pastry, and white), 500 g = £5.31
For gluten-sensitive enteropathies including steatorrhoea due to gluten sensitivity, coeliac disease, and dermatitis herpetiformis

Gluten-free, wheat-free, crisp bread, 2 × 125 g = £3.61; crisp roll, 220 g = £3.72. Fibre loaf (sliced or unsliced), 400 g = £2.73. Fibre rolls, 4 = £2.97. White loaf (sliced or unsliced), 400 g = £3.06. White rolls, 4 = £2.97. Mixes (fibre bread, bread, white or fibre), 500 g = £5.31; cake or pastry mix, 500 g = £5.31.
For gluten-sensitive enteropathy with co-existing established wheat sensitivity

Glutano® (Gluten Free Foods Ltd)
Gluten-free, wheat-free. Tea biscuits, net price 125 g = £1.58; wheat-free digestive biscuit, 200 g = £1.58. Shortcake rings, 125 g = £1.12. Crispbread, 125 g = £1.58. Crackers, 150 g = £1.58. Flour mix, 750 g = £4.12. Pasta (animal shapes, spaghetti, spirals, tagliatelle), 250 g = £1.58; macaroni, 500 g = £3.16. White sliced bread (par-baked), 300 g = £1.86. Wholemeal bread (sliced), 500 g = £2.24. Baguette or rolls (par-baked), 200 g = £1.49.
For gluten-sensitive enteropathies including steatorrhoea due to gluten sensitivity, coeliac disease, and dermatitis herpetiformis

Juvela® (SHS)
Gluten-free. Harvest mix, fibre mix, and flour mix, net price 500 g = £5.47. Bread (whole or sliced), 400-g loaf = £2.72; part-baked loaf (with or without fibre), 400g = £2.83. Fibre bread (sliced and unsliced), 400-g loaf = £2.64. Bread rolls, 5 × 85 g = £3.56, fibre bread rolls, 5 × 85 g = £3.56, part-baked rolls (with or without fibre), 5 × 75 g = £3.67. Crispbread, 210 g = £3.45. Pasta (fusilli, macaroni, spaghetti), 500 g = £5.36; lasagne, 250 g = £2.47; tagliatelle, 250 g = £2.74. Pizza bases, 2 × 180 g = £6.53. Digestive biscuits, 160 g = £2.27. Savoury biscuits, 150 g = £2.84. Tea biscuits, 160 g = £2.27.
For gluten-sensitive enteropathies including steatorrhoea due to gluten sensitivity, coeliac disease, and dermatitis herpetiformis

Lifestyle® (Ultrapharm)
Gluten-free. Brown bread (sliced and unsliced), net price 400 g = £2.63. White bread (sliced and unsliced), 400 g = £2.63. High fibre bread (unsliced), 400 g = £2.63. Bread rolls, 400 g = £2.63.
For gluten-sensitive enteropathies including steatorrhoea due to gluten sensitivity, coeliac disease, and dermatitis herpetiformis

Orgran® (Community)
Gluten-free. Pasta: lasagne (corn, rice and maize), 150 g = £2.89; shells (split pea and soya), 200 g = £2.25; spaghetti (corn, rice, rice and maize), 250 g = £2.25; spirals (buckwheat, corn, rice, rice and millet, rice and maize), 250 g = £2.25, spirals (organic brown rice), 250 g = £2.60. Crispbread (corn or rice), 200 g = £2.39. Pizza and pastry mix, 375 g = £3.33.
For gluten-sensitive enteropathies including steatorrhoea due to gluten sensitivity, coeliac disease, and dermatitis herpetiformis

Pleniday® (TOL)
Gluten-free. Bread: loaf (sliced) net price 350 g = £1.80; country loaf (sliced), 500 g = £2.85; rustic loaf (par-baked

baguette), 400 g = £2.09; petit pain, 2 × 150 g = £2.02. Pasta (penne), 250 g = £1.27; (rigate), 250 g = £1.50

For gluten-sensitive enteropathies including steatorrhoea due to gluten sensitivity, coeliac disease, and dermatitis herpetiformis

Polial® (Ultrapharm)
Biscuits. Gluten- and lactose-free. Net price 200-g pack = £2.85.

For gluten-sensitive enteropathies including steatorrhea due to gluten sensitivity, coeliac disease, and dermatitis herpetiformis

Rite-Diet® Gluten-free (Nutricia Dietary)
Gluten-free. White bread (sliced or unsliced), 400 g = £2.75. White loaf (part-baked), 400 g = £3.09. Fibre bread (sliced or unsliced), 400 g = £2.75. Fibre loaf (part-baked), 400 g = £3.09. White rolls, 4 = £2.72; (part-baked) long, 2 = £3.04. Fibre rolls, 4 = £2.72 (part-baked) long, 2 = £2.95. Flour mix (white or fibre), 500 g = £5.22.

For gluten-sensitive enteropathies including steatorrhoea due to gluten sensitivity, coeliac disease, and dermatitis herpetiformis

Schar® (Nutrition Point)
Gluten-free. Bread.(white, sliced), net price 2 x 200 g = £2.65. Baguette (french bread), 400 g = £2.90. Bread rolls, 150 g = £1.60. Lunch rolls, 150 g = £1.85. White bread buns, 200 g = £2.30. Bread mix, 1 kg = £4.75. Ertha brown bread, 2 x 250 g = £3.00. Cake mix, 500 g = £4.50. Flour mix, 1 kg = £4.75. Breadsticks (Grissini), 150 g = £1.95. Cracker toast, 150 g = £2.10. Crackers, 200 g = £2.35. Crispbread, 250 g = £3.50. Pasta (fusilli, penne), 500 g = £3.30; lasagne, 250 g = £3.30; macaroni pipette, 500 g = £3.30; spaghetti, 500 g = £3.30. Pizza bases, 300 g (2 × 150 g) = £4.75. Biscuits, 200 g = £2.00. Savoy biscuits, 200 g = £2.25.

For gluten-sensitive enteropathies including steatorrhoea due to gluten sensitivity, coeliac disease, and dermatitis herpetiformis

Sunnyvale® (Everfresh)
Mixed grain bread, gluten-free. Net price 400 g = £1.79.

For gluten-sensitive enteropathies including steatorrhoea due to gluten sensitivity, coeliac disease and dermatitis herpetiformis

Tinkyada® (General Dietary)
Gluten-free. Brown rice pasta (elbows, fettucini, fusilli, penne, shells, spaghetti, spirals). Net price 454 g = £3.00.

For gluten-sensitive enteropathies including steatorrhoea due to gluten-sensitivity, coeliac disease and dermatitis herpetiformis

Tritamyl® (Gluten Free Foods Ltd)
Gluten-free. Flour, net price 1 kg = £5.60. Brown bread mix, 1 kg = £5.60. White bread mix, 1 kg = £5.60.

For gluten-sensitive enteropathies including steatorrhoea due to gluten sensitivity, coeliac disease and dermatitis herpetiformis

Ultra® (Ultrapharm)
Gluten-free. Baguette, net price 400 g = £2.46. Bread, net price 400 g = £2.46. High-fibre bread, 500 g = £3.26. Crackerbread, 100 g = £1.77. Pizza base, net price 400 g = £2.65.

For gluten-sensitive enteropathies including steatorrhoea due to gluten sensitivity, coeliac disease and dermatitis herpetiformis

Valpiform® (Gluten Free Foods Ltd)
Gluten-free. Bread mix, 2 × 500 g = £6.74; country loaf (sliced), 400 g = £3.74. Crac'form toast, 2 × 125 g = £3.52. Crisp rolls, 220 g = £3.60; Maxi baguettes, 2 × 200 g = £4.49. Pastry mix, 2 × 500 g = £6.74. Petites baguettes, 2 × 160 g = £2.99.

For gluten-sensitive enteropathies including steatorrhoea due to gluten sensitivity, coeliac disease and dermatitis herpetiformis

Low-protein foods

Aminex® (Gluten Free Foods Ltd)
Low-protein. Biscuits, net price 200 g = £3.75. Cookies, 150 g = £3.75. Rusks, 200 g = £3.75.

For inherited metabolic disorders, renal or liver failure requiring a low-protein diet

Aproten® (Ultrapharm)
Low protein. Low Na^+ and K^+. Net prices: biscuits 180 g (36) = £2.88; bread mix 250 g = £2.17; cake mix 300 g = £2.10; crispbread 260 g = £4.06; pasta (anellini, ditalini, rigatini, spaghetti) 500 g = £4.06; tagliatelle 250 g = £2.16.

For inherited metabolic disorders, renal or liver failure requiring a low-protein diet

Ener-G (General Dietary)
Low protein egg replacer, carbohydrate 94 g, energy 1574 kJ (376 kcal)/100 g. Egg-, gluten- and lactose-free, net price 454 g = £4.05.

For phenylketonuria, similar amino acid abnormalities, renal failure, liver failure and liver cirrhosis.

Low protein pasta (lasagne, macaroni, large shells, small shells, spaghetti), net price 454 g = £5.05.

For phenylketonuria, similar amino acid abnormalities, renal failure, liver failure requiring a low-protein diet

Low protein rice bread, net price 600 g = £4.39.

For inherited metabolic disorders, renal or liver failure requiring a low-protein diet

Fate® (Fate)
Low protein. All-purpose mix, net price 500 g = £5.63; Cake mix, 2 × 250 g = £5.63; Chocolate-flavour cake mix, 2 × 250 g = £5.63.

For inherited metabolic disorders, renal or liver failure requiring a low-protein diet

Juvela® (SHS)
Low Protein. Mix, net price 500 g = £5.81. Bread (whole or sliced), 400-g loaf = £2.72. Bread rolls, 5 × 70 g = £3.38. Biscuits, orange and cinnamon flavour, 125 g = £5.68; chocolate chip, 130 g = £4.89.

For inherited metabolic disorders, renal or liver failure requiring a low-protein diet

Loprofin® (SHS)
Low protein. Sweet biscuits, net price 150 g = £1.82; chocolate cream-filled biscuits, 125 g = £1.82; cookies (chocolate chip or cinnamon), 100 g = £4.82; crunch bar, 8 × 41 g = £1.09; wafers (orange, vanilla, or chocolate), 100 g = £1.76. Breakfast cereal, 375 g = £5.65. Egg replacer, 500 g = £10.59. Egg-white replacer, 100 g = £6.82. Bread (sliced or whole), 400-g loaf = £2.72. Rolls (part-baked) 4 × 65 g = £2.86. Mix, 500 g = £5.78. Crackers, 150 g = £2.48. Herb crackers, 150 g = £2.48. Pasta (lasagne, macaroni, pasta spirals, spaghetti), 500 g = £6.03. Pasta (vermicelli), 250 g = £3.00. Snack Pot, 47 g = £3.20. Rice, 500 g = £6.22.

For inherited metabolic disorders, renal or liver failure requiring a low-protein diet

Low protein drink (Milupa)
Powder, protein 0.4%, carbohydrate 5.1%, fat 2% when reconstituted. Net price 400 g = £7.23.

For inherited disorders of amino acid metabolism in childhood

Note Termed *Milupa® lpd* by manufacturer

PK Foods (Gluten Free Foods Ltd)
Bread, white (sliced), 550 g = £4.00. Crispbread, 75 g = £2.00. Pasta (spirals), 250 g = £2.00.

For phenylketonuria and similar amino acid abnormalities

Cookies (chocolate chip, orange, or cinnamon), 150 g = £3.75. Egg replacer, 350 g = £3.75. Flour mix, 750 g = £6.99. Jelly (orange or cherry flavour), 4 × 80 g = £5.76.

For phenylketonuria

Promin® (Firstplay Dietary)
Low protein. Cous Cous, 500 g = £5.70. Pasta (alphabets, macaroni, shells, shortcut spaghetti, spirals); Pasta tricolour (alphabets, shells, spirals), net price 500 g = £5.70; Lasagne sheets, 200 g = £2.45. Pasta shells in tomato, pepper and herb sauce, 4 x 72-g sachets = £6.30; Pasta elbows in cheese and broccoli sauce, 4 x 66- g sachets = £6.20. Pasta meal, 500 g = £5.70. Pasta imitation rice, 500 g = £5.70.
For inherited metabolic disorders, renal or liver failure requiring a low-protein diet

Rite-Diet® Low-protein (SHS)
Low protein. Baking mix. Net price 500 g = £5.78. Flour mix. 400 g = £4.95.
For inherited metabolic disorders, renal or liver failure requiring a low-protein diet

Sno-Pro® (SHS)
Drink, protein 220 mg (phenylalanine 12.5 mg), carbohydrate 8 g, fat 3.8 g, energy 280 kJ (67 kcal)/100 mL. Net price 200 mL = 85p.
For phenylketonuria, chronic renal failure, and other inborn errors of metabolism

Ultra® (Ultrapharm)
Low protein. PKU bread, 400 g = £2.16. PKU flour, 500 g = £3.07. PKU biscuits, 200 g = £2.21. PKU cookies, 250 g = £2.31. PKU pizza base, 400 g = £2.21. PKU savoy biscuits, 150 g = £2.06.
For inherited metabolic disorders, renal or liver failure requiring a low-protein diet

Vita Bite® (Vitaflo)
Bar, protein 30 mg (less than 2.5 mg phenylalanine), carbohydrate 15.35 g, fat 8.4 g, energy 572 kJ (137 kcal)/ 25 g. Chocolate flavoured, net price 25 g = 88p.
For inherited metabolic disorders, renal or liver failure requiring a low-protein diet. Not recommended for any child under 1 year

Flavouring preparations

FlavourPac® (Vitaflo)
Powder, flavours: blackcurrant, lemon, orange, tropical or raspberry, net price 4 × 30 × 4-g sachets = £40.10
For use in conjuntion with Vitaflo's Inborn Error range of protein substitutes

Flavour Sachets (SHS)
Powder, flavours: cherry-vanilla, grapefruit, lemon-lime, net price 20 × 5-g sachets = £8.32.
For use with SHS unflavoured amino acid and peptide products

SHS Modjul® Flavour System (SHS)
Powder, blackcurrant, orange and pineapple flavours. Net price 100 g = £8.32.
For use with any unflavoured products based on peptides or amino acids

Metabolic diseases

Glutaric aciduria (type 1)

[1]XLYS, Low TRY, Analog (SHS)
Powder, essential and non-essential amino acids 15.5% except lysine, and low tryptophan, with carbohydrate, fat, vitamins, minerals, and trace elements. Net price 400 g = £24.62.
For type 1 glutaric aciduria

[2]XLYS, Low TRY, Maxamaid (SHS)
Powder, essential and non-essential amino acids 30% except lysine, with carbohydrate, fat less than 0.5%, vitamins, minerals, and trace elements. Net price 500 g = £67.15.
For type 1 glutaric aciduria

Homocystinuria or hypermethioninaemia

HCU Express® (Vitaflo)
Powder, protein (essential and non-essential amino acids except methionine) 15 g, carbohydrate 3.8 g, fat 0.03 g, energy 315 kJ (75.3 kcal)/25 g with vitamins, minerals and trace elements. Unflavoured, net price 30 × 25- g sachets = £225.00
A methionine-free protein substitute for use as a nutritional supplement in patients over 8 years of age with homocystinuria

HCU gel® (Vitaflo)
Powder, protein (essential and non-essential amino acids except methionine) 8.4 g, carbohydrate 8.6 g, fat 0.03 g, energy 286 kJ (68 kcal)/20 g with vitamins, minerals and trace elements. Unflavoured, net price 30 × 20- g sachets = £129.50
For the dietary management of homocystinuria in children between 12 months and 10 years of age

[1]XMET Analog (SHS)
Powder, essential and non-essential amino acids 15.5% except methionine, with carbohydrate, fat, vitamins, minerals, and trace elements. Net price 400 g = £24.62.
For hypermethioninaemia; homocystinuria

XMET Homidon (SHS)
Powder, essential and non-essential amino acids 93%, except methionine. Net price 200 g = £49.59.
For homocystinuria or hypermethioninaemia

[2]XMET Maxamaid (SHS)
Powder, essential and non-essential amino acids 30% except methionine, with carbohydrate, fat less than 0.5%, vitamins, minerals, and trace elements. Net price 500 g = £67.15
For hypermethioninaemia, homocystinuria

[3]XMET Maxamum® (SHS)
Powder, essential and non-essential amino acids 47% except methionine, with carbohydrate, fat less than 0.5%, vitamins, minerals, and trace elements. Unflavoured, see also Flavour Sachets. Net price 500 g = £107.65.
For hypermethioninaemia, homocystinuria

1. Analog products are generally intended for use in children up to 1 year
2. Maxamaid products are generally intended for use in children aged 1 to 8 years, see also Flavour Sachets, for use with unflavoured amino acid and peptide products from SHS
3. Maxamum products are generally intended for use in children aged over 8 years

Hyperlysinaemia

[1]**XLYS Analog** (SHS)
Powder, essential and non-essential amino acids 15.5% except lysine, with carbohydrate, fat, vitamins, minerals, and trace elements. Net price 400 g = £24.62.
For hyperlysinaemia

[2]**XLYS Maxamaid** (SHS)
Powder, essential and non-essential amino acids 30% except lysine, with carbohydrate, fat less than 0.5%, vitamins, minerals, and trace elements. Net price 500 g = £67.15.
For hyperlysinaemia

Isovaleric acidaemia

[1]**XLEU Analog** (SHS)
Powder, essential and non-essential amino acids 15.5% except leucine, with carbohydrate, fat, vitamins, minerals, and trace elements. Net price 400 g = £24.62.
For isovaleric acidaemia
Ingredients: include arachis oil (peanut oil)

XLEU Faladon (SHS)
Powder, essential and non-essential amino acids 93%, except leucine. Net price 200 g = £50.87.
For isovaleric acidaemia

[2]**XLEU Maxamaid** (SHS)
Powder, essential and non-essential amino acids 28.6% except leucine, with carbohydrate, fat less than 0.5%, vitamins, minerals, and trace elements. Net price 500 g = £67.15.
For isovaleric acidaemia

Maple syrup urine disease

Isoleucine Amino Acid Supplement (Vitaflo)
Powder, isoleucine 0.05 g, carbohydrate 4 g, fat nil, energy 64 kJ (15 kcal)/4 g, net price 30 × 4-g sachets = £37.50
For use in conjunction with a protein supplement for maple syrup urine disease in children over 1 year

Mapleflex® (SHS)
Powder, essential and non-essential amino acids 35% except isoleucine, leucine, and valine, with carbohydrate 38%, fat 13.5%, vitamins, minerals, and trace elements. Unflavoured. Net price 30 × 29-g sachets = £142.10.
For maple syrup urine disease in children aged 1–10 years

MSUD Aid III® (SHS)
Powder, containing full range of amino acids except isoleucine, leucine, and valine, with vitamins, minerals, and trace elements. Net price 500 g = £127.20.
For maple syrup urine disease and related conditions where it is necessary to limit the intake of branched chain amino acids

[1]**MSUD Analog** (SHS)
Powder, essential and non-essential amino acids 15.5% except isoleucine, leucine and valine, with carbohydrate, fat, vitamins, minerals, and trace elements. Net price 400 g = £24.62.
For maple syrup urine disease

MSUD express® (Vitaflo)
Powder, protein equivalent (essential and non-essential amino acids except leucine, isoleucine, and valine) 15 g, carbohydrate 3.8 g, fat less than 0.1 g, energy 315 kJ (75 kcal)/25 g with vitamins, minerals, and trace elements. Unflavoured (see FlavourPac® for available flavouring sachets), net price 30 × 25-g sachets = £231.75.
For maple syrup urine disease in children over 8 years and adults

MSUD Gel® (Vitaflo)
Powder, protein equivalent (essential and non-essential amino acids except leucine, isoleucine, and valine) 8.4 g, carbohydrate 8.6 g, fat less than 0.1 g, energy 286 kJ (68 kcal)/20 g with vitamins, minerals, and trace elements. Unflavoured (see FlavourPac® for available flavouring sachets), net price 30 × 20-g sachets = £129.50.
For maple syrup urine disease in children aged 1 to 10 years

[2]**MSUD Maxamaid®** (SHS)
Powder, essential and non-essential amino acids 30% except isoleucine, leucine, and valine, with carbohydrate, fat less than 0.5%, vitamins, minerals, and trace elements. Net price 500 g = £67.15.
For maple syrup urine disease

[3]**MSUD Maxamum®** (SHS)
Powder, essential and non-essential amino acids 47% except isoleucine, leucine, and valine, with carbohydrate, fat less than 0.5%, vitamins, minerals, and trace elements. Flavours: orange, unflavoured, see also Flavour Sachets. Net price 500 g = £107.65.
For maple syrup urine disease

Valine Amino Acid Supplement (Vitaflo)
Powder, valine 0.05 g, carbohydrate 4 g, fat nil, energy 64 kJ (15 kcal)/4 g, net price 30 × 4-g sachets = £37.50
For use in conjunction with a protein supplement for maple syrup urine disease in children over 1 year

Methylmalonic or propionic acidaemia

[1]**XMTVI Analog** (SHS)
Powder, essential and non-essential amino acids 15.5% except methionine, threonine, valine and low isoleucine, with carbohydrate, fat, vitamins, minerals, and trace elements. Net price 400 g = £24.62.
For methylmalonic acidaemia or propionic acidaemia

XMTVI Asadon (SHS)
Powder, essential and non-essential amino acids 93% except methionine, threonine, and valine, with trace amounts of isoleucine. Net price 200 g = £50.87.
For methylmalonic acidaemia or propionic acidaemia

1. Analog products are generally intended for use in children up to 1 year
2. Maxamaid products are generally intended for use in children aged 1 to 8 years, see also Flavour Sachets, for use with unflavoured amino acid and peptide products from SHS
3. Maxamum products are generally intended for use in children aged over 8 years

[1]**XMTVI Maxamaid** (SHS)
Powder, essential and non-essential amino acids 30% except methionine, threonine, valine and low isoleucine, with carbohydrate, fat less than 0.5%, vitamins, minerals, and trace elements. Net price 500 g = £67.15.
For methylmalonic acidaemia or propionic acidaemia

[2]**XMTVI Maxamum** (SHS)
Powder, essential and non-essential amino acids 47% except methionine, threonine, valine, and low isoleucine, with carbohydrate, fat less than 0.5%, vitamins, minerals, and trace elements. Unflavoured, see also Flavour Sachets. Net price 500 g = £107.65.
For methylmalonic acidaemia or propionic acidaemia

Phenylketonuria

Aminogran® (UCB Pharma)
Food Supplement, powder, containing all essential amino acids except phenylalanine, net price 500 g = £39.78. Aminogran PKU tablet (≡ 1 g powder), net price 150-tab pack = £30.00.
For the dietary management of phenylketonuria. Tablets not to be prescribed for any child under 8 years

Easiphen® (SHS)
Liquid, protein (containing essential and non-essential amino acids, phenylalanine-free) 6.7 g, carbohydrate 5.1 g, fat 2 g, energy 275 kJ (65 kcal)/100 mL with vitamins, minerals, and trace elements. Forest berries, grapefruit, orange, or tropical flavour, net price 250-mL carton = £6.60.
For the dietary management of proven phenylketonuria. Not to be prescribed for children under 8 years

Lophlex® (SHS)
Powder, protein (containing essential and non-essential amino acids, phenylalanine-free) protein equivalent 20 g, carbohydrate 1.4 g, fat 60 mg, fibre 220 mg, energy 366 kJ (86 kcal)/27.8 g with vitamins, minerals, and trace elements. Flavours: berry, orange or unflavoured, net price 30 x 27.8-g sachets = £198.00.
For use in the dietary management of proven phenylketonuria in older children (over 8 years) and adults (includes use in pregnant women)

Loprofin® PKU Drink (SHS)
PKU Drink, protein 0.4 g (phenylalanine 10 mg), lactose 9.4 g, fat 2 g, energy 165 kJ (40 kcal)/100 mL. Net price 200-mL Tetrapak® = 52p.
For phenylketonuria

Minaphlex® (SHS)
Liquid, protein equivalent 8.4 g, carbohydrate 9.9 g, fat 3.9 g, energy 455 (108 kcal)/29-g sachet, with vitamins, minerals, and trace elements. Phenylalanine-free. Chocolate, pineapple, and vanilla. Unflavoured version also available (contains an extra 5 kcal of carbohydrate per sachet), net price 30 × 29 g sachets = £86.33.
For the dietary management of phenylketonuria. Not recommended for children under 1 year

Phlexy-10® Exchange System (SHS)
Bar, essential and non-essential amino acids except phenylalanine 8.33 g, carbohydrate 20.5 g, fat 4.5 g/42-g bar. Citrus fruit flavour. Net price per bar = £4.16

Capsules, essential and non-essential amino acids except phenylalanine 500 mg/capsule. Net price 200-cap pack = £29.09

Tablets, essential and non-essential amino acids except phenylalanine, 1 g tablet. Net price 75-tab pack = £18.85

Drink Mix, powder, containing essential and non-essential amino acids except phenylalanine 10 g, carbohydrate 8.8 g/20-g sachet. Apple and blackcurrant, citrus, or tropical flavour. Net price 20-g sachet = £2.92
All for phenylketonuria

PK Aid 4® (SHS)
Powder, containing essential and non-essential amino acids except phenylalanine. Net price 500 g = £97.78.
For phenylketonuria

PKU 2® (Milupa)
Granules, containing essential and non-essential amino acids except phenylalanine; with vitamins, minerals, trace elements, 7.1% sucrose. Flavour: vanilla. Net price 500 g = £44.75.
For phenylketonuria

PKU 3® (Milupa)
Granules, containing essential and non-essential amino acids except phenylalanine, vitamins, minerals, and trace elements, with 3.4% sucrose. Flavour: vanilla. Net price 500 g = £44.75.
For phenylketonuria, not recommended for children under 8 years

PKU express® (Vitaflo)
Powder, protein (containing essential and non-essential amino acids, phenylalanine-free) 72 g, carbohydrate 15.1 g, energy 1260 kJ (301.5 kcal)/100 g with vitamins, minerals, and trace elements. Lemon, orange, tropical or unflavoured, net price 30 x 25 g sachets = £140.50.
For phenylketonuria, not recommended for children under 8 years

PKU express cooler® (Vitaflo)
Liquid, protein equivalent 15 g, carbohydrate 7.8 g, energy 386 kJ (92 kcal)/130-mL pouch, with vitamins, minerals, and trace elements. Phenylalanine-free. Orange or purple option, net price 30 x 130 mL = £151.93.
For the dietary management of phenylketonuria, not recommended for children under 8 years

PKU gel® (Vitaflo)
Powder, protein (containing essential and non-essential amino acids, phenylalanine-free) 8.4 g, carbohydrate 8.6 g, fat 0.03 g, energy 285.5 kJ (68 kcal)/20 g with vitamins, minerals and trace elements. Orange or unflavoured, net price 30 × 20-g sachets = £80.85.
For use as part of the low-protein dietary management of phenylketonuria in children aged 1 to 10 years. Not recommended for children under 1 year

L-Tyrosine (SHS)
Powder, net price 100 g = £12.53.
For use as a supplement in maternal phenylketonurics who have low plasma tyrosine concentrations

[3]**XP Analog** (SHS)
Powder, essential and non-essential amino acids 15.5% except phenylalanine, with carbohydrate, fat, vitamins, minerals, and trace elements. Net price 400 g = £19.67.
For phenylketonuria

XP LCP Analog (SHS)
Powder, essential and non-essential amino acids except phenylalanine 15.5%, with carbohydrate, fat, vitamins, minerals and trace elements. Gluten- and lactose-free. Net price 400 g = £22.38.
For phenylketonuria in infants and children under 2 years of age

[1]**XP Maxamaid** (SHS)
Powder, essential and non-essential amino acids 30% except phenylalanine, with carbohydrate, vitamins, minerals, and trace elements. Net price powder (unfla-

1. Maxamaid products are generally intended for use in children aged 1 to 8 years, see also Flavour Sachets, for use with unflavoured amino acid and peptide products from SHS
2. Maxamum products are generally intended for use in children aged over 8 years
3. Analog products are generally intended for use in children up to 1 year

voured), 500 g = £39.73; (orange-flavoured), 500 g = £39.73.

For phenylketonuria. Not to be prescribed for children under 2 years

[1]XP Maxamaid Concentrate (SHS)

Powder, essential and non-essential amino acids 65% except phenylalanine, with carbohydrate, fat less than 0.5%, vitamins, minerals, and trace elements. Unflavoured. Net price 500 g = £101.72.

For phenylketonuria. Not to be prescribed for children under 2 years

Note See also Flavour Sachets, for use with unflavoured amino acid and peptide products from SHS

[2]XP Maxamum® (SHS)

Powder, essential and non-essential amino acids 47% except phenylalanine, with carbohydrates, vitamins, minerals, and trace elements. Flavours: orange, unflavoured, see also Flavour Sachets. Net price 30 × 50-g sachets = £190.17, 500 g = £61.42.

For phenylketonuria. Not to be prescribed for children under 8 years

Tyrosinaemia

TYR Gel® (Vitaflo)

Gel, essential and non-essential amino acids (except tyrosine and phenylalanine) 10.1 g, protein equivalent 8.4 g, carbohydrate 8.6 g, fat 0.03 g, energy 285.5 kJ (68 kcal)/ 20 g, with vitamins, minerals and trace elements. Unflavoured, net price 30 × 20-g sachets = £129.50

A tyrosine- and phenylalanine-free protein substitute for use in the dietary management of tyrosinaemia in children between 12 months and 10 years

[3]XPHEN TYR Analog (SHS)

Powder, essential and non-essential amino acids 15.5% except phenylalanine and tyrosine, with carbohydrate, fat, vitamins, minerals and trace elements. Net price 400 g = £24.62.

For tyrosinaemia

[1]XPHEN TYR Maxamaid (SHS)

Powder, essential and non-essential amino acids 30% except phenylalanine and tyrosine, with carbohydrate, fat less than 0.5%, vitamins, minerals, and trace elements. Unflavoured. Net price 500 g = £67.15.

For tyrosinaemia

XPHEN TYR Tyrosidon (SHS)

Powder, essential and non-essential amino acids 93%, except phenylalanine and tyrosine. Net price 500 g = £127.20

For tyrosinaemia where plasma methionine concentrations are normal

[3]XPTM Analog (SHS)

Powder, essential and non-essential amino acids 15.5% except phenylalanine, tyrosine and methionine, with carbohydrate, fat, vitamins, minerals and trace elements. Net price 400 g = £24.62.

For tyrosinaemia

XPTM Tyrosidon (SHS)

Powder, essential and non-essential amino acids 93%, except methionine, phenylalanine, and tyrosine. Net price 500 g = £127.20.

For tyrosinaemia type I where plasma concentrations are above normal

Urea cycle disorders (other than arginase deficiency)

L-Arginine (SHS)

Powder, net price 100 g = £8.39.

For use as a supplement in urea cycle disorders other than arginase deficiency, such as hyperammonaemia types I and II, citrullaemia, arginosuccinic aciduria, and deficiency of N-acetyl glutamate synthetase

Conditions for which toilet preparations may be prescribed on FP10, GP10 (Scotland), WP10 (Wales)

Note This is a list of clinical conditions for which the ACBS has approved toilet preparations. For details of the preparations see Chapter 13.

Birthmarks

See disfiguring skin lesions.

Dermatitis

Aveeno Bath Oil; Aveeno Cream; Aveeno Colloidal; Aveeno Baby Colloidal ; E45 Emollient Bath Oil; E45 Emollient Wash Cream; E45 Lotion; Vaseline Dermacare Cream and Lotion

Dermatitis herpetiformis

See gluten-sensitive enteropathies.

Disfiguring skin lesions (birthmarks, mutilating lesions, scars, vitiligo)

Covermark classic foundation and finishing powder; Dermacolor Camouflage cream and fixing powder; Keromask masking cream and finishing powder; Veil Cover cream and Finishing Powder. (Cleansing Creams, Cleansing Milks, and Cleansing Lotions are excluded)

Disinfectants (antiseptics)

May be prescribed on an FP10 only when ordered in such quantities and with such directions as are appropriate for the treatment of patients, but not for general hygenic purposes.

Eczema

See dermatitis.

Photodermatoses (skin protection in)

Coppertone Ultrashade 23; Delph Sun Lotion SPF 15, SPF 20, SPF 25, and SPF 30; E45 Sun Block SPF 25, and 50; RoC Total Sunblock Cream SPF 25; Spectraban 25, and Ultra; Sunsense Ultra; Uvistat Sun Block Cream Factor 20, and Ultrablock Suncream Factor 30.

Pruritus

See dermatitis.

1. Maxamaid products are generally intended for use in children aged 1 to 8 years, see also Flavour Sachets, for use with unflavoured amino acid and peptide products from SHS
2. Maxamum products are generally intended for use in children aged over 8 years
3. Analog products are generally intended for use in children up to 1 year

A3 Cautionary and advisory labels for dispensed medicines

Preparations in the *BNF for Children* include code numbers of the cautionary labels that pharmacists are recommended to add when dispensing. It is also expected that, when necessary, pharmacists will counsel children or their carers.

Counselling needs to be related to the age, experience, background, and understanding of the child or carer. The pharmacist should ensure understanding of how to take or use the medicine and how to follow the correct dosage schedule. Any effects of the medicine on co-ordination, performance of skilled tasks, any foods or medicines to be avoided, and what to do if a dose is missed should also be explained. Other matters, such as the possibility of staining of the clothes or skin, or discoloration of urine or stools by a medicine should also be mentioned.

For some preparations there is a special need for counselling, such as an unusual method or time of administration or a potential interaction with a common food or domestic remedy, and this should be mentioned where necessary.

Original packs Most preparations are now dispensed in unbroken original packs (see Patient Packs, p. vii) that include further advice for the patient in the form of patient information leaflets. The advice in patient information leaflets may be less appropriate when the medicine is for a child, particularly for unlicensed medicines or indications. Pharmacists should explain discrepancies to carers, if necessary. The patient information leaflet should only be withheld in exceptional circumstances because it contains other information that should be provided. Label 10 may be of value where appropriate. More general leaflets advising on the administration of preparations such as eye drops, eye ointments, inhalers, and suppositories are also available.

Scope of labels In general, no label recommendations are provided for injections on the assumption that they will be administered by a healthcare professional or a well-instructed child or carer. The labelling is not exhaustive and pharmacists are recommended to use their professional discretion in labelling new preparations and those for which no labels are shown.

Individual labelling advice is not given on the administration of the large variety of antacids. In the absence of instructions from the prescriber, and if on enquiry the patient has had no verbal instructions, the directions given under 'Dose' should be used on the label.

It is recognised that there may be occasions when pharmacists will use their knowledge and professional discretion and decide to omit one or more of the recommended labels for a particular child. In this case counselling is of the utmost importance. There may also be an occasion when a prescriber does not wish additional cautionary labels to be used, in which case the prescription should be endorsed 'NCL' (no cautionary labels). The exact wording that is required instead should then be specified on the prescription.

Pharmacists label medicines with various wordings in addition to those directions specified on the prescription. Such labels include 'Shake the bottle', 'For external use only', and 'Store in a cool place', as well as 'Discard . . . . days after opening' and 'Do not use after . . . .', which apply particularly to antibiotic mixtures, diluted liquid and topical preparations, and to eye-drops. Although not listed in the *BNF for Children* these labels should continue to be used when appropriate; indeed, 'For external use only' is a legal requirement on external liquid preparations, while 'Keep out of the reach of children' is a legal requirement on all dispensed medicines. Care should be taken not to obscure other relevant information with adhesive labelling.

It is the usual practice for patients to take standard tablets with water or other liquid and for this reason no separate label has been recommended.

The label wordings recommended by the *BNF for Children* apply to medicines dispensed against a prescription. Children and carers should be made aware that a dispensed medicine should never be taken by, or shared with, anyone other than for whom the prescriber intended it. Therefore, the *BNF for Children* does not include warnings against the use of a dispensed medicine by persons other than for whom it was specifically prescribed.

The label or labels for each preparation are recommended after careful consideration of the information available. However, it is recognised that in some cases this information may be either incomplete or open to a different interpretation. The Executive Editor will therefore be grateful to receive any constructive comments on the labelling suggested for any preparation.

Recommended label wordings

Wordings which can be given as separate warnings are labels 1-19 and labels 29-33. Wordings which can be incorporated in an appropriate position in the directions for dosage or administration are labels 21-28. A label has been omitted for number 20.

If separate labels are used it is recommended that the wordings be used without modification. If changes are made to suit computer requirements, care should be taken to retain the sense of the original.

1 **Warning. May cause drowsiness**
To be used on *preparations for children* containing antihistamines, or other preparations given to children where the warnings of label 2 on driving or alcohol would not be appropriate.

2 **Warning. May cause drowsiness. If affected do not drive or operate machinery. Avoid alcoholic drink**
To be used on *preparations for adults that can cause drowsiness*, thereby affecting coordination and the ability to drive and operate hazardous machinery; label 1 is more appropriate for children. *It is an offence to drive while under the influence of drink or drugs*. It should be remembered that children and adolescents do, on occasion, consume alcohol and should be made aware of potential problems.
Some of these preparations only cause drowsiness in the first few days of treatment and some only cause drowsiness in higher doses.
In such cases the patient should be told that the advice applies until the effects have worn off. However many of these preparations can produce a slowing of reaction time and a loss of mental concentration that can have the same effects as drowsiness.
Avoidance of alcoholic drink is recommended because the effects of CNS depressants are enhanced by alcohol. Strict prohibition however could lead to some patients not taking the medicine. Pharmacists should therefore explain the risk and encourage compliance, particularly in patients who may think they already tolerate the effects of alcohol (see also label 3). Queries from patients with epilepsy regarding fitness to drive should be referred back to the patient's doctor.
Side-effects unrelated to drowsiness that may affect a patient's ability to drive or operate machinery safely include *blurred vision, dizziness, or nausea*. In general, no label has been recommended to cover these cases, but the patient should be suitably counselled.

3 **Warning. May cause drowsiness. If affected do not drive or operate machinery**
To be used on *preparations containing monoamine-oxidase inhibitors*; the warning to avoid alcohol and dealcoholised (low alcohol) drink is covered by the patient information leaflet.
Also to be used as for label 2 but where alcohol is not an issue.

4 **Warning. Avoid alcoholic drink**
To be used on *preparations where a reaction such as flushing may occur if alcohol is taken* (e.g. metronidazole and chlorpropamide). Alcohol may also enhance the hypoglycaemia produced by some oral antidiabetic drugs but routine application of a warning label is not considered necessary.

5 **Do not take indigestion remedies at the same time of day as this medicine**
To be used with label 25 on *preparations coated to resist gastric acid* (e.g. enteric-coated tablets). This is to avoid the possibility of premature dissolution of the coating in the presence of an alkaline pH.
Label 5 also applies to drugs such as ketoconazole *where the absorption is significantly affected by antacids*; the usual period of avoidance recommended is 2 to 4 hours.

6 **Do not take indigestion remedies or medicines containing iron or zinc at the same time of day as this medicine**
To be used on *preparations containing ofloxacin and some other quinolones, doxycycline, lymecycline, minocycline, and penicillamine*. These drugs chelate calcium, iron and zinc and are less well absorbed when taken with calcium-containing antacids or preparations containing iron or zinc. These incompatible preparations should be taken 2-3 hours apart.

7 **Do not take milk, indigestion remedies, or medicines containing iron or zinc at the same time of day as this medicine**
To be used on *preparations containing ciprofloxacin, norfloxacin or tetracyclines that chelate, calcium, iron, magnesium, and zinc* and are thus less available for absorption; these incompatible preparations should be taken 2-3 hours apart. Doxycycline, lymecycline and minocycline are less liable to form chelates and therefore only require label 6 (see above).

8 **Do not stop taking this medicine except on your doctor's advice**
To be used on *preparations that contain a drug which is required to be taken over long periods without the patient necessarily perceiving any benefit* (e.g. antituberculous drugs).
Also to be used on *preparations that contain a drug whose withdrawal is likely to be a particular hazard* (e.g. clonidine for hypertension). Label 10 (see below) is more appropriate for corticosteroids.

9 **Take at regular intervals. Complete the prescribed course unless otherwise directed**
To be used on *preparations where a course of treatment should be completed* to reduce the incidence of relapse or failure of treatment.
The preparations are antimicrobial drugs given by mouth. Very occasionally, some may have severe side-effects (e.g. diarrhoea in patients receiving clindamycin) and in such cases the patient may need to be advised of reasons for stopping treatment quickly and returning to the doctor.

10 **Warning. Follow the printed instructions you have been given with this medicine**
To be used particularly on *preparations containing anticoagulants, lithium and oral corticosteroids*. The appropriate treatment card should be given to the patient and any necessary explanations given.
This label may also be used on other preparations to remind the patient of the instructions that have been given.

11 **Avoid exposure of skin to direct sunlight or sun lamps**
To be used on *preparations that may cause phototoxic or photoallergic reactions* if the patient is exposed to ultraviolet radiation. Many drugs other than those listed (e.g. phenothiazines and sulphonamides) may, on rare occasions, cause reactions in susceptible patients. Exposure to high intensity ultraviolet radiation from sunray lamps and sunbeds is particularly likely to cause reactions.

12 **Do not take anything containing aspirin while taking this medicine**
To be used on *preparations containing probenecid and sulfinpyrazone* whose activity is reduced by aspirin.
Label 12 should not be used for anticoagulants since label 10 is more appropriate.

13 **Dissolve or *mix with water* before taking**
To be used on *preparations that are intended to be dissolved in water* (e.g. soluble tablets) or *mixed with water* (e.g. powders, granules) before use. In a few cases other liquids such as fruit juice or milk may be used.

14 **This medicine may colour the urine**
To be used on *preparations that may cause the patient's urine to turn an unusual colour*. These include phenolphthalein (alkaline urine pink), triamterene (blue under some lights), levodopa (dark reddish), and rifampicin (red).

15 **Caution flammable: keep away from fire or flames**
To be used on *preparations containing sufficient flammable solvent to render them flammable if exposed to a naked flame.*

16 **Allow to dissolve under the tongue. Do not transfer from this container. Keep tightly closed. Discard eight weeks after opening**
To be used on *glyceryl trinitrate tablets* to remind the patient not to transfer the tablets to plastic or less suitable containers.

17 **Do not take more than . . . in 24 hours**
To be used on *preparations for the treatment of acute migraine* except those containing ergotamine, for which label 18 is used. The dose form should be specified, e.g. tablets or capsules.
It may also be used on preparations for which no dose has been specified by the prescriber.

18 **Do not take more than . . . in 24 hours or . . . in any one week**
To be used on preparations containing ergotamine. The dose form should be specified, e.g. tablets or suppositories.

19 **Warning. Causes drowsiness which may continue the next day. If affected do not drive or operate machinery. Avoid alcoholic drink**
To be used on *preparations containing hypnotics (or some other drugs with sedative effects) prescribed to be taken at night.* On the rare occasions (e.g. nitrazepam in epilepsy) when hypnotics are prescribed for daytime administration this label would clearly not be appropriate. Also to be used as an *alternative to the label 2 wording* (the choice being at the discretion of the pharmacist) *for anxiolytics prescribed to be taken at night.*
It is hoped that this wording will convey adequately the problem of residual morning sedation after taking 'sleeping tablets'.

21 **. . . with or after food**
To be used on *preparations that are liable to cause gastric irritation, or those that are better absorbed with food.*
Patients should be advised that a *small amount of food is sufficient.*

22 **. . . half to one hour before food**
To be used on some preparations *whose absorption is thereby improved.*
Most oral antibacterials require label 23 instead (see below).

23 **. . . an hour before food or on an empty stomach**
To be used on *oral preparations whose absorption may be reduced by the presence of food and acid in the stomach.*

24 **. . . sucked or chewed**
To be used on *preparations that should be sucked or chewed.*
The pharmacist should use discretion as to which of these words is appropriate.

25 **. . . swallowed whole, not chewed**
To be used on *preparations that are enteric-coated or designed for modified-release.*
Also to be used on *preparations that taste very unpleasant or may damage the mouth* if not swallowed whole.

26 **. . . dissolved under the tongue**
To be used on *preparations designed for sublingual use.* Patients should be advised to hold under the tongue and avoid swallowing until dissolved. The buccal mucosa between the gum and cheek is occasionally specified by the prescriber.

27 **. . . with plenty of water**
To be used on *preparations that should be well diluted* (e.g. chloral hydrate), *where a high fluid intake is required* (e.g. sulphonamides), or *where water is required to aid the action* (e.g. methylcellulose). The patient should be advised that 'plenty' means at least 150 mL (about a tumblerful). In most cases fruit juice, tea, or coffee may be used.

28 **To be spread thinly . . .**
To be used on *external preparations* that should be applied sparingly (e.g. corticosteroids, dithranol).

29 **Do not take more than 2 at any one time. Do not take more than 8 in 24 hours**
To be used on containers of dispensed *solid dose preparations containing paracetamol for adults when the instruction on the label indicates that the dose can be taken on an 'as required' basis.* The dose form should be specified, e.g. tablets or capsules.
This label has been introduced because of the serious consequences of overdosage with paracetamol.

30 **Do not take with any other paracetamol products**
To be used on all containers of dispensed *preparations containing paracetamol.*

31 **Contains aspirin and paracetamol. Do not take with any other paracetamol products**
To be used on all containers of dispensed *preparations containing aspirin and paracetamol.*

32 **Contains aspirin**
To be used on containers of dispensed *preparations containing aspirin when the name on the label does not include the word 'aspirin'.*

33 **Contains an aspirin-like medicine**
To be used on containers of dispensed *preparations containing aspirin derivatives.*

Dental Practitioners' Formulary

List of Dental Preparations

The following list has been approved by the appropriate Secretaries of State, and the preparations therein may be prescribed by dental practitioners on form FP10D (GP14 in Scotland, WP10D in Wales).

Sugar-free versions, where available, are preferred.

Aciclovir Cream, BP
Aciclovir Oral Suspension, BP, 200 mg/5 mL
Aciclovir Tablets, BP, 200 mg
Amoxicillin Capsules, BP
Amoxicillin Oral Powder, DPF[1]
Amoxicillin Oral Suspension, BP
Amphotericin Lozenges, BP
Amphotericin Oral Suspension, BP
Ampicillin Capsules, BP
Ampicillin Oral Suspension, BP
Artificial Saliva, DPF[2]
Artificial Saliva Substitutes as listed below (to be prescribed only for indications approved by ACBS[3]):
- AS Saliva Orthana®
- Glandosane®
- Biotene Oralbalance®
- BioXtra®
- Saliveze®
- Salivix®

Ascorbic Acid Tablets, BP
Aspirin Tablets, Dispersible, BP[4]
Azithromycin Oral Suspension, 200 mg/5 mL, DPF
Benzydamine Mouthwash, BP 0.15%
Benzydamine Oromucosal Spray, BP 0.15%
Carbamazepine Tablets, BP
Carmellose Gelatin Paste, DPF
Cefalexin Capsules, BP
Cefalexin Oral Suspension, BP
Cefalexin Tablets, BP
Cefradine Capsules, BP
Cefradine Oral Solution, DPF
Chlorhexidine Gluconate 1% Gel, DPF
Chlorhexidine Mouthwash, BP
Chlorhexidine Oral Spray, DPF
Chlorphenamine Tablets, BP
Choline Salicylate Dental Gel, BP
Clindamycin Capsules, BP
Diazepam Oral Solution, BP, 2 mg/5 mL
Diazepam Tablets, BP
Diflunisal Tablets, BP
Dihydrocodeine Tablets, BP, 30 mg
Doxycycline Capsules, BP, 100 mg
Doxycycline Tablets, 20 mg, DPF
Ephedrine Nasal Drops, BP
Erythromycin Ethyl Succinate Oral Suspension, BP
Erythromycin Ethyl Succinate Tablets, BP
Erythromycin Stearate Tablets, BP
Erythromycin Tablets, BP
Fluconazole Capsules, 50 mg, DPF
Fluconazole Oral Suspension, 50 mg/5 mL, DPF
Hydrocortisone Cream, BP, 1%
Hydrocortisone Oromucosal Tablets, BP
Hydrocortisone and Miconazole Cream, DPF
Hydrocortisone and Miconazole Ointment, DPF
Hydrogen Peroxide Mouthwash, BP
Ibuprofen Oral Suspension, BP, sugar-free
Ibuprofen Tablets, BP
Lidocaine 5% Ointment, DPF
Menthol and Eucalyptus Inhalation, BP 1980[5]
Metronidazole Oral Suspension, DPF
Metronidazole Tablets, BP
Miconazole Oromucosal Gel, BP
Mouthwash Solution-tablets, DPF
Nitrazepam Tablets, BP
Nystatin Ointment, BP
Nystatin Oral Suspension, BP
Nystatin Pastilles, BP
Oxytetracycline Tablets, BP
Paracetamol Oral Suspension, BP[6]
Paracetamol Tablets, BP
Paracetamol Tablets, Soluble, BP
Penciclovir Cream, DPF
Pethidine Tablets, BP
Phenoxymethylpenicillin Oral Solution, BP
Phenoxymethylpenicillin Tablets, BP
Promethazine Hydrochloride Tablets, BP
Promethazine Oral Solution, BP
Sodium Chloride Mouthwash, Compound, BP
Sodium Fluoride Mouthwash, BP
Sodium Fluoride Oral Drops, BP
Sodium Fluoride Tablets, BP
Sodium Fluoride Toothpaste 0.619%, DPF
Sodium Fusidate Ointment, BP
Temazepam Oral Solution, BP
Temazepam Tablets, BP
Tetracycline Tablets, BP
Triamcinolone Dental Paste, BP
Vitamin B Tablets, Compound, Strong, BPC

1. Amoxicillin Dispersible Tablets are no longer available
2. Supplies may be difficult to obtain
3. Indications approved by the ACBS are: patients suffering from dry mouth as a result of having (or having undergone) radiotherapy or sicca syndrome
4. The BP directs that when soluble aspirin tablets are prescribed, dispersible aspirin tablets should be dispensed
5. This preparation does not appear in subsequent editions of the BP
6. The BP directs that when Paediatric Paracetamol Oral Suspension or Paediatric Paracetamol Mixture is prescribed and no strength stated Paracetamol Oral Suspension 120 mg/5 mL should be dispensed

Nurse Prescribers' Formulary

Nurse Prescribers' Formulary for Community Practitioners

Nurse Prescribers' Formulary Appendix (Appendix NPF). List of preparations approved by the Secretary of State which may be prescribed on form FP10P (form HS21(N) in Northern Ireland, form GP10(N) in Scotland, forms FP10(CN) and FP10(PN) in Wales or, when available, WP10CN and WP10PN in Wales) by Nurses for National Health Service patients.

Community practitioners who have completed the necessary training may only prescribe items appearing in the nurse prescribers' list set out below.

Medicinal Preparations

Almond Oil Ear Drops, BP
Arachis Oil Enema, NPF
[1]Aspirin Tablets, Dispersible, 300 mg, BP
Bisacodyl Suppositories, BP (includes 5-mg and 10-mg strengths)
Bisacodyl Tablets, BP
Cadexomer-Iodine Ointment, NPF
Cadexomer-Iodine Paste, NPF
Cadexomer-Iodine Powder, NPF
Catheter Maintenance Solution, Chlorhexidine, NPF
Catheter Maintenance Solution, Sodium Chloride, NPF
Catheter Maintenance Solution, 'Solution G', NPF
Catheter Maintenance Solution, 'Solution R', NPF
Chlorhexidine Gluconate Alcoholic Solutions containing at least 0.05%
Chlorhexidine Gluconate Aqueous Solutions containing at least 0.05%
Choline Salicylate Dental Gel, BP
Clotrimazole Cream 1%, BP
Co-danthramer Capsules, NPF
Co-danthramer Capsules, Strong, NPF
Co-danthramer Oral Suspension, NPF
Co-danthramer Oral Suspension, Strong, NPF
Co-danthrusate Capsules, BP
Co-danthrusate Oral Suspension, NPF
Crotamiton Cream, BP
Crotamiton Lotion, BP
Dimeticone barrier creams containing at least 10%
Docusate Capsules, BP
Docusate Enema, NPF
Docusate Enema, Compound, BP
Docusate Oral Solution, BP
Docusate Oral Solution, Paediatric, BP
Econazole Cream 1%, BP
Emollients as listed below:
- Aqueous Cream, BP
- Arachis Oil, BP
- Cetraben® Emollient Cream
- Decubal® Clinic
- Dermamist®
- Diprobase® Cream
- Diprobase® Ointment
- Doublebase®
- E45® Cream
- Emulsifying Ointment, BP
- [2]Epaderm®
- Gammaderm® Cream
- Hydromol® Cream
- Hydromol® Ointment
- Hydrous Ointment, BP
- Keri® Therapeutic Lotion
- Lipobase®
- Liquid and White Soft Paraffin Ointment, NPF
- Neutrogena® Dermatological Cream
- Oilatum® Cream
- Paraffin, White Soft, BP
- Paraffin, Yellow Soft, BP
- Ultrabase®
- Unguentum M®
- Zerobase® Cream

Emollient Bath Additives as listed below:
- Alpha Keri® Bath Oil
- Ashbourne Emollient Medicinal Bath Oil
- [3]Balneum®
- Cetraben® Emollient Bath Additive
- Dermalo® Bath Emollient
- Diprobath®
- Hydromol® Emollient
- Imuderm® Bath Oil
- Oilatum® Emollient
- Oilatum® Fragrance Free Junior
- Oilatum® Gel

Folic Acid 400 micrograms/5 mL Oral Solution, NPF
Folic Acid Tablets 400 micrograms, BP
Glycerol Suppositories, BP
[4]Ibuprofen Oral Suspension, BP
[4]Ibuprofen Tablets, BP
Ispaghula Husk Granules, BP

1. Max. 96 tablets; max. pack size 32 tablets
2. Included in the Drug Tariff, Scottish Drug Tariff, and Northern Ireland Drug Tariff
3. Except pack sizes that are not to be prescribed under the NHS (see Part XVIIIA of the Drug Tariff, Part XI of the Northern Ireland Drug Tariff)
4. Except for indications and doses that are PoM

Ispaghula Husk Granules, Effervescent, BP
Ispaghula Husk Oral Powder, BP
Lactulose Solution, BP
Lidocaine Gel, BP
Lidocaine Ointment, BP
Lidocaine and Chlorhexidine Gel, BP
Macrogol Oral Powder, NPF
Macrogol Oral Powder, Compound, NPF
Macrogol Oral Powder, Compound, Half-strength, NPF
Magnesium Hydroxide Mixture, BP
Magnesium Sulphate Paste, BP
Malathion alcoholic lotions containing at least 0.5%
Malathion aqueous lotions containing at least 0.5%
Mebendazole Oral Suspension, NPF
Mebendazole Tablets, NPF
Methylcellulose Tablets, BP
Miconazole Cream 2%, BP
Miconazole Oromucosal Gel, BP
Mouthwash Solution-tablets, NPF
Nicotine Inhalation Cartridge for Oromucosal Use, NPF
Nicotine Lozenge, NPF
Nicotine Medicated Chewing Gum, NPF
Nicotine Nasal Spray, NPF
Nicotine Sublingual Tablets, NPF
Nicotine Transdermal Patches, NPF
Nystatin Oral Suspension, BP
Nystatin Pastilles, BP
Olive Oil Ear Drops, BP
Paracetamol Oral Suspension, BP (includes 120 mg/5 mL and 250 mg/5 mL strengths—both of which are available as sugar-free formulations)
[1]Paracetamol Tablets, BP
[1]Paracetamol Tablets, Soluble, BP (includes 120-mg and 500-mg tablets)
Permethrin Cream, NPF
Phenothrin Alcoholic Lotion, NPF
Phenothrin Aqueous Lotion, NPF
Phosphates Enema, BP
Phosphate suppositories, NPF
Piperazine and Senna Powder, NPF
Povidone–Iodine Solution, BP
Senna Granules, Standardised, BP
Senna Oral Solution, NPF
Senna Tablets, BP
Senna and Ispaghula Granules, NPF
Sodium Chloride Solution, Sterile, BP
Sodium Citrate Compound Enema, NPF
Sodium Picosulfate Capsules, NPF
Sodium Picosulfate Elixir, NPF
Spermicidal contraceptives as listed below:
- Ortho-Creme® Cream
- Orthoforms® Pessaries

Sterculia Granules, NPF
Sterculia and Frangula Granules, NPF
Streptokinase and Streptodornase Topical Powder, NPF
Titanium Ointment, BP
Water for Injections, BP
Zinc and Castor Oil Ointment, BP
Zinc Cream, BP
Zinc Ointment, BP
Zinc Oxide and Dimeticone Spray, NPF
Zinc Oxide Impregnated Medicated Stocking, NPF
Zinc Paste Bandage, BP 1993
Zinc Paste and Calamine Bandage
Zinc Paste, Calamine and Clioquinol Bandage BP 1993
Zinc Paste and Ichthammol Bandage, BP 1993

Appliances and Reagents (including Wound Management Products)

In the Drug Tariff Appliances and Reagents which may **not** be prescribed by Nurses are annotated Ⓝ (**Nx** in the Scottish Drug Tariff and N in the Northern Ireland Drug Tariff)

Applicators, Vaginal as listed in Part IXA of the Drug Tariff (Part 3 of the Scottish Drug Tariff, not prescribable by nurses in Northern Ireland)
Atomizers, Hand Operated as listed in Part IXA of the Drug Tariff (Part 3 of the Scottish Drug Tariff, not prescribable by nurses in Northern Ireland)
Auto Inflation Device (for treatment of glue ear) as listed in Part IXA of the Drug Tariff (Part 3 of the Scottish Drug Tariff, Part III of the Northern Ireland Drug Tariff)
Breast Reliever as listed in Part IXA of the Drug Tariff (Part 3 of the Scottish Drug Tariff, not prescribable by nurses in Northern Ireland)
Breast Shields as listed in Part IXA of the Drug Tariff (not prescribable by nurses in Scotland or Northern Ireland)
Catheter Accessories as listed in Part IXA of the Drug Tariff (Part 3 of the Scottish Drug Tariff, Part III of the Northern Ireland Drug Tariff)
Catheter Maintenance Solutions as listed in Part IXA of the Drug Tariff (Part 3 of the Scottish Drug Tariff, Part III of the Northern Ireland Drug Tariff)
Catheters, Urethral Sterile as listed under Catheters in Part IXA of the Drug Tariff (Part 3 of the Scottish Drug Tariff, Part III of the Northern Ireland Drug Tariff)
Cervical Collar, Soft Foam as listed in Part IXA of the Drug Tariff (Part 3 of the Scottish Drug Tariff, not prescribable by nurses in Northern Ireland)

1. Max. 96 tablets; max. pack size 32 tablets

Chemical Reagents
The following as listed in Part IXR of the Drug Tariff (Part 9 of the Scottish Drug Tariff, Part II of the Northern Ireland Drug Tariff):
- Detection Strips for Glycosuria
- Detection Strips for Ketonuria
- Detection Strips for Proteinuria
- Detection Strips for Blood Glucose
- Detection Strips for Blood Ketones (not prescribable by nurses in Northern Ireland)
- Detection strips for determination of International Normalised Ratio (INR) (not prescribable by nurses in Northern Ireland)

Chiropody Appliances as listed in Part IXA of the Drug Tariff (Part 2 of the Scottish Drug Tariff (except for Corn Plasters), not prescribable by nurses in Northern Ireland)

Contraceptive Devices as listed in Part IXA of the Drug Tariff (Part 3 of the Scottish Drug Tariff, Part III of the Northern Ireland Drug Tariff (fertility (ovulation) thermometers only))

Douches (with vaginal and rectal fittings) as listed in Part IXA of the Drug Tariff (Part 3 of the Scottish Drug Tariff, not prescribable by nurses in Northern Ireland)

Droppers as listed in Part IXA of the Drug Tariff (Part 3 of the Scottish Drug Tariff, not prescribable by nurses in Northern Ireland)

Dry Mouth Products as listed in part IXA of the Drug Tariff (Part 3 of the Scottish Drug Tariff, not prescribable by nurses in Northern Ireland)

Ear Wax Softening Medical Devices as listed in Part IXA of the Drug Tariff (Part 3 of the Scottish Drug Tariff, Part III of the Northern Ireland Drug Tariff)

Elastic Hosiery including accessories as listed in Part IXA of the Drug Tariff (Part 4 of the Scottish Drug Tariff, Part III of the Northern Ireland Drug Tariff)

Emollients as listed in Part IXA of the Drug Tariff (Part 3 of the Scottish Drug Tariff, Part III of the Northern Ireland Drug Tariff)

Eye Baths as listed in Part IXA of the Drug Tariff (Part 3 of the Scottish Drug Tariff, not prescribable by nurses in Northern Ireland)

Eye-drop Dispensers as listed in Part IXA of the Drug Tariff (Part 3 of the Scottish Drug Tariff, Part III of the Northern Ireland Drug Tariff)

Eye Shades as listed in Part IXA of the Drug Tariff (Part 3 of the Scottish Drug Tariff, not prescribable by nurses in Northern Ireland)

Finger Cots as listed in Part IXA of the Drug Tariff (Part 3 of the Scottish Drug Tariff, not prescribable by nurses in Northern Ireland)

Finger Stalls as listed in Part IXA of the Drug Tariff (Part 3 of the Scottish Drug Tariff, not prescribable by nurses in Northern Ireland)

Head Lice Device as listed in Part IXA of the Drug Tariff (Part 3 of the Scottish Drug Tariff, Part III of the Northern Ireland Drug Tariff)

Hypodermic Equipment as listed in Part IXA of the Drug Tariff (Part 3 of the Scottish Drug Tariff, Part III of the Northern Ireland Drug Tariff (with some exceptions))

Incontinence Appliances as listed in Part IXB of the Drug Tariff (Part 5 of the Scottish Drug Tariff, Part III of the Northern Ireland Drug Tariff)

Inhaler, Spare Tops as listed in Part IXA of the Drug Tariff (Part 3 of the Scottish Drug Tariff, not prescribable by nurses in Northern Ireland)

Insufflators as listed in Part IXA of the Drug Tariff (Part 3 of the Scottish Drug Tariff, not prescribable by nurses in Northern Ireland)

Irrigation Fluids as listed in Part IXA of the Drug Tariff (Part 2 of the Scottish Drug Tariff, Part III of the Northern Ireland Drug Tariff)

Latex Foam, Adhesive as listed in Part IXA of the Drug Tariff (not prescribable by nurses in Scotland or Northern Ireland)

Lubricating Jelly as listed in Part IXA of the Drug Tariff (Part 2 of the Scottish Drug Tariff, not prescribable by nurses in Northern Ireland)

Nasal Device (nasal dilator) as listed in Part IXA of the Drug Tariff (Part 3 of the Scottish Drug Tariff, Part III of the Northern Ireland Drug Tariff)

Nasal Drops, Sodium Chloride 0.9% as listed in Part IXA of the Drug Tariff (Part 3 of the Scottish Drug Tariff)

Nipple Shields, Plastic as listed in Part IXA of the Drug Tariff (Part 3 of the Scottish Drug Tariff, not prescribable by nurses in Northern Ireland)

Oral Film Forming Agents as listed in Part IXA of the Drug Tariff (Part 3 of the Scottish Drug Tariff, not prescribable by nurses in Northern Ireland)

Peak Flow Meters as listed in Part IXA of the Drug Tariff (Part 3 of the Scottish Drug Tariff, not prescribable by nurses in Northern Ireland)

Pessaries as listed in Part IXA of the Drug Tariff (Part 3 of the Scottish Drug Tariff, Part III of the Northern Ireland Drug Tariff (with some exceptions))

Protectives as listed in Part IXA of the Drug Tariff (Part 2 of the Scottish Drug Tariff, Part III of the Northern Ireland Drug Tariff (EMA Disposable Film Gloves only))

Stoma Appliances and Associated Products as listed in Part IXC of the Drug Tariff (Part 6 of the Scottish Drug Tariff, Part III of the Northern Ireland Drug Tariff)

Suprapubic Belts (replacements only) as listed in Part IXA of the Drug Tariff (Part 3 of the Scottish Drug Tariff, not prescribable by nurses in Northern Ireland)

Suprapubic Catheters as listed in Part IXA of the Drug Tariff (Part 3 of the Scottish Drug Tariff, not prescribable by nurses in Northern Ireland)

Synovial Fluid as listed in Part IXA of the Drug Tariff (Part 3 of the Scottish Drug Tariff, not prescribable by nurses in Northern Ireland)

Syringes (Bladder/Irrigating, Ear, Enema, Spare Vaginal Pipes) as listed in Part IXA of the Drug Tariff (Part 3 of the Scottish Drug Tariff, not prescribable by nurses in Northern Ireland)

Test Tubes as listed in Part IXA of the Drug Tariff (Part 3 of the Scottish Drug Tariff, not prescribable by nurses in Northern Ireland)

Tracheostomy and Laryngectomy Appliances as listed in Part IXA of the Drug Tariff (Part 2 of the Scottish Drug Tariff, not prescribable by nurses in Northern Ireland)

Trusses as listed in Part IXA of the Drug Tariff (Part 3 of the Scottish Drug Tariff, not prescribable by nurses in Northern Ireland)

Vacuum Pumps and Constrictor Rings for Erectile Dysfunction as listed in Part IXA of the Drug Tariff (Part 3 of the Scottish Drug Tariff, Part III of the Northern Ireland Drug Tariff)—prescribing restrictions may apply (see Drug Tariff)

Vaginal Moisturisers as listed in Part IXA of the Drug Tariff (Part 3 of the Scottish Drug Tariff)

Wound Management and Related Products (including bandages, dressings, gauzes, lint, stockinette, etc)

The following as listed in Part IXA of the Drug Tariff (Part 2 of the Scottish Drug Tariff, Part III of the Northern Ireland Drug Tariff):

- Absorbent Cellulose Dressing with Fluid Repellent Backing
- Absorbent Cottons
- Absorbent Cotton Gauzes
- Absorbent Cotton and Viscose Ribbon Gauze, BP 1988
- Absorbent Dressing Pads, Sterile
- Absorbent Lint, BPC
- Absorbent Perforated Dressing with Adhesive Border
- Absorbent Perforated Plastic Film Faced Dressing
- Arm Slings
- Belladonna Adhesive Plaster BP 1980
- Boil Dressing Pack
- Cellulose Wadding, BP 1988
- Chlorhexidine Gauze Dressing, BP
- Conforming Bandage (Synthetic)
- Cotton Conforming Bandage, BP 1988
- Cotton Crêpe Bandage, BP 1988
- Cotton Crêpe Bandage, Hospicrepe 239
- Cotton, Polyamide and Elastane Bandage
- Cotton Stretch Bandage, BP 1988
- Crêpe Bandage, BP 1988
- Elastic Adhesive Bandage, BP
- Elastic Web Bandages
- Elastomer and Viscose Bandage, Knitted
- Gauze and Cotton Tissues
- Heavy Cotton and Rubber Elastic Bandage, BP
- High Compression Bandages (Extensible)
- Knitted Polyamide and Cellulose Contour Bandage, BP 1988
- Knitted Viscose Primary Dressing, BP, Type 1
- Multi-layer Compression Bandaging
- Multiple Pack Dressing No. 1
- Open-wove Bandage, BP 1988, Type 1
- Paraffin Gauze Dressing, BP
- Plaster of Paris Bandage BP 1988
- Polyamide and Cellulose Contour Bandage, BP 1988
- Polyester Primary Dressing with Neutral Triglycerides, Knitted
- Povidone–Iodine Fabric Dressing, Sterile
- Short Stretch Compression Bandage
- Skin Adhesive, Sterile
- Skin Closure Strips, Sterile
- Standard Dressings
- Sterile Dressing Packs
- Stockinettes
- Sub-compression Wadding Bandage
- Surgical Adhesive Tapes
- Surgical Sutures (absorbable and non-absorbable)
- Suspensory Bandages, Cotton
- Swabs
- Triangular Calico Bandage, BP 1980
- Vapour-permeable Adhesive Film Dressing, BP (including with absorbent pad)
- Vapour-permeable Waterproof Plastic Wound Dressing, BP, Sterile
- Venous Ulcer Compression System
- Wound Drainage Pouch
- Wound Management Dressings (including activated charcoal, alginate, capillary-action, cavity, collagen, honey-based application, hydrocolloid, hydrogel, foam, polyurethane matrix, protease modulating matrix, silicone, silver-coated and silver-impregnated, and soft polymer dressings)
- Zinc Paste Bandages (including both plain and with additional ingredients)—see also under Medicinal Preparations

> In the Drug Tariff Appliances and Reagents which may **not** be prescribed by Nurses are annotated Ⓝ (**Nx** in the Scottish Drug Tariff and ₦ in the Northern Ireland Drug Tariff)

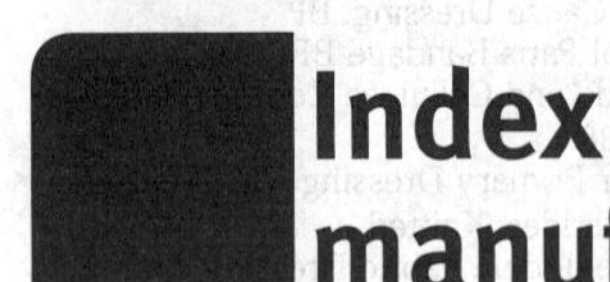

Index of manufacturers

3M
3M Health Care Ltd
3M House
Morley St
Loughborough
Leics, LE11 1EP.
tel: (01509) 611611
fax: (01509) 237288

A&H
Allen & Hanburys Ltd
See GSK

Abbott
Abbott Laboratories Ltd
Abbott House
Norden Rd, Maidenhead
Berks, SL6 4XE.
tel: (01628) 773 355
fax: (01628) 644 185
ukmedinfo@abbott.com

Acorus
Acorus Therapeutics Ltd
High Crane Lodge
Hamsterley, Bishop Auckland
Durham, DL13 3QS.
tel: (01388) 710 505
fax: (01388) 710 770
enquiries@acorus-therapeutics.com

Actelion
Actelion Pharmaceuticals UK Ltd
BSi Building, 13th Floor
389 Chiswick High Rd, London, W4 4AL.
tel: (020) 8987 3333
fax: (020) 8987 3322

Activa
Activa Healthcare
1 Lancaster Park
Newborough Rd, Needwood
Burton-upon-Trent, Staffs, DE13 9PD.
tel: (0845) 060 6707
fax: (01283) 576 808
advice@activahealthcare.co.uk

Adams Hlth.
Adams Healthcare Ltd
Lotherton Way
Garforth, Leeds, LS25 2JY.
tel: (0113) 232 0066
fax: (0113) 287 1317
enquiries@adams-healthcare.co.uk

ADL
ADL Healthcare Diagnostics
Pitcairn House
Crown Square
1st Avenue, Centrum 100
Burton-on-Trent, Staffs, DE14 2WW.
tel: (01283) 494 300
fax: (01283) 494 304
truetrak@adlhealthcare.co.uk

Advancis
Advancis Medical Ltd
Lowmoor Business Park
Kirkby-in-Ashfield, Nottingham, NG17 7JZ.
tel: (01623) 751 500
fax: (01623) 757 636
info@advancis.co.uk

Aguettant
Aguettant Ltd
Bishops House
Bishops Rd, Claverham
Somerset, BS49 4NF.
tel: (01934) 835 694
fax: (01934) 876 790
info@aguettant.co.uk

Air Products
Air Products plc
Medical Group
2 Millennium Gate
Westmere Drive, Crewe
Cheshire, CW1 6AP.
tel: (0800) 373 580
fax: (0800) 214 709

Alcon
Alcon Laboratories (UK) Ltd
Pentagon Park
Boundary Way
Hemel Hempstead, Herts, HP2 7UD.
tel: (01442) 341 234
fax: (01442) 341 200

Alembic Products
Alembic Products Ltd
River Lane
Saltney, Chester, Cheshire, CH4 8RQ.
tel: (01244) 680 147
fax: (01244) 680 155

ALK-Abelló
ALK-Abelló (UK) Ltd
1 Tealgate
Hungerford, Berks, RG17 0YT.
tel: (01488) 686 016
fax: (01488) 685 423
info@uk.alk-abello.com

Allergan
Allergan Ltd
1st Floor Marlow International
The Parkway
Marlow
Bucks, SL7 1YL.
tel: (01628) 494 026
fax: (01628) 494 057

Allergy
Allergy Therapeutics Ltd
Dominion Way
Worthing, West Sussex, BN14 8SA.
tel: (01903) 844 702
fax: (01903) 844 744
infoservices@allergytherapeutics.com

Alliance
Alliance Pharmaceuticals Ltd
Avonbridge House
2 Bath Rd
Chippenham, Wilts, SN15 2BB.
tel: (01249) 466 966
fax: (01249) 466 977
info@alliancepharma.co.uk

Alpharma
Alpharma Ltd
Whiddon Valley
Barnstaple, Devon, EX32 8NS.
tel: (01271) 311 257
fax: (01271) 346 106
med.info@alpharma.co.uk

Alphashow
Alphashow Ltd
PO Box 1009
Hemel Hempstead, HP3 0XN.
tel: (0870) 240 2775
fax: (0870) 240 2775
info@alphashow.co.uk

Altana
Altana Pharma Ltd
Three Globeside Business Park
Fieldhouse Lane
Marlow, Bucks, SL7 1HZ.
tel: (01628) 646 400
fax: (01628) 646 401
medinfo@altanapharma.co.uk

Amdipharm
Amdipharm plc
Regency House
Miles Gray Rd
Basildon, Essex, SS14 3AF.
tel: (0870) 777 7675
fax: (0870) 777 7875
medinfo@amdipharm.com

Amgen
Amgen Ltd
240 Cambridge Science Park
Milton Rd, Cambridge, CB4 0WD.
tel: (01223) 420 305
fax: (01223) 426 314
infoline@uk.amgen.com

Anglian
Anglian Pharma Sales & Marketing
Titmore Court
Titmore Green
Little Wymondley, Hitchin
Herts, SG4 7XJ.
tel: (01438) 743 070
fax: (01438) 743 080
mail@anglianpharma.com

Anpharm
See Goldshield

Antigen
See Goldshield

APS
See TEVA UK

Ardana
Ardana Bioscience Ltd
58 Queen St
Edinburgh, EH2 3NS.
tel: (0131) 226 8550
fax: (0131) 226 8551
info@ardana.co.uk

Ardern
Ardern Healthcare Ltd
Pipers Brook Farm
Eastham
Tenbury Wells, Worcs, WR15 8NP.
tel: (01584) 781 777
fax: (01584) 781 788
info@ardernhealthcare.com

AS Pharma
AS Pharma Ltd
PO Box 181
Polegate, East Sussex, BN26 6WD.
tel: (08700) 664 117
fax: (08700) 664 118
info@aspharma.co.uk

Ashbourne
Ashbourne Pharmaceuticals Ltd
Victors Barns
Northampton Rd
Brixworth, Northampton, NN6 9DQ.
tel: (01604) 883 100
fax: (01604) 881 640

Astellas
Astellas Pharma Ltd
Lovett House, Lovett Rd
Staines, TW18 3AZ.
tel: (01784) 419 615
fax: (01784) 419 401

AstraZeneca
AstraZeneca UK Ltd
Horizon Place
600 Capability Green
Luton, Beds, LU1 3LU.
tel: 0800 7830 033
fax: (01582) 838 003
medical.informationuk@astrazeneca.com

Auden Mckenzie
Auden Mckenzie (Pharma Division) Ltd
30 Stadium Business Centre
North End Rd
Wembley, Middx, HA9 0AT.
tel: (020) 8900 2122
fax: (020) 8903 9620

Aurum
Aurum Pharmaceuticals Ltd
Hubert Rd
Brentwood
Essex, CM14 4LZ.
tel: (01277) 266600
fax: (01277) 848 976
info@martindalepharma.co.uk

Aventis Pasteur
See Sanofi Pasteur

Aventis Pharma
See Sanofi-Aventis

Ayrton Saunders
Ayrton Saunders Ltd
Ayrton House
Commerce Way
Parliament Business Park
Liverpool, Merseyside, L8 7BA.
tel: (0151) 709 2074
fax: (0151) 709 7336
info@ayrtons.com

Bailey, Robert
Robert Bailey Healthcare Ltd
Unit 6
Heapham Rd Industrial Estate
Gainsborough, Lincs, DN21 1RZ.
tel: (01427) 677 559
fax: (01427) 677 654
rbsales@cottonwool.uk.com

Bard
Bard Ltd
Forest House
Brighton Rd
Crawley, West Sussex, RH11 9BP.
tel: (01293) 527 888
fax: (01293) 552 428

Bausch & Lomb
Bausch & Lomb UK Ltd
106 London Rd
Kingston-upon-Thames
Surrey, KT2 6TN.
tel: (020) 8781 2900
fax: (020) 8781 2901

Baxter
Baxter Healthcare Ltd
Wallingford Rd
Compton
Newbury
Berks, RG20 7QW.
tel: (01635) 206 345
fax: (01635) 206 071
surecall@baxter.com

Baxter BioScience
See Baxter

Bayer
Bayer plc
Pharmaceutical Division
Bayer House, Strawberry Hill
Newbury, Berks, RG14 1JA.
tel: (01635) 563 000
fax: (01635) 563 393
medical.science@bayer.co.uk

Bayer Consumer Care
See Bayer

Bayer Diagnostics
See Bayer

BCM Specials
BCM Specials Manufacturing
D10 First 114
Nottingham, NG90 2PR.
tel: 0800 952 1010
fax: 0800 085 0673
bcm-specials@bcm-ltd.co.uk

Beacon
Beacon Pharmaceuticals Ltd
85 High St
Tunbridge Wells, TN1 1YG.
tel: (01892) 600 930
fax: (01892) 600 937
info@beaconpharma.co.uk

Becton Dickinson
Becton Dickinson UK Ltd
Between Towns Rd
Cowley, Oxford, Oxon, OX4 3LY.
tel: (01865) 748 844
fax: (01865) 717 313

Beiersdorf
Beiersdorf UK Ltd
2010 Solihull Parkway
Birmingham Business Park
Birmingham, B37 7YS.
tel: (0121) 329 8800
fax: (0121) 329 8801

Bell and Croyden
John Bell and Croyden
50-54 Wigmore St
London, W1U 2AU.
tel: (020) 7935 5555
fax: (020) 7935 9605
jbc@johnbellcroyden.co.uk

Berk
See TEVA UK

BHR
BHR Pharmaceuticals Ltd
41 Centenary Business Centre
Hammond Close
Attleborough Fields, Nuneaton
Warwickshire, CV11 6RY.
tel: (024) 7635 3742
fax: (024) 7632 7812
info@bhr.co.uk

Bioaccelerate
Bioaccelerate Ltd
11-12 Charles II St
Savanah House
London, SW1Y 4QU.
tel: (020) 7451 2488
fax: (020) 7451 2469
info@bioaccelerate.com

Biogen
Biogen Ltd
5d Roxborough Way
Foundation Park
Maidenhead
Berks, SL6 3UD.
tel: (01628) 501 000
fax: (01628) 501 010

Biolitec
Biolitec Pharma Ltd
Unit 2, Broomhill Business Park
Broomhill Rd
Tallaght
Dublin 24, Ireland.
tel: (00353) 14637415
fax: (00353) 14637411
medical.info@biolitec.com

Biosurgical Research
Biosurgical Research Unit
See ZooBiotic

Blackwell
Blackwell Supplies Ltd
Medcare House
Centurion Close
Gillingham Business Park, Gillingham
Kent, ME8 0SB.
tel: (01634) 877 620
fax: (01634) 877 621

Blake
Thomas Blake & Co
The Byre House
Fearby
Nr. Masham
North Yorks, HG4 4NF.
tel: (01765) 689 042
fax: (01765) 689 042
sales@veilcover.com

BOC
BOC Medical
The Priestley Centre,
10 Priestley Rd
Surrey Research Park
Guildford, Surrey, GU2 7XY.
tel: 0800 111 333
fax: 0800 111 555

Boehringer Ingelheim
Boehringer Ingelheim Ltd
Ellesfield Ave
Bracknell
Berks, RG12 8YS.
tel: (01344) 424 600
fax: (01344) 741 444
medinfo@bra.boehringer-ingelheim.com

Boots
Boots The Chemists
Medical Services
Thane Rd
D90 East S10
Nottingham, NG90 1BS.
tel: (0115) 959 5168
fax: (0115) 959 2565

Borg
Borg Medicare
PO Box 99
Hitchin
Herts, SG5 2GF.
tel: (01462) 442 993
fax: (01462) 441 293

BPC 100
The Bolton Pharmaceutical 100 Ltd
2 Chapel Drive
Ambrosden
Oxfordshire, OX25 2RS.
tel: (0845) 602 3907
fax: (0845) 602 3908
info@bpc100.com

BPL
Bio Products Laboratory
Dagger Lane
Elstree, Herts, WD6 3BX.
tel: (020) 8258 2200
fax: (020) 8258 2601

Braun
B Braun (Medical) Ltd
Brookdale Rd
Thorncliffe Park Estate
Chapeltown, Sheffield, S35 2PW.
tel: (0114) 225 9000
fax: (0114) 225 9111
info.bbmuk@bbraun.com

Braun Biotrol
See Braun

Bray
Bray Health & Leisure
1 Regal Way
Faringdon
Oxon, SN7 7BX.
tel: (01367) 240 736
fax: (01367) 242 625
info@bray.co.uk

Bristol
Bristol Laboratories Ltd
Unit 3, Canalside
Northbridge Rd
Berkhamsted
Herts, HP4 1EG.
tel: (01442) 200 922
fax: (01442) 873 717
info@bristol-labs.co.uk

Bristol-Myers Squibb
Bristol-Myers Squibb Pharmaceuticals Ltd
Uxbridge Business Park
Sanderson Rd
Uxbridge
Middx, UB8 1DH.
tel: (01895) 523 000
fax: (01895) 523 010
medical.information@bms.com

Britannia
Britannia Pharmaceuticals Ltd
41-51 Brighton Rd
Redhill
Surrey, RH1 6YS.
tel: (01737) 773 741
fax: (01737) 762 672
medicalservices@forumgroup.co.uk

British Biocell
British Biocell International
Golden Gate, Ty Glas Avenue
Llanishen, Cardiff, CF14 5DX.
tel: (02920) 747 232
fax: (02920) 747 242
info@bbigold.co.uk

BSIA
See Torbet

BSN Medical
BSN Medical Ltd
PO Box 258
Willerby
Hull, HU10 6WT.
tel: (0845) 1223 600
fax: (0845) 1223 666

C D Medical
C D Medical Ltd
Aston Grange
Oker, Matlock, DE4 2JJ.
tel: (01629) 733 860
fax: (01629) 733 414

Cambridge
Cambridge Laboratories
Deltic House, Kingfisher Way
Silverlink Business Park, Wallsend
Tyne & Wear, NE28 9NX.
tel: (0191) 296 9300
fax: (0191) 296 9368
customer.services@camb-labs.com

Cardinal
Cardinal Health Martindale Products
Hubert Rd
Brentwood
Essex, CM14 4JY.
tel: (01277) 266 600
fax: (01277) 848 976
info@martindalepharma.co.uk

Castlemead
Castlemead Healthcare Ltd
2nd Floor
The Maltings
Bridge St
Hitchin, Herts, SG5 2DE.
tel: (01462) 454 452
fax: (01462) 435 684

Cell Therapeutics
Cell Therapeutics (UK) Ltd
100 Pall Mall
London, SW1Y 5HP.
tel: (0031) 6 5164 1765
fax: (0031) 24360 8075
celltherapeuticseurope@vwbintermedical.com

Celltech
See UCB Pharma

Centrapharm
See Derma UK

Cephalon
Cephalon UK Ltd
11-13 Frederick Sanger Rd
Surrey Research Park
Guildford
Surrey, GU2 7YD.
tel: 0800 783 4869
fax: (01483) 453 324
ukmedinfo@cephalon.com

Ceuta
Ceuta Healthcare Ltd
Hill House
41 Richmond Hill
Bournemouth
Dorset, BH2 6HS.
tel: (01202) 780 558
fax: (01202) 780 559

Chauvin
Chauvin Pharmaceuticals Ltd
106 London Rd
Kingston-Upon-Thames
Surrey, KT2 6TN.
tel: (020) 8781 2900
fax: (020) 8781 2901

Chefaro UK
Chefaro UK Ltd
Unit 1, Tower Close
St. Peter's Industrial Park
Huntingdon
Cambs, PE29 7DH.
tel: (01480) 421 800
fax: (01480) 434 861

Chemical Search
Chemical Search International Ltd
29th floor
1 Canada Square
Canary Wharf
London, E14 5DY.
tel: (020) 7712 1758
fax: (020) 7712 1759
info@chemicalsearch.co.uk

Chemidex
Chemidex Pharma Ltd
Chemidex House
Egham Business Village
Crabtree Rd, Egham
Surrey, TW20 8RB.
tel: (01784) 477 167
fax: (01784) 471 776
info@chemidex.co.uk

Chiron
Chiron Corporation Ltd
See Derma UK
tel: (020) 8580 4000
fax: (020) 8580 4001
medicalinfo-europe@chiron.com

Chiron Vaccines
See Novartis Vaccines

CHS
Cambridge Healthcare Supplies Ltd
14D Wendover Rd
Rackheath Industrial Estate
Rackheath
Norwich, NR13 6LH.
tel: (01603) 735 200
fax: (01603) 735 217
customerservices@typharm.com

Chugai
Chugai Pharma UK Ltd
Mulliner House, Flanders Rd
Turnham Green
London, W4 1NN.
tel: (020) 8987 5680
fax: (020) 8987 5661

Clement Clarke
Clement Clarke International Ltd
Edinburgh Way
Harlow
Essex, CM20 2TT.
tel: (01279) 414 969
fax: (01279) 456 304
resp@clement-clarke.com

CliniMed
CliniMed Ltd
Cavell House, Knaves Beech Way
Loudwater
High Wycombe
Bucks, HP10 9QY.
tel: (01628) 850 100
fax: (01628) 850 331
enquires@clinimed.co.uk

Clinisupplies
Clinisupplies Ltd
9 Crystal Way
Elmgrove Rd
Harrow
Middx, HA1 2HP.
tel: (020) 8863 4168
fax: (020) 8426 0768
info@clinisupplies.co.uk

Clonmel
Clonmel Healthcare Ltd
Waterford Rd
Clonmel
Co. Tipperary
Ireland
tel: (00353) 52 77777
fax: (00353) 52 77799
info@clonmelhealthcare.com

Colgate-Palmolive
Colgate-Palmolive Ltd
Guildford Business Park
Middleton Rd
Guildford
Surrey, GU2 5LZ.
tel: (01483) 302 222
fax: (01483) 303 003

Coloplast
Coloplast Ltd
Peterborough Business Park
Peterborough, PE2 6FX.
tel: (01733) 392 000
fax: (01733) 233 348
gbcareteam@coloplast.com

Community
Community Foods Ltd
Micross, Brent Terrace
London, NW2 1LT.
tel: (020) 8450 9411
fax: (020) 8208 1803
email@communityfoods.co.uk

Concord
Concord Pharmaceuticals Ltd
Bishops Weald House
Albion Way
Horsham, RH12 1AH.
tel: (0870) 241 2330
fax: 0870 241 2335
enquiries@concordpharma.com

ConvaTec
ConvaTec Ltd
Harrington House, Milton Rd
Ickenham
Uxbridge
Middx, UB10 8PU.
tel: (01895) 628 400
fax: (01895) 628 456

Cow & Gate
See Nutricia Clinical
tel: (01225) 768 381
fax: (01225) 768 847

CP
See Wockhardt

Crawford
Crawford Pharmaceuticals
Cheshire House
164 Main Rd
Goostrey
Cheshire, CW4 8NP.
tel: (01477) 537 596
fax: (01477) 534 262

Crookes
Crookes Healthcare Ltd
D6 Building
Nottingham, NG90 6BH.
tel: (0115) 968 8922
fax: (0115) 968 8722
medicalinfo@crookes.co.uk

DDD
DDD Ltd
94 Rickmansworth Rd
Watford
Herts, WD18 7JJ.
tel: (01923) 229 251
fax: (01923) 220 728

De Vilbiss
De Vilbiss Health Care UK Ltd
High Street
Wollaston
West Midlands, DY8 4PS.
tel: (01384) 446 688
fax: (01384) 446 699

De Witt
E C De Witt & Co Ltd
Tudor Rd
Manor Park
Runcorn
Cheshire, WA7 1SZ.
tel: (01928) 579 029
fax: (01928) 579 712
ecdewitt@ecdewitt.com

Denfleet
Denfleet Pharmaceuticals Ltd
260 Centennial Park
Elstree Hill South
Elstree
Herts, WD6 3SR.
tel: (020) 8236 0000
fax: (020) 8236 3501
medical.information@denfleet.com

Dental Health
Dental Health Products Ltd
60 Boughton Lane
Maidstone
Kent, ME15 9QS.
tel: (01622) 749 222
fax: (01622) 744 672

Dentsply
Dentsply Ltd
Hamm Moor Lane
Addlestone
Weybridge
Surrey, KT15 2SE.
tel: (01932) 837 279
fax: (01932) 858 970

Derma UK
Derma UK Ltd
ARC Progress
Mill Lane
Stotfold
Beds, SG5 4NY.
tel: (01462) 733 500
fax: (01462) 733 600
info@dermauk.co.uk

Dermal
Dermal Laboratories Ltd
Tatmore Place
Gosmore
Hitchin
Herts, SG4 7QR.
tel: (01462) 458 866
fax: (01462) 420 565

Dexcel
Dexcel-Pharma Ltd
1 Cottesbrooke Park
Heartlands Business Park
Daventry
Northamptonshire, NN11 8YL.
tel: (01327) 312 266
fax: (01327) 312 262
office@dexcelpharma.co.uk

DiagnoSys
DiagnoSys Medical
Cams Hall
Fareham
Hants, PO16 8AB.
tel: 0800 085 8808
fax: (01329) 227 599

Dimethaid
Dimethaid International
c/o Benoliel Partners
Linden House, Ewelme
Oxfordshire, OX10 6HQ.
tel: (01491) 825 016
fax: (01491) 834 592
medinfo@dimethaid.com

Dr Falk
Dr Falk Pharma UK Ltd
Bourne End Business, Cores End Rd
Bourne End, Bucks, SL8 5AS.
tel: (01628) 536 600

DuPont
See Bristol-Myers Squibb

Durbin
Durbin plc
180 Northolt Rd
South Harrow
Middx, HA2 0LT.
tel: (020) 8869 6500
fax: (020) 8869 6565
info@durbin.co.uk

Easigrip
Easigrip Ltd
Unit 13, Scar Bank
Millers Rd
Warwick
Warwickshire, CV34 5DB.
tel: (01926) 497 108
fax: (01926) 497 109
enquiry@easigrip.co.uk

Egis
Egis Pharmaceuticals UK Ltd
127 Shirland Rd
London, W9 2EP.
tel: (020) 7266 2669
fax: (020) 7266 2702
enquiries@medimpexuk.com

Eisai
Eisai Ltd
3 Shortlands
Hammersmith
London, W6 8EE.
tel: (020) 8600 1400
fax: (020) 8600 1401
Lmedinfo@eisai.net

Elida Fabergé
Elida Fabergé Ltd
Coal Rd
Seacroft
Leeds, LS14 2AR.
tel: (0113) 222 5000
fax: (0113) 222 5362

ENTACO
ENTACO Ltd
Royal Victoria Works,
Birmingham Rd, Studley
Warwickshire, B80 7AP.
tel: (01527) 852 306
fax: (01527) 857 447
sales@entaco.com

Epiderm
Epiderm Ltd
Wass Lane
Sotby
Market Rasen, LN8 5LR.
tel: (01507) 343 091
fax: (01507) 343 092
djjcovermarkcryo@aol.com

Espire
Espire Healthcare Ltd
The Search Offices
Main Gate Road
The Historic Dockyard
Chatham, ME4 4TE.
tel: (01634) 812 144
fax: (01634) 813 601
info@espirehealth.com

Essential Generics
Essential Generics
7 Egham Business Village
Thorpe Industrial Estate
Egham
Surrey, TW20 8RB.
tel: (01784) 477 167
fax: (01784) 471 776

Ethicon
Ethicon Ltd
P.O. Box 1988
Simpson Parkway
Kirkton Campus
Livingston, EH54 0AB.
tel: (01506) 594 500
fax: (01506) 460 714

Eumedica
Eumedica S.A.
Winston Churchill Avenue 67
1180 Brussels
Belgium
tel: (0208) 444 3377
fax: (0208) 444 6866
enquiries@eumedica.com

Everfresh
Everfresh Natural Foods
Gatehouse Close
Aylesbury
Bucks, HP19 3DE.
tel: (01296) 425 333
fax: (01296) 422 545

Exelgyn
Exelgyn Laboratories
PO Box 4511
Henley-on-Thames
Oxon, RG9 5ZQ.
tel: (01491) 642 137
fax: (0800) 731 6120

Fabre
Pierre Fabre Ltd
Hyde Abbey House
23 Hyde St
Winchester
Hampshire, SO23 7DR.
tel: (01962) 856 956
fax: (01962) 874 413
PFabreUK@aol.com

Farillon
See Healthcare Logistics

Fate
Fate Special Foods
Unit E2
Brook Street Business Centre
Brook St, Tipton
West Midlands, DY4 9DD.
tel: (01215) 224 433
fax: (01215) 224 433

Fenton
Fenton Pharmaceuticals Ltd
4J Portman Mansions
Chiltern St
London, W1U 6NS.
tel: (020) 7224 1388
fax: (020) 7486 7258
mail@Fent-Pharm.co.uk

Ferndale
Ferndale Pharmaceuticals Ltd
Unit 605, Thorp Arch Estate
Wetherby
West Yorks, LS23 7BJ.
tel: (01937) 541 122
fax: (01937) 849 682
info@ferndalepharma.co.uk

Ferraris
Ferraris Medical Ltd
4 Harforde Court
John Tate Rd
Hertford
Herts, SG13 7NW.
tel: (01992) 526 300
fax: (01992) 526 320
info@fre.ferrarisgroup.com

Ferring
Ferring Pharmaceuticals (UK)
The Courtyard
Waterside Drive
Langley
Berks, SL3 6EZ.
tel: (01753) 214 800
fax: (01753) 214 801

Firstplay Dietary
Firstplay Dietary Foods Ltd
338 Turncroft Lane
Offerton
Stockport
Cheshire, SK1 4BP.
tel: (0161) 474 7576
fax: (0161) 474 7576

Flynn
Flynn Pharma Ltd
2nd Floor, The Maltings
Bridge St
Hitchin
Herts, SG5 2DE.
tel: (01462) 458 974
fax: (01462) 450 755

Foodlink
Foodlink (UK) Ltd
2B Plymouth Rd
Plympton
Plymouth, PL7 4JR.
tel: (01752) 344 544
fax: (01752) 342 412
info@foodlinkltd.co.uk

Ford
Ford Medical Associates Ltd
8 Wyndham Way
Orchard Heights
Ashford
Kent, TN25 4PZ.
tel: (01233) 633 224
fax: (01223) 646 595
enquiries@fordmedical.co.uk

Forest
Forest Laboratories UK Ltd
Bourne Rd
Bexley
Kent, DA5 1NX.
tel: (01322) 550 550
fax: (01322) 555 469
medinfo@forest-labs.co.uk

Fournier
See Solvay

Fox
C. H. Fox Ltd
22 Tavistock St
London, WC2E 7PY.
tel: (020) 7240 3111
fax: (020) 7379 3410

FP
Family Planning Sales Ltd
Maerdy Industrial Estate
Rhymney
Gwent, NP22 5PY.
tel: (0870) 4444 620
fax: (0870) 4444 621

Fresenius Kabi
Fresenius Kabi Ltd
Cestrian Court
Eastgate Way
Manor Park, Runcorn
Cheshire, WA7 INT.
tel: (01928) 533 533
fax: (01928) 533 534
med.info-uk@fresenius-kabi.com

Frontier
Frontier Multigate
Newbridge Rd Industrial Estate
Blackwood
South Wales, NP12 2YL.
tel: (01495) 233 050
fax: (01495) 233 055
multigate@frontier-group.co.uk

Fujisawa
See Astellas

Galderma
Galderma (UK) Ltd
Meridien House
69-71 Clarendon Rd
Watford
Herts, WD17 1DS.
tel: (01923) 208 950
fax: (01923) 208 998

Galen
Galen Ltd
Seagoe Industrial Estate
Craigavon
Northern Ireland, BT63 5UA.
tel: (028) 3833 4974
fax: (028) 3835 0206

Garnier
Laboratoires Garnier
255 Hammersmith Rd, London, W6 8AZ.
tel: (020) 8762 4000
fax: (020) 8762 4001

GBM
GBM Healthcare Ltd
Beechlawn House
Hurtmore Rd
Godalming
Surrey, GU7 2RA.
tel: (01483) 860 881
fax: (01483) 425 715
mba_gbm@compuserve.com

GE Healthcare
GE Healthcare
The Grove Centre, White Lion Rd
Amersham, Bucks, HP7 9LL.
tel: (01494) 544 000

Geistlich
Geistlich Pharma
Newton Bank
Long Lane
Chester, CH2 2PF.
tel: (01244) 347 534
fax: (01244) 319 327

General Dietary
General Dietary Ltd
PO Box 38
Kingston upon Thames
Surrey, KT2 7YP.
tel: (020) 8336 2323
fax: (020) 8942 8274

Generics
Generics (UK) Ltd
Albany Gate
Darkes Lane
Potters Bar
Herts, EN6 1AG.
tel: (01707) 853 000
fax: (01707) 643 148

Genus
Genus Pharmaceuticals
Benham Valence
Newbury
Berks, RG20 8LU.
tel: (01635) 568 400
fax: (01635) 568 401
enquiries@genuspharma.com

Genzyme
Genzyme Biosurgery
4620 Kingsgate
Cascade Way
Oxford Business Park South
Oxford, OX4 2SU.
tel: (01865) 405 200
fax: (01865) 774 172

Gilead
Gilead Sciences
The Flowers Building
Granta Park
Great Abington
Cambs, CB1 6GT.
tel: (01223) 897 300
fax: (01223) 897 282
ukmedinfo@gilead.com

GlaxoSmithKline
See GSK

Glenwood
Glenwood Laboratories Ltd
Jenkins Dale
Chatham
Kent, ME4 5RD.
tel: (01634) 830 535
fax: (01634) 831 345
g.wooduk@virgin.net

Gluten Free Foods Ltd
Gluten Free Foods Ltd
Unit 270 Centennial Park
Centennial Ave
Elstree, Borehamwood
Herts, WD6 3SS.
tel: (020) 8953 4444
fax: (020) 8953 8285
info@glutenfree-foods.co.uk

Goldshield
Goldshield Pharmaceuticals Ltd
NLA Tower
12-16 Addiscombe Rd
Croydon, CR0 0XT.
tel: (020) 8649 8500
fax: (020) 8686 0807

GP Pharma
See Derma UK

Grünenthal
Grünenthal Ltd
Aston Court
Kingsmead Business Park
Frederick Place
High Wycombe, Bucks, HP11 1LA.
tel: (0870) 351 8960

Grifols
Grifols UK Ltd
72 St Andrew's Rd
Cambs, CB4 1GS.
tel: (01223) 446 900
fax: (01223) 446 911
reception.uk@grifols.com

GSK
GlaxoSmithKline
Stockley Park West
Uxbridge
Middx, UB11 1BT.
tel: 0800 221 441
fax: (020) 8990 4328
customercontactuk@gsk.com

GSK Consumer Healthcare
GlaxoSmithKline Consumer Healthcare
GSK House
980 Great West Rd
Brentford
Middx, TW8 9GS.
tel: (0500) 888 878
fax: (020) 8047 6860
customer.relations@gsk.com

Hameln
Hameln Pharmaceuticals Ltd
Nexus
Gloucester Business Park
Gloucester, GL3 4AG.
tel: (01452) 621 661
fax: (01452) 632 732
enquiries@hameln.co.uk

Hartmann
Paul Hartmann Ltd
Unit P2, Parklands
Heywood Distribution Park
Pilsworth Rd, Heywood
Lancs, OL10 2TT.
tel: (01706) 363 200
fax: (01706) 363 201
info@uk.hartmann.info

Hawgreen
Hawgreen Ltd
The Maltings, 2nd Floor
Bridge St
Hitchin
Herts, SG5 2DE.
tel: (01462) 441 831
fax: (01462) 435 868

Healthcare Logistics
Healthcare Logistics Ltd
1 Progress Park
Elstow
Bedford, MK42 9XE.
tel: (01234) 248 606
fax: (01234) 248 705
nhsvaccines@healthcarelogistics.co.uk

Heinz
H. J. Heinz Company Ltd
South Building
Hayes Park
Hayes, UB4 8AL.
tel: (020) 8573 7757
fax: (020) 8848 2325
Farleys_Heinz@Heinz.co.uk

Henleys
Henleys Medical Supplies Ltd
Brownfields
Welwyn Garden City
Herts, AL7 1AN.
tel: (01707) 333 164
fax: (01707) 334 795

Hillcross
AAH Pharmaceuticals Ltd
Sapphire Court
Walsgrave Triangle
Coventry, CV2 2TX.
tel: (024) 7643 2000
fax: (024) 7643 2001

HK Pharma
HK Pharma Ltd
PO Box 105
Hitchin
Herts, SG5 2GG.
tel: (01462) 433 993
fax: (01462) 450 755

Hoechst Marion Roussel
See Sanofi-Aventis

HRA Pharma
Laboratoire HRA Pharma
15 rue Beranger
75003
Paris
France
tel: (0033) 1 40 33 11 30
fax: (0033) 1 40 33 12 31
info@lysodren-europe.com

Hybrand
Hybrand Ltd
Eagle House, The Ring
Bracknell, Berks, RG12 1HB.
tel: (08700) 114 545
fax: (08700) 114 646
customer.services@hybrand.com

Hypoguard
Hypoguard Ltd
Dock Lane
Melton
Woodbridge
Suffolk, IP12 1PE.
tel: (01394) 387 333
fax: (01394) 380 152
enquiries@hypoguard.com

IDIS
IDIS World Medicines
IDIS House
Churchfield Rd
Weybridge
Surrey, KT13 8DB.
tel: (01932) 824 000
fax: (01932) 824 200
idis@idispharma.com

Infai
Infai UK Ltd
Innovation Centre
University of York Science Park
University Rd
Heslington, York, YO10 5DG.
tel: (01904) 435 228
fax: (01904) 435 229
paul@infai.co.uk

Intrapharm
Intrapharm Laboratories Ltd
60 Boughton Lane
Maidstone
Kent, ME15 9QS.
tel: (01622) 749 222
fax: (01622) 744 672
sales@intraphamlabs.com

Invicta
See Pfizer

Ipsen
Ipsen Ltd
190 Bath Rd
Slough
Berks, SL1 3XE.
tel: (01753) 627 777
fax: (01753) 627 778
medical.information@ipsen.com

IVAX
IVAX Pharmaceuticals UK Ltd
IVAX Quay, Albert Basin
Royal Docks
London, E16 2QJ.
tel: (08705) 020 304
fax: (08705) 323 334
medinfo@actavis.co.uk

J&J
Johnson & Johnson Ltd
Foundation Park
Roxborough Way
Maidenhead
Berks, SL6 3UG.
tel: (01628) 822 222
fax: (01628) 821 222

J&J Medical
Johnson & Johnson Medical
Coronation Rd
Ascot
Berks, SL5 9EY.
tel: (01344) 871 000
fax: (01344) 872 599

J&J MSD
Johnson & Johnson MSD
See McNeil
tel: (01494) 450 778
fax: (01494) 450 487

Janssen-Cilag
Janssen-Cilag Ltd
PO Box 79
Saunderton
High Wycombe
Bucks, HP14 4HJ.
tel: (01494) 567 567
fax: (01494) 567 568

JHC
JHC Healthcare Ltd
The Maltings, 2nd Floor
Bridge St
Hitchin
Herts, SG5 2DE.
tel: (01462) 432 533
fax: (01462) 432 535

JLB
B. Braun JLB Ltd
Unit 2A
St Columb Industrial Estate
St Columb Major
Cornwall, TR9 6SF.
tel: (01637) 880 065
fax: (01637) 881 549

K/L
K/L Pharmaceuticals Ltd
21 Macadam Place
South Newmoor
Irvine
Ayrshire, KA11 4HP.
tel: (01294) 215 951
fax: (01294) 221 600

Kestrel
Kestrel Ltd
Ashfield House
Resolution Rd
Ashby de la Zouch
Leics, LE65 1HW.
tel: (01530) 562 301
fax: (01530) 562 430
kestrel@ventiv.co.uk

King
King Pharmaceuticals Ltd
3 Ash Street
Leicester, LE5 0DA.
tel: (01462) 434 366
fax: (01462) 450 755

KoGEN
KoGEN Ltd
Seagoe Industrial Estate
Craigavon, BT63 5UA.
tel: (028) 383 33933
fax: (028) 383 33665
info@kogen.co.uk

KoRa
KoRa Healthcare Ltd
Frans Maas House
Swords Business Park, Swords
Co. Dublin
Ireland
tel: (00353) 1890 0406
fax: (00353) 1890 3016
Kora@ireland.com

Kyowa Hakko
Kyowa Hakko UK Ltd
258 Bath Rd
Slough
Berks, SL1 4DX.
tel: (01753) 566 020
fax: (01753) 566 030

LAB
Laboratories for Applied Biology
91 Amhurst Park
London, N16 5DR.
tel: (020) 8800 2252
fax: (020) 8809 6884
enquiries@cerumol.com

Lederle
See Wyeth

LEO
LEO Pharma
Longwick Rd
Princes Risborough
Bucks, HP27 9RR.
tel: (01844) 347 333
fax: (01844) 342 278
medical-info.uk@leo-pharma.com

LifeScan
LifeScan
50-100 Holmers Farm Way
High Wycombe
Bucks, HP12 4DP.
tel: (01494) 658 750
fax: (01494) 658 751

Lilly
Eli Lilly & Co Ltd
Lilly House
Priestley Rd
Basingstoke
Hampshire, RG24 9NL.
tel: (01256) 315 999
fax: (01256) 775 858

Linderma
Linderma Ltd
Canon Bridge House
Canon Bridge
Madley
Hereford, HR2 9JF.
tel: (01981) 250 124
fax: (01981) 251 412
linderma@virgin.net

Link
Link Pharmaceuticals Ltd
Bishops Weald House
Albion Way
Horsham
West Sussex, RH12 1AH.
tel: (01403) 272 451
fax: (01403) 272 455
medical.information@linkpharm.co.uk

LPC
LPC Medical (UK) Ltd
30 Chaul End Lane
Luton, Beds, LU4 8EZ.
tel: (01582) 560 393
fax: (01582) 560 395
info@lpcpharma.com

Lundbeck
Lundbeck Ltd
Lundbeck House
Caldecotte Lake Business Park
Caldecotte, Milton Keynes
Bucks, MK7 8LF.
tel: (01908) 649 966
fax: (01908) 647 888
ukmedicalinformation@lundbeck.com

Mölnlycke
Mölnlycke Health Care Ltd
The Arenson Centre
Arenson Way
Dunstable
Beds, LU5 5UL.
tel: (0870) 606 0766
fax: (0870) 608 1888
info.uk@molnlycke.net

Mandeville
Mandeville Medicines
Stoke Mandeville Hospital
Ayelsbury
Bucks, HP21 8AL.
tel: (01296) 394 142
fax: (01296) 397 223

Manx
Manx Healthcare
Taylor Group House
Wedgnock Lane
Warwick, CV34 5YA.
tel: (01926) 482 511
fax: (01926) 498 711
info@manxhealthcare.com

Martindale
See Cardinal

MASTA
MASTA
Moorfield Rd
Yeadon
Leeds, LS19 7BN.
tel: (0113) 238 7500
fax: (0113) 238 7501
medical@masta.org

Mayne
Mayne Pharma plc
Queensway
Royal Leamington Spa
Warwickshire, CV31 3RW.
tel: (01926) 820 820
fax: (01926) 821 041
medinfouk@uk.maynepharma.com

McNeil
McNeil Ltd
Enterprise House, Station Rd
Loadwater, High Wycombe, Bucks,
HP10 9UF.
tel: (01494) 450 778
fax: (01494) 450 487

MDE
MDE Diagnostics Europe Ltd
The Surrey Technology Centre
40 Occam Rd
Surrey Research Park, Guildford
Surrey, GU2 7YG.
tel: (01483) 688 400
info@mdediagnostic.co.uk

Mead Johnson
Mead Johnson Nutritionals
Uxbridge Business Park
Sanderson Rd
Uxbridge
Middx, UB8 1DH.
tel: (00800) 8834 2568
fax: (01895) 523 103

Meadow
Meadow Laboratories Ltd
18 Avenue Rd
Chadwell Heath
Romford
Essex, RM6 4JF.
tel: (020) 8597 1203
enquiries@meadowlabs.fsnet.co.uk

Meda
Meda Pharmaceuticals Ltd
Regus House, Herald Way
Pegasus Business Park
Castle Donnington
Derbyshire, DE74 2TZ.
tel: (01332) 638 033
fax: (01332) 638 192
information@uk.meda.se

Medac
Medac (UK)
Scion House, Stirling University
Stirling, FK9 4NF.
tel: (01786) 458 086
fax: (01786) 458 032
info@medac-uk.co.uk

Medical House
The Medical House plc
199 Newhall Rd
Sheffield, S9 2QJ.
tel: (0114) 261 9011
fax: (0114) 243 1597
info@themedicalhouse.com

Medigas
Medigas Ltd
Enterprise Drive
Four Ashes
Wolverhampton, WV10 7DF.
tel: (01902) 791 944
fax: (01902) 791 125

MediSense
MediSense
Abbott Laboratories Ltd
Mallory House
Vanwall Business Park
Maidenhead, Berks, SL6 4UD.
tel: (01628) 678 900
fax: (01628) 678 805

Medix
See Clement Clarke

Medlock
Medlock Medical Ltd
Tubiton House
Medlock St.
Oldham, OL1 3HS.
tel: (0161) 621 2100
fax: (0161) 627 0932
medical.information@medlockmedical.com

MedLogic
MedLogic Global Ltd
Western Wood Way
Langage Science Park
Plympton
Plymouth, Devon, PL7 5BG.
tel: (01752) 209 955
fax: (01752) 209 956
enquiries@mlgl.co.uk

Menarini
A. Menarini Pharma UK SRL
Menarini House
Mercury Park
Wycombe Lane, Wooburn Green
Bucks, HP10 0HH.
tel: (01628) 856 400
fax: (01628) 856 402

Menarini Diagnostics
A. Menarini Diagnostics
Wharfedale Rd
Winnersh
Wokingham
Berks, RG41 5RA.
tel: (0118) 944 4100
fax: (0118) 944 4111

Merck
Merck Pharmaceuticals
Harrier House
High St
West Drayton
Middx, UB7 7QG.
tel: (01895) 452 307
fax: (01895) 452 286
medinfo@merckpharma.co.uk

Merck Consumer Health
See Seven Seas

Merck Sharp & Dohme
See MSD

Micro Medical
Micro Medical Ltd
Quayside
Chatham Maritime
Chatham
Kent, ME4 4QY.
tel: (01634) 893 500
fax: (01634) 893 600
sales@micromedical.co.uk

Milupa
Milupa Ltd
White Horse Business Park
Trowbridge
Wilts, BA14 0XQ.
tel: (01225) 711 511
fax: (01225) 711 970

Molar
Molar Ltd
The Borough Yard
The Borough
Wedmore
Somerset, BS28 4EB.
tel: (01934) 710 022
fax: (01934) 710 033
info@molar.ltd.uk

Morningside
Morningside Healthcare Ltd
115 Narborough Rd
Leicester, LE3 OPA.
tel: (0116) 204 5950
fax: (0116) 247 0756

MSD
Merck Sharp & Dohme Ltd
Hertford Rd
Hoddesdon
Herts, EN11 9BU.
tel: (01992) 467 272
fax: (01992) 451 066

Myogen
Myogen GmbH
PO Box 122
Richmond
North Yorks, DL10 5YA.
tel: (01748) 828 812
fax: (01748) 828 801
info@myogen.de

Nagor
Nagor Ltd
PO Box 21, Global House
Isle of Man Business Park
Douglas
Isle of Man, IM99 1AX.
tel: (01624) 625 556
fax: (01624) 661 656
enquiries@nagor.com

Napp
Napp Pharmaceuticals Ltd
Cambridge Science Park
Milton Rd
Cambs, CB4 0GW.
tel: (01223) 424 444
fax: (01223) 424 441

Neolab
Neolab Ltd
57 High St
Odiham, Hampshire, RG29 1LF.
tel: (01256) 704 110
fax: (01256) 701 144
info@neolab.co.uk

Neomedic
Neomedic Ltd
2a Crofters Rd
Northwood
Middx, HA6 3ED.
tel: (01923) 836 379
fax: (01923) 840 160
marketing@neomedic.co.uk

Nestlé
Nestlé UK Ltd
St. George's House
Park Lane
Croydon
Surrey, CR9 1NR.
tel: (020) 8686 3333
fax: (020) 8686 6072

Nestlé Clinical
Nestlé Clinical Nutrition
St George's House
Park Lane
Croydon
Surrey, CR9 1NR.
tel: (020) 8667 5130
fax: (020) 8667 6061
nutrition@uk.nestle.com

Network
Network Health & Beauty
Network House
41 Invincible Rd
Farnborough
Hants, GU14 7QU.
tel: (01252) 533 333
fax: (01252) 533 344
networkm@globalnet.co.uk

Neutrogena
See J&J

Nordic
Nordic Pharma UK Ltd
Abbey House
1650 Arlington Business Park
Theale
Reading, RG7 4SA.
tel: (0118) 929 8233
fax: (0118) 929 8234
info@nordicpharma.co.uk

Norgine
Norgine Pharmaceuticals Ltd
Chaplin House
Moorhall Rd
Harefield
Middx, UB9 6NS.
tel: (01895) 826 600
fax: (01895) 825 865

Nova
Nova Laboratories Ltd
Martin House
Gloucester Crescent
Wigston
Leicester, LE18 4YL.
tel: (0116) 223 0099
fax: (0116) 223 0120
sales@novalabs.co.uk

Novartis
Novartis Pharmaceuticals UK Ltd
Frimley Business Park
Frimley
Camberley
Surrey, GU16 7SR.
tel: (01276) 692 255
fax: (01276) 692 508

Novartis Consumer Health
Novartis Consumer Health
Wimblehurst Rd
Horsham
West Sussex, RH12 5AB.
tel: (01403) 210 211
fax: (01403) 323 939
medicalaffairs.uk@ch.novartis.com

Novartis Vaccines
Novartis Vaccines Ltd
Gaskill Rd
Speke
Liverpool, L24 9GR.
tel: (08457) 451 500
fax: (0151) 7055 669
serviceuk@chiron.com

Novo Nordisk
Novo Nordisk Ltd
Broadfield Park
Brighton Rd
Crawley
West Sussex, RH11 9RT.
tel: (01293) 613 555
fax: (01293) 613 535
customercareuk@novonordisk.com

Nutricia Clinical
Nutricia Clinical Care
Nutricia Ltd
White Horse Business Park
Trowbridge
Wilts, BA14 0XQ.
tel: (01225) 711 688
fax: (01225) 711 798
cndirect@nutricia.co.uk

Nutricia Dietary
Nutricia Dietary Care
see Nutricia Clinical
tel: (01225) 711 801
fax: (01225) 711 567

Nutrition Point
Nutrition Point Ltd
13 Taurus Park
Westbrook
Warrington
Cheshire, WA5 7ZT.
tel: (07041) 544 044
fax: (07041) 544 055
info@nutritionpoint.co.uk

Nycomed
Nycomed UK Ltd
The Magdalen Centre
Oxford Science Park, Oxford, UX4 4GA.
tel: (01865) 784 500
fax: (01865) 784 501
nycomed.uk@nycomed.com

Octapharma
Octapharma Ltd
6 Elm Court
Copse Drive, Meriden Green
Coventry, CV5 9RG.
tel: (01676) 521 000
fax: (01676) 521 200
octapharma@octapharma.co.uk

Omron
Omron Healthcare (UK) Ltd
Opal Drive
Fox Milne
Milton Keynes, MK15 0DG.
tel: (0870) 750 2771
fax: (0870) 750 2772
info.omronhealthcare.uk@eu.omron.com

OPi
OPi Ltd
2nd Floor, Titan Court
3 Bishop Square
Hatfield
Herts, AL10 9NA.
tel: (01707) 226 094
fax: (01707) 226 194
OPi.UK@orphan-opi.com

Opus
See Trinity-Chiesi

Oral B Labs
Oral B Laboratories Ltd
Gillette Corner
Great West Rd
Isleworth
Middx, TW7 5NP.
tel: (020) 8847 7800
fax: (020) 8847 7828

Organon
Organon Laboratories Ltd
Cambridge Science Park
Milton Rd
Cambs, CB4 0FL.
tel: (01223) 432 700
fax: (01223) 424 368
medrequest@organon.co.uk

Orion
Orion Pharma (UK) Ltd
Oaklea Court
22 Park Street
Newbury
Berks, RG14 1EA.
tel: (01635) 520 300
fax: (01635) 520 319
medicalinformation@orionpharma.com

Orphan Europe
Orphan Europe (UK) Ltd
Isis House
43 Station Rd
Henley-on-Thames
Oxon, RG9 1AT.
tel: (01491) 414 333
fax: (01491) 414 443
info.uk@orphan-europe.com

Ortho Biotech
Ortho Biotech
PO Box 79
Saunderton
High Wycombe
Bucks, HP14 4HJ.
tel: (0800) 389 2926
fax: (01494) 567 568

Otsuka
Otsuka Pharmaceutical (UK) Ltd
BSi Tower
389 Chiswick High Rd, London, W4 4AJ.
tel: (020) 8742 4300
fax: (020) 8994 8548
medinfo@otsuka.co.uk

Owen Mumford
Owen Mumford Ltd
Brook Hill
Woodstock
Oxford, OX20 1TU.
tel: (01993) 812 021
fax: (01993) 813 466
customerservices@owenmumford.co.uk

Paines & Byrne
Paines & Byrne Ltd
Lovett House
Lovett Rd
Staines
Middx, TW18 3AZ.
tel: (01784) 419 620
fax: (01784) 419 401

Parema
See Urgo

Pari
PARI Medical Ltd
Enterprise House
Station Approach
West Byfleet
Surrey, KT14 6NE.
tel: (01932) 341 122
fax: (01932) 341 134
parimedical@compuserve.com

Parke-Davis
See Pfizer

Parkside
Parkside Healthcare
12 Parkside Ave
Salford, M7 4HB.
tel: (0161) 795 2792
fax: (0161) 795 4076

Peckforton
Peckforton Pharmaceuticals Ltd
Crewe Hall
Crewe
Cheshire, CW1 6UL.
tel: (01270) 582 255
fax: (01270) 582 299
info@peckforton.com

Penn
Penn Pharmaceuticals Services Ltd
Unit 23 & 24, Tafarnaubach Industrial Estate
Tredegar
Gwent, NP22 3AA.
tel: (01495) 711 222
fax: (01495) 711 225
penn@pennpharm.co.uk

Pfizer
Pfizer Ltd
Walton Oaks
Dorking Rd
Walton-on-the-Hill
Surrey, KT20 7NS.
tel: (01304) 616 161
fax: (01304) 656 221

Pfizer Consumer
See Pfizer

Pharma-Global
Pharma-Global Ltd
SEQ Ltd, Nerin House
26 Ridgeway St
Douglas, Isle of Man, IM1 1EL.
tel: (01624) 692 999
fax: (01624) 613 998

Pharmacia
see Pfizer

Pharmasol
Pharmasol Ltd
North Way, Walworth Industrial Estate
Andover, Hampshire, SP10 5AZ.
tel: (01264) 363 117
fax: (01264) 332 223
info@pharmasol.co.uk

Pharmion
Pharmion Ltd
Riverside House
Riverside Walk
Windsor
Berks, SL4 1NA.
tel: (01753) 240 600
fax: (01753) 240 656
info-UK@pharmion.com

Pickles
J. Pickles Healthcare
Beech House
62 High St
Knaresborough
N. Yorks, HG5 0EA.
tel: (01423) 867 314
fax: (01423) 869 177

Pinewood
Pinewood Healthcare
Ballymacabry
Clonmel, Co Tipperary, Eire
tel: (00353) 523 6253
fax: (00353) 523 6311
info@pinewood.ie

PLIVA
PLIVA Pharma Ltd
Vision House
Bedford Rd
Petersfield
Hampshire, GU32 3QB.
tel: (01730) 710900
fax: (01730) 710901
medinfo@pliva-pharma.co.uk

Procter & Gamble
Procter & Gamble UK
The Heights
Brooklands
Weybridge
Surrey, KT13 0XP.
tel: (01932) 896 000
fax: (01932) 896 200

Procter & Gamble Pharm.
Procter & Gamble Technical Centres
Medical Dept
Rusham Park
Whitehall Lane
Egham, Surrey, TW20 9NW.
tel: (01784) 474 900
fax: (01784) 474 705

Profile
Profile Pharma Ltd
Heath Place
Bognor Regis
West Sussex, PO22 9SL.
tel: (0870) 770 2025
fax: (0870) 770 2224
info@profilepharma.com

Profile Respiratory
Profile Respiratory Systems Ltd
Heath Place
Bognor Regis
West Sussex, PO22 9SL.
tel: (0870) 770 3434
fax: (0870) 770 3433
info@profilehs.com

ProStrakan
ProStrakan Ltd
Galabank Business Park
Galashiels, TD1 1QH.
tel: (01896) 664 000
fax: (01896) 664 001
medinfo@prostrakan.com

Provalis
See KoGEN

R&C
See Reckitt Benckiser

Ransom
Ransom Consumer Healthcare
104 Bancroft
Hitchin
Herts, SG5 1LY.
tel: (01462) 437 615
fax: (01462) 443 512
info@williamransom.com

Reckitt Benckiser
Reckitt Benckiser Healthcare
Dansom Lane
Hull, HU8 7DS.
tel: (01482) 326 151
fax: (01482) 582 526
miu@reckittbenckiser.com

Recordati
Recordati Pharmaceuticals Ltd
Ash House
Fairfield Avenue
Staines
Middx, TW18 4AB.
tel: (01784) 224 237
fax: (01784) 224 312

Rhône-Poulenc Rorer
See Sanofi-Aventis

Richardson
Richardson Healthcare
Richardson House
Crondal Rd
Coventry
Warwickshire, CV7 9NH.
tel: (08700) 111 126
fax: (08700) 111 127

Robinsons
Robinson Healthcare Ltd
Lawn Rd
Carlton-in-Lindrick Industrial Estate
Worksop
Notts, S81 9LB.
tel: (01909) 735 001
fax: (01909) 731 103
enquiries@robinsoncare.com

Roche
Roche Products Ltd
Hexagon Place
6 Falcon Way, Shire Park
Welwyn Garden City
Herts, AL7 1TW.
tel: (0800) 328 1629
fax: (01707) 384 555
medinfo.uk@roche.com

Roche Consumer Health
See Bayer

Roche Diagnostics
Roche Diagnostics Ltd
Bell Lane
Lewes
East Sussex, BN7 1LG.
tel: (01273) 480 444
fax: (01273) 480 266

Rosemont
Rosemont Pharmaceuticals Ltd
Rosemont House
Yorkdale Industrial Park
Braithwaite St
Leeds, LS11 9XE.
tel: (0113) 244 1999
fax: (0113) 246 0738
infodesk@rosemontpharma.com

Rowa
Rowa Pharmaceuticals Ltd
Bantry
Co Cork
Ireland
tel: (00 353 27) 50077
fax: (00 353 27) 50417
rowa@rowa-pharma.ie

Rybar
See Shire

S&N Hlth.
Smith & Nephew Healthcare Ltd
Healthcare House
Goulton St
Hull, HU3 4DJ.
tel: (01482) 222 200
fax: (01482) 222 211
advice@smith-nephew.com

Sallis
Sallis Healthcare Ltd
Vernon Works
Waterford St
Basford
Nottingham, NG6 0DH.
tel: (0115) 978 7841
fax: (0115) 942 2272

Sandoz
Sandoz Ltd
Unit 37
Woolmer Way
Bordon
Hants, GU35 9QE.
tel: (01420) 478 301
fax: (01420) 474 427

Sankyo
Sankyo Pharma UK Ltd
Sankyo House
Repton Place
White Lion Rd, Amersham
Bucks, HP7 9LP.
tel: (01494) 766 866
fax: (01494) 766 557
medinfo@sankyo.co.uk

Sanochemia
Sanochemia Diagnostics UK Ltd
Argentum
510 Bristol Business Park
Coldharbour Lane
Bristol, BS16 1EJ.
tel: (0117) 906 3562
fax: (0117) 906 3709

Sanofi Pasteur
Sanofi Pasteur MSD Ltd
Mallards Reach
Bridge Avenue
Maidenhead
Berks, SL6 1QP.
tel: (01628) 785 291
fax: (01628) 671 722

Sanofi-Aventis
Sanofi-Aventis Ltd
1 Onslow St
Guildford
Surrey, GU1 4YS.
tel: (01483) 505 515
fax: (01483) 535 432
uk-medicalinformation@sanofi-aventis.com

Sanofi-Synthelabo
See Sanofi-Aventis

Schering Health
Schering Health Care Ltd
The Brow
Burgess Hill
West Sussex, RH15 9NE.
tel: (0845) 609 6767
fax: (01444) 465 878
customer.care@schering.co.uk

Schering-Plough
Schering-Plough Ltd
Shire Park
Welwyn Garden City
Herts, AL7 1TW.
tel: (01707) 363 636
fax: (01707) 363 763
medical.info@spcorp.com

Schwarz
Schwarz Pharma Ltd
Schwarz House
East St
Chesham
Bucks, HP5 1DG.
tel: (01494) 797 500
fax: (01494) 774 960
medinfo@schwarzpharma.co.uk

Searle
See Pfizer

Serono
Serono Pharmaceuticals Ltd
Bedfont Cross
Stanwell Rd
Feltham
Middx, TW14 8NX.
tel: (020) 8818 7200
fax: (020) 8818 7222
serono_uk@serono.com

Servier
Servier Laboratories Ltd
Gallions
Wexham Springs
Framewood Rd
Wexham, SL3 6RJ.
tel: (01753) 662 744
fax: (01753) 663 456

Seven Seas
Seven Seas Ltd
Hedon Rd
Marfleet
Hull, HU9 5NJ.
tel: (01482) 375 234
fax: (01482) 374 345

Shiloh
Shiloh Healthcare Ltd
Lion Mill
Fitton St
Royton
Oldham, OL2 5JX.
tel: (0161) 624 5641
fax: (0161) 627 0902
enquiry@shiloh.co.uk

Shire
Shire Pharmaceuticals Ltd
Hampshire International Business Park
Chineham
Basingstoke
Hants, RG24 8EP.
tel: (01256) 894 000
fax: (01256) 894 708
medinfo@uk.shire.com

SHS
SHS International Ltd
100 Wavertree Boulevard
Wavertree Technology Park
Liverpool, L7 9PT.
tel: (0151) 228 8161
fax: (0151) 230 5365
seve@shsint.co.uk

Sigma
Sigma Pharmaceuticals plc
PO Box 233
Unit 1-7 Colonial Way
Watford
Herts, WD24 4YR.
tel: (01923) 444 999
fax: (01923) 444 998
info@sigpharm.co.uk

Sinclair
Sinclair Pharmaceuticals Ltd
Borough Rd
Godalming
Surrey, GU7 2AB.
tel: (01483) 426 644
fax: (01483) 860 927
info@sinclairpharma.com

SMA Nutrition
See Wyeth

SNBTS
Scottish National Blood Transfusion Service
Protein Fractionation Centre
Ellen's Glen Rd
Edinburgh, EH17 7QT.
tel: (0131) 536 5700
fax: (0131) 536 5781

Solvay
Solvay Healthcare Ltd
Mansbridge Rd
West End
Southampton, SO18 3JD.
tel: (023) 8046 7000
fax: (023) 8046 5350
medinfo.shl@solvay.com

Sovereign
See Amdipharm

Special Products
Special Products Ltd
Unit 25
Boundary Business Centre
Surrey, GU21 5DH.
tel: (01483) 736 950
fax: (01483) 721 926
graham.march@specprod.co.uk

Specials Laboratory
The Specials Laboratory Ltd
Unit 1, Regents Drive
Lower Prudhoe Industrial Estate
Northumberland, NE42 6PX.
tel: (0800) 028 4925
fax: (0800) 083 4222

Squibb
See Bristol-Myers Squibb

SSL
SSL International plc
Venus, 1 Old Park Lane
Trafford Park
Urmston
Manchester, M41 7HA.
tel: (08701) 222 690
fax: (08701) 222 692
medical.information@ssl-international.co

STD Pharmaceutical
STD Pharmaceutical Products Ltd
Plough Lane
Hereford, HR4 0EL.
tel: (01432) 373 555
fax: (01432) 373 556
enquiries@stdpharm.co.uk

Sterling Health
See GSK Consumer Healthcare

Sterwin
See Winthrop

Stiefel
Stiefel Laboratories (UK) Ltd
Holtspur Lane
Wooburn Green
High Wycombe
Bucks, HP10 0AU.
tel: (01628) 524 966
fax: (01628) 810 021
general@stiefel.co.uk

Strakan
See ProStrakan

Sutherland
Sutherland Health Ltd
Unit 1, Rivermead
Pipers Way
Thatcham
Berks, RG19 4EP.
tel: (01635) 874 488
fax: (01635) 877 622

Swedish Orphan
Swedish Orphan International (UK) Ltd
The White House
Wilderspool Park, Greenalls Ave
Stockton Heath, Warrington
Cheshire, WA4 6HL.
tel: (01925) 438 028
fax: (01925) 438 001

Syner-Med
Syner-Med (Pharmaceutical Products) Ltd
Beech House
840 Brighton Rd
Purley, CR8 2BH.
tel: (0845) 634 2100
fax: (0845) 634 2101
mail@syner-med.com

Takeda
Takeda UK Ltd
Takeda House, Mercury Park
Wycombe Lane
Wooburn Green
High Wycombe, Bucks, HP10 0HH.
tel: (01628) 537 900
fax: (01628) 526 615

Taro
Taro Pharmaceuticals (UK) Ltd
1st Floor, Prince of Wales House
3 Bluecoats Ave
Hertford, SG14 1PB.
tel: (01992) 557 445
fax: (01992) 557 447
customerservice@taropharma.co.uk

Tarus
See Chemidex

Teofarma
Teofarma S.r.l.
c/o Professional Information Ltd
The Aske Stables
Richmond, DL10 5HG.
tel: (01748) 828 857

Teva
Teva Pharmaceuticals Ltd
The Gate House
Gatehouse Way
Aylesbury
Bucks, HP19 8DB.
tel: (01296) 719 768
fax: (01296) 719 769
med.info@tevapharma.co.uk

TEVA UK
TEVA UK Ltd
Brampton Rd
Hampden Park, Eastbourne
East Sussex, BN22 9AG.
tel: (01323) 501 111
fax: (01323) 520 306

TheraSense
TheraSense UK
Centaur House
Ancells Business Park, Ancells Rd
Fleet
Hants, GU51 2UJ.
tel: (01252) 761 392
fax: (01252) 761 393

Thornton & Ross
Thornton & Ross Ltd
Linthwaite Laboratories
Huddersfield, HD7 5QH.
tel: (01484) 842 217
fax: (01484) 847 301
mail@thorntonross.com

Tillomed
Tillomed Laboratories Ltd
3 Howard Rd
Eaton Socon, St Neots
Cambs, PE19 3ET.
tel: (01480) 402 400
fax: (01480) 402 402
info@tillomed.co.uk

TOL
Tree of Life
Coaldale Rd
Lymedale Business Park
Newcastle Under Lyme
Staff, ST5 9QX.
tel: (01782) 567 100
fax: (01782) 567 199
health@tol-europe.com

Torbet
Torbet Laboratories Ltd
14D Wendover Rd
Rackheath Industrial Estate
Rackheath
Norwich, NR13 6LH.
tel: (01603) 735 200
fax: (01603) 735 217
torbet@typharm.com

Transdermal
Transdermal Ltd
35 Grimwade Ave
Croydon
Surrey, CR0 5DJ.
tel: (020) 8654 2251
fax: (020) 8654 2252
transdermal@transdermal.co.uk

Trinity
Trinity Pharmaceuticals Ltd
See Trinity-Chiesi

Trinity-Chiesi
Trinity-Chiesi Pharmaceuticals Ltd
Cheadle Royal Business Park
Highfield
Cheadle, SK8 3GY.
tel: (0161) 488 5555
fax: (0161) 488 5565

TSL
Tissue Science Laboratories plc
Victoria House
Victoria Rd
Aldershot
Hants, GU11 1EJ.
tel: (01252) 333 002
fax: (01252) 333 010
enquiries@tissuescience.com

Tyco
Tyco Healthcare
154 Fareham Rd
Gosport
Hants, PO13 0AS.
tel: (01329) 224 000

Typharm
Typharm Ltd
14D Wendover Rd
Rackheath Industrial Estate
Rackheath
Norwich, NR13 6LH.
tel: (01603) 735 200
fax: (01603) 735 217
customerservices@typharm.com

UCB Pharma
UCB Pharma Ltd
208 Bath Rd
Slough, SL1 3WE.
tel: (01753) 534 655
fax: (01753) 536 632
medicalinformationuk@ucb-group.com

Ultrapharm
Ultrapharm Ltd
Centenary Business Park
Henley-on-Thames
Oxon, RG9 1DS.
tel: (01491) 578 016
fax: (01491) 570 001
orders@glutenfree.co.uk

Univar
Univar Ltd
International House
Zenith, Paycocke Rd
Basildon
Essex, SS14 3DW.
tel: (01268) 594 400
fax: (01268) 594 481
trientine@univareurope.com

Unomedical
Unomedical Ltd
Thornhill Rd
Redditch, B98 7NL.
tel: (01527) 587 700
fax: (01527) 592 111

Urgo
Urgo Ltd
Sullington Rd
Shepshed
Loughborough
Leics, LE12 9JJ.
tel: (01509) 502 051
fax: (01509) 650 898
medical@parema.com

Valeant
Valeant Pharmaceuticals Ltd
Cedarwood
Chineham Business Park
Crockford Lane, Basingstoke
Hants, RG24 8WD.
tel: (01256) 707 744
fax: (01256) 707 334
valeantuk@valeant.com

Vernon-Carus
Vernon-Carus Ltd
Penwortham Mills
Preston
Lancs, PR1 9SN.
tel: (01772) 744 493
fax: (01772) 748 754
mail@vernon-carus.co.uk

Viatris
Viatris Pharmaceuticals Ltd
Building 2000, Beach Drive
Cambridge Research Park
Waterbeach, Cambs, CB5 9PD.
tel: (01223) 205 999
fax: (01223) 205 998
info@viatrisuk.co.uk

Viridian
Viridian Pharma Ltd
Seales Barn
School Lane
Shuttington, Tamworth
Staffs, B79 0DX.
tel: (01827) 896 996
fax: (0870) 705 8153
info@viridianpharma.co.uk

Vitaflo
Vitaflo Ltd
11 Century Building
Brunswick Business Park
Liverpool, L3 4BL.
tel: (0151) 709 9020
fax: (0151) 709 9727
vitaflo@vitaflo.co.uk

Vitaline
Vitaline Pharmaceuticals UK Ltd
8 Ridge Way
Drakes Drive
Crendon Business Park
Long Crendon, Bucks, HP18 9BF.
tel: (01844) 202 044
fax: (01844) 202 077
vitalineinfo@aol.com

Vitalograph
Vitalograph Ltd
Maids Moreton
Buckingham, MK18 1SW.
tel: (01280) 827 110
fax: (01280) 823 302
sales@vitalograph.co.uk

W-L
Warner Lambert UK Ltd
See Pfizer

Wallace Mfg
Wallace Manufacturing Chemists Ltd
Wallace House
New Abbey Court
51-53 Stert St, Abingdon
Oxon, OX14 3JF.
tel: (01235) 538 700
fax: (01235) 538 800
info@alinter.co.uk

Wanskerne
Wanskerne Ltd
44 Broomfield Drive
Billingshurst, RH4 9TN.
tel: (01403) 783 214
fax: (01403) 783 214

Warner Lambert
See Pfizer

Winthrop
Winthrop Pharmaceuticals UK Ltd
PO Box 611
Guildford, Surrey, GU1 4YS.
tel: (01483) 554 101
fax: (01483) 554 810
winthropsales@sanofi-aventis.com

Wockhardt
Wockhardt UK Ltd
Ash Rd North
Wrexham Industrial Estate
Wrexham, LL13 9UF.
tel: (01978) 661 261
fax: (01978) 660 130

Wyeth
Wyeth Pharmaceuticals
Huntercombe Lane South
Taplow
Maidenhead
Berks, SL6 0PH.
tel: (01628) 604 377
fax: (01628) 666 368
ukmedinfo@wyeth.com

Wynlit
Wynlit Laboratories
153 Furzehill Rd
Borehamwood
Herts, WD6 2DR.
tel: (07903) 370 130
fax: (020) 8292 6117

Wyvern
Wyvern Medical Ltd
PO Box 17
Ledbury
Herefordshire, HR8 2ES.
tel: (01531) 631 105
fax: (01531) 634 844

Yamanouchi
See Astellas

Zeal
G. H. Zeal Ltd
Deer Park Rd
London, SW19 3UU.
tel: (020) 8542 2283
fax: (020) 8543 7840
scientific@zeal.co.uk

Zeneus
Zeneus Pharma Ltd
Abel Smith House
Gunnels Wood Rd
Stevenage, Herts, SG1 2BT.
tel: (01438) 731 731
fax: (01438) 765 080
medinfo@zeneuspharma.com

Zeroderma
Zeroderma Ltd
The Manor House
Victor Barns
Northampton Rd, Brixworth
Northampton, NN6 9DQ.
tel: (01604) 889 855
fax: (01604) 883 199
info@ixlpharma.com

ZLB Behring
ZLB Behring UK Ltd
Hayworth House
Market Place
Haywards Heath
West Sussex, RH16 1DB.
tel: (01444) 447 400
fax: (01444) 447 401
medinfo@zlbbehring.com

ZooBiotic
ZooBiotic Ltd
Biosurgical Research Unit
Surgical Materials Testing Laboratory
Princess of Wales Hospital, Coity Rd
Bridgend, Mid Glamorgan, South Wales, CF31 1RQ.
tel: (0845) 230 1810
fax: (01656) 752 830
maggots@smtl.co.uk

Zurich
See Trinity-Chiesi

Special-order Manufacturers

The following **companies** manufacture 'special-order' products: BCM Specials, Fresenius, Martindale, Nova Laboratories, Phoenix, Rosemont, Special Products, The Specials Laboratory (see Index of Manufacturers for contact details). **Hospital manufacturing units** also manufacture 'special-order' products, details may be obtained from any of the centres listed below.

> It should be noted that when a product has a licence the *Department of Health recommends that the licensed product should be ordered* unless a specific formulation is required

England

East Anglian and Oxford

Mr Con Hanson
Production Manager
Pharmacy Manufacturing Unit
The Ipswich Hospital NHS Trust
Heath Rd

Ipswich, IP4 5PD.
tel: (01473) 703 603
fax: (01473) 703 609
con.hanson@ipsh-tr.anglox.nhs.uk

London

Mr M. Lillywhite
Director of Technical Services
Barts and the London NHS Trust, St. Bartholomew's Hospital
West Smithfield
London, EC1A 7BE.
tel: (020) 7601 7491
fax: (020) 7601 7486
mike.lillywhite@bartsandthelondon.nhs.uk

Mr P. Forsey
Production Manager
Guy's and St. Thomas' NHS Foundation Trust
Pharmacy Department
St. Thomas' Hospital
Lambeth Palace Rd
London, SE1 7EH.
tel: (020) 7188 5003
fax: (020) 7188 5013
paul.forsey@gstt.nhs.uk

Mr C. Evans
Production Manager
Pharmacy Department
St. George's Hospital
Blackshaw Rd
Tooting
London, SW17 0QT.
tel: (020) 8725 1770
fax: (020) 8725 3690
chris.evans@stgeorges.nhs.uk

Mr A. Krol
Managing Director
Moorfield Pharmaceuticals
25 Provost St
London, N1 7NG.
tel: (020) 7684 8555
fax: 0800 328 8191
alan.krol@moorfields.nhs.uk

North West

Mr M.D. Booth
Principal Pharmacist, Production & Aseptic Services Manager
Stockport Pharmaceuticals
Stepping Hill Hospital
Poplar Grove
Stockport
Cheshire, SK2 7JE.
tel: (0161) 419 5657
fax: (0161) 419 5664
mike.booth@stockport-tr.nwest.nhs.uk

Northern

Ms Stephanie Klein
Production Manager
Pharmacy Production Unit
Royal Victoria Infirmary
Queen Victoria
Newcastle-upon-Tyne, NE1 4LP.
tel: (0191) 282 0389
fax: (0191) 282 0376
stephanie.klein@nuth.northy.nhs.uk

South East

Mr F. Brown
Production Manager
Pharmacy Production Unit
St Peter's Hospital
Guildford Rd
Chertsey
Surrey, KT16 OPZ.
tel: (01932) 722 520
fax: (01932) 873 632
fraser.brown@asph.nhs.uk

Ms G. Middlehurst
Quality Assurance and Business Manager
Pharmacy Manufacturing Unit
Queen Alexandra Hospital
Southwick Hill Rd
Cosham
Portsmouth
Hants, PO6 3LY.
tel: (02392) 286 335
fax: (02392) 378 288
gillian.middlehurst@porthosp.nhs.uk

South Western

Mr P. S. Bendell
Pharmacy Manufacturing Services Manager
Torbay PMU
South Devon Healthcare
Kemmings Close
Long Rd
Paignton
Devon, TQ4 7TW.
tel: (01803) 664 707
fax: (01803) 664 354
phil.bendell@.nhs.net

Trent

Mr R.W. Brookes
Production Pharmacist
Royal Hallamshire Hospital
Glossop Rd
Sheffield, S10 2JF.
tel: (0114) 271 3104
fax: (0114) 271 2783
roger.brookes@sth.nhs.uk

West Midlands

Mr A. Broad
Principal Pharmacist
Sterile Fluids Manufacturing Unit
Queen Elizabeth Medical Centre
Edgbaston
Birmingham, B15 2TH.
tel: (0121) 627 2326
fax: (0121) 627 2168
alan.broad@uhb.nhs.uk

Mr P.G. Williams
Principal Pharmacist
Pharmacy Manufacturing Unit
Queens Hospital
Burton Hospitals NHS Trust
Belvedere Rd
Burton-on-Trent, DE13 0RB.
tel: (01283) 566 333/511 511 Extn 5138
fax: (01283) 593 036
paul.williams@queens.burtonh-tr.wmids.nhs.uk

Yorkshire

Dr J. Harwood
Production Manager
Pharmacy Manufacturing Unit
Huddersfield Royal Infirmary
Lindley
Huddersfield
West Yorks, HD3 3EA.
tel: (01484) 342 421
fax: (01484) 342 074
john.harwood@cht.nhs.uk

Northern Ireland

Mr Eamon Mullaney
Assistant Director of Pharmaceutical Services
Victoria Pharmaceuticals
Royal Group of Hospitals
77 Boucher Crescent
Belfast, BT12 6HU.
tel: (028) 9055 3407
fax: (028) 9055 3498
eamon.mullaney@royalhospitals.n-i.nhs.uk

Scotland

Mr Baxter W. Millar
General Manager
Tayside Pharmaceuticals
Ninewells Hospital
Dundee, DD1 9SY.
tel: (01382) 632 183
fax: (01382) 632 060
baxter.w.millar@tuht.scot.nhs.uk

Wales

Mr P. Spark
Principal Pharmacist
Sterile Production Services
Cardiff and Vale NHS Trust
Heath Park
Cardiff, CF14 4XW..
tel: (029) 2074 4828
fax: (029) 2074 3114
paul.spark@cardiffandvale.wales.nhs.uk

Index

Principal page references are printed in **bold** type. Proprietary (trade) names are printed in *italic* type; where the BNF for children does not include a full entry for a branded product, the non-proprietary name is shown in brackets. Names of organisms are also shown in *italic* type.

A

For marketing authorisation and BNFC advice, see p. 2

Index

Information on dose adjustment in children with hepatic and renal impairment is included in drug entries

Index

For information on excipients in medicines, see p. 3

B

Information on administration is included in drug entries

C

Index

Index

For general information on doses for children, see p. 11

E

G

For prescription requirements of Controlled Drugs, see p. 17

H

For information on excipients in medicines, see p. 3

I

Information on dose adjustment in children with hepatic and renal impairment is included in drug entries

J

K

L

M

N

Index

Information on administration is included in drug entries

O

For marketing authorisation and BNFC advice, see p. 2

P

Index

Index

For general information on doses for children, see p. 11

Q

R

Index

S

For information on excipients in medicines, see p. 3

Information on dose adjustment in children with hepatic and renal impairment is included in drug entries

U

Index

For marketing authorisation and BNFC advice, see p. 2

V

Index

COMMISSION ON
HUMAN MEDICINES

In Confidence

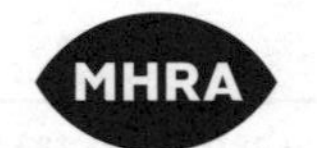

SUSPECTED ADVERSE DRUG REACTIONS

If you suspect that an adverse reaction may be related to a drug, or a combination of drugs, you should complete this Yellow Card or complete a report on the website at www.yellowcard.gov.uk. For *intensively monitored medicines* (identified by ▼) report **all** suspected reactions (including any considered not to be serious). For *established drugs* and *herbal remedies* report **all serious** adverse reactions in adults; report **all serious and minor** adverse reactions in **children** (under 18 years). You do not have to be certain about causality: if in doubt, please report. Do not be put off reporting just because some details are not known. See BNF (page 10) or the MHRA website (www.yellowcard.gov.uk) for additional advice.

PATIENT DETAILS Patient Initials: ________ Sex: M / F Weight if known (kg): ________

Age (at time of reaction): ________ Identification (Your Practice / Hospital Ref.)*: ________

SUSPECTED DRUG(S)

Give brand name of drug and batch number if known	Route	Dosage	Date started	Date stopped	Prescribed for

SUSPECTED REACTION(S)

Please describe the reaction(s) and any treatment given:

Outcome

- Recovered ☐
- Recovering ☐
- Continuing ☐
- Other ☐

Date reaction(s) started: ________ Date reaction(s) stopped: ________

Do you consider the reaction to be serious? Yes / No

If *yes*, please indicate why the reaction is considered to be serious (please tick all that apply):

- Patient died due to reaction ☐
- Life threatening ☐
- Congenital abnormality ☐
- Involved or prolonged inpatient hospitalisation ☐
- Involved persistent or significant disability or incapacity ☐
- Medically significant; please give details:

* This is to enable you to identify the patient in any future correspondence concerning this report

Please attach additional pages if necessary

Please list other drugs taken in the last 3 months prior to the reaction (including self-medication & herbal remedies)

Was the patient on any other medication? Yes / No If *yes*, please give the following information if known:

Drug (Brand, if known)	Route	Dosage	Date started	Date stopped	Prescribed for

Additional relevant information e.g. medical history, test results, known allergies, rechallenge (if performed), suspected drug interactions. For congenital abnormalities please state all other drugs taken during pregnancy and the date of the last menstrual period.

REPORTER DETAILS

Name and Professional Address: ______

Post code: ______ Tel No: ______

Speciality: ______

Signature: Date:

CLINICIAN (if not the reporter)

Name and Professional Address: ______

Post code: ______

Tel No: ______ Speciality: ______

If you would like information about other adverse reactions associated with the suspected drug, please tick this box ☐

If you report from an area served by a Yellow Card Centre, MHRA may ask the Centre to communicate with you, on its behalf, about your report. If you want only MHRA to contact you, please tick this box. ☐

Send to **Medicines and Healthcare Products Regulatory Agency, CHM FREEPOST, LONDON SW8 5BR**

Yellowcard

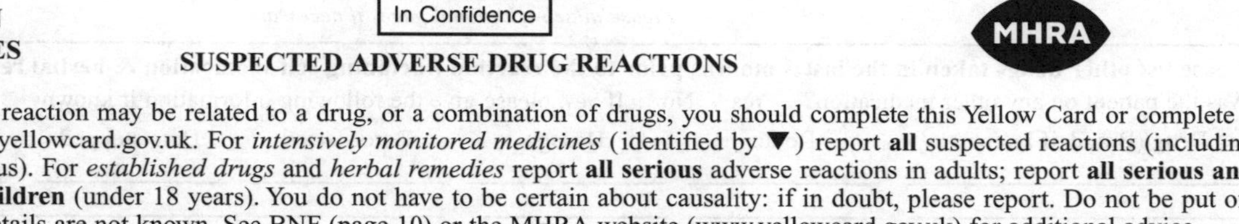

COMMISSION ON HUMAN MEDICINES

In Confidence

MHRA

SUSPECTED ADVERSE DRUG REACTIONS

If you suspect that an adverse reaction may be related to a drug, or a combination of drugs, you should complete this Yellow Card or complete a report on the website at www.yellowcard.gov.uk. For *intensively monitored medicines* (identified by ▼) report **all** suspected reactions (including any considered not to be serious). For *established drugs* and *herbal remedies* report **all serious** adverse reactions in adults; report **all serious and minor** adverse reactions in **children** (under 18 years). You do not have to be certain about causality: if in doubt, please report. Do not be put off reporting just because some details are not known. See BNF (page 10) or the MHRA website (www.yellowcard.gov.uk) for additional advice.

PATIENT DETAILS Patient Initials: ______ Sex: M / F Weight if known (kg): ______

Age (at time of reaction): ______ Identification (Your Practice / Hospital Ref.)*: ______

SUSPECTED DRUG(S)

Give brand name of drug and batch number if known	Route	Dosage	Date started	Date stopped	Prescribed for

SUSPECTED REACTION(S)

Please describe the reaction(s) and any treatment given:

Outcome

Recovered ☐

Recovering ☐

Continuing ☐

Other ☐

Date reaction(s) started: ______ Date reaction(s) stopped: ______

Do you consider the reaction to be serious? Yes / No

If *yes*, please indicate why the reaction is considered to be serious (please tick all that apply):

Patient died due to reaction ☐ Involved or prolonged inpatient hospitalisation ☐

Life threatening ☐ Involved persistent or significant disability or incapacity ☐

Congenital abnormality ☐ Medically significant; please give details:

* This is to enable you to identify the patient in any future correspondence concerning this report

Please attach additional pages if necessary

Please list other drugs taken in the last 3 months prior to the reaction (including self-medication & herbal remedies)

Was the patient on any other medication? Yes / No If *yes*, please give the following information if known:

Drug (Brand, if known)	Route	Dosage	Date started	Date stopped	Prescribed for

Additional relevant information e.g. medical history, test results, known allergies, rechallenge (if performed), suspected drug interactions. For congenital abnormalities please state all other drugs taken during pregnancy and the date of the last menstrual period.

REPORTER DETAILS

Name and Professional Address: ________

Post code: ________ Tel No: ________

Speciality: ________

Signature: Date:

CLINICIAN (if not the reporter)

Name and Professional Address: ________

Post code: ________

Tel No: ________ Speciality: ________

If you would like information about other adverse reactions associated with the suspected drug, please tick this box ☐

If you report from an area served by a Yellow Card Centre, MHRA may ask the Centre to communicate with you, on its behalf, about your report. If you want only MHRA to contact you, please tick this box. ☐

Send to **Medicines and Healthcare Products Regulatory Agency, CHM FREEPOST, LONDON SW8 5BR**

Yellowcard

COMMISSION ON HUMAN MEDICINES

In Confidence

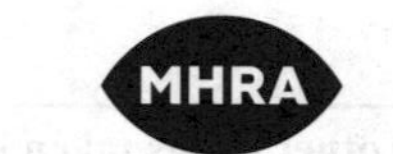

SUSPECTED ADVERSE DRUG REACTIONS

If you suspect that an adverse reaction may be related to a drug, or a combination of drugs, you should complete this Yellow Card or complete a report on the website at www.yellowcard.gov.uk. For *intensively monitored medicines* (identified by ▼) report **all** suspected reactions (including any considered not to be serious). For *established drugs* and *herbal remedies* report **all serious** adverse reactions in adults; report **all serious and minor** adverse reactions in **children** (under 18 years). You do not have to be certain about causality: if in doubt, please report. Do not be put off reporting just because some details are not known. See BNF (page 10) or the MHRA website (www.yellowcard.gov.uk) for additional advice.

PATIENT DETAILS Patient Initials: ______ Sex: M / F Weight if known (kg): ______

Age (at time of reaction): ______ Identification (Your Practice / Hospital Ref.)*: ______

SUSPECTED DRUG(S)

Give brand name of drug and batch number if known	Route	Dosage	Date started	Date stopped	Prescribed for

SUSPECTED REACTION(S)

Please describe the reaction(s) and any treatment given:

Outcome

Recovered ☐
Recovering ☐
Continuing ☐
Other ☐

Date reaction(s) started: ______ Date reaction(s) stopped: ______

Do you consider the reaction to be serious? Yes / No

If *yes*, please indicate why the reaction is considered to be serious (please tick all that apply):

Patient died due to reaction ☐ Involved or prolonged inpatient hospitalisation ☐

Life threatening ☐ Involved persistent or significant disability or incapacity ☐

Congenital abnormality ☐ Medically significant; please give details:

* This is to enable you to identify the patient in any future correspondence concerning this report

Please attach additional pages if necessary

Please list other drugs taken in the last 3 months prior to the reaction (including self-medication & herbal remedies)

Was the patient on any other medication? Yes / No If *yes*, please give the following information if known:

Drug (Brand, if known)	Route	Dosage	Date started	Date stopped	Prescribed for

Additional relevant information e.g. medical history, test results, known allergies, rechallenge (if performed), suspected drug interactions. For congenital abnormalities please state all other drugs taken during pregnancy and the date of the last menstrual period.

REPORTER DETAILS

Name and Professional Address: ________

Post code: ________ Tel No: ________

Speciality: ________

Signature: Date:

CLINICIAN (if not the reporter)

Name and Professional Address: ________

Post code: ________

Tel No: ________ Speciality: ________

If you would like information about other adverse reactions associated with the suspected drug, please tick this box ☐

If you report from an area served by a Yellow Card Centre, MHRA may ask the Centre to communicate with you, on its behalf, about your report. If you want only MHRA to contact you, please tick this box. ☐

Send to **Medicines and Healthcare Products Regulatory Agency, CHM FREEPOST, LONDON SW8 5BR**

Yellowcard

COMMISSION ON HUMAN MEDICINES

In Confidence

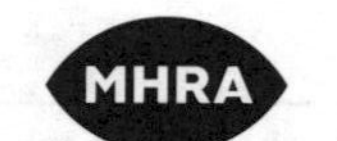

SUSPECTED ADVERSE DRUG REACTIONS

If you suspect that an adverse reaction may be related to a drug, or a combination of drugs, you should complete this Yellow Card or complete a report on the website at www.yellowcard.gov.uk. For *intensively monitored medicines* (identified by ▼) report **all** suspected reactions (including any considered not to be serious). For *established drugs* and *herbal remedies* report **all serious** adverse reactions in adults; report **all serious and minor** adverse reactions in **children** (under 18 years). You do not have to be certain about causality: if in doubt, please report. Do not be put off reporting just because some details are not known. See BNF (page 10) or the MHRA website (www.yellowcard.gov.uk) for additional advice.

PATIENT DETAILS Patient Initials: ______ Sex: M / F Weight if known (kg): ______

Age (at time of reaction): ______ Identification (Your Practice / Hospital Ref.)*: ______

SUSPECTED DRUG(S)

Give brand name of drug and batch number if known	Route	Dosage	Date started	Date stopped	Prescribed for

SUSPECTED REACTION(S)

Please describe the reaction(s) and any treatment given:

Outcome

- Recovered ☐
- Recovering ☐
- Continuing ☐
- Other ☐

Date reaction(s) started: ______ Date reaction(s) stopped: ______

Do you consider the reaction to be serious? Yes / No

If *yes*, please indicate why the reaction is considered to be serious (please tick all that apply):

- Patient died due to reaction ☐
- Life threatening ☐
- Congenital abnormality ☐
- Involved or prolonged inpatient hospitalisation ☐
- Involved persistent or significant disability or incapacity ☐
- Medically significant; please give details:

* This is to enable you to identify the patient in any future correspondence concerning this report

Please attach additional pages if necessary

Please list other drugs taken in the last 3 months prior to the reaction (including self-medication & herbal remedies)

Was the patient on any other medication? Yes / No If *yes*, please give the following information if known:

Drug (Brand, if known)	Route	Dosage	Date started	Date stopped	Prescribed for

Additional relevant information e.g. medical history, test results, known allergies, rechallenge (if performed), suspected drug interactions. For congenital abnormalities please state all other drugs taken during pregnancy and the date of the last menstrual period.

REPORTER DETAILS

Name and Professional Address: ______________________

Post code: ____________ Tel No: ____________

Speciality: ______________________

Signature: Date:

CLINICIAN (if not the reporter)

Name and Professional Address: ______________________

Post code: ____________

Tel No: ____________ Speciality: ____________

If you would like information about other adverse reactions associated with the suspected drug, please tick this box ☐

If you report from an area served by a Yellow Card Centre, MHRA may ask the Centre to communicate with you, on its behalf, about your report. If you want only MHRA to contact you, please tick this box. ☐

Send to **Medicines and Healthcare Products Regulatory Agency, CHM FREEPOST, LONDON SW8 5BR**

Yellowcard

NEWBORN LIFE SUPPORT

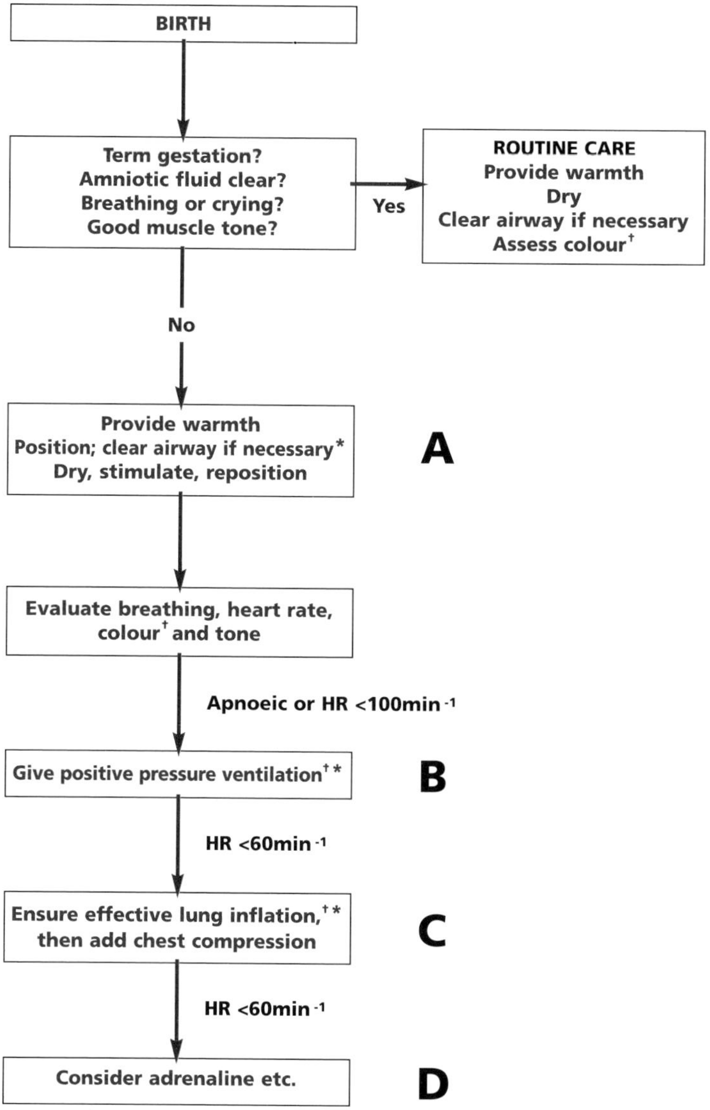

BIRTH

↓

Term gestation?
Amniotic fluid clear?
Breathing or crying?
Good muscle tone?

→ Yes → **ROUTINE CARE**
Provide warmth
Dry
Clear airway if necessary
Assess colour†

↓ No

Provide warmth
Position; clear airway if necessary*
Dry, stimulate, reposition

A

↓

Evaluate breathing, heart rate, colour† and tone

↓ Apnoeic or HR $<100min^{-1}$

Give positive pressure ventilation†*

B

↓ HR $<60min^{-1}$

Ensure effective lung inflation,†*
then add chest compression

C

↓ HR $<60min^{-1}$

Consider adrenaline etc.

D

*Tracheal intubation may be considered at several steps
†Consider supplemental oxygen at any stage if cyanosis persists

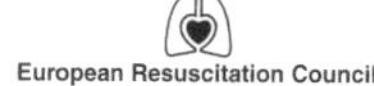

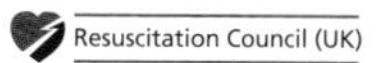

PAEDIATRIC BASIC LIFE SUPPORT

(Healthcare professionals with a duty to respond)

UNRESPONSIVE?

↓

Shout for help

↓

Open airway

↓

NOT BREATHING NORMALLY?

↓

5 rescue breaths

↓

STILL UNRESPONSIVE?
(no signs of a circulation)

↓

15 chest compressions
2 rescue breaths

After 1 minute call resuscitation team then continue CPR

European Resuscitation Council

Resuscitation Council (UK)

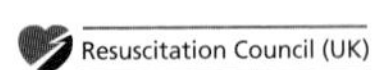

PAEDIATRIC ADVANCED LIFE SUPPORT

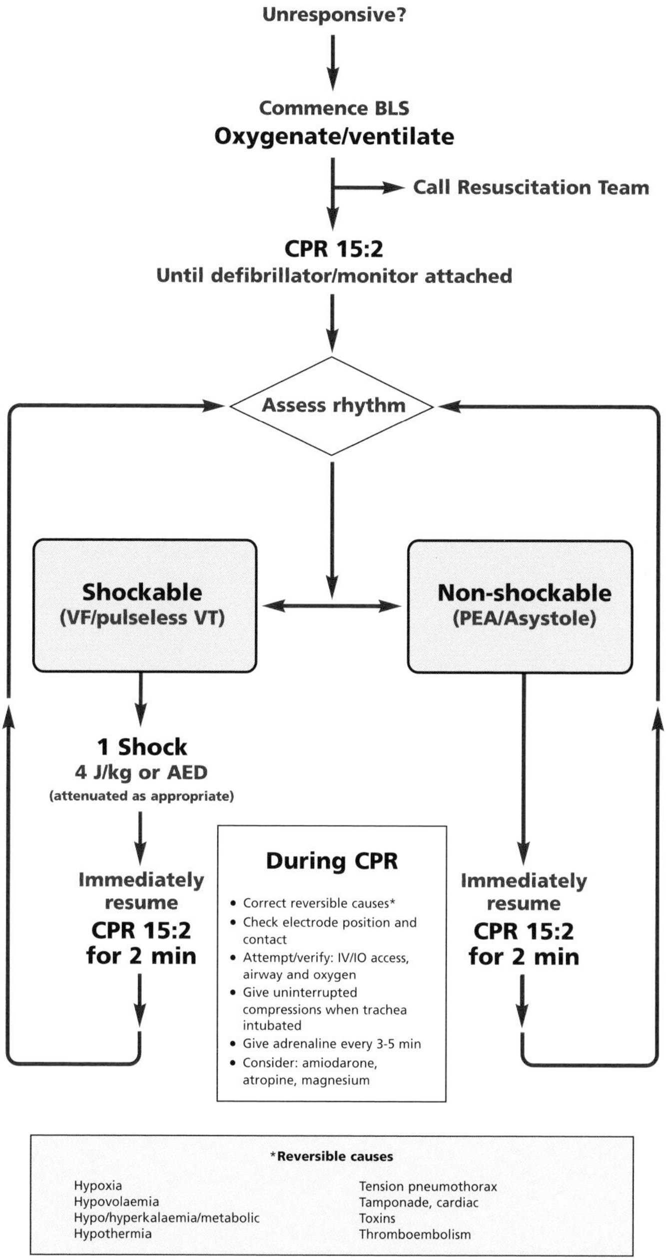

Unresponsive?

Commence BLS
Oxygenate/ventilate

→ **Call Resuscitation Team**

CPR 15:2
Until defibrillator/monitor attached

Assess rhythm

Shockable
(VF/pulseless VT)

1 Shock
4 J/kg or AED
(attenuated as appropriate)

Immediately resume
CPR 15:2
for 2 min

Non-shockable
(PEA/Asystole)

Immediately resume
CPR 15:2
for 2 min

During CPR

- Correct reversible causes*
- Check electrode position and contact
- Attempt/verify: IV/IO access, airway and oxygen
- Give uninterrupted compressions when trachea intubated
- Give adrenaline every 3-5 min
- Consider: amiodarone, atropine, magnesium

***Reversible causes**

Hypoxia	Tension pneumothorax
Hypovolaemia	Tamponade, cardiac
Hypo/hyperkalaemia/metabolic	Toxins
Hypothermia	Thromboembolism

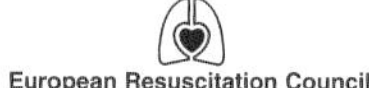

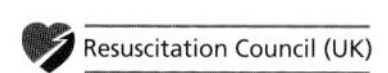

BODY SURFACE AREA NOMOGRAM – INFANTS

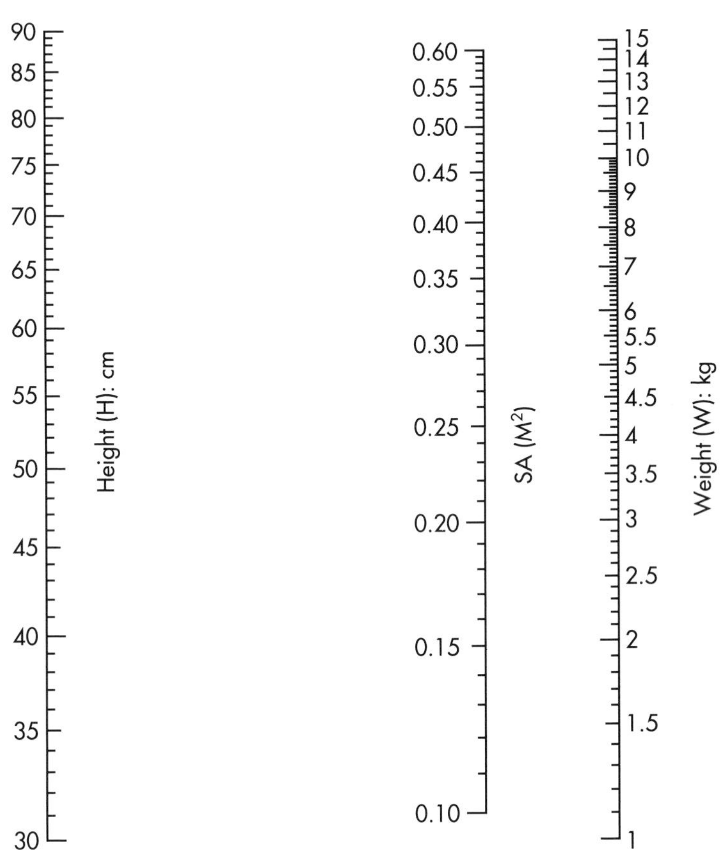

$$SA = W^{0.5378} \times H^{0.3964} \times 0.024265$$

Reprinted from Haycock GB et al, Journal of Pediatrics 1978: 98; 62–66 with permission from Elsevier Science.

BODY SURFACE AREA NOMOGRAM – CHILDREN AND ADOLESCENTS

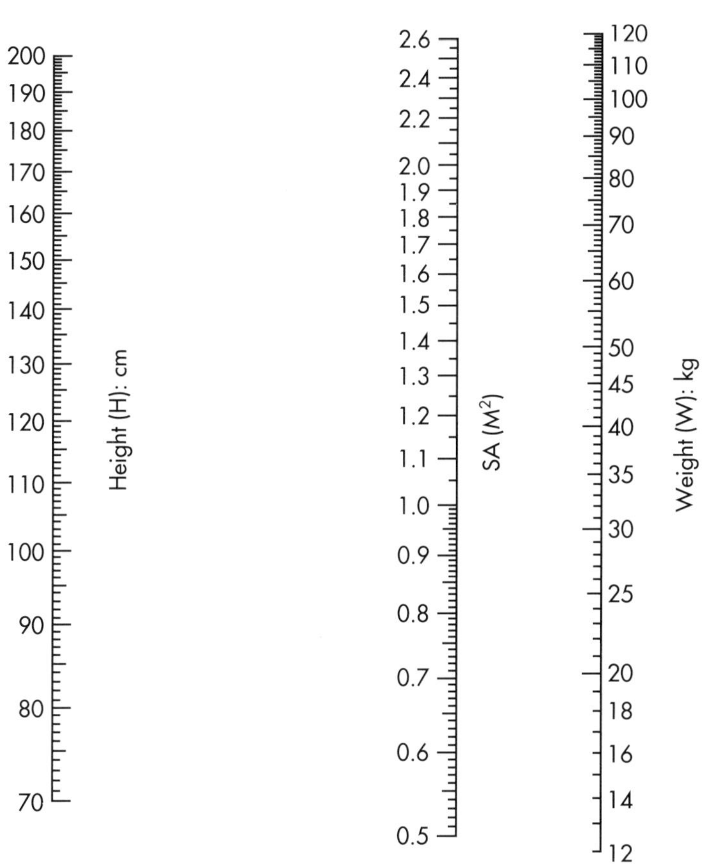

$$SA = W^{0.5378} \times H^{0.3964} \times 0.024265$$

Medical emergencies in the community

Drug treatment outlined below is intended for use by community healthcare professionals. Only drugs that are used for immediate relief are shown; advice on supporting care is not given. Where the child's condition requires investigation and further treatment, the child should be transferred to hospital promptly.

Anaphylaxis

(section 3.4.3)

Adrenaline injection 1 mg/mL (1 in 1000)

- By intramuscular injection
  Child 1–6 months 50 micrograms (0.05 mL), repeated every 5 minutes if necessary
  Child 6 months–6 years 120 micrograms (0.12 mL), repeated every 5 minutes if necessary
  Child 6–12 years 250 micrograms (0.25 mL), repeated every 5 minutes if necessary
  Child 12–18 years 500 micrograms (0.5 mL), repeated every 5 minutes if necessary

Chlorphenamine injection 10 mg/mL

- By intravenous injection over 1 minute
  Child 1 month–1 year 250 micrograms/kg (max. 2.5 mg) up to 4 times in 24 hours
  Child 1–6 years 2.5–5 mg up to 4 times in 24 hours
  Child 6–12 years 5–10 mg up to 4 times in 24 hours
  Child 12–18 years 10–20 mg up to 4 times in 24 hours (max. 40 mg in 24 hours)

Oxygen should be given if required.
Hydrocortisone by intravenous injection (section 6.3.2) has delayed action but it should be given to severely affected children to prevent further deterioration.

Asthma: mild to moderate exacerbation

(section 3.1)

Salbutamol aerosol inhaler 100 micrograms/metered inhalation

- By aerosol inhalation
  Child 1 month–5 years 1 puff every 15–30 seconds through a close-fitting facemask with a spacer, up to max. 10 puffs; repeat after 20–30 minutes if necessary
  Child 5–18 years 1 puff every 15–30 seconds through a spacer, up to max. 10 puffs; repeat after 20–30 minutes if necessary

A short course of **prednisolone** (section 6.3.2) should also be prescribed.

Asthma: severe or life-threatening

(section 3.1)

Either **salbutamol** aerosol inhaler as described above
or **salbutamol** nebuliser solution 1 mg/mL, 2 mg/mL

- By inhalation of nebulised solution
  Child 1 month–5 years 2.5 mg every 20–30 minutes if necessary
  Child 5–18 years 5 mg every 20–30 minutes if necessary

or **terbutaline** nebulised solution 2.5 mg/mL

- By inhalation of nebulised solution
  Child 1 month–5 years 5 mg every 20–30 minutes if necessary
  Child 5–18 years 10 mg every 20–30 minutes if necessary

If response to beta$_2$ agonist is poor (while awaiting transfer to hospital) **ipratropium** nebuliser solution 250 micrograms/mL

- By inhalation of nebulised solution
  Child under 2 years 125–250 micrograms every 20–30 minutes if necessary
  Child 2–18 years 250 micrograms every 20–30 minutes if necessary

Plus (in all cases)

Either **prednisolone** soluble tablets 5 mg

- By mouth
  Child 2–18 years 1–2 mg/kg (max. 20 mg for child under 5 years, max. 40 mg for child 5–18 years) once daily for 3–5 days

or **hydrocortisone**

- By intramuscular or intravenous injection
  Child 1 month–1 year 25 mg
  Child 1–6 years 50 mg
  Child 6–12 years 100 mg
  Child 12–18 years 100–500 mg

Croup

(section 3.1)

Dexamethasone oral solution 2 mg/5 mL

- By mouth
  Child 1 month–2 years 150 micrograms/kg as a single dose

Convulsions

(section 4.8.2)

Either **midazolam** buccal solution 10 mg/mL or injection solution given by buccal route

- By buccal administration
  Neonate 300 micrograms/kg
  Child 1–6 months 300 micrograms/kg
  Child 6 months–1 year 2.5 mg
  Child 1–5 years 5 mg
  Child 5–10 years 7.5 mg
  Child 10–18 years 10 mg

or **diazepam** rectal solution 2 mg/mL, 4 mg/mL

- By rectum, repeated after 5 minutes if necessary
  Neonate 1.25–2.5 mg
  Child 1 month–2 years 5 mg
  Child 2–12 years 5–10 mg
  Child 12–18 years 10 mg

Febrile convulsions lasting longer than 15 minutes

(section 4.8.3)

Diazepam rectal solution 2 mg/mL, 4 mg/mL

- By rectum, repeated after 5 minutes if necessary
  Neonate 1.25–2.5 mg
  Child 1 month–2 years 5 mg
  Child over 2 years 5–10 mg

Diabetic hypoglycaemia

(section 6.1.4)

Glucose or **sucrose**

- By mouth

  Child 2–18 years approx. 10–20 g (2–4 teaspoonfuls of sugar or 3–6 sugar lumps or 50–100 mL *Lucozade® Sparkling Glucose Drink* or 90–180 mL *Coca-Cola®*—both non-diet versions), repeated after 10–15 minutes if necessary

or if hypoglycaemia unresponsive *or* if oral route cannot be used

Glucagon injection 1 mg/mL

- By subcutaneous, intramuscular or intravenous injection

  Child body-weight under 25kg 500 micrograms (0.5 mL)

  Child body-weight over 25kg 1 mg (1 mL)

or if hypoglycaemia prolonged *or* unresponsive to glucagon after 10 minutes

Glucose intravenous infusion 10%

- By intravenous injection into large vein

  Child 1 month–18 years 2–5 mL/kg (glucose 200–500 mg/kg)

Meningococcal disease

(Table 1, section 5.1)

Benzylpenicillin injection 600 mg, 1.2 g

- By intravenous injection (or by intramuscular injection if venous access not available)

  Neonate 300 mg

  Child 1 month–1 year 300 mg

  Child 1–10 years 600 mg

  Child 10–18 years 1.2 g

  Note Give single dose and transfer urgently to hospital

or if history of delayed allergy to penicillin

Cefotaxime injection 1 g

- By intravenous injection (or by intramuscular injection if venous access not available)

  Neonate 50 mg/kg

  Child 1 month–12 years 50 mg/kg (max. 1 g)

  Child 12–18 years 1 g

  Note Give single dose and transfer urgently to hospital

or if history of immediate allergy (including anaphylaxis, angioedema or urticarial reaction) to penicillin or cephalosporins

Chloramphenicol injection 1 g

- By intravenous injection

  Child 1 month–18 years 12.5–25 mg/kg

  Note Give single dose and transfer urgently to hospital

Pneumonia: uncomplicated

(Table 1, section 5.1)

Amoxicillin oral suspension 125 mg/5 mL, 250 mg/5 mL; capsules 250 mg

- By mouth

  Child 6 months–1 year 125 mg 3 times daily

  Child 1–5 years 250 mg 3 times daily

  Child 5–18 years 500 mg 3 times daily

or if allergic to penicillin *or* atypical organism suspected

Erythromycin oral suspension 125 mg/5 mL, 250 mg/5 mL; tablets 250 mg

- By mouth

  Child 6 months–2 years 125 mg 4 times daily

  Child 2–8 years 250 mg 4 times daily

  Child 8–18 years 250–500 mg 4 times daily

Prescribing for children

Weight, height and body surface area

The table below shows the **mean values** for weight, height and body surface area by age; these values may be used to calculate doses in the absence of actual measurements. However, the child's actual weight and height might vary considerably from the values in the table and it is important to see the child to ensure that the value chosen is appropriate. In most cases the child's actual measurement should be obtained as soon as possible and the dose re-calculated.

Age	Weight	Height	Body surface
	kg	cm	m^2
Full-term neonate	3.5	50	0.23
1 month	4.2	55	0.26
2 months	4.5	57	0.27
3 months	5.6	59	0.32
4 months	6.5	62	0.34
6 months	7.7	67	0.40
1 year	10	76	0.47
3 years	15	94	0.62
5 years	18	108	0.73
7 years	23	120	0.88
10 years	30	132	1.05
12 years	39	148	1.25
14 years	50	163	1.50
Adult male	68	173	1.80
Adult female	56	163	1.60

Approximate conversions and units

lb	kg	stones	kg	mL	fl oz
1	0.45	1	6.35	50	1.8
2	0.91	2	12.70	100	3.5
3	1.36	3	19.05	150	5.3
4	1.81	4	25.40	200	7.0
5	2.27	5	31.75	500	17.6
6	2.72	6	38.10	1000	35.2
7	3.18	7	44.45		
8	3.63	8	50.80		
9	4.08	9	57.15		
10	4.54	10	63.50		
11	4.99	11	69.85		
12	5.44	12	76.20		
13	5.90	13	82.55		
14	6.35	14	88.90		
		15	95.25		

Length

1 metre (m)		= 1000 millimetres (mm)
1 centimetre (cm)		= 10 mm
1 inch (in)		= 25.4 mm
1 foot (ft)	=12 inches	= 304.8 mm

Mass

1 kilogram (kg)	= 1000 grams (g)
1 gram (g)	= 1000 milligrams (mg)
1 milligram (mg)	= 1000 micrograms
1 microgram	= 1000 nanograms
1 nanogram	= 1000 picograms

Volume

1 litre	= 1000 millilitres (mL)
1 millilitre (1 mL)	= 1000 microlitres
1 pint	≈ 568 mL

Other units

1 kilocalorie (kcal)	= 4186.8 joules (J)
1000 kilocalories (kcal)	= 4.1868 megajoules (MJ)
1 megajoule (MJ)	= 238.8 kilocalories (kcal)
1 millimetre of mercury (mmHg)	= 133.3 pascals (Pa)
1 kilopascal (kPa)	= 7.5 mmHg (pressure)

Plasma-drug concentrations in *BNF for Children* are expressed in mass units per litre (e.g. mg/litre). The approximate equivalent in terms of amount of substance units (e.g. micromol/litre) is given in brackets.

Recommended wording of cautionary and advisory labels

For details see Appendix 3

1 Warning. May cause drowsiness
2 Warning. May cause drowsiness. If affected do not drive or operate machinery. Avoid alcoholic drink
3 Warning. May cause drowsiness. If affected do not drive or operate machinery
4 Warning. Avoid alcoholic drink
5 Do not take indigestion remedies at the same time of day as this medicine
6 Do not take indigestion remedies or medicines containing iron or zinc at the same time of day as this medicine
7 Do not take milk, indigestion remedies, or medicines containing iron or zinc at the same time of day as this medicine
8 Do not stop taking this medicine except on your doctor's advice
9 Take at regular intervals. Complete the prescribed course unless otherwise directed
10 Warning. Follow the printed instructions you have been given with this medicine
11 Avoid exposure of skin to direct sunlight or sun lamps
12 Do not take anything containing aspirin while taking this medicine
13 Dissolve or mix with water before taking
14 This medicine may colour the urine
15 Caution flammable: keep away from fire or flames
16 Allow to dissolve under the tongue. Do not transfer from this container. Keep tightly closed. Discard 8 weeks after opening
17 Do not take more than ... in 24 hours
18 Do not take more than ... in 24 hours or ... in any one week
19 Warning. Causes drowsiness which may continue the next day. If affected do not drive or operate machinery. Avoid alcoholic drink
21 ... with or after food
22 ... half to one hour before food
23 ... an hour before food or on an empty stomach
24 ... sucked or chewed
25 ... swallowed whole, not chewed
26 ... dissolved under the tongue
27 ... with plenty of water
28 To be spread thinly ...
29 Do not take more than 2 at any one time. Do not take more than 8 in 24 hours
30 Do not take with any other paracetamol products
31 Contains aspirin and paracetamol. Do not take with any other paracetamol products
32 Contains aspirin
33 Contains an aspirin-like medicine